THIRD EDITION

PART A

GARNER AND KLINTWORTH'S

PATHOBIOLOGY OF OCULAR DISEASE

Edited by

Gordon K. Klintworth

Duke University, Durham, North Carolina, USA

Alec Garner

Institute of Ophthalmology, Moorfields Eye Hospital, London, UK

Associate Editors

J. Godfrey Heathcote

Dalhousie University, Halifax, Nova Scotia, Canada

J. Douglas Cameron

Mayo Clinic, Rochester, Minnesota, USA

Victor M. Elner

Kellogg Eye Institute, University of Michigan, Ann Arbor, Michigan, USA

Narsing A. Rao

Doheny Eye Institute, Keck School of Medicine, University of Southern California, Los Angeles, California, USA

informa
healthcare

New York London

Informa Healthcare USA, Inc.
52 Vanderbilt Avenue
New York, NY 10017

Printed in the United States of America on acid-free paper
10 9 8 7 6 5 4 3 2 1

International Standard Book Number-10: 0-8493-9816-9 (Hardcover)
International Standard Book Number-13: 978-0-8493-9816-2 (Hardcover)
Part A: ISBN-10: 1-4200-7975-1; ISBN-13: 978-1-4200-7975-3
Part B: ISBN-10: 1-4200-7976-X; ISBN-13: 978-1-4200-7976-0

Library of Congress Cataloging-in-Publication Data

Garner and Klintworth's pathobiology of ocular disease/edited by Gordon K. Klintworth, Alec Garner.—3rd ed.
p. ; cm.
Rev. ed. of: Pathobiology of ocular disease/edited by Alec Garner, Gordon K. Klintworth. 2nd ed. c1994.
Includes bibliographical references and index.
ISBN-13: 978-0-8493-9816-2 (hardcover: alk. paper)
ISBN-10: 0-8493-9816-9 (hardcover: alk. paper)
1. Eye—Pathophysiology. 2. Eye—Diseases—Pathophysiology. I. Klintworth, Gordon K. II. Garner, Alec. III. Pathobiology of ocular disease. IV. Title: Pathobiology of ocular disease.
[DNLM: 1. Eye Diseases—pathology. 2. Eye Diseases—physiopathology. 3. Eye Diseases—etiology. WW 140 G234 2007]
RE67.P38 2007
617.7′1—dc22
2007030661

For Corporate Sales and Reprint Permissions call 212-520-2700 or write to: Sales Department, 52 Vanderbilt Avenue, 16th floor, New York, NY 10017.

Visit the Informa Web site at
www.informa.com

and the Informa Healthcare Web site at
www.informahealthcare.com

GARNER AND KLINTWORTH'S

PATHOBIOLOGY OF OCULAR DISEASE

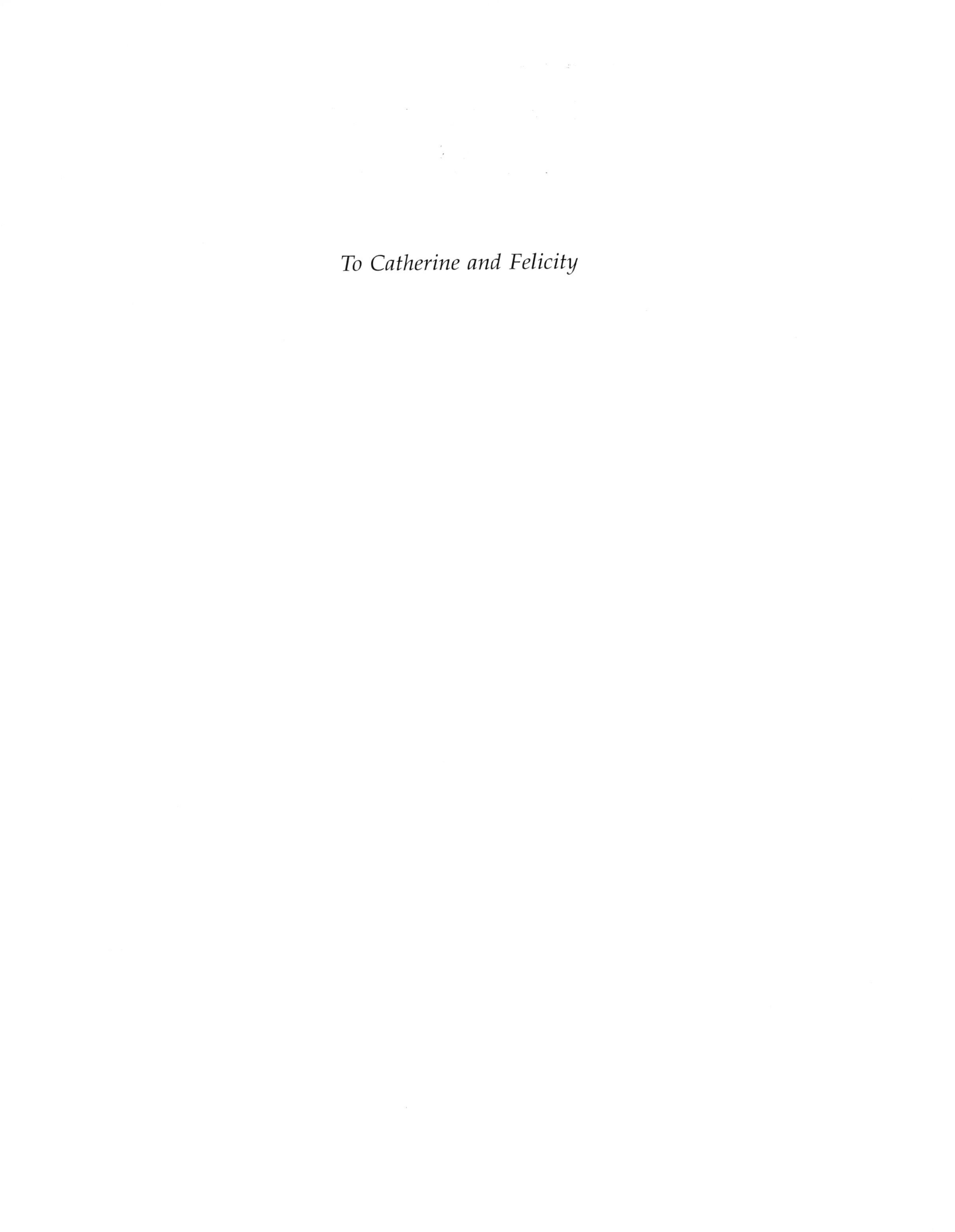

To Catherine and Felicity

Foreword to the Third Edition

A quarter of a century has passed since the first edition of *Pathobiology of Ocular Disease: A Dynamic Approach* was published. This successful, unique text, which is edited by two of the very few pathologists who have devoted major portions of their careers to ophthalmic pathology, has now gone into a third edition after a lapse of more than a decade. Unlike most books on ophthalmic pathology, this one devotes a large amount of space to a consideration of the etiology and pathogenesis of the diseases that afflict the tissues of the eye and its adnexa, as well as the visual pathways within the central nervous system. The current status of knowledge about the common blinding diseases of cataract, glaucoma, age-related maculopathy, and diabetic retinopathy is reviewed, but the vast numbers of infectious, immunologic, metabolic, toxic, degenerative, neoplastic, vascular, traumatic, and genetic diseases are also considered. By covering the embryologic development of the eye, the nature of ocular developmental anomalies can be appreciated.

Because this ambitious undertaking is multi-disciplinary, the chapters were prepared by almost one hundred contributors with variable backgrounds from different parts of the world.

An understanding of the causes, variable behavior, and mechanisms underlying specific diseases is essential to their rational therapy. Although the editors decided not to cover therapy because of space restrictions and uncertainties about the ideal treatment of diseases, the text provides a background for the development of rational therapeutic approaches.

The third edition is vastly different from the second edition because of the amazing amount of new information that has emerged as a result of the combined research efforts of numerous individuals, involving, in particular, molecular genetic techniques. The Human Genome Project, completed in 2003 after thirteen years, was a major factor in the exponential increase in information, and it is not surprising that the current edition contains so much new information about mutated genes and the newly discovered metabolic pathways, such as those involved in programmed cell death (apoptosis). This body of information has necessitated an increase in the number of chapters from 54 to 72.

I congratulate the editors in bringing together this group of respected contributors to provide a comprehensive overview of the current status of knowledge about the diseases that affect the eye and vision. The book will undoubtedly be a valuable asset to those desiring information about the enormous array of ophthalmic disorders.

Lorenz E. Zimmerman, MD
Emeritus Chairman,
Department of Ophthalmic Pathology
Armed Forces Institute of Pathology,
Walter Reed Army Medical Center
Washington, DC, U.S.A.

Foreword from the Second Edition

Over a decade has passed since I contributed a foreword to the first edition of this scholarly work, and in that short time biomedical research has advanced further than could have been imagined. This second edition is accordingly expanded, and the fifty-four chapters, covering a wide range of disciplines, illustrate in a striking way the influence of this progress in the field of ophthalmology. The advances derive in the main from highly sophisticated developments in research technology, providing new concepts rather than etiological revelations. Thus, many blinding diseases, as from cataract, glaucoma, diabetes, and age-related maculopathy, still await definitive explanations of their cause, but our increasing appreciation of the many factors apparently playing a role in their pathogenesis, so well expounded here, provide a sure foundation for tomorrow's achievements in rational therapy.

Whether the authors are clinicians, pathologists, or other scientists, they are all authorities in their subjects and together present, to a standard equal to the best in medical literature, our latest knowledge of eye disease, within the context of cognate progress in general pathology. It is a most impressive work and surely unequalled in its particular approach to diseases of the eye, not as an organ sequestered in the orbit, but as one vulnerable to diseases of the body as a whole.

In congratulating the authors I express my hope that this second edition will continue to provide both pleasure and profit to the wide readership it will undoubtedly attract.

Norman Ashton, CBE, FRS
Emeritus Professor of Pathology
University of London and
The Royal College of Surgeons of England

Foreword from the First Edition

No systematized presentation of the pathology of the eye existed in any language until 1808 when James Wardrop, a Scotsman then aged 26, published his first edition of *Essays on the Morbid Anatomy of the Human Eye*, followed the next year by *Fungus Haemotodes or Soft Cancer* which established retino-blastoma as a recognized entity. Although these books were not the first to describe or illustrate specimens or ocular disease, and in fact contained little morbid anatomy as now defined, they introduced, by dissections and macroscopical studies, an area of investigation eventually to become the specialty of ophthalmic pathology.

The subsequent development of microscopy in the late nineteenth century and early twentieth century and its wider use throughout all aspects of laboratory science led to an immense and still expanding increase in knowledge. The revelations of histology and histopathology had as dramatic an impact as those of electron microscopy in modern times, and ophthalmic pathology in its turn became largely concerned with the documentation of macroscopical and microscopical features of diseased ocular tissues. There followed many textbooks dealing exclusively or predominantly with these aspects; the most widely admired are beautifully illustrated first with superb paintings and drawings and later by photographic reproductions, which in the last two decades reached the highest quality. These remain classic textbooks in ophthalmology and are of inestimable value, but curiously ophthalmic pathology continued to be confined to morbid anatomy long after pathology itself had branched out to found the present main disciplines of histopathology, chemical pathology, hematology, medical microbiology, and immunopathology. Even today ophthalmic pathology is usually equated with histopathology of the eye; that is certainly the main interest of American, Canadian, and European ophthalmic pathology societies. This has been at least partly due to the fact that for many years ophthalmic pathology was a part-time pursuit of ophthalmologists engaged in exacting clinical practice, and perhaps it would be as reasonable to expect them to have had the time to become conversant with the many developments in pathology as it would be to expect a general pathologist to be skilled, for instance, in the latest methods of cataract extraction or the management of glaucoma. Thus while freely acknowledging that the present sum of knowledge in ophthalmic pathology is much indebted to them, I have always been convinced that future progress must be more widely based. In 1957, I wrote …

"If in the future, eye pathology is to be taught and practised in the traditional way, as an elaborate recording of histologic minutiae, then the subject is not too demanding and may well be undertaken as a part-time pursuit, and probably best by the ophthalmologist who is most able to extract the greatest clinical value from the findings. But if the study of ocular pathology is to have its full meaning, the eye must be regarded as a unit of an entire organism, and its behavior in disease must as far as possible be related to that of the whole. Research in this field, in common with the general tendency, should concern itself with disease mechanisms rather than with disease patterns, and for this purpose the widest possible knowledge of pathologic processes is desirable and the whole armamentarium of modern scientific method should be available. To establish ocular pathology on this broad basis will demand the full and concentrated attention of workers trained and experienced in the appropriate disciplines."*

Nearly a quarter of a century later I have nothing to add to these convictions and I warmly welcome this monumental work in two volumes planned and executed on the lines I had so hopefully visualized, and I am proud that such a notable work should have been assembled by Professor Alec Garner, my successor as director of the Department of Pathology at the Institute of Ophthalmology in London, and Professor Gordon Klintworth, some-time visiting professor there. With their able collaborators they present in these comprehensive volumes exactly the approach to ocular disease that is essential both for its immediate elucidation and for the whole future development of the subject, not in isolation but within the context of pathology as a whole.

With this conviction I warmly commend this book to everyone interested and involved in this fascinating field of learning, and wish all those concerned in its production the success so richly deserved.

Norman Ashton, CBE, FRS
Emeritus Professor of Pathology
University of London and
The Royal College of Surgeons of England

* Am. J. Ophthalmol. 44:5-6, 1957.

Preface to the Third Edition

Pathology at the clinical level is principally concerned with diagnosis, and rightly so. But it has an even deeper significance, which stems from its very definition. Pathology is the study of disease. In other words, it is fundamentally concerned with the processes underlying the clinical manifestations of disease. This is the principle we have tried to uphold in putting the present compilation together.

What is unique about this book? Before providing an answer, let us consider other books on ophthalmic pathology. Several are designed for the trainee in clinical ophthalmology and focus on clinically relevant information that examiners require of persons taking professional examinations. Such books are valuable to persons intent on persuading their examiners that they know enough pathology to be allowed to practice clinical ophthalmology. Other books provide a manual of diagnostic ophthalmic pathology and concentrate on descriptive morphology and are often extensively illustrated. *Garner and Klintworth's Pathobiology of Ocular Disease, Third Edition*, contains some elements of both of these types of books, but it goes far beyond material necessary to pass examinations or diagnose disorders based on morphologic criteria. Morphology continues to be the bedrock in defining the pathology of any disorder and, where appropriate, our contributors have not shied away from spelling out the clinical and histological aspects of the conditions they describe. But because pathology goes far beyond morbid anatomy, they have sought, where possible, to use these definitions as a basis for describing the underlying cellular events at a molecular level.

Back in the 1960s, when the editors were learning the trade, knowledge about eye diseases was proving elusive, largely from lack of appropriate methods of investigation. But since then the introduction of such techniques as electron microscopy, precise histochemical stains, and tissue and cell culture revolutionized the functional appreciation of a multitude of diseases. The revolution has continued unabated with the application of extremely sophisticated molecular biology techniques able to exploit an ever-expanding understanding of cytogenetics and immunology.

In the preface to the first edition of a much-valued textbook on pathology that was current when the editors of this book were medical students (1), we were reminded that, "Pathology is the elucidation of the vital processes which underlie the end-results studied by the morbid anatomist. It is the study of disease from the physiological point of view." Indeed, this has always been the real goal of the pathologist, a point purportedly made more than a hundred years ago by the distinguished surgeon, scientist, and one-time professor of pathology, Sir Victor Horsley (1857–1916), who was intent on pushing back the limitations of clinical practice when he wrote, "What is currently thought of as pathology is nothing of the sort—it is morbid anatomy. The pathologist should be a student of disordered function." It is to this understanding of ophthalmic pathology that we and our contributors have been committed in this multi-disciplinary book purposely titled, *Pathobiology of Ocular Disease*.

As with the two earlier editions, the book was designed with the ophthalmic practitioner in mind to provide, as far as is possible, an appreciation of the processes responsible for producing the disorders observed in hospital clinics and consulting rooms. While therapy is not considered because of space restrictions and the fact that it is often empirical, the information provided about the cause and basic mechanisms of specific diseases provides insight into potential therapeutic approaches. The effective rational therapy of any disease must be derived from a sound understanding of the underlying basic mechanisms.

In the decade that has intervened since the last edition, major advances have been made, particularly in the realms of molecular biology, cytogenetics, computerized databases, and, more recently, in molecular genetics. The ability to amplify DNA with the polymerized chain reaction, to sequence the human genome, and to identify specific proteins in different tissues with the highly sensitive matrix-assisted laser desorption ionization–time of flight mass spectrometry has played an important role in furthering knowledge. The study of ocular disease has shared in this advance, and the findings have impinged on the etiology and pathogenesis of many ocular diseases. This knowledge has expanded exponentially, largely as a result of research by scientists with a wide variety of techniques and the rapid dissemination of information on the Internet.

Such has been the increase in knowledge that several chapters were completely revamped and several new chapters added. The vast increase in knowledge about the genetics of many ocular diseases spawned specific chapters dealing with molecular genetic aspects of glaucoma and cataracts, as well as corneal, retinal, and optic nerve disease. Other new chapters focus on the molecular pathways of apoptosis, wound healing, the vasculitides, aging, age-related maculopathy, the aging lens, myopia, and amblyopia.

In the first edition we diligently avoided abbreviations, despite their emerging popularity in biomedical publications. By the second edition, abbreviations were unavoidable, and in this new edition the number increased immensely, largely due to the use of acronyms and conventions that have arisen regarding the nomenclature of the vast number of identified genes and their encoded proteins. When possible, we used accepted abbreviations that have come into common usage among experts who are furthering knowledge about diseases. For example, for consistency we used italicized uppercase letters for human genes and non-italicized letters for the protein products. Mouse genes that are involved in many animal models of ocular diseases are designated according to the accepted format of lowercase italicized letters. For readers not familiar with abbreviations, we have insisted that they be defined the first time that they are used in each chapter, and for the ease of finding the definition, the separate section on abbreviations has been retained. Hopefully, the large number of abbreviations in some chapters is not a chaotic alphabet soup.

So many human genetic diseases are now recognized that each has a Mendelian Inheritance in Man (MIM) number (2). Information about these diseases is freely available on the Internet, with links to information about the involved genes and their protein products. To facilitate the reader's access to this material, the Mendelian Inheritance in Man number for specific inherited diseases that are discussed in the book is provided when possible.

Another significant editorial change in the book is the rejection of the possessive form of eponyms for diseases, syndromes, anatomic structures, and other eponymous terms. This was done for multiple reasons, as outlined elsewhere (3), and the trend is gradually gaining momentum in medical writings.

We are fortunate to have been able to enlist the services of some of the most highly qualified investigators in their respective fields who provide authoritative accounts of the current understanding of the enormous spectrum of ocular diseases. To assist us in the critical evaluation of the text and the editing process we also recruited four highly respected ophthalmic pathologists as associate editors (Drs. J. Godfrey Heathcote, J. Douglas Cameron, Victor M. Elner, and Narsing A. Rao). We are most grateful to these individuals, who have expertise in different areas of the subject, for their constructive comments and editorial suggestions. We would also like to acknowledge several other individuals who helped bring this book to fruition: Mr. Geoffrey Greenwood, who convinced us to embark on a third edition, and Ms. Sandra Beberman, Ms. Dana Bigelow, Ms. Beth Campbell, Ms. Mary Drabot, and Mr. Christopher DiBiase of Informa Healthcare, as well as Ms. Paula Garber, Ms. Joanne Jay, and Mr. Peter Compitello of The Egerton Group Ltd., who were most helpful in bringing this book to fruition. As with the previous two editions, we wish to acknowledge the support and encouragement provided by our wives, Felicity and Catherine, and have great pleasure in dedicating this third edition to them.

The preparation of each edition of this book has aptly confirmed the impression of the great British soldier, statesman, author, and first honorary citizen of the United States, Sir Winston Churchill (1874–1965), who stated, "Writing a book is an adventure. To begin with it is a toy, then an amusement. Then it [becomes] a mistress, and then it becomes a master, and then it becomes a tyrant and, in the last stage, just as you are about to be reconciled to your servitude, you kill the monster and fling him to the public" (Grosvenor House, London, November 2, 1949) (4).

Gordon K. Klintworth
Alec Garner

REFERENCES

1. Boyd W. A Textbook of Pathology: An Introduction to Medicine. 1st ed. Philadelphia: Lea and Febiger, 1932.
2. http://www.ncbi.nlm.nih.gov/entrez/query.fcgi?db=OMIM
3. Iverson C, Flanagin A, Fontanarosa PB, et al. American Medical Association Manual of Style: A Guide for Authors and Editors. 9th ed. Baltimore: Williams and Wilkins, 1998.
4. The words from the original speaking notes for Churchill's address after receiving the Times Literary Award. Churchill Archives Centre Cambridge, CHUR 5/28A, paragraph 4, page 2.

Preface from the Second Edition

A knowledge of pathology is the basis of sound medicine, and the thinking ophthalmologist is keen to understand, as well as may be, the forces responsible for the clinical manifestations of eye disease. Only then can management be pursued in a rational manner. The descriptive elements of ophthalmic pathology are fundamental and need to be precisely defined in the interests of accurate diagnosis. But beyond that utilitarian function is their importance as building blocks in comprehending the nature of the disease processes per se, and it is to this second objective in particular that the present text is directed. Correspondingly, we have not sought to provide a detailed manual of diagnostic pathology—there are now a number of excellent texts and atlases available that achieve this purpose far better than we could ever have hoped to do. Instead, where possible, we have tried to interpret the facts and to provide a feeling for the dynamic aspects of ophthalmic pathology.

As noted in the preface to the first edition, laudable though such a purpose may be, it is difficult to succeed. Firstly, depending on the particular disease state under consideration, it requires a sound knowledge of a range of complementary disciplines such as molecular biology, biochemistry, immunology, and genetics. In this regard, we have been fortunate in having the services of many recognized experts in these various fields capable of writing with authority. Secondly, not all the necessary building blocks are yet identified, let alone in position. Nevertheless, an incredible body of new information has accrued in almost every field in the twelve years since the first edition, especially in the understanding of disease at the molecular level, and an update of our text had become imperative if it was to remain relevant. We were encouraged to take up the challenge by the favorable reception of the first edition and because, despite the welcome increase in textbooks related to the pathology of eye disease, ours remains the only reasonably comprehensive attempt to address the functional aspects of the subject.

As with the first edition, this has been a daunting task, and we are more than grateful to our contributors, who have responded to their briefs quite magnificently. For one reason or another, we have had to enlist the help of a number of new authors, and such has been the enormous volume of new material to be covered that even existing authors have had to engage in extensive revision of their chapters, amounting in some cases to a complete rewrite.

Again, we very much hope that the attraction of the book will extend beyond the precious but small number of practicing ophthalmic pathologists to pathologists working in other fields, because study of the eye has relevance far beyond its own orbit. Clinical ophthalmologists too will, we trust, find much to assist them in the evaluation and treatment of their patients. We hope that others outside the medical community—those employed in related disciplines of biology, immunology, and genetics—will also discover something of value.

We are very conscious of and more than happy to acknowledge the enormous assistance provided by our secretaries, Pat Goodwin, Carmen Quarrie, Wanda Dietze, Elizabeth Barnard, Karen Alliume, and Kristina Boewe. We are also indebted to Allan T. Summers for his painstaking role in verifying and completing countless references. Finally, as before, we want to thank our wives, Catherine and Felicity, who have been most supportive, and we hope they will find pleasure in the outcome which we take great delight in dedicating to them.

Alec Garner
Gordon K. Klintworth

Preface from the First Edition

Such is the volume of ophthalmologic and pathological writing that only by stepping aside completely from one's commitment to engage actively in these disciplines would it be possible to absorb all that might profitably be read. It would be irresponsible of any potential author or editor to unleash on the busy student yet more reading matter should it not fill a real need. There are in existence already several excellent treatises relating to the pathological anatomy of the eye, and it would have been redundant for us to seek to emulate them; rather we have sought to direct attention to dynamic considerations and disease mechanisms, and so complement the emphasis on descriptive pathology to be found in other writings on the subject. Hence the title *Pathobiology of Ocular Disease: A Dynamic Approach.*

It is our belief that knowing the appearance of a lesion and being able to recognize it is only the beginning of the story. If appropriate and rational treatment is to be instituted, it is also necessary to understand what is happening and, where possible, why. For instance, from the practicing clinician's standpoint, more important than to recognize granulomatous inflammation when seen in a microscopical preparation is to have some idea of what that means in terms of causative factors and likely behavior. That is not to say we decry descriptive pathology—far from it, for morphology and function are but the two sides of the same coin and are patently interdependent. But the job of the pathologist is both to identify disease processes and to interpret them in behavioral terms. It was with this dual role of pathology in mind that we invited the various contributors to compose their chapters.

However, success is an elusive goal when the brief is so demanding. To state what and where is one thing; to ask how and why is quite another. Nevertheless, as editors, we feel that our contributors have responded magnificently and it is our fervent hope that the result will meet the needs of serious students of ophthalmology, be they trainees or more experienced practitioners, who are keen to understand the nature of the disorders they are called on to treat. The emphasis on dynamic disease processes inevitably encompasses the whole gamut of pathological disciplines—microbiology, immunology, and biochemistry, as well as histopathology, and this all-embracing interpretation of pathology serves further to distinguish our book from existing texts.

For a variety of reasons, which need not be spelt out here, ophthalmic pathology is commonly viewed with suspicion by other pathologists. Trained as general pathologists ourselves, we as editors hope that, by relating the specific matters of ocular pathology to the basic and more general aspects of disease processes, we will have gone some way towards persuading our colleagues that study of the eye is both fascinating and rewarding.

Inevitably, to assemble a multiauthor compendium of the sort we have compiled, such that there is not too much diversity of approach, has involved a great deal of effort, not only for the editors, but also for the gallant contributors who have had to contend with a seemingly endless stream of queries and comments. We want to thank them for their cooperation and forbearance.

Other people whose assistance has been invaluable are acknowledged elsewhere but we would also put on record our appreciation of the unstinting advice and practical help provided by the staff of our publisher, Marcel Dekker, Inc., and of the colossal support we have received from our secretaries, Catherine Thornton, Pat Goodwin, Louise Hart, Frances Slocum, Candiss Weaver, Pat Burks, Bonnie Lynch, Diane Evans, Linda Brogan, Marge Penny, and Virginia Hotelling. Lastly, if for no other reason than that they are the ones who at the end of the day have had to bear with us when the task of preparing the book weighed overheavily on our shoulders, we want to thank our wives and children for their tolerance and encouragement.

This book would not have been possible without the assistance of many individuals. Aside from the vital role of the authors and the editorial staff of Marcel Dekker, Inc., numerous individuals provided critical reviews of chapters. In this regard, we wish to thank the following:

Mathea R. Allansmith
Douglas R. Anderson
Norman Ashton
Elaine R. Berman
Stanley Braverman
Robert P. Burns
R. Jean Campbell
Leo T. Chylack
David G. Cogan
Byron P. Croker, Jr.
Anthony J. Dark
D. Doniach
Roberta Meyers Elliot
Bernard F. Fetter
Ben S. Fine
Ramon L. Font

Robert Y. Foos
Doyle G. Graham
Donald B. Hackel
Hal K. Hawkins
Hannah Kinney
Jin H. Kinoshita
John F. R. Kuck, Jr.
Robert Machemer
Kenneth S. McCarty, Jr.
Don Minckler
Ralph Muller
G. Richard O'Connor
M. Bruce Shields
James Tiedeman
Robert Trelstad
F. Stephen Vogel
Lorenz E. Zimmerman

Allan Summers, Susan Feinglos, Ginger Reeves, Betty Adams, Mary Ann Brown, and Janet Shields were most helpful in checking and completing the innumerable references.

The following assisted authors with specific chapters: Nancy L. Robinson, Glenn P. Kimball, and Karen A. Pelletier (Chapter 49), David Andrews (Chapter 48), Joseph Hackett (Chapter 40).

Alec Garner
Gordon K. Klintworth

Contents of Part A

DISORDERS OF THE VITREOUS

DISORDERS OF THE ANTERIOR SEGMENT

METABOLIC AND GENETIC DISORDERS

Contents of Part B

Contributors

Anthony P. Adamis Eyetech Pharmaceuticals, New York, New York, U.S.A.

D. Cory Adamson Departments of Neurosurgery and Neurobiology, Duke University, Durham, North Carolina, U.S.A.

Daniel M. Albert Department of Ophthalmology and Visual Sciences, University of Wisconsin, Madison, Wisconsin, U.S.A.

Thomas Albini Bascom Palmer Eye Institute, Miller School of Medicine, University of Miami, Miami, Florida, U.S.A.

R. Rand Allingham Department of Ophthalmology, Duke University, Durham, North Carolina, U.S.A.

Fahd Anzaar Massachusetts Eye Research and Surgery Institute and Harvard University, Boston, Massachusetts, U.S.A.

Pelin Atmaca-Sönmez Kellogg Eye Institute, University of Michigan, Ann Arbor, Michigan, U.S.A.

William Robert Bell Wilmer Eye Institute, Johns Hopkins University, Baltimore, Maryland, U.S.A.

Elaine R. Berman (deceased) Hadassah-Hebrew University Medical School, Jerusalem, Israel

Paul N. Bishop Faculty of Medical and Human Sciences and Wellcome Trust Centre for Cell-Matrix Research, University of Manchester, Manchester, U.K.

Zita F. H. M. Boonman Department of Ophthalmology, Leiden University Medical Center, Leiden, The Netherlands

Ray P. Boot-Handford Faculty of Life Sciences, Wellcome Trust Centre for Cell Matrix Research, University of Manchester, Manchester, U.K.

Edward H. Bossen Department of Pathology, Duke University, Durham, North Carolina, U.S.A.

Rose-Mary Boustany Departments of Pediatrics and Neurobiology, Duke University, Durham, North Carolina, U.S.A. and Abu-Haidan Neuroscience Institute, American University of Beirut, Beirut, Lebanon

Harry H. Brown Harvey and Bernice Jones Eye Institute, University of Arkansas for Medical Sciences, Little Rock, Arkansas, U.S.A.

Matthew J. Burton International Centre for Eye Health, London School of Hygiene and Tropical Medicine, London, U.K.

J. Douglas Cameron Department of Ophthalmology, Mayo Clinic, Rochester, Minnesota, U.S.A.

George M. Cherian Departments of Pathology, Pharmacology, and Toxicology, University of Western Ontario, London, Ontario, Canada

Chung-Jung Chiu Department of Ophthalmology and the Jean Mayer USDA Human Nutrition Research Center on Aging, Tufts University, Boston, Massachusetts, U.S.A.

M. Joseph Costello Department of Cell and Developmental Biology, University of North Carolina, Chapel Hill, North Carolina, U.S.A.

J. Oscar Croxatto Departments of Teaching and Research and Laboratory of Ophthalmic Pathology, Fundación Oftalmológica Argentina Jorge Malbran, Buenos Aires, Argentina

Thomas J. Cummings Departments of Pathology and Ophthalmology, Duke University, Durham, North Carolina, U.S.A.

Karim F. Damji University of Ottawa Eye Institute, Ottawa, Ontario, Canada

Hakan Demirci Kellogg Eye Institute, University of Michigan, Ann Arbor, Michigan, U.S.A.

Erin Demo Divison of Genetics and Metabolism, University of North Carolina, Chapel Hill, North Carolina, U.S.A.

Susan G. Elner Kellogg Eye Institute, University of Michigan, Ann Arbor, Michigan, U.S.A.

Victor M. Elner Kellogg Eye Institute, University of Michigan, Ann Arbor, Michigan, U.S.A.

Geoffrey G. Emerson Casey Eye Institute, Oregon Health and Science University, Portland, Oregon, U.S.A.

Jan J. Enghild Department of Molecular Biology, University of Aarhus, Aarhus, Denmark

Andrew Flint Department of Pathology, University of Michigan, Ann Arbor, Michigan, U.S.A.

C. Stephen Foster Massachusetts Eye Research and Surgery Institute and Harvard University, Boston, Massachusetts, U.S.A.

Peter J. Francis Casey Eye Institute, Oregon Health and Science University, Portland, Oregon, U.S.A.

Anne B. Fulton Department of Ophthalmology, Children's Hospital, Boston, Massachusetts, U.S.A.

David M. Gamm Department of Ophthalmology and Visual Sciences, University of Wisconsin, Madison, Wisconsin, U.S.A.

Alec Garner Institute of Ophthalmology, Moorfields Eye Hospital, London, U.K.

Devin M. Gattey Casey Eye Institute, Oregon Health and Science University, Portland, Oregon, U.S.A.

Jennifer B. Green Division of Endocrinology, Department of Medicine, Duke University, Durham, North Carolina, U.S.A.

W. Richard Green Wilmer Eye Institute, Johns Hopkins University, Baltimore, Maryland, U.S.A.

Ian Grierson Unit of Ophthalmology, School of Clinical Sciences, University of Liverpool, Liverpool, U.K.

Hans E. Grossniklaus Departments of Ophthalmology and Pathology, Emory University, Atlanta, Georgia, U.S.A.

Duane L. Guernsey Departments of Pathology, Ophthalmology and Visual Sciences, Surgery, Physiology, and Biophysics, Dalhousie University, Halifax, Nova Scotia, Canada

Avinash Gurbaxani Kings College Hospital, London, U.K.

Robyn H. Guymer Centre for Eye Research Australia, University of Melbourne, East Melbourne, Victoria, Australia

John R. Guyton Department of Medicine, Duke University, Durham, North Carolina, U.S.A.

Sarah Hale University Hospital of Wales, Cardiff, U.K.

John J. Harding Nuffield Laboratory of Ophthalmology, University of Oxford, Oxford, U.K.

J. Godfrey Heathcote Departments of Pathology and Ophthalmology and Visual Sciences, Dalhousie University, Halifax, Nova Scotia, Canada

John R. Heckenlively Kellogg Eye Institute, University of Michigan, Ann Arbor, Michigan, U.S.A.

Mitchell T. Heflin Center for Aging and Human Development, Duke University, Durham, North Carolina, U.S.A.

Paul Hiscott Unit of Ophthalmology, School of Clinical Sciences, University of Liverpool, Liverpool, U.K.

David N. Howell Department of Pathology, Duke University and Durham Veterans Administration Medical Center, Durham, North Carolina, U.S.A.

Martine J. Jager Department of Ophthalmology, Leiden University Medical Center, Leiden, The Netherlands

Henrik Karring Department of Experimental Medical Science, Lund University, Lund, Sweden

Cay M. Kielty Faculty of Life Sciences, Wellcome Trust Centre for Cell Matrix Research, University of Manchester, Manchester, U.K.

Priya S. Kishnani Division of Medical Genetics, Duke University, Durham, North Carolina, U.S.A.

Mary K. Klassen-Fischer Armed Forces Institute of Pathology, Washington, D.C., U.S.A.

Gordon K. Klintworth Departments of Pathology and Ophthalmology, Duke University, Durham, North Carolina, U.S.A.

Dwight D. Koeberl Division of Medical Genetics, Duke University, Durham, North Carolina, U.S.A.

Amol D. Kulkarni Department of Ophthalmology and Visual Sciences, University of Wisconsin, Madison, Wisconsin, U.S.A.

Jerome R. Kuszak Department of Ophthalmology, Rush University Medical Center, Chicago, Illinois, U.S.A.

Anand Shreeram Lagoo Department of Pathology, Duke University, Durham, North Carolina, U.S.A.

Susan Lightman Department of Clinical Ophthalmology, Moorfields Eye Hospital, London, U.K.

Lyndell L. Lim Centre for Eye Research Australia, University of Melbourne, East Melbourne, Victoria, Australia

Ming Lu Vantage Eye Center, Monterey, California, U.S.A.

Helen Lum Durham Veterans Administration Medical Center, Durham, North Carolina, U.S.A.

Curtis E. Margo University of South Florida, Tampa, Florida, U.S.A.

Suzanne P. McKee Smith-Kettlewell Eye Research Institute, San Francisco, California, U.S.A.

Stuart J. McKinnon Departments of Ophthalmology and Neurobiology, Duke University, Durham, North Carolina, U.S.A.

Janine D. Mendola Center for Advanced Imaging, West Virginia University School of Medicine, Morgantown, West Virginia, U.S.A.

Ravikanth Metlapally Duke Center for Human Genetics and Duke Eye Center, Duke University, Durham, North Carolina, U.S.A.

Sara E. Miller Department of Pathology, Duke University, Durham, North Carolina, U.S.A.

David Millington Division of Medical Genetics, Duke University, Durham, North Carolina, U.S.A.

Torben Møller-Pedersen Department of Molecular Biology, University of Aarhus, Aarhus, Denmark

Anne Moskowitz Department of Ophthalmology, Children's Hospital, Boston, Massachusetts, U.S.A.

Ronald C. Neafie Armed Forces Institute of Pathology, Washington, D.C., U.S.A.

Thomas T. Norton Department of Vision Sciences, University of Alabama at Birmingham, Birmingham, Alabama, U.S.A.

Terrence P. O'Brien Bascom Palmer Eye Institute of the Palm Beaches, Palm Beach Gardens, Florida, U.S.A.

Alan D. Proia Department of Pathology, Duke University, Durham, North Carolina, U.S.A.

Narsing A. Rao Doheny Eye Institute, Keck School of Medicine, University of Southern California, Los Angeles, California, U.S.A.

Johane M. Robitaille Departments of Ophthalmology and Visual Sciences and Pathology, Dalhousie University, Halifax, Nova Scotia, Canada

Diva R. Salomão Department of Pathology, Mayo Clinic, Mayo Foundation, and Mayo Medical School, Rochester, Minnesota, U.S.A.

Ursula Schlötzer-Schrehardt University of Erlangen-Nürnberg, Erlangen, Germany

Bryan J. Schwent Department of Ophthalmology, Emory University, Atlanta, Georgia, U.S.A.

Alan Shiels Department of Ophthalmology and Visual Sciences, Washington University School of Medicine, St. Louis, Missouri, U.S.A.

Brian S. F. Shine Department of Clinical Biochemistry, John Radcliffe Hospital, and Oxford Centre for Diabetes, Endocrinology, and Metabolism, Oxford, U.K.

Barbara A. W. Streeten State University of New York Upstate Medical University, Syracuse, New York, U.S.A.

Allen Taylor Department of Ophthalmology and the Jean Mayer USDA Human Nutrition Research Center for Aging, Tufts University, Boston, Masssachusetts, U.S.A.

René E. M. Toes Department of Rheumatology, Leiden University Medical Center, Leiden, The Netherlands

Julie H. Tsai University of South Carolina School of Medicine, Columbia, South Carolina, U.S.A.

Richard Vander Heide Wayne State University Medical School and John D. Dingell Veterans Administration Medical Center, Detroit, Michigan, U.S.A.

Bret M. Wehrli Department of Pathology, University of Western Ontario, London, Ontario, Canada

Janey L. Wiggs Department of Ophthalmology, Harvard Medical School, and Massachusetts Eye and Ear Infirmary, Boston, Massachusetts, U.S.A.

David J. Wilson Casey Eye Institute, Oregon Health and Science University, Portland, Oregon, U.S.A.

Carolyn S. Wu Department of Ophthalmology, Children's Hospital, Boston, Massachusetts, U.S.A.

Hai Yan Department of Pathology, Duke University, Durham, North Carolina, U.S.A.

Sarah Young Division of Medical Genetics, Duke University, Durham, North Carolina, U.S.A.

Terri L. Young Duke Eye Center and Duke Center for Human Genetics, Duke University, Durham, North Carolina, U.S.A.

1

The Cell in Health and Disease

Richard Vander Heide
Wayne State University Medical School and John D. Dingell Veterans Administration Medical Center, Detroit, Michigan, U.S.A.

INTRODUCTION

The primary goal of this chapter is to acquaint the reader with the cell types encountered in the ocular tissues in health and disease and to point out the changes in cellular structure and function that result from disease. This discussion focuses on basic concepts and is not intended to be comprehensive—for that the reader is referred to several excellent textbooks on cell biology and pathology (2,50,71).

THE NORMAL CELL

Most mammalian cells are surrounded by a plasma membrane and contain a nucleus and cytoplasm.

Nucleus

The nuclei of most cells are more or less spherical, although certain normal cells such as polymorphonuclear leukocytes (PMNs) exhibit pronounced lobulations. The nucleus is surrounded by two membranes which constitute the nuclear envelope. These two membranes are fused at multiple foci, forming nuclear pores (Fig. 1) (13). Nuclear pores represent sites of two-way communication between the nucleus and cytoplasm. Both RNA efflux from the nucleus and the import of proteins such as nucleoplasmin into the nucleus have been documented to occur through the pores (25). The chromatin in the nucleus is either relatively electron-dense (heterochromatin) or comparatively electron-lucent (euchromatin) (Fig. 1). The nucleolus is composed of several different components, including small granules about the size and shape of ribosomes (15–20 nm), and very fine fibrillar material (27): hence the cytologic terms *pars granulosa* and *pars fibrosa*.

Cytoplasm

The cytoplasm contains glycogen, an endoplasmic reticulum (ER), ribosomes, the Golgi apparatus, lyosomes, mitochondria, and various other constituents based on the nature of the cell type.

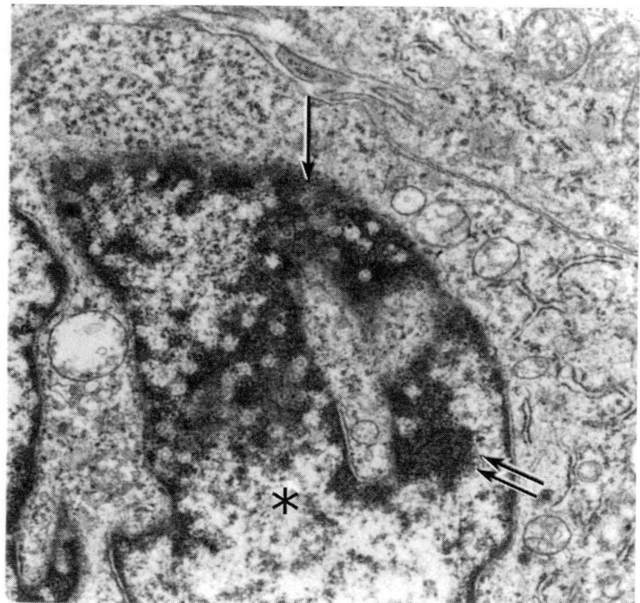

Figure 1 The nucleus of this tumor cell exhibits numerous nuclear pores, which appear as small clear circles (*arrow*), sometimes with a central dot. Presumably, this represents a grazing or en face section of the nucleus. Heterochromatin (*double arrow*) and euchromatin (*asterisk*) are also identified. It is important that nuclear pores not be confused with viral particles (×14,300). *Source*: Courtesy of Dr. John D. Shelburne.

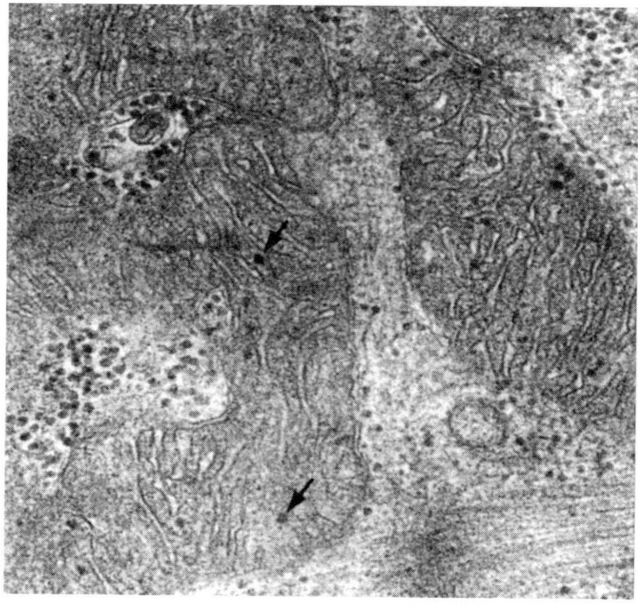

Figure 2 Normal human myocardial mitochondria. The normal mitochondrial matrix granules (*arrows*) are easily distinguishable from the flocculent densities of Figure 5. An early sign of cell injury is *loss* of these normal granules (×48,000). *Source*: Courtesy of Dr. John D. Shelburne.

Mitochondria

Mitochondria, which provide adenosine triphosphate (ATP) for cellular activity, are normally bound by a double membrane with the inner membrane exhibiting deep invaginations into the central compartment or matrix space (68). These invaginations of the inner membrane are referred to as cristae. The mitochondrial matrix space of normal cells contains amorphous protein and often electron-dense granules which are distinct from the densities characteristic of cell injury (see later discussion). Normal cells contain at least two different forms of mitochondria; condensed or orthodox. As implied by the name, the "orthodox" configuration is more common. Condensed mitochondria are common in the corneal endothelium and are occasionally seen in biopsied tissue. Condensed mitochondria are obtained in vitro with isolated mitochondria or in intact cells when the adenosine diphosphate (ADP)/ATP ratio is high (32,35,72).

The brain, retina, striated muscle, and many other tissues derive their main source of energy from the generation of ATP by oxidative phosphorylation within mitochondria (Figs. 2–6). The complex generation of this energy, which is under the control of both nuclear DNA and mitochondrial DNA genes (see Chapter 31) (89) involves five multiple subunit enzyme

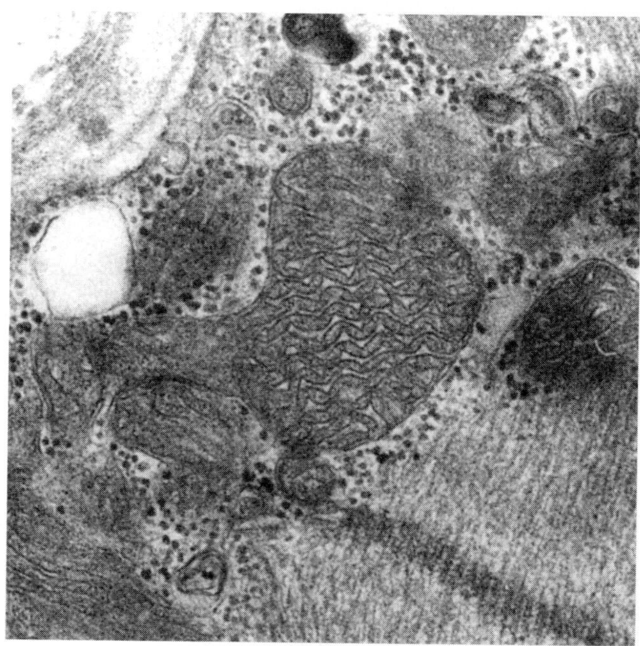

Figure 3 Normal human myocardial cell mitochondria sometimes exhibit jagged cristae (×49,900). *Source*: Courtesy of Dr. John D. Shelburne.

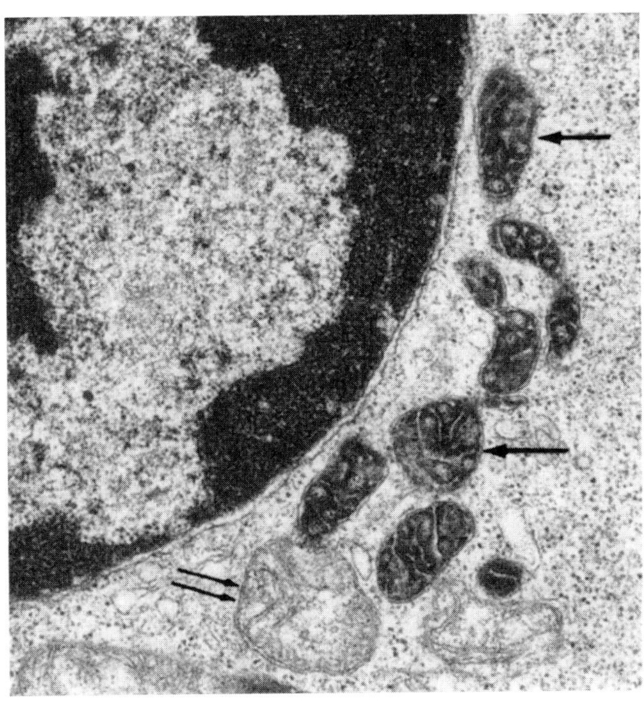

Figure 4 This circulating lymphocyte exhibits within the cytoplasm of this single cell *both* condensed (*arrows*) and slightly swollen orthodox (*double arrows*) mitochondria (×23,900). *Source*: Courtesy of Dr. John D. Shelburne.

complexes (designated complex I through V) in addition to the adenine nucleotide translocator (all situated within the mitochondrial inner membrane). Complexes I through IV make up the electron transport chain. In complex I, reduced nicotinamide adenine dinucleotide (NADH) is oxidized by NADH dehydrogenase to nicotinamide adenine dinucleotide. This complex consists of more than 30 polypeptides. In complex II, which involves four nuclear DNA-encoded polypeptides, succinate dehydrogenase oxidizes succinate to fumarate, while electrons are transferred to ubiquinone [coenzyme Q (CoQ)] to yield ubiquinol (reduced CoQ). Electrons are then transferred to cytochrome *c* by way of complex III (ubiquinol: cytochrome *c* oxireductase), which consists of 10 polypeptides, and finally to oxygen in the 13 polypeptide-containing complex IV (cytochrome *c* oxidase). Complex V (ATP synthetase), which embraces 12 polypeptides, forms ATP by condensing ADP and inorganic phosphate (see the section entitled Mitochondrial Pathway of Apoptosis in Chapter 2).

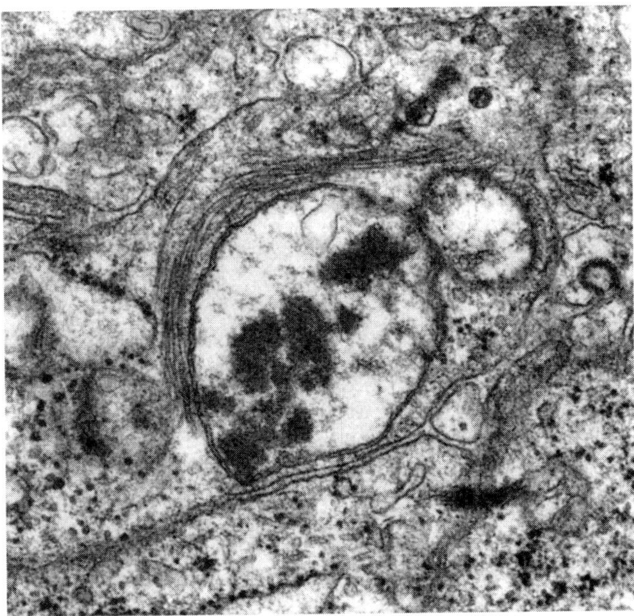

Figure 5 Typical flocculent or amorphous matrical densities in a mitochondrion of a neoplastic squamous cell (×39,100). *Source*: Courtesy of Dr. John D. Shelburne.

Rough ER

The space between the two membranes of the nuclear envelope (the perinuclear cisterna) is continuous with cisternae of the rough ER. Proteins destined for secretion are synthesized in the rough ER prior to their passage through the Golgi apparatus and subsequent packing in secretory vacuoles (69). Conversely, proteins destined for intracellular use are believed to be synthesized on intracellular-free polyribosomes not connected to cisternae of the ER. Consequently, cisternae of the rough ER are especially prominent in cells that synthesize proteins for export, e.g., fibroblasts, plasma cells, hepatocytes, and epithelial glandular cells (lacrimal gland).

Lysosomes

Primary lysosomes bud directly from the Golgi apparatus and are thus a form of secretory vacuole (20). Their primary function is in the turnover and processing of proteins. Heterophagy refers to the phagocytosis (or "endocytosis") of extracellular material foreign to the cell in question. This process is to be distinguished from autophagocytosis or autophagy, in which the cell digests a portion of its own cytoplasm. In autophagy, organelles, such as mitochondria, bud into the lysosomal space of the same cell and become degraded (5,64,73,74). Pinocytosis designates the formation of very small vacuoles which appear devoid of recognizable material but likely contain fluid and/or protein. Both phagocytic and autophagic vacuoles fuse with primary lysosomes to form secondary lysosomes in which hydrolytic enzymes partly degrade the contents. The fusion of primary lysosomes with phagocytic vacuoles usually occurs rapidly.

Golgi Apparatus

The Golgi complex consists of flattened slightly curved sacks which are stacked together. Their outer, or convex,

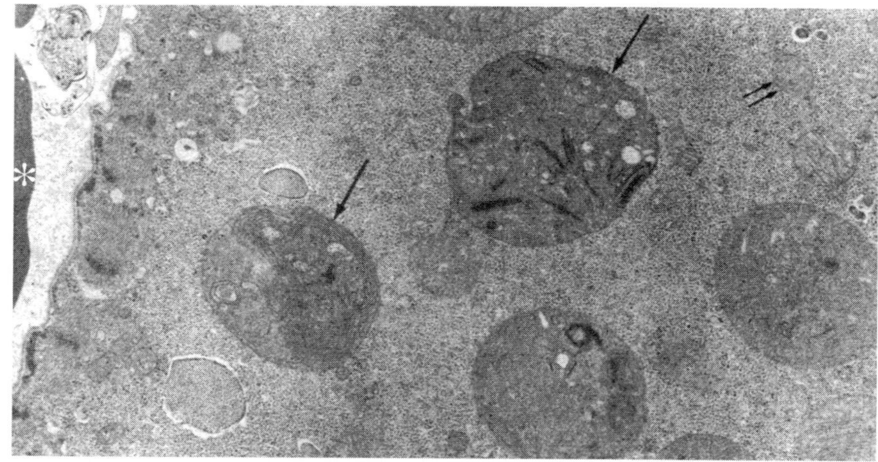

Figure 6 Several enlarged mitochondria (*arrows*) are visible in the cytoplasm of this myocardial cell. Compare their size with the normal mitochondrion shown at the *double arrows*, and with a portion of an erythrocyte (*asterisk*). Large amounts of glycogen are present in the cyto-plasm (×10,300). *Source*: Courtesy of Dr. John D. Shelburne.

surface is sometimes referred to as the "forming" face since it is thought to be proximal in terms of chemical flow through the synthetic machinery of the cell (10). Secretory vacuoles bud off the "inner" or "concave" face, which is also known as the "maturing" face. The Golgi apparatus is considered to be the site of glycosylation of glycoproteins and of polysaccharide synthesis. It is thought that most proteins synthesized in the rough ER move through the Golgi before being "packaged" into secretory vacuoles.

Peroxisomes

Peroxisomes are ubiquitous self-replicating organelles within the cytosol that rid cells of toxic substances. They are surrounded by a plasma membrane that is critical for importing substances into the organelle.

Ribosomes

Ribosomes are large, complex structures that are composed of RNA and protein in a two-thirds to one-third ratio. Ribosomes are the structures upon which the coordinated synthesis of proteins occurs.

Single-Membrane-Limited Structures of Diagnostic Interest

Dense core granules. Dense core granules are present in an incredible variety of normal and abnormal tissues (especially carcinoid tumors and paragangliomas). These are often referred to as "neurosecretory" granules because of their presence in many neural tissues, including the adrenal medulla (29). Unless associated with confirmatory evidence of a neurosecretory activity it is best to avoid the term "neurosecretory" granules and to refer to them as dense core granules or single-membrane-limited dense granules. They are usually (but not always) distinguishable from lysosomes because of their small size, the homogeneity and extreme electron density of the included material, and the relative uniformity of size and shape. In many tissues dense core granules are thought to contain amines, such as serotonin, and indeed this has been established in the case of the dense core granules of platelets (18).

Birbeck granules. Characteristic rod- and racquet-shaped cytoplasmic organelles known as Birbeck granules (9) occur in the normal Langerhans cell (Fig. 7).

Melanosomes. Melanosomes are single-membrane-limited organelles with a characteristic 9-nm periodic paracrystalline structure (Fig. 8) which is the tyrosinase enzyme. These are discussed in Chapter 59.

Weibel–Palade bodies. Capillary endothelial cells in many tissues contain peculiar cigar-shaped single-membrane-limited bodies first described by Weibel and Palade (87). These so-called Weibel–Palade bodies can be distinguished from premelanosomes, which they resemble in size, through the use of transmission electron microscopy (TEM) because they exhibit a unique inner structure (Fig. 9). Functionally, Weibel–Palade bodies contain Factor VIII, and serve as a valuable marker of capillary endothelial cells.

Glycogen. Glycogen is often seen in the cytoplasm in many cell types, including liver, skeletal muscle, and the myocardium.

Cylinder organelles. Strange crystalline structures known as "cylinder organelles" have been described in the cytosol in the outer plexiform layer of the retina in normal and pathologic conditions, including Alexander disease (83).

Cilia

Cilia are present in large numbers in certain epithelium such as the upper respiratory tract where they function in the removal of mucus and bacterial organisms thereby reducing the risk of lung infection. Cilia contain microtubules with the characteristic 9 + 2 arrangement (Fig. 10).

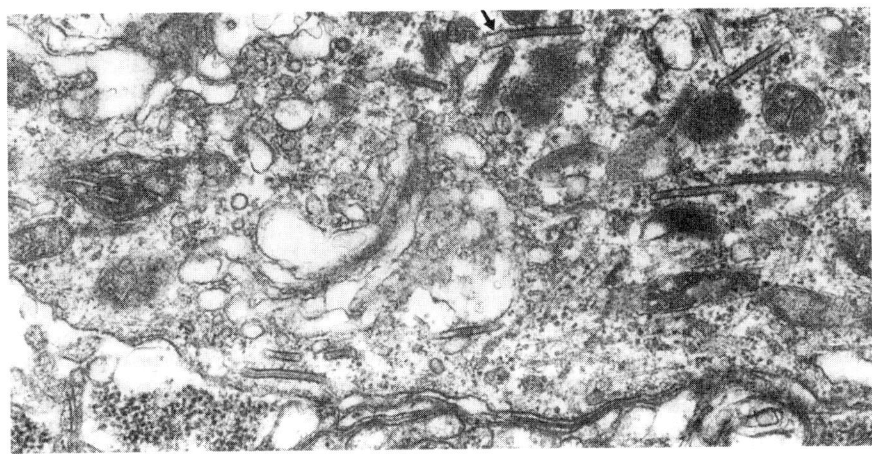

Figure 7 Typical Birbeck granules in the cytoplasm of a normal Langerhans cell of human epidermis. Note the "drumstick" configuration of some of these granules (*arrow*) (×35,400). *Source*: Courtesy of Dr. John D. Shelburne.

Microtubules and Cell Filaments

Microtubules. Microtubules measure about 25 nm in diameter and appear as hollow cylinders on routine electron microscopy. They are composed of the protein tubulin (see Chapter 36). Microtubules are present in most cells, and thus documentation of their presence is rarely of diagnostic value.

Cytoplasmic filaments. Cell filaments belong to one of three major groups—thick filaments, intermediate filaments, or microfilaments. The myosin filaments of normal or neoplastic skeletal muscle cells measure approximately 15 nm in diameter, and are termed "thick" filaments, easily distinguished from the approximately 6 nm actin "microfilaments." Microfilaments are as ubiquitous as microtubules and measure approximately 5 to 7 nm in diameter. Just as in smooth muscle cells, at least some microfilaments of most cells are composed of actin or actin-like proteins (77,78). Many epithelial cells have a dense feltwork of filaments in the apical cytosol ("terminal bar") (42), and the basal bodies of cilia if cilia are present. Tumors that derive from muscle cells (such as leiomyosarcomas) may exhibit

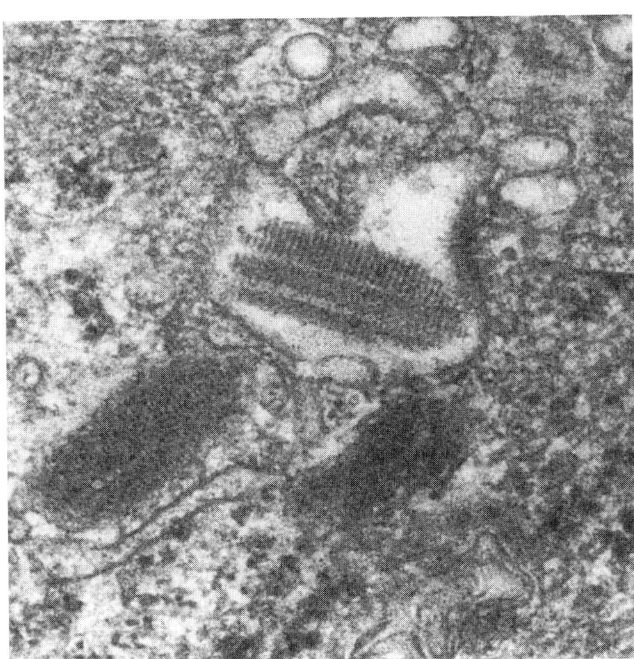

Figure 8 A typical premelanosome in the cytoplasm of an amelanotic melanoma cell. The paracrystal in the single-membrane-limited vacuole has a characteristic 9 nm periodicity (×106,700). *Source*: Courtesy of Dr. John D. Shelburne.

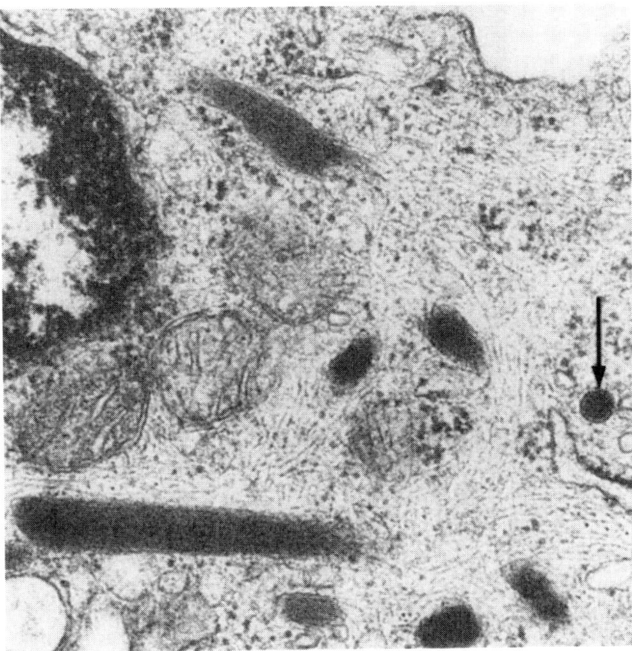

Figure 9 Weibel–Palade bodies in a normal vascular endothelial cell. Note that the tubular array is *parallel* to the long axis of this organelle, not at right angles to it as is true for melanosomes (Fig. 8). Note also that cross-sections of these cigar-shaped bodies may appear as single-membrane-limited dense core granules (*arrow*). It is important not to confuse these with true dense core granules (×50,500). *Source*: Courtesy of Dr. John D. Shelburne.

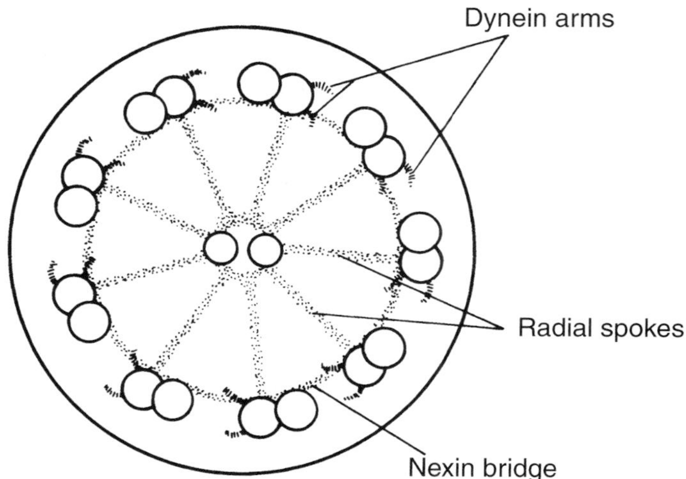

Figure 10 A cross-section of a typical cilium showing the idealized ultrastructure of a normal cilium. Recent ultrastructural studies of humans with a variety of clinical disorders have shown absent radial spokes or dynein arms. Note that the outer dynein arm is visualized better than the inner arm. *Source*: Courtesy of Dr. John D. Shelburne.

numerous fine cytoplasmic filaments with interspersed small fusiform densities.

Intermediate filaments refer to fibrous proteins typically between 7 and 11 nm in diameter, and thus intermediate in size between the actin and myosin filaments of skeletal muscle. Currently five major types of intermediate filaments are recognized including: glial filaments, neurofilaments, keratins, vimentin, and desmin (see Chapter 36). Glial filaments (89,91) measure approximately 7 to 8 nm in diameter and are composed of glial fibrillary acidic protein. The demonstration of glial filaments is useful in the diagnosis of astrocytomas (17). Neurofilaments present in neurons are slightly thicker (10 nm). Keratin is composed in part of masses of fine filaments known as tonofibrillar aggregates or bundles. These aggregates are seen in normal keratinizing epidermis, in abnormal keratinized conjunctival and corneal epithelium, and in squamous cell carcinomas and thus are of diagnostic value. Other intermediate filaments are generally identified with immunocytochemistry. Vimentin is present in a variety of mesenchymal cells, whereas desmin is a marker for skeletal, smooth or cardiac muscle cells.

Cell Junctions

Normal cells are connected to one another through six major types of cell junctions (10,61), namely desmosomes, intermediate junctions, tight junctions, gap junctions, complex interdigitations and hemidesmosomes.

Desmosomes. Desmosomes (maculae adherentes) are button-like firm attachments that connect epithelial cells, including squamous epithelial cells, such as those of the cornea and conjunctiva, and certain mesodermal tissues. The maculae adherentes are often referred to as "spot desmosomes" or "spot welds" because of their shape and strength. Desmosomes characteristically exhibit a central dense line and numerous 10-nm filaments are attached to the cytoplasmic side and stream outward into the cytosol. Desmosomes are common in epithelial neoplasms but uncommon in sarcomas.

Intermediate junctions. Frequently, the term "desmosome" is misapplied to intermediate junctions, which lack a central dense line and have far less fibrillar material in the associated cytoplasm. At 7 nm, the fibrils are thinner than the 10-nm fibrils associated with desmosomes. In many normal epithelial cells this type of junction extends as a band all the way around the cell apex (just beneath the tight junction) and therefore has been called zonula adherens or "belt desmosomes." Intermediate junctions are extremely common and are not usually of value in distinguishing between carcinomas and sarcomas. In the retina zonulae adherentes are present at the apex of photoreceptor cells and correspond to the outer limiting membrane of the retina as recognized by light microscopy. These junctions are also present in the rosettes of retinoblastomas (1).

Tight junctions. Tight junctions are present at the apex of many epithelial cells and are a continuous, crisscrossing network of ridges at points of fusion between two adjacent plasma membranes. In normal tissues these junctions are referred to as a single zonula occludens, or as multiple zonulae occludentes since they form an impermeable band all the way around the entire apex of these cells. In the retina such junctions unite the cell bodies of the retinal pigment epithelium (RPE). In these cells and in most normal epithelial cells, intermediate junctions are usually visible just beneath the tight junction and desmosomes are present below the intermediate junctions. This arrangement of a tight junction followed by an intermediate junction and then a desmosome is referred to as a junctional complex. This characteristic combination of junctions is helpful in establishing the diagnosis of adenocarcinoma using TEM when the diagnosis is uncertain by light microscopy.

Gap junctions. Gap junctions (also termed fasciae communicantes or nexus) form low-resistance pathways connecting many different types of cells. They are not of great value in the diagnosis of specific neoplasms. In this type of cell junction the two plasma membranes are separated only by a small *constant* space approximately 2 to 3 nm wide. Gap junctions are important in cardiac myocytes as they are thought to provide the pathway for ionic communication between individual myocytes and therefore underlie the coordinated electrical activity characteristic of the normal heart beat. The square arrays seen in the lens fiber cells are thought to be related to gap junctions (Fig. 11) (19).

Complex interdigitations. Complex interdigitations between cells may be regarded as a type of cell junction. Histiocytes in inflammatory (e.g., granulomas) and neoplastic conditions (e.g., fibrous histiocytomas) frequently exhibit complex interdigitations. In granulomas interdigitation probably precedes cell fusion in the formation of multinucleated giant cells. The individual cells in meningiomas also exhibit numerous complex interdigitations (16).

Hemidesmosomes. Epithelial cells that attach to a basement membrane ("basal lamina"), such as those of the cornea or epidermis, exhibit half-desmosomes or hemidesmosomes at the cell base. These vary in morphology somewhat from cell to cell, with fine filaments being seen at very high magnification connecting the plasma membrane of the cell to the basement membrane (16). It has been postulated that a lack of these filaments is responsible for the poor adhesion of epidermal hemidesmosomes to the basement membranes in patients with the recurrent epithelial erosion syndrome of the cornea (discussed in Chapter 30) and in cutaneous diseases such as epidermolysis lethalis hereditaria (a blistering disorder) (67).

The basement membrane is itself connected to the underlying stroma in some tissues, such as skin, by focally periodic anchoring fibrils. The fact that these are uniquely absent in the skin of patients with epidermolysis bullosa dystrophica-recessive suggests that they are important in maintaining the normal integrity of epithelia (11).

Newer Cell Structures

In the past few years, in vitro studies have revealed the presence of unique cellular structures called podosomes and invadopodia (60). Both structures have an actin core and contain other proteins usually associated with actin polymerization and are seen in macrophages and in invading cancer cells. Podosomes are somewhat smaller than invadopodia (1–2 μM vs. 8–10 μM, respectively) and some have suggested that podosomes form first and then evolve into invadopodia. It has been suggested that the defect in Wiskott–Aldrich syndrome may be due to dysfunctional podosomes but much work remains to be done to confirm a role for podosomes in human disease.

CELL CYCLE

Cells capable of replication and division pass through a cell cycle (Fig. 12). Before describing the cell cycle, it will be useful to define the context in which it exists. Cells can be divided into three major categories: continuously cycling or labile cells, quiescent or stable cells, and permanent cells. Most tissue and therefore organs consist of mixtures of the various cell types. In

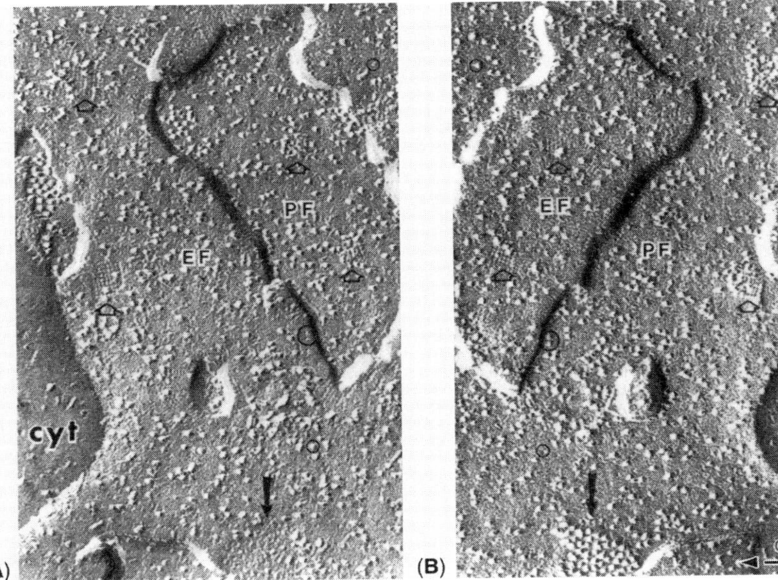

Figure 11 Freeze fracture replica of bovine lens outer cortex. This "double replica" illustrates both sides of the fracture plane through fiber cells. Note that the two images, (**A**) and (**B**), fit together perfectly. A gap junction (*solid arrows*) is visible at the bottom of the figure. Open circles refer to complementary pairs of isolated pits and particles. The *open arrows* mark the curious square arrays characteristic of these cells. These square arrays help maintain extremely close contact between adjacent cells, and are related to ion and water movement. The cytoplasm (cyt) is convex in (**A**) and concave in (**B**). The E-face (EF) and P-face (PF) are complementary surfaces. *Source*: Adapted from Ref. 19.

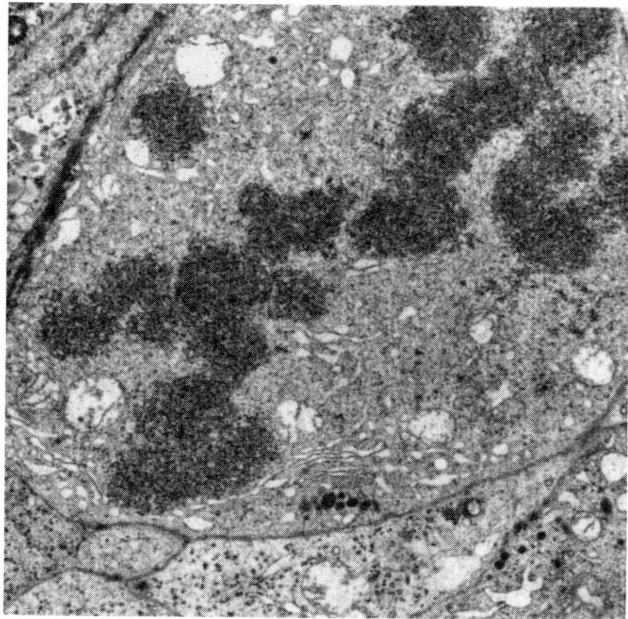

Figure 12 Note that there is no nuclear envelope around the chromatin of this dividing cell. Reorganization of the nucleus into the two daughter cells occasionally leads to the inclusion of organelles (×5,300). *Source*: Courtesy of Dr. John D. Shelburne.

labile tissues, cells proliferate (i.e., enter the cell cycle) throughout their life cycle. These tissues are represented by organs such as the cervix and uterus which contain surface epithelium that is constantly turning over, the lining of the gut (constant turnover of lining and absorptive cells), and hematopoietic cells/bone marrow. Resident stem cells are normally present in these tissues and are thought to be the precursors to the mature cells. Quiescent tissue normally exhibits a low level of resting cell replication but are capable of being stimulated to "rebuild" the underlying tissue if necessary. Examples of quiescent cells include hepatocytes, renal tubular cells, and pancreatic parenchymal cells as well as smooth muscle cells, endothelial cells, lymphocyte/inflammatory cells, and fibroblasts. Permanent tissues, the final type, contain cells that can no longer enter the cell cycle and therefore cannot undergo replication and division. Classic examples include myocytes, neurons, and skeletal muscle cells. Recent data question whether the central nervous system and the heart may indeed possess a population of stem cells that, under extremely defined conditions, may be able to regenerate some normal tissue constituents but the evidence is incomplete.

The cell cycle consists of four phases. Before cells can enter the cell cycle, they must undergo transition from the resting or quiescent state (G0) to G1, or the presynthetic phase (permanent cells are thought to exist in the G0 phase). During G1, cells increase in mass. The critical gate point is the transition between G1 and the next phase, synthesis (S). Because this is a critical check point for cell replication, the cell has multiple control mechanisms in place at this juncture. Once past this restriction point, cells are thought to be committed to replication. In S phase, cells replicate their DNA which is manifest as duplication or doubling of their chromosomes. After the S phase, replicating cells enter the G2 phase before entering mitosis, or M stage, the final stage where the cell divides. Similar to the G1 to S transition, the transition from G2 to M is highly regulated. At this point, the newly replicated DNA is checked for errors to determine if it is "safe" to enter mitosis. Newly divided cells return to G1 phase to enter a new replicative cycle (continuously dividing cells) or become quiescent (i.e., stable cells).

CELL TYPES

Multicellular organisms are composed of numerous specialized cells with exclusive functions. The eye and its adnexa normally contain a wide variety of unique specialized cells. These specialized cells are found in the cornea (corneal epithelium, keratocytes, corneal endothelium), conjunctiva (conjunctival epithelium, mucous-secreting goblet cells), lens (lens epithelium, lens fibers), vitreous (hyalocytes) retina [ganglion cells, Müller cells, amacrine cells, bipolar cells, horizontal cells, photoreceptors (rods and cones), RPE], uvea (pigment epithelium, non-pigmented epithelium) and orbit (lacrimal gland, lacrimal duct). Other cell types that are widely dispersed throughout the body are also found within the ocular tissues and some of them become particularly abundant in particular pathologic states.

Leukocytes

Inflammatory cells are important in many processes in the body, most importantly in acute and chronic inflammation. PMNs (Fig. 13), monocytes, eosinophils (Fig. 14), lymphocytes, basophils (Fig. 15), and platelets are all important constituents of the cellular phase of inflammation and all circulate through the vascular system to the area of damage/irritation. Each circulating leukocyte has unique components and/or structure that allow proper specific function in the inflammatory response. Other cells are also important in the inflammatory reaction including mast cells (Figs. 16 and 17) (which surround blood vessels) and resident macrophages and lymphocytes. These resident cells are important in engulfing offending infectious organisms (macrophages) and/or in the generation of the growth factors/cytokines

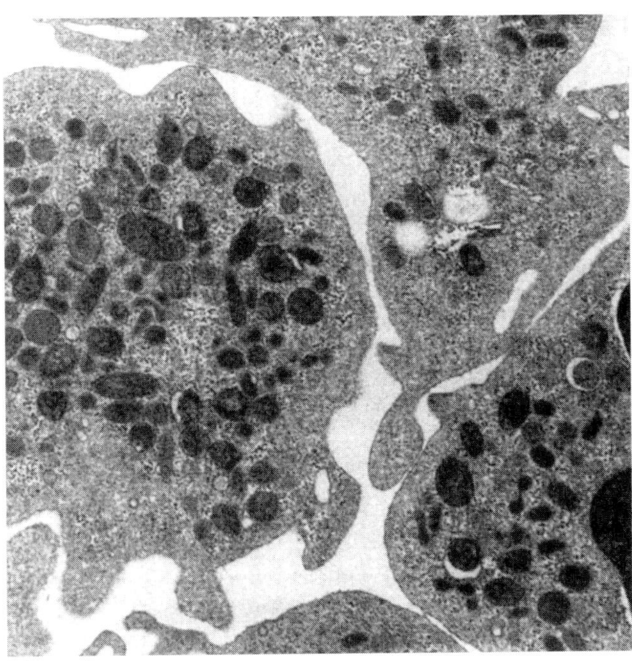

Figure 13 Typical polymorphonuclear leukocyte granules (×12,500). *Source*: Courtesy of Dr. John D. Shelburne.

important in the amplification and containment of the inflammatory response (lymphocytes). Different types of lymphocytes are recognized on the basis of specific cell surface markers. They include the B lymphocytes (B cells) and several subsets of T lymphocytes (T cells) [two types of T helper cells (T helper cell type 1 and T helper cell type 2), natural killer cells, suppressor T cells] (see Chapter 3). In addition to acute and chronic inflammatory responses, leukocytes play an important role in clinical disease states such as autoimmune diseases (i.e., hypersensitivity reactions), drug reactions, allergic reactions, tissue necrosis, and physical injury. Finally, defects in leukocyte function (either inherited or acquired) are not uncommon and can be associated with the inability to kill organisms and resulting life threatening infections. Full discussion of the specific roles of the individual inflammatory cells and the leukocyte deficiencies are beyond the scope of this chapter but leukocytes will be mentioned in connection with disease processes as appropriate.

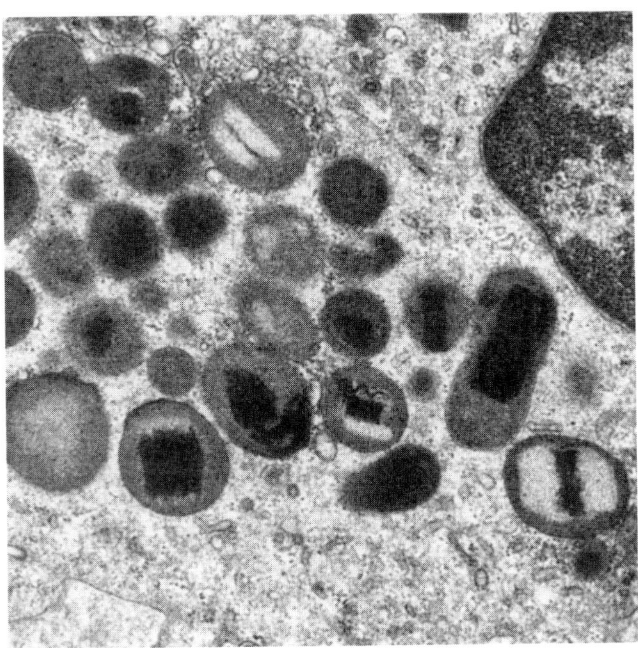

Figure 14 Typical eosinophil granules, with characteristic electron-dense crystalline core in several granules (×19,700). *Source*: Courtesy of Dr. John D. Shelburne.

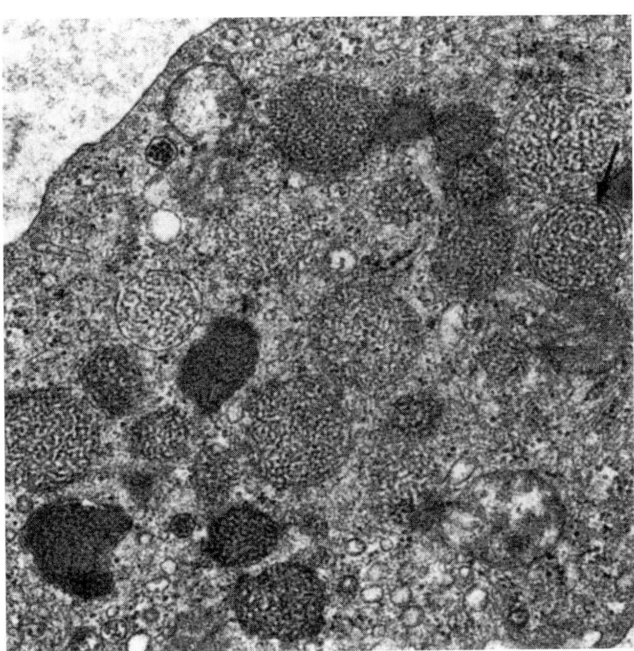

Figure 15 Typical basophil granules which are finely stippled and sometimes exhibit a concentric array (×9,000). *Source*: Courtesy of Dr. John D. Shelburne.

Plasma Cells

Once presented with an antigen, B lymphocytes differentiate into effector B cells. Effector B cells manufacture and secrete antibody in response to recognition of the presented antigen. Plasma cells are the most mature effector B cells and because they synthesize large amounts of protein (i.e., antibody), exhibit an extensive rough ER. In contrast, effector T cells do not secrete antibodies and therefore do not contain an extensive rough ER.

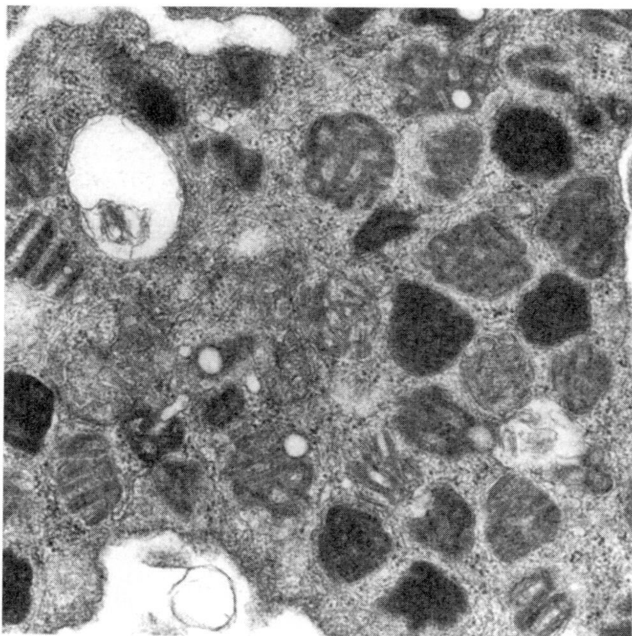

Figure 16 Typical scroll-like inclusions in a human mast cell viewed at low magnification (×27,800). *Source*: Courtesy of Dr. John D. Shelburne.

Dendritic Cells

Dendritic cells are derived from circulating monocytes once the monocytes enter the interstitial space. Similar to macrophages, dendritic cells are capable of ingesting foreign substances and organisms which is central to their function as antigen-presenting cells. However, the sole function of dendritic cells is antigen presentation to activate T lymphocytes; they are less active in phagocytosis than macrophages.

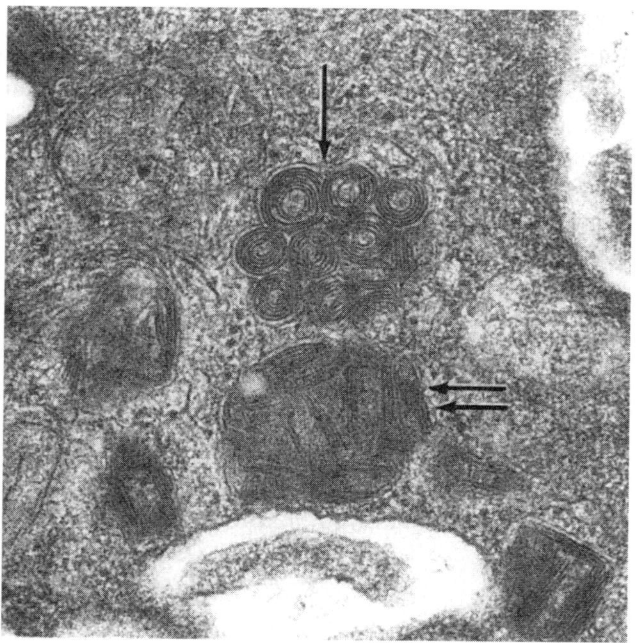

Figure 17 Higher-magnification view of the same cell as Figure 16, showing clearly the scroll-like inclusions in cross (*arrow*) and longitudinal (*double arrow*) sections (×58,800). *Source*: Courtesy of Dr. John D. Shelburne.

Langerhans Cells

Langerhans cells contain prominent dendritic processes and the characteristic organelles called Birbeck granules (Fig. 7). These cells are thought to be immature dendritic cells and important in antigen presentation which is key to a normal inflammatory response. They usually reside in the epidermis.

Melanocytes

Melanocytes are found in many organs but they are most commonly located in the skin as single dendritic cells that perform the important function of making melanin; a pigment which provides important protection against harmful ultraviolet rays from the sun especially in fair-skinned populations. Melanosome formation/maturation has been described in four stages from more primitive, oval cells containing protein material and little pigment to a stage 4 mature dendritic melanosome. Premelanosomes are usually classified as stage 3 (partially melanized) (2).

Vascular Endothelial Cells

Vascular endothelial cells are a single layer lining the entire cardiovascular system. Historically endothelial cells were thought to provide a physical barrier to activation of hemostasis and therefore the formation of blood clots. However, over the past 25 years, it has become increasingly apparent that endothelium is a dynamic, synthetic cell type that plays an important role in maintaining appropriate blood–tissue interaction. Endothelial cells contain a unique identifying structures (at the level of TEM) called Weibel–Palade bodies (87) that contain von Willebrand factor (Fig. 9).

Pericytes

Pericytes are perivascular mesenchymal cells that surround capillaries and postcapillary venules. A similar cell is present in larger vessels where they are called veil cells. Pericytes can form extensive regions of membrane contact with endothelial cells.

Smooth Muscle Cells

Smooth muscle cells are spindle-shaped and have single, cigar-shaped nuclei. They are contractile cells and therefore contain both thick (myosin) and thin (actin) contractile elements as well as cytoskeletal filaments. Thin filaments (actin) predominate over thick and insert into condensations of electon-dense material (called dense bodies) located underneath and adjacent to the plasma membrane. It is thought that dense bodies are analogous structures to the Z band present in striated cardiac muscle.

Striated Muscle Cells

Skeletal muscle fibers are derived from the fusion of many embryonic myoblasts and therefore, in contrast to smooth muscle cells, are multinucleated. Satellite cells, a stem cell population, are present adjacent to the cell membrane of the fiber. In contrast to smooth muscle cells, the myofilaments are arranged in highly organized units called sarcomeres. The sarcomeres consist of overlapping thick (myosin) and thin (actin) filaments and perpendicularly arranged Z bands. Similar to smooth muscle cells, the myofibrils interact with the sarcolemma (cell membrane). However, in keeping with the more structured organization of the myofibrils, the interaction between the myofibrils and the sarcolemma takes place through a highly organized series of cytoskeletal proteins including dystrophin, dystroglycan, and sarcoglycan.

Lymphatic Channels

Lymphatic channels are thin-walled, endothelial-lined channels that exist nearly everywhere in the body and function to return the interstitial tissue fluid and inflammatory cells to the blood. Because of their connection with the vascular system, lymphatics play an important role in the spread of infection and malignant tumors to other distant areas of the body. Lymphatics are absent in the lamina propria of the gut mucosa and most parts of the eye and its adnexa. Only the eyelids and conjunctiva contain lymphatic channels.

Schwann Cells

Schwann cells are specialized glial or support cells that are responsible for the synthesis of myelin in peripheral nerves. The counterpart in the central nervous system is called an oligodendrocyte. These cells wrap their own cytoplasm around the nerve axon to form an insulating layer that is important in the rapid conduction of nerve impulses.

Fibroblasts

Fibroblasts are a member of the large family of cells known as connective tissue cells. The members of the family are diverse and have the ability to convert their phenotypes under the appropriate conditions. Fibroblasts are considered to be the least specialized of the connective tissue cells and are responsible for the secretion of extracellular matrix rich in collagen type I and/or type III. Fibroblasts are present nearly everywhere in the body and are important in the repair of tissue following injury.

Myofibroblasts

Myofibroblasts are fibroblasts that, under conditions of wound repair, alter actin expression such that the contractile activity of the fibroblast is more similar to smooth muscle cells. In this state of differentiation, the fibroblasts aid in "pulling" the edges of a healing wound together.

CELLULAR PHYSIOLOGICAL AND PATHOLOGIC RESPONSES

Overview

The normal cell has several relationships that are critical to its overall structure and function including its association with neighboring cells, the surrounding connective tissue matrix, and other cell types within the resident organ. The individual cell exists normally in equilibrium with its surroundings (homeostasis) and when in this state, is capable of performing its defined task. However, when physiological demand or other stresses arise, the cell must respond to maintain equilibrium with its new altered environment. The increase in demand or stress results in changes in the cells which together are called cellular adaptations. The adaptive response may result in an increase in the number of cells (hyperplasia), or an increase in the size of individual cells (hypertrophy). It is also possible for a cell to undergo a decrease in size (atrophy), when the cell is exposed to a reduction in demand or stimulation. When the stress causing the adaptive response is persistent or chronic, cells can completely change from one type of differentiated cell to another differentiated cell (metaplasia), or accumulate endogenous or exogenous substances (intracellular storage), or even undergo transformation to a less differentiated cell type (dysplasia).

When an adverse, altered environment and/or prolonged stress causes a failure of cellular adaptation, the cell undergoes a complex series of subcellular reactions which together can be called cell injury. Cell injury and the associated changes are reversible up to a certain point depending upon the type and duration of the offending stimulus, but if the offending stimulus is not abated, the cell will eventually undergo irreversible cell injury, or cell death. Cell death can result from many different stimuli (discussed later), but its occurrence is critical to the initiation and progression of disease in virtually every tissue and organ of the human body.

Cellular Adaptation

Hypertrophy

Hypertrophy is defined as an increase in the size of a cell and/or organ and it can be divided into two basic types: physiologic and pathologic. Physiologic hypertrophy results from an increase in functional demand or an increase in organ-specific hormone stimulation. Physiologic hypertrophy results in larger cells that operate at a higher functional capacity. The increased cell size is associated with a proportionate increase in protein synthesis and content. Examples of physiologic hypertrophy include the increased size of the uterus during pregnancy and the increase sized and capacity of the leg muscles of a marathon runner. Hypertrophy can also be a response to a pathologic stimulus as in cardiac hypertrophy resulting from the heart having to eject against abnormal hemodynamic loads imposed by systemic hypertension and/or poorly functioning cardiac valves. In the eye the RPE can undergo hypertrophy.

Hyperplasia

Hyperplasia results in an *increase in the number of cells* present in a tissue or organ in response to a stimulus. Hyperplasia is similar to hypertrophy in that it results in an increased size/volume of the affected organ and it can be divided into physiologic and pathologic subtypes.

Physiologic hyperplasia. Physiologic hyperplasia results from either hormonal stimulation or increased functional demand. The designation physiologic hyperplasia is also used to describe the regeneration of an organ in response to partial loss of function. For example, if a significant portion of the liver is removed, the function of the liver may be compromised. In response to the loss of tissue/function, the remaining hepatocytes undergo hyperplasia to restore function toward normal. Similarly, if one kidney is removed, the remaining kidney will undergo compensatory hyperplasia to restore renal function toward normal.

Pathologic hyperplasia. Pathologic hyperplasia is best exemplified by endometrial hyperplasia. In this process, an unchecked excess of estrogen results in stimulation of the growth and number of glandular epithelial cells in the endometrium. The male counterpart of this process is benign prostatic hyperplasia where excess androgen stimulation results in increased glandular epithelium in the prostate gland. There is one more important difference between hyperplasia and hypertrophy; hyperplasia, especially pathologic hyperplasia, provides an important backdrop for the development of dysplasia and/or carcinoma (cancer). This is discussed in more detail later in the chapter.

Neoplasia

Neoplasia is strictly defined as new ("neo") tissue growth ("plasia"). However, in common practice it refers to the formation of an abnormal growth or tumor which can be either benign or malignant (see Chapter 53). Important ocular cells that give rise to malignant neoplasms are melanocytes in the uvea (see Chapter 59) and primitive retinal neurons (see Chapter 60). It is noteworthy that despite the fact the RPE frequently reacts in many pathologic states it very rarely gives rise to benign or malignant neoplasms. A spontaneous neoplasm derived from the epithelial cell of the lens has not been documented in humans or in any animal. However, malignant neoplasms can be created in the crystalline lens with genetic engineering (60).

Atrophy

Atrophy is defined as a reduction in the size of a cell or organ. Although it is important to note that organ atrophy can result from an irreversible loss of cells (i.e., cell death), in this section, the discussion will be confined to cellular atrophy. Cellular atrophy can result from a number of non-lethal stimuli and when it does, it is considered reversible. In other words, if the stimulus for the cellular atrophy is removed, the cell is capable of resynthesizing the appropriate proteins to fully resume its normal physiologic function. Common causes of atrophy include decreased use/reduced functional demand, loss of innervation, inadequate nutrient supply, loss of trophic/hormonal signals, aging, and inadequate blood supply (ischemia). Examples of each are listed below.

An excellent example of reduced demand leading to atrophy is the muscle atrophy of a limb that is immobilized in a cast. Once the cast is removed and full use of the limb is restored, there is rapid reversal of the muscle atrophy. Nerves provide trophic substances for the muscles they innervate. Therefore, loss of innervation can lead to muscle atrophy. Ischemia can reduce blood flow to a critical level such that tissue viability is threatened. The resulting relentless loss of individual cell viability can result in atrophy of the tissue in the vascular distribution of the affected vessel. An example of this is the brain atrophy observed in patients with severe long-standing atherosclerosis of the cerebral vascular system. Inadequate nutrition is somewhat similar to ischemia in that a loss of normally available nutrients can result in atrophy of the affected tissue. An example of this process is the cachexia found in patients with severe chronic diseases such as cancer or inflammatory bowel disease. In some cases, lack of adequate caloric intake can also lead to atrophy of adipose and/or muscle tissue as seen in persons suffering from starvation. In hormonally responsive tissue, a loss of endocrine stimulation can result in atrophy. This response is exemplified by the changes seen in the breast and uterine tissue of postmenopausal females but also occurs in response to intentional hormonal-based therapy for certain cancers such as androgen ablation therapy for prostate cancer. Retinal atrophy is a manifestation of age-related macular degeneration (see Chapter 18), many genetically determined diseases (see Chapter 35) and retinal ischemia (see Chapter 67).

Metaplasia

As mentioned above, when the environmental stress causing the adaptive response is persistent or chronic, cells can undergo a complete phenotypic change from one type of differentiated cell to another differentiated cell. The corneal endothelium commonly becomes transformed into fibroblast-like cells in conditions that result in a loss of this cell type. In the eye, the RPE commonly gives rise to ossification as in phthisis bulbi. The source of the bone remains to be determined, but the RPE is closely involved in the process and either undergoes transformation into bone or induces another yet-to-be-identified cell type to undergo metaplasia. Although the cell type appears to "change" from one to another, the actual mechanism of metaplasia involves reprogramming stem cells or uncommitted reserve cells that are normally present in most normal tissue to differentiate in a different final direction. An example of squamous metaplasia occurs in the cornea when the endothelial cells become transformed into a stratified squamous epithelium as in posterior polymorphous corneal dystrophy (see Chapter 32). Some forms of metaplasia are considered to reversible; if the offending stimulus is removed, the metaplastic cell type will revert to the cell type normally present in that location.

Dysplasia

When a cell undergoes transformation to a less differentiated cell type, it is called dysplasia. Similar to metaplasia, dysplasia is a response that certain cells undergo to a chronic injurious stimulus and it is reversible upon abolishment of the injurious stimulus. However, there is one critical difference between metaplasia and dysplasia. Dysplasia consists of disordered growth and maturation of tissue that is considered to be a preneoplastic process; i.e., it is considered to be a step on the way to the development of a tumor; usually a malignant tumor. Similar to the prevailing theory of carcinogenesis, dysplasia results from a series of genetic mutations in a population of cells capable of cell division. The accumulation of mutations in some cells provides them with a selective survival advantage over non-mutated cells. The cells with the selective advantage acquire morphologic features different from surrounding cells exhibiting variations in cell size and shape, hyperchromatic, irregularly shaped nuclei, and disorderly arrangement of the cells. Dysplasia is a common lesion in the conjunctiva (see Chapter 57).

Dyskeratosis

Dyskeratosis is defined as early keratinization in cells that are not part of the normal, keratinized surface of the skin. Intraepithelial dyskeratosis is a striking feature of benign intraepithelial dyskeratosis which affects the bulbar and oral mucous membranes (see Chapter 32).

Cellular Accumulations

One manifestation of a dysfunctional cell can be the intracellular accumulation of various substances ranging from normal constituents to exogenous pigments. The accumulation of these substances can have a wide variety of effects on the cell ranging from no apparent effect to a severe toxicity resulting in cell death. Some accumulations involve normal nutrients like fat, glycogen, or vitamins. An example is steatosis, or fat accumulation seen in liver cells in certain clinical conditions such as diabetes mellitus or alcoholism. In both cases, normal triglyceride metabolism is altered such that they accumulate inside the individual hepatocyte. This change is reversible and generally not toxic to the cell. Glycogen is also a normal constituent of liver and muscle cells where it is an important storage component for energy and metabolism. A group of inborn errors of metabolism involving deficiencies in the enzymes necessary for glycogen catabolism results in glycogen accumulation (see Chapter 39). Excess glycogen can also be seen in diabetes mellitus due to poor regulation of serum glucose concentrations. Within the iris such glycogen storage results in the lacy vacuolation of the iris pigment epithelium (90). Lysosomes are subcellular organelles containing enzymes that are responsible for the breakdown of complex lipids and glycosaminoglycans (Fig. 1). Inherited defects in these enzymes lead to a series of disease called lysosomal storage diseases (see Chapter 38) which include the sphingolipidoses and neuronal ceroid lipofuscinoses (see Chapter 41), mucolipidoses (see Chapter 42), and mucopolysaccaridodoses (see Chapter 40). In addition to normal substances, cells can accumulate abnormal proteins as well (see Chapter 36). Cells can also accumulate exogenous pigments such as the accumulation of carbon particles seen in the macrophages of the lung. This is primarily the result of air pollution which is a large problem in industrialized cities across the globe. A variety of foreign substances may accumulate in the tissues of the eye and its adnexa (see Chapter 15). Iron and other metals also can accumulate. Accumulations of metals can lead to well known and clinically significant disease such as hemochromatosis (accumulation of iron) and Wilson disease (copper accumulation) (see Chapter 48). Hemochromatosis can result from too much exogenous iron (usually seen in repeated red blood cell transfusions for hereditary anemias) or from inherited defects in iron metabolism.

CELLULAR PATHOLOGY

Cell Injury

When an adverse altered environment and/or stress causes a cell to adapt beyond its ability the cell undergoes a complex series of subcellular reactions which together can be called cell injury. Cell injury and the associated changes are reversible up to a certain point depending upon the type and duration of the offending stimulus, but if the offending stimulus is not abated, the cell will eventually undergo irreversible cell injury, or cell death. Cell death can result from many different stimuli (discussed later) but its occurrence is critical to the initiation and progression of disease in virtually every tissue and organ of the human body. Cell injury is traditionally divided into two phases: reversible and irreversible. The subcellular changes associated with reversible cell injury resolve when the stimulus ceases or is removed. Cell death occurs when the injurious stimulus persists beyond the point of irreversibility. By definition, the cell cannot live at this point if it is returned to its native environment. Once irreversibly injured, a cell undergoes a series of morphologic changes that is recognized as cell death. The classic form of cell death is called necrosis and depending upon the nature of the injury and the specific tissue involved the pattern differs somewhat. A different pattern of morphologic changes associated with cell death is called apoptosis (see Chapter 2). The morphologic hallmarks and mechanisms of apoptosis are distinct from necrosis. Apoptosis differs significantly from necrosis in both the pattern of changes seen in the tissue and in the fact that apoptosis functions in the normal physiologic pathways of development. For example, apoptosis is involved in the immune and inflammatory responses, the hormone-dependent involution of tissue, and the programmed involution of certain cells during normal embryogenesis. A detailed description of the pathways involved in apoptosis is provided in Chapter 2. Apoptosis takes place in numerous degenerative diseases of the retina.

Causes of Cell Injury

As might be expected, the potential causes of cell injury are as diverse as the environment in which the organism exists. Some causes are endogenous to the organism while others are imposed upon from the external environment. Examples of endogenous insults include reduction in blood flow to a critical level, accumulation of endogenous substances to high levels, or genetic derangements. The external causes can be physical or chemical agents as well as biologic organisms such as bacteria, viruses, and fungi as well as other, less common organisms. A more thorough discussion of each of the major categories of cell injury is presented in the next section. However, regardless of the origin of the initiating insult, almost all agents cause cell injury ultimately acting through a small group of common mechanisms. We will discuss these common mechanisms in the next section.

Mechanisms of Cell Injury

Certain mechanisms of cell injury provide common threads that tie together the myriad causes of cell injury. These mechanisms include: (*i*) depletion of high-energy phosphates (HEP) (i.e., ATP); (*ii*) loss of calcium homeostasis; (*iii*) generation of reactive oxygen species (i.e., free radicals); and (*iv*) membrane damage.

ATP depletion. HEP are usually depleted under two circumstances: oxygen deprivation and chemical injury. The best studied example of HEP depletion is ischemic cell death associated with the occlusion of a coronary artery supplying muscle in the heart. Soon after the blood flow in the artery stops, the ATP levels in the myocardium rapidly decline. HEP are critical to overall homeostasis of the myocytes and critically important to a number of energy-dependent membrane pumps. Once HEP is reduced to a critical level (5–10% of normal), the individual cell is no longer capable of maintaining normal ionic homeostasis and cell death begins. It is noteworthy that HEP loss has many effects on the myocyte in addition to the energy-requiring membrane pumps including effects on the source of energy (i.e., switch to anaerobic glycolysis from oxidative phosphorylation), loss of intracellular ion homeostasis (see below), protein structure and function (specifically cytoskeletal proteins), and protein degradation pathways. The sum of the changes invoked by depletion of HEP leads to cell death. The critical step or change that ultimately leads to cell death is still not known with certainty. Ischemic cell death also occurs in neural tissue including retina, glial cells, and neurons. Studies of ischemic injury in these tissues confirm that there is a complex relationship between HEP, tissue pH, and oxygen levels that leads to cell injury in the various tissues which is ultimately dependent upon factors that need further investigation.

Loss of calcium homeostasis. Calcium is a cofactor for many intracellular enzymes and plays an important role in living cells. Calcium is also necessary for normal muscle contraction and is hence critical for the functioning of the extraocular muscles. Because too much calcium leads to cell death, cells have developed sophisticated mechanisms to strictly control the level of intracellular calcium ions. Certain intracellular organelles are important in calcium homeostasis including the ER (sarcoplasmic reticulum in muscle tissue) and the mitochondria. Ischemia (as mentioned above) as well as certain toxins can lead to alterations of calcium levels through increased influx from the extracellular space or release from intracellular storage sites. When calcium rises above a critical level, it activates enzymes which can catalyze cell membrane damage as well as other critical intracellular proteins, such as enzymes and cytoskeletal proteins. Loss of calcium regulation resulting from changes in mitochondrial structure and/or function plays a major role in apoptosis.

Generation of reactive oxygen species. Oxygen is critical to the generation of the HEP necessary for normal cellular function as well as cell survival. The basic reaction used to generate energy involves the reduction of oxygen in the presence of hydrogen to water. One byproduct of this reaction is the formation of three major subspecies of oxygen that contain unpaired electrons. These species are called oxygen-derived free radicals (ODFR) and include the superoxide anion (O_2^-), hydrogen peroxide (H_2O_2), and hydroxyl radical (OH). ODFR, like all free radical species, are extremely reactive and have relatively short half lives in the cell and therefore have the potential to cause damage to any protein or lipid that they contact. ODFR are important in the normal killing process associated with inflammation (i.e., used by PMNs to kill invading organisms) but are also seen in many clinically important diseases such as oxygen toxicity, radiation, reperfusion injury, and chemical toxicity. When not associated with inflammation, ODFR are usually produced in small quantities by the mitochondria as a result of "electron transport leak."

Defense mechanisms exist that prevent ODFR from causing unchecked cellular damage under normal conditions. Both endogenous and exogenous scavengers of free radicals exist. Scavengers can either block the initiation of free radical generation or terminate the continued generation of ODFR. Examples of exogenous antioxidants include vitamin E, vitamin C, and the vitamin A precursor, retinol. Vitamin E and retinol are fat soluble and therefore can function to inhibit the chain reactions that can form in lipid membranes that are under free radical attack. Endogenous enzymes also exist that can either scavenge or inhibit the continued production of ODFR. These enzymes usually exist within the cell near the sites of free radical generation. Superoxide dismutase is the first line of defense against superoxide by catalyzing the conversion of two molecules of superoxide anion into oxygen and hydrogen peroxide. Catalase is located primarily in the peroxisomes. It acts to decompose two molecules of hydrogen peroxide into two molecules of water and oxygen. Glutathione peroxidase exists in both the cytosol and the mitochondria and catalyzes the reduction of hydrogen peroxide and lipid peroxides into water and reduced glutathione. In most circumstances, the combination of endogenous and exogenous defense mechanisms prevents cell injury and/or death resulting from ODFR. However, when either the production of ODFR is increased or the cell defense mechanisms are compromised (or both together), the potential exists for an excess concentration of ODFR inside the cell. This excess can be called oxidative stress. Oxidative stress, when present in at a high enough level or for a long enough time, can cause cell injury and/or cell death. It apparently plays an important role in certain disorders of aging, such as cataract formation (see Chapter 23) and age-related maculopathy (see Chapter 18).

One important characteristic of ODFR that make them potentially dangerous to cells is that they are capable of undergoing autocatalytic chain reactions whereby a small initial amount of ODFR results in the generation of a much larger burden of potentially more harmful species of free radicals. Free radicals can cause cell injury and death through three major pathways. First, they cause lipid peroxidation. Since lipids are a major component of cell membranes, peroxidation breaks down and eventually destroys cell membranes. Loss of cell membrane integrity is incompatible with life. Secondly, free radicals alter and/or damage cellular proteins (see Chapter 36). Oxidative stress can cause damage to the amino acid backbone as well as the side chains and results in cross-linking, fragmentation, aggregation, or degradation of proteins. Since proteins are involved in a multitude of critical cellular processes including structural support and enzymes for metabolism, alteration/destruction of proteins can have catastrophic consequences for cell survival. Finally, free radicals can damage DNA. Oxidative damage to DNA is known to be important in the malignant transformation of cells and is thought to play an important role in cellular aging (see Chapter 17).

Increased membrane permeability. All cell membranes are critical to the survival of the cell including the external cell membrane and membranes of intracellular organelles such as mitochondria and lysosomes. The loss of membrane integrity results in the loss of homeostasis and ultimately to cell death. Defects can develop in cell membranes in response to a variety of insults including severe, prolonged loss of HEP as in ischemia, bacterial toxins, viral proteins, components of the serum complement system, or physical/chemical agents. Therefore, this category represents a final common pathway of many diverse insults including mitochondrial dysfunction, protein aggregation/breakdown, and direct oxidative stress. Loss of plasma membrane integrity results in an immediate loss of ionic homeostasis, loss of energy-generating enzymes and cofactors, calcium overload and cell death. Mitochondrial membrane integrity can be compromised from a variety of causes (i.e., calcium overload, oxidative stress, lipid peroxidation) and when it occurs, it leads to activation of the apoptotic signaling pathway which leads to apoptotic cell death. Cell death due to viral infection can be a direct result of virus replication causing host cell lysis or due to immunologically mediated killing. A more detailed discussion of immunologically mediated killing is discussed in Chapter 3. Disorders that cause a loss of lysosomal membrane integrity will release the digestive enzymes (RNAses, DNAases, proteases, phosphatases, and other degradative enzymes) that are normally within these membrane-bound organelles and the cells die through necrosis.

Major Categories of Cell Injury

Oxygen deprivation. Obviously the depletion or loss of oxygen will eventually lead to cell death. This can occur from a reduction in oxygen content despite a normal blood flow to the affected tissue (hypoxia) or from both a reduction in oxygen and a critical decrease in blood flow to the affected tissue (ischemia). Therefore, ischemia imposes an additional stress on the cells because exchange and efflux of metabolic waste products are impaired in addition to the lack of oxygen supply. As a consequence, ischemic tissue suffers cell death much quicker than hypoxic tissue. The most common cause of clinically significant ischemia is the blockage/obstruction of an arterial vessel usually due to significant atherosclerosis. This is particularly important in occlusovascular disease of the retina (see Chapter 67). Hypoxia in the absence of ischemia is less common and is best represented by the hypoxia associated with severe anemia or carbon monoxide poisoning.

Physical injury. Physical causes of cell injury are obvious and myriad and include trauma, electrical shock, temperature extremes, radiation exposure, and barotraumas (see Chapter 15).

Chemical agents. The list of chemicals that can cause cell injury is extremely large and grows larger each year. Common examples include poisons such as arsenic and cyanide as well as historical examples such as lead and mercury. Even essential molecules like oxygen can be toxic if given at inappropriate levels as in the retinopathy of prematurity (see above discussion and Chapter 67). One important category that should be mentioned is therapeutic drugs (see Chapter 50). Nearly all therapeutic drugs have some potential for harmful side effects including cell death especially if given in the presence of a comorbid condition, such as liver and/or renal disease, or with another drug with which it interacts.

Infectious agents. Biologic organisms that cause cell injury and cell death are extensive and include viruses (see Chapter 8), bacteria (see Chapter 9), fungi (see Chapter 11), prions (see Chapter 70), protozoa (see Chapter 12), helminths (see Chapter 13), and arthropods (see Chapter 14).

Genetic derangements. Alterations in the genetic code can cause a wide range of injury ranging from identifiable physical abnormalities such as Down syndrome to alterations in single enzymes necessary for the phototransduction needed for vision (see Chapter 35). Moreover, some genetic mutations are responsible for the increased risk of cancer seen in retinoblastoma (see Chapter 60). Some inherited syndromes such as neurofibromatosis types 1 and 2, tuberous sclerosis, von Hippel–Lindau disease, and familial adenomatous polyposis (see Chapter 55) have been postulated to be responsible for the difference in life expectancy between individuals and/or susceptibility to the development of disease in response to an environmental toxin (i.e., smoking and variability to the development of lung cancer). A full discussion of the genetic disorders is provided elsewhere (see Chapter 31), and in specific chapters covering the genetic aspects of disorders of cornea (see Chapter 32), retina and optic nerve (see Chapter 35) as well the genetics of cataracts (see Chapter 33), and glaucoma (see Chapter 34). Other chapters also discuss the importance of genetic derangements in myopia (see Chapter 26) and ocular developmental anomalies (see Chapter 52).

Disorders Involving Specific Cellular Components

Disorders of the Nucleus

Abnormalities of nuclear size and shape. Enlargement of nuclei is a common cellular abnormality. For example, in malignant neoplasms the nuclei of cells are often larger than those of the parent tissue. Nuclear enlargement, as viewed in routine histologic sections, can be seen as an increase in volume, surface area, or both. The nuclear shape becomes complex and tortuous if the surface area of the nucleus increases far more than its volume. Spherical nuclei have the lowest nuclear surface area/nuclear volume ratio. This ratio increases in the normal maturation of neutrophils and in humans is very high in the so-called Sézary cell, a specific circulating malignant lymphoid cell (28,38,50), and in anaplastic carcinomas (Fig. 18) (21).

Nuclear inclusions. There are various types of nuclear inclusions. Viral inclusions in cells infected with herpes simplex (as in herpetic keratitis), varicella zoster, adenovirus, papilloma virus,

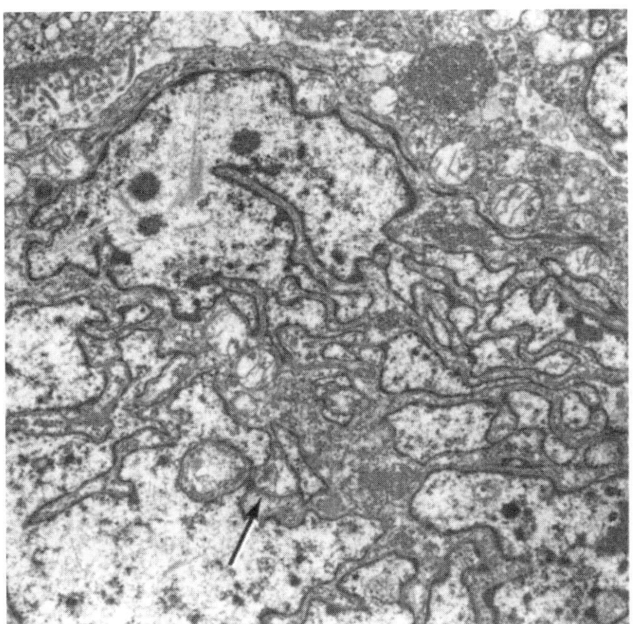

Figure 18 Transmission electron micrograph showing only part of the nucleus of an anaplastic epithelial cell. Note the incredible complexity of the nucleus. Often two nuclear envelopes are separated from one another only by a thin bridge or stand of chromatin (*arrow*). This nucleus obviously has an extremely high nuclear surface area/nuclear volume ratio (×6,000). *Source*: Courtesy of Dr. John D. Shelburne.

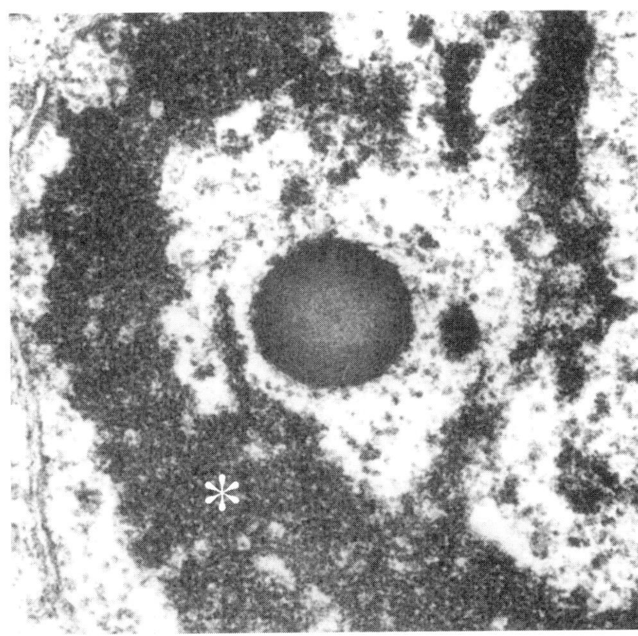

Figure 19 This concentric, lamellar nuclear inclusion within a rabbit alveolar macrophage contains cadmium sequential to in vitro incubation with cadmium chloride. This severely injured cell also exhibits clumping of heterochromatin in the nucleus (*asterisk*) (×39,100). *Source*: Courtesy of Dr. John D. Shelburne.

cytomegalovirus, and measles virus are well known (see Chapter 8) (51,62,63,92). There are, however, many non-viral nuclear inclusions which should be considered in the differential diagnosis of nuclear inclusion bodies. Heavy metals such as lead (30), bismuth (7), and cadmium (Fig. 19) (8) all produce nuclear inclusions, some of which are visible by light microscopy and consist of the metal plus associated proteins.

All the aforementioned inclusions are actually within the nucleus ("true" nuclear inclusions). However, with abnormally shaped nuclei, the cytoplasm may deeply invaginate the nucleus and appear by light microscopy to be within the nucleus. These "pseudoinclusions" can be easily recognized by TEM since the two membranes of the nuclear envelope surround them and establish their cytoplasmic topography as being outside the nucleus (Fig. 20). The cells in malignant neoplasms are particularly prone to such nuclear pseudoinclusions. Pseudoinclusions at the edge of a nucleus are referred to as "nuclear pockets" (Fig. 21). These are present in lymphocytes in normal germinal centers but are rare in peripheral blood except in leukemia. Thus, their presence in the peripheral blood can have diagnostic value. Occasionally, TEM reveals nuclear inclusions which are surrounded by a single unit membrane (Fig. 22) (15,56). Single-membrane-limited nuclear inclusions are often seen in malignant plasma cells (Dutcher bodies). Retinoblastoma cells also frequently exhibit a flattened single-membrane-limited cisterna immediately adjacent to the nuclear envelope (Fig. 20) (46).

Multinucleation. Multinucleation occurs in the giant cells of granulomatous inflammation, in many regenerating tissues (Fig. 23), and in neoplastic cells (Fig. 24).

Disorders of the Cytoplasm

Peroxisomal disorders. The characteristic phi body in the circulating malignant myeloid cell in myelogenous leukemia is a type of peroxisome (Fig. 25). The adrenoleukodystrophies are caused by mutations in genes that affect peroxisomes and hence can be considered as peroxisomal disorders (see Chapter 70).

Lysosomal disorders. Lysosomal hydrolases can be released extracellularly during phagocytosis; presumably "leaking" out of the phagocytic vacuole before it closes its connection to the extracellular space (70). The "old" secondary lysosomes of neurons, myocardial cells, and hepatocytes contain lipofuscin-indigestible brown–black lipid plus protein (80). Lipofuscin is a prominent constituent of the RPE (24). More importantly, lysosomes are associated with a variety of diseases, usually inherited deficiencies of

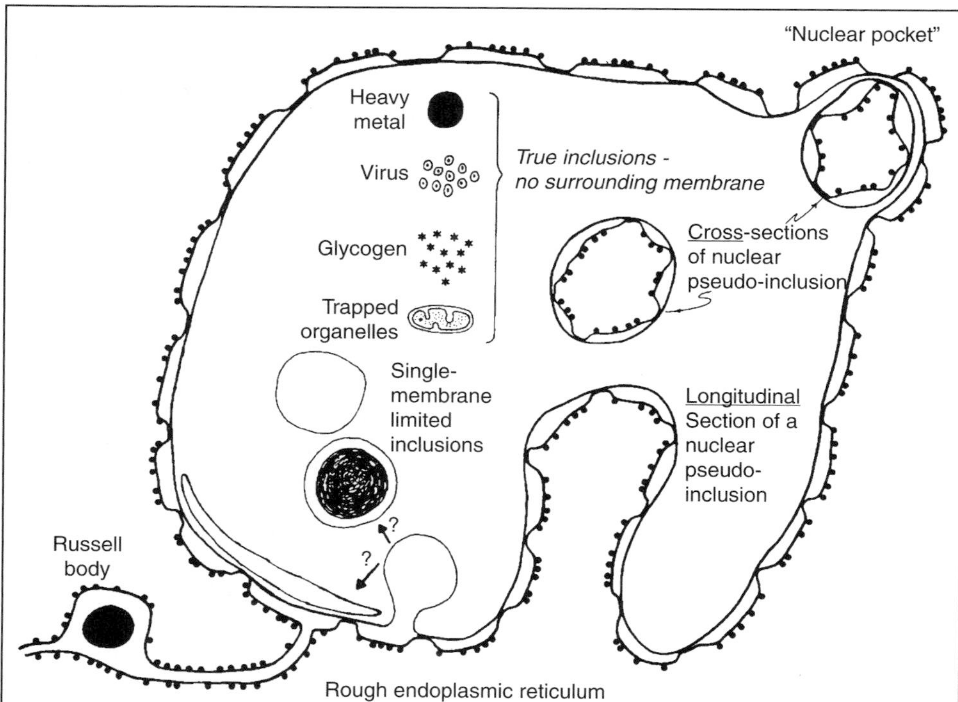

Figure 20 This diagram summarizes some important changes seen in nuclei. Note particularly the topology of nuclear inclusions. An examples of a true nuclear inclusion is present in Figure 19. A "nuclear pocket" is seen in Figure 21. An example of a single-membrane-limited nuclear inclusion is shown in Figure 22. The diagram shows why it is not surprising that single-membrane-limited nuclear inclusions form in plasma cells which also exhibit Russell body formation. *Source*: Courtesy of D. Powell.

certain lysosomal enzymes, and are therefore associated with accumulations of endogenous or exogenous materials. In glycogenosis type II (Pompe disease) (MIM #23200), an inherited deficiency of the lysosomal enzyme acid maltase (α-1,4-glucosidase) the lysosomal accumulation of large amounts of glycogen results

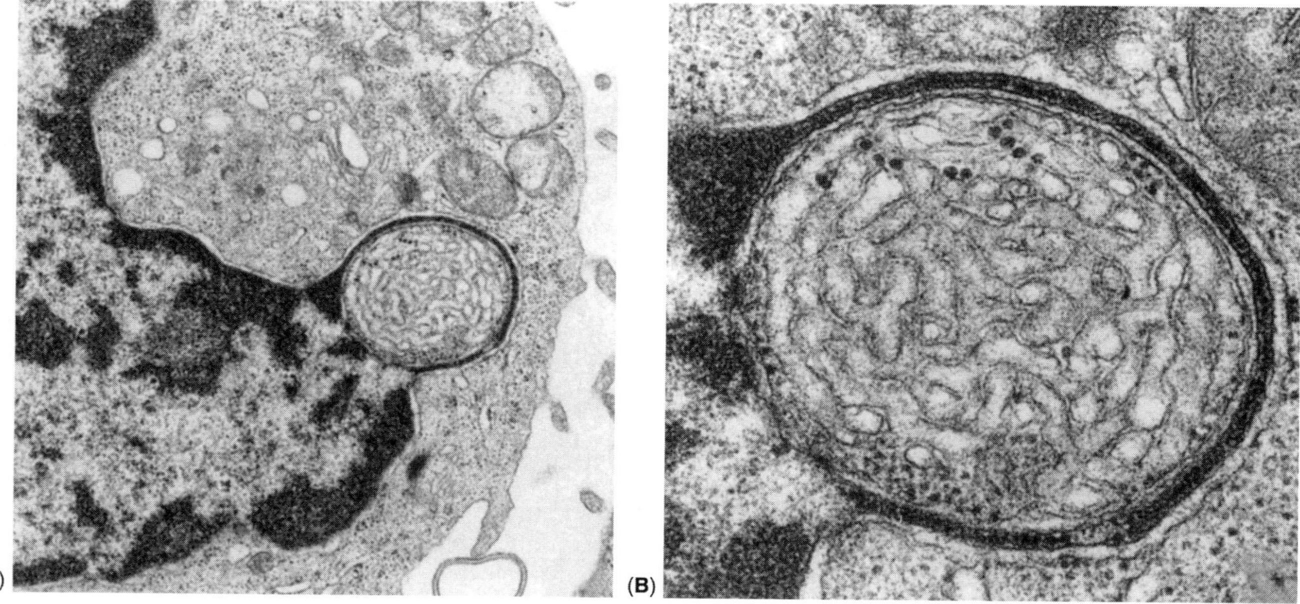

Figure 21 (**A**) This nuclear pseudoinclusion is present at the very edge of the nucleus; hence, it is termed a "nuclear pocket" (×22,900). (**B**) At higher magnification, the "nuclear pocket" of (**A**) is seen to be a nuclear pseudoinclusion, as revealed by the presence of nuclear envelope on *both* sides of a thin strand of heterochromatin. Note that there is an excess of cisternae of smooth endoplasmic reticulum within this pseudoinclusion (×67,900). *Source*: Courtesy of Dr. John D. Shelburne.

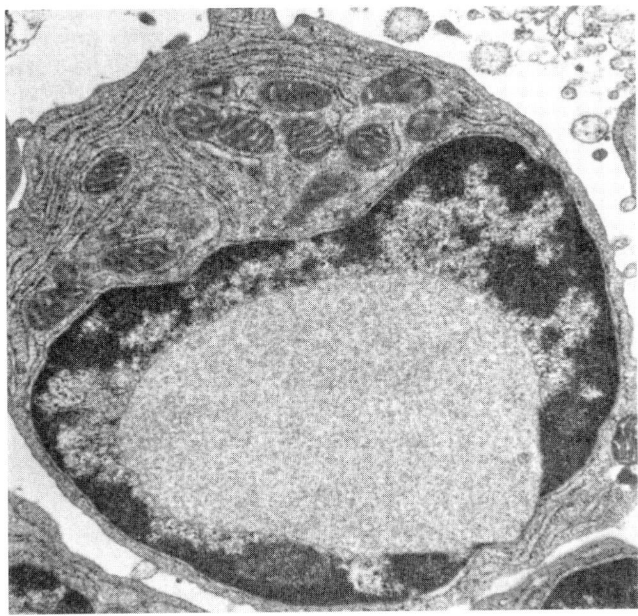

Figure 22 This large single-membrane limited-inclusion within a myeloma cell contains fine, flocculent material that presumably is protein (×6,100). *Source*: Courtesy of Dr. John D. Shelburne.

because a normal degradative pathway is blocked (see Chapter 39). Fabry disease (MIM #301500) is caused by the lack of a critical enzyme (α-galactosidase A) (Fig. 26) (see Chapter 41). Many lysosomal storage diseases are known and the list continues to grow as new entities become recognized (see Chapter 38) (67). Hemosiderin (Fig. 27) accumulates in macrophages at sites where hemoglobin is actively phagocytosed, as occurs with intraocular hemorrhage. The RPE phagocytize the shed outer segments of photoreceptor cells (36). Exogenous material also accumulates within macrophages when it is not degraded. This can become manifest when foreign substances enter ocular tissues accidentally, following the topical application of medications, or when it is intentionally introduced into the eye of experimental animals (49). Bacteria accumulate in secondary lysosomes in numerous infections, including Whipple disease (59) and malakoplakia (54).

DeDuve and Wattiaux (20) postulated that the rupture of lysosomes with the intracellular release of powerful lysosomal hydrolases would kill the cell. This "suicide bag" concept of cell death appears to be applicable to at least two human diseases: silicosis and gout (3,39). Ingested silica or uric acid crystals may rupture secondary lysosomes to cause cell death. However, the suicide bag hypothesis is probably not valid for all types of cell death.

Mitochondrial disorders. Swollen mitochondria, often with a broken outer membrane, are seen in lethally injured cells. These frequently exhibit amorphous, flocculent densities in the matrix. Microcrystalline or granular calcium phosphate deposits can also form around the cristae in lethally injured cells (Fig. 28), but it is unusual to see these crystals in surgically excised or postmortem material. The presence of either type of density in many mitochondria is proof of cell death (9).

Mitochondria are easily visible by light microscopy (44,53,82) and under certain pathologic conditions the matrix space may contain crystals, spherical densities (26), iron (14,84), and glycogen (45). For example, in progressive familial ophthalmoplegia (see Chapter 72), large numbers of subsarcolemmal mitochondria in skeletal muscle exhibit complex paracrystalline arrangements of their cristae (43). It is noteworthy that certain normal cells (parathyroid oxyphil cells) and some tumors (called oncocytomas) contain so many mitochondria that there seems little room for any other organelles (Fig. 29). Oncocytomas

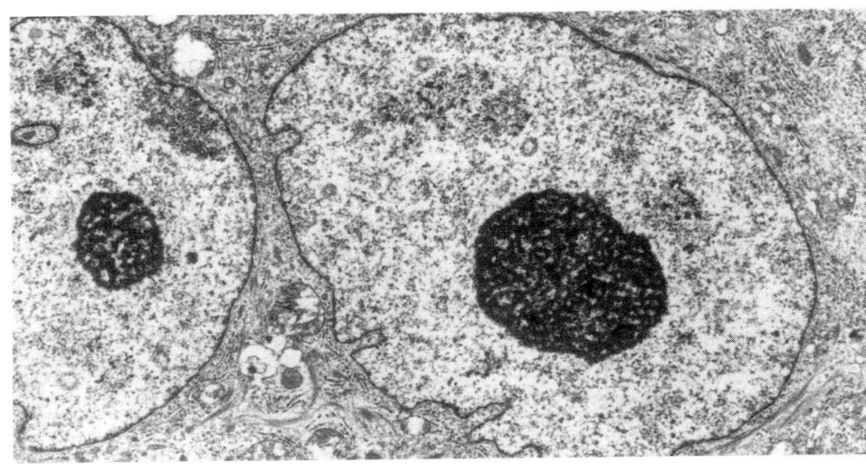

Figure 23 Each of the nuclei in this binucleated regenerating type II cell in the lung contains large prominent nucleoli. (×7,900). *Source*: Courtesy of Dr. John D. Shelburne.

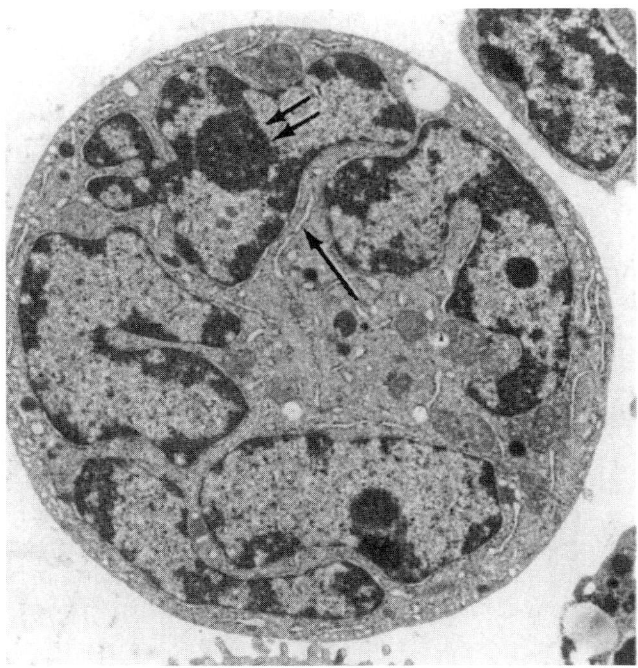

Figure 24 This anaplastic multinucleated plasma cell exhibits prominent cisternae of the rough endoplasmic reticulum (*arrow*) and prominent nucleoli (*double arrow*) (×8,700). *Source*: Courtesy of Dr. John D. Shelburne.

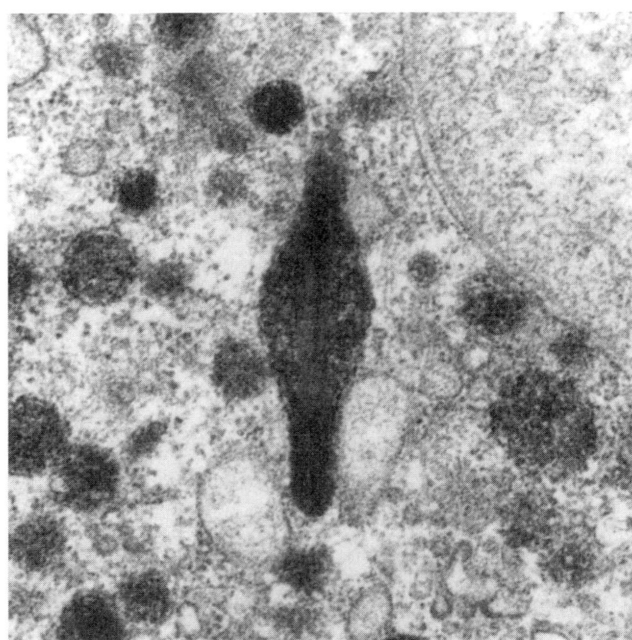

Figure 25 A typical phi body in a circulating malignant myeloid cell in myelogenous leukemia. The nucleus is visible at the top right. The tissue has been stained for catalase to enhance the visibility of the phi body. Phi bodies are a type of peroxisome (×32,500). *Source*: Adapted from Hanker JS, Romanovitz DK. Phi bodies: peroxidatic particles that produce crystalloidal cellular inclusions. Science 1977; 197:895–8.

have been described in virtually every organ including conjunctiva (see Chapter 57) or lacrimal gland (6,52).

A heterogenous group of disorders exist which affect the central nervous system, skeletal muscle and many other organs which specifically interfere with normal oxidative phosphorylation. The so-called mitochondrial encephalomyopathies comprise several distinct syndromes: Leigh disease (see Chapter 70), Alper syndrome, Kearns–Sayre syndrome, myoclonus epilepsy with "ragged-red fibers" (Figs. 30 and 31), mitochondrial myopathy, encephalopathy, lactic acidosis, stroke-like episodes (see Chapter 72) and Leber hereditary optic neuropathy (see Chapter 35).

Disorders of cilia. Subtle abnormalities may occur in cilia which can result in clinically evident disease. For example, patients with Kartagener syndrome (situs inversus viscerum, chronic sinusitis, bronchiectasis) and the immotile-cilia syndrome (immotile spermatozoa and chronic airway infections) (22,23,55). High-resolution TEM has revealed the partial or complete absence of dynein arms on the microtubules of the cilia in respiratory epithelium and spermatozoa of patients with these conditions. Presumably, the absence of dynein arms, which contain an adenosine triphosphatase, causes the cilia to function poorly, resulting in decreased fertility as well as recurrent respiratory infections. These patients also have abnormalities in the arrangement of cilia. Cilia with defective radial spokes have also been documented in certain patients with chronic respiratory disease (81). A high incidence of abnormal nasal cilia has been noted in patients with retinitis pigmentosa in Usher syndrome (see Chapter 35) (4). It is noteworthy that the rudimentary cilia of the photoreceptor cells of the retina normally lack the two central microtubules and only exhibit the outer nine doublets, an attribute that is also characteristic of the rosettes in retinoblastomas (85). Documentation of the presence of cilia can be of diagnostic value in certain tumors (e.g., retinoblastomas and ependymomas) (12). However, cilia can be seen occasionally in non-epithelial cells such as non-pigmented stromal cells in the iris (41).

Disorders of the ER and Golgi apparatus. Proteins can accumulate within the rough ER both in normal and abnormal cells (10). For example, the rough ER is distended with such material in normal fibroblasts. When large amounts of immunoglobin are present in plasma cells these aggregates are visible by light microscopy and are referred to as Russell bodies. This tendency for proteins to accumulate in cisternae

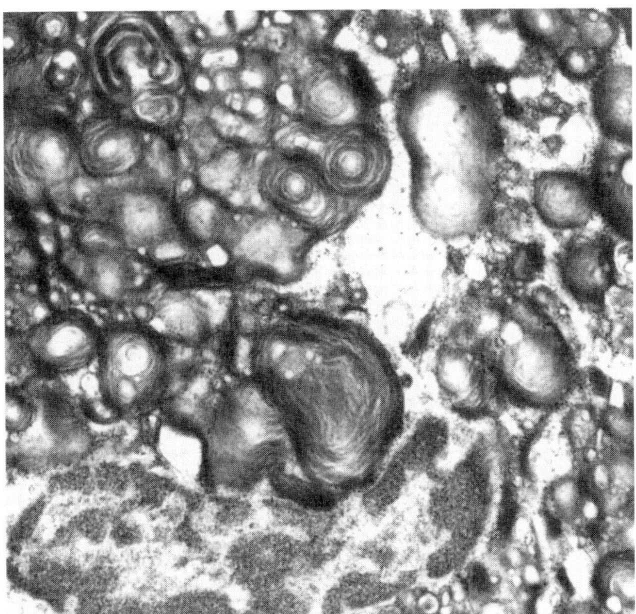

Figure 26 Large accumulations of lipid dominate the cytoplasm of this capillary endothelial cell from a patient with Fabry disease. This biopsy was fixed with 2% osmium tetroxide only, resulting in excellent preservation of the lipid in secondary lysosomes (×14,000). *Source*: Courtesy of Dr. John D. Shelburne.

of the rough ER can be seen in multiple myeloma and chronic lymphocytic leukemia, where their presence in circulating lymphocytes can be a helpful diagnostic marker. The ER can exhibit a wide variety of other abnormalities, including a whorled pattern (Fig. 32) and more complex arrangements. Paired cisternae or confronting cisternae (Fig. 33) appear as two fused cisternae of the rough ER or of the nuclear envelope. These are associated with a breakdown of the nuclear envelope; hence, they are fairly common in rapidly dividing cells, including human neoplasms (37) and in viral infections (see Chapter 8) (75). In some viral conditions including the acquired immunodeficiency syndrome (AIDS), paired or confronting cisternae may be arranged in a cylindrical pattern. The cytoplasmic tubular aggregates "tubuloreticular inclusions" or "paramyxovirus-like particles" (Fig. 34) seen in endothelial cells in patients with systemic lupus erythematosus, polymyositis, and other systemic immune disorders are also considered by some investigators to be a degeneration product of the ER (31). More recently, these have been seen in capillary endothelial cells and in circulating lymphocytes of patients with AIDS (76,88), and are known to correlate with elevated levels of gamma-interferon (IFNγ). IFNγ stimulates the formation of both tubuloreticular inclusions and annulate lamellae in cultured hairy cell leukemia cells (40). Proliferations of the rough and smooth ER have been observed in a wide variety of conditions (82) and can occasionally be of diagnostic value, as in tumors of steroid-producing organs (e.g., adrenal gland) or of the RPE (46).

Defects in the Golgi apparatus could theoretically give rise to accumulations of protein in the rough ER (56). Neoplasms such as adenocarcinomas exhibit a prominent rough ER and Golgi complex since they are normally engaged in synthetic activity.

Filament abnormalities. Filament abnormalities may be associated with pathologic states. For example, it has been argued that certain forms of cholestasis are caused by microfilament deficiencies. Mallorys alcoholic hyaline in hepatocytes is composed of dense masses of keratin intermediate filaments arranged in a complex mat (44,50). Neurofibrillary tangles are one of the diagnostic features of Alzheimer disease (see Chapter 70) and are composed of microtubule-associated proteins and neurofilaments in a complex, haphazard arrangement reflective of the disruption of the neuronal cytoskeleton (50).

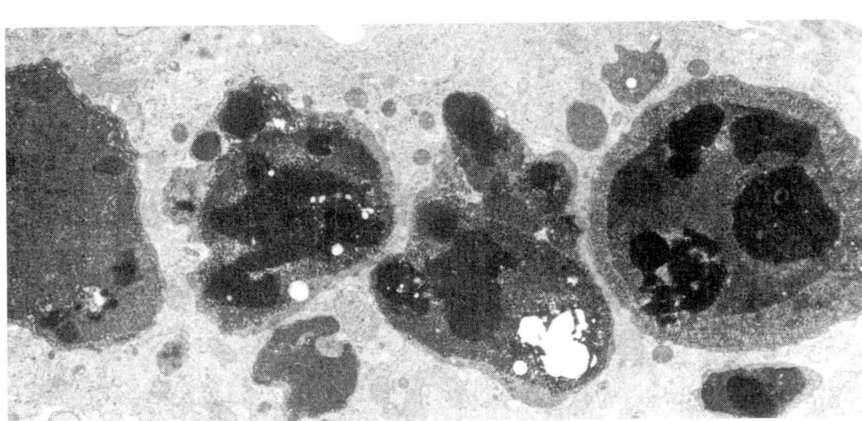

Figure 27 Typical hemosiderin containing residual bodies in a macrophage. At high magnification ferritin is visible in some regions of these secondary lysosomes. However, most of the iron is present in large, extremely electron-dense clumps (×7,600). *Source*: Courtesy of Dr. John D. Shelburne.

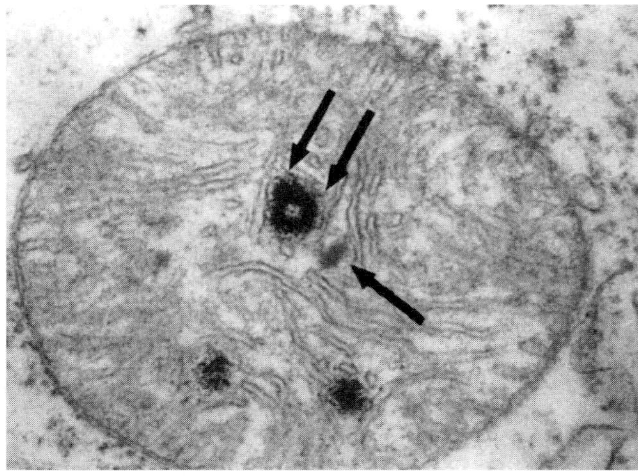

Figure 28 Examples of both flocculent or amorphous matrical densities (*single arrow*) and the more electron-dense granular or microcrystalline densities (*double arrows*) are visible in this mitochondrion from a necrotic cell (×52,500). *Source*: Adapted from Ref. 72.

Diseases of Specific Cell Types

Smooth Muscle Cells

Tumors of smooth muscle occur in many organs and can be benign (leiomyoma) or malignant (leiomyosarcoma) (see Chapter 64).

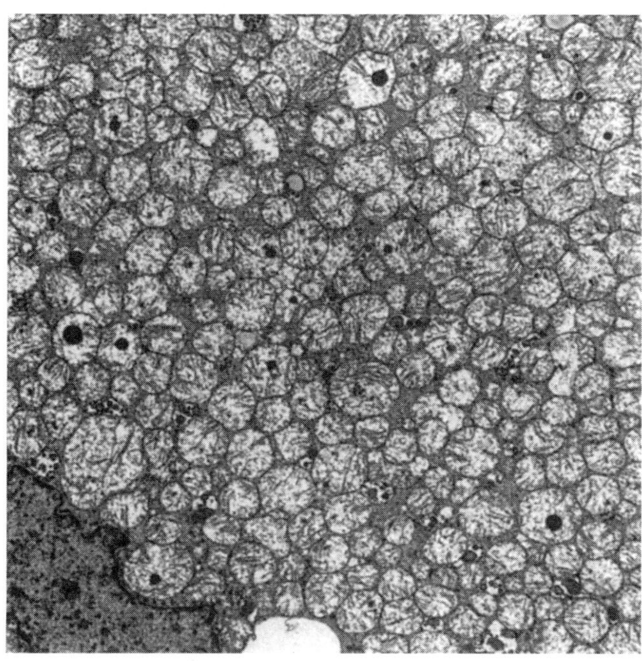

Figure 29 Note the incredible proliferation of mitochondria in the cytoplasm of this oncocytic renal cell carcinoma cell. These mitochondria are markedly swollen and exhibit spherical electron-dense inclusions (×16,800). *Source*: Courtesy of Dr. John D. Shelburne.

Striated Muscle Cells

The importance of the cytoskeletal proteins in linking or anchoring proteins in striated muscle is seen in muscular dystrophy. Duchenne and Becker muscular dystrophy involve a congenital absence of dystrophin, one of the important anchoring proteins that provide structure to the highly differentiated skeletal muscle fiber. Many other types of muscular dystrophy and myopathies occur some of which specifically affect the ocular muscles (see Chapter 72). Tumors of skeletal muscle occur in many organs and can be benign (rhabdomyoma) or malignant (rhabdomyosarcoma). Rhabdomyosarcoma is an important malignant neoplasm of the orbit, but it is believed to be derived from primitive mesenchymal tissue rather than from mature striated muscle (see Chapter 64).

Langerhans Cells

Aside from playing a role in antigen presentation as part of an immunologic process in the normal inflammatory response Langerhans cells can also be involved in a neoplastic process called *histiocytosis*. Histiocytosis is characterized by a proliferation of immature dendritic cells (i.e., Langerhans cells) and usually presents in one of three clinicopathologic entities: (*i*) multifocal multisystem Langerhans cell histiocytosis (old term Letterer–Siwe disease); (*ii*) unifocal and multifocal unisystem Langerhans cell histiocytosis (old term eosinophilic granuloma); or (*iii*) unifocal lesions. The triad of calvarial bone defects, diabetes insipidus, and exophthalamus is a presentation of multifocal unisystem Langerhans cell histiocytosis disease previously known at Hand–Schüller–Christian disease. The identification of Birbeck granules by TEM can be diagnostic in all of these entities.

Vascular Endothelial Cells

Loss of vascular endothelium and/or endothelial function in arteries is important in the genesis of atherosclerosis. New blood vessels sprout from the endothelium of postcapillary venules in many pathologic states. This angiogenesis is particularly common in association with inflammation or neoplasia (see Chapter 68). The vascular endothelium sometimes gives rise to a neoplasm (hemangioendothelioma) (see Chapter 62).

Pericytes

A loss of pericytes in the retinal capillaries is a characteristic feature of diabetic retinopathy (see Chapter 67).

Melanocytes

When melanocytes cluster, they are referred to as a nevus. A melanocytic nevus refers to a neoplasm of

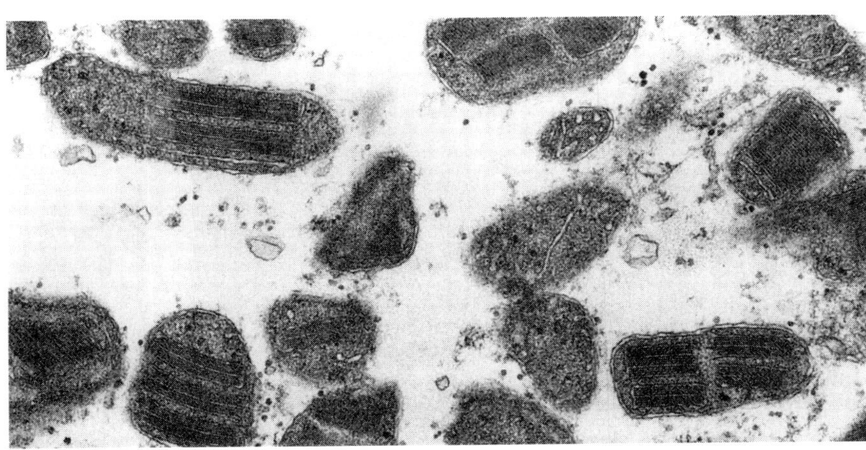

Figure 30 Typical mitochondrial paracrystals in the mitochondria of muscle with "red ragged fiber disease" (×34,600). *Source*: Courtesy of Dr. John D. Shelburne.

melanocytes which can be benign or transform into a malignant neoplasm known as malignant melanoma. Malignant melanoma is most common in the skin but it is also an important primary intraocular tumor and sometimes it arises from the ocular adnexal tissues (see Chapter 59).

Lymphatic Channels

Tumors of lymphatics occur usually in infants and are called lymphangiomas, but they do not usually involve the ocular tissue. However, orbital lymphangioma has been documented (38,47,48,68), but they are currently believed to be venous vascular abnormalities (see Chapter 62). Conjunctival lymphatic channels may become dilated as the draining lymphatics become obstructed.

Schwann Cells

Benign tumors of Schwann cells are called schwannomas and are usually seen in association with neurofibromatosis type 2. Sporadic schwannomas are associated with mutations in the gene for neurofibromatosis type 2 (*NF2*) on chromosome 22 (see Chapter 63). Malignant schwannomas are usually termed malignant peripheral nerve sheath tumors and are considered high-grade sarcomas. They do not

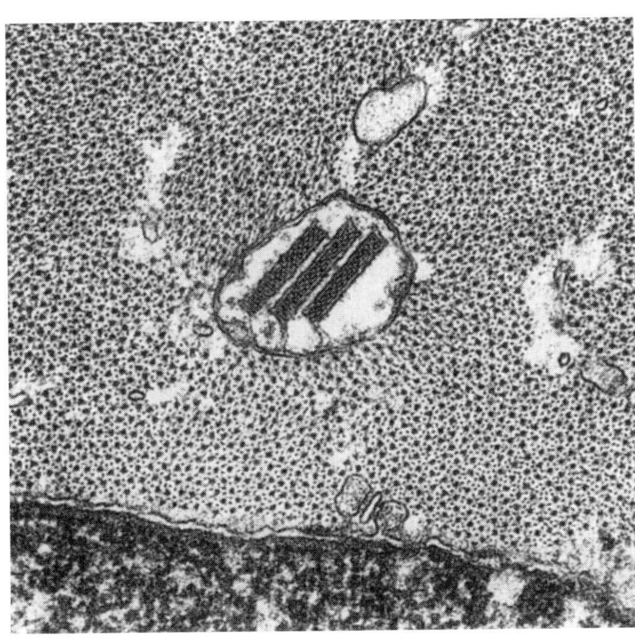

Figure 31 These mitochondrial paracrystals are clearly derived from the inner mitochondrial membrane or cristae (×54,600). *Source*: Courtesy of Dr. B. Alexander.

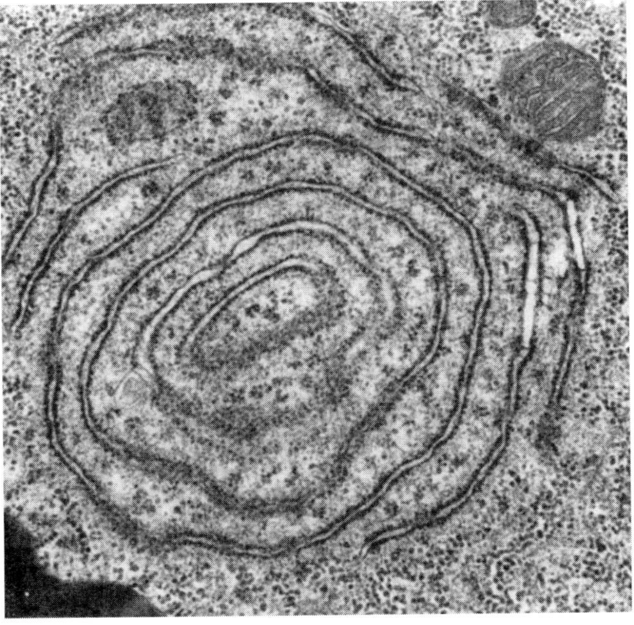

Figure 32 Note the swirled arrangement of the rough endoplasmic reticulum in this myocardial cell. Large amounts of glycogen surround this region (×26,500). *Source*: Courtesy of Dr. John D. Shelburne.

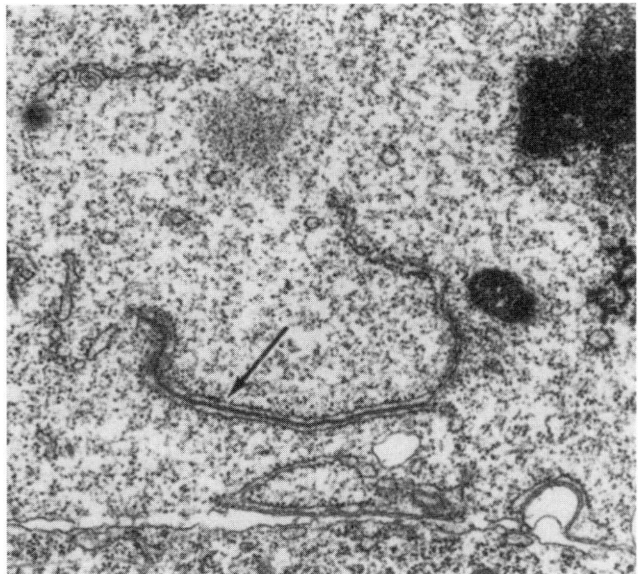

Figure 33 Fusion of two cisternae of the rough endoplasmic reticulum result in the formation of paired cisternae (*arrow*). Paired cisternae are most commonly seen in rapidly dividing cells (×19,000). *Source*: Courtesy of Dr. S. Walker.

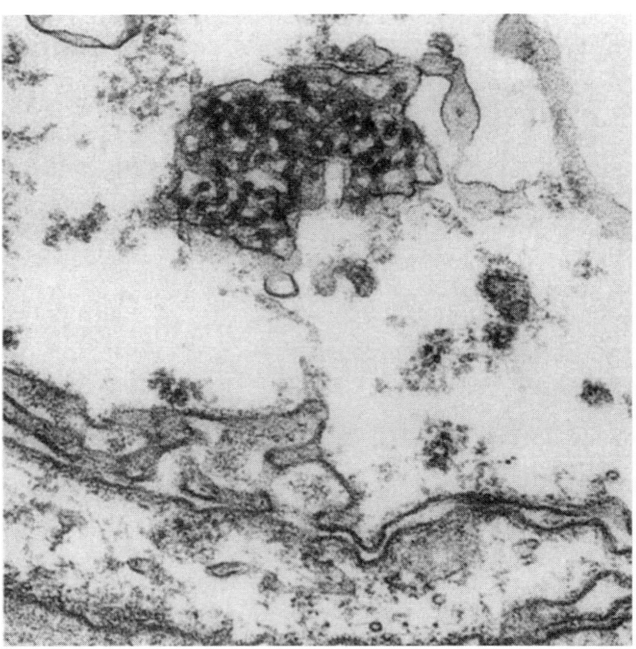

Figure 34 Tubuloreticular inclusions are visible in the cytoplasm of this swollen capillary endothelial cell in the kidney of a patient with systemic lupus erythematosus (×49,800). *Source*: Courtesy of Dr. John D. Shelburne.

arise from benign schwannomas but rather as de novo lesions or from a preexisting plexiform neurofibroma (see Chapter 63).

Fibroblasts

Benign tumors of fibroblasts are called fibromas. Fibromas are a relatively common lesion and can be seen in many different organs. The malignant counterpart, fibrosarcoma, is rare and can occur in any organ but is most commonly diagnosed in the retroperitoneum, the thigh and the distal extremities (see Chapter 64).

Myofibroblasts

Myofibroblasts are present in preretinal membranes (see Chapters 27 and 28) and anterior subcapsular cataracts (see Chapter 23). Keratocytes in the corneal stroma become transformed into myofibroblasts in corneal wounds and certain pathologic states. This transformation is reversible and can be induced with transforming growth factor beta (TGFβ) (58).

Cell Death

Once a cell undergoes an irreversible cell injury, it inevitably dies. However, cell death is not a singular event, but a series of steps and/or reactions that lead to different morphologic appearances when the insult is complete. Cells generally die through one of two processes: necrosis or apoptosis. Necrosis is the best known and best described form of cell death. It results from an exogenous cell injury and often is referred to as pathologic cell death. In contrast, apoptosis is important in normal development and therefore is often referred to as physiological cell death. However, there is considerable overlap between the two kinds of cell death depending upon the type of insult causing the cell injury.

Necrosis

In general, necrosis is associated with cell death from an external insult. Cells undergoing necrosis exhibit a series of structural and functional changes primarily as the result of energy depletion and the progressive digestion of the dying cells by degradative enzymes (i.e., lysosomal enzymes). The end result is loss of membrane integrity and leakage of intracellular constituents into the extracellular space. However, before the cell dies, subcellular changes occur that are considered essential features of necrosis including (*i*) cell swelling and (*ii*) loss of membrane integrity. Cell swelling results from HEP (ATP) depletion, which leads to loss of homeostatic ionic gradients due to decreased function of the energy-dependent ion pumps. The result of HEP depletion is swelling of subcellular organelles such as the ER and mitochondria as well as an overall increase in cellular volume. Other structural changes associated with necrosis include clumping and random dissolution of the nucleus, disruption of cytoskeletal–membrane connections often associated with large, free-floating membrane blebs, and loss of external membrane integrity. Some structural changes in dying cells are used in the clinical laboratory to aid in the diagnosis of cell death. An example of this is the release of creatine kinase and troponin I from dying myocardial cells which is useful in the laboratory diagnosis of acute myocardial infarction. Necrosis can be further divided into subtypes which can be classified based upon the morphologic pattern of the necrotic tissue.

Coagulation necrosis. This term is used when degradation is the primary pattern and typically occurs in ischemic cell death. In coagulation necrosis, the outline/membrane of the dead cells can readily be discerned at the light microscopic level for up to several days after the cells have died. However, after the plasma membrane ruptures and intracellular constituents are released into the extracellular space, the dead tissue elicits an acute inflammatory response, which results in complete digestion of the dead cells as well as some of the surrounding non-affected tissue resulting in a loss of tissue volume. As time passes and depending upon the specific tissue, the digested area becomes repaired with either an ingrowth of new resident cells or replacement by collagen (i.e., scar tissue). The inflammatory reaction in response to necrosis is ordered and sequential. Indeed, when associated with infarction, as in the heart, it is so reproducible that pathologists can determine with a relatively high degree of certainty when the actual infarct occurred. The timing of similar events in other tissues, such as the retina, is presumably comparable.

Liquefactive necrosis. This type of necrosis is characterized by an early, total destruction of the dead cells usually culminating in a cystic cavity. Simply put, the rate of cell death and resorption/destruction of the dead cells exceeds that of any potential repair process. This variety of necrosis usually follows deep-seated bacterial infections (i.e., abscesses), some fungal infections, or ischemia/hypoxia in the brain.

Fat necrosis. Fat necrosis is not a specific pattern of necrosis but rather necrosis of adipose tissue. Common clinical examples of fat necrosis include traumatic fat necrosis and fat necrosis resulting from pancreatitis. From the standpoint of the ocular tissues, fat necrosis is most frequently caused by infarction of the orbital fat in fungal infections such as *mucormycosis*. The unique feature of fat necrosis is the presence of triglycerides in the dying adipose tissue which are further broken down into free fatty acids. The free fatty acids then undergo saponification whereby they are precipitated as calcium soaps.

Caseous necrosis. Caseous necrosis occurs in the center of a tubercle or tuberculous granuloma and is diagnostic of tuberculosis. The natural history of mycobacterial infection involves engulfment by macrophages and the containment of the organism initially in regional lymph nodes. However, presumably due to the nature of the mycobacterial cell wall, it is extremely difficult to eradicate the offending organism and a chronic granulomatous inflammatory process ensues. However, the necrosis is neither coagulative (the cell outlines are obliterated) nor liquefactive (there is not dissolution of the tissue) but rather caseous necrosis is in between these two types. Grossly, this type of necrosis resembles the food cottage cheese in appearance hence the designation "caseous" necrosis.

Fibrinoid necrosis. Fibrinoid necrosis occurs exclusively in the walls of blood vessels. This type of necrosis was historically seen in patients with malignant (i.e., uncontrolled) hypertension but today it is most commonly observed in certain types of vasculitis (see Chapter 69). The nature of the necrosis is not specific but rather refers to the histologic appearance of the involved blood vessel wall, which is infiltrated with plasma proteins as it undergoes injury and takes on a very eosinophilic appearance when viewed by routine light microscopy.

Apoptosis

Apoptosis (programmed cell death) is a highly regulated and tightly controlled process that is involved in physiologic cell death and is distinctly different from necrosis. Apoptosis is discussed in detail in Chapter 2. Important differences exist in the fundamental nature of the two processes at the level of the dying cell. For example, necrosis is never an intentional action but rather occurs in response to a noxious external insult and necrosis is by nature a swelling process. Many of the subcellular events taking place in the context of necrosis involve swelling and dissolution of organelles and the cytoplasm of the entire cell. In contrast, a cell undergoing apoptosis undergoes shrinkage as it dies. This difference is also seen with respect to the fate of the cell membrane. In necrosis, the cell membrane ruptures or develops breaks in response to the underlying insult. In apoptosis, the cell membrane remains intact and does not generally rupture. Also, necrosis elicits a reactive inflammatory response that may contribute to additional cell damage resulting from release of hydrolases from PMNs. Apoptosis, in contrast, is not associated with a significant inflammatory reaction. Apoptosis usually affects individual cells or small groups of cells whereas necrosis generally involves large zones or regions of the affected tissue.

Despite the many well-established differences between apoptosis and necrosis, the two entities probably share some features and pathogenetic mechanisms. Indeed, in some situations, apoptosis and necrosis may coexist in the same tissue and apoptotic cells may even undergo secondary necrosis. In these situations, it appears that the severity of the insult stimulating cell death may play an important role. For example, in patients with severe chronic atherosclerotic coronary artery disease, it is thought that apoptosis is responsible for the progressive loss of individual myocytes and small groups of myocytes. In contrast, an acute myocardial infarct resulting from the occlusion of a large coronary artery exhibits large areas of zonal necrosis even though some apoptosis may be measured in the infarct zone.

REFERENCES

1. Albert DM, Lahav M, Lesser R, Craft T. Recent observations regarding retinoblastoma: 1. Ultrastructure, tissue culture growth, incidence and animal models. Trans Ophthalmol Soc U K 1974; 94:909–28.
2. Alberts B, Johnson A, Lewis J, et al. Molecular Biology of the Cell. 4th ed. New York: Garland Science, 2002.
3. Allison AC, Harrington JC, Birbeck M. An examination of the cytotoxic effects of silica on macrophages. J Exp Med 1966; 124:141–54.
4. Arden GB, Fox B. Increased incidence of abnormal nasal cilia in patients with retinitis pigmentosa. Nature 1979; 279:534–6.
5. Arstila AU, Shelburne JD, Trump BF. Studies on cellular autophagocytosis: a histochemical study on sequential alterations of mitochondria in the glucagon-induced autophagic vacuoles of rat liver. Lab Invest 1972; 27: 317–23.
6. Bauserman SC, Hardman JM, Schochet SS, Earle KM. Pituitary oncocytoma: indispensable role of electron microscopy in its identification. Arch Pathol Lab Med 1978; 102:456–9.
7. Beaver DL, Burr RE. Electron microscopy of bismuth inclusions. Am J Pathol 1963; 42:609–18.
8. Bell SW, Masters SK, Ingram P, et al. Ultrastructure and x-ray microanalysis of macrophages exposed to cadmium chloride. In: Johari O, Becker RP, eds. Scanning Electron Microscopy, AMF O'Hare, Illinois. Scanning Electron Microscopy Inc., 1979:111–22.
9. Birbeck MS, Breathnach AS, Evarall JD. An electron microscopic study of basal melanocytes and high-level clear cells (Langerhans cells) in vitiligo. J Invest Dermatol 1961; 37:51–64.
10. Bloom W, Fawcett DW. A Textbook of Histology. 11th ed. Philadelphia: W.B. Saunders, 1986.
11. Briggaman RA. Wheeler CE. Epidermolysis bullosa dystrophica-recessive: a possible role of anchoring fibrils in the pathogenesis. J Invest Dermatol 1975; 65:203–11.
12. Burger PC, Scheithauer BW, Vogel FS. Surgical Pathology of the Nervous System and Its Coverings. 4th ed. New York: Churchill Livingstone, 2002.
13. Busch H. The Cell Nucleus. New York: Academic Press, 1974.
14. Cartwright GE, Deiss A. Sideroblasts, siderocytes and sideroblastic anemia. N Engl J Med 1975; 292:185–93.
15. Cohen HJ, Lefer LG. Intranuclear inclusions in Bence Jones lambda plasma cell myeloma. Blood 1975; 45:131–9.
16. Copeland DD, Bell SW, Shelburne JD. Hemidesmosome-like intercellular specialization in human meningiomas. Cancer 1978; 41:2242–9.
17. Copeland DD, Talley FA, Bigner DD. The fine structure of intracranial neoplasms induced by the inoculation of avian sarcoma virus in neonatal and adult rats. Am J Pathol 1976; 83:149–76.
18. Costa JL, Joy DC, Maher DM, et al. Fluorinated molecule as a tracer: difluoroserotonin in human platelets mapped by electron energy-loss spectroscopy. Science 1978; 200:537–9.
19. Costello MJ, McIntosh TJ, Robertson JD. Membrane specializations in mammalian lens fiber cells: distribution of square arrays. Curr Eye Res 1985; 4:1183–201.
20. DeDuve C, Wattiaux R. Functions of lysosomes. Annu Rev Physiol 1966; 28:435–92.
21. Elias H, Fong BB. Nuclear fragmentation in colon carcinoma cells. Hum Pathol 1978; 9:679–84.
22. Eliasson R, Mossberg B, Camner P, Afzelius BA. The immotile-cilia syndrome: a congenital ciliary abnormality as an etiologic factor in chronic airway infections and male sterility. N Engl J Med 1977; 297:1–6.
23. Fawcett DW. What makes cilia and sperm tails beat? N Engl J Med 1977; 297:46–8.
24. Feeney L. Lipofuscin and melanin of human retinal pigment epithelium: fluorescence enzyme cytochemical and ultrastructural studies. Invest Ophthalmol Vis Sci 1978; 17:583–600.
25. Feldherr CM, Akin D. EM visualization of nucleocytoplasmic transport processes. Electron Microsc Rev 1990; 3: 73–86.
26. Ghadially FN. Ultrastructural Pathology of the Cell and Matrix. 3rd ed. London: Butterworths, 1988.
27. Ghosh S. The nucleolar structure. Int Rev Cytol 1976; 44: 1–28.
28. Gold JH, Shelburne JD, Bossen EH. Meningeal mycosis fungoides: cytologic and ultrastructural aspects. Acta Cytol 1976; 20:349–55.
29. Gould VE. Neuroendocrinomas and neuroendocrine carcinomas: APUD cell system neoplasms and their aberrant secretory activities. Pathol Annu 1977; 12:33–62.
30. Goyer RA, May P, Cates MM, Krigman MR. Lead and protein content of isolated intranuclear inclusion bodies from kidneys of lead-poisoned rats. Lab Invest 1970; 22: 245–51.
31. Grimley PM, Schaff Z. Significance of tubuloreticular inclusions in the pathobiology of human diseases. Pathobiol Annu 1976; 6:221–58.
32. Hackenbrock CR. Ultrastructural basis for metabolically linked mechanical activity in mitochondria. I. Reversible ultrastructure changes with change in metabolic steady state in isolated liver mitochondria. J Cell Biol 1966; 30: 269–97.
33. Hackenbrock CR. Ultrastructural basis of metabolically linked mechanical activity in mitochondria. II. Electron transport-linked ultrastructural transformations in mitochondria. J Cell Biol 1968; 37:345–69.
34. Hackenbrock CR. Energy-linked ultrastructural transformations in isolated liver mitochondria and mitoplasts: preservation of configurations by freeze-cleaving as compared to chemical fixation. J Cell Biol 1972; 53: 450–65.
35. Hackenbrock CR, Rehn TG, Weinbach EL, LeMasters JJ. Oxidative phosphorylation and ultrastructural transformation in mitochondria in the intact ascites tumor cell. J Cell Biol 1971; 51:123–37.

36. Hall MO. Phagocytosis of light- and dark-adapted rod outer segments by cultured pigment epithelium. Science 1978; 202:526–8.
37. Hanaoka H, Friedman B. Paired cisternae in human tumor cells. J Ultrastruct Res 1970; 32:323–33.
38. Harris GJ, Sakol PJ, Bonovolonta G, de Conciliis C. An analysis of thirty cases or orbital lymphangioma: pathophysiologic considerations and management recommendations. Ophthalmology 1990; 97:1583–92.
39. Hawkins HK. Reactions of lysosomes to cell injury. In: Arstila AU, Trump BF, eds. Pathology of Membranes. Vol. 3. New York: Academic Press, 1980:251–89.
40. Hiraoka A, Golomb HM. Responses of hairy cell leukemia cells to a recombinant alpha-2 interferon in vitro and in vivo: correlation between formation of tubuloreticular structures and clinical parameters. J Biol Response Modif 1986; 5:270–81.
41. Hogan MJ, Alvarado JA, Weddell JE. Histology of the human eye: an atlas and textbook. Philadelphia: W.B. Saunders, 1971.
42. Hull BE, Staehelin LA. The terminal web: a reevaluation of its structure and function. J Cell Biol 1979; 81:67–82.
43. Iannaccone ST, Griggs RC, Markesbery WR, Joynt RJ. Familial progressive external ophthalmoplegia and red-ragged fibers. Neurology 1974; 24:1033–8.
44. Iseri OA, Gottlieb LS. Alcoholic hyalin and megamitochondria as separate and distinct entities in liver disease associated with alcoholism. Gastroenterology 1971; 60: 1027–35.
45. Ishikawa T, Pei YF. Intramitochondrial glycogen particles in rat retinal receptor cells. J Cell Biol 1965; 25:402–8.
46. Jakobiec FA, Font RC, Iwamoto T. Diagnostic ultrastructural pathology of ophthalmic tumors. In: Jakobiec FA, ed. Ocular and Adnexal Tumors. Birmingham, AL: Aesculapius, 1978:359–453.
47. Jones IS. Lymphangiomas of the ocular adnexa. An analysis of 62 cases. Trans Am Ophthalmol Soc 1959; 57: 602–65.
48. Jones IS. Lymphangiomas of the ocular adnexa. An analysis of 62 cases. Am J Ophthalmol 1961; 51:481–509.
49. Klintworth GK. Experimental studies on the phagocytic capability of the corneal fibroblast. Am J Pathol 1969; 55: 283–94.
50. Kumar V, Abbas AK, Fausto N. Robbins and Cotran Pathologic Basis of Disease. 7th ed. Philadelphia: Elsevier Saunder, 2005.
51. Landers MB III, Klintworth GK. Subacute sclerosing parencephalitis (SSPE). Arch Ophthalmol 1971; 86:156–63.
52. Lee SC, Roth LM. Malignant oncocytoma of the parotid glands: a light and electron microscopic study. Cancer 1976; 37:1607–14.
53. Lindal S, Lund I, Torbergsen T, et al. Mitochondrial diseases and myopathies: a series of muscle biopsy specimens with ultrastructural changes in the mitochondria. Ultrastruct Pathol 1992; 16:263–75.
54. Lou TY, Teplitz C. Malacoplakia: pathogenesis and ultrastructural morphogenesis: a problem of altered macrophage (phagolysosomal) response. Hum Pathol 1974; 5:192–207.
55. Lurie M, Rennert G, Goldenberg S, et al. Ciliary ultrastructure in primary ciliary dyskinesia and other chronic respiratory conditions: the relevance of microtubular abnormalities. Ultrastruct Pathol 1992; 16:547–53.
56. Mabry RJ, Shelburne JD, Cohen HJ. In vitro kinetics of immunoglobulin synthesis and secretion by non-secretory human myeloma cells. Blood 1977; 50:1031–8.
57. Mahon KA, Chepelinsky AB, Khillan JS et al. Oncogenesis of the lens in transgenic mice. Science 1987; 35:1622–5.
58. Maltseva O, Folger P, Zekaria D, et al. Fibroblast growth factor reversal of the corneal myofibroblast phenotype. Invest Ophthalmol Vis Sci 2001; 42:2490–5.
59. Mansbach CM II, Shelburne JD, Stevens RD, Dobbins WO III. Lymph-node bacilliform bodies resembling those of Whipple's disease in a patient without intestinal involvement. Ann Intern Med 1978; 89:64–6.
60. Marx J. Podosomes and invadopodia help mobile cells step lively. Science 2006; 312:1868–9.
61. McNutt NS, Weinstein RS. Membrane ultrastructure at mammalian intercellular junctions. Prog Biophys Mol Biol 1973; 26:45–101.
62. Miller SE. Detection and identification of viruses by electron microscopy. J Electron Microsc Tech. 1986; 4: 265–301.
63. Miller SE. Diagnosis of viral infection by electron microscopy. In: Schmidt NJ, Lennette EH, Lennette DA, Lennette ET, Emmons RW, eds. Laboratory Diagnostic Procedures for Viral, Rickettsial, and Chlamydial Infections. Chapter 3. 7th ed. Washington, D.C.: American Public Health Association, 1995: 37–78.
64. Mitchener JS, Shelburne JD, Bradford WD, Hawkins HK. Cellular autophagocytosis induced by deprivation of serum and amino acids in HeLa cells. Am J Pathol 1976; 83:485–98.
65. Muscatello U, Pasquali-Ronchetti I. The relation between structure and function in mitochondria: its relevance in pathology. Pathobiol Annu 1972; 2:1–46.
66. Palade G. Intracellular aspects of protein synthesis. Science 1975; 189:347–58.
67. Papadimitriou JM, Henderson DW, Spagnolo DV. Diagnostic Ultrastructure of Non-Neoplastic Diseases. New York: Churchill Livingstone, 1992.
68. Reese AB, Howard GM. Unusual manifestations of ocular lymphangioma and lymphangiectasis. Surv Ophthalmol 1973; 18:226–31.
69. Reimer KA, Jennings RB. Myocardial ischemia, hypoxia and infarction. In: Fozzard HA, Harber E, Jennings RB, Katz AM, Morgan HE, eds. The Heart and Cardiovascular System. Chapter 75. 2 ed. New York: Raven Press, Ltd., 1992:1875–973.
70. Roos B, Keller HU, Hess MW, Cottier H. Alveolar macrophages: phagocytosis induced release of neutrophil chemotactic activity. In: Sanders CL, Schneider RP, Dagle GE, Ragan HA, eds. Pulmonary Macrophage and Epithelial Cells. Springfield, VA: Technical Information Center, Energy Research and Development Administration, 1976: 78–84.
71. Rubin E, Gorstein F, Rubin R, Schwarting R, Strayer D. Rubin's Pathology. Clinicopathologic Foundations of Medicine. Baltimore, MD: Lippincott, Williams, and Wilkins, 2005.
72. Scalettar BE, Abney JR, Hackenbrock CR. Dynamics, structure and function are coupled in the mitochondrial matrix. Proc Natl Acad Sci U S A 1991; 88:8057–61.
73. Shelburne JD, Arstila AU, Trump BF. Studies on cellular autophagocytosis: cyclic AMP and dibutyryl cyclic AMP stimulated autophagy in rat liver. Am J Pathol 1973; 72: 521–40.
74. Shelburne JD, Arstila AU, Trump BF. Studies on cellular autophagocytosis: the relationship of autophagocytosis to protein synthesis and to energy metabolism of the rat liver and in flounder kidney tubules in vitro. Am J Pathol 1973; 73:641–70.
75. Shimizu YK, Feinstone SM, Purcell RH, Alter HJ, London WT. Non-A, non-B hepatitis: ultrastructural evidence for two agents in experimentally infected chimpanzees. Science 1979; 205:197–200.

76. Sidhu GS, Stahl RE, El-Sadr W, Cassai ND, Forrester EM, Zolla-Pazner S. The acquired immunodeficiency syndrome: an ultrastructural study. Hum Pathol 1985; 16: 377–86.
77. Small JV, Sobiescek A. Studies on the function and composition of the 10 nm (100 Å) filaments of vertebrate smooth muscle. J Cell Sci 1977; 23:243–68.
78. Somlyo AP, Somlyo AV, Ashton FT, Vallieres J. Vertebrate smooth muscle: ultrastructure and function. In: Goldman RD, ed. Cell Motility, Cold Spring Harbor Symposium. Cold Spring Harbor, NY: Cold Spring Harbor Laboratory, 1976:165–83.
79. Staubli W, Hess R, Weibel ER. Correlated morphometric and biochemical studies on the liver cell. II. Effects of phenobarbital on rat hepatocytes. J Cell Biol 1969; 42:92–112.
80. Strehler BL. On the histochemistry and ultrastructure of age pigment. Adv Gerontol Res 1964; 1:343–84.
81. Sturgess JM, Chao J, Wong J, et al. Cilia with defective radial spokes: a cause of human respiratory disease. N Engl J Med 1979; 300:53–6.
82. Suzuki T, Furusato M, Takasaki S, Ishikawa E. Giant mitochondria in the epithelial cells of the proximal convoluted tubules of diseased human kidneys. Lab Invest 1975; 33:578–90.
83. Towfighi J, Young R, Sassani J, et al. Alexander's disease: further light-, and electron-microscopic observations. Acta Neuropathol 1983; 61:36–42.
84. Trump BF, Berezesky IK, Jiji RM, et al. Energy dispersive x-ray microanalysis of mitochondrial deposits in sideroblastic anemia. Lab Invest 1978; 39:375–80.
85. Tso MOM., Zimmerman LE, Fine BS. The nature of retinoblastoma, II. Photoreceptor differentiation: an electron microscopic study. Am J Ophthalmol 1970; 69:350–9.
86. Wallace DC. Mitochondrial genetics: a paradigm for aging and degenerative disease? Science 1992; 256:628–32.
87. Weibel ER, Palade GE. New cytoplasmic components in arterial endothelia. J Cell Biol 1964; 23:101–12.
88. Wills EJ. Infectious agents: fungi, bacteria and viruses. In: Papadimitriou JM, Henderson DW, Spagnolo DV, eds. Diagnostic Ultrastructure of Non-Neoplastic Diseases. New York: Churchill Livingstone, 1992:46–83.
89. Wuerker RB. Neurofilaments and glial filaments. Tissue Cell 1970; 1:1–9.
90. Yanoff M, Fine BS, Berkow JW. Diabetic lacy vacuolation of iris pigment epithelium. Am J Ophthalmol 1970; 69: 201–10.
91. Yen SH, Dahl D, Schachner M, Shelanski ML. Biochemistry of the filaments of brain. Proc Natl Acad Sci U S A 1976; 73: 529–33.
92. Yunis EJ, Hashida Y, Haas JE. The role of electron microscopy in the identification of viruses in human diseases. In: Sommers SC, Rosen PP, eds. Pathology Annual, Part 1. Vol. 12. New York: Appleton-Century-Crofts, 1977:311–30.

2

Apoptosis

Victor M. Elner, Hakan Demirci, and Susan G. Elner
Kellogg Eye Institute, University of Michigan, Ann Arbor, Michigan, U.S.A.

INTRODUCTION

Cell death is an important process that regulates dynamic balances in living systems during development, growth, homeostasis, disease, and repair (see Chapter 1) (48). Three types of cell death are known: (*i*) apoptosis (programmed cell death), (*ii*) autophagy, and (*iii*) necrosis (69). Apoptosis is a highly regulated mechanism by which cells die in response to defined internal or external stimuli. Autophagy is characterized by bulk degradation of cellular components, principally proteins that are essential for maintaining cellular integrity when nutrients are scarce. Necrosis is a passive process characterized by disruption of cell membranes and a progressive breakdown of organelles in response to severe environmental perturbations such as hypoxia/ischemia, temperature variations, and mechanical trauma.

The morphologic differences between these different types of cell death are presented in Table 1. In this chapter, we will focus on apoptosis.

Apoptosis is a major control mechanism by which cells undergo self-destruction. Whatever its initiating stimulus, the end target of apoptosis is irreparable DNA damage. Apoptosis can cause or contribute to various diseases, including those with uncontrolled cell proliferation or accumulation as seen in neoplasms, failure to eradicate aberrant cells that occurs in autoimmune diseases, or inappropriate loss of cells that is seen in degenerative diseases and aging.

There are two major apoptotic pathways that may be triggered by a wide variety of external or internal signals (49). The extrinsic pathway, also known as the death receptor pathway, is activated by the binding of ligands derived from other cells to death-inducing cell surface receptors on the cells targeted for apoptosis. The intrinsic pathway, also known as the mitochondrial pathway, may be initiated by a wide variety of extrinsic or intrinsic stress-inducing signals that are ultraviolet- or γ-irradiation, toxins, chemotherapeutic drugs, growth factor deprivation, or reactive oxygen metabolites (49). Mitochondrial destabilization is the primary and key initial target of the intrinsic pathway (49).

Table 1 Comparison Between Different Types of Cell Death

Factor	Apoptosis	Autophagy	Necrosis
Nucleus	Chromatin condensation	Partial chromatin condensation	Karyolysis
	DNA laddering and fragmentation	No DNA laddering and fragmentation	Karyorrhexis
	Pyknosis	Sometimes pyknosis	Pyknosis
Cytoplasm	Cytoplasmic condensation	Many large autophagic vacuoles	Cytoplasmic condensation
	Fragmentation to apoptotic bodies	Many autophagosomes	Cell swelling and lysis
	Increase in MMP	Potential involvement of MMP	Matrix swelling, lipid peroxidation, and decrease in membrane integrity
	Activation of caspase cascade	Caspase independent	Caspase independent
	Potential release of lysosomal enzymes	Lysosomal activation	Lysosomal leakage
	No swelling of organelles		Organelle swelling
Membrane	Blebbing	Blebbing	Loss of membrane integrity

Abbreviation: MMP, mitochondrial membrane permeability.

HISTORY OF THE CONCEPT OF APOPTOSIS

Cell death occurring during physiologic processes was observed by several scientists as early as the 18th century, first in plants and later in animals. In 1940, Rita Levi-Montalcini described neuronal death that occurs during normal chick embryo morphogenesis (30). Later, in 1949, Hamburger and Levi-Montalcini postulated that neuronal growth factors released from tissues targeted by migrating neurons act to select and regulate the number of neurons that survive at each stage of development (42). Other investigators later showed that cell death is an integral part of normal embryonic development (30). In 1965, the phrase, programmed cell death, was first used by Lockshin to describe cell death during the physiologic process of eliminating unwanted cells during insect metamorphosis (30). The term "apoptosis" was first used in 1972 by Kerr et al. (54) to describe the morphological features of an active and programmed phenomenon that leads to cellular elimination and is complementary to mitosis in regulating cell populations. The term "apoptosis" was coined, originating from the combination of the Greek words "apo," meaning separation, and "ptosis," meaning falling off, as it pertains to the seasonal shedding of leaves from trees or of petals from flowers (30,37). When co-opted for its use in medical biology, apoptosis is used to signify this process of programmed cell death (37). Later, apoptotic programmed cell death was shown to be an active process of self-destruction resulting from either the overexpression of specific inducing signals or the absence of specific survival signals, thereby eliminating unneeded or damaged cells, regulating cell numbers, and selecting the fittest cells (93,114,122). These observations have led to the concept that cells have energy-dependent intrinsic machinery that is tightly regulated during diverse processes of morphogenesis, homeostasis, and response to pathologic stimuli.

EXTRINSIC APOPTOTIC PATHWAY

The extrinsic pathway of apoptosis is mediated by death receptors expressed on the cell surface (Fig. 1). Eight members of the death receptor family have been characterized so far: tumor necrosis factor receptor 1 (TNFR1), Fas, death receptor 3 (DR3), TNF-related apoptosis-inducing ligand receptor 1 (TRAILR1), TRAILR2, DR6, ectodysplasin A receptor (EDAR) and nerve growth factor receptor (35,60,118).

All contain a cytoplasmic tail of about 80 amino acid residues termed the death domain. Stimulation of death receptors by their corresponding death ligands results in oligomerization of the receptors and recruitment of the adaptor proteins—Fas-associated death domain (FADD) and TNFR-associated death domain (TRADD) proteins—and caspase-8, forming a death-inducing signaling complex. When aggregated in the signaling complex, caspase-8 is activated. Its activation initiates a downstream cascade that activates effector caspases, including caspase-3, -6, and -7, which mediate the cell death program (44). Death ligands also interact with decoy receptors displayed on the cell surface. These decoys do not possess cytoplasmic death domains and are unable to form signaling complexes. Four decoy receptors have been recognized: TRAIL3 (DcR1), TRAIL4 (DcR2), DcR3, and osteoprotegerin (OPG) (60).

Activation of either Fas or TRAIL receptors induces recruitment of death-inducing signaling complexes with similar compositions (60,92). This type of death-inducing signaling complex results in the activation of caspase-8, which plays the central role in transduction of the apoptotic signal. However, some TRAIL receptors are decoys and bind ligands that would otherwise stimulate death-inducing complex formation. Activation of TNFR1, DR3, DR6 and EDAR receptors recruits a different set of molecules to form a second type of death-inducing signaling complex that transduces both apoptotic and survival signals (60,92).

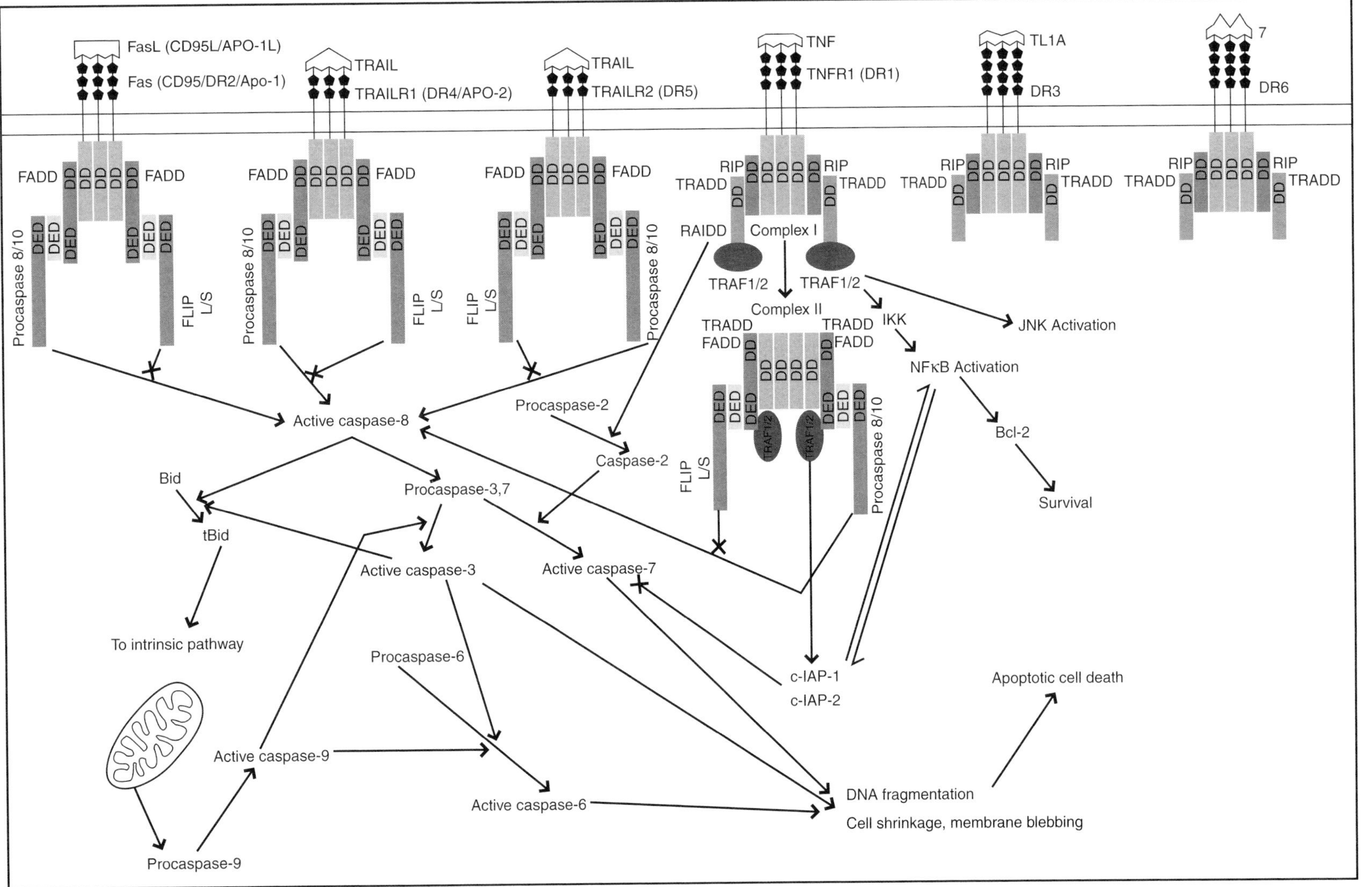

Figure 1 Extrinsic apoptotic pathway. Binding of ligands to specific cell surface receptors induces intracellular signaling that may lead directly to apoptotic cell death. Indirect stimulation of the intrinsic pathway may also occur. Stimulation of survival pathways may mitigate apoptosis (see text for definitions of abbreviations).

Fas and TRAIL Receptor Pathway

Fas Signaling

Binding of Fas ligand (FasL) to Fas leads to Fastrimerization and recruitment of specific adaptor proteins to the cytoplasmic tail death domain of Fas, which interacts with the FADD protein. FADD then binds to isoforms a and b of procaspases-8 and -10 which form the death effector domain. The regulatory protein, FLICE-inhibitory protein (FLIP), then binds to the aggregate to complete the Fas death-inducing signaling complex (92). Activation of procaspase-8 is believed to follow an induced proximity model, in which high local concentrations of procaspase-8 at the death-inducing signaling complex lead to autoproteolytic activation of caspase-8. This involves a multi-step cleavage process resulting in the formation of an activated caspase-8 heterotetramer containing two large subunits (p18) and two small subunits (p10). The activated enzyme is then released into the cytosol to propagate the apoptotic signal. Procaspase-10 is also activated at the death-inducing signaling complex, also forming an active heterotetramer. However, the role of caspase-10 remains unclear since activated caspase-10 appears to be unable to trigger apoptotic cell death in the absence of caspase-8 activation. The inhibitory protein, FLIP, is an important regulator of death receptor-mediated apoptosis. Two types of FLIP have been found: $FLIP_S$ (Short) and $FLIP_L$ (Long). The role of FLIP in death receptor-mediated apoptosis remains controversial. FLIP can be recruited to the death-inducing signaling complexes of DR2 and TRAIL receptors, disabling the activation and release of caspase-8 (57). FLIP may also activate nuclear factor kappa B (NFκB) which may modulate cell death by pro- and anti-apoptotic effects (50).

According to their requirement for the mitochondrial pathway in Fas-induced apoptosis cells can be divided into two types (99). Type I cells are characterized by high levels of death-inducing signaling complex formation and activated caspase-8. The high levels of activated caspase-8 that are generated in these cells lead directly to the activation of downstream caspases, whose action on the protein and DNA of cellular targets results in the execution phase of apoptosis. In type II cells, Fas signaling results in lower levels of complex formation and caspase-8 activation. This more modest initial signaling requires an amplification loop that involves cleavage of the Bcl-2 family protein, Bid, by caspase-8 to generate a truncated form designated tBid. tBid translocates to the outer membrane of the mitochondia, causing their permeabilization and release of cytochrome *c* that results in apoptosome formation. The apoptosome activates procaspase-9, which in turn cleaves downstream effector caspases. Fas signaling in type II cells may be inhibited by anti-apoptotic Bcl-2 family members, including Bcl-2 and Bcl-x.

TRAIL Receptor Signaling

Five distinct TRAIL receptors have been identified. Two are death-inducing receptors (TRAILR1 and TRAILR2) and three are death-inhibitory receptors (TRAILR3, TRAILR4 and OPG) (49). Both TRAILR1 and TRAIL2 contain a C-terminal death domain that signals downstream caspase activation to mediate TRAIL-induced apoptosis. In contrast to TRAILR1 and TRAILR2, TRAIL3 and TRAIL4 lack a functional cytoplasmic death domain. These two receptors serve as decoys and protect cells from TRAIL-induced apoptosis by competing with the death-inducing TRAIL receptors for TRAIL ligands (49). OPG also is a decoy that does not transduce apoptotic signals; it has low affinity for TRAIL ligands at physiologic temperatures and is less effective at competing with the death-inducing receptors. These decoy receptors also antagonize the stimulation of Fas by competing for FasL.

The TRAIL-induced apoptotic signaling is similar to that induced by Fas–FasL binding. When bound by TRAIL ligands, TRAILR1 and TRAILR2 trigger the formation of a death-inducing signaling complex by recruiting FADD, caspase-8, -10 and FLIP, followed by activation of caspases-8 and -3. Like Fas-mediated apoptosis in type II cells, TRAIL-induced signaling causes mitochondia to release second mitochondria-derived activator of caspase (Smac), a protein that antagonizes the X-linked inhibitory apoptotic protein (XIAP). Antagonizing XIAP, the most powerful inhibitor of caspase-3, is a major pro-apoptotic response to TRAIL (21). TRAIL is also a weak activator of the NFκB pathway that has pro- and anti-apoptotic effects.

FLIP is an important negative regulator of TRAIL-induced apoptosis (55,95). Overexpression of FLIP protects cells from TRAIL-induced apoptosis, and suppression of FLIP by silencing RNA sensitizes cells to TRAIL-induced apoptosis. Inhibitory apoptotic proteins (IAP) can mitigate TRAIL-induced apoptosis by directly reducing caspase activity. Other cell signaling pathways may also be involved in the regulation of TRAIL sensitivity, including the *AKT1*, Myc, NFκB, or p53 pathways. Constitutive activation of AKT1 in several types of cancer cells has been shown to confer resistance to TRAIL (76). This inhibition of TRAIL-induced apoptosis by activated AKT may occur due to cleavage of the pro-apothis protein, Bid. Suppression of AKT activity in tumor cells sensitizes them to TRAIL-induced apoptosis. Myc is a positive regulator of TRAIL sensitivity and has been shown to upregulate TRAIL receptor expression in some tumor cells while repressing

FLIP gene expression in others (121). p53 is another important regulator of TRAIL sensitivity and sensitizes cells to TRAIL through a mitochondrial amplification loop.

TNF Receptor Pathway

There are two major TNF receptors, tumor necrosis factor receptor superfamily member 1A (TNFRSF1A) and tumor necrosis receptor superfamily member 1B (TNFRSF1B) (49,119). TNFRSF1A is expressed in most tissues and is the major mediator of TNF apoptotic signaling. TNFRSF1B is mainly found in the immune system and is only fully activated by membrane bound, and not soluble, TNF. TNFRSF1A binding to its ligand, TNFα, is thought to result in the formation of two sequential signaling complexes (77). Complex I, the initial plasma membrane-bound complex, comprises TNFRSF1A, TRADD adaptor protein, receptor-interacting protein kinase 1 (RIP1) kinase, TNF receptor-associated factors 1 and 2 (TRAF1 and TRAF2), and other yet unidentified molecules. Complex I signals activation of modulators of apoptosis: NFκB through the recruitment of IκB kinase (IKK) complex and c-Jun N-terminal protein kinase (JNK) through a TRAF2-dependent mechanism. These modulators act through diverse mechanisms chiefly by activating transcription factors for genes involved in many cell functions and by modulating oxidative pathways affecting the intrinsic apoptotic pathway. TRADD, bound to the cytoplasmic tail of DR1, serves as a common assembly platform for binding TRAF2 and RIP1 kinase. In contrast to the Fas and TRAIL receptor pathway, complex I lacks FADD and procaspase-8. However, the complex I assembly separates from TNFRSF1A and translocates to associate with the FADD, procaspases-8 and -10, and $FLIP_S$ and $FLIP_L$ in the cytoplasm. This cytoplasmic complex is termed the traddosome, or complex II. Activation of procaspase-8 takes place in the traddosome and is followed by activation of downstream death signaling. All death receptors investigated so far appear to depend on FADD and caspase-8 to induce cell death (109). However, in contrast to Fas and TRAILR1 and TRAILR2, TNFRSF1A is indirectly linked to FADD by TRADD which is also responsible for bridging TNFRSF1A to TRAF2 and the IKK complex.

In the TNF pathway, the balance between survival and death depends on the efficacy of complex II formation, caspase-8 activation, and the amount of FLIP in the cells that blocks procaspase-8 activation at complex II. Unlike Fas and TRAIL receptor signaling, TNFα binding to TNFRSF1A also induces strong cell survival signals. The binding of TRAF1 or TRAFT2 to TRADD recruits cellular inhibitor of apoptosis 1 (c-IAP1) and c-IAP2. RIP binding to TRADD in complex I leads to activation of NFκB, resulting in transcription of anti-apoptotic genes that promote cell survival. When NFκB is activated by complex I, complex II also harbors the caspase-8 inhibitor $FLIP_L$ and the cell survives. Otherwise, cells undergo apoptosis through the complex II-mediated signaling pathway (77). Thus, the TNF receptor pathway includes a check point, resulting in cell death via complex II when the initial signal via complex I and NFκB is not sufficiently activated. TNF-R2 mitigates TNFRSF1A-induced apoptosis by forming a heterocomplex with TNFRSF1A. The complex recruits TRAF1 and TRAF2, c-IAP1, and c-IAP2, stimulating anti-apoptotic pathways, including inactivation of caspase-7.

TNFRSF1A is also able to mediate apoptosis through the recruitment of an adaptor molecule called: RIP-associated caspase-2 (ICH-1)/cell death abnormality (CED-3) homologous protein with a death domain (RAIDD) (29). RAIDD associates with RIP1 in the death domain and recruits caspase-2 through an interaction with a motif, similar to the death effector domain, known as the caspase activation and recruitment domain (CARD). Recruitment of caspase-2 leads to activation of caspase-7 which activates terminal apoptotic pathways with degradation of cellular and nuclear constituents (49). Alternatively, and in contrast to RIP1 stimulation of NFκB that mediates pro- and anti-apoptotic signaling, necrosis can be induced directly by RIP1 kinase activity.

The DR3 and DR6 signaling pathways are less well characterized. RIP and TRADD are recruited to the receptor complex; DR3 and DR6 also promote activation of survival genes (49).

THE INTRINSIC APOPTOTIC PATHWAY

The intrinsic pathway of apoptosis is mediated by diverse apoptotic stimuli, which converge at the mitochondria (Fig. 2) (79). The apoptotic stimuli increase mitochondrial outer membrane permeability, precipitating cell death either through the release of molecules involved in apoptosis, or by loss of mitochondrial energy production that is essential for cell survival. Release of cytochrome *c* from the mitochondria into the cytoplasm initiates a caspase cascade. Cytosolic cytochrome *c* binds to apoptosis protease-activating factor 1 (Apaf-1) and procaspase-9, generating a death-inducing signaling complex known as the apoptosome. Within the apoptosome, caspase-9 is activated, leading to activation of the same effector caspases activated by the death-inducing signaling complex of the extrinsic pathway (49). The intrinsic apoptotic pathway is initiated by diverse stimuli which affect cellular homeostasis, including oxidative stress, growth factor deprivation, ionizing radiation, and toxic agents. Loss of mitochondrial integrity is

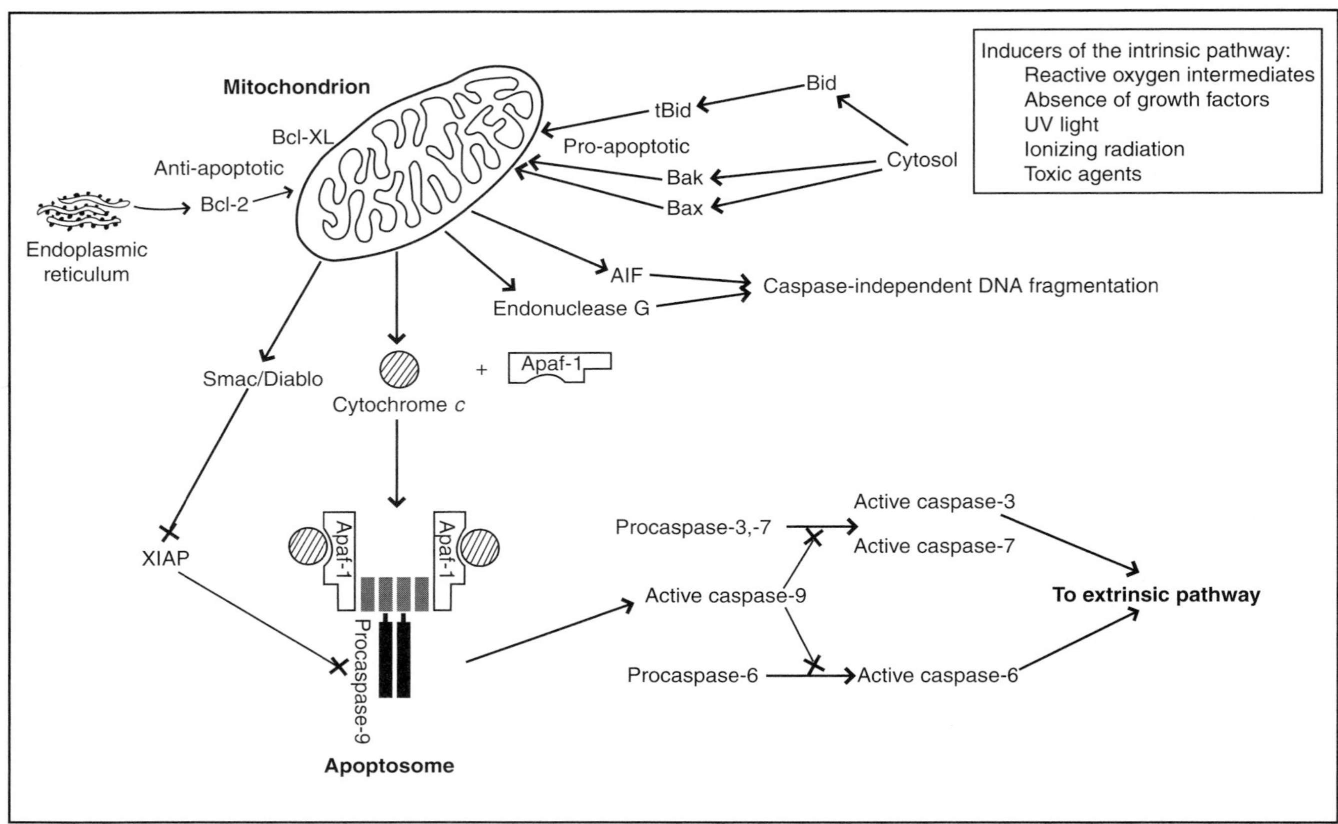

Figure 2 Intrinsic apoptotic pathway. Inducers, including reactive oxygen intermediates and toxic agents, stimulate mediators that destabilize mitochondrial membrane polarization, resulting in release of pro-apoptotic molecules into the cytosol. The pro-apoptotic molecules congregate to form the apoptosome, which activates downstream caspases, resulting in apoptotic cell death, characterized by DNA fragmentation, cell shrinkage, and cell membrane blebbing (see text for definitions of abbreviations).

the key factor involved in the intrinsic apoptotic pathway. The pivotal event is an increase in mitochondrial outer membrane permeability (47,79) triggered by opening of the mitochondrial permeability transition pores (PTPs) located at contact sites between the inner and outer mitochondrial membranes. The main components of mitochondrial PTP include the adenine translocator (ANT) at the inner membrane and the voltage-dependent anion channel (VDAC), also called porin, at the outer membrane. The mitochondrial PTP also includes other proteins such as hexokinase II, mitochondrial creatine kinase, cyclophilin D, and peripheral benzodiazepine receptor, all playing roles in modulating the activity of the PTP (33). Pore opening is influenced by numerous endogenous effectors such as ions (Ca^{2+}, Mg^{2+}, H^{+}), local ADP/ATP concentrations, mitochondrial membrane potential, and changes in composition or functions of the Bcl-2 complex (33). PTP opening induced by pro-apoptotic Bcl proteins, reactive oxygen metabolites, and ions allow passage of molecules up to 1.5 kDa with loss of inner mitochondrial membrane integrity and loss of transmembrane potential required for ATP generation.

PTP opening causes water to enter the mitochondrial matrix which swells, rupturing the outer membrane to release proteins from the mitochondrial intermembranous space. This precipitates cell death through either the release into the cytosol of caspase-activating molecules involved in apoptosis, or the loss of mitochondrial functions, most notably the generation of ATP, essential for cell survival (39). Release of cytochrome *c* from the mitochondrial intermembranous space is the main event that leads to caspase activation. Once in the cytosol, cytochrome *c* binds to an adaptor molecule, Apaf-1, and activates it. In the presence of cytochrome *c* and ATP, the CARD of Apaf-1 binds with the CARD domain of procaspase-9, forming the mitochondrial death-inducing signaling complex, called the apoptosome. The apoptosome activates caspase-9 which then activates the downstream caspases-3, -6, and -7 (67).

Mitochondrial outer membrane permeabilization is strongly regulated by Bcl-2 protein family members, which modulate the permeability of the PTP (1). Members of the Bcl-2 family proteins are located on or translocated to the outer mitochondrial membrane from the cytosol. They can be divided into at least three groups (49). They all contain at least one of four relatively conserved Bcl-2-homology (BH) domains: B, BH2, BH3, and/or BH4. Two groups are pro-apoptotic and induce cell death. One group has multiple BH domains (multi-BH domain proteins); the other contains only BH3 domains (BH3-only domains). The multi-BH domain group members include Bax, Bak, and Bok. These proteins are normally located in the cytosol and translocate to the outer mitochondrial membrane in response to apoptotic signaling. Upon activation in the cytosol, the multi-BH domain proteins change conformation, translocate, insert into the mitochondrial outer membrane, oligomerize, and form openings in the membrane independent of the PTP. The BH3-only members, which include Bid, Bad and Bim, are also found in the cytoplasm and undergo activation by modifications such as cleavage or dephosphorylation, before translocating to the outer mitochondrial membrane. Active BH3-only members may activate multi-BH domain members, such as Bax and Bak, leading to the oligomerization of the multi-domain members, and the formation of openings in the outer membrane sufficient for PTP-independent release of pro-apoptotic proteins from the intermembranous mitochondrial space (39,83). The different family members of the multi-BH domain and BH3-only domain groups can undergo homotypic or heterotypic aggregation, and the relative ratios of the pro-apoptotic proteins and anti-apoptotic proteins determine the susceptibility of cells to death from the intrinsic apoptotic pathway. Other regulators of this process include VDAC binding to Bak that prevents its allosteric conformational activation, reducing susceptibility to apoptotic death (16).

The third group of Bcl-2 family proteins is anti-apoptotic. Its members include Bcl-2, Bcl-3, Bcl-XL, Bcl-w, A1 and Mcl-1, all of which promote cell survival. The two best characterized members, Bcl-2 and Bcl-XL, contain all four BH domains. Bcl-2 is found in the endoplasmic reticulum (ER) and nuclear membranes; it translocates to the outer mitochondrial membrane in response to apoptotic signals. Bcl-XL is only present in the outer mitochondrial membrane. The anti-apoptotic members antagonize the actions of the multi-BH domain and BH3-only domain pro-apoptotic proteins. Because of the anti-apoptotic group members are present in the outer mitochondrial membrane, they can interact with pro-apoptotic proteins to prevent their aggregation. Anti-apoptotic Bcl-2 family proteins inhibit multi-BH proteins by sequestering them; BH3-only proteins can act indirectly to promote apoptosis by releasing multi-BH proteins from their anti-apoptotic captors. One example of this is the induced failure of Bcl-2 and Bcl-XL to prevent pro-apoptotic oligomerization of multi-BH Bax. Another mechanism involves BH3-only member, Bad, which is dephosphorylated in the absence of survival factors and binds and antagonizes Bcl-2 or Bcl-XL on the outer mitochondrial membrane, promoting apoptosis. In the presence of survival factors, however, Bad is phosphorylated and remains in the cytoplasm. Moreover, phosphorylation of Bad, even after translocation to the outer mitochondrial membrane, results in its dissociation from Bcl-2 and Bcl-XL, promoting survival.

Bcl-2 family proteins also appear to have the capacity to release cytochrome *c* by increasing inner and/or outer mitochondrial membranes permeability by a combination of the PTP-dependent and the PTP-independent mechanisms (78). The activated BH3-only proteins in conjunction with oligomerized multi-BH domain proteins themselves induce PTP-independent permeability of the outer mitochondrial membrane causing the release of intermembranous cytochrome *c*, which constitutes 15% of the total amount of the mitochondrial enzyme. Then, by a PTP-dependent mechanism involving cyclophilin D, the mitochondria release the other 85% of mitochondrial cytochrome *c* from the cristae. PTP formation is inhibited by cyclosporin A that targets cyclophilin D, bonkrekic acid that target ANT, and bcl-2 and bcl-XL.

Bcl-2 family proteins also appear to control the release of other pro-apoptotic proteins upon increasing the permeability of the mitochondrial outer membrane. These proteins include certain caspases-2, -3, and -9, apoptosis inducing factor (AIF), Smac/direct IAP-binding protein, Omi/HtrA2, and endonuclease G (28,74,106,116). Smac can interact with inhibitors of IAPs, such as XIAP, to prevent their activity (28). The caspase coactivator Smac/Diablo is released along with cytochrome *c* during apoptosis to neutralize the inhibitory action of IAPs and promote cytochrome *c*-dependent caspase activation. Smac/Diablo also plays an important protective role in death receptor-mediated apoptosis (21). Omi/HtrA2 is a serine protease that contributes to caspase-dependent and caspase-independent cell death and that interacts with IAPs (113). Endonuclease G is released from the mitochondria into the cytosol where it translocates to the nucleus during apoptosis and induces caspase-independent DNA fragmentation (65). The effect of AIF is caspase independent. Once released into the cytosol, AIF translocates to the nucleus in response to death-promoting stimuli, including bacterial products, ultraviolet radiation, chemical toxins, reactive oxygen metabolites, and p53 (49). In the nucleus, AIF induces peripheral chromatin condensation and DNA fragmentation. AIF in association with a heat-labile cytosolic factor may also make mitochondrial membranes permeable (107).

A molecular link between the extrinsic death receptor pathways and the mitochondrial apoptosis pathway is present at the level of caspases-3 and -8, both of which cleave cytosolic Bid, a member of the BH3 domain-only subgroup of Bcl-2 family (70). Cleaved Bid, also known as tBid then translocates from the cytosol to the mitochondrial outer membrane, opening the PTP to induce cytochrome *c* release, amplifying apoptosis through the mitochondrial pathway (70).

During apoptosis, elongated and branching mitochondria fragment to yield smaller, rounder, and more numerous mitochondria (123). This process requires the integral outer mitochondrial membrane protein, fission 1 (FIS1), which recruits dynanim-related protein 1 (DRP1) from the cytosol (63,123). FIS1/DRP1 then concentrates at foci on the outer mitochondrial membrane at sites where mitochondrial fission is initiated. Inhibition of FIS1 or DRP1 prevents mitochondrial fragmentation and impairs apoptosis (34). Counteracting the tendency of FIS1 and DRP1 to mediate mitochondrial fission are mitochondrial fusion proteins that also belong to the dynamin-family, namely the encoded protein product that causes optic atrophy type 1 (OPA1) (see Chapter 35), mitofusin 1 (MFN1), and mitofusin 2 (MFN2) (14). These fusion proteins inhibit mitochondrial fission and cell death, indicating their importance in apoptosis. OPA1 is a large GTPase located in the mitochondrial intermembranous space. Loss-of-function OPA1 mutations result in mitochondrial fragmentation, release of cytochrome *c*, and apoptosis (86). Mutated OPA1 also results in hereditary dominant optic atrophy via retinal ganglion cell death (2,20). OPA1 GTPase activity is required for MFN1 and MFN2 function (47). These proteins form homotypic and heterotypic complexes that promote mitochondrial fusion by docking and fusing the outer membranes of adjacent mitochondria to one another, promoting the elongated and branching mitochondrial forms normally present in healthy cells (14,56). Overexpression of MFN1 and MFN2 has also been shown to inhibit apoptosis, presumably by stabilizing mitochondrial membranes (105).

Mitochondrial fragmentation is initiated when Bax translocates from the cytosol to the outer mitochondrial membrane and complexes with Bak which is normally distributed on the membrane (34,53). These complexes then associate with DRP1 at sites where mitochondrial fission is initiated (52,82). Inhibition of DRP1 inhibits mitochondrial fragmentation and cytochrome *c* release that normally occurs within 15 minutes of Bax translocation (34,53). Thus, Bax and Bak are important for mitochondrial fission as well as their established roles in mitochondrial pore formation and cytochrome *c* release of the intrinsic apoptotic pathway. Upon exposure to BH3-only, Bcl-2 family members, Bid and Bik, mitochondrial cristae undergo widening that is associated with cytochrome *c* release (36). Cristal widening is exacerbated by loss of OPA1 expression and reduced by DRP1 inhibition (87,123). Initiators of mitochondrial fragmentation and apoptosis include ischemia and release of Ca^{2+} into the cytosol during ER stress response, both of which are known initiators of the intrinsic apoptotic pathway (123). Taken together, these findings suggest that mitochondrial fission and fusion are likely to be related to cytochrome *c* release by dynamic remodeling of mitochondrial membranes.

CONVERGENCE OF APOPTOTIC PATHWAYS

The two pathways of apoptosis, extrinsic/death receptor and intrinsic/mitochondrial, converge on caspase-3 and subsequently on other proteases and nucleases that drive the terminal events of programmed cell death.

The cellular targets of these enzymes are diverse, including protein kinases, structural proteins, DNA repair proteins, cell cycle proteins, and nuclear DNA. The last steps of apoptosis include packaging of fragmented cell contents into apoptotic cell bodies which then undergo phagocytosis (49,101). The recognition of apoptotic cells by neighboring cells or macrophages has been studied intensively. Apoptotic cells display signals to induce phagocytosis. One of these is exposure of phosphatidylserine (PtdSer) on the cell surface. PtdSer is normally present on the cytoplasmic side of the cell membrane, but is externalized on the cell membrane during apoptosis. This event triggers phagocytosis by scavenger cells (98). Another phagocytosis-inducing signal is a lipid attractant that is released by apoptotic cells through caspase-mediated cleavage of calcium-independent phospholipase A_2 (61).

Apoptosis is tightly controlled by a complex regulatory network. Pro-survival signals enhance the expression and/or activity of anti-apoptotic regulatory molecules thereby keeping in check the activation of pro-apoptotic factors. A set of various anti-apoptotic molecules and mechanisms has been identified, such as NFκB, AKT, Bcl-2, and the IAP family of proteins. Every step in the apoptotic cascade is monitored and controlled by certain pro-survival signals (117). Pro-apoptotic factors can counteract those inhibitory molecules when apoptotic demise is initiated.

THE FINAL APOPTOTIC PATHWAY: CASPASES

Caspases (cysteine-*asp*artic acid-prote*ases*) are a family of cysteine proteases that cleave proteins after aspartic acid that are the effectors of the apoptotic pathways. They are involved in the regulation and execution of cell death in each of the described pathways. Apoptotic signaling mainly converges on the activation of intracellular caspases, a family of cysteine-dependent, aspartate-directed proteases which propagate death signaling by cleaving key cellular proteins (84). Caspases are synthesized as inactive proenzymes containing prodomains followed by p20 (large) and p10 (small) subunits. They are rapidly activated after the induction of apoptosis by autoproteolytic cleavage or cleavage by other caspases. All caspases cleave their substrates at aspartic acid bonds with other amino acids (110).

Based on their function, the caspases can be classified into three groups (8). The first group consists of inflammatory caspases, including caspases-1, -4, -5, -12, -13, and -14. The second group contains apoptosis-initiating caspases possessing long domains with either death effector domains (caspases-8 and -10) or CARD (caspases-2 and -9). These domains interact with upstream cytoplasmic adaptor molecules of extrinsic receptor pathway death-inducing signaling complexes or of intrinsic pathway apoptosome complex initiated by mitochondrial outer membrane permeablization. The third group includes apoptosis effector caspases-3, -6, and -7. They are characterized by the presence of short prodomains, and typically processed and activated by upstream caspases. Once they are activated, they perform the downstream execution steps of apoptosis by cleaving multiple cellular substrates (8).

Apoptosis-initiating and -effector caspases are activated by different mechanisms. The apoptosis-initiating caspases are autoproteolytically activated when bought into close proximity of each other, a phenomenon designated as the induced proximity activation (4). This type of activation appears to involve dimerization model. In the intrinsic pathway, caspase-9 homodimerization is promoted by mitochondrial cytochrome *c* release-induced apoptosome formation which binds the caspase and increases its local concentration. Similarly, in the extrinsic pathway, the death-inducing signaling complex induces dimerization and subsequent autoactivation of caspase-8 (8,24). The activated conformation of the initiating caspases is also stabilized in the complexes of the intrinsic and extrinsic pathways. Initiating caspases-8 and -10 each contain death effector domains in their long prodomains; they interact with the extrinsic and intrinsic pathway adaptor proteins and their complexes. Regions with affinity for the CARD on adaptor molecules, including Apaf-1, are found on caspases-2 and -9 (110). These regions are an important link in the extrinsic and intrinsic apoptotic pathways, binding to adaptor molecules and activating effector caspases.

Effector procaspases, cleaved and activated by initiating caspases, in turn cleave and activate various death substrates to induce cell death. Most procaspases are activated by proteolytic cleavage at two sites. All these cleavage sites are located at aspartate bonds with other amino acids, making autocatalytic activation possible (111). This autocatalytic cascade mode of activation is prominent for the three downstream effector caspases, caspases-3, -6, and -7 (103). These caspases are usually more abundant and active than the upstream initiator caspases like caspases-8 and -9. Caspase-3 is recognized as the critical executioner caspase. The remaining executioner caspases seem to play redundant roles in most apoptotic pathways.

Effector caspases act on a variety of substrates resulting in proteolysis of cellular proteins and death by apoptosis. One key target of caspase proteolysis is poly-(ADP-ribose) polymerase (PARP), a nuclear protein required for DNA repair (31). PARP is activated by DNA breaks and catalyzes the attachment of ADP-ribose polymers to multiple nuclear factors, facilitating repair. When activated, this DNA repair process consumes large amounts of NAD^+, thereby indirectly depleting the cellular ATP stores. Profound loss of cellular ATP results in the induction of necrosis, while caspase-mediated inactivation of PARP is associated with retention of relatively higher levels of cellular ATP and death by apoptosis. DNA repair proteins, such as DNA-dependent protein kinase, Rad51, and ATM, are additional targets of the effector caspases during apoptosis (44). Other targets of effector caspases are nuclear lamins, the cleavage of which results in nuclear shrinkage; cytoskeletal proteins like fodrin and gelsolin, the cleavage of which disrupts the actin filament network, contributing to loss of cell shape and detachment from the extracellular matrix during apoptosis; cleavage of intermediate proteins (keratin 18, keratin 19, vimentin) and adherence proteins of junctional complexes (β-catenin and plakoglobin γ-catenin), which result in the disruption of cell–cell interactions (58). Also targeted are cell cycle regulators, including retinoblastoma susceptibility protein, and cell cycle inhibitors, such as Cdc27, Wee1, p21, and p27 (64).

The proteolytic activity of caspases is a major regulator of caspase activity. Apoptosis is generally not dependent on protein synthesis, but modulation of the expression of the various genes that encode caspases can affect the sensitivity of cells to apoptosis. Deregulation of E2F by adenovirus E1A or RB1 gene loss may lead to the accumulation of procaspases through a direct transcriptional mechanism (81). The increased concentration of caspases promotes apoptosis in the presence of p53-generated signals that trigger caspase activation (71,81). p53 itself can target transcription of caspases-6 and -10, enhancing the propensity for apoptosis (71,96). Post-translational modifications of caspases and their proenzyme forms, such as nitrosylation, oxidation, ubiquination, and phosphorylation (see Chapter 36), also appear to play roles in regulating caspase activity.

Inhibitors of Apoptosis

IAPs are key negative regulators of caspase activation. They were originally found in baculoviruses and mammalian cells retain one to three baculoviral IAP repeats (BIR). Several IAPs have been identified and include: XIAP, c-IAP1, c-IAP2, BIR-containing ubiquitin-conjugating enzyme, neuronal apoptosis inhibitory protein, livin, and survivin. IAPs inhibit apoptosis by binding and inhibiting certain caspases (62). For example, XIAP, c-IAP1, and c-IAP2 bind to caspases-3, -7, and -9. Regions closely related to the third BIR domain (BIR3) specifically inhibit caspase-9, while the linker region close to BIR2 targets caspases-3 and -7 (13,108). Most IAPs bind and directly suppress caspase catalytic activity, but some inhibit apoptosis by direct caspase cleavage. For example, XIAP, the most powerful caspase inhibitor (23), has ubiquitin-protein ligase activity that promotes proteosomal degradation of caspase-3. The activity of IAPs is finely regulated during apoptosis. XIAP and c-IAP1 may be themselves inactivated by specific cleavage by effector caspases to ensure the induction of apoptosis. The Smac and Omni/Htra2 are released from the mitochondria upon apoptotic stimuli (28). They promote caspase activation by inhibition of IAPs (28). Although Smac is a target for the ubiquitin-protein ligase activity of XIAP, Smac/Diablo promotes apoptosis by antagonizing this ubiquitin-protein ligase activity as well as other IAP–caspase interactions. Tumor-upregulated CARD-containing antagonist inhibits caspase-9 activation induced by the Apaf-1 that is formed following cytochrome *c* release from the mitochondria (88). Heat shock proteins (Hsp) (see Chapter 36), synthesized in response to stress, facilitate cell survival by inhibiting apoptosis. Hsp27 can protect mitochondria during apoptosis by inhibiting the activity of pro-apoptotic Bcl-2 family proteins or they can disrupt apoptosome formation (7).

ENDOPLASMIC RETICULUM AND APOPTOSIS

Endoplasmic reticulum (see Chapter 1) is the second cellular compartment participating in the intrinsic apoptotic pathway (49,116). In the ER, control mechanisms ensure that only properly folded proteins are passed along the secretory pathway. Stress factors including oxidative stress, toxins, Ca^{2+} ionophores, and inhibitors of glycosylation can all cause protein misfolding. This leads to a protective unfolded protein response that is characterized by a compensatory reduction in protein synthesis, induction of proteins that assist other proteins in achieving proper folding (chaperones) in the ER and catalysts, and degradation of the abnormal proteins. Persistent or severe stresses affect Ca^{2+} homeostasis. Ca^{2+} released from the ER lumen into the cytosol may initiate apoptosis by either of two mechanisms (9). First, released Ca^{2+} may directly promote the opening of the mitochondrial PTP. Second, released Ca^{2+} may directly activate caspase-12 on the surface of ER membrane (9). This mechanism probably involves both a calpain-dependent removal of the caspase-12 prodomain and autocatalytic activation. Once activated, caspase-12 may cleave procaspase-9 which then activates caspase-3. When efflux of Ca^{2+} from the ER is associated with mitochondrial PTP opening, outer membrane permeabilization, and cytochrome *c* release, Ca^{2+} enters the mitochondria. This establishes an apoptosis-promoting amplification loop between the dysfunctional mitochondria and ER. Small amounts of cytochrome *c* released from the mitochondria diffuse into the adjacent ER and bind to $InsP_3$ receptors, thereby enhancing Ca^{2+} release from the ER. The increasing concentrations of Ca^{2+} released into the cytosol affect increasing numbers of mitochondria causing a cascade of massive cytochrome *c* loss from the mitochondria and apoptotic cell death.

Bcl-2 protein members appear to regulate ER involvement in apoptosis. Bcl-2 interrupts the apoptosis-promoting amplification loop between the ER and mitochondria. Bax and Bak, localized on the cytoplasmic surface membrane of ER, may be necessary to promote ER stress-induced apoptosis (49,100,116). These pro-apoptotic molecules promote Ca^{2+} efflux from the ER while acting on the mitochondrial outer membrane to permeabilize it, enhancing the apoptotic amplification loop between the ER and mitochondria. Bax and Bak also function by directly activating caspase-12 on the ER surface.

REGULATORY MECHANISMS

There are four main pathways that regulate apoptosis: Myc, NFκB, JNK, and AKT pathways.

Myc Pathway

Myc family members, including, c-Myc, N-Myc, and L-Myc, are important to cell proliferation (see

Chapter 53) and death (38,51). These functions rely on coordinated effects of the family members on many genes (89). Activation or overexpression of Myc can promote apoptosis by sensitizing cells to other pro-apoptotic stimuli (51). A prominent pro-apoptotic function of c-Myc is its stimulation of Fas receptor and ligand expression and suppression of FLIP expression, sensitizing cells to death receptor-induced apoptosis of the extrinsic pathway. Myc also enhances the intrinsic pathway mainly by suppressing Bcl-2 and Bcl-XL and inducing Bax. However, c-Myc also stimulates the formation of reactive oxygen metabolites that promote apoptosis via the intrinsic pathway. Myc-induced apoptosis is modulated by p53 in complex interactions (124). Myc activates p53 by transcriptionally upregulating ARF; ARF protein then inhibits mouse double-minute 2 homolog (MDM2), which would otherwise downregulate p53 transcription and degrade p53. The net effect is to promote p53 pro-apoptotic activity. ARF also is extremely effective at blocking transcriptional activity promoted, but not antagonized by c-Myc, enhancing the pro-apoptotic functions of c-Myc. ARF thus regulates a balance between c-Myc-induced proliferation and apoptosis. This ARF mechanism appears to be independent of p53. p53 functions as a transcription factor regulating downstream genes important in cell cycle arrest, DNA repair, and apoptosis (38). Once DNA damage occurs, p53 arrests the cell at a checkpoint in its cycle until DNA repair is effected. However, if the damage is too severe or irreversible, apoptosis is triggered. The events by which p53 promotes apoptosis under these conditions is not yet evident.

NFκB Pathway

NFκB is a nuclear transcription factor that is activated by growth factors, cytokines, inflammatory mediators, radiation, and toxins. It is present in its inactive form within the cytoplasm where it is bound to IκB inhibitor proteins. Stimuli that phosphorylate IκB cause NFκB to be released and activated by degradation that exposes nuclear homing signals on NFκB subunits. It then translocates to the nucleus and regulates expression of genes involved in the regulation of apoptosis, viral replication, tumorigenesis, inflammation, and autoimmune diseases (38,73). NFκB has several family members including Rel A (p65), Rel B, c-Rel, p50 (NFκB1), and p52 (NFκB2). NFκB has both pro-apoptotic and anti-apoptotic functions depending on the stimuli and cell context (59,90). Under physiologic conditions, NFκB behaves as an anti-apoptotic mediator by activating factors, including IAP, XIAP, Bcl-XL, FLIP, and TNF receptor-associated factor. When it is activated by cytokine withdrawal, chemotherapeutic agents, ischemia, p53, and viral proteins, it behaves as a pro-apoptotic mediator by activating interferon-regulated factor-1, c-Myc, p53, and caspase-1. NFκB also represses DNA transcription when it is induced by DNA damaging chemotherapeutic agents.

JNK Pathway

c-Jun N-terminal protein kinase/stress-activated protein kinase (SAPK), a member of the mitogen-activated protein kinase (MAPK) superfamily, is activated by phosphorylation through a MAP kinase module, MAPK3–MAPK2–MAPK. JNK is downregulated by NFκB and is the main regulator of c-Jun activity, a transcription factor. JNK signaling pathway has both anti- and pro-apoptotic functions depending on cell type, nature of stimulus, duration of activation, and activity of other signaling pathways, mainly NFκB and p53 (38). In neurons, JNK plays a pro-apoptotic role by inactivating Bcl-2 and Bcl-XL, and activating the BH3-only protein BIM (5,6,22). It also induces expression of p53 and FAS/FASL molecules (38). In T cells, JNKK1 is an anti-apoptotic mediator that inhibits the phosphorylation of BAD, a pro-apoptotic Bcl-2 family protein. Recently, it was shown that the JNK pathway is required for TNF-induced apoptosis (22). TNF activates the JNK pathway through Mkk7 by inducing the cleavage of Bid to j-Bid. j-Bid translocates to the mitochondria and causes the release of Smac, leading to apoptosis. Activation of the JNK pathway also inhibits p53-induced cell cycle arrest, promoting apoptosis.

AKT Pathway

The AKT pathway is an anti-apoptotic signaling pathway that is activated under different circumstances such as withdrawal of extracellular signaling factors, oxidative and osmotic stress, radiation, chemotherapeutic drugs, and ischemia (26). Activation of cell surface receptor protein tyrosine kinase leads to the production of second messengers such as phoshatidylinositol 4,5-biphosphate 3 and phosphodylinositol 3,4,5-triphosphate in the cytoplasm. Phosphatidylinositol 4,5-biphosphate 3 signals activate kinase 3-phosphoinositide-dependent protein kinase-1 and 2 that activate AKT. AKT activation promotes phosphorylation of certain proteins that induce cell survival mechanisms (27). Phosphorylation of IκB by AKT leads to activation of NFκB and hence, cell survival. Similarly, phosphorylation of Bad by AKT inhibits its pro-apoptotic function (18). The other proteins inactivated by the anti-apoptotic AKT pathway by phosphorylation are caspase-9 and the Forkhead family of transcription factors, which induce expression of pro-apoptotic FasL and Bim (10,12,49).

REMOVAL OF APOPTOTIC CELLS

Elimination of apoptotic cells before loss of cell membrane integrity is very important to prevent cytotoxic effects on surrounding cells and antigenic immune responses to autoantigens (Fig. 3). The most common and well-known alteration on the surfaces of apoptotic cells are the loss of phospholipid asymmetry in the plasma membrane and the translocation of PtdSer from the inner layer to outer layer. PtdSer and annexin I form discrete patches on the surface of plasma membrane which function as phagocytic signals for recognition and uptake (32). Accessory serum-derived molecules form extracellular bridges to increase the numbers of receptors engaged in the recognition and engulfment of the apoptotic cells. These molecules include: milk-fat-globule-EGF-factor 8 (MFG-E8), β2 glycoprotein I, serum protein S, and growth arrest-specific 6 (Gas6). Similar additional molecules, such as mannose-binding lectin and C1q, facilitate receptor-mediated apoptotic cell removal by binding to altered sugar molecules on the surface of apoptotic cells.

MFG-E8, a protein secreted by mononuclear phagocytes, binds to apoptotic cells and stimulates their phagocytosis, in part by initiating the cytoskeletal rearrangements required for phagocytosis (32). The MFG-E8 bridge between the phagocyte and the apoptotic cell simultaneously inhibits mononuclear phagocyte activation and prevents the initiation of autoimmune responses against apoptotic cell antigens.

A variety of receptors on the surfaces of phagocytes are responsible for the binding and phagocytosis of apoptotic cells. Scavenger receptors, including CD36, CD68, and lectin-like oxidized low-density lipoprotein receptor-1, recognize PtdSer. $\alpha_V\beta3$ integrin, the vitronectin receptor, can bind to MFG-E8 that forms bridges to PtdSer. A tyrosine kinase known as MER binds to Gas6 that also forms bridges to PtdSer. CD91 binds indirectly mannose-binding lectin and C1q. The lipopolysaccharide receptor, CD14, binds to intercellular adhesion molecule-3 and PtdSer receptors. All these receptor interactions require close proximity of the phagocytes and apoptotic cells. Assisting in achieving the required approximation are chemoattractants for mononuclear phagocytes that are secreted by apoptotic cells.

APOPTOSIS IN DISEASE

Apoptosis is involved in the pathophysiology of many ophthalmic diseases, including autoimmune, neoplastic, and degenerative processes. The roles and mechanisms of apoptosis in these disorders are complex, but emerging themes have developed.

Apoptosis is a prominent outcome of immune and inflammatory effector pathways (72). Apoptosis provides antigens that are processed to promote

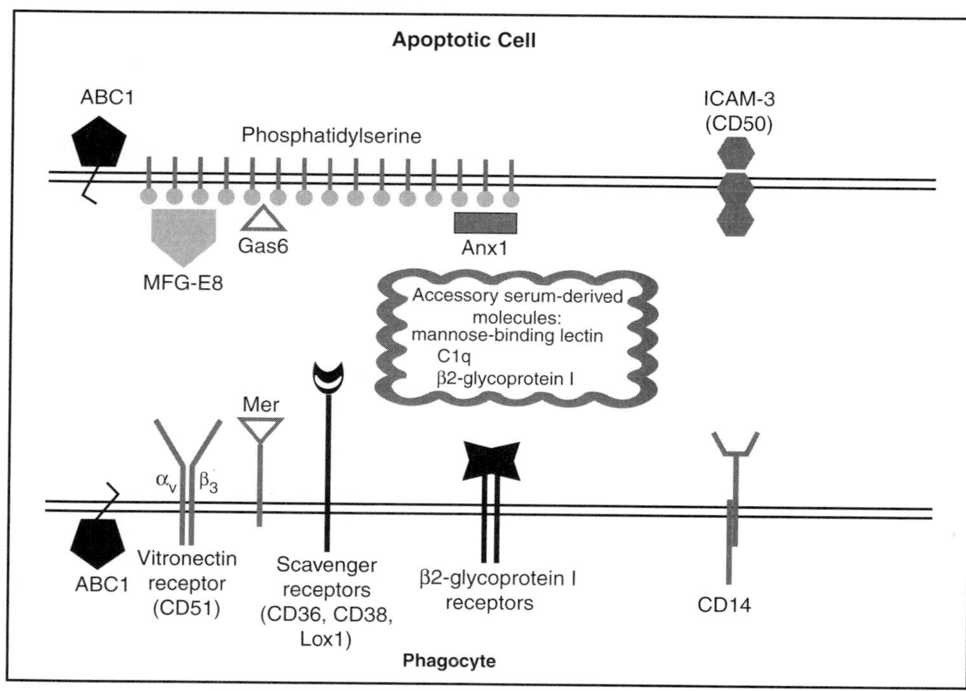

Figure 3 Elimination of apoptotic cells by phagocytes. Molecules expressed on the cell surfaces of apoptotic cells are bound by specific receptors on phagocytes, a process that may be facilitated by accessory serum-derived molecules (see text for definitions of abbreviations).

tolerance, thereby limiting immune responses to potential autoantigens. It is also required for the selection or elimination of lymphocyte subsets required for the development and fine tuning of immune responses. Impaired apoptotic mechanisms may result in autoimmunity to antigens that are usually tolerated (see Chapter 3). Thus, autoimmune disease with the production of self-reactive antibodies may occur when lymphocytes normally destined for elimination fail to express apoptotic surface receptors such as MFG-E8 (49,97). In this circumstance and other contexts, autoimmunity appears to result, at least in part, from the impaired clearance of apoptotic cells because the uncleared cells undergo secondary necrosis. The necrotic cellular debris, in contrast to inducing tolerance, instead stimulates immune reactivity. Dysregulation of Fas- or TRAIL-mediated apoptosis of lymphocytes may also contribute to autoimmunity by permitting the accumulation of lymphocytes which cause enhanced cellular and humoral immune responses to self-antigens and impaired apoptosis of T lymphocytes (102,104). In Sjögren syndrome, for example, several types of autoantibodies contribute to the development of the disease (see Chapter 6) (19). Reduced apoptosis and aberrant maturation of B lymphocytes may result in autoreactive and hyperreactive B lymphocytes. This dysregulation may not only result in autoimmunity to glandular tissue, but also result in the development of lymphoma that occurs in 5% of the patients with Sjögren syndrome.

In neoplasia, inactivating or downregulating mutations in pro-apoptotic genes and overexpression or upregulation of anti-apoptotic genes appear to result in insufficient apoptosis, and favor proliferation and accumulation of tumor cells. One of the important alterations is overexpression of genes responsible for anti-apoptotic pathway mediators including Bcl-2 family members, IAPs, and AKT and NFκB pathway members (49). For example, in follicular B-cell lymphoma, chromosomal translocation t(14;18) results in immunoglobulin heavy chain locus linkage to the Bcl-2 gene, causing enhanced Bcl-2 expression (see Chapter 66) (11). The AKT pathway, a pro-survival pathway, is overexpressed by a loss-of-function mutation in the *PTEN* tumor suppressor gene or gain-of-function mutation of oncogenes Ras and BCR-ABL (25,80). The downregulation of pro-apoptotic pathways, especially the p53 pathway, facilitates tumorigenesis. p53 regulates the transcription of several genes in cell cycle arrest (p21, Gadd45) or induction of apoptosis (Bax, Apaf-1, caspase-9, Fas, DR5, p53-inducible gene, Noxa). The p53 mutations play roles in more than 50% of human cancers. One example is the Li-Fraumeni syndrome in which mutations inactivating p53 function predisposes to the risks of breast cancer and soft tissue sarcomas, including rhabdomyosarcoma. These mechanisms subserve many type of neoplasia (see Chapter 53). Overexpression of Bcl-2 and inactivating mutations of p53 enhance the formation of basal and squamous cell carcinomas of the skin (see Chapter 56) (112). IAPs also enhance tumorigenesis. One IAP, surviving, is often overexpressed in tumors in which it inhibits apoptosis at the G_2/M checkpoint, contributing to aberrant mitotic activity (22). In mucosal-associated lymphoid tumors, the lymphomas demonstrate translocations of the c-IAP2 gene (41). Apoptotic mechanisms also are important to chemotherapy, sensitivity and resistance. Reduction or loss of Fas from cell surfaces and overexpression of Bcl-2 and Bcl-XL causes resistance to drugs such as dexamethasone, etiposide, vincristine, doxorubicin, and actinomycin D (66,75).

Apoptotic mechanisms have been shown to participate in degenerative diseases, including those involving the central nervous system, retina, and cornea (Fuchs dystrophy and keratoconus) (see Chapter 32). Alterations in the expression of extrinsic pathway death receptors by neuronal cells suggest involvement of this mechanism in Alzheimer disease, Huntington disease, Parkinson disease and motor neuron disease (see Chapter 70) (43,91,115). Involved in these neurodegenerative diseases are Fas–FasL and TNFα–TNFR interactions as well as ER stress-mediated apoptosis due to the presence of abnormal, misfolded proteins (49). In the retina, neuronal cell death appears to be controlled by complex interactions among numerous stimuli including extracellular mediators, intracellular pathways, and downstream executioner pathways (45,68). In addition to classical extrinsic death pathway interactions, such as Fas–FasL induction of photoreceptor apoptosis in retinal detachment, extrinsic release of neurotransmitters (e.g., glutamate and dopamine), neuropeptides [e.g., pituitary adenylate cyclase-activating peptide (PACAP) and vasoactive intestinal peptide (VIP)], and growth factors [e.g., brain-derived neurotrophic factor (BDNF) and pigment epithelium-derived growth factor (PEDF)] appear to modulate neuronal susceptibility to apoptosis. Intracellular mediators of retinal neuronal cell apoptosis include the intrinsic apoptotic pathway which is subject to mediators such as Ca^{2+}, reactive oxygen metabolites, and other stress metabolites classically involved in this pathway, as well as mediators that are of particular relevance to the retinal stress, including cyclic AMP-protein kinase A, nitric oxide, and ultraviolet light. A recently described gene product, OPA1, has been implicated in dominant optic atrophy (2,20,123). Loss of OPA1 expression causes mitochondrial fission and fragmentation that is an early hallmark of apoptosis induced via the intrinsic pathway.

Apoptotic mechanisms are also key to normal reparative responses, such as inflammation and wound healing (94). Neutrophils, the first of the leukocytes to arrive at sites of inflammation, perform their tasks, undergo rapid apoptosis that is enhanced by TNFα and β2 integrins (CD11b/CD18), and are efficiently eliminated by mononuclear phagocytes (85,120). Mononuclear phagocytes subsequently arrive and then undergo apoptosis, by mechanisms which appear to involve transforming growth factor (TGF) β1 (3). p53 also is involved in leukocyte apoptosis while controlling the proliferation of fibroblasts and other connective tissue cells involved in fibrovascular proliferative responses (3,94). Early in the fibrovascular response, growth factors, particularly vascular endothelial growth factor, promote vascular endothelial proliferation and impairs apoptosis of this cell type. This is followed by a scripted process of vascular endothelial cell and myofibroblast apoptosis (15). Fibroblast proliferation is promoted by insulin-like growth factor-1 and TGFβ1 and TGFβ2 that block apoptosis pathways in the fibroblasts (94). Ultimately, however, fibroblast proliferation is downregulated by regulatory mechanisms, including c-myc which potentiates fibroblast apoptosis that is initiated by Fas/FasL interactions of the extrinsic apoptotic pathway (40,46). With reduced growth factor expression, fibroblast and vascular endothelial cell apoptosis is favored and wound healing becomes quiescent (17). Aberrant apoptosis during inflammation and wound healing is likely to be an important component of tissue alterations in important ocular diseases such as keratitis sicca, autoimmune conjunctival scarring, corneal allograft rejection, diabetic retinal neovascularization, age-related macular degeneration, and proliferative vitreoretinopathy.

REFERENCES

1. Adams JM, Cory S. The Bcl-2 protein family: arbiters of cell survival. Science 1998; 281:1322–6.
2. Alexander C, Votruba M, Pesche UE, et al. OPA1, encoding a dynamin-related GTPase, is mutated in autosomal dominant optic atrophy linked to chromosome 3q28. Nat Genet 2000; 26:211–5.
3. Antoniades HN, Galanopoulous T, Neville-Golden J, et al. P53 expression during normal tissue regeneration in response to acute cutaneous injury in sweine. J Clin Invest 1994; 93:2206–14.
4. Ashkenazi A, Dixit VM. Death receptors: signaling and modulation. Science 1998; 281:1305–8.
5. Basu A, Haldar S. Identification of a novel Bcl-XL phosphorylation site regulating the sensitivity of taxol- or 2-methoxyestradiol-induced apoptosis. FEBS Lett 2003; 538:41–7.
6. Becker EB, Howell J, Kodama Y, et al. Characterization of the c-Jun N-terminal kinase-bimel signaling pathway in neuronal apoptosis. J Neurosci 2004; 24:8762–70.
7. Beere HM, Wolf BB, Cain K, et al. Heat shock protein 70 inhibits apoptosis by preventing recruitment of procaspase-9 to the Apaf-1 apoptosome. Nat Cell Biol 2000; 2: 469–75.
8. Boatright KM, Renatus M, Scott FL, et al. A unified model for apical caspase activation. Mol Cell 2003:11:529–41.
9. Breckendridge DG, Germain M, Mathai JP, et al. Regulation of apoptosis by endoplasmic reticulum pathways. Oncogene 2003; 22:8608–18.
10. Brunet A, Bonni A, Zigmond MJ, et al. Akt promotes cell survival by phosphorylating and inhibiting a Forkhead transcription factor. Cell 1999; 96:857–68.
11. Cantley LC, Neel BG. New insights into tumor suppression; PTEN suppresses tumor formation by restraining the phosphoinositide 3-kinase/AKT pathway. Proc Natl Acad Sci U S A 1999; 96:4240–5.
12. Cardone MH, Roy N, Stennicke HR, et al. Regulation of cell death protease caspase-9 by phosphorylation. Science 1998; 282:1318–21.
13. Chai J, Shiozaki E, Srinivasula SM, et al. Structural basis of caspase-7 inhibition by XIAP. Cell 2001; 104:769–80.
14. Chen H, Detmer SA, Ewald AJ, et al. Mitofusins MFN1 and MFN2 coordinately regulate mitochondrial fusion and are essential for embryonic development. J Cell Biol 2003; 160:189–200.
15. Compton CC, Gill JM, Bradford DA, et al. Skin regenerated from cultured epithelial autografts on full-thickness burn wounds from 6 days to 5 years after grafting. A light, electron microscope and immunohistochemical study. Lab Invest 1989; 60:600–12.
16. Danial NN, Korsmeyer SJ. Cell death: critical control points. Cell 2004; 116:205–19.
17. Darby IA, Bisucci T, Pittet B, et al. Skin flap-induced regression of granulation tissue correlates with reduced growth factor and increased metalloproteinase expression. J Pathol 2002; 197:117–27.
18. Datta SR, Dudek H, Tao X, et al. AKT phosphorylation of bad couples survival signals to the cell-intrinsic death machinery. Cell 1997; 91:231–41.
19. Delaleu N, Jonsson R, Koller MM, et al. Sjogren's syndrome. Eur J Oral Sci 2005; 113:101–13.
20. Delettre C, Lenaers G, Griffoin JM, et al. Nuclear gene OPA1, encoding a mitochondrial dynamin-related protein, is mutated in dominant optic atrophy. Nat Genet 2000; 26:207–10.
21. Deng Y, Lin Y, Wu X. TRAIL-induced apoptosis requires bax-dependent mitochondrial release of Smac/Diablo. Genes Dev 2002; 16:33–45.
22. Deng Y, Ren X, Yang L, et al. A JNK-dependent pathway is required TNFα-induced apoptosis. Cell 2003; 115:61–70.
23. Deveraux QL, Takahashi R, Salvesen GS, et al. X-linked IAP is a direct inhibitor of cell death proteases. Nature 1997; 388:300–4.
24. Donepudi M, Sweeney AM, Briand C, et al. Insights into the regulatory mechanism for caspase-8 activation. Mol Cell 2003; 11:543–9.
25. Douma S, Van Laar T, Zevenhoven J, et al. Suppression of anoikis and induction of metastasis by the neurotrophic receptor TrKB. Nature 2004; 430:1034–9.
26. Downward J. Mechanisms and consequences of activation of protein kinase B/Akt. Curr Opin Cell Biol 1998; 10: 262–7.
27. Downward J. PI 3-kinase, Akt and cell survival. Semin Cell Dev Biol 2004; 15:177–82.

28. Du C, Fang M, Li Y, et al. Smac, a mitochondrial protein that promotes cytochrome *c*-dependent caspase activation by eliminating IAP inhibition. Cell 2000; 102:33–42.
29. Duan H, Dixit VM. RAIDD is a new death adaptor molecule. Nature 1997; 385:86–9.
30. Duque-Parra JE. Note on the origin and history of the term "Apoptosis." Anat Rec (B: New Anat.) 2005; 283B:2–4.
31. Duriez PJ, Shah GM. Cleavage of poly-(ADP-ribose) polymerase: a sensitive parameter to study cell death. Biochem Cell Biol 1997; 75:337–49.
32. Fadok VA, Voelker DR, Campbell PA, et al. Exposure of phosphatidylserine on the surface of apoptotic lymphocytes triggers specific recognition and removal by macrophages. J Immunol 1992; 148:2207–16.
33. Festjens N, van Gurp M, Van Loo G, et al. Bcl-2 family members as sentinels of cellular integrity and role of mitochondrial intermembrane space proteins in apoptotic cell death. Acta Haematol 2004; 111:7–27.
34. Frank S, Gaume B, Bergmann-Leitner ES, et al. The role of dynamin-related protein a mediator of mitochondrial fission, in apoptosis. Dev Cell 2001; 1:515–25.
35. French LE, Tschopp J. Protein-based therapeutic approaches targeting death receptors. Cell Death Differ 2003; 10:117–23.
36. Germain M, Mathai JP, McBride HM, et al. Endoplasmic reticulum BIK initiates DRP1-regulated remodeling of mitochondrial cristae during apoptosis. EMBO J 2005; 24: 1546–56.
37. Gerschenson LE, Rotello RJ. Apoptosis: a different type of cell death. FASEB J 1992; 6:2450–5.
38. Ghobrial IM, Witzig TE, Adjel AA. Targeting apoptosis pathways in cancer therapy. CA Cancer J Clin 2005; 55: 178–94.
39. Green DR, Kroemer G. The pathophysiology of mitochondrial cell death. Science 2004; 305:626–9.
40. Green DR. A Myc-induced apoptosis pathway surfaces. Science 1997; 278:1246–7.
41. Griffith TS, Chin WA, Jackson GC, et al. Intracellular regulation of TRAIL-induced apoptosis in human melanoma cells. J Immunol 1998; 161:2833–40.
42. Hamburger V, Levi-Montalcini R. Proliferation, differentiation and degeneration in the spinal ganglia of the chick embryo under normal and experimental conditions. J Exp Zool 1949; 111:457–502.
43. Hartmann A, Hirsch EC. Parkinson's disease. The apoptosis hypothesis revisited. Adv Neurol 2001; 86: 143–53.
44. Hotti A, Jarvinen K, Siivola P, et al. Caspases and mitochondria in c-Myc-induced apoptosis: identification of Atm as a new target of caspases. Oncogene 2000; 19: 1272–82.
45. Hueber AO, Zornig M, Lyon D, et al. Requirement for the CD95 receptor-ligand pathway in c-Myc-induced apoptosis. Science 1997; 278:1305–9.
46. Huehn MH, Fingert JH, Kwon YH. Retinal ganglion cell death in glaucoma: mechanisms and neuroprotective strategies. Ophthalmol Clin N Am 2005; 18:383–95.
47. Ishihara N, Eura Y, Mihara K. Mitofusin 1 and 2 play distinct roles in mitochondrial fusion reactions via GTPase activity. J Cell Sci 2004; 117:6535–46.
48. Jaattela M. Multiple cell death pathways as regulators of tumor initiation and progression. Oncogene 2004; 36: 2746–56.
49. Jin Z, El-Deiry WS. Overview of cell death signaling pathways. Cancer Biol Ther 2005; 4:139–63.
50. Jin Z, McDonald ER III, Dicker DT, et al. Deficient tumor necrosis factor-related apoptosis-inducing ligand (TRAIL) death receptor transport to the cell surface in human colon cancer cells selected for resistance to TRAIL-induced apoptosis. J Biol Chem 2004; 279: 35829–39.
51. Juin P, Junt A, Littlewood T, et al. c-Myc functionally cooperates with Bax to induce apoptosis. Mol Cell Biol 2002; 22:6158–69.
52. Karbowski M, Lee YJ, Gaume B, et al. Spatial and temporal association of Bax with mitochondrial fission sites, Drp1, and MFN2 during apoptosis. J Cell Biol 2002; 159:931–8.
53. Karbowski M, Amoult D, Chen H, et al. Quantitation of mitochondrial dynamics by photolabeling of individual organelles shows that mitochondrial fusion is blocked during the Bax activation phase of apoptosis. J Cell Biol 2004; 164:493–9.
54. Kerr JF, Wyllie AH, Currie AR. Apoptosis: a basic biological phenomenon with wide-ranging implications in the tissue kinetics. Br J Cancer 1972; 26:239–57.
55. Kim JH, Ajaz M, Lokshin A, et al. Role of antiapoptotic proteins in tumor necrosis factor-related apoptosis-inducing ligand and cisplatin-augmented apoptosis. Clin Cancer Res 2003; 9:3134–41.
56. Koshiba T, Detmer Sa, Kaiser JT, et al. Structural basis of mitochondrial tethering by mitofusin complexes. Science 2004; 305:858–62.
57. Krueger A, Schmitz I, Baumann S, et al. Cellular flice-inhibitory proteinsplice variants inhibit different steps of caspase-8 activation at the CD95 death-inducing signaling complex. J Biol Chem 2001; 276:20633–40.
58. Ku NO, Liao J, Omary MB. Apoptosis generates stable fragments of human type 1 keratins. J Biol Chem 1997; 272:33197–203.
59. Kuhnel F, Zender L, Paul Y, et al. NfkappaB mediates apoptosis through transcriptional activation of Fas (CD95) in adenoviral hepatitis. J Biol Chem 2000; 275: 6421–7.
60. Lauber K, Bohn E, Krober SM, et al. Apoptotic cells induce migration of phagocytes via caspase-3-mediated release of a lipid attraction signal. Cell 2003; 113:717–30.
61. Lavrik I, Golks A, Krammer PH. Death receptor signaling. J Cell Sci 2005; 118:265–7.
62. Leblanc AC. Natural cellular inhibitors of caspases. Prog Neuropyschopharmacol Biol Psychiatry 2003; 27: 215–29.
63. Lee YJ, Jeong SY, Karbowski M, et al. Roles of the mammalian mitochondrial fission and fusion mediators Fis 1, Drp 1, and Opa1 in apoptosis. Mol Biol Cell 2004; 15:5001–11.
64. Levkau B, Koyama H, Raines EW, et al. Cleavage of P21cip1/Waf1 and P27kip1 mediates apoptosis in endothelial cells through activation of Cdk2: role of a caspase cascade. Mol Cell 1998; 1:553–63.
65. Li LY, Luo X, Wang X. Endonuclease G is an apoptotic DNase when released from mitochondria. Nature 2001; 412:95–9.
66. Li L, Thomas RM, Suzuki H, et al. A small molecule smac mimic potentiates TRAIL- and TNFalpha-mediated cell death. Science 2004; 305:1471–4.
67. Li P, Nijhawan D, Budihardjo I, et al. Cytochrome *c* and dATD-dependent formation of Apaf-1/caspase-9 complex initiates an apoptotic protease cascade. Cell 1997; 91: 479–89.
68. Linden R, Martins RAP, Silveira MS. Control of programmed cell death by neurotransmitters and neuropeptides in the developing mammalian retina. Prog Retin Eye Res 2005; 24:457–91.

69. Lockshin RA, Zakeri Z. Apoptosis, autophagy or more. Int J Biochem Cell Biol 2004; 36:2405–19.
70. Luo X, Budihardjo I, Zou H, et al. Bid, a Bcl-2 interacting protein, mediates cytochrome *c* release from mitochondria in response to activation of cell surface death receptors. Cell 1998; 94:481–90.
71. Maclachan TK, El-Deiry WS. Apoptotic threshold is lowered by p53 transactivation of caspase-6. Proc Natl Acad Sci U S A 2002; 99:9492–7.
72. Mahoney JA, Rosen A. Apoptosis and autoimmunity. Curr Opin Immunol 2005; 17:583–8.
73. Maldonado V, Melendez-Zajgla J, Ortega A. Modulation of NF-kappa B, and Bcl-2 in apoptosis induced by cisplatin in HeLa cells. Mutat Res 1997; 381:67–75.
74. Mancini M, Nicholson DW, Roy S, et al. The caspase-3 precursor has a cytosolic and mitochondrial distribution: implications for apoptotic signaling. J Cell Biol 1998; 140: 1485–95.
75. Mandruzzato S, Brasseur F, Andry G, et al. A casp-8 mutation recognized by cytolytic T lymphocytes on a human head and neck carcinoma. J Exp Med 1997; 186: 785–93.
76. Martelli AM, Tazzari PL, Tabellini G, et al. A new selective AKT pharmacological inhibitor reduces resistance to chemotherapeutic drugs, TRAILs, all-trans-retinoic acid, and ionizing radiation of human leukemia cells. Leukemia 2003; 17:1794–805.
77. Micheau O, Tschopp J. Induction of TNF receptor I-mediated apoptosis via two sequential signaling complexes. Cell 2003; 114:181–90.
78. Mignotte B, Vayssiere JL. Mitochondria and apoptosis. Eur J Biochem 1998; 252:1–15.
79. Mohamad N, Gutierrez A, Nunez M, et al. Mitochondrial apoptotic pathways. Biocell 2005; 29:149–61.
80. Nagle JA, Ma Z, Byrne MA, et al. Involvement of insulin receptor substrate 2 in mammary tumor metastasis. Mol Cell Biol 2004; 24:9726–35.
81. Nahle Z, Polakoff J, Davuluri RV, et al. Direct coupling of the cell cycle and cell death machinery by E2f. Nat Cell Biol 2002; 4:859–64.
82. Nechushtan A, Smith CL, Lamensdorf I, et al. Bax and Bak coalesce into novel mitochondria-associated clusters during apoptosis. J Cell Biol 2001; 153:1265–76.
83. Newmeyer DD, Ferguson-Miller S. Mitochondria: releasing power for life and unleashing machineries of death. Cell 2003; 112:481–90.
84. Nicholson DW, Thornberry NA. Caspases: killer proteases. Trends Biochem Sci 1997; 22:299–306.
85. Ohata H, Yatomi Y, Sweeney EA, et al. A possible role of sphinogosine in induction of apoptosis by tumor necrosis factor-alpha in human neutrophils. FEBS Lett 1994; 355: 267–70.
86. Olichon A, Baricault L, Gas N, et al. Loss of OPA1 perturbates the mitochondrial inner membrane structure and integrity, leading to cytochrome *c* release and apoptosis. J Biol Chem 2003; 278:7743–6.
87. Olichon A, Emorine LJ, Descoins E, et al. The human dynamin-related protein OPA1 is anchored to the mitochondrial inner membrane facing the inter-membrane space. FEBS Lett 2002; 523:171–6.
88. Pathan N, Marusawa H, Krajewska M, et al. TUCAN, antiapoptotic caspase recruitment domain family protein overexpressed in cancer. J Biol Chem 2001; 276:32220–9.
89. Pelengaris S, Khan M, Evan GI. Suppression of Myc-induced apoptosis in beta cells exposes multiple oncogenic properties of Myc and triggers carcinogenic progression. Cell 2002; 109:321–34.
90. Perkins ND. NF-kappaB: tumor promoter and suppressor. Trends Cell Biol 2004; 14:64–9.
91. Perry SW, Dewhurst S, Bellizzi MJ, et al. Tumor necrosis factor-alpha in normal and diseased brain: conflicting effects via intraneuronal receptor crosstalk? J Neurovirol 2002; 8:611–24.
92. Peter ME, Krammer PH. The CD95(APO-1/Fas) DISC and beyond. Cell Death Differ 2003; 10:26–35.
93. Raff MC. Social controls on cell survival and cell death. Nature 1992; 356:397–400.
94. Rai NK, Tripathi K, Sharma D, et al. Apoptosis: a basic physiologic process in would healing. Int J Low Extrem Wounds 2005; 4:138–44.
95. Ricci MS, Jin Z, Dews M, et al. Direct repression of flip expression by c-Myc is a major determinant of TRAIL sensitivity. Mol Cell Biol 2004; 24:8541–55.
96. Rikhof B, Corn PG, El-Deiry WS. Caspase-10 levels are increased following DNA damage in a p53-dependent manner. Cancer Biol Ther 2003; 2:707–12.
97. Sambrano GR, Steinberg D. Recognition of oxidatively damaged and apoptotic cells by an oxidized low density lipoprotein receptor on mouse peritoneal macrophages: role of membrane phosphatidylserine. Proc Natl Acad Sci U S A 1995; 92:1396–400.
98. Savill J, Fadok V. Corpse clearance defines the meaning of cell death. Nature 2000; 407:784–8.
99. Scaffidi C, Fulda S, Srinivasan A, et al. Two CD95 (Apo-1/FAS) signaling pathways. EMBO J 1998; 17: 1675–87.
100. Scorrano L, Oakes SA, Opferman JT, et al. Bax and Bak regulation of endoplasmic reticulum Ca^{2+}: a control point for apoptosis. Science 2003; 300:135–9.
101. Shi Y. Mechanisms of cascapase activation and inhibition during apoptosis. Moll Cell 2002; 9:459–70.
102. Siegel RM, Chan FK, Chun HJ, et al. The multifaceted role of Fas signaling in immune cell homeostasis and autoimmunity. Nat Immunol 200; 1:469–74.
103. Slee EA, Harte MT, Kluck RM, et al. Ordering the cytochrome *c*-initiated caspase-cascade: hierarchical activation of caspases-2, -3, -6, -7, -8 and -10 in a caspase-9-dependent manner. J Cell Biol 1999; 144: 281–92.
104. Song K, Chen Y, Goke R, et al. Tumor necrosis factor-related apoptosis-inducing ligand (TRAIL) is an inhibitor of autoimmune inflammation and cell cycle progression. J Exp Med 200; 191:1095–104.
105. Sugioka R, Shimizu S, Tsujimoto Y. Fzo1, a protein involved in mitochondrial fusion, inhibits apoptosis. J Biol Chem 2004; 279:52726–34.
106. Susin SA, Lorenzo HK, Zamzami N, et al. Mitochondrial release of caspase-2 and -9 during the apoptotic process. J Exp Med 1999; 189:381–94.
107. Susin SA, Daudas E, Ravagan L, et al. Two distinct pathways leading to nuclear apoptosis. J Exp Med 2000; 192:571–80.
108. Takahashi R, Deveraux Q, Tamm I, et al. A single bir domain of XIAP sufficient for inhibiting caspases. J Biol Chem 1998; 273:7787–90.
109. Thorbourn A. Death receptor-induced cell killing. Cell Signal 2004; 16:139–44.
110. Thornberry NA, Lazebnik Y. Caspases: enemies within. Science 1998; 28:1312–6.
111. Thornberry NA, Rano TA, Peterson EP, et al. A combinational approach defines specificities of members of the caspase family and granzyme B. Functional relationships established for key mediators of apoptosis. J Biol Chem 1997; 272:17907–11.

112. Tilli CMLJ, Van Steensel MAM, Krekels GAM, et al. Molecular aetiology and pathogenesis of basal cell carcinoma. Br J Dermatol 2005; 152:1108–24.
113. Van Loo G, van Gurp M, Depuydt B, et al. The serine protease Omi/HtrA2 is released from mitochondria during apoptosis. Omi interacts with caspase-inhibitor XIAP and induces enhanced caspase activity. Cell Death Differ 2002; 9:20–6.
114. Vaux DL, Korsmeyer SJ. Cell death in development. Cell 1999; 96:245–54.
115. Verkhratsky A, Toescu EC. Endoplasmic reticulum CA2+ homeostasis and neuronal death. J Cell Mol Med 2003; 7: 351–61.
116. Vermeulen K, Van Bockstaele DR, Berneman ZN. Apoptosis: mechanisms and relevance in cancer. Ann Hematol 2005; 84:627–39.
117. Vogelstein B, Kinzler KW. Cancer genes and the pathways they control. Nat Med 2004; 10:789–99.
118. Wajant H. Death receptors. Essays Biochem 2003; 39: 53–71.
119. Wajant H, Pfizenmaier K, Scheurich P. Tumor necrosis factor signaling. Cell Death Differ 2003; 10:45–65.
120. Walzog B, Jeblonski F, Zakrewicz A, et al. β2 integrins promote apoptosis of human neutrophils. FASEB J 1997; 11:1177–86.
121. Wang Y, Engels IH, Knee DA, et al. Synthetic lethal targeting of Myc by activation of the DR5 death receptor pathway. Cancer Cell 2004; 5:501–12.
122. Williams GT, Smith CA, Spooncer E, et al. Haemopoietic colony stimulating factors promote cell survival by suppressing apoptosis. Nature 1990; 343:76–9.
123. Youle RJ, Karbowski. Mitochondrial fission in apoptosis. Mol Cell Biol 2005; 6:657–63.
124. Zindy F, Eischen CM, Randle DH, et al. Myc signaling via the ARF tumor suppressor regulates p53-dependent apoptosis and immortalization. Genes Dev 1998; 12:2424–33.

3

Immunologic Processes in Disease

Thomas Albini
Bascom Palmer Eye Institute, Miller School of Medicine, University of Miami, Miami, Florida, U.S.A.

Narsing A. Rao
Doheny Eye Institute, Keck School of Medicine, University of Southern California, Los Angeles, California, U.S.A.

INTRODUCTION

Many eye diseases represent the interaction of the immune system with ocular or periocular tissues. A good knowledge of the immune system and its interaction with the eye is necessary to understand the several ocular and ocular adnexal inflammatory diseases. This chapter outlines the general principles of immunology, discusses specific ocular manifestations of the immune response, and finally considers immunologic processes in ocular infections. A full discussion of immunology is beyond the scope of this text and many excellent reviews exist (1,21,531–3).

CELLS AND CELL SURFACE MARKERS OF THE IMMUNE SYSTEM

All the cells making up the immune system are derived from the hemopoietic stem cells of the bone marrow. Differentiation of the many cell types that make up the immune system has been greatly enhanced by the development of monoclonal and polyclonal antibodies that specifically react with surface glycoproteins on certain cell subtypes. These surface markers often help differentiate the status of a given cell as well. For example, many cells express certain surface molecules only when they are activated. These markers have been standardized and systematized by international workshops into a system of clusters of differentiation (CD) (Table 1). A group of glycoproteins called major histocompatibility complex (MHC) molecules—known as human leukocyte antigen (HLA) molecules in humans—have been identified as extremely important in predicting rejection following tissue transplantation. These surface molecules present antigens to immunocompetent cells, primarily T lymphocytes. Two classes of MHC molecules exist: class I molecules are found on all nucleated cells and present antigen derived from the intracellular components, such as tumor or viral

Table 1 List of Selected CD Antigens

CD antigen	Cellular expression	Functions	Synonyms
CD1	Cortical thymocytes, Langerhans cells, dendritic cells, B cells, intestinal epithelium, smooth muscle, blood vessels	MHC class I-like molecule with special role in presentation of lipid molecules	
CD2	T cells, thymocytes, NK cells	Adhesion molecule binding CD58 (LFA-3)	T11, LFA-2
CD3	Thymocytes, T cells	Associated with the T-cell antigen receptor (TCR). Required for surface expression and activation TCR	T3
CD4	Thymocyte subsets, Th1 cells, Th2 cells, monocytes, macrophages	Co-receptor of MHC class II molecule	T4, L3T4
CD8	Thymocyte subsets, cytotoxic T cells	Co-receptor of MHC class I molecule	T8, Lyt2,3
CD11a	Leukocytes	Subunit of integrin LFA-1	LFA-1
CD11b	Granulocytes, macrophages	Binds CD54, complement component iC3b, and extracellular matrix proteins	Mac-1
CD11c	Granulocytes, macrophages, lymphocytes		Adhesion molecule, binds fibrinogen
CD16	Neutrophils, NK cells, macrophages	Low-affinity Fc receptor, mediates phagocytosis and antibody-dependent cell-mediated cytotoxicity	FcγRIII
CD23	Mature B cells, activated macrophages, eosinophils, follicular dendritic cells, platelets	Low-affinity receptor for IgE	FcεRIII
CD28	T-cell subsets, activated B cells	Activation of naïve T cells, receptor for costimulatory signal. Binds CD80 (B7.1) and CD86 (B7.2)	
CD40	B cells, macrophages, dendritic cells, basal epithelial cells	Binds CD154 (CD40L); receptor for costimulatory signal for B cells; promotes growth, differentiation, and isotype switching of B cells	
CD45	All hematopoietic cells	Tyrosine phosphatase	Leukocyte common antigen

Note: For a complete list visit the Website of the human leukocyte differentiation antigens/human cell differentiation molecules at http://www.hlda8.org or protein reviews provided by the NIH at http://ww.ncbi.nlm.gov/prow/.

antigens, to cytotoxic CD8+ T lymphocytes; class II molecules are found predominantly on professional antigen-presenting cells (APCs), such as dendritic cells, macrophages and B cells, and these cells present extracellular antigens that have been endocytosed, such as fungal or bacterial antigens, to helper CD4+ T lymphocytes.

Polymorphonuclear leukocytes (PMNs), eosinophilic leukocytes, mast cells, macrophages, dendritic cells, and microglia (4) are derived from the myeloid progenitor cell in the bone marrow. Among these, the cells containing intracytoplasmic granules are divided into PMNs, eosinophils and basophils based on differential staining of their granules. Most circulating granulocytes are PMNs. These cells express surface receptors for immunoglobulin (Ig)G and certain complement components. Following upregulation of adhesion molecules on vascular endothelial cells in an inflamed tissue, chemotactic agents such as complement components, fibrinolytic and kinin system components, and leukocyte, platelet or bacterial products cause circulating PMNs to migrate into the involved tissue and release inflammatory mediators into the surrounding tissue. Eosinophils possess surface receptors for IgE, IgG and complement components. These cells are commonly found in allergic and parasitic conditions. Like PMNs eosinophils degranulate when activated. Mast cells reside near small blood vessels and they are distributed in the human conjunctiva, uvea, and other ocular tissues. These cells are numerous in the conjunctiva and 5000 to 6000 cells/mm^2 are present around the vascular elements (3). These cells are important activators of the allergic response and mucosal immunity. When antigen binds to two adjacent IgE molecules on the mast cell surface, the mast cell degranulates releasing vasoactive amines, such as histamine, which increase vascular permeability and allow immune complexes to deposit in the vessel wall. Basophils express surface receptors for IgE, IgG and complement components and their function appears to be similar to that of mast cells.

Dendritic cells and macrophages are typical APCs since they constitutively express MHC class II molecules, which present antigen to CD4+ T lymphocytes (Fig. 1). They also express IgG receptors which can be used to engulf extracellular antigens after they are coated with IgG, a reaction specifically known as opsonization. Moreover, APCs stimulate lymphocytes by cytokine production, such as

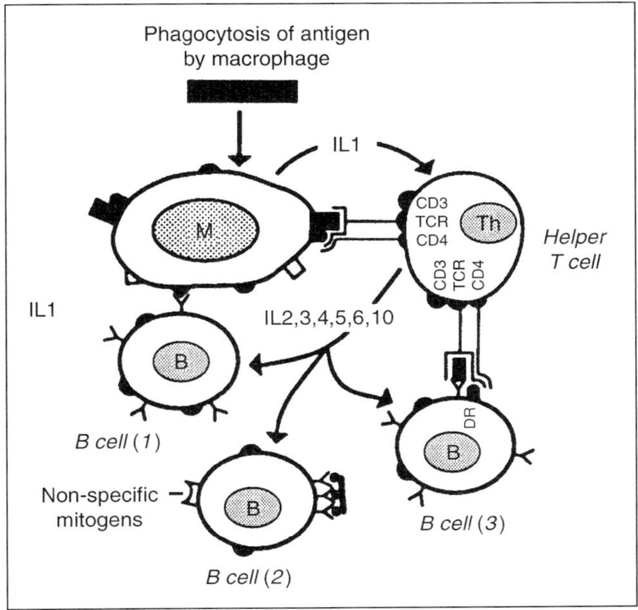

Figure 1 Network of cellular interactions in immune regulation. Antigen taken up by macrophages (M) is broken into fragments, linked with class II HLA, and presented to a helper T cell (Th). T-cell receptor (TCR) and the CD4 molecules recognize the modified antigen on the surface of the macrophage. In addition to CD3, which stabilizes the TCR, other accessory molecules on helper T cells bind to corresponding receptors on the macrophage. These interactions are a prerequisite for T-cell activation. Subsequent B-cell activation can develop in three ways: (*i*) antigen can be presented directly by a macrophage in the presence of T cell-derived IL3, IL4, IL5, IL6, and IL10; (*ii*) alternatively, antigen, particularly a polymer with repeating peptide units, even when it is unprocessed, can sometimes bind directly and promote B-cell activation; or (*iii*) B cells may also express class II HLA and therefore behave as antigen-presenting cells and stimulate TH to initiate an immune response. *Source*: Courtesy of Dr. Amjad H.S. Rahi.

interleukin (IL) 1 and tumor necrosis factor-alpha (TNFα), and by surface expression of costimulatory molecules required for successful antigen presentation (discussed in greater detail later in this section). These cells secrete a host of other immune mediators including proteases, collagenases, angiotensin-converting enzyme, lysozyme, IL6, and macrophage colony-stimulating factor and reactive oxygen and nitrogen species. Specialized macrophages exist in many tissues such as the Kupffer cells of the liver, denditic histiocytes of lymphoid organs and uveal tissue, Langerhans cells of the skin, lymph nodes, conjunctiva and cornea, and microglia of the retina and central nervous system (CNS).

A common lymphoid progenitor gives rise to lymphocytes. Lymphocytes are 7 to 8 μm, round mononuclear cells (Fig. 2). A subset of them, B cells, mature in the bone marrow and produce antibodies. They are the primary cells responsible for adaptive humoral immunity. B lymphocytes can recognize extracellular antigens not processed or presented by other immune cells by means of surface antibody receptors and the antibody which the cell itself produces and secretes. Antibodies are divided into five classes by the characteristics of the constant regions of the antibody molecule. IgM is the first antibody class produced to a specific antigen. Typically during a second exposure to the same antigen, the B cell is activated either by the surrounding cytokine milieu or by some bacterial polysaccharides and lipopolysaccharides, known as T-cell–independent antigens, and the cell switches class production to either IgG, IgA or IgE class antibodies. IgG is the major antibody component and can neutralize toxins, activate the complement system (Fig. 3), and react with pathogens. IgA is the principal antibody of mucosal immunity and is found in external secretions such as tears, milk, nasal and intestinal secretions. IgE is the principal antibody of allergic responses and immune reactions to parasites. IgD is found on the surface of immature B cells but its function remains obscure.

Any particular B cell produces one specific antibody, whose variable region recognizes one specific antigen (Fig. 4). The fact that an almost infinite range of specificities can be encoded by a finite number of genes is explained by the fact that during B-cell development in the bone marrow, gene segments are randomly irreversibly joined so as to encode the variable region of the antibody for that particular B cell. Through the recombination of various germline gene segments—grouped into V, D and J segments—one of over 10^{14} potential different genetic combinations is produced in each individual B lymphocyte. When a particular B-cell antibody molecule binds antigen, it is engulfed and presented to other lymphocytes by means of the MHC class II molecule of the B lymphocyte. Since B cells can present antigen to T lymphocytes in their MHC class II molecule peptide groove, B cells are considered to be a type of APC. With the right response from the interacting "helper" T cell, the B cell undergoes clonal expansion and begins to secrete antibody with the same specificity.

Another subset of lymphocytes matures in the thymus and carries the T-cell receptor (CD3), which allows these cells to recognize specific peptides presented by APCs within the peptide groove of either MHC class I or II molecules. T cells are responsible for adaptive cellular immunity. Like antibodies, T-cell receptors that recognize over 10^{18} specific peptides in specific MHC molecules are produced by random combinations of the germline V, D, and J segment genes that make up the variable regions of the T-cell receptor. These cells undergo

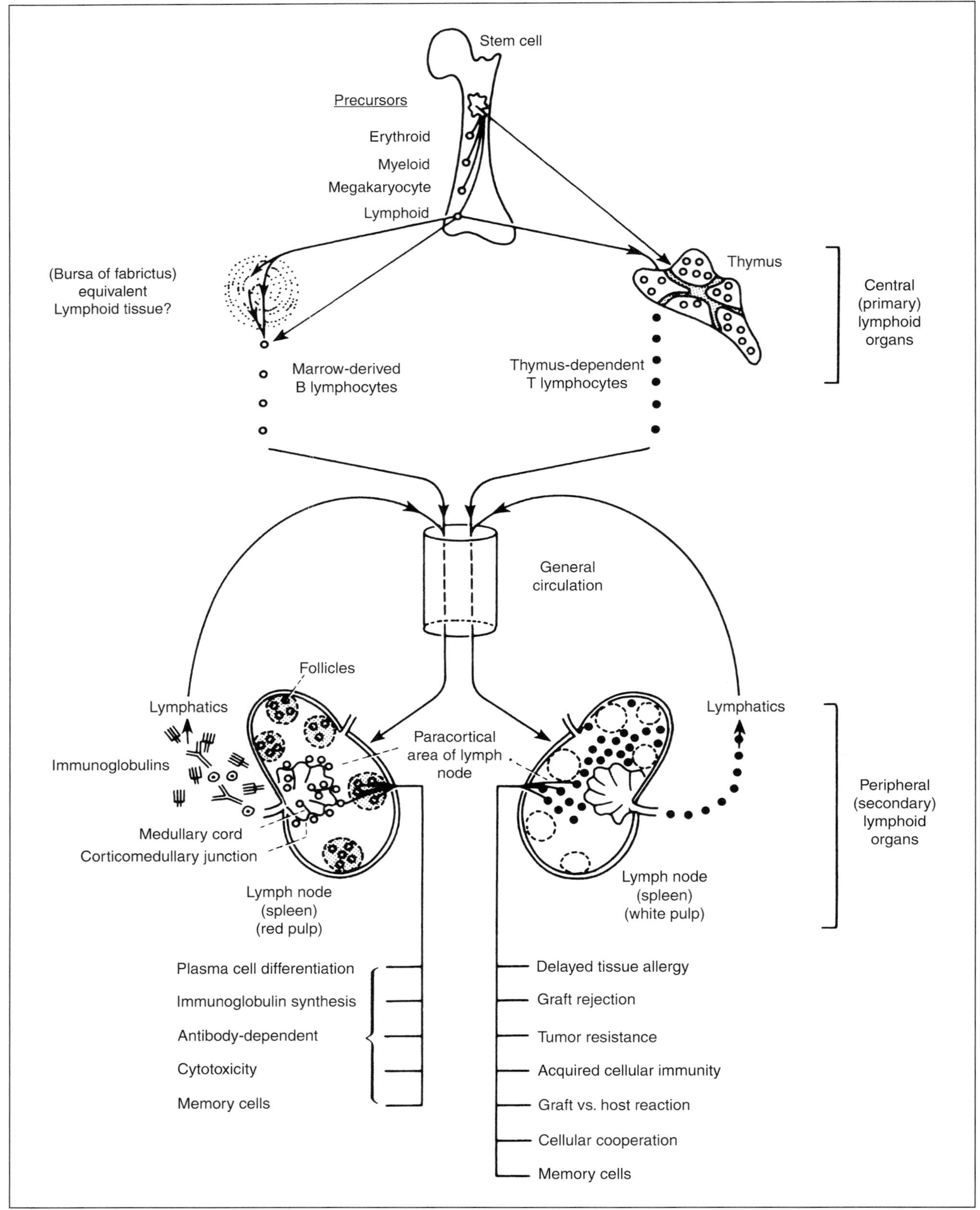

Figure 2 Origin and development of the lymphoid system. The peripheral lymphoid organs include, in addition to lymph nodes, the spleen and lymphocyte aggregates in the submucosal tissue of the gut and elsewhere in the body. *Source*: Courtesy of Dr. Amjad H.S. Rahi.

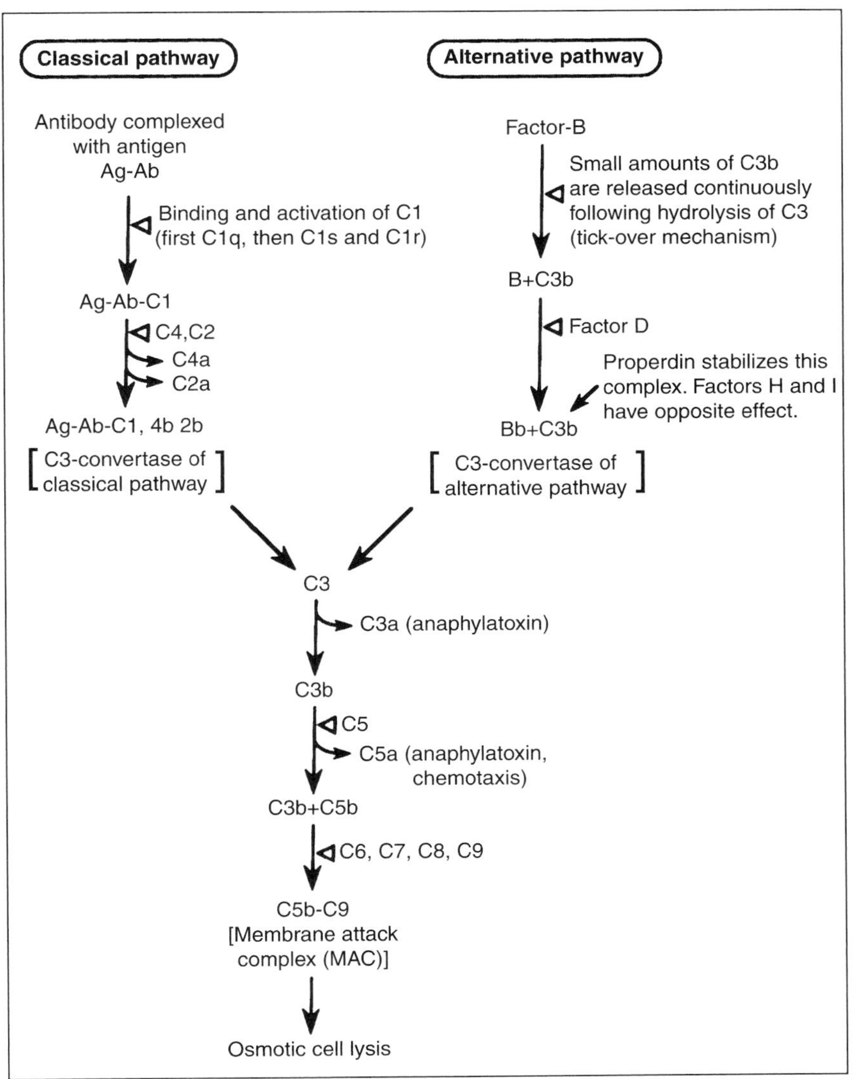

Figure 3 Complement activation. The classic pathway generally requires an antigen–antibody reaction on the surface of the target cell (although C-reactive protein can also be effective), whereas the alternative pathway can be activated by aggregated immunoglobulins (such as IgG) and proteolytic enzymes. C3-convertase generated by either of the pathways leads to the sequential activation of C3 through C9. The production of a membrane attack complex results in permeability damage to the phospholipid layer of the cell membrane by inserting molecules of C9 in a concentric fashion to create a tunnel. This predisposes to osmotic lysis of the target cell by permitting the entry of sodium ions. *Source*: Courtesy of Dr. Amjad H. S. Rahi.

clonal deletion during maturation in the thymus which is thought to remove all T cells that react with the host's own antigens, so as to preclude potentially self-destructive T-cell activation (i.e., autoimmunity). When mature T cells are presented with an antigen for which they have a specific T-cell receptor (CD3) by APCs, the T cells undergo clonal expansion, initiating an immune response targeted at the specific antigen. CD3 was first identified using monoclonal antibodies that bound only one cloned T-cell line but not others thereby inhibiting antigen recognition by that clone of T cells, or specifically activating them. Each receptor consists of two different polypeptide chains, termed the T-cell receptor α and β chains, linked by a disulfide bond. These heterodimers are analogous in structure to the Fab fragment of an Ig molecule, and they account for antigen recognition by most T cells. A minority of T cells bear an alternative, but structurally similar, receptor made up of a different pair of polypeptide chains designated γ and δ. These T-cell receptors appear to have different antigen-recognition properties from the α and β T-cell receptors, although the function of γ and δ T cells in immune responses is not yet well understood. Each T cell caries approximately 30,000 CD3 molecules, but all CD3 molecules on any given cell express only one of over 10^{18} V, D and J segment combinations, rendering each T cell specific for a single antigen presented in the context of an MHC molecule. The CD3 molecule is the only antigen-specific molecule on the T cell. Subsets of T cells react to antigen in two different ways depending on the co-receptor molecule (either CD4 or CD8) associated with their T-cell receptor (CD3). Cells bearing the CD4 co-receptor promote the immune response through secreted cytokines that activate surrounding lymphocytes and/or macrophages. These cells recognize extracellular antigens that have been processed in intracellular vesicles following

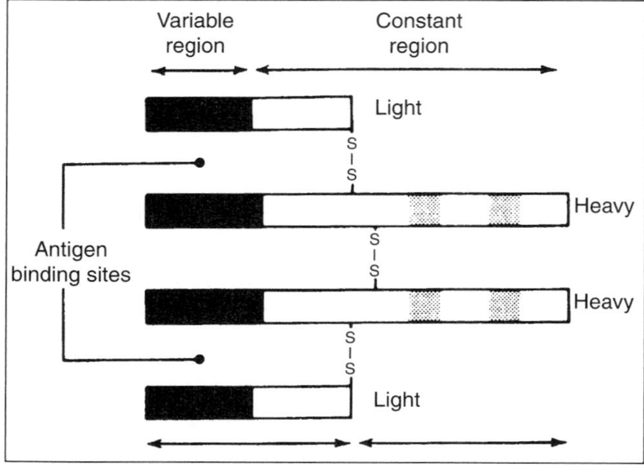

Figure 4 Immunoglobulin G (IgG) molecule. The antigen-binding site is located at the amino termini of the light and heavy chains and has a variable composition. The chains are linked together by disulfide bonds; similar internal bonds form loops that in the Fc region of the heavy chain provide sites for the several biological activities of the molecule. In the IgG molecule there are two such sites on the constant region of the heavy chain: C_H2 is concerned with complement fixation and regulation of catabolism and C_H3 with macrophage binding. C_H1 is located on the constant region of the heavy chain within the Fab part of the molecule. *Source*: Adapted from Garner A. The immune response. In: Scadding JG, Cumming G, eds. Scientific Foundations of Respiratory Medicine. Heinemann: London, 1981.

ingestion by an APC and presented as peptide in the groove of MHC class II molecules. T cells bearing the CD8 co-receptor are cytocidal, destroying the cells harboring the antigen. These cells recognize cytotoxic antigens, such as viral antigens, presented in the groove of MHC class I molecules and are called cytotoxic T cells. In addition to antigen-specific signals mediated through the T-cell receptor and co-receptor molecules, T cells also require antigen-nonspecific costimulation for activation. The B7 family of molecules on APCs, which include B7-1 (CD80) and B7-2 (CD86), play important roles in providing costimulatory signals required for development of antigen-specific immune responses.

A third type of lymphocyte is the natural killer (NK) cell which plays an important role in innate or antigen-nonspecific cytotoxic responses to tumor cells or virus-infected cells. The cells are large granular lymphocytes and are characterized by the lack of CD3 and Ig on their surface. NK cells can kill a variety of targets, including tumor cells, without the need of specific antigen interaction. Recent reports suggest that the NK-cell population is heterogeneous, for although most are CD3–, CD16+, and CD56+, a small proportion may also express CD3 antigen (28). They do not require IgG to kill the target. It has been demonstrated that the granules of NK cells contain a protein called perforin, which resembles the ninth component of complement (C9) and produces anatomical holes (i.e., permeability defects) in the target cells (70). NK cells are CD56+ and are activated in the presence of interferon gamma (IFNγ) (28,30).

ANTIGEN

An antigen is classically defined as any substance that can bind to a specific antibody; this includes proteins, carbohydrates and nucleic acids. All antigens by definition have the potential to react with specific antibodies, but some need to be attached to a protein to successfully elicit an immune response. Any substance that elicits an immune response is termed immunogenic and is called an immunogen. Many non-protein antigens are not immunogenic unless they are presented in conjunction with a protein immunogen carrier and it is the immunogenicity of the protein antigens that determines the immune response in most cases. Furthermore, although almost any molecule can be recognized by antibody as an antigen, usually only proteins elicit fully developed adaptive immune responses, because proteins have the unique ability to be recognized by CD3 of T cells, which contribute to most antibody responses and are required for immunologic memory. An adaptive immune response that includes immunologic memory can be induced by non-protein antigens, only if these antigens are attached to a protein carrier which can engage the T cell.

Most proteins are poorly immunogenic or non-immunogenic when administered by themselves in experimental models. Significant adaptive immune responses to protein antigens usually require that the antigen be injected in a mixture known as an adjuvant, defined simply as any substance that enhances the immunogenicity of substances mixed with it. Unlike protein carriers, adjuvants do not form stable linkages with the antigen. Many adjuvants increase macrophage phagocytosis of antigens and delay their release so as to increase the duration of immune exposure. These are thought to be the main functions of the oil-in-water emulsion produced by the use of incomplete Freund adjuvant. Complete Freund adjuvant additionally contains dead mycobacteria which induce IL12 and costimulatory molecules and thereby render macrophages more effective APCs (24). The magnitude of the immune response to an immunogen also depends on the dose of immunogen administered. At very low doses, too few immune competent cells are engaged to produce a significant response. As the dose of immunogen is increased, the immune response increases in severity until a plateau level is reached. At very high doses of immunogen the immune response is often inhibited by a process

A proportion of the IgG in tears is derived from the circulation and may target antigens encountered systemically. It has also been found that some of the locally produced IgA targets antigens presented at non-ocular sites. Increased lymphocytic infiltration of the lacrimal gland and subsequent atrophy of the lacrimal epithelium are seen in autoimmune causes of dry eye such as Sjögren syndrome (SS) (see Chapter 6) (31). A majority of these infiltrating lymphocytes are CD4+ T cells, resulting in a rise of the CD4+ T-cell/CD8+ T-cell ratio from 0.3 in normal lacrimal glands to 3.0 in SS (42). The cause of this infiltration is not clearly understood, but is thought to possibly involve viral infections in genetically predisposed individuals. It is noteworthy that the lymphocytic infiltration of the lacrimal gland increases with age. Inhibition of T-cell function, via cyclosporine, has proven useful in increasing tear production in animal models and in one clinical trial, resulting in topical cyclosporine therapy for dry eye (50). More specific immunomodulating targets have been recently explored as well. For example, adenovirus-mediated transfer of a TNFα inhibitor in a rabbit autoimmune dacryoadenitis resulted in increased tear production and tear stability, as well as a decrease in the CD4+ T-cell/CD8+ T-cell ratio (61).

IMMUNOLOGIC PROCESSES AND OCULAR INFECTIONS

All clinical infections represent the interactions of the pathogenic organism and the host immune system according to the mechanisms that have outlined above. Specific insights into the better studied ocular infections are provided below.

Viral Infection

Virus infections are discussed in Chapter 8 and immunologic processes play an important role in these diseases. Peptide derivatives of intracellular viral antigens are processed in the endoplasmic reticulum and presented to T lymphocytes on the host cell surface in the peptide groove of MHC class I molecules. CD8+ T lymphocytes with the appropriate CD3 for that specific peptide/MHC combination are then activated, undergo clonal expansion and elicit an adaptive, antigen specific cytotoxic response, destroying all cells displaying the same peptide. Similarly, extracellular viral particles are either phagocytosed, endocytosed in a receptor (IgG receptor)-mediated process, or pinocytosed. The antigens are then processed in the endosomal–lysosomal compartment of the cell, and expressed on the cell surface as peptides. When these cells interact with CD4+ T lymphocyte bearing the appropriate T-cell receptor, the T cell is activated, undergoes clonal expansion, and drives a Th1 or Th2 response. Th2 responses drive class switching and lead to IgG, IgM and or IgE production. These antibodies can neutralize virus infectivity or lead to lysis of infected host cells by means of complement. Antibody binding to viral capsid or envelope prevents or causes conformational changes that preclude the virus' normal functions. Viruses that bud from the cell surface also bear viral surface antigens, to which antibody-mediated responses can be mounted. Viruses that are readily released and spread into the extracellular space, such as hepatitis and enteroviruses, are more susceptible to humoral immunity and patients with antibody deficiencies are more susceptible to these infections. In contrast viruses that tend to be more intracellular, such as herpes viruses or human immunodeficiency virus (HIV) are less susceptible to humoral immunity. Cellular responses to viruses include antigen-specific cytotoxic T-cell cytotoxicity, antibody-dependent cell-mediated cytolysis, NK cell cytotoxicity, and macrophage activation. Viruses that bind antibody can be cleared by different leukocytes that bear IgG receptors on their surface, including NK cells and macrophages. Additionally, NK cells can destroy virus-infected cells in an antibody-independent manner, by means of a variety of NK-cell receptors. Three types of IFN play important roles in viral infections. IFNα is secreted by lymphocytes and macrophages in response to viral and bacterial products, polynucleotides, tumor cells and allogenic cells. IFNβ is produced by fibroblasts, epithelial cells, and leukocytes. T lymphocytes are capable of producing IFNγ when activated, promoting a Th1 response. When the IFNs interact with the infected cell, they induce intracellular protein production that inhibits translation of the viral genome. IFNs enhance T-cell cytotoxicity, enhance or depress antibody production, enhance macrophage phagocytosis, oxidative metabolism, and upregulate MHC class I and II expression. IFNs upregulate MHC class I expression on numerous cell types, and IFNγ upregulates MHC class II expression, even on cells that do not normally express it, such as RPE.

Viruses cause host damage by means of: (*i*) lyzing host cells; (*ii*) transforming host cells; (*iii*) altering cell function; (*iv*) inducing inflammation; and (*v*) inciting autoimmune disease. An example of a virus-induced autoimmune disease is the immune destruction of myelin within the CNS following the experimental infection of the mouse with picornavirus (40). Similarly, Coxsackie viruses induce antibodies cross-reacting with myosin (molecular mimickry) that result in myositis (22).

Bacterial Infection

The conjunctiva and eyelid are colonized with numerous nonpathogenic bacteria as well as with bacteria capable of causing disease (see Chapter 9).

Many of these organisms produce disease because of immunologic hypersensitivities elicited in response to their antigens. For example, ribitol teichoic acid from *Staphylococcus* sp. may elicit antibody formation which forms immune complexes that are deposited typically at the corneoscleral limbus, where antibody and antigen concentrations and vascularity favor their deposition (33). These depositions can result in an infiltration of PMNs that leads to the formation of necrotic ulcers. The deposition of immune complexes and the subsequent lesions occur as an example of a hypersensitivity type III reaction.

Another immune-mediated manifestation of Staphylococcal blepharoconjunctivitis is the formation of phlyctenules, elevated limbal lesions that extend toward the central cornea with accompanying blood vessels (47). These represent a cell-mediated hypersensitivity type IV reaction, responding to Staphylococcal antigens. In the developing world this is more commonly seen with tuberculosis. These lesions typically occur in younger patients and run a self-limited 14-day course.

Chlamydia trachomatis, the causal agent of trachoma, causes a blinding chronic scarring follicular keratoconjunctivitis, afflicting over 500 million people worldwide (see Chapter 10). The disease is progressive, with the first exposure resulting typically in a mild self-limiting infection. Immunity is short-lived and following repeated exposure more severe inflammation and scarring develop. Conjunctival cultures during chronic disease often do not yield the infectious organism, suggesting that the chronic form may result from immune mechanisms. *Chlamydia psittaci* naturally infects guinea pigs producing an animal model of trachoma. In this model, repeated exposure to viable, but not replicating organisms results in clinical and histologic evidence of a hypersensitivity type IV (64). A prominent lymphocytic infiltrate accompanied by monocytes occurs in the conjunctiva not only after re-exposure of the conjunctiva to organism, but also after other non-ocular mucosal surfaces are inoculated. These findings strongly argue for the role of delayed type hypersensitivity in the pathogenesis of trachoma.

Fungal Infection

Fungal infections of the ocular tissues are discussed in Chapter 11. In some of these infections immunologic processes play an important role. For example, several components of the immune system and inflammatory response are important in ocular candidiasis. Several lines of evidence suggest that PMNs play a central role in the host response to *Candida* (14). The growth of *C. albicans* in vitro is inhibited by PMNs, granulocytopenic mice are highly susceptible to disseminated candidiasis, and stimulation of PMN function by IFNγ is protective (14). Furthermore, TNFα knock-out animals exhibited increased mortality in response to experimental candidiasis, associated with a 10- to 1000-fold increase in yeast outgrowth in internal organs, delay in PMN recruitment, and a decreased ability to phagocytoze *Candida* blastospores (36). Th1 responses are protective and are found to be important in the development of responses to reinfection, and important in driving phagocyte-dependent mucosal immunity (10). Antibodies have also been shown to be important in enhancing phagocytosis of *Candida* organisms (9). These studies indicate that immunity to *Candida* is complex and involves the interplay of multiple immune pathways; deficiency in one or more of these pathways results in increased susceptibility to infection. These experimental findings help explain, for example, why some patients without neutropenia develop chronic mucocutaneous candidiasis associated with decreased Th1 cytokine profiles (25).

PMNs are similarly essential in the host defense against *Aspergillus*. The clinical observation that *Aspergillus* endophthalmitis tends to occur only in the setting of granulocytopenia, while *Candida* endophthalmitis often occurs in the absence of granulocytopenia, suggests a greater role for PMNs in *Aspergillus* infection than in *Candida* infection (43). Tissue studies of eyes with *Aspergillus* endophthalmitis have revealed an almost exclusive growth of these organisms in the subretinal and the subretinal pigment epithelial spaces. This histopathologic finding is consistent with the finding that RPE contains numerous antioxidant proteins, such as superoxide dismutase, catalase, glutathione peroxidase, and other antioxidant enzymes, that inhibit the function of oxidants produced by PMNs. These antioxidant proteins likely hinder the PMNl mediated clearance of *Aspergillus* by such oxidants as superoxide, hydrogen peroxide, and related metabolites.

Parasitic Infection

The interaction between parasites and the immune system is complex and parasites have evolved mechanisms so that they can survive the immunologic processes of the host that normally protect against foreign invaders (see Chapters 12 and 13). In cases where parasites are recognized by the immune system, a characteristic histopathologic finding of amorphous eosinophilic material surrounded by granulomatous inflammation with an abundance of eosinophils occurring in response to parasitic infections as well as other infectious and non-infectious processes has been termed the Splendore–Hoeppli phenomenon (46). This phenomenon has been observed in the conjunctiva; however, an organism has been found in only a minority of cases, suggesting that often the inflammatory process is successful in eliminating the pathogenic parasite. An imunohistochemical analysis of the amorphous central eosinophilic material found in the conjunctiva has revealed predominantly complement proteins in some specimens and the major basic protein of eosinophils in other cases. Eosinophil major protein, one of four cationic proteins found in cytoplasmic granules of eosinophils, is toxic to helminths. A histopathologic study of two cases has suggested that the immune response and formation of eosinophilic granuloma consists first of antibody deposition, immune complex formation and complement fixation in the early stages, followed by recruitment and degranulation of eosinophils in later stages (46).

The protozoan obligate intracellular parasite *Toxoplasma gondii* commonly infects humans and is a leading cause of posterior uveitis (see Chapter 12). Infection results in IgM and IgG antibodies but these are insufficient to provide immunity because the organism persists intracellularly. As one would expect, the intracellular parasite elicits a predominantly CD8+ T-cell response. The T cells in turn release cytokines particularly IFNγ that activate macrophages, recruiting them to sites of infection where they function both as effector and APCs. *Toxoplasma* actively invades both phagocytic and nonphagocytic cells, forming a non-fusogenic compartment, called the parasitophosphorous vacule, within the host cell cytosol (49). This compartment lacks many host cell membrane proteins and is unable to fuse with cell lysosmes. In contrast dead or opsonized parasites are taken up by phagocytes into normally functioning intracellular vacules which fuse with lysosomes thereby introducing the pathogens to an acidified hydrolytic environment. By blocking fusion with lysosomes the organism prevents pathogen-derived peptides from being expressed on the host cell's MHC molecules and evade the host immune system. Hence *Toxoplasma* may remain dormant within intracytoplasmic vesicles without exciting an immune response. Intracellular *Toxoplasma* has also been shown to actively interfere with transcription factors necessary for cytokine expression, including IL12, IFNγ, TNFα, and others (49). Furthermore, induced apoptotic pathways in macrophages infected with *Toxoplasma* are strongly inhibited, allowing intracellular parasites to survive longer in the host cell.

Once *Toxoplasma* replicates, the host cell becomes destroyed and the pathogen is opsonized and engulfed by macrophages which can then present antigen to both CD4+ T cells that typically produce Th1 cytokines and CD8+ T cells that eliminate infected cells and further drive the inflammatory process. Hypersensitivity reactions have also been implicated in toxoplasmosis. Results from monkey studies (65) have suggested that while retinochoroiditis results from an immune response directed toward heat-inactivated organism, vitritis, vasculitis, anterior uveitis and neuritis may result from hypersensitivity reactions. The immune mechanisms of these reactions have not been well characterized.

REFERENCES

1. Abbas AK, Lichtman AH. Basic Immunology: Functions and Disorders of the Immune System. 2nd ed. Philadelphia: Saunders, 2006.
2. Adamus G, Chan CC. Experimental autoimmune uveitides: multiple antigens, diverse diseases. Int Rev Immunol 2002; 21:209–29.
3. Allansmith MR, Greiner JV, Baird RS. Number of inflammatory cells in the normal conjunctiva. Am J Ophthalmol 1978; 86:250–9.
4. Barron KD. The microglial cell. A historical review. J Neurol Sci 1995; 134(Suppl. 27):57–68.
5. Bonini S, Micera A, Iovieno A, et al. Expression of Toll-like receptors in healthy and allergic conjunctiva. Ophthalmology 2005; 112:1528.e1–1528.e8.
6. Brix TH, Kyvik KO, Christensen K, Hegedus L. Evidence for a major role of heredity in Graves' disease: a population-based study of two Danish twin cohorts. J Clin Endocrinol Metab 2001; 86:930–4.
7. Camelo S, Kezic J, McMenamin PG. Anterior chamber-associated immune deviation: a review of the anatomical evidence for the afferent arm of this unusual experimental model of ocular immune responses. Clin Exp Ophthalmol 2005; 33:426–32.
8. Caspi RR. Th1 and Th2 responses in pathogenesis and regulation of experimental autoimmune uveoretinitis. Int Rev Immunol 2002; 21:197–208.
9. Cassone A, De Bernardis F, Torososantucci A. An outline of the role of anti-*Candida* antibodies within the context of passive immunization and protection from candidiasis. Curr Mol Med 2005; 5:377–82.
10. Cenci E, Mencacci A, Fe d'Ostiani C, et al. Cytokine- and T-helper-dependent immunity in murine aspergillosis. Res Immunol ????; 149:445–54.
11. Davidson A, Diamond B. Autoimmune diseases. N Engl J Med 2001; 345:340–50.
12. Dick AD, Cheng YF, Liversidge J, Forrester JV. Intranasal administration of retinal antigens suppresses retinal antigen-induced experimental autoimmune uveoretinitis. Immunology 1994; 82:625–31.
13. Espinosa-Heidmann DG, Suner IJ, Hernandez EP, et al. Macrophage depletion diminishes lesion size and severity in experimental choroidal neovascularization. Invest Ophthalmol Vis Sci 2003; 44:3586–92.
14. Fidel PL Jr. Immunity to *Candida*. Oral Dis 2002; 8(Suppl. 2): 69–75.
15. Franklin RM, Remus LE. Conjunctival-associated lymphoid tissue: evidence for a role in the secretory immune system. Invest Ophthalmol Vis Sci 1984; 25:181–7.
16. Gell PGH, Coombs RRA. The classification of allergic reactions underlying disease. In: Coombs RRA, Gell PGH, eds. Clinical Aspects of Immunology. Philadelphia: FA Davis Co., 1963; 317–37.
17. Hageman GS, Mullins RF. Molecular composition of drusen as related to subretinal phenotype. Mol Vis 1999; 5:28–37.
18. Hall JM. Specificity of antibody formation after intravitreal immunization with bovine gamma globulin and

ovalbumin. I. Primary response. Invest Ophthalmol Vis Sci 1971; 10:775–83.

19. Heiligenhaus A, Dutt JE, Foster CS. Histology and immunopathology of systemic lupus erythematosus affecting the conjunctiva. Eye 1996; 10:425–32.
20. Hembry RM, Playfair J, Watson PG, Dingle JT. Experimental model for scleritis. Arch Ophthalmol 1979; 97:1337–40.
21. Janeway C. Immunobiology: The Immune System in Health and Disease. 6th ed. New York: Garland Science, 2005.
22. Jongen PJ, Heessen FW, Bergmann I, et al. Coxsackie B1 virus-induced murine myositis: a correlative study of muscular lesions and serological changes. J Autoimmun 1994; 7:727–37.
23. Kasp E, Graham EM, Stanford MR, et al. A point prevalence study of 150 patients with idiopathic retinal vasculitis: 2. Clinical relevance of antiretinal autoimmunity and circulating immune complexes. Br J Ophthalmol 1989; 73:722–30.
24. Lassmann S, Kincaid C, Asensio VC, Campbell IL. Induction of type 1 immune pathology in the brain following immunization without central nervous system autoantigen in transgenic mice with astrocyte-targeted expression of IL-12. J Immunol 2001; 167:5485–93.
25. Lilic D. New perspectives on the immunology of chronic mucocutaneous candidiasis. Curr Opin Infect Dis 2002; 15: 143–7.
26. Liu H, Meagher CK, Moore CP, Phillips TE. M cells in the follicle-associated epithelium of the rabbit conjunctiva preferentially bind and translocate latex beads. Invest Ophthalmol Vis Sci 2005; 46:4217–23.
27. Marak GE Jr, Font RL, Johnson MC, Alepa FP. Lymphocyte-stimulating activity of ocular tissues in sympathetic ophthalmia. Invest Ophthalmol 1971; 10:770–4.
28. McKenzie J, King A, Hare J, et al. Immunocytochemical characterization of large granular lymphocytes in normal cervix and HPV associated disease. J Pathol 1991; 165: 75–80.
29. Medzhitov R, Janeway C Jr. Innate immunity. N Engl J Med 2000; 343:338–44.
30. Merigan TC. Human interferon as a therapeutic agent: a decade passes. N Engl J Med 1988; 318:1458–60.
31. Mircheff AK, Gierow JP, Wood RL. Autoimmunity of the lacrimal gland. Int Ophthalmol Clin 1994; 34:1–18.
32. Modlin RL. Th1–Th2 paradigm: insights from leprosy. J Invest Dermatol 1994; 102:828–32.
33. Mondino BJ, Laheji AK, Adamu SA. Ocular immunity to *Staphylococcus aureus*. Invest Ophthalmol Vis Sci 1987; 28: 560–4.
34. Mullins RF, Aptsiauri N, Hageman GS. Structure and composition of drusen associated with glomerulonephritis: implications for the role of complement activation in drusen biogenesis. Eye 2001; 15:390–5.
35. Murphy CC, Duncan L, Forrester JV, Dick AD. Systemic CD4(+) T cell phenotype and activation status in intermediate uveitis. Br J Ophthalmol 2004; 88:412–6.
36. Netea MG, van Tits LJ, Curfs JH, et al. Increased susceptibility of TNF-alpha lymphotoxin-alpha double knockout mice to systemic candidiasis through impaired recruitment of neutrophils and phagocytosis of *Candida albicans*. J Immunol 1999; 163:1498–505.
37. Newport MJ, Huxley CM, Huston S, et al. A mutation in the interferon-gamma-receptor gene and susceptibility to mycobacterial infection. N Engl J Med 1996; 335:1941–9.
38. Nussenblatt R. Orally and nasally induced tolerance studies in ocular inflammatory disease: guidance for future interventions. Ann N Y Acad Sci 2004; 1029: 278–85.
39. O'Garra A, Vieira P. Regulatory T cells and mechanisms of immune system control. Nat Med 2004; 10:801–5.
40. Oleszak EL, Kuzmak J, Good RA, Platsoucas CD. Immunology of Theiler's murine encephalomyelitis virus infection. Immunol Res 1995; 14:13–33.
41. Patel N, Ohbayashi M, Nugent AK, et al. Circulating anti-retinal antibodies as immune markers in age-related macular degeneration. Immunology 2005; 115:422–30.
42. Pflugfelder SC. Lacrimal gland epithelium and immunopathology. In: Homma M, ed. Proceedings of the IV International Sjögren Syndrome Symposium. Amsterdam: Kugler, 1994:9–12.
43. Rao NA, Hidayat AA. Endogenous mycotic endophthalmitis: variations in clinical and histopathologic changes in candidiasis compared with aspergillosis. Am J Ophthalmol 2001; 132:244–51.
44. Rao NA, Wacker WB, Marak GE Jr. Experimental allergic uveitis: clinicopathologic features associated with varying doses of S antigen. Arch Ophthalmol 1979; 97:1954–8.
45. Rao NA, Robin J, Hartmann D, et al. The role of the penetrating wound in the development of sympathetic ophthalmia experimental observations. Arch Ophthalmol 1983; 101:102–4.
46. Read RW, Zhang J, Albini T, et al. Splendore-Hoeppli phenomenon in the conjunctiva: immunohistochemical analysis. Am J Ophthalmol 2005; 140:262–6.
47. Rohatgi J, Dhaliwal U. Phlyctenular eye disease: a reappraisal. Jpn J Ophthalmol 2000; 44:146–50.
48. Rose NR. Mechanisms of autoimmunity. Semin Liver Dis 2002; 22:387–94.
49. Sacks D, Sher A. Evasion of innate immunity by parasitic protozoa. Nat Immunol 2002; 3:1041–7.
50. Sall K, Stevenson OD, Mundorf TK, Reis BL. Two multicenter, randomized studies of the efficacy and safety of cyclosporine ophthalmic emulsion in moderate to severe dry eye disease. CsA Phase 3 Study Group. Ophthalmology 2000; 107:631–9.
51. Sawatzki G, Rich IN. Lactoferrin stimulates colony stimulating factor production in vitro and in vivo. Blood Cells 1989; 15:371–85.
52. Shao H, Sun SL, Kaplan HJ, Sun D. Characterization of rat CD8+ uveitogenic T cells specific for interphotoreceptor retinal-binding protein 1177–91. J Immunol 2004; 173: 2849–54.
53. Silverstein AM. A History of Immunology. San Diego, CA: Academic Press, 1989.
54. Smolin G, Hyndiuk RA. Lymphatic drainage from vascularized rabbit cornea. Am J Ophthalmol 1971; 72: 147–51.
55. Smolin G. The role of tears in the prevention of infections. Int Ophthalmol Clin 1987; 27:25–6.
56. Smolin G, Friedlaender MH. Immunology of ocular tissues. In: Tasman W, ed. Duane's Foundations of Clinical Ophthalmology. Chapter 26. Vol. 2. New York: Lippincott Williams and Wilkins, 1995; 1–8.
57. Sonoda KH, Sakamoto T, Qiao H, et al. The analysis of systemic tolerance elicited by antigen inoculation into the vitreous cavity: vitreous cavity-associated immune deviation. Immunology 2005; 116:390–9.
58. Streilein JW, Dana MR, Ksander BR. Immunity causing blindness: five different paths to herpes stromal keratitis. Immunol Today 1997; 18:443–9.
59. Streilein JW. Ocular immune privilege: the eye takes a dim but practical view of immunity and inflammation. J Leukoc Biol 2003; 74:179–85.

60. Tomer Y. Unraveling the genetic susceptibility to autoimmune thyroid diseases: CTLA-4 takes the stage. Thyroid 2001; 11:167–9.
61. Trousdale MD, Zhu Z, Stevenson D, et al. Expression of TNF inhibitor gene in the lacrimal gland promotes recovery of tear production and tear stability and reduced immunopathology in rabbits with induced autoimmune dacryoadenitis. J Autoimmune Dis 2005; 2:6.
62. Wacker WB. Experimental allergic uveitis. Studies on characterization and isolation of the pathogenic retina antigen. Int Arch Allergy Appl Immunol 1973; 45(5):639–56.
63. Wacker WB. Retinal autoimmunity: two decades of research. Jpn J Ophthalmol 1987; 31:188–96.
64. Watkins NG, Hadlow WJ, Moos AB, Caldwell HD. Ocular delayed hypersensitivity: a pathogenetic mechanism of chlamydial-conjunctivitis in guinea pigs. Proc Natl Acad Sci USA 1986; 83:7480–4.
65. Webb RM, Tabbara KF, O'Connor GR. Retinal vasculitis in ocular toxoplasmosis in nonhuman primates. Retina 1984; 4:182–8.
66. Wenkel H, Streilein JW. Analysis of immune deviation elicited by antigens injected into the subretinal space. Invest Ophthalmol Vis Sci 1998; 39:1823–34.
67. Wu GS, Sevanian A, Rao NA. Detection of retinal lipid hydroperoxides in experimental uveitis. Free Radic Biol Med 1992; 12:19–27.
68. Wu GS, Lee TD, Moore RE, Rao NA. Photoreceptor mitochondrial tyrosine nitration in experimental uveitis. Invest Ophthalmol Vis Sci 2005; 46:2271–81.
69. Yamaki K, Gocho K, Hayakawa K, et al. Tyrosinase family proteins are antigens specific to Vogt-Koyanagi-Harada disease. J Immunol 2000; 165:7323–9.
70. Young RA. Stress proteins and immunology. Annu Rev Immunol 1990; 8:401–20.

4

Intraocular Manifestations of Immune Disorders

Julie H. Tsai
University of South Carolina School of Medicine, Columbia, South Carolina, U.S.A.

Narsing A. Rao
Doheny Eye Institute, Keck School of Medicine, University of Southern California, Los Angeles, California, U.S.A.

INTRODUCTION

Uveitis is an intraocular inflammation involving primarily the uveal tract, an intraocular structure derived from embryonic mesoderm and neural crest. The iris, ciliary body, and choroid of the eye can have various degrees of involvement. Visual loss often depends on the affected intraocular structure(s) and the type and severity of uveitis. Inflammation in these individual regions can be induced by autoimmune disease, malignancy, infection or trauma to the eye. Most forms of idiopathic uveitis appear to be immune-mediated. Posterior and panuveitis may involve T cells, but inflammatory conditions presenting with anterior uveitis may be B-cell mediated. For instance, sympathetic ophthalmia (SO) and Vogt–Koyanagi–Harada disease (VKH) show features consistent with T-cell disorders; phacoantigenic uveitis (PU) seems to occur secondary to immune complex formation; and Fuchs heterochromic iridocyclitis (FHI) may be B-cell mediated.

All of these entities are characterized by inflammatory cell infiltration in the uvea; choroidal involvement is prominent in SO and VKH disease, whereas inflammatory infiltration of the iris and ciliary body is the main feature in FHI and PU. In contrast, the inflammatory process in pars planitis is mainly observed in the pars plana ciliaris and adjacent peripheral retina with infiltration of the anterior part of the vitreous by chronic inflammatory cells. As the interactions between humoral and cellular immunity are often complex, animal models of uveitis have been developed in order to study the clinical course of these diseases as well as emerging therapies that may ameliorate the signs and symptoms of these diseases.

FUCHS HETEROCHROMIC IRIDOCYCLITIS

Overview

Fuchs heterochromic iridocyclitis, also known as Fuchs uveitis syndrome, primarily involves anterior chamber cell infiltration and iris heterochromia. The disease begins insidiously, affecting young adults and accounting for 1.2% to 4.5% of referrals to ophthalmologists in uveitis practice. However, FHI has a variable presentation and may be under diagnosed because of the subtleties of its clinical presentation (6,13,19,55,87).

Clinical Features

Fuchs heterochromic iridocyclitis is characterized by low-grade anterior uveitis with iris heterochromia, as well as a fine neovascularization, often seen bridging the angle on gonioscopy. These blood vessels tend to bleed during paracentesis of the anterior chamber. Patients with FHI typically have no complaints of pain, redness or photophobia. Inflammatory cells may spill over into the anterior vitreous, occasionally causing a mild to moderate reaction. Many patients are diagnosed incidentally and may have excellent visual acuity. However, some present with blurred vision secondary to cataract or vitreous floaters.

The disease is usually unilateral, although bilateral disease has been reported in 15% of cases (20). The initial findings include iris stromal atrophy and heterochromia iridis, with the involved eye being lighter in color and having a "moth-eaten" appearance, with transillumination of patchy segments of the iris. In blue-eyed individuals, the affected eye may be darker since atrophy of the anterior iris stroma reveals the underlying pigmented epithelium (reverse heterochromia). Fine, stellate keratic precipitates (KPs) can be seen scattered over the entire endothelial surface of the cornea but all types of precipitates, including the granulomatous "mutton-fat" type, have been described (55). Cataract is seen in >80% of cases and glaucoma affects 25% to 60% of patients, arising either from the inflammation or from corticosteroid therapy (20,36). Most importantly, the chronic inflammation of FHI does not usually cause posterior synechiae or cystoid macular edema, unlike other causes of anterior uveitis. Anterior segment fluorescein angiography reveals peripupillary dye leakage, delayed iris filling and areas of ischemia associated with neovascularization. A characteristic filiform hemorrhage occurs with anterior chamber paracentesis (Amsler sign), which occurs due to fine neovascular vessels with gonioscopy that can be seen crossing the angle (1).

Histopathology

A chronic, non-granulomatous inflammatory reaction is seen on light microscopy in the iris, ciliary body and trabecular meshwork. The iris stroma contains blood vessels with endothelial cell proliferation and hyalinized walls, and plasma cells, which often contain Russell bodies. In longstanding cases the iris stroma atrophies and the sphincter pupillae muscle becomes fibrotic. Inflammatory membranes may be seen on the anterior surface of the iris and ciliary body. Fine neovascularization of the anterior surface of the iris and the anterior chamber angle are also present. There are no distinctive light or transmission electron microscopic (TEM) features that differentiate FHI from other types of anterior uveitis.

Etiology and Pathogenesis

Several hypotheses have been proposed to explain the cause and pathogenesis of FHI, including neurogenic, vascular, infectious and inflammatory-immunologic mechanisms. The discoloration of the iris was originally thought to derive from a congenital paralysis of the sympathetic system; however, Loewenfeld and Thompson found no convincing evidence to support such an explanation (44,45). Other neurogenic associations include isolated cases of FHI found concomitantly with hemifacial atrophy and Moebius syndrome, although neither entity presents with intraocular inflammation (20,23,32,37).

The presence of irregular iris blood vessels and neovascularization has been suggested as a possible pathogenetic factor of FHI (5,77). Immune complexes may also be implicated in hyalinization and endothelial proliferation of iris vessel walls (24).

In some individuals, FHI has been noted in conjunction with chorioretinal scars resembling those seen in ocular toxoplasmosis, indicating an infectious etiology. Antibodies against *Toxoplasma gondii* in the blood and aqueous humor of patients with FHI have been reported but causality has never been firmly established (42,55,84). *Herpes simplex* virus (HSV) has also been considered as a possible causal agent and this virus has been detected in the aqueous humor in one case of FHI (55). Other studies have failed to detect HSV DNA or local antibody formation (4,55,64).

Patients with FHI have circulating immune complexes, which can deposit in the iris vessels, leading to their occlusion, ischemia and neovascularization of the iris as described above. Moreover, deposits of these complexes can activate the complement cascade, and lead to the generation of various cytokines and the recruitment of inflammatory cells. Experimental uveitis models induced by various ocular antigens, cytokines and endotoxin have not revealed clinical and histological features similar to FHI, suggesting that the cause of the inflammatory response in FHI remains unknown.

Lymphocytes, plasma cells, mast cells and eosinophils are observed in the irides of patients with FHI indicates that an inflammatory reaction is part of the disease. Some reports indicate normal numbers and function of B cells and T cells in the peripheral blood, while others note activation of these cells. Receptors for interleukin 2 (IL2), a marker for early

T-lymphocyte activity, have been reported to be high in the peripheral blood (3,59). High levels of interleukin 6 (IL6) have also been noted in the anterior chamber compared with peripheral blood (55,60). Increased B-lymphocyte activity and immunoglobulin G (IgG) levels in the anterior chamber may be a result of increased IL6 levels, suggesting that FHI may be B-cell driven (61). Despite such cytokine and activated B-cell and T-cell activity, these findings do not allow a comprehensive explanation of the disease process.

INTERMEDIATE UVEITIS

Overview

Intermediate uveitis is an intraocular inflammatory disorder that primarily involves the anterior vitreous, pars plana and peripheral retina. Such inflammation is seen in patients with sarcoidosis, multiple sclerosis (see Chapter 70), human T-cell leukemia virus I (HTLV-I) infection, tuberculosis and inflammatory bowel disease (7,17,54,65,100). However, the vast majority of patients have no known infectious disease or systemic disorder associated with their intermediate uveitis, and such idiopathic cases are recognized as pars planitis.

Clinical Features

Pars planitis is a fairly common form of bilateral uveitis that accounts for about 15% of all cases seen in referral uveitis clinics (28). Patients are usually between the ages of 5 and 40 years, with a bimodal age distribution (younger group: 5–15 yrs, older group: 20–40 yrs) (30). There is no overall sex or racial predilection. The clinical course can be divided into three categories: a self-limited, benign course; a chronic, indolent course; and a chronic course with remissions and exacerbations. Patients usually report blurred vision, floaters and distorted central vision. Up to 80% of cases are bilateral at presentation (27,82) with organized exudates on the pars plana.

Only mild anterior segment inflammation is usually noted upon clinical examination. KPs, if present, are sparse and most often found in the inferior quadrant of the corneal endothelium. The hallmark of the disease is vitritis, which consists of vitreous cells that form aggregates, commonly referred to as "snowballs." The pars plana inflammation may progress to form organized exudates called "snowbanks." Vascular sheathing and retinal neovascularization can also be observed in the inferior peripheral retina. The neovascular areas can bleed, resulting in vitreous hemorrhage and peripheral tractional and rhegmatogenous retinal detachments (8). Cystoid macular edema is the most frequent complication, leading to visual loss (46,65). The optic disc may also manifest hyperemia, edema and neovascularization (38).

Histopathology

The classic snowbank typically involves the area surrounding the vitreous base of the inferior retina. Histological examination of this area demonstrates fibroglial and vascular proliferation with an infiltration of lymphocytes. Although this material appears clinically as an exudate, it is composed of an organized inflammatory cell infiltration. Lymphocytic cuffing surrounds the peripheral retinal veins, and an infiltration of lymphocytes has been noted in the peripheral choroid. The vascular component of the snowbank is presumably related to preretinal neovascularization. Pederson et al. found that the blood vessels involved in the snowbank are sometimes continuous with the retina, and these retinal vessels can extend through breaks in the inner limiting membrane (ILM) (63). Furthermore, inflammation of the choroid or ciliary body is mild in the inflammatory process appearing to involve primarily the peripheral retina and vitreous base (63).

The snowballs in intermediate uveitis contain B cells with a smaller number of T cells, phagocytic cells and cellular debris. Occasionally, the epithelioid cells and multinucleated giant cells may be seen in the vitreous and such cells are not found in the uvea, suggesting that the vitreous is the primary site of inflammation (26).

An ultrastructural evaluation of the snowbank by Yoser et al. revealed condensed and collapsed vitreous, along with fibrous astrocytes with fibroglial membranes, collagen production and non-pigmented ciliary epithelial cell inclusions (98). In addition, the authors noted high endothelial venules and experimental animal studies suggest that the endothelial cells of such vessels play a role in lymphocyte traffic, attachment and migration through the vessel wall into the extracellular matrix. The presence of the high endothelial venules within the fibrous organization of the pars plana may play a role in the recurrence of the inflammatory process and in recruitment of cells at the site of fibrovascular proliferation.

Etiology and Pathogenesis

Other studies have noted no significant choroidal inflammation; supporting the hypothesis that intermediate uveitis does not originate from the choroid (89). The cause of pars planitis remains unknown. Numerous studies have reported human leukocyte antigen (HLA) associations and several subtypes are more frequent in these patients, including HLA-B8, HLA-B51, HLA-DR17, HLA-DR51 and HLA-DR2. HLA-DR15, a suballele of HLA-DR2, has been shown to have the highest association with intermediate uveitis/pars planitis, since it is present in 64.3% to 72% of patients (17). This same allele is associated with multiple sclerosis and may serve to explain the relationship between the two disorders. This HLA association suggests an autoimmune process in the pathogenesis of pars planitis.

SYMPATHETIC OPHTHALMIA

Overview

Sympathetic ophthalmia, also known as sympathetic uveitis, is a rare, bilateral granulomatous panuveitis that occurs after a penetrating injury to one eye. The injured eye is referred to as the exciting eye. The uninjured, or sympathizing, eye usually develops clinical signs and symptoms after a latent period of anywhere from a few days to several decades after the initial injury (25,99). In general, the interval between the time of injury and the onset of symptoms is rarely less than two weeks. The majority of cases (70–80%) occur within 3 months, and 90% within 1 year; the peak incidence occurs 4 to 8 weeks after the original injury (12). Historically, various authors have reported incidences ranging from 0.28 to 12% following penetrating injury (25). In 1972, Liddy and Stuart reported an incidence of 0.19% following penetrating trauma and 0.07% following intraocular surgery (43). Currently, SO occurs in about 0.2% to 0.5% of patients with eye injuries and 0.01% of those who undergo intraocular surgery (12). The risk of SO increases when surgical procedures are accompanied or followed by additional operations, particularly those involving the posterior segment (25). There is a slight male predilection; but this likely reflects the difference in frequency of ocular injury between the sexes.

Clinical Features

The most prominent clinical feature of SO is its diffuse, intraocular granulomatous inflammatory response. After the inciting injury, whether traumatic or surgical, patients may present with symptoms ranging from mild blurring of vision to significant visual loss in the sympathizing eye. There may also be decreased vision and increased photophobia in the exciting eye. Typically, bilateral posterior and/or anterior uveitis with cells, flare and "mutton-fat" KPs are seen. Inflammatory nodules may be noted in the iris stroma. Complete posterior synechiae may form, possibly resulting in secondary glaucoma. In the posterior segment, the severity of inflammation may vary and can include vitritis, choroiditis, and papillitis. Serous retinal detachment, edema of the optic nerve head and hyperemia may be observed. Whitish-yellow lesions, known as Dalen–Fuchs nodules, can be seen at the level of the retinal pigment epithelium (RPE). Chronic intraocular inflammation can lead to a number of vision-limiting complications, including cataract, glaucoma, subretinal neovascularization and fibrosis, and atrophy of the retina, choroid and optic nerve. Rarely, extraocular findings such as poliosis, vitiligo, alopecia and dysacusis can be demonstrated in the patient with SO (25).

Before the use of systemic corticosteroids, the visual prognosis for patients with SO was generally poor, with approximately 70% of the affected eyes becoming permanently blind. With corticosteroid therapy, 65% of patients can maintain a visual acuity of 20/60 or better, and 93% maintain vision of 20/400 or better. The prognosis of SO has improved since the introduction of cyclosporine and other immunomodulatory agents (25).

Histopathology

The histologic features of SO are similar in the exciting and sympathizing eye, with the exception of the wound site. The uvea is diffusely thickened by non-necrotizing granulomatous inflammation. The uveal infiltrate consists of lymphocytes, nests of epithelioid cells and variable proportions of multinucleated giant cells. The cytoplasm of both epithelioid cells and giant cells contains melanin granules. The uveal thickening is more prominent in the peripapillary region. In the majority of cases, the inflammatory process does not involve the choriocapillaris or the retina; this is because most of the globes enucleated for SO are removed during the acute phase of the disease (Fig. 1). Lastly, typical Dalen-Fuchs nodules reveal clusters of proliferated RPE cells, histiocytes and epithelioid mononuclear cells on Bruch membrane.

Etiology and Pathogenesis

The cause of SO is still obscure and early theories of infection as the initiating event have not been substantiated. The autoimmune hypothesis, on the other hand, is increasingly supported by both clinical and experimental studies. The penetrating trauma is believed to initiate the immune cascade generated against uveal self-antigens. Also, the association of peripheral signs, such as discoloration and depigmentation of integumentary structures (e.g., poliosis, vitiligo and alopecia) may suggest a more generalized response against melanocytes. The original animal experiment that produced intraocular inflammation resembling SO was performed by sensitizing guinea pigs with whole uvea and a retinal homogenate in complete Freund adjuvant (14,15). Three immunogenic proteins were identified in these preparations: retinal soluble protein (S-antigen, now known as arrestin), rhodopsin, and uveal antigen.

Rao et al. showed variations in the clinical and histopathological features in guinea pigs injected with varying doses of S-antigen (49,70). These animals developed acute necrotizing panuveitis when injected with a high dose (50 μg) of arrestin and a mild

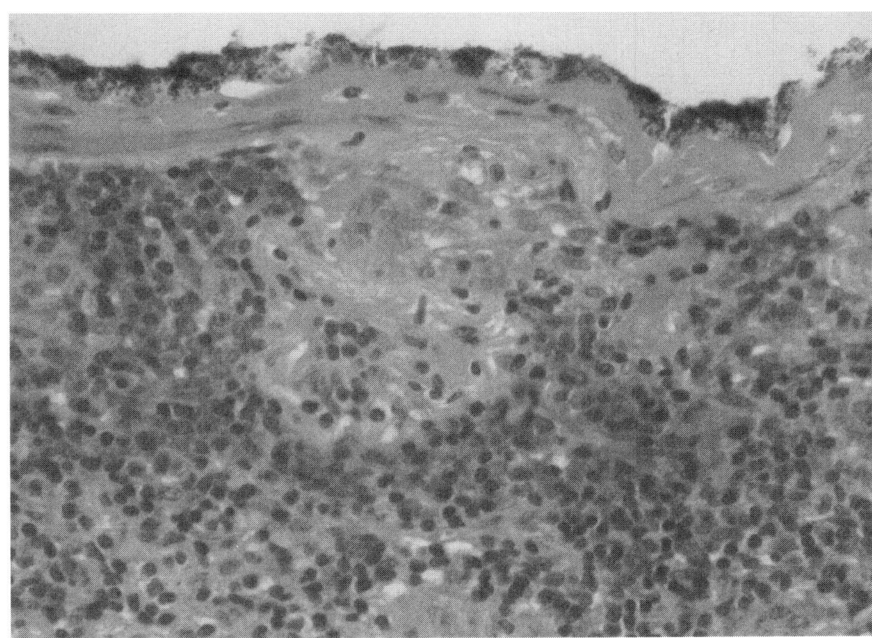

Figure 1 Sympathetic ophthalmia showing granulomatous choroiditis with preservation of choriocapillaris (hematoxylin and eosin, ×320).

non-granulomatous choroiditis with a low dose (1 μg). With an intermediate dose of 10 to 25 mcg of arrestin they developed non-necrotizing granulomatous panuveitis with Dalen–Fuchs nodules, virtually identical to those seen in human SO. Moreover, the experimental animals had melanosomes in the epithelioid and giant cells.

Inflammation limited to the uvea can be produced in rats immunized with partially purified melanin, as reported by Broekhuyse et al. (9), and spontaneous recurrent uveitis has been reported in the same model. Caspi et al. were able to reproduce uveitis in two mouse strains by immunizing the animals with arrestin or interphotoreceptor binding protein (IRBP) (10). A relatively high dose of antigen and an intensified immunization protocol produced disease that occurred later, was of longer duration, and had a less acute course. Damage to the retina and uvea was focal rather than diffuse. It was suggested that this model appeared to be better, approximating some types of human uveitis with respect to its pathologic manifestations and its more chronic course (10). Based on these observations, it appears that retinal or uveal antigens may be uveitogenic in SO. However, the retinal antigens induce primarily retinitis (Fig. 2), which is rarely seen in human SO.

Further studies conducted by Rao et al. revealed the importance of penetrating injury in exposing the uveitogenic intraocular antigens to the conjunctival lymphatics drainage for the development of SO (69). In their experimental study an intraocular injection of arrestin into one eye did not produce uveitis in the contralateral eye; however, subconjunctival injections of the antigen readily caused inflammation in the contralateral eye. These observations suggest that extrusion of uveal or retinal antigens into the surrounding ocular tissues may be a key in sensitization to the antigen; the rich lymphatic drainage of the conjunctiva along with possible bacterial contamination of the wound may reinforce the sensitization and subsequent development of bilateral uveitis. Despite such findings, the low rate of SO is yet to be accounted for, despite the fact that extruded intraocular tissue is often encountered in cases of trauma. Moreover, the rare incidence of SO in patients with filtering blebs cannot be explained, despite the possible exposure of retinal/uveal antigens to the conjunctival lymphatics.

Genetic predisposition may explain the low rates of SO after traumatic or surgical injury. Several HLA haplotypes (HLA-A11, HLA-B40, HLA DR4/DRw53, and HLA-DR4/DQw3) have known associations with SO (18,40,73,79). Genetic susceptibility may be a prerequisite for the development of SO.

In SO, the uveitis typically reveals pigment-containing epithelioid and giant cells in the absence of apparent uveal necrosis by light microscopy. Immunohistochemical studies show that the pigment-containing epithelioid cells express markers of histiocytes. The presence of phagocytosed pigment in these cells suggests that the choroidal melanocytes could undergo necrosis or apoptosis. Moreover, transformation of histiocytes to epithelioid cells requires T helper cell cytokines, particularly those involved in the Th1 immune response. Such observations, along with the detection of T-cell infiltration in the choroidal infiltrates of SO, suggest that SO is a

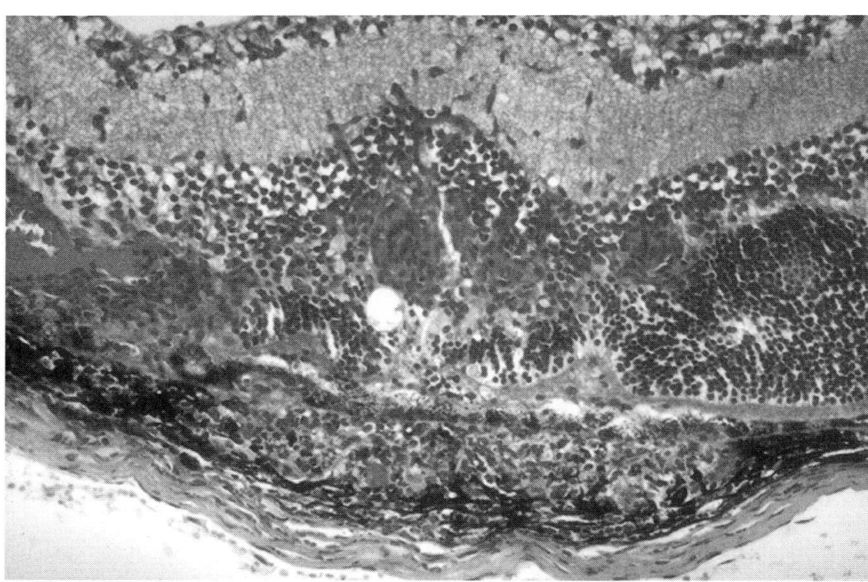

Figure 2 B10A mouse immunized with IRBP reveals retinitis with thickening of pigmented choroid from inflammatory cell infiltration (hematoxylin and eosin, ×240).

helper T-cell type 1 (Th1)-mediated process resulting from altered tolerance to intraocular proteins, in particular uveal melanin peptides (tyrosinase peptides).

Another typical feature of SO is the preservation of the choriocapillaris in the presence of a heavy infiltration of the choroid by inflammatory cells. The RPE generates several cytokines and proteins that could suppress the inflammatory cell infiltration into the choriocapillaris and one of these proteins suppresses the generation of oxidants by the inflammatory cells, possibly protecting the choriocapillaris in SO (91,92). Despite the presence of macrophages in Dalen-Fuchs nodules, the choriocapillaris and overlying retina at the sites of these nodules are not damaged, perhaps because of the presence of proliferating RPE cells within the nodules.

The combination of the animal studies, the HLA haplotype association, bilateral granulomatous uveitis with inflammatory cells at the sites of melanocytes and the response of the uveitis to the specific T-cell inhibitor cyclosporine suggests that SO is a T-cell–mediated process that develops from altered tolerance to uveal melanocyte protein. Penetrating injury, allowing exposure of the intraocular antigen to lymphatics in genetically susceptible individuals, may play a role in altering the tolerance and inducing the uveitis.

VOGT–KOYANAGI–HARADA DISEASE

Overview

Vogt–Koyanagi–Harada disease is a systemic disorder that involves the eye, skin, ear, and central nervous system (CNS). It is characterized by bilateral granulomatous uveitis associated with exudative retinal detachment and by extraocular manifestations, including pleocytosis of the cerebrospinal fluid (CSF), dysacusis and, in some cases, poliosis, alopecia, and vitiligo. The entity has become better characterized and the First International Workshop on VKH adopted the term VKH disease (67).

While VKH disease is relatively common among pigmented races, it is rarely seen in whites. It accounts for 6.8% to 9.2% of patients with uveitis in Japan and 1% to 4% in the United States (56). It generally affects adults, primarily between the ages of 20 and 50 years, without a clear sex predilection, although some reports indicate that the majority of patients are women (67).

Clinical Features

Typical clinical features include bilateral panuveitis associated with exudative retinal detachments; meningismus associated with headache and CSF pleocytosis; dysacusis ranging from tinnitus to hearing loss; and cutaneous changes such as vitiligo, poliosis, and alopecia (Fig. 3). The clinical features vary with the stage of the disease and all of them are rarely seen during the initial presentation. Symptoms during the prodromal stage may be limited to headaches, nausea, dizziness, orbital pain, fever, and meningismus. Tearing and light sensitivity may occur 1 to 2 days after the onset of the initial symptoms. Rarely, specific neurological signs, such as cranial nerve palsy or optic neuritis, may occur. CSF analysis during this stage often reveals a lymphocytic pleocytosis.

In the acute uveitic stage, the initial symptoms involve the posterior segment and include a thickened

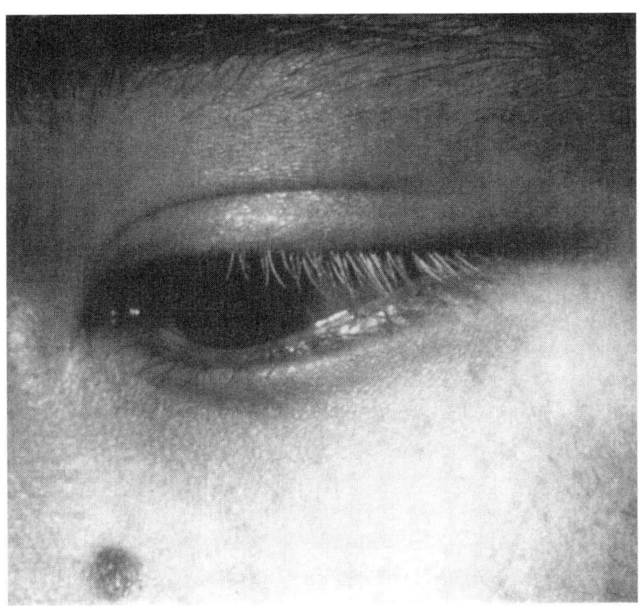

Figure 3 Vogt–Koyanagi–Harada syndrome. Vitiligo and poliosis are illustrated. *Source*: Courtesy of Dr. C.S. Foster.

posterior choroid, elevated peripapillary retinochoroidal layer, multiple serous retinal detachments, as well as hyperemia and edema of the optic nerve head. The inflammation then becomes more diffuse, extending into the anterior segment and manifesting as anterior chamber cells and a flare. Inflammation of the ciliary body can also occur and may result in forward displacement of the lens iris diaphragm, leading to acute angle-closure glaucoma or annular choroidal detachment (39,96).

Chronic cases often have a characteristic depigmentation of the eye, the earliest sign of which can be seen in the perilimbal area (Sugiura sign). Depigmentation of the choroid results in a mottled appearance with a bright orange-red color described as a "sunset glow" fundus. Multiple small areas of chorioretinal atrophy can be seen in the inferior midperiphery. These lesions do not coincide with Dalen-Fuchs nodules as described in cases of SO. Rather, they appear more punched out due to a focal loss of the RPE and the formation of chorioretinal adhesions (33).

Extraocular signs and symptoms are important in diagnosing VKH disease, but these extraocular manifestations are more common in Asians than in white or Hispanic patients. Meningeal signs are often noted, and a CSF lymphocytic pleocytosis is seen in >80% of patients (41,95). Dysfunction of the inner ear often results in cochlear hearing loss in the high frequency range, rather than in vestibular symptoms. Increased sensitivity to touch of hair and skin may also be noted. Lastly, poliosis of the eyebrows, eyelashes and hair and varying degrees of alopecia can be observed. Vitiligo is another characteristic manifestation and it is often symmetric in distribution. These hair and skin findings are usually found during the late stages of disease and are noted concurrently with depigmentation of the ocular tissues. Cataract, secondary glaucoma, subretinal neovascularization and subretinal fibrosis often complicate recurrent inflammation (56,72).

Histopathology

The inflammatory process consists primarily of a diffuse thickening of the uveal tract with non-necrotizing granulomatous inflammation. Just as the clinical features of VKH differ at each stage of the disease, so do the histopathologic findings. In the acute stage, the sensory retina is detached from the RPE by a subretinal eosinophilic exudate containing proteinaceous material. The choroid is diffusely infiltrated by lymphocytes, intermixed with focal aggregates of epithelioid histiocytes and multinucleated giant cells. Although uveal necrosis is apparently absent, the macrophages, epithelioid cells, and giant cells contain intracytoplasmic uveal pigment granules. These changes are almost identical to those found in SO (68).

Focal disruptions of the RPE can be detected on fluorescein angiography during the acute uveitic phase (Fig. 4). Although, at the level of light microscopy, the RPE appears intact during this acute

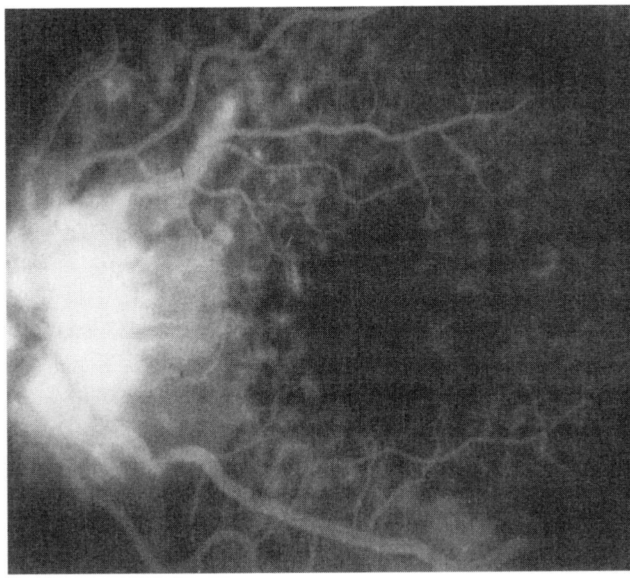

Figure 4 Fluorescein angiogram, patient with Vogt–Koyanagi–Harada (VKH) syndrome. Early pinpoint leakage of fluorescein dye at the level of the retinal pigment epithelium, followed by late staining at that level, are the features characteristic of VKH. Optic nerve inflammation in this eye is reflected by late staining of the nerve head. *Source*: Courtesy of Dr. C.S. Foster.

phase, and occasional lymphocytes can be seen under the RPE. Focal collections of mononuclear inflammatory cells under the elevated mounds of RPE represent Dalen–Fuchs nodules, similar to those noted in SO. Despite an extensive inflammatory cell infiltration in the choroid during the acute phase of VKH, these inflammatory cells do not involve the choriocapillaris or retina, a feature also observed in SO.

The number of inflammatory cells in the vitreous may vary. These cells probably enter the vitreous in the pars plana region of the ciliary body. Both pigmented and non-pigmented ciliary epithelial layers exhibit diffuse infiltration of inflammatory cells. The iris may reveal either granulomatous inflammation or a diffuse lymphocytic infiltration, predominantly in the stroma.

The convalescent stage of VKH is characterized by a mild to moderate non-granulomatous inflammation. The choroid is depigmented at this stage, displaying spindle-shaped melanocytes devoid of melanin granules, and presenting clinically as the "sunset glow" fundus. The RPE remains intact with the normal complement of melanin granules. Numerous small atrophic peripheral lesions are noted with choroidal depigmentation and atrophy involving the overlying choriocapillaris and the outer retina. At these sites the RPE is absent (33).

The chronic recurrent stage of VKH is characterized by a diffuse cellular infiltration of the uvea consisting of a granulomatous process similar to that seen in the acute stage. However, the uveal thickening in the chronic recurrent stage is less prominent and eyes enucleated at this stage tend to lack a retinal detachment. Chorioretinal adhesions, with RPE atrophy and/or proliferation, are common in the chronic recurrent stage. The hyperplastic RPE is hyperpigmented on ophthalmoscopic examination, although metaplastic proliferated RPE may also present as subretinal fibrosis. In association with the RPE changes, photoreceptor degeneration and gliosis is found in the overlying neural retina. At this stage the choriocapillaris is involved in the degenerative process and these sites manifest chorioretinal adhesions.

Etiology and Pathogenesis

The overlap of clinical findings and histopathologic changes in VKH disease and SO suggests that these two diseases represent similar immunologic processes. Inflammation can be found concomitantly with loss of melanocytes in the uvea and skin on histologic examination and presumably similar changes may be found in the meninges of the CNS and the inner ear. The exact cause of these findings has yet to be discerned, but recent findings suggest that an autoimmune process driven by T lymphocytes is directed against an as yet unidentified ligand associated with melanocytes or tyrosinase peptides. This process is not linked to any known mechanism, but sensitization to the melanocytic peptides may occur as a result of viral infection.

Immunohistochemical studies conducted on the eyes of patients with active VKH found an increased ratio of T-helper to T-suppressor cells, as well as the presence of activated T-lymphocytes expressing CD25, an antigen to the IL2 receptor and a marker of early T-lymphocyte activation. Another antigenic marker, CD26, was also observed on the cell surface, indicative of late T-lymphocyte activation (75). In the acute stage of VKH, these T-lymphocytes are seen in close proximity to uveal melanocytes, which express class II major histocompatibility complex (MHC), as noted in the convalescent stage of the disease. Ongoing inflammation consists mainly of T-lymphocytes, and the disappearance of choroidal melanocytes during this phase suggests that the melanocytes are likely target cells of the immune process. The melanocytes may play an active immunologic role in the uveitis, potentially serving as antigen-presenting cells. Experimental studies by Yamaki et al. indicate that tyrosinase peptides derived from the melanocytes could be the inciting antigen in the induction of VKH (94).

There are strong associations with the HLA-DR4 in Japanese patients diagnosed with VKH. Pre-dominant alleles of DRB1*0405 and HLA-DRB1*0410 have been noted in these patients and in a subset of individuals with VKH from Korea (80). In other ethnic groups with a high prevalence of VKH, other loci were more prominent. In the Hispanics of Southern California and the majority of Mexican Mestizo patients, HLA-DR1 and HLA-DR4 were found in 84% and 89% of patients with VKH, respectively (2,88). A higher relative risk with HLA-DR1 and HLA-DR4 was also noted by Weisz et al., 4.11 versus 1.96, respectively (88). These studies suggest that these specific HLA genes may confer increased risk for VKH.

PHACOANTIGENIC UVEITIS

Overview

Phacoantigenic uveitis is an intraocular inflammation induced by lens crystallins that occurs after surgical or traumatic rupture of the lens capsule. It accounts for <1% of all cases of uveitis and usually develops within days to weeks of the disruption of the lens capsule, although some cases have been reported to occur months later (28,74). It may occur within 24 hours of cataract surgery in a patient who has been previously sensitized to lens protein. In the past, several terms have been used to describe this entity, including phacoanaphylactic endophthalmitis or phacogenic ("phacotoxic") uveitis. These terms may be misleading, however, as the response is neither anaphylactic nor toxic; there is no

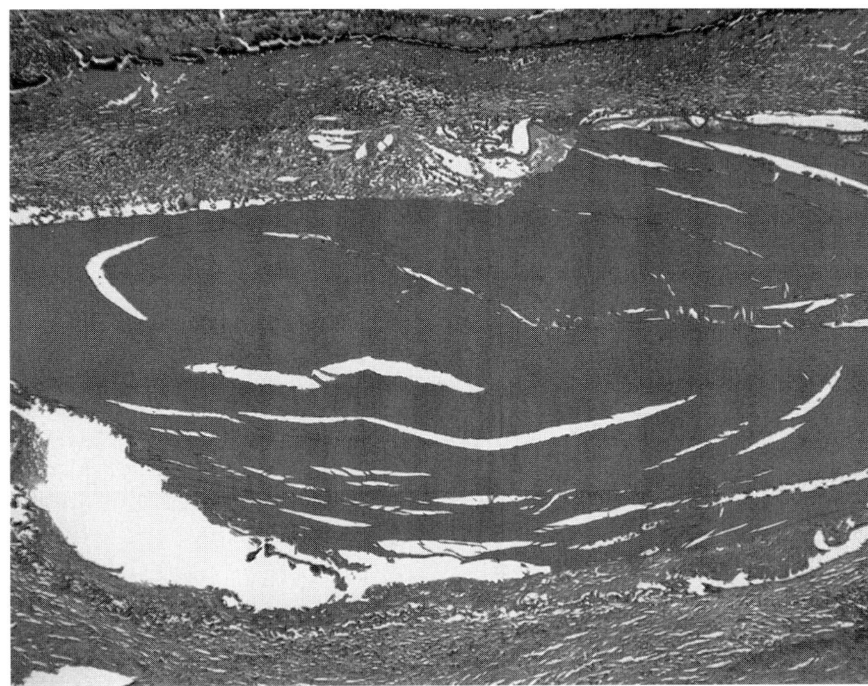

Figure 5 Phacoantigenic uveitis exhibits disrubuted lens cortex surrounded by inflammatory cells (hematoxylin and eosin, ×100).

evidence that immunoglobulin E, mast cells, and basophils are present in PU or that lens proteins are directly toxic to ocular tissues. It is more likely these subsets describe a difference in severity of response in patients previously sensitized to lens proteins.

Clinical Features

The more severe form, previously termed phacoanaphylactic endophthalmitis, typically presents with a sudden onset of a granulomatous inflammatory response. "Mutton-fat" KPs and posterior synechiae are commonly observed, and there is often a moderate to severe anterior chamber reaction. Hypopyon formation may be noted, along with lens debris floating in the anterior chamber. Obstruction of the trabecular meshwork may cause elevated intraocular pressure (IOP). The retina, choroid and optic nerve are not usually involved but there may be an associated vitritis. Visual acuity is usually decreased but there is generally less pain associated with this entity than with acute infectious endophthalmitis.

A less severe nongranulomatous response may also occur. Findings in these cases are generally less acute. The disrupted retained lens material may stimulate an inflammatory response with cells and flare in the anterior chamber and formation of posterior synechiae. Intraocular pressures may also become elevated from an obstruction of the trabecular meshwork by inflammatory cells or lens fragments.

Histopathology

PU is characterized by inflammation centered on the damaged lens with a zonal type of granulomatous inflammation surrounding it. Polymorphonuclear leukocytes (PMNs) are present around the lens (Fig. 5). These, in turn, are surrounded by epithelioid cells and occasional giant cells. An outer zone consisting of lymphocytes and plasma cells surrounds these epithelioid cells. Although the choroid is mildly inflamed, the inflammatory reaction is more marked in the anterior uvea.

Etiology and Pathogenesis

The cause of PU was once believed to be an immunological response to lens proteins occurring after surgical or non-surgical trauma to the lens capsule. The lens proteins were thought to be organ-specific and sequestered from the immune system in normal individuals by an intact lens capsule. However, subsequent studies have shown that the lens capsule does not absolutely sequester the lens proteins and crystallins have been identified in the aqueous humor of normal individuals (76). Moreover, the crystallins are expressed in tissues such as retina, heart, and skeletal muscle, indicating that they are not specific to the lens (31). Fifty percent of normal subjects, and a greater percentage of patients with cataracts or diabetic mellitus, have preoperative antibodies to lens proteins in the serum. Titers of antibodies to lens proteins often increase after extracapsular cataract surgery despite minimal postoperative inflammation (90).

Experiments performed in rats, mice, and rabbits demonstrate that spontaneous inflammation after lens capsule rupture is rare (58). Intravitreal injection of lens protein after prior immunization also produces only minimal inflammation (16,52). Thus, it is now believed that the development of inflammation around the lens depends more upon altered tolerance to the lens protein than on an immune reaction to previously sequestered antigens (47,48).

Animal models of experimental lens-induced granulomatous endophthalmitis demonstrate that the autoimmune response can be transferred with hyperimmune antisera (50,51). However, cutaneous delayed hypersensitivity reactions can be seen after immunization with lens proteins from other species (xenogeneic lens material) and not homologous lens (70). B-cell activation and antibody production to lens protein requires activation of T-helper cells or polyclonal B-cell activation with bacterial lipopolysaccharide.

Studies by Marak and associates have indicated that complement-fixing antibodies specific for lens protein are sufficient to cause PU in animals (51) and prevention of this complement cascade decreases the level of inflammation. Complement-dependent inflammatory mediators, such as the fragment of the fifth component of complement (C5a), may explain the PMN infiltration at the site of exposed lens material. Widespread complement activation is suggested as a cause for those cases with a severe uveitis. Activated macrophages may also play a role, given the presence of both epithelioid cells and giant cells on histologic examination. The animal models require pre-immunization with crystallins mixed with complete Freund adjuvant followed by lens capsule disruption. Such immunization leads to the generation of high anti-lens antibody titers, a prerequisite for the induction of the uveitis. The adjuvants contain either heat killed *Mycobacterium tuberculosis* or *Propionibacterium acnes*. At the time of traumatic lens disruption, *P. acnes* may be introduced into the disrupted lens where the bacteria may act as an adjuvant in the induction of the uveitis (78). Currently no single mechanism satisfactorily explains the pathogenesis of PU; however, disruption of the lens capsule along with altered tolerance to the crystallins is required for its development.

EXPERIMENTAL AUTOIMMUNE UVEITIS

Overview

Experimental autoimmune uveitis (EAU) is a useful, organ-specific animal model of human autoimmune uveitic diseases. EAU closely mimics immune-mediated human uveitic conditions, such as SO, and provides a method for elucidating the immunopathogenic factors associated with posterior uveitis (85,86). The mechanism is based on T-cell–mediated intraocular inflammation induced in susceptible species by the inoculation of ocular-specific proteins including S-antigen, rhodopsin, recoverin, phosducin, and IRBP (10,29,34,85,86). Immunization of these animals can occur in one of two methods: active immunization, which involves purifying the retinal antigens or peptides and mixing them with mycobacterium emulsified in complete Freund adjuvant prior to injection of these antigens in the footpad of the animal; or adoptive transfer, which involves transfer of lymphocytes from an animal with EAU to a naïve recipient (53). Signs of intraocular inflammation are typically seen within 9 to 14 days in animals actively immunized with the ocular proteins, whereas those inoculated via adoptive transfer exhibit signs and symptoms of uveitis in as few as 3 to 4 days (11,81).

Clinical Features

The initial changes seen in EAU are similar to findings in human cases of retinal vasculitis, with perivasculitis, sheathing of retinal vessels, and creamy white to yellow lesions deep in the retina. Dalen-Fuchs nodules can be seen in monkeys and mice immunized with uveitogenic antigens, particularly IRBP (62). Immunization with various antigens can produce a spectrum of disease findings ranging from acute inflammatory changes in susceptible animals, to chronic changes usually seen in the mouse model (10). Clinically, these lesions simulate findings most often seen in posterior uveitides such as VKH disease, ocular sarcoidosis and SO; thus EAU becomes a useful model for studying the pathogenesis of these autoimmune disorders.

Histopathology

In general, the histologic manifestations of EAU are characterized by cellular infiltration of the aqueous and vitreous, as well as inflammation of the uvea and retina with damage and disruption of the photoreceptors. The specific features can vary based on the type of antigen used, the dosage, and as the genetic susceptibility of the animal included in the model. For instance, S-antigen at a dose of 1 to 50 mcg can induce a wide spectrum of histopathologic changes in the guinea pig (70). Rao et al. noted that with increasing dose of S-antigen, the onset of disease occurred sooner, and the clinical findings were more severe. At the highest dose of 50 mcg, a hyperacute reaction developed and was associated with massive infiltration of neutrophils, eosinophils, and mononuclear cells. Marked thickening of the choroid was observed, as well as hemorrhage and fibrinoid necrosis of the choroidal vessels. At a lower dose (25 mcg), the clinical findings were more consistent with endophthalmitis, with a primary infiltrate of mononuclear cells. A granulomatous reaction can be observed in the choroid, accompanied by infiltrates of lymphocytes, epithelioid cells and occasional giant cells grouped between Bruch membrane and the RPE. These lesions are similar to Dalen-Fuchs nodules. Collins et al. described a mild, non-granulomatous posterior uveitis in those guinea pigs immunized with 1 mcg of S-antigen (14). In those eyes, the primary infiltrate consisted of lymphocytes and were thought to resemble SO.

Immunization with IRBP produces a disease picture with an accelerated onset and more localized response in comparison to S-antigen induced uveoretinitis, with total destruction of the photoreceptor layer (10). These findings have been described in rats and primates, but a newer model of chronic disease, termed murine EAU, was developed in mice immunized with IRBP. The mice, immunized with 20 mcg of IRBP, were observed to have a delayed onset of disease; however, the findings were focal rather than diffuse, and the disease course was longer in duration in comparison to their counterparts inoculated with 20 mcg of S-antigen. The most prominent histologic findings include retinal vasculitis, perivasculitis, retinal and choroidal granuloma formation, and serous detachments with localized photoreceptor dropout. Caspi et al. surmise that the focal involvement of posterior segment structures, along with the relatively longer duration of this disease process may allow the testing of therapeutic intervention (10).

Etiology and Pathogenesis

The essential component in the pathogenesis of EAU is the response of the animal to the Th-1 subset of helper T cells, but the complexity of the T-cell–mediated response is beyond the scope of this chapter. The central theory notes that susceptibility is characterized by conversion of Th-0 and Th-2 responses to Th1-cell responses. In general, the higher percentage of Th1 cells in the T-cell population, the more is uveitogenic (11). Th1 cells promote production of opsonizing and complement-fixing antibodies and activation of macrophages and neutrophils, and these activated cells are the major effectors of the observed tissue damage in EAU (21,22). Antibody-dependent cell cytotoxicity and type IV (delayed type) hypersensitivity reactions are also components of a Th1-cell response (22,57). Also, uveitogenic T-cell lines that are capable of adoptively transferring disease have a predominantly Th1 phenotype and produce elevated levels of IFNγ and low levels of IL4 (11).

In contrast, the Th-2 provides for components of the humoral immune response, particularly of the IgE type and mucosal immunity through facilitation of IgA synthesis (57). The Th2 response is known to be counter-regulatory to Th1 (11). Experimentally, rats treated with mercuric chloride develop a Th2 response that inhibits the lesions, and in mice, treatment with a combination of cytokines that skew the immune response away from Th1 also limits the histopathologic changes (11). Cytokines associated with a Th2 response include IL4, IL13 and IL10, and these act to inhibit the Th1-cell response by preventing recruitment of new cells into the Th1 pathway and inhibiting existing mature Th1 effector cells (11,81).

The Th1 response is initiated by endogenous levels of IL12, the central cytokine that promotes differentiation of Th0 cells into Th1 cells producing IFNγ (11,57). Antigen presenting cells such as dendritic cells, B cells and Langerhans cells produce IL12. Several authors have noted that anti-IL12 therapy at the time of immunization with uveitogenic antigens prevented development of EAU and pathogenic Th1 cells, and also induced a Th2 response that appeared to be protective when the animals were further challenged with the same antigen. Also, IL12 deficient mice did not develop EAU after immunization, despite maximizing the disease inducing regimen, and actually the animals developed a Th2-like antigen specific response (83,97). Note, however, that cells primed for EAU in the presence of IL12 prior to adoptive transfer can induce full-blown disease due to the fact that such cells respond by producing severalfold more IFNγ in response to antigen, and become more polarized toward the Th1 phenotype.

Interestingly, the Th2 response has been described not only as a preventer of pathology, but also as an inducer of pathology in EAU. Interferon γ (IFNγ) knockout (KO) mice were studied to determine if IFNγ at the local level could enhance disease by upregulating proinflammatory cytokines such as tumor necrosis factor (TNF) and IL6 (11). These IFNγ KO mice were found to develop EAU, with disease severity equal or greater than those found in wild type mice. The Th2 response was the effector phenotype, and a Th2-like cytokine profile was noted upon immunohistochemical staining and examination of the cellular composition of the inflammatory infiltrate (11).

Other theories on the pathogenesis of EAU describe oxidative stress in the early phases of EAU. In S-antigen induced disease, a recent study by Wu et al. found nitration of photoreceptor mitochondria-related proteins on day 5 post injection, before the macrophage and neutrophil infiltration of the retina (early EAU) that occurs on days 9 to 11 (93). These observations suggest that early damage may be induced by oxidative stress, through the production of nitric oxide, superoxide, and peroxynitrite (35,71)

The authors noted that proinflammatory cytokines such as TNFα, IFNγ, IL1α, and CD28 were found to be upregulated by day 5 post immunization with the antigen, and that inducible nitric oxide synthase was also upregulated. Furthermore, this oxidative stress was localized to the mitochondria of the photoreceptor inner segments and found prior to infiltration of inflammatory cells into the retinal tissues (66). The presence of the other upregulated cytokines were attributed to the few activated T cells noted in the retina by day 5. These new studies suggest that other aspects of inflammation unrelated to T-cell response may play a role in the early stages of EAU. This work has also provided further insight into the complexity of cytokine interaction as well as the effect of both Th1 and Th2 responses in EAU, though a comprehensive mechanism has yet to be elucidated.

ACKNOWLEDGMENTS

Supported in part by NIH grant EY03040 and a grant from Research to Prevent Blindness, Inc., New York, New York, U.S.A.

REFERENCES

1. Amsler M, Verrey F. Heterochromic de Fuchs et fragilite vasculaire. Ophthalmologica 1946; 111:177–81.
2. Arellanes-Garcia L, Bautista N, Mora P, et al. HLA-DR is strongly associated with Vogt-Koyanagi-Harada disease in Mexican Mestizo patients. Ocul Immunol Inflamm 1998; 6:93–100.
3. Arocker-Mettinger E, Asenbauer T, Ulbrich S, et al. Serum interleukin 2-receptor levels in uveitis. Curr Eye Res 1990; Suppl 9:25–9.
4. Barequet IS, Li Q, Wang Y, et al. *Herpes simplex* virus DNA identification from aqueous fluid in Fuchs heterochromic iridocyclitis. Am J Ophthalmol 2000; 129:672–3.
5. Berger BB, Tessler HH, Kottow MH. Anterior segment ischemia in Fuchs' heterochromic cyclitis. Arch Ophthalmol 1980; 98:499–501.
6. Bloch-Michel E. Physiopathology of Fuchs' heterochromic cyclitis. Trans Ophthalmol Soc UK 1981; 101:384–6.
7. Breeveld J, Rothova A, Kuiper H. Intermediate uveitis and Lyme borreliosis. Br J Ophthalmol 1992; 76:181–2.
8. Brockhurst RJ, Schepens CL. Uveitis. IV. Peripheral uveitis: the complications of retinal detachment. Arch Ophthalmol 1968; 80:747–53.
9. Broekhuyse RM, Kuhlmann ED, Winkens HJ. Experimental autoimmune posterior uveitis accompanied by epithelioid cell accumulations (EAPU). A new type of experimental ocular disease induced by immunization with PEP-65, a pigment epithelial polypeptide preparation. Exp Eye Res 1992; 55:819–29.
10. Caspi RR, Roberge FG, Chan CC, et al. A new model of autoimmune disease. Experimental autoimmune uveoretinitis induced in mice with two different retinal antigens. J Immunol 1988; 140:1490–5.
11. Caspi RR. Th1 and Th2 responses in pathogenesis and regulation of experimental autoimmune uveoretinitis. Intern Rev Immunol 2002; 21:197–208.
12. Chu DS, Foster CS. Sympathetic ophthalmia. Int Ophthalmol Clin 2002; 42:179–85.
13. Chung YM, Yeh TS, Liu JH. Endogenous uveitis in Chinese—an analysis of 240 cases in a uveitis clinic. Jpn J Ophthalmol 1988; 32:64–9.
14. Collins RC. Experimental studies on sympathetic ophthalmia. Am J Ophthalmol 1949; 32:1687–99.
15. Collins RC. Further experimental studies on sympathetic ophthalmia. Am J Ophthalmol 1953; 36:150–62.
16. Cousins SW, Kraus-Mackiw E. Lens-associated uveitis. In: Pepose JS, Holland GN, Wilhelmus KR, eds. Ocular Infection & Immunity. 1st ed. St. Louis: Mosby, 1996: Chapter 42, 507–28.
17. Davis JL, Chan CC, Nussenblatt RB. Immunology of intermediate uveitis. Dev Ophthalmol 1992; 23:71–85.
18. Davis JL, Mittal KK, Freidlin V, et al. HLA associations and ancestry in Vogt-Koyanagi-Harada disease and sympathetic ophthalmia. Ophthalmology 1990; 97:1137–42.
19. Dernouchamps JP. Fuchs' heterochromic cyclitis: an IUSG study about 550 cases. In: Saari KM, ed. Uveitis Update. Amsterdam: Elsevier, 1984:129–35.
20. Fearnley IR, Rosenthal AR. Fuchs' heterochromic iridocyclitis revisited. Acta Ophthalmol Scand 1995; 73: 166–70.
21. Forrester JV, Huitinga I, Lumsden L, et al. Marrow-derived activated macrophages are required during the effector phase of experimental autoimmune uveoretinitis in rats. Curr Eye Res 1998; 17:426–37.
22. Fowell D, McKnight AJ, Powrie F, Dyke R, Mason D. Subsets of CD4[+] T cells and their roles in the induction and prevention of autoimmunity. Immunol Rev 1991; 123: 37–64.
23. Fulmek R. Hemiatrophia progressiva faciei (Romberg-syndrome) associated with heterochromia complicata (Fuchs-syndrome). Klin Monatsbl Augenheilkd 1974; 164:615–28.
24. Goldberg MF, Erozan YS, Duke JR, et al. Cytopathologic and histopathologic aspects of Fuchs' heterochromic iridocyclitis. Arch Ophthalmol 1965; 74:604–9.
25. Goto H, Rao NA. Sympathetic ophthalmia and Vogt-Koyanagi-Harada syndrome. Int Ophthalmol Clin 1990; 30:279–85.
26. Green WR, Kincaid MC, Michels RG, et al. Pars planitis. Trans Ophthalmol Soc UK 1981; 101:361–7.
27. Henderly DE, Genstler AJ, Rao NA, et al. Pars planitis. Trans Ophthalmol Soc UK 1986; 105:227–32.
28. Henderly DE, Genstler AJ, Smith RE, et al. Changing patterns of uveitis. Am J Ophthalmol 1987; 103:131–6.
29. Hirose S, Kuwabara T, Nussenblatt RB, Wiggert B, Redmond TM, Gery I. Uveitis induced in primates by interphotoreceptor retinoid binding protein. Arch Ophthalmol 1986; 104:1698–702.
30. Hogan MJ, Kimura SJ, O'Connor GR. Peripheral retinitis and chronic cyclitis in children. Trans Ophthalmol Soc UK 1965; 85:39–52.
31. Horwitz J. Proctor lecture. The function of alpha-crystallin. Invest Ophthalmol Vis Sci 1993; 34:10–22.
32. Huber A, Kraus-Mackiw E. Fuchs's heterochromic cyclitis in Moebius' syndrome (author's transl). Klin Monatsbl Augenheilkd 1981; 178:182–5.
33. Inomata H, Rao NA. Depigmented atrophic lesions in "sunset glow" fundi of Vogt-Koyanagi-Harada disease. Am J Ophthalmol 2001; 131:607–14.
34. Inoue H, Takeuchi M, Tanaka T, et al. Analysis of the uveitopathogenic determinant in repeat structure of retinal interphotoreceptor retinoid-binding protein (IRBP). Clin Exp Immunol 1994; 97:219–25.

35. Ito S, Wu GS, Kimoto T, et al. Peroxynitrite-induced apoptosis in photoreceptor cells. Curr Eye Res 2004; 28: 17–24.
36. Jones NP. Fuchs' heterochromic uveitis: a reappraisal of the clinical spectrum. Eye 1991; 5:649–61.
37. Jones NP. Cataract surgery in Fuchs' heterochromic uveitis: past, present, and future. J Cataract Refract Surg 1996; 22:261–8.
38. Kalina PH, Pach JM, Buettner H, et al. Neovascularization of the disc in pars planitis. Retina 1990; 10:269–73.
39. Kawano Y, Tawara A, Nishioka Y, et al. Ultrasound biomicroscopic analysis of transient shallow anterior chamber in Vogt-Koyanagi-Harada syndrome. Am J Ophthalmol 1996; 121:720–3.
40. Kilmartin DJ, Dick AD, Forrester JV. Prospective surveillance of sympathetic ophthalmia in the UK and Republic of Ireland. Br J Ophthalmol 2000; 84:259–63.
41. Kitamura M, Takami K, Kitachi N, et al. Comparative study of two sets of criteria for the diagnosis of Vogt-Koyanagi-Harada's disease. Am J Ophthalmol 2005; 139: 1080–5.
42. La Hey E, de Jong PT, Kijlstra A. Fuchs' heterochromic cyclitis: review of the literature on the pathogenetic mechanisms. Br J Ophthalmol 1994; 78:307–12.
43. Liddy L, Stuart J. Sympathetic ophthalmia in Canada. Can J Ophthalmol 1972; 7:157–9.
44. Loewenfeld IE, Thompson HS. Fuchs's heterochromic cyclitis: a critical review of the literature. I. Clinical characteristics of the syndrome. Surv Ophthalmol 1973; 17:394–457.
45. Loewenfeld IE, Thompson HS. Fuchs's heterochromic cyclitis: a critical review of the literature. II. Etiology and mechanisms. Surv Ophthalmol 1973; 18:2–61.
46. Malinowski SM, Pulido JS, Folk JC. Long-term visual outcome and complications associated with pars planitis. Ophthalmology 1993; 100:818–24, discussion 825.
47. Marak GE Jr. Phacoanaphylactic endophthalmitis. Surv Ophthalmol 1992; 36:325–39.
48. Marak GE Jr, Lim LY, Rao NA. Abrogation of tolerance to lens proteins. II. Allogeneic effect. Ophthalmic Res 1982; 14:176–81.
49. Marak GE Jr, Rao NA. Retinal 's' antigen disease in rats. Ophthalmic Res 1982; 14:29–39.
50. Marak GE Jr, Rao NA, Antonakou G, et al. Experimental lens-induced granulomatous endophthalmitis in common laboratory animals. Ophthalmic Res 1982; 14:292–7.
51. Marak GE, Font RL, Alepa FP. Experimental lens-induced granulomatous endophthalmitis. Mod Probl Ophthalmol 1976; 16:75–9.
52. Misra RN, Rahi AH, Morgan G. Immunopathology of the lens. II. Humoral and cellular immune responses to homologous lens antigens and their roles in ocular inflammation. Br J Ophthalmol 1977; 61:285–96.
53. Mochizuki M, Kuwabara T, McAllister C, Nussenblatt RB, Gery I. Adoptive transfer of experimental autoimmune uveoretinitis in rats: Immunopathogenic mechanisms and histologic features. Invest Ophthalmol Vis Sci 1985; 26:1–9.
54. Mochizuki M, Watanabe T, Yamaguchi K, et al. Uveitis associated with human T-cell lymphotropic virus type I. Am J Ophthalmol 1992; 114:123–9.
55. Mohamed Q, Zamir E. Update on Fuchs' uveitis syndrome. Curr Opin Ophthalmol 2005; 16:356–63.
56. Moorthy RS, Inomata H, Rao NA. Vogt-Koyanagi-Harada syndrome. Surv Ophthalmol 1995; 39:265–92.
57. Mosmann TR, Cherwinski II, Bond MW, Giedlin MA, Coffman RL. Two types of murine helper T cell clone. I. Definition according to profiles of lymphokine activities and secreted proteins. J Immunol 1986; 136: 2348–57.
58. Mueller H. Phacolytic glaucoma and phacogenic ophthalmia (lens-induced uveitis). Trans Ophthalmol Soc UK 1963; 83:689–704.
59. Murray PI, Dinning WJ, Rahi AH. T-lymphocyte subpopulations in uveitis. Br J Ophthalmol 1984; 68:746–9.
60. Murray PI, Hoekzema R, van Haren MA, et al. Aqueous humor interleukin-6 levels in uveitis. Invest Ophthalmol Vis Sci 1990; 31:917–20.
61. Murray PI, Mooy CM, Visser-de Jong E, et al. Immunohistochemical analysis of iris biopsy specimens from patients with Fuchs' heterochromic cyclitis. Am J Ophthalmol 1990; 109:394–9.
62. Nussenblatt RB. Proctor lecture: experimental autoimmune uveitis: mechanisms of disease and clinical therapeutic indications. Invest Ophthalmol Vis Sci 1991; 32:3131–41.
63. Pederson JE, Kenyon KR, Green WR, et al. Pathology of pars planitis. Am J Ophthalmol 1978; 86:762–74.
64. Quentin CD, Reiber H. Fuchs heterochromic cyclitis: rubella virus antibodies and genome in aqueous humor. Am J Ophthalmol 2004; 138:46–54.
65. Raja SC, Jabs DA, Dunn JP, et al. Pars planitis: clinical features and class II HLA associations. Ophthalmology 1999; 106:594–9.
66. Rajendram R, Saraswathy S, Rao NA. Photoreceptor mitochondrial oxidative stress in early experimental autoimmune uveoretinitis. Br J Ophthalmol 2007; 91: 531–7.
67. Rao PK, Rao NA. Chapter 107: Vogt-Koyanagi-Harada disease. In: Ryan SJ, ed. Retina, 4th ed. Elsevier, 2005: 1827–37.
68. Rao NA, Marak GE Jr. Experimental granulomatous uveitis: an electron microscopic study of pigment containing giant cells. Invest Ophthalmol Vis Sci 1985; 26:1303–5.
69. Rao NA, Robin J, Hartmann D, et al. The role of the penetrating wound in the development of sympathetic ophthalmia experimental observations. Arch Ophthalmol 1983; 101:102–4.
70. Rao NA, Wacker WB, Marak GE Jr. Experimental allergic uveitis: clinicopathologic features associated with varying doses of S antigen. Arch Ophthalmol 1979; 97: 1954–8.
71. Rao NA, Wu GS. Free radical mediated photoreceptor damage in uveitis. Prog Retin Eye Res 2000; 19:41–68.
72. Read RW, Rechodouni A, Butani N, et al. Complications and prognostic factors in Vogt-Koyanagi-Harada disease. Am J Ophthalmol 2001; 131:599–606.
73. Reynard M, Shulman IA, Azen SP, et al. Histo-compatibility antigens in sympathetic ophthalmia. Am J Ophthalmol 1983; 95:216–21.
74. Rodriguez A, Calonge M, Pedroza-Seres M, et al. Referral patterns of uveitis in a tertiary eye care center. Arch Ophthalmol 1996; 114:593–9.
75. Sakamoto T, Murata T, Inomata H. Class II major histocompatibility complex on melanocytes of Vogt-Koyanagi-Harada disease. Arch Ophthalmol 1991; 109: 1270–4.
76. Sandberg HO. The alpha-crystallin content of aqueous humour in cortical, nuclear, and complicated cataracts. Exp Eye Res 1976; 22:75–84.
77. Schwab IR. The epidemiologic association of Fuchs' heterochromic iridocyclitis and ocular toxoplasmosis. Am J Ophthalmol 1991; 111:356–62.

78. Semel J, Bowe B, Guo A, et al. Propionibacterium acnes-enhanced lens-induced granulomatous uveitis in the rat. Invest Ophthalmol Vis Sci 1992; 33:1766–70.
79. Shindo Y, Ohno S, Usui M, et al. Immunogenetic study of sympathetic ophthalmia. Tissue Antigens 1997; 49: 111–5.
80. Shindo Y, Ohno S, Yamamoto T, et al. Complete association of the HLA-DRB1*04 and -DQB1*04 alleles with Vogt-Koyanagi-Harada's disease. Hum Immunol 1994; 39:169–76.
81. Singh VK, Rai G, Agarwal SS. Role of cytokines in experimental and clinical uveitis. Indian J Ophthalmol 2001; 49:81–90.
82. Smith RE, Godfrey WA, Kimura SJ. Complications of chronic cyclitis. Am J Ophthalmol 1976; 82:277–82.
83. Tarrant TK, Silver PB, Chan CC, Wiggert B, Caspi RR. Endogenous IL-12 is required for the induction and expression of experimental autoimmune uveitis. J Immunol 1998; 161:122–7.
84. Teyssot N, Cassoux N, Lehoang P, et al. Fuchs heterochromic cyclitis and ocular toxocariasis. Am J Ophthalmol 2005; 139:915–6.
85. Wacker WB, Lipton MM. Experimental allergic uveitis. I. Homologous retina as uveitogenic antigen. Nature 1965; 206:253–4.
86. Wacker WB, Lipton MM. Experimental allergic uveitis. I. Production in the guinea-pigs and rabbit by immunization with retina in adjuvant. J Immunol 1968; 101:151–6.
87. Weiner A, BenEzra D. Clinical patterns and associated conditions in chronic uveitis. Am J Ophthalmol 1991; 112: 151–8.
88. Weisz JM, Holland GN, Roer LN, et al. Association between Vogt-Koyanagi-Harada syndrome and HLA-DR1 and -DR4 in Hispanic patients living in southern California. Ophthalmology 1995; 102:1012–5.
89. Wetzig RP, Chan CC, Nussenblatt RB, et al. Clinical and immunopathological studies of pars planitis in a family. Br J Ophthalmol 1988; 72:5–10.
90. Wirostko E, Spalter HF. Lens-induced uveitis. Arch Ophthalmol 1967; 78:1–7.
91. Wu GS, Rao NA. A novel retinal pigment epithelial protein suppresses neutrophil superoxide generation. I. Characterization of the suppressive factor. Exp Eye Res 1996; 63:713–25.
92. Wu GS, Rao NA. Activation of NADPH oxidase by docosahexaenoic acid hydroperoxide and its inhibition by a novel retinal pigment epithelial protein. Invest Ophthalmol Vis Sci 1999; 40:831–9.
93. Wu GS, Lee TD, Moore RE, et al. Photoreceptor mitochondrial tyrosine nitration in experimental uveitis. Invest Ophthalmol Vis Sci 2005; 46:2271–81.
94. Yamaki K, Gocho K, Hayakawa K, et al. Tyrosinase family proteins are antigens specific to Vogt-Koyanagi-Harada disease. J Immunol 2000; 165:7323–9.
95. Yamaki K, Hara K, Sakuragi S. Application of revised diagnostic criteria for Vogt-Koyanagi-Harada disease in Japanese patients. Jpn J Ophthalmol 2005; 49:143–8.
96. Yamamoto N, Naito K. Annular choroidal detachment in a patient with Vogt-Koyanagi-Harada disease. Graefes Arch Clin Exp Ophthalmol 2004; 242:355–8.
97. Yokoi H, Kato K, Kezuka T, Sakai J, Usui M, Yagita H, et al. Prevention of experimental autoimmune uveoretinitis by monoclonal antibody to interleukin-12. Eur J Immunol 1997; 27:641–66.
98. Yoser SL, Forster DJ, Rao NA. Pathology of intermediate uveitis. Dev Ophthalmol 1992; 23:60–70.
99. Zaharia MA, Lamarche J, Laurin M. Sympathetic uveitis 66 years after injury. Can J Ophthalmol 1984; 19:240–3.
100. Zierhut M, Foster CS. Multiple sclerosis, sarcoidosis and other diseases in patients with pars planitis. Dev Ophthalmol 1992; 23:41–7.

5

Extraocular Manifestations of Immune Disorders

C. Stephen Foster and Fahd Anzaar
Massachusetts Eye Research and Surgery Institute and Harvard University, Boston, Massachusetts, U.S.A.

INTRODUCTION

The eye can be affected by almost any of the immunological disorders associated with autoimmunity. Understanding the primary mechanism of a particular patient's inflammatory problem lays the groundwork for the correct treatment. The diagnostic pursuit of mechanistic understanding of the patient's inflammatory problem will be sight saving, at the very least, and may be responsible for the diagnosis of a disease that, undiagnosed, would have been fatal. This chapter is organized along the lines of the classic Gell, Coombs, and Lachmann hypersensitivity reactions (71). The four types of hypersensitivity reactions rarely exist in pure form in human pathological states, in isolation from each other; it is typical for hypersensitivity reactions to include more than one of the Gell and Coombs responses as participants in the inflammatory problem. When it is known, this combination of types of mechanisms is pointed out in the various ocular diseases presented and discussed in this chapter. The ophthalmic complications of the connective tissue, collagen vascular, and vasculitic diseases that comprise many of the type III hypersensitivity reactions typical of autoimmunity are covered in Chapter 6.

HAY FEVER

Clinical Features

Hay fever or allergic rhinitis is an immediate hypersensitivity reaction to environmental antigens. Hay fever conjunctivitis, or seasonal allergic conjunctivitis (SAC), is the chief ocular manifestation of this atopic disease. Mucous membranes, including the nasal mucosa and conjunctiva, are generally affected in such reactions, which are a manifestation of type I hypersensitivity mediated by immunoglobulin E (IgE)-triggered mast cell degranulation and the varied actions of a multitude of cytokines (34,87). SAC is the most common allergic disease affecting the eye (10).

A typical attack of allergic rhinitis consists of watery rhinorrhea, sneezing, and nasal obstruction, with itching of the nose and eyes. These episodes are usually seasonal, but with perennial allergens, such as house dust, symptoms may occur year-round. The conjunctiva is edematous, pale, and boggy, and the eyelids may be edematous and hyperemic.

The most common allergens responsible for hay fever are chemically complex substances derived from plants or animals. In many parts of the United States, ragweed, which pollenates between July and mid-October, is the most common allergen to incite SAC. Pollens of grasses, trees, weeds, fungi, house dust, animal danders, industrial chemicals, some foods, and certain airborne particles in the home may also be allergenic. Symptoms related to some allergens occur year-round, but other antigens, such as most pollens and fungi, provoke recurrent allergic reactions that have a characteristic seasonal peak.

Immunopathology

Increased eotaxin-1 levels have been detected in the tears of SAC patients, which leads to chemotaxis, recruitment and activation of eosinophils, which liberate IgE. Eotaxin binds to its CCR3 receptor not only on eosinophils, but also on mast cells and T helper 2 (Th2) cells that express it, drawing them in also (57). Allergens cause increased mucosal synthesis from epithelial cells (95). IgE released by eosinophils binds to mast cells, and on subsequent exposure and cross-linking of IgE by allergen, mast cells release both preformed and newly synthesized mediators such as histamine, tryptase, chymase, carboxypeptidase, cathepsin G, leukotriene C_4 leukotriene D_4, prostaglandin D_2 and cytokines [interleukin (IL) 4, IL5, IL6, IL8, and IL13, tumor necrosis factor alpha (TNFα)], that play a direct role in the allergic response. The MC_{TC} subset (containing both tryptase and chymase granules) release IL4 and IL13 (stimulating Th2 cells and IgE production), while the MC_T subset (containing tryptase granules, a minority subset) release IL5 and IL6 (11). Th2 cells produce cytokines such as IL4, IL5 (among others) that lead to further recruitment of eosinophils and the production of IgE, establishing a vicious cycle. Fortunately, this process relents when the seasonal allergy trigger disappears, unlike those unfortunate patients who are perenially allergic or have atopic keratoconjunctivitis (AKC) or vernal keratoconjunctivitis (VKC) (see sections below). IL4, IgE, histamine, tryptase, chymase, CD45RO+ cells, EG2+ cells have all been found at higher levels in SAC patients than normal controls.

Histopathology

The histopathological characteristics of SAC include a normal conjunctival epithelium with increased goblet cells, a scanty mononuclear cell infiltrate in the substantia propria, and (as highlighted by alkaline Giemsa staining) abundant mast cells and eosinophils in the substantia propria; many of these are seen to be degranulating. Mast cells are also usually present in the epithelium. This feature alone is of great diagnostic importance, since few diseases other than those that involve a type I hypersensitivity mechanism are associated with the presence of mast cells in the epithelium. The increased mast cell numbers do not return to normal even out of the allergy season (122). Stem cell factor, a chemotactic and growth factor for mast cells which also enhances cytokine release, has been shown to be increased fourfold in SAC patients (197). In SAC, only the mast cell numbers are raised while in the other allergic eye disease such as VKC and AKC, both mast and T cell numbers are raised (128).

Diagnosis

The diagnosis of SAC is not difficult and is typically based securely on the medical review of systems and the historical relationship of allergen exposure and symptoms. Instillation of the offending allergen into the conjunctival sac provokes the signs and symptoms of hay fever conjunctivitis, but this test is rarely necessary or indicated. Cutaneous tests may help determine the allergens to which a patient is sensitive. Scratch or prick tests may be applied to the lower surface of the forearms or back; an immediate wheal-and-flare skin response indicates atopic sensitivity. In questionable or negative responses to strongly suspected allergens, an intracutaneous injection may be given. These are usually administered in lower dilutions since systemic (anaphylactic) reactions are more likely to develop with intracutaneous testing. The finding of a few eosinophils in a Giemsa-stained scraping of the nasal mucosa or conjunctiva may be helpful if a diagnosis of hay fever is in question, and biopsied mucosa or conjunctiva would show the histopathological characteristics just described in those rare instances when this step might be required to establish the diagnosis.

DRUG ALLERGY

Clinical Features

Drug reactions are among the most commonly encountered problems in medical practice, including ophthalmology (59). It may sometimes be difficult to separate the toxic from the allergic side effects of a particular drug. Drug-induced allergy can be caused by various immunological reactions, but the type IV delayed hypersensitivity reaction is the most common mechanism responsible for this inflammatory reaction.

The clinical manifestations of drug reactions are protean. Dermatitis is almost always present. Other skin reactions that may develop include urticaria (penicillin), exanthematous eruptions (ampicillin), exfoliative dermatitis (barbiturates, heavy metals, and sulfonamides), bullae (iodides and bromides), erythema multiforme (EM) (sulfonamides and barbiturates), lichenoid eruptions (gold salts, thiazides, and antimalarials), and fixed drug eruptions (phenolphthalein, barbiturates, and sulfonamides).

Allergic reactions, including urticaria, wheezing, respiratory arrest, pruritus, shock, laryngeal edema, and exanthemata, have been reported following the intravenous diagnostic drug fluorescein (163).

Adverse side effects of the systemically administered β-adrenergic blocker practolol (now withdrawn) include rash, a lupus erythematosus-like syndrome, secretory otitis, sclerosing peritonitis leading to small bowel obstruction (54,194), and an oculomucocutaneous syndrome characterized by rash, dry eyes, and cicatrizing conjunctivitis similar to cicatricial pemphigoid. This syndrome, which appears to be unrelated to toxicity, has several immunological features, with patients manifesting an increased incidence of autoantibodies, including antinuclear antibodies and antibodies to thyroid cytoplasm (94). The conjunctival lesions associated with practolol administration include loss of goblet cells and subepithelial fibrosis. An inflammatory reaction affecting the conjunctiva, lacrimal gland, iris, and ciliary body may occur (148).

Allergic keratitis is an extremely rare side effect of medication with chlordiazepoxide (55). Even topical medications can cause significant allergic reactions (see the section entitled Contact Dermatitis). Of particular importance to the ophthalmologist are anti-glaucoma agents, corticosteroids, and anesthetics. Patients may become sensitized either to the therapeutic agents or to the preservatives used (benzalkonium chloride). Such patients may be exposed to the offending agent by multiple routes, including during routine eye evaluations, after surgery, in the treatment of their ophthalmic condition, and of course by the use of a contact lens solution (76). Some authors have even suggested that allergic sensitization to topical anesthetics is an occupational hazard for ophthalmologists and ophthalmic technicians, after observing cross-sensitization with proparacaine and tetracaine (46).

Immunopathology

Type I (anaphylactic) hypersensitivity reactions are potentially fatal. They occur within minutes after the administration of a drug and are mediated by IgE-triggered mast cell degranulation. Typical manifestations include urticaria and morbilliform skin eruptions (which can involve the eyelids), hypotension, shock, asthma, and laryngeal edema. Type I reactions may be triggered by antibiotics, such as penicillin and streptomycin. Penicillin can also cause adverse side effects through types II, III, and IV hypersensitivity mechanisms.

Type II (cytotoxic) hypersensitivity occurs when antibody interacts with antigen attached to a target cell, the latter commonly being a leukocyte or platelet. These reactions are complement dependent, and usually a complex of drug, antibody, and complement becomes fixed to the cell membrane to cause lysis of the target cell. Type II reactions can be induced by penicillin, methyldopa, sulfonamides, or quinidine or by incompatible blood transfusions.

Type III hypersensitivity drug reactions may lead to urticaria, serum sickness, or a multisystemic complement-dependent vasculitis. Immune complexes deposit within the tissues, including blood vessels, and the complement pathways are activated to produce foci of local inflammation. Bilateral iritis has been described in a patient who developed serum sickness following a series of injections of horse antipneumococcal serum for pneumonia (171), and a similar type of uveitis was produced experimentally in the rabbit.

Type IV hypersensitivity reactions are commonly encountered as a contact allergy to topical medications, and in the ocular context this occurs with topical antibiotics, anesthetics, dilating agents, and certain preservatives.

Diagnosis

Tests for the diagnosis of drug allergy include the basophil degranulation test, lymphocyte activation test, and radioallergosorbent test, with the practicality and usefulness of these procedures depending on the condition under investigation.

ATOPIC DERMATITIS AND KERATOCONJUNCTIVITIS

Clinical Features

Atopic dermatitis, one of the eczematous skin eruptions, often occurs in childhood but may occur in adolescents and adults. The incidence in children under 5 years of age is estimated as about 3% (73). Frequently, patients with atopic dermatitis have a history of respiratory allergy (allergic rhinitis, asthma), hay fever or allergic reactions to certain foods. Although immunological abnormalities are invariably present, an abnormal reactivity of the skin to various stimuli, which may be due to a genetically determined metabolic defect, seems to coexist, and despite extensive allergic testing, a relationship between atopic dermatitis and a known allergen is sometimes not found. House dust, mites, mite feces, and foods or chemicals in foods are common allergens to which atopic dermatitis patients are sensitive.

The skin of patients with atopic dermatitis is easily irritated by nonspecific irritants, such as harsh soaps and detergents, frequent bathing, chapping in cold weather, and fabrics such as wool and nylon (191). Typical distributions of skin lesions have been described for different ages; e.g., in infants, the neck and face are most commonly affected while in adults, cubiteal and popliteal fossae involvement is seen.

Ocular Manifestations

Ocular complications are seen in 32% to 67% of AKC patients (198). The eyelids of patients with AKC are affected by the patient's eczema, with resultant scaly dermatitis, eyelid thickening, loss of eyelashes (madurosis), and meibomian gland dysfunction. Secondary staphylococcal blepharitis may occur as well. Ocular manifestations include conjunctival hyperemia, chemosis, a stringy mucous discharge, and a corneal epitheliopathy (Fig. 1). Large papillae resembling cobblestones may develop on the tarsal conjunctiva, but in contrast to vernal conjunctivitis, the lower rather than the upper tarsus is more frequently involved in AKC (161). Localized deposits of eosinophils can occur at the corneoscleral limbus (Trantas dots), as in VKC. Linear or stellate scars in the tarsal conjunctiva, fornix foreshortening, and symblepharon, similar to that in ocular cicatricial pemphigoid (OCP), can occur.

Numerous small defects in the corneal epithelium may develop and appear as spots after the cornea is stained with fluorescein, and if the disease is severe, stromal ulcers, scarring and vascularization may ensue. The keratopathy is the main cause of visual impairment, and may lead to herpes simplex or other microbial keratitis. Patients are also prone to severe herpetic skin eruptions (eczema herpeticum) due to a deficiency in cellular immunity (see later section). Keratoconus is sometimes associated with atopic dermatitis. Copeman reviewed 100 patients with keratoconus and found 32 to have some form of eczema (42). The incidence of atopic eczema in the general population is about 3%, compared with 16% in patients with keratoconus. Karseras and Ruben (99) also found a strong association between keratoconus and atopic conditions and suggested that the irritation of the eyelids due to eczema or hay fever leads to excessive eye rubbing. This, coupled with a congenitally thinned and weakened cornea, was postulated to play a role in the pathogenesis of keratoconus.

Cataracts designated as "atopic cataracts" occur mainly in the severe chronic forms of atopic dermatitis, especially in children and young adults, usually appearing at least 10 years after the onset of the skin disease (23). Once detected the cataract may evolve rapidly to complete opacification of the lens within 6 months. Typically, atopic cataracts are bilateral and often symmetrical, manifesting as a shield-like opacification of the anterior lens cortex, but sometimes the cataract begins as a posterior subcapsular opacity.

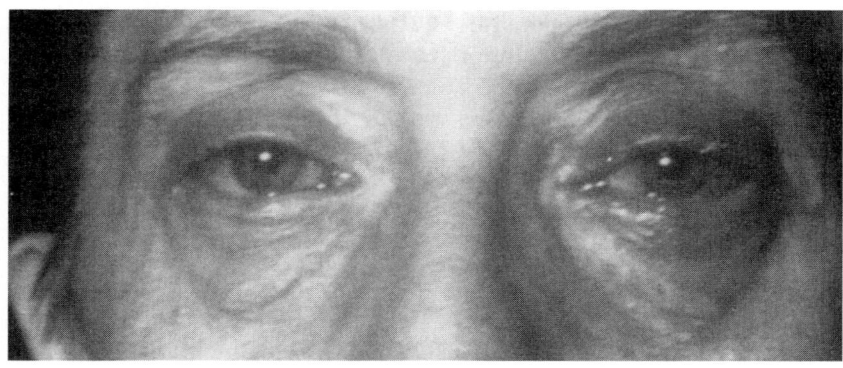

Figure 1 Atopic keratoconjunctivitis, showing dermatitis and conjunctivitis (including chemosis).

Aside from the usual complications of cataract extraction, a relatively high incidence of pre- and postoperative retinal detachment has been reported (89). Spontaneous retinal detachment is probably more common in patients with atopic dermatitis than in the general population (40,89), but the question of whether this results from continued rubbing of the eyes, degenerative changes in the vitreous, or other factors is unanswered.

Immunopathology

Abnormal and paradoxical skin responses are observed in patients with atopic dermatitis (191). A response known as "white dermographism" occurs after stroking the skin with a blunt instrument. Thus, although the formation of erythema and wheal characteristic of the triple response of Lewis normally develops, in individuals with atopic dermatitis the erythema is often replaced by a white line surrounded by an area of blanching. After the injection of acetylcholine or methylcholine into the skin of normal individuals, vasodilation and erythema develop, but in patients with atopic dermatitis a white, spreading reaction appears 5 to 30 minutes after the injection and persists for up to 1 hour. This delayed blanch phenomenon of atopy, which was originally thought to be due to paradoxical vasoconstriction (118), is now believed to represent vasodilation, the erythema being obscured by edema resulting from an excessive transudation into the skin. Patients with atopic dermatitis have decreased levels of circulating plasma norepinephrine but higher concentrations than normal in affected areas of skin (160).

Serum IgE concentrations are generally elevated in individuals with atopic dermatitis (165), and upon remission of the clinical manifestations of the disease, the level may decline markedly (97). Usually, the serum IgA, IgM, and IgD are normal (100). IgG levels may be normal or elevated but IgG_4 is often high. Despite an elevated serum IgE, most persons with atopic dermatitis have normal numbers of peripheral blood lymphocytes bearing IgE and other immunoglobulins, but an increase in the number of lymphocytes with complement receptors may be found.

Recent evidence suggests a deficiency of cellular immunity in patients with atopic dermatitis. Delayed hypersensitivity skin responses to ubiquitous antigens, including *Candida* and streptokinase–streptodornase, may be poor (129). This form of delayed cutaneous anergy is most marked in children with severe dermatitis, who may also fail to become sensitized by the topical application of dinitrochlorbenzene. Furthermore, the mean percentage of T cells in the peripheral blood of patients with eczema is often lower than in normal control subjects. The response of T lymphocytes to low concentrations of the mitogen phytohemagglutinin may also be significantly depressed. Perhaps because of a defective cellular immunity, atopic patients have an increased susceptibility to viral and fungal infections (119,188). Perhaps the reason for this deficiency is related to preferential apoptosis of T helper (Th1) cells in atopic patients, and the resultant excess of Th2 cells, which drives the cytokine profile toward humoral immunity rather than cell-mediated immunity (3). Overexpression of suppressor of cytokine signaling (SOCS3) is also seen; which downregulates Th1 cells (124).

T helper 2 (Th2) cells are considered central to the pathogenesis of allergic conjunctival diseases such as SAC, AKC and VKC and giant papillary conjunctivitis (GPC) (see below). Excess numbers are found in biopsies, tears and peripheral blood [much higher proportions than Th1 cells (196)] and the cytokines and chemokines they produce recruit other, 'effector' cell types such as basophils, mast cells, and eosinophils, which are the hallmarks of allergic inflammation. When activated, they release their toxic, tissue damaging granule contents such as histamine, major basic protein, cationic protein, protein X, neurotoxin, peroxidase, tryptase and chymase and many others. All these, and their conjugate receptors, have been detected in conjunctival biopsy specimens, tears and also in resected papillae themselves, lending credence to this hypothesis (120). The Th2 cytokines include IL1, IL3 and IL4 (eosinophil and Th2 differentiation, maturation, IgE synthesis, eotaxin production), IL5 (eosinophil chemotaxis), IL9, and IL13. Eotaxin (chemokinetic for eosinophils) and its receptors (CCR3 and CCR4) has been shown to have abnormally high expression in the papillae of AKC, along with the resulting eosinophil infiltration. The chemokine receptor CXCR4 and its ligands (SDF-1/CXCL12) mediate chemotaxis of T cells and B cells, activation of T cells and angiogenesis/neovascularization. Demonstrated high levels of these may underlie the recruitment of, and release of cytokines from activated T cells, causing the conjunctival remodeling associated with the formation of papillae. The corneal damage is thought to result from the eosinophilic proteins secreted by eosinophils in the papilla. Blockade of CXCR4, SDF-1/CXCL12 may be a novel treatment strategy (12). The Th2 cytokines IL1, IL4, IL5, IL13, and transforming growth factor β (TGFβ) (from eosinophils) increase vascular endothelial growth factor (VEGF) production from subepithelial fibroblasts (also increasing eotaxin production), resulting in a self-perpetuating cycle and the formation of new capillaries characteristic of papillae (177). Neutrophils have also been suggested to play a role in pathogenesis, as elastase deposition (released from the primary or azurophilic granules) has been seen in AKC and VKC patients; and myelin basic protein (MBP) from the eosinophils already present has been shown to activate neutrophils (12). Recent studies have shown that there is preferential apoptosis of Th1 T cells (3), which showed procaspase degradation and active caspase 8 formation; and overexpression of SOCS3 in AKC, a cytokine which downregulates Th1 cells.

Cytokine liberation from inflammatory cells induces pronounced upregulation of class II glycoprotein expression on the surface of fibroblasts and epithelial cells, along with other adhesion molecules, which no doubt play a role in the cellular infiltration seen in AKC.

Other abnormalities in atopic patients include an eosinophilia of the peripheral blood and an increase in the absolute number of B lymphocytes (177).

Since T lymphocytes are important regulators of the synthesis of IgE and other antibodies, a disorder of T regulator cells could be responsible for the failure to terminate IgE-mediated responses of certain antigens (147). IgE then binds to skin mast cells, initiating a release of histamine and other chemical mediators during antigenic stimulation. The overly reactive skin of atopic patients may respond excessively to the effects of histamine and other chemical mediators. They have a decreased itch threshold, and a prolonged response of the neural endings to histamine, causing them to itch earlier, for a longer time, than non-atopics. This may be from lower intracellular cAMP levels due to increased activity of cAMP phophodiesterases. Cytotoxic T cells were shown to release their various granule contents (including perforin) twice as fast as and much more completely than those of controls.

Tissue sections of skin with atopic dermatitis contain intraepithelial vesicles, dilated dermal blood vessels, and a perivascular infiltration by lymphocytes, eosinophils, and mast cells. Hyperkeratosis and acantholysis occur in chronic skin lesions.

Histopathology

The histopathological and immunopathological characteristics of conjunctiva affected by AKC are typical of chronic type I and type IV immunologically mediated inflammatory reactions (62). The number of B cells and T cells, neutrophils, plasma cells, basophils, dendritic cells and macrophages in the conjunctival substantia propria is vast, and fibroblast proliferation and new collagen formation are obvious. Mast cells and eosinophils are present in the epithelium and are more abundant in the substantia propria than normal; a large proportion are degranulating (196). Helper (CD4) T lymphocytes far outnumber suppressor (CD8) T cells, and the T cells are activated, a large proportion of them expressing the IL2 receptor. This influx of T cells, producing IL2 and interferon gamma (IFNγ) suggests a type IV reaction, with the resultant conjunctival structural alterations mentioned earlier from the liberated cytokines (4,112,113).

VERNAL KERATOCONJUNCTIVITIS

Clinical Features

Vernal keratoconjunctivitis, a bilateral, interstitial conjunctival allergic disease occurring primarily in young males, is characterized clinically by a stringy, mucous discharge, giant papillae of the upper palpebral conjunctiva, and extreme itching (Fig. 2) (66). Other symptoms include lacrimation, photophobia, foreign body sensation, and burning (53). It begins as early as age 4 years, reaching a peak incidence between 11 and 13 years of age. During childhood the disease is much more common in males than in females (183) (perhaps pointing to an androgen-driven pathogenesis) but after the age of 20 years the incidence in the two sexes is about the same; after the third decade the condition is uncommon. Perennial forms occur, but as the name implies, the disease is most prominent in the spring of each year. VKC develops more frequently in warm climates than in temperate zones and is rarely seen in cold environments. Because of this geographical pattern, heat, airborne allergens, such as pollens, and other physical factors are thought to contribute to the pathogenesis of the disease. Palpebral, limbal and mixed forms of the disease have been described (53).

Giant papillae, which are polygonal and flat topped "cobblestones" and contain tufts of capillaries on the upper palpebral conjunctiva are the hallmark of VKC (Fig. 3); other portions of the conjunctiva have a milky appearance, with many fine papillae sometimes present on the lower palpebral conjunctiva. A pseudo-membrane may be present in severe cases.

Corneal abnormalities include keratoconus, keratoglobus, superficial punctate keratitis, epithelial defects, superficial ulcers, micropannus, neovascularization, degenerative corneal changes such as pellucid marginal degeneration (176), and pseudogerontoxon (often adjacent to a limbal papilla or previously inflamed segment of the corneoscleral limbus). Limbal papillae located at the limbus and topped by white dots on the apices (Trantas dots) containing numerous eosinophils are most commonly seen in VKC in deeply pigmented individuals (183) while the tarsal and corneal signs predominate in light skinned individuals.

Immunopathology

Many features of VKC suggest an allergic/atopic cause, and the majority (but not all) affected individuals have a personal or family history of atopic disease, such as hay fever, atopic dermatitis (eczema), or asthma. Increased levels of IgE, IL5 (induces eosinophil

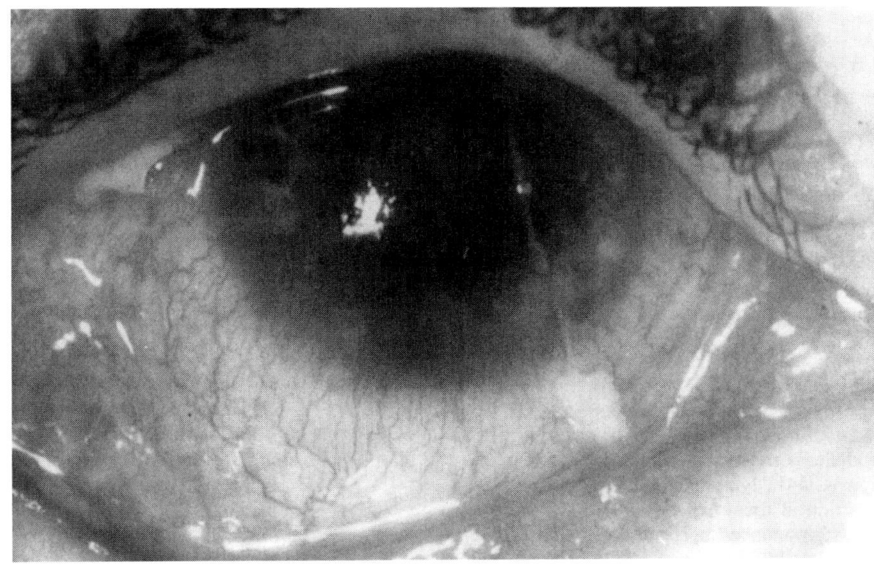

Figure 2 Vernal keratoconjunctivitis. The conjunctiva is edematous and hyperemic and has ropy yellow mucus.

differentiation, recruitment, and activation), eotaxins 1 and 2 (chemokinetic for eosinophils) activated eosinophils and their products [eosinophil cationic protein (ECP), eosinophil protein X, eosinophil major basic protein], tryptase, and chymase (mast cell products) (53) are found in the tears and serum of patients with VKC (5,33,146). In this disease, local synthesis of IgA, IgD, and IgE by conjunctival plasma cells occurs in a ratio of approximately 4:1:2, respectively (5).

The conjunctiva of patients with VKC contains many eosinophils, Th2 lymphocytes, plasma cells, neutrophils, and mast cells. A Th2-driven mechanism is postulated with activation of mast cells and eosinophils; and they have been shown to be present in the conjunctival epithelium. They produce the fibrogenic growth factors TGFβ [fibroblast proliferation/extracellular matrix (ECM) component synthesis], basic fibroblast growth factor and platelet-derived growth factor (mitogens). Elevated levels of these, along with VEGF (neovascularization), mucous membrane pemphigoid (MMP) (ECM degrading enzymes made by eosinophils and other cells), granulocyte/macrophage colony-stimulating factor, TNFα, and plasminogen activators (both tissue and urokinase)

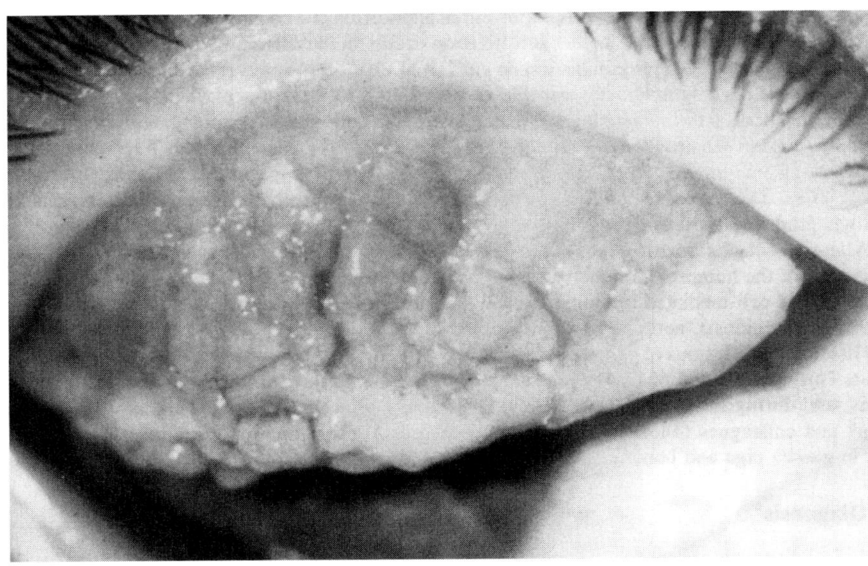

Figure 3 Vernal keratoconjunctivitis. Numerous giant papillary excrescences are present on the upper tarsal conjunctiva.

have been found (32,112). Abberrant and upregulated expression of epithelial integrins (adhesion molecules), laminin, and the epidermal growth factor receptor are also reported, signifying a proliferative state associated with epithelial wound healing (1). All these mediators are thought to account for the extensive conjunctival remodeling (subepithelial fibrosis/thickening, mucous hyperplasia/metaplasia, ingrowths and breakdown of connective tissue septae in the giant papillae) seen in VKC. TNFα, ECP levels, chymase and MMP9 levels are all significantly correlated with disease severity, number of tarsal papillae and corneal lesions (113); the corneal complications are thought to result directly from the latter toxic eosinophil products (114).

Although VKC is generally thought of as a type I hypersensitivity reaction (defined in Chapter 3), basophils, neutrophils, vascular endothelial cell hypertrophy and hyperplasia, and deposits of fibrin in the substantia propria, such as those that occur in cutaneous basophil hypersensitivity reactions, have been recognized (41), indicating that both type I and type IV hypersensitivity reactions participate in this disease. Also, many patients are not atopic and IgE is no longer considered to be the main player in pathogenesis (32).

Similar but milder histopathological changes occur in the GPC associated with the wearing of hard or soft contact lenses (6). This condition is also seen in association with chronic exposure to other foreign bodies, such as ocular prostheses, sutures, filtering blebs, and scleral buckles (167). Itching is considerably milder than in VKC. The inciting antigen in this entity is thought to be material that accumulates with time on the surface of the contact lens and that may produce a hypersensitivity reaction having both humoral and cellular immune components.

CONTACT DERMATITIS

Clinical Features

Contact dermatitis, one of the most common immunological disorders, results from the exposure of the skin to a wide variety of substances commonly found in the environment, including drugs, dyes, plant resins, preservatives, cosmetics, and metals. There are two varieties of contact dermatitis: irritant and allergic.

Irritant Contact Dermatitis

Irritant contact dermatitis is caused by excessive moisture or by damage to the skin induced by acids, alkalis, resins, or chemicals capable of injuring any person's skin if persistent contact is allowed. Allergy or hypersensitivity plays no known role in irritant contact dermatitis.

Allergic Contact Dermatitis

Allergic contact dermatitis, on the other hand, occurs only in individuals sensitized to a particular antigenic substance and upon reexposure to the same agent. Erythematous, delayed-onset skin reactions develop as a result of cell-mediated immune mechanisms. This is considered to be the most common cause of acute eyelid dermatitis, with prevalences ranging from 46% to 74% (76).

Contact dermatitis is characterized by erythema, exudation, edema, and vesiculation during the acute phase, and scaling, eczema, crusting, and lichenification predominate in chronic lesions. The diagnosis is often suggested by the site of the lesions, because they are localized to areas exposed to the offending substances, such as the hands, face, neck, or legs. Clinically, irritant dermatitis and allergic dermatitis may appear similar, but irritant lesions generally occur 1 to 2 hours after contact with the provoking agent and allergic contact dermatitis develops over a 48-hour period.

The eye is frequently involved in contact dermatitis (49), with such drugs as neomycin sulfate, atropine and its derivatives, chloramphenicol, penicillin, and related compounds all acting as contact sensitizers: antazoline, an ophthalmic antihistamine solution, is also a potential sensitizer. Like the skin elsewhere, the eyelids typically become erythematous, with scaling and crusting. Primary irritant conjunctivitis may accompany contact allergy and cause conjunctival injection and a fine epithelial punctate keratitis. It must be kept in mind that patients presenting with eyelid dermatitis may have a variety of other conditions that may be related to their dermatits, e.g., seborrheic-, atopic- and neuro-dermatitis, urticaria, respiratory allergies, drug eruptions, infections, collagen diseases, such as Sjögren syndrome or dermatomyositis, sarcoidosis and tumors (sebaceous adenoma, squamous and basal cell carcinoma, cutaneous T-cell lymphoma) (76). It is noteworthy that females account for 90% of patients presenting with eyelid dermatitis, a finding that has been consistently reported.

Parabens, used in many lotions, creams, and cosmetics, are excellent antimicrobial agents that prevent spoilage as well as bacterial and fungal growth. Paraben allergy was first reported in 1966 (156) and is now thought to be one of the leading causes of contact dermatitis. Metals, such as nickel in jewelry, undergarments, and makeup: cobalt (usually co-existing with nickel as an impurity), chromates (in costume jewelry), lead, arsenic, and gold (ubiquitous enough to be named "allergen of the year") (65); leather products, bleaches, industrial chemicals, fabrics, and automobile products are common sensitizers. Cosmetics (fragrances and lanolin in creams), cocamidopropyl betaine in shampoos and soaps, shellac, thiomersalate, colophony and balsam of Peru in eyeliner, eye shadow, mascara, makeup brushes and applicators, and nail products (lacquer with toluene, sulfonamide, formaldehyde, methacrylate, cyanoacrylate) are frequent causes. Reasons postulated for the dermatitis are that the skin of the eyelids is thin, with potential for percutaneous absorption; some agents like metals are water soluble and so moist skin may potentiate this systemic absorption; the sharp-edged particles in eye makeup causing mechanical damage to the thin eyelid skin; the co-existence of other atopies and disease mentioned above; and a combined irritant and allergic effect after long-term use (152). Paraphenylenediamine, widely used in hair dyes, clothing, and shoes, contains a "benzamine" nucleus and may cross-react with a variety of therapeutic agents, including sulfonamides, ethylaminobenzoate, and hydrochlorothiazide.

Immunopathology

In allergic contact dermatitis, the sensitizing substances are generally low-molecular-weight nonantigenic compounds (haptens) that bind to dermal proteins to form complete antigens without significantly altering the configuration of the carrier proteins. Upon initial application of a contact sensitizer, most of the applied chemical is rapidly absorbed. Whether sensitization occurs in the draining lymph nodes, at a peripheral site in the skin, or elsewhere remains unknown. Initial exposure, however, results in the production of specifically sensitized lymphocytes capable of responding to the antigen when reexposure occurs. A second application of the sensitizing substance leads to a cell-mediated inflammatory response. In the guinea pig, contact sensitivity can be transferred to unsensitized guinea pigs with T lymphocytes or with cells isolated from lymph nodes. This was first demonstrated in the experiments of Landsteiner and Chase in 1942 (111). The chemical substances that mediate these erythematous cutaneous reactions may be cytokines produced by sensitized lymphocytes on exposure to a specific antigen.

Allergic contact dermatitis does not depend on humoral antibodies and can occur in individuals with deficiencies of the humoral immune system. Contact sensitivity is absent or diminished in patients with deficiencies of cell-mediated immunity, however, such as occurs in individuals with certain malignant neoplasms, sarcoidosis, and cellular immunodeficiency states.

Histologically, lesions of contact dermatitis are characterized by a mononuclear cell infiltration of the dermis. During the acute phase, spongiosis followed by intraepidermal vesiculation occurs in the epidermis, and during the chronic stage, irregular epidermal thickening and hyperkeratosis may develop. Dvorak and colleagues (51,52) have drawn attention to the prominent infiltration of basophilic leukocytes in guinea pigs and humans.

Diagnosis

The clinical diagnosis of contact sensitivity is established by applying the suspected allergen to the skin and covering it with a patch for 48 hours. An erythematous reaction, delayed in onset, indicates a positive patch test and a strong suspicion of previous sensitization. To interpret the findings it is important to realize that substances with primary irritant properties may also produce a positive response, but this occurs within a few hours of application and can be avoided by using low doses of testing substances. Conversely, sometimes a true allergic response is not maximal until 72 hours after application of the antigen.

For irritant substances, cutaneous microcirculation measurements and the transepidermal water loss rate have been used; as the positive patch reaction is typically absent.

PEMPHIGUS

Clinical Features

Several forms of the chronic progressive bullous disorder known as pemphigus are recognized. The most common and best studied is pemphigus vulgaris. Pemphigus affects Jewish persons more frequently than others but has been documented in all ethnic groups. Before the advent of corticosteroids, the disease was almost invariably fatal, owing to fluid and electrolyte imbalance, cachexia, and sepsis.

The thin and flaccid intraepidermal blisters of pemphigus form on any part of the body, and slight pressure over areas of normal-appearing skin may cause dislodgement of the epidermis, leaving a denuded raw area (Nikolsky sign). Any age group, with the possible exception of early childhood, may be affected, but the disease is more common in persons between the 50 and 70 years of age. Cutaneous bullae may become pustular before rupturing, and once ruptured, the blisters show little tendency to heal.

Ocular Manifestations

The mucous membranes, particularly the oral mucosa, may be involved, and the most common type of ocular involvement in pemphigus is a catarrhal or purulent conjunctivitis (150). Vesicles, which rapidly rupture and erode, may involve the inner canthus or palpebral conjunctiva. These are acutely painful but generally disappear within 1 week to 10 days, leaving no scar. Some ophthalmologists consider that the formation of repeated bullae may lead to conjunctival cicatrization with progressive contraction of the conjunctival sac, especially the lower fornix (175).

Pemphigus foliaceus can involve the eyelids and a mild conjunctivitis may occur (9,21,131), the palpebral conjunctiva usually being affected and the bulbar conjunctiva remaining normal.

Immunopathology

Direct immunofluorescence studies in pemphigus have shown that immunoglobulins, particularly IgG, localize in the intercellular spaces of the epidermis (67,91). Complement components (C1, C4, and C3), properdin factor B (C3 proactivator), and, to a lesser extent, properdin (factor P) have also been found in the intercellular spaces (98). In addition, levels of complement in the blister fluid are markedly decreased, suggesting tissue deposition and utilization of complement. Intercellular IgG is detected in the conjunctiva of patients with pemphigus vulgaris (Fig. 5) (21).

Most patients with pemphigus also possess circulating IgG antibodies, which have an affinity for material in the intercellular spaces of squamous epithelium. This antibody, found in over 95% of patients with pemphigus vulgaris (92), is believed to be directed against the intercellular cement substance (27,28); the specific relevant antigen within the intercellular cement is cadherin (8). A strong binding of this antibody to intercellular cement suggests that it is a true autoantibody but may form after damage to the intercellular space caused by some other mechanism. The injection of circulating antiepithelial antibodies (induced in rabbits) facilitates acantholysis (192). Serum from humans with pemphigus causes normal human skin epithelial cells to separate from each other (acantholysis) in vitro, and the injection of such serum into rabbits and primates induces acantholytic lesions characteristic of pemphigus (26). The antibody localizes in the epidermal intercellular spaces (151). It is possible that the autoantibodies in pemphigus initiate a pathological process that is followed by complement deposition, influx of leukocytes, and destructive changes leading to blister formation. Thus, the disease may be viewed as occurring primarily as the result of a type II hypersensitivity reaction.

Histologically, the intercellular cement material is lost before any morphological alteration in desmosomal attachments. After losing the desmosomes, the cells separate from each other, become rounded, and form the intraepithelial blister cavity characteristic of pemphigus.

OCULAR CICATRICIAL PEMPHIGOID

Clinical Features

Ocular cicatricial pemphigoid (benign MMP or ocular pemphigoid) is a chronic cicatrizing condition primarily affecting not only the mucous membranes of the mouth and eye but also the nasal, genital, laryngeal, and esophageal mucosa and the skin (60). It too probably occurs primarily on the basis of a type II hypersensitivity reaction. OCP is a subset of a family of autoimmune blistering dermatoses recently dubbed MMP. Members of this disease spectrum occur as a consequence of the production of autoantibody directed against one or more glycoproteins in or associated with the epithelial basement membrane zone. We have identified the predominant target autoantigen in patients with OCP as the β4 peptide of α6β4 integrin (179), and specifically an epitope within the cytoplasm of the basal epithelial cells; binding of autoantibody to this epitope affects signal transduction between the cell and the underlying hemidesmosome and the molecules in the basement membrane zone with which the extracellular part of α6β4 integrin interacts (36,110,179). A cascade of events then ensues which results in an influx of a variety of inflammatory cells, stimulation of fibroblass, production of collagen and cicatrization. OCP most often affects persons after the fifth decade, and women are afflicted twice as often as men, although no ethnic predilection exists. The oral bullae usually begin on the gingival or buccal mucosa, often after a dental procedure. The hard and soft palate can be affected, but lesions of the uvula, tonsillar pillars, and tongue are infrequent. Esophageal lesions cause recurrent strictures; these strictures and laryngeal involvement can be life threatening. The bullae ulcerate and heal with scarring.

The incidence of neoplasia is not higher in OCP patients than in age- and sex-matched control subjects (81,166).

Ocular Manifestations

The conjunctiva is involved in 50% to 75% of OCP cases, according to several large series (81,139), the ocular lesions beginning 1 to 20 years after the onset of other mucosal or cutaneous bullae. Cases of isolated ocular involvement are not rare, however. Initially, a nonspecific conjunctivitis may affect one or both eyes, with early symptoms that include burning, foreign body sensation, excessive tearing, encrusting of the eyelids, and photophobia. Occasionally, blisters are alleged to form on the bulbar conjunctiva or margins of the eyelids (149), but the author has never seen this in his experience of over 200 patients with OCP. Hyperemia and thickening of the conjunctiva occur, and a ropy mucoid discharge often develops. Subtle

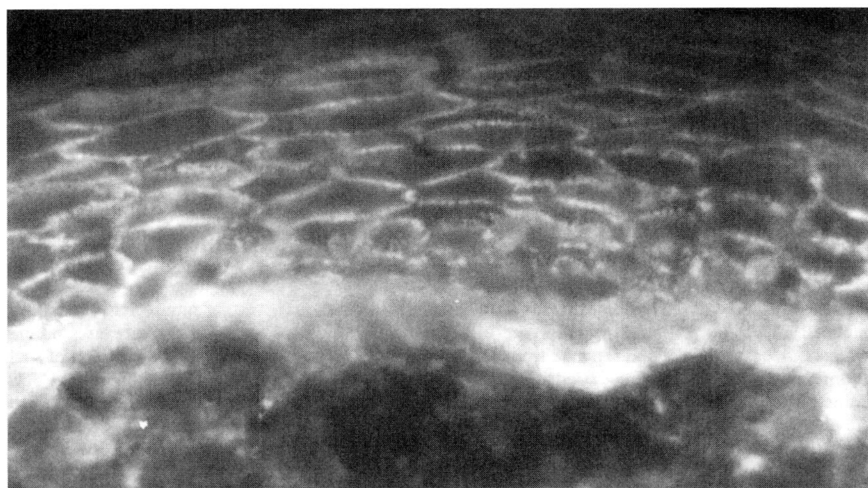

Figure 4 Conjunctival biopsy of a patient with pemphigus vulgaris. The fluoresceinated antibody used on this specimen was anti-immunoglobulin G (IgG). Note the basket weave pattern of IgG deposition at the sites of the intercellular junctions.

striae of new collagen (subepithelial fibrosis) are first observable under the lower and upper tarsal conjunctival epithelium.

As the inflammation-driven cicatrizing process progresses, fornix foreshortening and symblepharon become evident, especially in the inferior cul-de-sac. Unless the patient is treated systemically with immunomodulating regimens, the disease may progress relentlessly to obliteration of the fornices, with extensive adhesions between the bulbar and palpebral conjunctivae. Cicatricial entropion, trichiasis. distichiasis, meibomian duct obstruction, lacrimal ductule obstruction, superficial punctate epithelial keratitis, epithelial defect formation, corneal scarring, and neovascularization are seen (Fig. 4). Total dryness and epidermalization of the cornea may follow (Figs. 5 and 6). Corneal ulceration secondary to trichiasis or severe dry eye can lead to corneal perforation. Ocular involvement in this severe debilitating and blinding disease may be asymmetric but is usually bilateral, and most affected individuals become blind, usually in both eyes, unless treated systemically with immunosuppressive chemotherapeutic agents (60).

Immunopathology

Early investigators failed to detect antibodies to tissue antigens in OCP (84) but studies employing more sensitive immunological techniques have disclosed basement membrane zone antibodies in tissue and sometimes in the serum (22,25,68,84). With direct immunofiuorescence or immunoperoxidase amplifi-

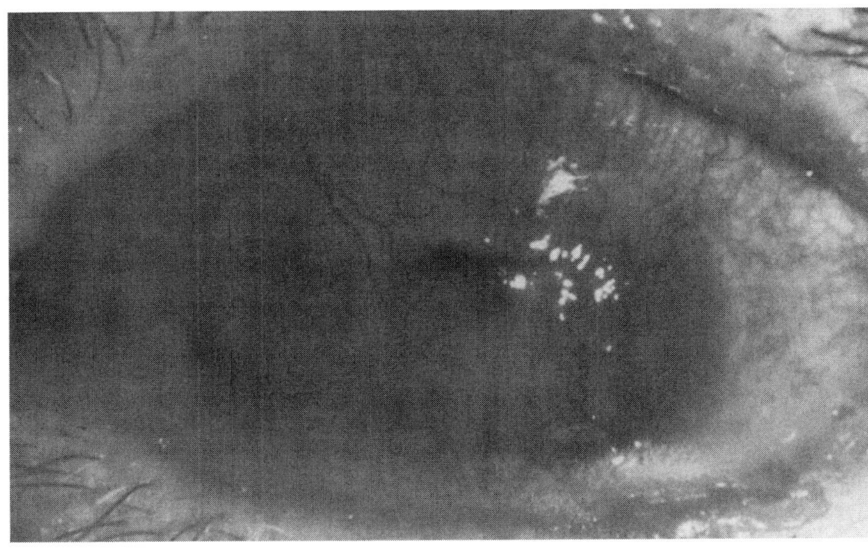

Figure 5 Cicatricial pemphigoid. Conjunctivitis, an associated keratopathy with stromal scarring, and neovascularization are present.

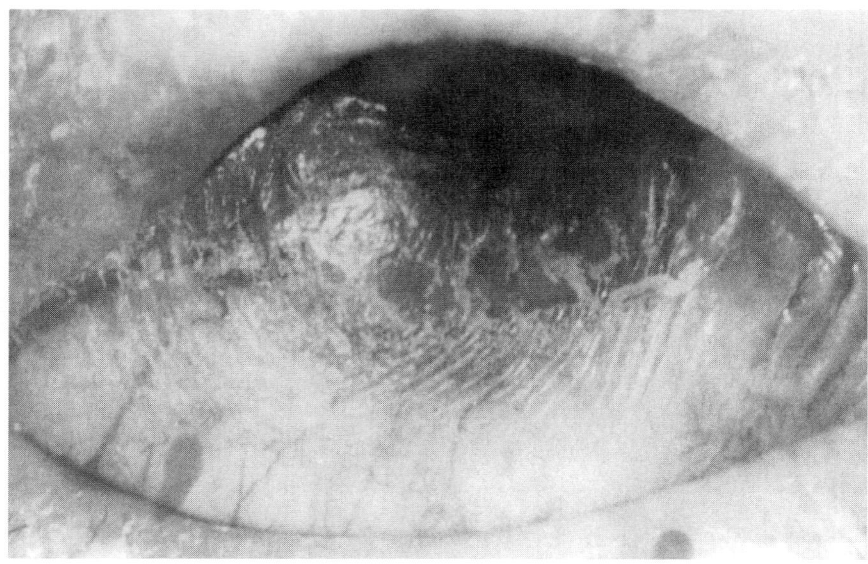

Figure 6 Cicatricial pemphigoid, stage 4. Note the ankyloblepharon and the profound sicca syndrome, with keratinization of the surface of the globe.

cation techniques, immunoglobulin and/or complement components can be detected at the basement membrane zone of the conjunctiva in approximately 90% of patients with OCP (Fig. 7) (20–22,60). The deposition of the components of the alternative pathway of complement activation is believed to occur through the C3b amplification mechanism rather than by direct activation of the complement system. Some individuals with OCP, especially patients with extensive disease, possess circulating IgG antibodies directed against the basement membrane of normal conjunctiva. The antibodies are usually in low titers and manifest more specificity for the patient's own tissues than tissue from either normal control subjects or other individuals. More sensitive techniques now exist for the detection of these autoantibodies, and it is now clear that they are much more commonly present than was earlier imagined. In general, circulating antibodies are less common in OCP than in bullous pemphigoid, in which antibodies to basement membrane are detected by indirect immunofluorescence in 85% to 90% of patients.

Antinuclear antibodies occur in variable numbers of patients with OCP (185), but the serum levels do not correlate with the clinical course of the disease. The circulating "intercellular" antibodies of pemphigus have occasionally been demonstrated in OCP.

OCP clearly has a genetic predisposition, the gene that confers this predisposition having been localized to the human leukocyte antigen (HLA)-DQβ*0301

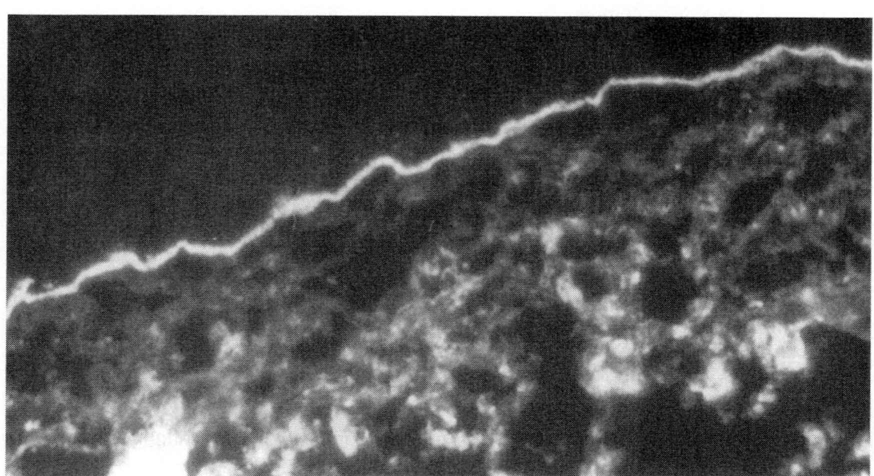

Figure 7 Conjunctival biopsy from a patient with cicatricial pemphigoid A continuous, linear, bright apple-green fluorescence at the level of the epithelial basement membrane zone, indicating the deposition of immunoglobulin A (IgA) at this patient's epithelial basement membrane zone. IgA-positive plasma cells are also present in the substantia propria (immunofluorescence microscopy; fluoresceinated antibody, ×33).

locus (2). The relevant target antigen in the basement membrane zone in OCP is distinctly different from the target antigen in bullous pemphigoid (2). Specifically, the target autoantigen in OCP is an intracytoplasmic domain of the beta 4 peptide integrin (29).

Light microscopy discloses squamous metaplasia of the affected conjunctiva in OCP, and the substantia propria contains a mononuclear cell infiltrate and numerous mast cells, many degranulated. In a substantial proportion of patients there is a microscopic angiopathy with mononuclear cell perivascular infiltrates, the blood vessels show transmission electron microscopic evidence of basement membrane damage. The immunopathological characteristics of biopsied conjunctiva from patients with OCP include an increase in class II HLA glycoproteins, which are abnormally expressed throughout the epithelium. There is also a reversal of the helper/suppressor T-cell ratio, with a dramatic influx of helper T cells into the substantia propria (Fig. 8) and the presence of the activation marker, the IL2 receptor, on the surface of a large proportion of the T lymphocytes in the infiltrate.

DERMATITIS HERPETIFORMIS

Clinical Features

Dermatitis herpetiformis is a chronic bullous cutaneous disease in which one finds increased serum IgA and the deposition of IgA along the epidermal basement membrane and an increased incidence of the HLA-B8 histocompatibility antigen in affected individuals (39,180).

An intense burning pruritus is characteristic of dermatitis herpetiformis. At any age, symmetric, polymorphous papulovesicular lesions erupt on the extensor surfaces of the buttocks, elbows, knees, back, or head. Lesions on the hands are often hemorrhagic. They generally heal without scarring unless there is superimposed bacterial infection (135). The eyelids may be involved, but the conjunctiva is only rarely affected (50). Although the untreated disease can persist for several years with chronic low-grade activity and acute exacerbations, the prognosis of dermatitis herpetiformis is excellent and no fatalities have been documented. It is part of a spectrum of gluten-sensitive disorders, the others being celiac disease (CD), gluten-sensitive ataxia and possibly IgA nephropathy (135). Both are associated with the HLA DQB1*0201 and DQA1*0501 antigens (115).

There is a well documented association with other autoimmune diseases [such as thyroid, insulin-dependent diabetes mellitus, systemic lupus erythematosus, Sjögren syndrome, rheumatoid arthritis (RA), pernicious anemia], splenic atrophy and with malignancies in patients on a gluten-containing diet (T-cell and B-cell lymphomas, small bowel and esophageal adenocarcinomas) (43).

Immunopathology

Direct immunofluorescence studies disclose a granular deposition of IgA at the dermal–epidermal junction (with accentuation at the tips of dermal papilaae) (187) and, less frequently, IgG, IgM, and the third component of complement (C3) in the same location. Normally, however, the complement components C1q and C4 only rarely deposit at the junction

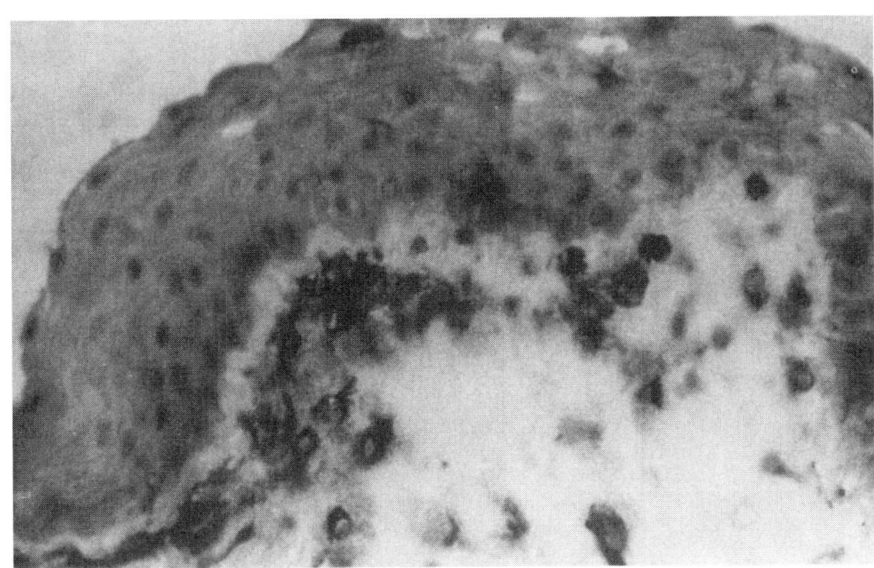

Figure 8 Conjunctival biopsy from a patient with cicatricial pemphigoid. The primary antibody used on this specimen was anti-CD4 (helper T cells). Numerous CD4-positive dark-rimmed helper T cells are present in the substantia propria (avidin–biotin–immunoperoxidase technique, ×21).

between the dermis and epidermis, suggesting activation of the complement system. In some patients, Clq has been detected with IgG or IgM (145). The relationship between IgA and the complement system in dermatitis herpetiformis is poorly understood. IgA is incapable of activating the classic complement sequence but can activate the alternative complement pathway. Thus, IgA and the alternative complement pathway may be important in dermatitis herpetiformis.

Anti-basement membrane antibodies can be detected by indirect immunofluorescence in the serum of these patients, as can endomysial antibodies. The specific target antigen has been shown to be tissue transglutimanse 3 (153). Serum complement levels are normal.

Approximately 90% of patients with dermatitis herpetiformis have the histocompatibility antigen HLA-B8, in contrast to a frequency of less than 30% in the normal population. Interestingly, 90% of persons with adult celiac disease (CD) also have this antigen, suggesting a genetic predisposition to develop these diseases (70). In this regard it is noteworthy that gastrointestinal abnormalities occur in some patients with dermatitis herpetiformis (93), including intestinal malabsorption and lesions of the jejunal mucosa. IgA and IgM may be increased in the gastrointestinal fluid, and gluten induces an increased synthesis of IgA in the tissues of the gastrointestinal tract of these patients in vitro. This has raised speculation about the coincidence of dermatitis herpetiformis and gluten sensitivity in genetically susceptible individuals. The initiating event is unknown, but ingested wheat antigen somehow interacts with the enzyme tissue transglutaminase 2 and leads to activation of T cells in the gut. Subsequent liberation of cytokines and the activation of metalloproteinases lead to a patchy intestinal atrophy. The humoral response produces IgM and IgA antibodies directed against the gliadin component of gluten (a wheat peptide) and also against autoantigens like transglutaminase 2. These IgA immune complexes then enter the systemic circulation, recognize an autoantigen in the skin, deposit there, and activate the complement system, causing damage to the basement membrane. Perhaps this is elastin, which is similar to glutenin, another wheat peptide. Another hypothesis speculates that there is cross-reactivity between the inciting antigen and normal cutaneous structures. Epidermal transglutimanse 3, of the transglutaminase family, has recently been identified as the skin antigen; it is conceivable that the IgA antibodies cross react to this (15,77).

Some investigators found the presence of the J-chain ('joining' chain of dimeric IgA, signifying mucosal origin) but others have not; the mucosal origin of the IgA deposits seems weak. However, the gut associated lymphoid tissue (GALT) system is required for disease manifestation, as direct application of gluten in skin does not cause lesions whereas oral or rectal administration does.

Histologically, the lesions of dermatitis herpetiformis are characterized by subepidermal bullae and neutrophilic microabscesses containing numerous eosinophils, characteristically within the dermal papillae. The tips of dermal papillae separate from the overlying epidermis forming clefts; these coalesce and form the blisters seen clinically. Intestinal biopsies have disclosed a patchy duodenal or jejunal atrophy indistinguishable from that in adult CD, but a frank malabsorption syndrome is rare. The numbers of intraepithelial lymphocytes and gamma delta T cells are increased.

ACUTE DISSEMINATED EPIDERMAL NECROSIS

Clinical Features

The cause of acute disseminated epidermal necrosis (ADEN), an acute, self-limited vasculitic bullous eruption of the skin and mucous membranes, is unknown but is considered to be related to a drug reaction or an infection. Over 50% of the cases are idiopathic. Three types of ADEN are recognized. Type I is used to describe drug-associated Stevens–Johnson syndrome (SJS), type II for drug-associated transitional cases (previously EM), and type III for drug-associated toxic epidermal necrosis. Histopathology shows only limited involvement at the dermo/epidermal junction. The more severe major form (SJS) is of greater concern to the ophthalmologist because the conjunctiva is very frequently involved (164). SJS can progress further into toxic epidermal necrolysis (TEN); both characterized by full thickness epidermal necrosis (85). EM, SJS and TEN are considered by some to be increasingly severe representations of a single disease entity (58).

ADEN can manifest at any age but occurs most frequently in children and young male adults. The cutaneous lesions appear several days after prodromal symptoms of fever, malaise, headache, transient arthralgia, and often evidence of an upper respiratory infection. In the minor form of ADEN, the skin lesions are red, with a symmetrical distribution that is most apparent on the extensor surfaces and distal parts of the extremities. Typically, the skin eruptions contain concentric red and white zones ("iris" or "target" lesions).

In SJS, tense bullae form beneath these characteristic lesions. Two or more mucus membrane surfaces are affected (e.g., the lips and oral mucosa); the blisters become confluent. Raw, painful, crusted areas appear where bullae rupture and liberate a serosanguineous exudate. This process may extend to the pharynx, trachea, and bronchi, gastrointestinal and genitourinary tracts, and the disease can be fatal. The mortality rate in SJS is about 5%, whereas that of TEN approaches 30%; with secondary sepsis (perhaps predisposed to by steroid treatment) being a frequent cause of death (58).

Ocular Manifestations

Ocular involvement is typical of SJS. Lesions develop on the eyelids as part of a generalized eruption, sometimes with a hemorrhagic crusting. A mild conjunctivitis may resolve without complications, but severe conjunctival involvement with blister formation leads to conjunctival infarction, pseudomembranes, fibrosis and symblepharon. Deformities of the eyelids and trichiasis result from the scarring, and a loss of conjunctival goblet cells and lacrimal duct scarring lead to a deficiency of tears and the dry eye syndrome. Conversely, punctal obstruction may cause epiphora. Corneal complications are the most serious ocular manifestations of the disease, ulceration, perforation, scarring, and vascularization sometimes developing.

Immunopathology

ADEN has long been suspected of being a type III hypersensitivity disease in which precipitating causes include infectious agents, drugs, sunlight, cold, x-irradiation for malignant neoplasms. Pediatric cases are related mostly to infection; adult cases to drugs or malignant neoplasms.

The most common infectious agent associated with ADEN is herpes simplex, which has been isolated from throat swabbings of affected individuals. Moreover, a rise in the serum herpes simplex antibody titer is sometimes detected in patients with ADEN, and additionally, the vesiculobullous lesions of ADEN can be reproduced by an intradermal injection of antigen prepared from killed herpes simplex viruses. *Mycoplasma pneumoniae,* which has been recovered from blister fluid in cases of ADEN, is another notable cause of ADEN in children, and the pneumonia caused by this microbe can be fatal if not diagnosed and treated. Complement-fixing antibodies to *M. pneumoniae* may be elevated in the serum of individuals with ADEN. Indeed, *Mycoplasma* must be considered in any child who develops ADEN. Other viruses (mumps, variola, vaccinia, and poliomyelitis), bacteria (*Mycobacterium tuberculosis* and *Neisseria gonorrhoeae*), fungi (*Histoplasma*), and protozoa have also been considered possible etiological agents (189).

The drugs most often associated with ADEN are long-acting sulfonamides, but tetracycline, penicillin, bromides, iodides, salicylates, barbiturates, phenylbutazone, cortisone, allopurinol, carbamazepine, non-steroidal anti-inflammatory drugs and vaccines against poliomyelitis, smallpox, influenza, diphtheria, and tetanus have also been implicated. ADEN typically develops within 2 weeks after starting therapy with the offending drug. Drugs blamed for ADEN have often been prescribed or taken for an upper respiratory infection, and in these instances the microbe causing this infection may be the responsible agent. Although many possible causes for ADEN have been proposed, none has been established clearly and with certainty, so that the disease could represent pathophysiological events that are precipitated by many different stimuli.

An IgA-mediated vasculitis, with release of necrotizing toxins within the epidermis, occurs in ADEN (Fig. 9). The early bullae form subdermally like those in pemphigoid. The basement membrane of the epidermis is external to the bullae, but necrosis of the overlying epidermis may accompany extensive dermal inflammation. Numerous inflammatory cells, including neutrophils and eosinophils, occur in conjunctival scrapings, which typically lack bacteria, although normal flora can be isolated in culture.

MOOREN ULCER

Clinical Features

Mooren ulcer is a rare idiopathic peripheral ulcerative keratitis that begins in clear cornea at the corneoscleral limbus and progresses centrally, circumferentially, and posteriorly through the corneal tissue, leaving a thinned, vascularized corneal residue in its wake. The edge of the progressive ulcer is undermined. Infiltrates in the corneal stroma in advance of the edge of the ulcer, presumably due to leukocytes, are characteristic (Fig. 10). The condition is painful, and the pain is usually out of proportion to clinical signs of ocular inflammation. A low-grade iritis may be present, and spontaneous or traumatic perforation of the cornea may occur. The corneal epithelium at the central edge of the ulcer remains intact; conjunctival epithelium covers the thinned, vascularized cornea left in the wake of the advancing ulcer, sometimes giving the impression of progressive corneal thinning with associated keratitis but without an epithelial defect. However, a narrow, crescent-shaped epithelial defect can be seen when the cornea is examined under cobalt blue light after the instillation of 2% fluorescein eye drops and subsequent forced closure of the eyelids for 30 seconds. The pathological process progresses slowly, with eventual destruction of the entire cornea, leaving a thinned, vascularized residua. The sometimes unbearable pain suddenly vanishes when the process finally sweeps over the entire cornea over a period that may take 4 to 18 months.

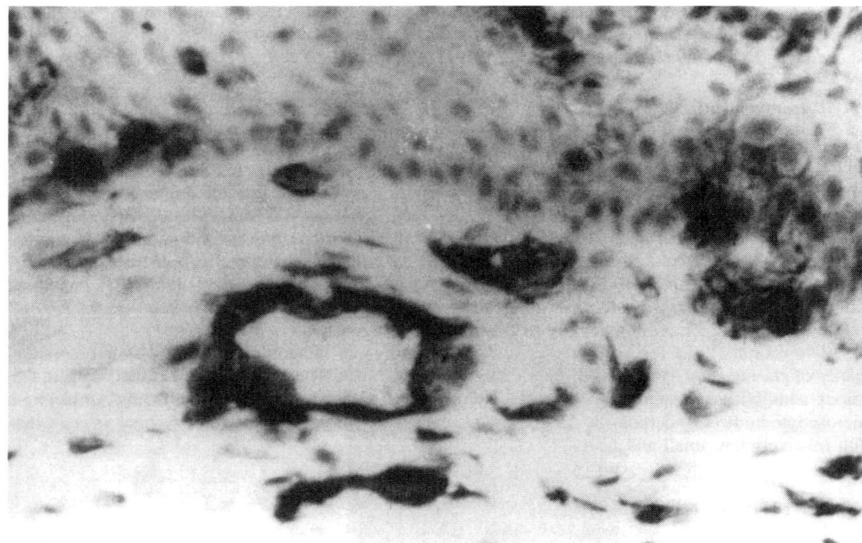

Figure 9 Conjunctival biopsy in acute disseminated epidermal necrosis. The primary antibody used on this specimen was anti-immunoglobulin A (IgA). IgA is deposited in the vascular basement membrane (avidin–biotin–immunoperoxidase technique, × 20).

There is no associated scleritis, and Mooren ulcer develops in the absence of any diagnosable systemic disorder (61). Fewer than 300 cases are documented in the literature; some cases included in reports of "Mooren ulcer" are not true Mooren ulcer but instances of peripheral ulcerative keratitis presenting clinically as the initial manifestation of an occult systemic disease.

Pathogenesis and Immunopathology

Mooren ulcer is included in this section because of circumstantial evidence that it involves a type III hypersensitivity reaction and because Mooren ulcer has some striking similarities to the peripheral ulcerative keratitis associated with some disorders, such as RA and polyarteritis nodosa that involve circulating immune complexes. However, the evidence for a type III hypersensitivity reaction is weak.

Immunoglobulins and complement are found in the peripheral cornea of patients with Mooren ulcer, suggesting the possibility of a type III immune complex deposition hypersensitivity reaction. As with all type III diseases, the predominant cell attracted to the site of immune complex deposition is the neutrophil, and this cell is abundant in the area of corneal destruction, which probably results from the liberation of proteinases and collagenase from the neutrophil granules. The substantia propria of the conjunctiva adjacent to the ulcerating cornea contains numerous plasma cells, which may account for the immunoglobulins found in the peripheral cornea. Circulating corneal autoantibodies (155) and

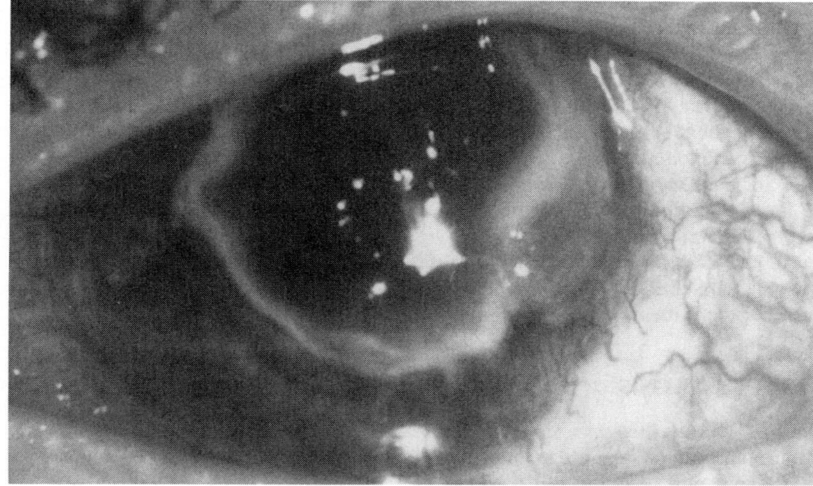

Figure 10 Mooren ulcer. The peripheral ulcerative keratitis with its inflammatory cell infiltration extends into the corneal stroma in advance of the circumferentially and centrally progressive corneal destruction.

immune complexes have been found in patients with Mooren ulcer (24). Removal of conjunctiva adjacent to the ulcerating cornea, combined with resection of the necrotic, ulcerating cornea and the application of a tissue adhesive to exclude neutrophils from access to the region, instantaneously stops the corneal destruction and cures most limited, unilateral Mooren ulcers. However, following such therapy the destructive process resumes in patients with the bilateral disease once the conjunctiva has regrown to the corneoscleral limbus and has been repopulated with the immunocompetent cells responsible for antibody and cytokine production. This suggests that in patients with bilateral disease, the antigen against which the antibodies are directed is inherently present in the cornea; and recently this 'target' has been found—corneal calgranulin C (CO-Ag, a cornea associated antigen). This is structurally identical to neutrophil calgranulin C (CaGC), a calcium-binding inflammatory mediator belonging to the S100 protein family (74). This subset of patients usually require systemic cytotoxic chemotherapy to stop the progressive corneal destruction.

Wood and Kaufman (193) emphasized the distinction between limited Mooren ulcer, usually occurring unilaterally in older individuals, and bilateral "malignant" Mooren ulcers, which mostly affect younger males and are typically relentlessly progressive despite treatment. Bilateral Mooren ulcer has been reported in young African and Indian males in whom there is evidence suggesting an association with helminthics (101). Some authors (154) have conjectured that the *Ascaris lumbricoides* and *Ancylostoma* cause Mooren ulcer, possibly through antigen–antibody reactions to toxins derived from helminths that deposit in the peripheral cornea. Another, more recent theory is as follows. CaGC is released by activated neutrophils as part of the immune response to microfilariae (123). It, in conjunction with the microbial surface, acts as an autoantigen, and initiates an immune response which subsequently cross-reacts with CO-Ag in the cornea. A self-perpetuating cycle occurs, with corneal damage, leukocyte (and neutrophil) recruitment, cytokine release (specifically IL1α and TNFα) which stimulate keratocytes to produce more CO-Ag (function unknown; postulated to be antimicrobial) (75). With this model of pathogenesis, it is easy to see why systemic chemotherapy is required. On the other hand, infestations with these nematodes are endemic in countries where young African males develop Mooren ulcer, but the disease is still rare in these areas, indicating that other mechanisms must be at play.

Other putative causes of Mooren ulcer include herpes simplex, hepatitis C, varicella zoster, trauma, and cataract extractions, but the evidence is not convincing.

The HLA subtypes DR17(3) and/or DQ2 have recently been shown to be present in 10 of 12 (83%) patients with Mooren ulcer, which is a significantly higher proportion than in ethnically matched controls (124). Another group found the DQ5 subtype to be present in 50% of patients (116). This suggests that a genetic predisposition, along with specific environmental factors (above), is required to cause the disease.

PHLYCTENULOSIS

Phlyctenulosis, which is thought to be caused by a type IV delayed hypersensitivity reaction to microbial antigens, is an uncommon type of keratoconjunctivitis usually associated with marked photophobia, lacrimation and blepharospasm, mostly seen in children (174). The entity is typified clinically by nodules (1–3 mm in diameter) in the bulbar conjunctiva, generally at or near the corneoscleral limbus (174). These vascularized nodules (phlyctenules) consist predominantly of densely packed small lymphocytes. The first phlyctenule generally appears at the corneoscleral limbus, but subsequent lesions may occur on either the conjunctiva or the cornea. The phlyctenules may extend toward the central cornea, followed by an invasion of blood vessels; the classic phlyctenular fascicular ulcer, which may become visually disabling. The phlyctenules themselves are immobile; the peripheral ulcer heals but the central margin remains active; essentially ulcerating its way through the cornea (170). Necrosis within the nodule may lead to ulceration of the overlying epithelium with subsequent regeneration. Phlyctenular keratoconjunctivitis was at one time most commonly associated with tuberculosis (referred to in the past as "scrofulous ophthalmia") (109), but now it is more commonly seen with staphylococcal antigens (140). Other causes of phlyctenulosis include *Candida albicans*, *Chlamydia trachomatis* serotypes L1, L2, and L3, the causal agent of lymphogranuloma venereum, nematodes (96), and the parasite *Hymenoleps nana* (7).

The phlyctenules run a self-limited course of 10 to 14 days, but stromal scarring produces a characteristic limbus-based triangular scar, and a wedge-shaped fascicular pannus may also occur. Corneal perforation, which is rare (136), has been observed, particularly in persons of African descent and Eskimos and is more frequently associated with tuberculosis than with *Staphylococcus* in developed societies (136).

CORNEAL TRANSPLANTATION

The mechanisms by which the host recognizes transplanted tissues as foreign or "self" are basic to an understanding of the body's immune system. For many years the cornea has been a popular site for the study of transplant rejection, owing largely to the normal clarity of the cornea and its "privileged" nature. The hypothesis initially advanced by the Nobel Laureate Sir Peter Medawar, that the cornea and anterior chamber are immunologically privileged sites (127,130,131,134,158) where antigen is invisible to the systemic immune system owing to the lack of blood vessels and lymphatics in the cornea and anterior chamber, is now known to be invalid. Rapid, potent systemic immune responses occur after foreign antigen presentation into the cornea or anterior chamber, but curiously the systemic immune response results predominantly in tolerance to the antigen rather than rejection of it, which produces the immunological privilege of these sites (63,121). Such immunological tolerance includes that usually enjoyed by the antigens on corneal allografts.

Corneal Allograft Antigens

The most important determinants for graft rejection or acceptance are products of a closely linked cluster of genes on a human chromosome 6 called the major histocompatibility complex (MHC) and designated the HLA region. These genes determine the histocompatibility antigens, which occur on the surface of all nucleated cells. The HLA region contains genes that encode for the class I (HLA A, B, and C) and for the class II HLA glycoproteins (HLA DR, DQ, and DP).

Since many alleles occur at each HLA locus, numerous potential phenotype combinations exist for the HLA glycoproteins that may be displayed on the cell surfaces of a given individual. The HLA phenotype of an individual can be determined serologically, and matching of HLA antigens can be carried out before tissue or organ transplantation. HLA typing is particularly useful in selecting appropriate donors for organ transplantation, and there is good correlation between the degree of HLA matching and the ultimate survival of the graft. Although it is not usually possible to match all four loci of the HLA region before transplantation, the best possible match is attempted. These principles apply to transplants of the kidney, heart, liver, lung, and bone marrow. Experience clearly shows that HLA matching is not necessary for successful corneal transplantation (56,181). However, such matching reduces the likelihood of graft rejection in individuals who have lost the normal immunological privilege of the cornea by virtue of corneal neovascularization or extreme alloantigen sensitization through prior transplant rejection (19,56,72,182). HLA matching in high risk patients has been shown to improve outcome by 40% compared to less-well-matched patients (102). It is also currently the only available intervention that can improve outcome for high risk patients without exposure to side effects, such as from systemic immunosuppression. The use of living live donors (used in kidney transplants) is also clearly unacceptable (44).

Several mechanisms account for the normal immune privilege of the cornea, almost all of which are overturned by the consequences of inflammation. Anitgen-presenting cells are rare in the cornea; recently bone marrow-derived Langerhans cells and three types of dendritic cells have been found, contrary to what was previously thought, but their MHC expression is limited (78,79,168). This limits the presentation of antigens to the immune system and the induction of an immune response. The corneal endothelial cells are resistant to T-cell lysis because they are unable to display endogenous antigenic peptides, unless they express the H3 minor histocompatibility antigen. Some authors have postulated that the presence or absence of this minor histocompatibility antigen is more important than those of the major ones, in contrast to other solid organ transplants (82). Fas ligand expression induces apoptosis in aberrant lymphocytes that reach the cornea (169), and the aqueous humor contains a unique immunosuppressive cytokine profile, with high levels of TGFβ, calcitonin gene-related peptide, vasoactive intestinal peptide, α melanocyte-stimulating hormone and complement regulating proteins such as decay accelerating factor, which downregulate the immune response should it occur. Blood vessels and lymphatics are absent (44). Inflammation increases the number of cells in the cornea, which remain there for years. MHC expression is increased; VEGF production results in neovascularization and lymphangiogenesis (45). Disruption of the blood–aqueous humor barrier leads to the influx of further proinflammatory cytokines. Thus inflammation in the cornea reduces its immune privilege, and also the likelihood of success of a corneal graft.

Graft Rejection

Grafts can be rejected by several mechanisms (30,88).

Hyperacute Rejection

Hyperacute rejection occurs within minutes or hours after transplantation owing to the presence of preexisting antibodies in the blood of the recipient that react with the donor tissue. The complement system and the clotting mechanisms become activated, and the resultant lesions are primarily vascular, although antibody-dependent cell-mediated cytotoxicity mechanisms may also damage cells of the graft.

Acute Rejection

Acute rejection is a term applied to an immunological rejection in a nonsensitized recipient, which may occur several days to several years after the transplant (162). Both cellular and humoral mechanisms probably play a role in acute rejection. In many animals cellular immune mechanisms appear to be most important, but humoral mechanisms may be more common in human allograft rejection. Direct destruction of donor cells by T lymphocytes and activation of macrophages, which in turn act as "aggressor cells," are the primary mechanisms in acute cellular rejection (157). Histologically, grafts become infiltrated, particularly around small and medium-sized blood vessels, by mononuclear cells, predominantly immature lymphocytes, but also by plasma cells and macrophages (140).

Chronic Rejection

The rejection of renal transplants may have a relatively late onset and be accompanied by a gradual loss of function in the transplanted kidney. This chronic rejection is associated with a progressive occlusion and ischemia of the graft (186). Histologically, cellular infiltration is not impressive and immunoglobulins cannot always be demonstrated in the lesions. Nevertheless, both sensitized T cells and antibody directed against donor cells may be present in the blood of the recipient, but since chronic rejection can occur in the T-cell-depleted animal, it is probably mediated primarily by humoral immune mechanisms (88).

Corneal Grafts

The early experiments of Medawar provided unequivocal evidence that corneal graft rejection results from an immunological reaction (131,138). Rejection of different layers of corneal grafts can occur independently under experimental conditions (103–107).

Epithelial Rejection

Epithelial rejection is characterized by congestion of pericorneal conjunctival vessels followed by the appearance of an epithelial rejection line, which is best observed if methylene blue is instilled into the eye (178). This linear abnormality forms at the edge of the graft adjacent to the vascularized portion of the cornea and migrates toward the center of the graft. It corresponds histopathologically to a zone of infiltration by lymphocytes and neutrophils. The rejected donor cells are rapidly replaced by epithelial cells of the recipient, so that the rejection may be subtle and missed clinically.

Rejection of the Corneal Stroma

Rejection of the corneal stroma also begins with congestion of the pericorneal blood vessels. A stromal haze appears at the edge of the graft, near the vessels, and an ill-defined whitish band sweeps across the donor tissue. When the rejection is completed, the haze resolves and the vessels in the graft regress. As with the epithelial rejection, the inflammatory cell infiltrate consists mainly of lymphocytes and neutrophils.

Rejection of the Corneal Endothelium

Rejection of the endothelium also starts with a pericorneal hyperemia but is followed by the appearance of keratic precipitates over the donor endothelium beginning nearest the blood vessels. The keratic precipitates enlarge over a few days and initially form a distinct line at the extreme periphery of the graft but then extend toward the center of the graft, leaving a residue of destroyed endothelial cells in their path (38,80,143). Endothelial rejection is the most important aspect of corneal graft rejection because of the crucial physiological role played by this layer of cells (Fig. 11) (90). Rejection and the consequent destruction of the corneal endothelium result in the entire graft becoming edematous, vascularized, and inflamed, whereas rejection of the stroma or epithelium can be transient and inconsequential (125–127).

Cellular Immune Mechanisms in Graft Rejection

The immunological mechanism by which acute rejection of corneal and other allografts takes place is considered to involve cellular rather than humoral immunity (type IV reaction) (13,16–18,141). This view is based on the destruction of grafts after passive transfer of cells, but not by serum, as well as the acceptance of grafts by treatment that interferes with cellular rather than humoral immunity (134). The transfer of sensitized lymphoid cells to the rabbit anterior chamber damages the corneal endothelium (108). Such observations support the idea that immunological rejection of corneal allografts is mediated by lymphoid cells contained in the passive transfer inoculum. The tendency for graft rejection is directly related to the number of antigen-presenting cells present in the cornea. MHC antigens shed from the transplant are taken up by host APCs and presented to T cells (indirect antigen presentation), or donor APCs may trigger host cells directly (direct antigen presentation) (31). Where this antigen presentation occurs is unknown, as the cornea supposedly lacks lymphatics. The resultant proliferation and activation of naïve T cells is promoted by IL2, whose action may be blocked with cyclosporine and FK 506 (35). Damage to the graft results mainly not only from CD4 T cells (CD8 T cells are not thought to play a role) (195), but also from macrophages, natural killer cells and granulocytes. Recently it has been suggested that macrophages function merely as APCs and not as effector cells that CD4 T cells function in both the afferent and efferent arms of the immune response, and that rejection may be Fas ligand independent (83). Rejection is also correlated with increased TNFα and IFNγ levels (133).

(A)

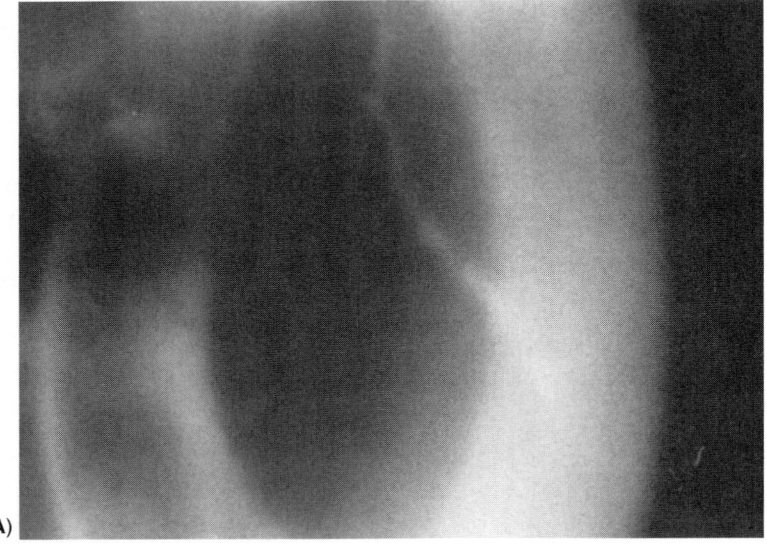

(B)

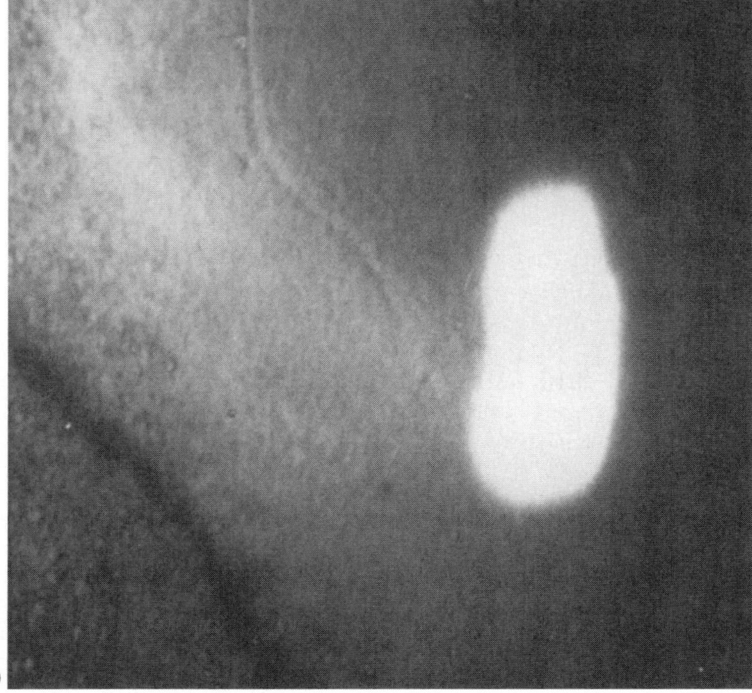

Figure 11 Corneal transplant endothelial graft rejection. A line is present (Khodadoust line) at the site where cytotoxic lymphocytes are present on the surface of the graft endothelium. (**B**) Higher magnification view of area of interest in (**A**).

Treatment of a grafted rabbit eye with topical corticosteroids is associated with fewer leukocytes infiltrating the endothelium and with destruction of lymphocytes, resulting in cessation of the rejection process. A direct cytolytic effect on the lymphocytes may be one mechanism by which corticosteroids abate cell-mediated immune rejection (69,86) but the proven effects of glucocorticoids on cell-mediated immunity include inhibition of expression of the IL2 gene in T cells by interfering with the interaction of IL2 with its receptors on T cells (86), interference with the activation of cytotoxic lymphocytes by IL2, and inhibition of natural killer cells (69,137). Corneal transplant rejection in rabbits can also be impeded by other methods that selectively impair cellular immunity, such as treatment with azathioprine (142), antilymphocyte serum (144,184), use of blocking antibody (37), or cyclosporin A (117). In contrast, complete Freund adjuvant administered intradermally or subconjunctivally can intensify graft reaction, possibly by a nonspecific stimulation of cellular immune mechanisms (159). Topically delivered antibody fragments have been shown to penetrate the cornea and enter the aqueous chamber; whole antibodies penetrate poorly after topical administration. CTLA4 antibody fragments (which bind to the costimulatory molecules B7-1 and B7-2, CD80 and 86, blocking their interaction with CD28) have been shown to prolong grafts in rodents and rabbits (172,173). Systemic anti-CD28 monoclonal antibodies have the same effect. The endothelium in humans does not divide and so it is also amenable to gene therapy. This has been done for corneal allografts in the mouse, rabbit, rat and sheep, with promising results (190).

The role of antibodies in corneal graft rejection is considered less important than that of cellular immune mechanisms. However, cytotoxic antibodies are believed to play a significant role in the hyperacute and chronic rejection of renal grafts and in the rejection of solid tissue xenografts. Although anticorneal antibodies are usually absent before keratoplasty, they can be demonstrated after grafting in both animals and humans but the relationship between anticorneal antibodies and corneal graft rejection is unclear. Some studies have detected cytotoxic antibodies against corneal tissues in graft recipients (47,48), and although these antibodies can appear in response to tissue injury, their importance in corneal graft rejection has not yet been determined. Nevertheless, lymphocytotoxic antibodies may develop if graft rejection cannot be reversed by therapy but rarely occur in patients when treatment of such reactions is successful. The presence of preoperative serum lymphocytotoxic antibodies can be considered an unfavorable prognostic sign since individuals with such antibodies may reject grafts despite immunosuppressive therapy. Evidence from our laboratory indicates that serum levels of soluble IL2 receptor (sIL2R) increase before the onset of clinical manifestations of corneal transplant rejection, increasing sometimes by several weeks. Failure of sIL2R levels to fall with transplant rejection therapy is associated with a poor prognosis for the graft (64).

ACKNOWLEDGMENTS

Portions of the material included in this chapter were originally presented in the first edition authored by Drs. Mitchell H. Friedlander and Martha R. Allansmith.

REFERENCES

1. Abu El-Asrar AM, Al-Mansouri S, Tabbara KF, et al. Immunopathogenesis of conjunctival remodelling in vernal keratoconjunctivitis. Eye 2006; 20:71–9.
2. Ahmed AR, Foster CS, Zaltas M, et al. Association of DQW7 (DQB1*0301) with ocular cicatricial pemphigoid. Proc Natl Acad Sci USA 1992; 88:11579–82.
3. Akdis M, Trautmann A, Klunker S, et al. T helper (Th) 2 predominance in atopic diseases is due to preferential apoptosis of circulating memory/effector Th1 cells. FASEB J 2003; 17:1026–35.
4. Akpek EK, Dart JK, Watson S, et al. A randomized trial of topical cyclosporin 0.05% in topical steroid-resistant atopic keratoconjunctivitis. Ophthalmology 2004; 111: 476–82.
5. Allansmith MR, Hahn GS, Simon MA. Tissue, tear, and serum IgE concentrations in vernal conjunctivitis. Am J Ophthalmol 1976; 81:506–11.
6. Allansmith MR, Korb DR, Greiner JV, et al. Giant papillary conjunctivitis in contact lens wearers. Am J Ophthalmol 1977; 83:697–708.
7. Al-Hussaini MK, Khalifa R, Al-Ansary AT, et al. Phlyctenular eye disease in association with Hymenolepis nana in Egypt. Br J Ophthalmol 1979; 63:627–31.
8. Amagi M, Klaus-Kovtun V, Stanley JR. Autoantibodies against a novel epithelial cadherin in pemphigus vulgaris, a disease of a cell adhesion. Cell 1991; 67: 869–77.
9. Amendola F. Ocular manifestations of pemphigus foliaceus. Am J Ophthalmol 1949; 32:35–44.
10. Anderson DF, MacLeod JD, Baddeley SM, et al. Seasonal allergic conjunctivitis is accompanied by increased mast cell numbers in the absence of leucocyte infiltration. Clin Exp Allergy 1997; 27:1060–6.
11. Anderson DF, Zhang S, Bradding P, et al. The relative contribution of mast cell subsets to conjunctival TH2-like cytokines. Invest Ophthalmol Vis Sci 2001; 42:995–1001.
12. Asano-Kato N, Fukagawa K, Okada N, et al. TGF-beta1, IL-1beta, and Th2 cytokines stimulate vascular endothelial growth factor production from conjunctival fibroblasts. Exp Eye Res 2005; 80:555–60.
13. Aviner Z, Henley WL, Okas S, et al. Leucocyte migration test in patients after corneal transplantation. Can J Ophthalmol 1976; 11:165–70.
14. Balas A, Vicario JL, Zambrano A, et al. Absolute linkage of celiac disease and dermatitis herpetiformis to HLA-DQ. Tissue Antigens 1997; 50:52–6.
15. Barghuthy FS, Kumar V, Valeski E, et al. Identification of IgA subclasses in skin of dermatitis herpetiformis patients. Int Arch Allergy Appl Immunol 1988; 85:268–71.
16. Barker CF, Billingham RE. Immunologically privileged sites and tissues. In: Corneal Graft Failure, Ciba Foundation Symposium. Amsterdam: Elsevier, 1973:79–99.
17. Basu PK, Miller I, Ormsby HL. Sex chromatin as a biologic cell marker in the study of the fate of corneal transplants. Am J Ophthalmol 1960; 49:513–5.
18. Basu PK, Ormsby H. Studies of the immunity with interlamellar corneal homografts in rabbits. Am J Ophthalmol 1957; 44:598–602.
19. Batchelor JR, Casey TA, Gibbs DC, et al. HLA matching and corneal grafting. Lancet 1976; 1:551–4.
20. Bean SF. Cicatrical pemphigoid. Int J Dermatol 1975; 14: 23–6.
21. Bean SF, Holubar K, Gillett RB. Pemphigus involving the eyes. Arch Dermatol 1975; 111:1484–6.
22. Bean SF, Waisman M, Michael B, et al. Cicatrical pemphigoid. Arch Dermatol 1972; 106:195–9.
23. Beetham WP. Atopic cataract. Arch Ophthalmol 1940; 24: 21–37.
24. Berkowitz PJ. Presence of circulating immune complexes in patients with peripheral corneal disease. Arch Ophthalmol 1983; 101:242–5.
25. Bettelheim H, Zehetbauer G, Kokoschka E, et al. Direkte immunofluorescenzoptische Untersuchungenheim Pemphigus ocularis (narbenbildendes Pemphigoid). Klin Monatsbl Augenheilkd 1973; 163:361–2.
26. Beutner EH, Chorzelski TP. Experimental studies on autosensitization in bullous diseases and on transfer of

pemphigus. In: Beutner EH, Chorzelski TP, Bean SI, Jordon RE, eds. Immunopathology of the Skin: Labeled Antibody Studies. Stroudsburg, PA: Dowden, Hutchinson & Ross, 1973:330–52.

27. Beutner EH, Jordon RE. Demonstration of skin antibodies in serum of pemphigus vulgaris patients by indirect immunoftuorescent staining. Proc Soc Exp Biol Med 1964; 117:505–10.
28. Beutner EH, Lever WF, Witebsky E, et al. Autoantibodies in pemphigus vulgaris. JAMA 1965; 192:682–8.
29. Bhol KC, Dans MJ, Simmons RK, et al. The autoantibodies to alpha 6 beta 4 integrin of patients affected by ocular cicatricial pemphigoid recognize predominantly epitopes within the large cytoplasmic domain of human beta 4. J Immunol 2000; 165:2824–9.
30. Billingham RE, Boswell T. Studies on the problem of corneal homografts. Proc R Soc Lond Biol. Sci 1953; 141: 392–406.
31. Boisgerault F, Liu Y, Anosova N, et al. Role of CD4+ and CD8+ T cells in allorecognition: lessons from corneal transplantation. J Immunol 2001; 167:1891–9.
32. Bonini S, Coassin M, Aronni S, Lambiase A. Vernal keratoconjunctivitis. Eye 2004; 18:345–51.
33. Brauninger GE, Centifanto YM. Immunoglobulin E in human tears. Am J Ophthalmol 1971; 72:558–61.
34. Buckle CF, Cohen AB. Nasal mucosal hyperpermeability to macromolecules in atopie rhinitis and extrinsic asthma. J Allergy Clin Immunol 1975; 55:213–21.
35. Camelo S, Shanley A, Voon AS, McMenamin PG. The distribution of antigen in lymphoid tissues following its injection into the anterior chamber of the rat eye. J Immunol 2004; 172:5388–95.
36. Chan RY, Bhol K, Tesavibul N, et al. The role of antibody to human beta4 integrin in conjunctival basement membrane separation: possible in vitro model for ocular cicatricial pemphigoid. Invest Ophthalmol Vis Sci 1999; 40:2283–90.
37. Chandler JW, Gebhardt BM, Kaufman HE. Immunologic protection of rabbit corneal allografts. 1. Preparation and in vitro testing of heterologous "blocking" antibody. Invest Ophthalmol 1973; 12:646–53.
38. Chi HH, Teng CC, Katzin HM. The fate of endothelial cells in corneal homografts. Am J Ophthalmol 1965; 59: 186–91.
39. Chorzelski TP, Beutner EH, Jablonska S, et al. Immunofluorescence studies in the diagnosis of dermatitis herpetiformis and its differentiation from bullous pemphigoid. J Invest Dermatol 1971; 56:373–80.
40. Coles RS, Laval J. Retinal detachments occurring in cataracts associated with neurodermatitis. Arch Ophthalmol 1952; 48:30–9.
41. Collin HB, Allansmith MR. Basophils in vernal conjunctivitis in humans: an electron microscopic study. Invest Ophthalmol Vis Sci 1977; 16:858–64.
42. Copeman PWM. Eczema and keratoconus. Br Med J 1965; 2:977–9.
43. Collin P, Pukkala E, Reunala T. Malignancy and survival in dermatitis herpetiformis: a comparison with coeliac disease. Gut 1996; 38:528–30.
44. Coster DJ, Williams KA. The impact of corneal allograft rejection on the long-term outcome of corneal transplantation. Am J Ophthalmol 2005; 140:1112–22.
45. Cursiefen C, Chen L, Borges LP, et al. VEGF-A stimulates lymphangiogenesis and hemangiogenesis in inflammatory neovascularization via macrophage recruitment. J Clin Invest 2004; 113:1040–50.
46. Dannaker CJ, Maibach HI, Austin E. Allergic contact dermatitis to proparacaine with subsequent cross-sensitization to tetracaine from ophthalmic preparations. Am J Contact Dermat 2001; 12:177–9.
47. D'Ermo F, Lanzieri M, Secchi AG. Anticorneal antibodies in rabbits after homologous and heterotogous corneal grafts. Acta Ophthalmol Copenh 1966; 44:233–45.
48. D'Ermo F, Lanzieri M, Secchi AG. Anticorneal antibodies in rabbits after homologous and heterologous corneal grafts. Transplantation 1966; 4:512–3.
49. Duke-Elder S. The ocular adnexa. In: System of Ophthalmology. Vol. 13, Part 1. London: Henry Kimpton, 1974:58–70.
50. Duke-Elder S. The ocular adnexa. In: System of Ophthalmology. Vol. 27. St. Louis. MO: Mosby, 1974:281.
51. Dvorak HF, Dvorak AM. Basophilic leukocytes: structure, function and the role in disease. Clin Hematol 1975; 4: 651–83.
52. Dvorak HF, Dvorak AM, Simpson BA, et al. Cutaneous basophil hypersensitivity. II. A light and electron microscopic study. J Exp Med 1970; 132:558–82.
53. Ebihara N, Funaki T, Takai S, et al. Tear chymase in vernal keratoconjunctivitis. Curr Eye Res 2004; 28:417–20.
54. Editorial. Beta-blockers and the eye. Br J Ophthalmol 1976; 60:311.
55. Efet VA. About allergic keratitis in patients treated with librium. Oftalmol Zh 1973; 28:108–10.
56. Ehlers N, Kissmeyer-Nielsen F. Influence of histocompatibility on the fate of the corneal transplant. In: Corneal Graft Failure, Ciba Foundation Symposium. Amsterdam: Elsevier, 1973:307–22.
57. Eperon S, Sauty A, Lanz R, et al. Eotaxin-1 (CCL11) upregulation in tears during seasonal allergic conjunctivitis. Graefes Arch Clin Exp Ophthalmol 2004; 242:966–70.
58. Forman R, Koren G, Shear NH. Erythema multiforme, Stevens–Johnson syndrome and toxic epidermal necrolysis in children: a review of 10 years' experience. Drug Saf 2002; 25:965–72.
59. Foster CS. Immunology: hypersensitivity reactions. In: Albert DM, Jokobiec FA, eds. Principles and Practices of Ophthalmology: Clinical Practice. Philadelphia: W.B. Saunders, 1993:318–26.
60. Foster CS. Cicatricial pemphigoid. Trans Am Ophthalmol Soc 1986; 84:527–663.
61. Foster CS, Kenyon KR, Greiner J, et al. The immunopathology of Mooren's ulcer. Am J Ophthalmol 1979; 88: 149–59.
62. Foster CS, Rice BA, Dutt J. Immunopathology of atopic keratoconjunctivitis. Ophthalmology 1991; 98:1190–6.
63. Foster CS, Wetzig RP. Immune reactions in the eye. Surv Immunol Res 1982; 1:93–108.
64. Foster CS, Wu HK, Merchant A. Soluble interleukin-2 receptor levels in corneal transplant recipients. Doc Ophthalmol 1993; 83:83–90.
65. Fowler JF Jr. Gold. Am J Contact Dermat 2001; 12:1–2.
66. Frankland AW, Easty D. Vernal keratoconjunctivitis: an atopie disease. Trans Ophthalmol Soc UK 1971; 91:479–82.
67. Freedman SO, Gold P. Clinical Immunology. 2nd ed. New York: Harper & Row, 1976.
68. Furey N, West C, Andrews T, et al. Immunofluorescent studies of ocular cicatricial pemphigoid. Am J Ophthalmol 1975; 80:825–31.
69. Gatti G, Cavallo R, Sartori ML, et al. Cortisol at physiological concentrations and prostaglandin E, are active inhibitors of human natural killer cell activity. Immunopharmacology 1986; 11:119–28.

70. Gebhard RL, Falchuk ZM, Katz SI, et al. Dermatitis herpetiformis: immunologic concomitants of small intestinal disease and relationship to histocornpatibility antigen HLA8. J Clin Invest 1974; 54:98–103.
71. Gell PGH, Coombs RRA, Lachmann PJ. Clinical Aspects of Immunology. 3rd ed. Oxford: Blackwell, 1975:761–81.
72. Gibbs DB, Batchelor JR, Casey TA. The influence of HLA compatibility on the fate of corneal grafts. In: Corneal Graft Failure, Ciba Foundation Symposium. Amsterdam: Elsevier, 1973:293–306.
73. Gigli I, Baer RL. Atopic dermatitis. In: Fitzpatrick TB, Eisen AZ, Wolff K, Freedberg IM, Austern KF, eds. Dermatology in General Medicine. Chapter 60. 2nd ed. New York: McGraw-Hill, 1987:520–8.
74. Gottsch JD, Liu SH. Cloning and expression of human corneal calgranulin C (CO-Ag). Curr Eye Res 1998; 17:870–4.
75. Gottsch JD, Li Q, Ashraf F, et al. Cytokine-induced calgranulin C expression in keratocytes. Clin Immunol 1999; 91:34–40.
76. Guin JD. Eyelid dermatitis: experience in 203 cases. J Am Acad Dermatol 2002; 47:755–65.
77. Hall RP, Lawley TJ. Characterization of circulating and cutaneous IgA immune complexes in patients with dermatitis herpetiformis. J Immunol 1985; 35:1760–5.
78. Hamrah P, Zhang Q, Liu Y, Dana MR. Novel characterization of MHC class II-negative population of resident corneal Langerhans cell-type dendritic cells. Invest Ophthalmol Vis Sci 2002; 43:639–46.
79. Hamrah P, Huq SO, Liu Y, et al. Corneal immunity is mediated by heterogeneous population of antigen-presenting cells. J Leukoc Biol 2003; 74:172–8.
80. Hanna C, Irwin ES. Fate of cells in the corneal graft. Arch Ophthalmol 1962; 68:810–7.
81. Hardy KM, Perry HO, Pingreee GC, Kirby TJ Jr. Benign mucous membrane pemphigoid. Arch Dermatol 1971; 104:467–75.
82. Haskova Z, Sproule TJ, Roopenian DC, Ksander AB. An immunodominant minor histocompatibility alloantigen that initiates corneal allograft rejection. Transplantation 2003; 75:1368–74.
83. Hegde S, Beauregard C, Mayhew E, Niederkorn JY. CD4 (+) T-cell-mediated mechanisms of corneal allograft rejection: role of Fas-induced apoptosis. Transplantation 2005; 79:23–31.
84. Herron BE. Immunologic aspects of cicatricial pemphigoid. Am J Ophthalmol 1975; 79:271–8.
85. Hockett KC. Stevens–Johnson syndrome and toxic epidermal necrolysis: oncologic considerations. Clin J Oncol Nurs 2004; 8:27–30, 55.
86. Horst HJ, Flad HD. Corticosteroid-interleukin 2 interactions: inhibition of binding of interleukin 2 receptors. Clin Exp Immunol 1987; 68:156–61.
87. Hubscher TT. Immune and biochemical mechanisms in the allergic disease of the upper respiratory tract: role of antibodies, target cells, mediators and eosinophils. Ann Allergy 1977; 38:83–90.
88. Hume DM. Organ transplants and immunity. In: Good RA, Fisher DW, eds. Immunobiology. Stamford, CT: Sinauer Associates, 1971:185–94.
89. Ingram RM. Retinal detachment associated with atopic dermatitis and cataract. Br J Ophthalmol 1965; 49:96–7.
90. Inomata H, Smelser GK, Polack FM. The fine structural changes in the corneal endothelium during graft rejection. Invest Ophthalmol 1970; 9:263–71.
91. Jablonska S. Immunopathology of bullous diseases. Ann Clin Res 1970; 2:7–12.
92. Jablonska S, Chorzelski TP, Beutner EH, Holubar K. Indications for skin and serum immunofluorescent studies in dermatology. In: Beutner EH, Chorzelski TP, Bean SF, Jordon RE, eds. Immunopathology of the Skin: Labeled Antibody Studies. Stroudsburg, PA: Dowden, Hutchinson and Ross, 1973:1–24.
93. Jablonska S, Chorzelski TP, Beutner EH, et al. Dermatitis herpetiformis and bullous pemphigoid: intermediate and mixed forms. Arch Dermatol 1976; 112:45–8.
94. Jachuk SJ, Bird T, Stephenson J, et al. Praetolol-induced autoantibodies and their relation to oculocutaneous complications. Postgrad Med J 1977; 53:75–7.
95. Jahnz-Rozyk K, Targowski T, Glodzinska-Wyszogrodzka E, Plusa T. Cc-chemokine eotaxin as a marker of efficacy of specific immunotherapy in patients with intermittent IgE-mediated allergic rhinoconjunctivitis. Allergy 2003; 58:595–601.
96. Jeffery MP. Ocular diseases caused by nematodes. Am J Ophthalmol 1955; 40:417–53.
97. Johansson SGO, Juhlin L. Immunoglobulin E in "healed" atopic dermatitis and after treatment with corticosteroids and azathioprine. Br J Dermatol 1970; 82:10–3.
98. Jordan RE, Schoeter AL, Rogers RS, III, Perry HO. Classical and alternate pathway activation of complement in pemphigus vulgaris lesions. J Invest Dermatol 1974; 63:256–9.
99. Karseras AG, Ruben M. Aetiology of keratoconus. Br J Ophthalmol 1976; 60:522–5.
100. Kaufman HS, Hobbs JR. Immunoglobulin deficiencies in an atopic population. Lancet 1970; 2:1061–3.
101. Keitzman B. Mooren's ulcer in Nigeria. Am J Ophthalmol 1968; 65:679–85.
102. Khaireddin R, Wachtlin J, Hopfenmuller W, Hoffmann F. HLA-A, HLA-B and HLA-DR matching reduces the rate of corneal allograft rejection. Graefes Arch Clin Exp Ophthalmol 2003; 241:1020–8.
103. Khodadoust AA, Silverstein AM. Studies on the heterotopic transplantation of cornea to the skin. Surv Ophthalmol 1966; 11:435–43.
104. Khodadoust AA, Silverstein AM. The survival and rejection of epithelium in experimental corneal grafts. Invest Ophthalmol 1969; 8:169–79.
105. Khodadoust AA, Silverstein AM. Transplantation and rejection of individual cell layers of the cornea. Invest Ophthalmol 1969; 8:180–95.
106. Khodadoust AA, Silverstein AM. Studies on the nature of the privilege enjoyed by corneal allografts. Invest Ophthalmol 1972; 11:137–48.
107. Khodadoust AA, Silverstein AM. Local graft-versus-host reactions within the anterior chamber of the eye: the formation of corneal endothelial pockets. Invest Ophthalmol 1975; 14:640–7.
108. Khodadoust AA, Silverstein AM. Induction of corneal graft rejection by passive cell transfer. Invest Ophthalmol 1976; 15:89–95.
109. Koppert HC, van Rij G. The phlycten, a come-back? Doc Ophthalmol 1982; 52:339–45.
110. Kumari S, Bhol KC, Simmons RK, et al. Identification of ocular cicatricial pemphigoid antibody binding site(s) in human beta4 integrin. Invest Ophthalmol Vis Sci 2001; 42: 379–85.
111. Landsteiner K, Chase MW. Experiments on transfer of cutaneous sensitivity to simple compounds. Proc Soc Exp Biol Med 1942; 49:688–90.
112. Leonardi A, Brun P, Sartori MT, et al. Urokinase plasminogen activator, uPa receptor, and its inhibitor in

vernal keratoconjunctivitis. Invest Ophthalmol Vis Sci 2005; 46:1364–70.
113. Leonardi A, Borghesan F, Faggian D, et al. Eosinophil cationic protein in tears of normal subjects and patients affected by vernal keratoconjunctivitis. Allergy 1995; 50:610–3.
114. Leonardi A, Brun P, Abatangelo G, et al. Tear levels and activity of matrix metalloproteinase (MMP)-1 and MMP-9 in vernal keratoconjunctivitis. Invest Ophthalmol Vis Sci 2003; 44:3052–8.
115. Lewis HM, Renaula TL, Garioch JJ, et al. Protective effect of gluten-free diet against development of lymphoma in dermatitis herpetiformis. Br J Dermatol 1996; 135:363–7.
116. Liang CK, Chen KH, Hsu WM, Chen KH. Association of HLA type and Mooren's ulcer in Chinese in Taiwan. Br J Ophthalmol 2003; 87:797–8.
117. Liu EY, Raizman MB, Rosner B, et al. Effects of blood transfusion and cyclosporin on rabbit corneal graft survival. Curr Eye Res 1989; 8:523–31.
118. Lobitz WC Jr, Campbell DJ. Physiologic studies in atopic dermatitis (disseminated neurodermatitis). 1. The local cutaneous response to intradermally injected acetylcholine and epinephrine. Arch Dermatol 1953; 67: 575–89.
119. Lobitz WC, Honeyman JF, Winkler NW. Suppressed cell-mediated immunity in two adults with atopic dermatitis. Br J Dermatol 1972; 86:317–28.
120. Lukacs NW, Berlin A, Schols D, et al. AMD3100, a CxCR4 antagonist, attenuates allergic lung inflammation and airway hyperreactivity. Am J Pathol 2002; 160: 1353–60.
121. MacDonald AL, Basu PK. Systemic sensitization of corneal allograft recipients before the clinical onset of graft reaction. Can J Ophthalmol 1977; 12:60–2.
122. Macleod JD, Anderson DF, Baddeley SM, et al. Immunolocalization of cytokines to mast cells in normal and allergic conjunctiva. Clin Exp Allergy 1997; 27: 1328–34.
123. Marti T, Erttmann KD, Gallin MY. Host–parasite interaction in human onchocerciasis: identification and sequence analysis of a novel human calgranulin. Biochem Biophys Res Commun 1996; 221:454–8.
124. Matsuura N, Uchio E, Nakazawa M, et al. Predominance of infiltrating IL-4-producing T cells in conjunctiva of patients with allergic conjunctival disease. Curr Eye Res 2004; 29:235–43.
125. Maumenee AE. The influence of donor-recipient sensitization on corneal grafts. Am J Ophthalmol 1951; 34:142–52.
126. Maumenee AE. The immune concept: its relation to corneal homotransplantation. Ann N Y Acad Set 1955; 59: 453–6l.
127. Maumenee AE. Clinical aspects of the corneal homograft reaction. Invest Ophthalmol 1962; 1:244–52.
128. McGill J. Conjunctival cytokines in ocular allergy. Clin Exp Allergy 2000; 30:1355–7.
129. McGready SJ, Buckley RH. Depression of cell-mediated immunity in atopic eczema. J Allergy Clin Immunol 1975; 56:393–406.
130. Medawar RB. Immunity to homologous grafted skin. 1. The suppression of cell division in grafts transplanted to immunized animals. Br J Exp Pathol 1946; 27:9–14.
131. Medawar PB. Behaviour and fate of skin autografts and skin homografts in rabbits. J Anat 1944; 78:176–99.
132. Michel B, Thomas C, Levine M, et al. Cicatricial pemphigoid and its relationship to ocular pemphigus and essential shrinkage of the conjunctiva. Ann Ophthalmol 1975; 7:11–20.
133. Niederkorn JY, Mayhew E, Mellon J, Hegde S. Role of tumor necrosis factor receptor expression in anterior chamber-associated immune deviation (ACAID) and corneal allograft survival. Invest Ophthalmol Vis Sci 2004; 45:2674–81.
134. Nelken E, Nelken D. Serologic studies in keratoplasty. Br J Ophthalmol 1965; 49:159–62.
135. Nicolas ME, Krause PK, Gibson LE, Murray JA. Dermatitis herpetiformis. Int J Dermatol 2003; 42:588–600.
136. Ostler HB, Lanier JD. Phlyctenular keratoconjunctivitis with special reference to the staphylococcal type. Trans Pac Coast Ophthalmol Soc 1974; 55:237–52.
137. Papa MZ, Vetto JT, Ettinghausen SE, et al. Effect of corticosteroid on the antitumor of lymphokine activated killer cells and interleukin 2 in mice. Cancer Res 1986; 46: 5618–23.
138. Paufique L, Sourdille GF, Offert G. Les Greffes de la cornee (Kerato-plasties). Paris: Masson, 1948.
139. Person J, Rogers RS. Bullous and cicatricial pemphigoid: clinical histopathologic and immunopathologic correlations. Mayo Clin Proc 1977; 52:54–66.
140. Polack FM. Histopathological and histochemical alterations in the early stages of corneal graft rejection. J Exp Med 1962; 116:709–17.
141. Polack FM. Modification of the immune graft response by azathioprine. Surv Ophthalmol 1966; 11:545–55.
142. Polack FM, Kanai A. Electron microscopic studies of graft endothelium in corneal graft rejection. Am J Ophthalmol 1972; 3:711–7.
143. Polack FM, Smelser GK, Rose J. Long-term survival of isotopically labeled stromal and endothelial cells in corneal homografts. Am J Ophthalmol 1964; 57:67–77.
144. Polack FM, Townsend WM, Waltman SR. Antilymphocyte serum and corneal graft rejection. Am J Ophthalmol 1972; 73:52–5.
145. Provost TT, Tomasi TB. Evidence for the activation of complement via the alternate pathway in skin disease. II. Dermatitis herpetiformis. Clin Immunol Immunopathol 1974; 3:178–86.
146. Pucci N, Novembre E, Lombardi E, et al. Atopy and serum eosinophil cationic protein in 110 white children with vernal keratoconjunctivitis: differences between tarsal and limbal forms. Clin Exp Allergy 2003; 33: 325–30.
147. Rachelefsky GS, Opelz G, Mickey MR, et al. Defective T cell function in atopic dermatitis. J Allergy Clin Immunol 1976; 57:569–76.
148. Rahi AHS, Chapman CM, Garner A, Wright P. Pathology of practolol induced ocular toxicity. Br J Ophthalmol 1976; 60:312–23.
149. Robin JB, Dugel R. Immunologic disorders of the cornea and conjunctiva. In: Kaufman HE, Barron BA, McDonald MB, Waltman SR, eds. The Cornea. Chapter 20. New York: Churchill Livingstone, 1988: 511–61.
150. Rook A, Wilkinson D, Ebling F, eds. Textbook of Dermatology. 2nd ed. Oxford: Blackwell, 1972.
151. Sanefuji M, Sugiura S. Cell mediated immunity in uveitis. 2. Leukocyte migration inhibition test in Harada disease. Acta Soc Ophthalmol Jpn 1974; 78: 306–10.
152. Sainio EL, Jolanki R, Hakala E, Kanerva L. Metals and arsenic in eye shadows. Contact Dermatitis 2000; 42:5–10.
153. Sardy M, Karpati S, Merkl B, et al. Epidermal transglutaminase (TGase 3) is the autoantigen of dermatitis herpetiformis. J Exp Med 2002; 195:747–57.

154. Schanzlin DJ. Mooren's ulceration. In: Smolin G, Thoft RA, eds. The Cornea: Scientific Foundations and Clinical Practice. Chapter 6, 2nd ed. Boston: Little, Brown, 1987:321–7.
155. Schapp OL, Feltkamp TEW, Breebaart AC. Circulating antibodies to corneal tissue in a patient suffering from Mooren's ulcer. Clin Exp Immunol 1969; 5:365–70.
156. Schorr WF, Mohajerin AH. Paraben sensitivity. Arch Dermatol 1966; 93:721–3.
157. Sher NA, Doughman DJ, Mindrup E, et al. Macrophage migration inhibition factor activity in the aqueous humor during experimental corneal xenograft and allograft rejection. Am J Ophthalmol 1976; 86:858–65.
158. Silverstein AM, Khodadoust AA. Transplantation immunobiology of the cornea. In: Corneal Graft Failure, Ciba Foundation Symposium. Amsterdam: Elsevier, 1973: 105–25.
159. Smolin G, Stein MR. Potentiation of the corneal graft reaction by complete Freund's adjuvant. Arch Ophthalmol 1972; 87:60–6.
160. Solomon LM, Nadler NJ. Radioautography of noradrenaline-^{14}C in atopic dermatitis. Can Med Assoc J 1967; 96:1147–50.
161. Spencer WH, Fisher JJ. The association of keratoconus with atopic dermatitis. Am J Ophthalmol 1959; 47: 332–40.
162. Stark WJ, Opelz G, Newsome D, et al. Sensitization to human lymphocyte antigens by corneal transplantation. Invest Ophthalmol 1973; 12:639–45.
163. Stein MR., Parker CW. Reactions following intravenous fluorescein. Am J Ophthalmol 1971; 72:861–8.
164. Stevens AM, Johnson FC. A new eruptive fever associated with stomatitis and ophthalmia: report of two cases in children. Am J Dis Child 1922; 24:526–33.
165. Stone SP, Muller SA, Gleich GJ. IgE levels in atopic dermatitis. Arch Dermatol 1973; 108:806–11.
166. Stone SP, Shroeter AL. Bullous pemphigoid and associated malignant neoplasms. Arch Dermatol 1975; 111: 991–4.
167. Strauss EC, Foster CS. Atopic ocular disease. Ophthalmol Clin North Am 2002; 15:1–5.
168. Streilein JW. New thoughts on the immunology of corneal transplantation. Eye 2003; 17:943–8.
169. Stuart PM, Griffith TS, Usui N, et al. CD95 ligand (FasL)-induced apoptosis is necessary for corneal allograft survival. J Clin Invest 1997; 99:396–402.
170. Taherian K, Shekarchian M, Taylor RH. Fascicular keratitis in children: can corneal phlycten be mobile? Clin Exp Ophthalmol 2005; 33:531–2.
171. Theodore FH, Lewson AC. Bilateral iritis complicating serum sickness. Arch Ophthalmol 1939; 21:828–32.
172. Thiel MA, Coster DJ, Standfield SD, et al. Penetration of engineered antibody fragments into the eye. Clin Exp Immunol 2002; 128:67–74.
173. Thiel MA, Steiger JU, O'Connell PJ, et al. Local or short-term systemic costimulatory molecule blockade prolongs rat corneal allograft survival. Clin Exp Ophthalmol 2005; 33:176–80.
174. Thygeson P. Observations on nontuberculous phlyctenular keratoconjunctivitis. Trans Am Acad Ophthalmol Otolaryngol 1954; 58:128–32.
175. Thygeson P. Dermatosis with ocular manifestations. In: Sorsby A, ed. Modern Ophthalmology. Vol. 2. London: Butterworths, 1963:559–86.
176. Totan Y, Hepsen IF, Cekic O, et al. Incidence of keratoconus in subjects with vernal keratoconjunctivitis: a videokeratographic study. Ophthalmology 2001; 108:824–7.
177. Trocme SD, Leiferman KM, George T, et al. Neutrophil and eosinophil participation in atopic and vernal keratoconjunctivitis. Curr Eye Res 2003; 26:319–25.
178. Tsutsui J, Watanabe S. Clinical evaluation of the precipitin test in the postoperative course of keratoplasty. Arch Ophthalmol 1961; 65:375–80.
179. Tyagi S, Bhol K, Natarajan K, et al. Ocular cicatricial pemphigoid antigen: partial sequence and biochemical characterization. Proc Natl Acad Sci USA 1996; 93: 14714–9.
180. Van Der Meer JB. Granular deposits of immunoglobulins in skin of patients with dermatitis herpetiformis: an immunofluorescent study. Br J Dermatol 1969; 81:493–503.
181. Vannas S. Histocompatibility in corneal grafting. Invest Ophthalmol 1975; 14:883–5.
182. Vannas S, Vannas A, Tilikainen A. Corneal transplantation reaction in avascular keratoconus patients due to HLA-associated immune aberration against infection. Invest Ophthalmol Vis Sci 1977; 16:644–6.
183. Vaughan D, Asbury T. General Ophthalmology. Los Altos, CA: Lange, 1977.
184. Waltman SR, Faulkner HW, Burde RM. Modification of the ocular immune response. 1. Use of antilymphocytic serum. Invest Ophthalmol 1969; 8:196–200.
185. Waltman S, Yarian D. Circulating autoantibodies in ocular pemphigoid. Am J Ophthalmol 1974; 77:891–4.
186. Wang HS, Basu PK,. Cellular immunity to xenogeneic corneal grafts in rabbits. Can J Ophthalmol 1975; 10: 263–70.
187. Warren SJ, Cockerell CJ. Characterization of a subgroup of patients with dermatitis herpetiformis with nonclassical histologic features. Am J Dermatopathol 2002; 24: 305–8.
188. Wenner HA. Complications of infantile eczema caused by the virus of herpes simplex. Am. J. Dis. Child. 67:247–264, 1944.
189. Whitmore PV. Skin and mucous membrane disorders. In: Duane T, ed. Clinical Ophthalmology. Vol. 5, Chapter 27. New York: Harper & Row, 1976:1–24.
190. Williams KA, Jessup CF, Coster DJ. Gene therapy approaches to prolonging corneal allograft survival. Expert Opin Biol Ther 2004; 4:1059–71.
191. Winkelman RK. Nonallergic factors in atopic dermatitis. J Allergy 1966; 37:29–37.
192. Wood GW, Beutner EH, Chorzelski TP. Studies in immunodermatology. II. Production of pemphigus-like lesions by intradermal injection of monkeys with Brazilian pemphigus foliaceous sera. Int Arch Allergy 1972; 42:556–64.
193. Wood TO, Kaufman HE. Mooren's ulcer. Am J Ophthalmol 1971; 71:417–22.
194. Wright P. Untoward effects associated with practolol administration: oculomucocutaneous syndrome. Br Med J 1975; 1:595–8.
195. Yamada J, Ksander BR, Streilein JW. Cytotoxic T cells play no essential role in acute rejection of orthotopic corneal allografts in mice. Invest Ophthalmol Vis Sci 2001; 42:386–92.
196. Yamagami S, Ebihara N, Amano SY. Chemokine receptor gene expression in giant papillae of atopic keratoconjunctivitis. Mol Vis 2005; 11:192–200.
197. Zhang S, Anderson DF, Bradding P, et al. Human mast cells express stem cell factor. J Pathol 1998; 186: 59–66.
198. Zierhut M, Stubiger N, Siepmann K, Deuter CM. MMF and eye disease. Lupus 2005; 14(Suppl. 1):s50–4.

6

The Eye in Systemic Immune Disorders

Avinash Gurbaxani
Kings College Hospital, London, U.K.

Sarah Hale
University Hospital of Wales, Cardiff, U.K.

Susan Lightman
Department of Clinical Ophthalmology, Moorfields Eye Hospital, London, U.K.

INTRODUCTION

A variety of systemic immune diseases affect the eye in different ways. Anterior uveitis is the most common ocular inflammatory disorder and it may be idiopathic or associated with a systemic disease (Table 1). Ocular inflammation can also be pathognomonic for the systemic immune condition, for example scleromalacia perforans and rheumatoid arthritis (RA). It may be the presenting complaint in a previously undiagnosed disorder such as necrotizing scleritis in Wegener granulomatosis.

There is increasing evidence to support the contribution of immunological processes in the systemic disorders included in this chapter, but it is still not clear why the eye should be involved in different ways in the different diseases. The pathogenesis of most non-infectious ocular inflammation of unknown cause is thought to be autoimmune, and that only a proportion of cases are a manifestation of a systemic condition. In this chapter we discuss those systemic diseases and their known pathologic mechanisms.

RHEUMATOID ARTHRITIS

General Remarks

Rheumatoid arthritis is a chronic inflammatory condition that involves all aspects of the immune response with the development of autoantibodies and immune complexes. It is a chronic multi-systemic inflammatory disorder that typically manifests as a symmetrical polyarthritis, with exacerbations and remissions. It is mainly characterized by synovitis and joint destruction. The prevalence is approximately 3%, with a female–male ratio of 3:1.

Clinical Features

Systemic

Rheumatoid arthritis is usually a disease of insidious onset with many patients complaining of ill-defined symptoms which may precede the arthritis in the form of fatigue, weight loss and diffuse pains. They are followed by a slow onset of polyarticular pain, stiffness and joint swelling. Approximately 15% of patients have a more acute illness. Many predisposing factors are said to be linked to disease onset, such as acute infections, stress, and depression but there is no clear cut evidence to support this. The diagnosis typically is made when four of seven qualifying criteria established by the American Rheumatism Association are met. These qualifying criteria are outlined below:

- Morning stiffness lasting longer than 1 hour before improvement
- Arthritis involving three or more joints
- Arthritis of the hand, particularly involvement of the proximal interphalangeal (PIP) joints, metacarpophalangeal (MCP) joints, or wrist joints
- Bilateral involvement of joint areas (i.e., both wrists, symmetric PIP, and MCP joints)
- Positive serum rheumatoid factor (RF)
- Rheumatoid nodules
- Radiographic evidence of RA

Other contributing history includes the following:

- General malaise
- Weakness
- Fever of undetermined etiology
- Weight loss
- Myalgias
- Tendonitis
- Bursitis

Joint involvement consists of pain, stiffness, and loss of function in the involved joints. Morning stiffness is characteristic and this symptom is a hallmark of the inflammatory activity. All joints can be affected, both large and small. The most commonly affected are the PIP, MCP, metatarsophalangeal, wrists, and knee joint.

Extra-articular involvement occurs in the form of rheumatoid nodules, cardiac problems (pericarditis, endocarditis, and myocarditis), pulmonary disease (pleurisy, pneumonitis, and fibrosing alveloitis), and peripheral neuropathy due to entrapment or mononeuritis multiplex, and lymph node and spleen enlargement.

Ocular

Ocular complications of RA are widespread and can affect most eye tissues. In a series of RA patients who were examined prospectively for ocular complications 17.1% had keratoconjunctivitis sicca, 0.9% had scleritis, 1.8% had a central retinal vein occlusion, and 2.7% had idiopathic retinal hemorrhages. Other lesions include episcleritis, marginal thinning of the cornea (peripheral ulcerative keratitis), and stromal corneal opacities with vascularization. Recognition of severe ocular inflammation such as necrotizing scleritis can herald the presence of associated systemic vasculitis with lesions in the bowel, heart, brain, and lung (76).

The diagnosis of RA is based on the clinical symptoms, signs, and some diagnostic tests. The diagnosis of RA is based on a persistent symmetrical polyarthritis with radiological evidence of an erosive arthritis. RA usually presents as an insidious polyarthritis initially affecting small joints of the hands and feet, excluding the distal interphalangeal joints, and progressing centrally. Subcutaneous nodules are present in one-third of patients and occur at pressure points, typically over the extensor surface of the forearm.

Table 1 Ocular Manifestation in Systemic Immune Diseases

Disease	Eyelids	Conjunctiva	Cornea	Episclera and sclera	Uvea	Retina	Others
Adult rheumatoid arthritis			Corneal furrows, sclerokeratitis	Episcleritis, various forms of scleritis	?		Sjögren syndrome
Juvenile rheumatoid arthritis			Band keratopathy		Anterior uveitis		Secondary cataract
Ankylosing spondylitis		Conjunctivitis	Keratitis, corneal	Episcleritis	Anterior uveitis	Retinitis (rare)	Optic neuritis (rare)
Sjögren syndrome		Keratoconjunctivitis sicca					
Systemic lupus erythematosus		Conjunctivitis (uncommon)		Episcleritis (rare)		Retinopathy	Papilledema
Polyarteritis nodosa			Ring ulcer	Sclerokeratitis		Retinopathy	Cogan syndrome
Wegener granulomatosis	Edema	Chemosis	Ring ulcer	Sclerokeratitis			Dacryocystitis proptosis
Giant cell arteritis			Ring ulcer			Central retinal artery occlusion	Ischemic optic neuropathy, extraocular muscle palsy, anterior segment ischemia
Relapsing polychondritis	Nodules	Conjunctivitis	Keratitis, corneal perforation	Episcleritis and scleritis	Anterior uveitis, chorioretinitis	Retinopathy	
Sarcoidosis	Nodules	Nodules	Band keratopathy		Anterior and posterior uveitis	Retinopathy	Dacryoadenitis, papilledema
Behçet disease			Keratitis (rare)	Scleritis (rare)	Anterior and posterior uveitis	Retinitis	
Scleroderma	Tightness			Episcleritis		Retinopathy	
Dermatomyositis	Erythematous lid discoloration and edema						
Colitic arthropathy					Anterior uveitis		

Source: Adapted in part from Ref. 100.

A rise in inflammatory markers such as the erythrocyte sedimentation rate (ESR) and C-reactive protein (CRP) are characteristic of RA and not seen in osteoarthritis. Other more specific tests aid the diagnosis as elucidated below.

Autoantibodies such as RF are detected in approximately 60% to 80% of patients with RA over the course of their disease, but are present in <40% of patients with early RA. This factor is a serum (auto) antibody to immunoglobulin M (IgM) with >80% specificity. RFs are autoantibodies directed against antigenic sites on the Fc portion of the heavy-chain of immunoglobulin G (IgG) and may be IgM, IgG, immunoglobulin E (IgE), or immunoglobulin A (IgA), although laboratory tests usually measure only the IgM factors. Their role is unclear, but they may be involved in complement fixation, the formation of immune complexes (particularly IgG RF), or facilitation of phagocytosis of immune complexes. They can be present in other conditions, such as systemic lupus erythematosus (SLE), and although they do not parallel disease activity, they correlate reasonably well with extra-articular manifestations.

A new diagnostic marker for RA is anti-cyclic citrullinated peptide (anti-CCP) antibodies, which has a specificity of 97% and a sensitivity of 81%. There is a strong association between anti-CCP and the presence of HLA-DR4 and a weaker one with HLA-DR1. When HLA-DRB1 was present 90% of the RA patients were anti CCP positive in one study (222). In a study of 315 patients, the comparison of RA-associated antibodies showed superior sensitivity of the anti-CCP antibody as compared to RF especially in the early detection of RA (60).

Histopathology

Systemic

The main feature of RA is inflammation primarily of the synovium, which becomes hyperplastic over time. There is an increased number of synoviocytes and infiltration with immune cells such as macrophages, B and T lymphocytes, plasma cells, and dendritic cells. Levels of tumor necrosis factor (TNFα), interleukin 6 (IL6), and other cytokines are also raised which play a key in the perpetuation of the inflammation and this ongoing inflammation causes joint destruction.

The proinflammatory cytokine TNFα plays a major role in the pathogenesis of RA. The mechanisms involved in the regulation of cytokine production are not fully understood but involve both soluble factors and cell/cell contact with other cell types (220).

The proposed stages in the development of RA include the initiation of inflammation with T cells produced in response to an antigen, localization of leukocytes to the joint and angiogenesis. With the accumulation of leukocytes there is proliferation of the synovial cells and synovitis. This causes joint erosion and a proliferation of chrondrocytes (38).

Rheumatoid nodules consist of a central nidus of fibrinoid necrosis surrounded by macrophages and fibroblasts. Vasculitis is a feature and it is thought to result from immune complex deposition in the blood vessel walls with subsequent complement activation and the attraction of polymorphonuclear leukocytes (PMNs) with the release of lysosomal enzymes (48). IgE-containing immune complexes have been identified and appear to correlate with disease activity (59). The progression from acute to chronic disease may be due to activated cells, rich in class II major histocompatibility complex (MHC) antigens that become the target of an autoimmune attack (281). An increase in the CD4/an CD8 ratio in peripheral blood and bone marrow and a higher percentage of T cells expressing class II antigens have been reported (43,64). Levels of serum interleukin 2 (IL2) receptors are also raised and appear to be good indicators of clinical disease activity (221,267).

It is the inappropriate immune mechanisms leading to immune complex deposition and microvasculitis in the joint that play a major role in the joint destruction seen in RA. Evidence has been found of immune complex mediated vasculitis in ocular tissues (74). Immune mechanisms triggered by the formation of antigen-antibody complexes attract PMNs with a production of proteolytic enzymes resulting in collagen breakdown and destruction of the cornea and sclera. It is thought that T-cell–mediated responses are important in necrotizing scleritis, high levels of T helper cells being found in the sclera and conjunctiva. In a series of patients with RA who presented with necrotizing scleritis or peripheral ulcerative keratitis biopsies showed micrangiopathy with fibrinoid necrosis, PMN invasion of blood vessels and/or vascular immunodeposits with IgA, IgG, IgM, the third component of complement (C3) and the fourth component of complement (C4). These features may herald systemic vasculitis (154).

Ocular

Scleritis

Scleritis may be classified as anterior or posterior. Anterior scleritis may be nodular, diffuse, necrotizing with inflammation, or necrotizing without a significant inflammatory cell infiltrate (scleromalacia perforans) (257).

With the exception of scleromalacia perforans, scleritis is very painful and often awakes the patient at night. In early diffuse disease, anterior segment fluorescein angiography (FA) demonstrates a rapid blood flow in the involved area. If the disease progresses to the necrotizing type, flow reduces and eventually ceases as the blood vessels thrombose. This can be reversed if inflammatory control can be achieved quickly (by the use of high-dose systemic corticosteroids), but scleral necrosis usually follows. On FA vascular closure is seen in the area of ischemic sclera, adjacent to vessels that manifest an increased permeability and that have lost their normal configuration. The sclera eventually becomes white or translucent or may resorb totally, exposing the underlying choroid.

In scleromalacia perforans, there is a nonpainful insidious necrosis of the sclera, often resulting in large areas of exposed choroid. Scleral perforation is unusual unless the condition is complicated by trauma or raised intraocular pressure (IOP). Scleromalacia perforans is usually bilateral in elderly females and nearly always associated with long-standing rheumatoid disease.

Scleritis posterior to the ocular equator may be associated with anterior scleritis. The patient usually presents with visual loss and a painful red eye, which rarely can be proposed with limited range of movement, although the mode of presentation is very variable (21). Posterior scleritis can present as angle-closure glaucoma (191) or with an apparent fundal mass that can be mistaken for a choroidal melanoma. Ultrasonography can confirm the considerable thickening of the posterior coats of the eye. Most ocular pathological specimens are of advanced necrotizing disease, obtained when a blind eye has been excised because of intractable pain. Some are removed at autopsy and others without any suspicion of scleritis. In one series, 12 of 30 eyes with histologically proven scleritis had been enucleated without a prior diagnosis of scleritis (78). Macroscopically, the affected sclera may be edematous, excavated, or ulcerated with undermined edge. Initially, necrotizing scleritis was thought to be primarily a passive destruction of the sclera without inflammation (203), although there was no clinical evidence to support this. The first pathological case reports suggested a primary scleral destruction that evoked a surrounding inflammatory reaction (247). However, the basic lesion in rheumatoid scleritis is now generally agreed to be a scleral zonal granuloma with a central area of fibrinoid necrosis, surrounded by macrophages, which may aggregate into giant cells (Fig. 1), plasma cells, and lymphocytes. PMNs and eosinophils are generally sparse, perhaps because of the high doses of systemic corticosteroids that most patients received previously (12). Mast cells are abundant and may act as local regulators of inflammation by controlling vascular permeability and the secretion of chemotactic factors (269).

Some pathologists believe that the different histopathological forms of scleritis reflect different clinical entities and pathogenetic mechanisms. Rao et al., in a histopathological study of 41 cases (195), divided scleritis into three groups: (*i*) scleritis associated with various systemic autoimmune disorders, including RA, (*ii*) postinfectious scleritis (following *Herpes zoster* and *Pseudomonas*), and (*iii*) idiopathic scleritis, without evidence of systemic disease. In the first group, the granulomatous inflammation was predominantly anterior to the ocular equator, with a marked vasculitis. There was no reactive proliferation of connective tissue or blood vessels, and lymphoid follicles were absent. The inflammation appeared to be zonal and to extend originally from adjacent episcleral and uveal tissue, a pattern Rao et al. attributed to immune complex-mediated vasculitis. The idiopathic cases, however, demonstrated a more diffuse cellular infiltration, affecting anterior and posterior sclera equally, with a predominance of lymphocytes and giant cells. There was a reactive proliferation of granulation tissue containing newly formed vascular channels, mixed with lymphocytes and macrophages

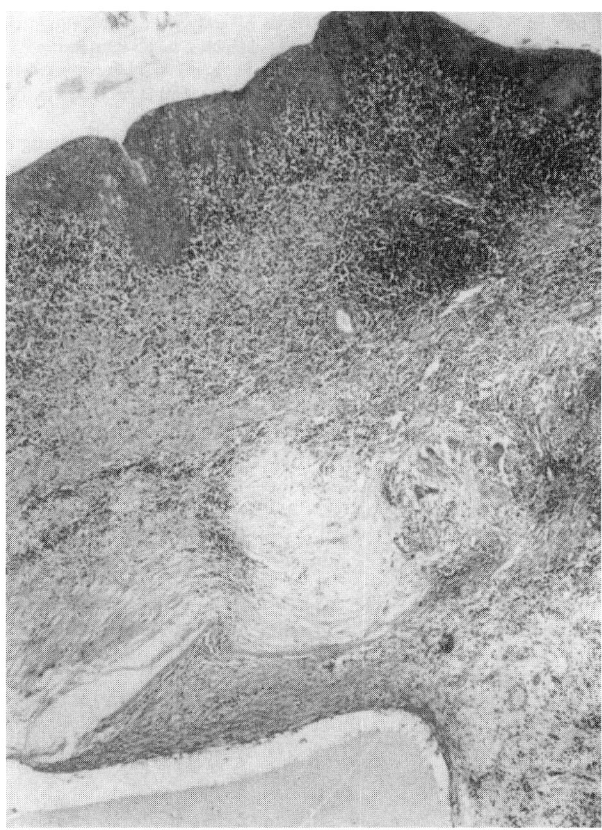

Figure 1 Necrotizing scleritis. The anterior sclera and corneoscleral junction are the site of a conspicuous chronic inflammatory cell infiltrate, which in places is granulomatous and includes multinucleated giant cells (hematoxylin and eosin, ×40). *Source*: Courtesy of Professor A. Garner.

(histiocytes), but no vasculitis. Rao et al. believed that this reactive proliferation and lack of vasculitis made an immune complex process unlikely and suggested that a delayed type of hypersensitivity to a scleral soluble antigen is involved.

A clinicopathologic study of 55 cases of scleritis looked at the various histopathological features and the causes. These were specimens from clinically diagnosed necrotizing scleritis. Twenty-five point four percent of cases were morphologically classified as zonal necrotizing granulomatous scleral inflammation. Of this group, 50% had evidence of autoimmune disease, including RA. They concluded that on the basis of histology autoimmune necrotizing scleritis can be differentiated from other idiopathic/infectious causes but the features seen in RA were not different from other autoimmune causes (201).

Inflammatory changes may be present in sclera that appears clinically normal. In patients with advanced necrotizing scleritis, numerous plasma cells and lymphocytes have been detected in the conjunctiva and episclera close to areas of scleral necrosis. Transmission electron microscopy (TEM) has disclosed active fibroblastic changes in the scleral stromal cells, together with early scleral matrix resorption, in sclera that appears normal by light microscopy. This observation led Young and Watson to conclude that extracellular matrix (ECM) resorption may precede granuloma formation and that granulomatous change is not the cause but the effect of increased tissue destruction. Collagen was seen to be degraded both extracellularly, with fibrils swollen, unraveled, and solubilized without close association with stromal cells, and intracellularly by cells resembling active fibroblasts and macrophages, which were observed phagocytosing collagen fibrils (274). Watson and Young also correlated light and TEM findings at sites peripheral to the area of scleral necrosis with FA and found that active scleral destruction in clinically normal areas can be indicated by vascular closure on FA (259). This is clinically important if surgery is to be performed since dissection must be extended to areas where the vascular pattern appears normal. In RA, anterior scleritis is more common than posterior scleritis. Watson (257) attributes this to the richer vascular supply anterior to the ocular equator. However, a study of the distribution of complement within the sclera found that, except for the first component of complement (C1), complement levels were higher in the posterior than anterior sclera, together with higher levels of immunoglobulin (Ig) and albumin, suggesting that the posterior sclera, by virtue of its underlying choroid, had a greater vascular supply (25). C1 is the recognition unit of the classic complement pathway, and perhaps in scleritis caused by immune complex deposition, the raised levels allow easier initiation of the complement cascade in the anterior sclera.

Corneal and Conjunctival Changes

The cornea can also be involved in RA. It may undergo peripheral thinning with relentless dissolution of the stroma. The cornea may also become edematous and then vascularize, eventually resolving to leave the deeper corneal layers opaque with an appearance like "candy floss" (sclerosing keratitis) (273). A stromal keratitis with dense white infiltrates resembling immune rings can result in permanent scarring, despite treatment. A more indolent form of guttering indicative of long-standing RA may also occur, with minimal inflammation; the cornea is thinned to about a third of its normal thickness peripherally, has a distinct edge, and resembles an eye wearing a microcorneal contact lens (231).

A secondary Sjögren syndrome is seen in 12% to 17% of patients with RA, who initially present with symptoms of keratoconjunctivitis sicca (see below).

Etiology and Pathogenesis

There is a genetic predisposition to RA such that 5% to 10% of people with a positive family history develop the disease (99). This link is associated with the human leukocyte antigen (HLA) DR4 subtype, which may be present in up to 70% of cases of RA (38).

Part of the genetic component arises from the HLA complex on chromosome 6 (6p21.3) (HLA-DRB1), where specific DRB1 alleles (shared epitopes) are located but additional telomeric genetic influences may exist, and that a non DRB1 susceptibility gene causes RA as well (126).

Another theory proposes an association between RA and primary hypothyroidism or pernicious anemia resulting from a defective cell mediated immune response (165). There is also some suggestion that RA is a toxic response to persistent foreign bacteria or viral antigen. In a prospective study of patients with synovitis (30% had RF positive RA and 16% negative RF RA) the prevalence of antibodies to *Proteus mirabilis* were examined and their association with RA. IgM and IgA anti-Proteus antibodies were significantly higher in patients with RF positive RA compared with all other patient groups (166).

SJÖGREN SYNDROME

General Remarks

Sjögren syndrome (SS) is a disorder characterized by salivary and lacrimal gland dysfunction, resulting in keratoconjunctivitis sicca and xerostomia associated with a lymphocytic infiltration of these secretory glands. Nasal and vaginal mucous membranes may be affected. Systemic manifestations, most commonly

RA and SLE, can be associated. The syndrome is named after Henrik Sjögren, a Swedish ophthalmologist who described the clinical and pathological findings of this entity affecting menopausal women in a classic monograph in 1933.

Sjögren syndrome is an autoimmune exocrine gland disease associated with multiple autoantibodies, a lymphocyte infiltration of various organs and a functional deficiency of T cells. The diagnosis of SS may be aided by a salivary gland biopsy and then further divided into primary or secondary based on the classification of the European study group on diagnostic criteria for SS (253). The condition usually presents as dryness of the mouth and eyes due to lacrimal and salivary gland involvement.

Primary Sjögren Syndrome

Primary SS (pSS) is a systemic autoimmune disorder with a prevalence of about 0.5% and a female–male ratio of 9:1 (33). There is overlap in an autoantibody profile with SLE.

The condition may be diagnosed on histopathological features. These are graded according to the Chisholm–Mason scale (47). Clinical and histopathological points are used for the American-European criteria for the diagnosis of pSS, a subgroup of SS patients who have lacrimal gland enlargement as a result of the lymphocytic infiltration (Fig. 2). This is relevant in view of the increased risk of lymphoma associated with pSS (177) (see Chapter 66). pSS can be associated with systemic complications such as pulmonary hypertension.

Tryptophan catabolism may regulate the immune response in pSS. In a series of 103 patients with pSS, the serum concentrations of tryptophan and its metabolite kynurenine were measured and compared to levels found in patients with symptoms of keratoconjunctivitis sicca. The kynurenine:tryptophan ratio reflects the activity of the indoleamine pyrrole 2,3 dioxygenase (IDO) an enzyme involved in tryptophan catabolism. Those with pSS had significantly higher serum kynurenine:tryptophan ratios compared to the two control groups. Patients with high IDO activity also had higher ESR, CRP, serum IgA, serum beta 2 microglobulin, creatinine, and more positive antinuclear antibodies compared to those with low IDO activity. This suggests that mechanisms dependent on tryptophan catabolism regulate immune responses in pSS. High IDO activity is associated with the severity of pSS (183).

Secondary Sjögren Syndrome

Secondary SS (sSS) is the presence of keratoconjuntivitis sicca superimposed on the background of a connective tissue disease, most commonly RA.

Other autoimmune diseases less commonly seen with SS are SLE, progressive systemic sclerosis, Hashimoto thyroiditis, polymyositis, polyarteritis nodosa, and Waldenström macroglobulinemia. There is usually a genetic predisposition. For example, sSS associated with RA usually coincides with a genetic background of HLA DR4. For diagnosis there needs to be a connective tissue disease, one sicca symptom and two positive tests for dry mouth and eyes (77).

Diagnosis

The diagnosis of SS is based on the clinical features and the presence of antinuclear antibodies (ANA) and antibodies to SS-A(Anti-Ro) or SS-B(Anti-La). In mild cases a specific diagnosis may be difficult to make

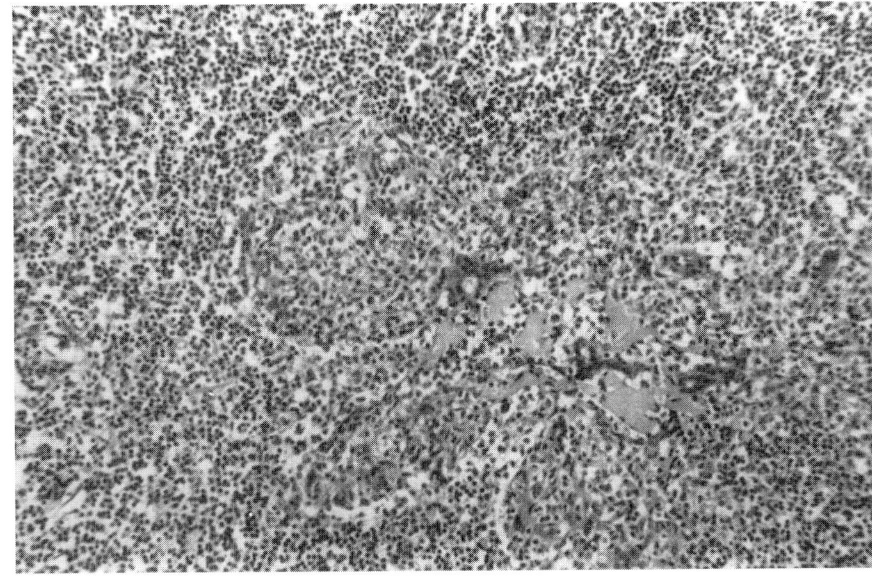

Figure 2 Sjögren syndrome. The lacrimal gland parenchyma is completely replaced by lymphoctyes and plasma cells (hematoxylin and eosin, ×160). *Source*: Courtesy of Professor A. Garner.

based on the international consensus criteria, for SS requires four of the six criteria to be positive for a diagnosis of pSS (77).

Clinical Features

Systemic

Secondary SS presents extraglandular manifestations which can involve joint and muscle (athritis/myositis), skin (Raynaud phenomenon, purpura, erythema multiforme, necrotizing vasculitis), head and neck (sinusitis, parotid swelling), lung (interstitial pneumonitis), heart (pericarditis), and renal (interstitial nephritis) (77).

Like RA, pSS is associated with an increase risk of non-Hodgkin lymphoma (see Chapter 66). The risk of lymphoma is 40 times that of the general population (146). Epstein–Barr virus (EBV) has been linked as a causative organism to lymphoma in both pSS and RA, but treatment with methotrexate in these conditions may also be implicated. In a review of tissue sections from 21 patients with RA and 6 with pSS with a history of lymphoma, only 26% of patients with RA and 1 patient with SS were positive for EBV (56). In another study, of 16 patients with lymphoma and SS, the lymphoma was mainly a low grade marginal zone lymphoma (MZL). These arise most commonly in mucosal extra nodal sites and are not associated with the viruses including EBV (146) (see Chapter 8).

Histopathology

Ocular Surface

The characteristic features of keratoconjunctivitis sicca include an abnormal proliferation and differentiation of the ocular surface epithelium, with decreased conjunctival goblet cells and an abnormal production of mucus (131).

Salivary Glands

Biopsy of a minor salivary gland in SS has become one of the diagnostic mainstays.

Etiology and Pathogenesis

The pathogenesis of SS appears to be multifactorial with possible triggering of an autoimmune response by environmental insults in a predisposed patient and may arise through dysfunction of the apoptotic pathway (see Chapter 2) in the salivary glands. The expression of *PDCD1*, a gene that encodes for a cell surface receptor belonging to the B7 superfamily and for its ligand PDL1 in salivary glands of patients with SS, is significantly higher than in healthy controls and in patients with RA or SLE. The expression of PDCD1 on T lymphocytes and PDL1 on epithelial cells from inflamed salivary glands with SS suggests that dysfunction of the PDCD1/PDL1 pathway may relate to tolerance for lymphocytes causing SS (128).

Biopsies of labial salivary glands from patients with SS there disclose destruction of acinar structures, which may be triggered by increased expression and activity of matrix metalloproteinases (MMPs), especially matrix metalloproteinase 3 (MMP-3) and matrix metalloproteinase 3 (MMP-9). Tissue inhibitors of MMPs (TIMPs) tightly control MMP activity. One study which evaluated the balance between MMPs and TIMPs in labial salivary glands found the MMP:TIMP ratio elevated and associated with acinar damage. As salivary gland acinar cells express both MMPs and TIMPs, these cells presumably contribute to ECM destruction in the pathobiology of SS (181).

A common finding in all affected tissues in SS is a progressive lymphocytic infiltration. A lympho-epithelial lesion consisting of lymphocytic replacement of the epithelium and the presence of epi-myoepithelial islands composed of keratin containing epithelial cells is a characteristic feature of salivary glands in SS. The predominant lymphocytes are T cells with a bias towards $CD4^+$ T cells rather than $CD8^+$ suppressor T cells. B cells make up about 20% of the infiltrating population and natural killer cells are less abundant (54).

The target of the immune system in pSS is the exocrine gland epithelial cells. Several viruses, primarily the herpes viruses, have been implicated in the pathophysiology of SS. In an analysis of tissue with the polymerase chain reaction (PCR), one study found that EBV and herpes simplex 1 may be implicated in a subset of SS cases (182). There is also evidence that coxsackie viruses may persistently infect the salivary glands of patients with pSS and play a permissive role for the perpetuation and induction of autoimmune disease in pSS (237). Studies have also shown sicca symptoms, positive ocular tests, lymphocyte infiltration of salivary glands, and autoantibodies in patients infected with hepatitis C virus (HCV) (193).

Lymphocytes

Several studies have analyzed the role of T-cell and B-cell dysfunctions in the pathogenesis of pSS. These have centered on the role of the cytotoxic T-lymphocyte-associated antigen 4 (CTLA4, also known as CD152) and possible alterations in the T-cell receptor. However, their specific role is still not clearly understood. SS is characterized by B-cell hyperreactivity and an altered distribution of circulating B-cell subpopulations may exist, as well as disturbances in the usage of the Ig-variable region genes from B cells. These B-cell alterations may play a role in the autoimmune/lymphoproliferative processes of pSS (192).

Changes in the Lacrimal Glands

Ectopic lymphoid follicles, the place of immune complex trapping and antigen presentation on dendritic cells, are often found in biopsies of labial salivary glands. In a series of 94 patients with pSS or sSS labial salivary gland biopsies, focal inflammatory infiltrates similar to lymphoid follicles were found in 64.9% of cases with pSS and in 23.1–49.6% of cases with sSS (187).

In addition to the role of lymphocyte-mediated epithelial cell destruction in the pathogenesis of SS, other mechanisms have been proposed. These include the role of other candidate antigens such as a family of integral membrane proteins, known as aquaporins. Because of the female preponderance, hormones such as estrogens are questioned, especially since estrogens are known to modulate immune responses and regulate apoptosis. Autonomic dysfunction is considered to be another relevant mechanism involved in pSS because, in some cases, histologically normal salivary acinar tissue may be detected that appears to be functional once removed from the patient (55,191).

The cause of SS is believed to be primarily autoimmune, with an abnormal immune response mounted against altered or abnormal self antigens expressed on the epithelium of the exocrine glands. This eventually leads to chronic inflammation and loss of function.

Genetic risk factors for pSS are linked to specific HLA alleles and the synthesis of anti-Ro/La autoantibodies. Other possibilities include single nucleotide polymorphisms (SNPs) of key cytokine genes, for example, the GCC haplotype in the *IL10* gene for interleukin 10 (IL10). Several studies have produced conflicting results regarding cytokine genes and this may be due to the different ethnic populations studied. However, it seems that SNPs in the *IL10* and *TNF* genes, which encode for IL10 and TNFα may be implicated (192).

SS is associated with anti-SSA (SS related antigen)/Ro antibody, but additional different antibodies may also be detected in patients with SS including anticentromere antibody (ACA), and autoantibodies against alpha-fodrin. A close association between fodrin and apoptotic mechanisms has been detected. Cases with ACA tend to have different laboratory features such as normal natural killer cell activity as compared to those who are anti-SSA/Ro positive (121). In a study evaluating the prevalence of IgA and IgG autoantibodies against alpha-fodrin in patients with pSS and sSS versus controls, IgA rather than IgG antibodies were found to be specific for, and frequently seen in, both pSS and sSS (266).

Some autoantibodies are subtypes that relate to the anti-Ro/SSA profile: anti-Ro52-kd/SSA, anti-Ro60-kd/SSA, and anti-La/SSB. In patients with both SS and SLE, anti-Ro60-kd/SSA autoantibodies occur more frequently than in pSS. The distribution of the subtypes of the anti-Ro/SSA autoantibodies and the disease type in pSS and sSS exists (79).

Autoantigens deposited as part of SS include the extracellular domains (ECD1) of the adenosine triphosphate binding cassette (ABCA7). ABCA7 is a member of the adenosine triphosphate binding cassette (ABC) proteins which mediates release of cellular cholesterol and phospholipid to form high density lipoprotein. A relationship between ABCA7 and SS seems to exist (235). Specific autoantigens are present in SS and autoantibodies against the antigens KLHL12 and KLHL7, which are specific for SS and not detected in RA or SLE, may be useful as serological markers for SS (243).

JUVENILE IDIOPATHIC ARTHRITIS (JUVENILE CHRONIC ARTHRITIS)

General Remarks

Juvenile arthritis (JA) can be divided into two main groups. The HLA-B27-related arthropathies, such as juvenile ankylosing spondylitis, Reiter syndrome, psoriatic arthritis, and the non HLA-B27 cases or JIA, which account for approximately 70% of all cases of JA (117).

Juvenile idiopathic arthritis (JIA) is an arthritis of at least 3 months duration, commencing before the sixteenth birthday that occurs in the absence of known causes of arthritis, such as SLE, scleroderma, polyarteritis nodosa and dermatomyositis, rheumatic fever, infections, neoplasia, and trauma.

Clinical Features

Systemic

Three subgroups of JIA are generally recognized (118): Systemic onset JIA, polyarticular onset JIA, and pauciarticular onset JIA.

Systemic Onset JIA

Systemic onset JIA, which occurs in about 20% of cases, presents with fever, a maculopapular rash, and generalized lymphadenopathy. Hepatosplenomegaly, pericarditis, and pleurisy can also occur. Initially, there may be only minimal joint symptoms, although most patients ultimately develop widespread polyarthritis. Less than 1% develops ocular manifestations.

Polyarticular Onset JIA

Polyarticular onset (five or more joints involved) in which joint symptoms and signs predominate. The knees, wrists, and ankles are most commonly involved. Approximately 25% of this group are seropositive for IgM RF and follow a clinical pattern similar to that in adults with RA.

Pauciarticular Onset JIA

Pauciarticular onset JIA (four or fewer joints involved), which accounts for approximately two-thirds of all cases of JA. The knee, ankle, and elbow are most commonly involved, although only a single finger or toe may be affected.

Ocular

The major ocular feature, anterior uveitis, is usually bilateral, and typically occurs in a girl who is RF negative and ANA positive, with pauciarticular JIA. The reported incidence of anterior uveitis in JIA varies from 2% to 21%. The differences in incidence can probably be attributed to the mode of detection because the onset of uveitis in most cases is insidious, occurring in a white eye and only detected on slit-lamp biomicroscopy. Posterior uveitis is uncommon and is usually secondary to anterior uveitis. Secondary glaucoma, usually caused by angle closure, posterior synechiae or trabecular damage, cataract, calcific band keratopathy, and macular edema, also occur, and all may contribute to visual loss. There is no parallel between the activity of uveitis and that of joint disease.

There is a distinctive pattern of abnormal cytokine production in children with active systemic onset JIA. TNFα is significantly overproduced, while interferon gamma (IFNγ) levels are markedly decreased (164). Elevated levels of interleukin 6 (IL6), interleukin 8 (IL8), monocyte chemoattractant protein-1 (MCP-1), E-selectin, and intracellular adhesion molecule (ICAM-1) are also found (58). The intercellular adhesion molecules (ICAM) are a family of receptors expressed on the surface of activated vascular endothelium.

Of all patients with JIA, 20% are seropositive for ANA, but this prevalence increases from 71% to 93% in those with arthritis plus uveitis. ANA are also more likely to be present in those with pauciarticular JIA (61). IgM RF is found in approximately 20% of the polyarticular group, and another study also demonstrated IgA RF, which appears to be specific for the same group and correlates with severe disease (62).

Histopathology

Joints

Microscopic examination of the synovium shows loss of its normally well-defined lining, with fibrin deposition on the surface and in the lining and subintimal layers. Other findings include hypertrophy and edema of the synovium, vascular congestion in the subsynovial tissue, and a marked infiltrate of plasma cells and lymphocytes, with variable numbers of macrophages, giant cells, and monocytes. PMNs are present but are not prominent (130).

Eye

The documented ocular histopathology is limited to a few reports. Merriam and collaborators described a case in which the iris and ciliary body architecture was entirely replaced by abundant plasma cells and lymphocytes, with destruction of the epithelium, blood vessels, processes of the ciliary body, and Bruch membrane (153). This specimen also had peripheral retinal vasculitis and serous retinal detachment with atrophy of all retinal layers, yet uveal inflammation ceased at the ocular equator. Granulomas with epithelioid and giant cells but without necrosis have also been described in the ciliary body and choroid (208).

Etiology and Pathogenesis

There is a positive correlation between HLA DR5 and DPW2 and pauciarticular JA with uveitis and HLA A2 and DRW8 and persistent arthritis (232). An association between JIA and allele 5 at the microsatellite D6S265 in the HLA class I region has been documented, independent of linkage disequilibrium (LD) with the DR8-DQ4 haplotype (226). Other alleles at D6S265 were investigated to determine if they modified the risk for JIA on different haplotypes (226). Allele 6 at D6S265 was significantly associated with JIA on the DRB1*1301-DQB1*0603 haplotype (odds ratio 5.5). In another study, 235 sporadic JIA families (82 pauciarticular, 153 polyarticular) and 639 controls were typed for 16 markers spanning the MHC region (207). Case-control and transmission disequilibrium test analyses demonstrated strong evidence for a susceptibility locus near D6S2447, a marker flanked by DQB1 and DRB1. HLA-DRB1*08 was strongly associated and overtransmitted to pauciarticular and polyarticular JIA probands. In pauciarticular probands, HLA-DRB1*11 was also associated and overtransmitted. Probands with polyarticular JIA showed association with a more extensive region compared with pauciarticular JIA probands. The above mentioned studies suggest the presence of additional JIA susceptibility locus/loci in the HLA class I region (207,226).

In another study HLA-DR3 alleles were investigated among 64 children with pauciarticular or polyarticular JIA and 64 controls (7). HLA-DR3 alleles were increased in children with pauciarticular JIA compared with controls. HLA-DRB1*0307 and *0308 were seen only in JIA probands. HLA-DR8 was increased in JIA patients. HLA-DR11 was increased in the controls compared with patients; however, this was not significant. This trend differs from the previously described increased frequency of HLA-DR5 (HLA-DR5 includes HLA-DR11 and HLA-DR12 alleles) among pauciarticular JIA probands (163).

Non-HLA Polymorphisms

In addition to the numerous associations between JIA and HLA variants, other non-HLA polymorphisms have been associated with JIA. The sibling recurrence risk, which is a commonly used genetic tool to determine the chance that a genetic disease may occur in siblings (or other relatives) of an affected child ([lambda]s) for JIA has been estimated to be approximately 15%, and the HLA-DR accounted for approximately 17% of the risk for JIA (186). This suggests that other loci both within and outside the MHC influence the genetic risk for JIA. Macrophage migration inhibitory factor (MIF) plays a role in the development of experimentally induced autoimmune disease. A single SNP at codon 173(G/C) of the *MIF* gene is associated with JIA. The functional relevance of this SNP was investigated in 136 patients and was found to be associated with systemic JIA (58). IL6 is another proinflammatory cytokine elevated in children with systemic JIA. Systemic JIA cohorts from three countries (United States, United Kingdom, and France) were typed for a SNP at position –174, and it was found that the IL6 174 nucleotide variant is significantly associated with systemic JIA (174).

The cause and pathogenesis of JIA remain unclear. No reliable evidence points to a single initiating infection or other event. Rubella virus has been isolated, but this may reflect an immunodeficiency state rather than the etiologic agent of JIA (184). A lack of suppressor/cytotoxic T cell response to EBV has also been demonstrated. Although an autoimmune mechanism is presumed, the exact process is unclear. Elevated levels of circulating immune complexes have been detected and appear most frequently in those with relatively severe disease. Some authors believe that the systemic form of the disease is characterized primarily by B-cell rather than T-cell abnormalities (241), although B-cell abnormalities may be related to defects in T-cell immunoregulation. An increase in the CD4/CD8 ratio has been demonstrated in the peripheral blood of patients with polyarticular disease, but this ratio is normal in individuals with pauciarticular disease (234). In patients with uveitis, deposits of IgM in iris stromal cells, raised levels of Ig in the aqueous humor, and serum antibodies to iris and retina have been detected (85).

Antibodies to soluble retinal antigens have been found more frequently in children with JA and uveitis than in those with JA alone, although this may be the result of damage rather than the pathogenetic mechanism per se (185).

Multiple factors have been considered as the cause of JA. A lack of suppressor/cytotoxic T cell response to EBV has also been demonstrated (241) Although an autoimmune mechanism is presumed, the exact process is unclear. Elevated levels of circulating immune complexes have been detected and appear most frequently in those with relatively severe disease (156). Some authors believe that the systemic form of the disease is characterized primarily by B-cell rather than T-cell abnormalities (244), although B-cell abnormalities may be related to defects in T-cell immunoregulation (16).

SARCOIDOSIS

General Remarks

Sarcoidosis is an idiopathic multisystem granulomatous disorder that can affect almost every organ in the body. The prevalence varies with different communities. It is three to four times more common in blacks than whites and less common in Asians. It usually occurs between 16 and 65 years of age, and in one worldwide survey, 68% of patients were below the age of 40 years at diagnosis (107). There is an equal sex distribution, although women suffer more skin disease.

Clinical Features

Systemic

The lungs are the most commonly affected organ. Chest roentgenograms reveal bilateral hilar lymphadenopathy (Fig. 3) and, less commonly, pulmonary infiltration, which may progress in a few to irreversible pulmonary fibrosis. Of all cases, however, 40% are asymptomatic at diagnosis. Erythema nodosum is the most frequent skin manifestation and almost always occurs in association with bilateral hilar lymphadenopathy, often with mild fever and arthralgia. Lupus pernio is also seen, more commonly in blacks. Two-thirds of patients eventually develop hepatic granulomas (246) although these are rarely symptomatic. About 5% of patients experience neurological manifestations, most frequently a facial nerve palsy, usually as part of a florid clinical picture. The joints (transient symmetrical arthropathy), heart, endocrine glands, lymph nodes, spleen, and kidney can also be involved.

Ocular

Ocular involvement occurs in 20% to 30% of cases, and uveitis accounts for 60% to 80% of the ocular

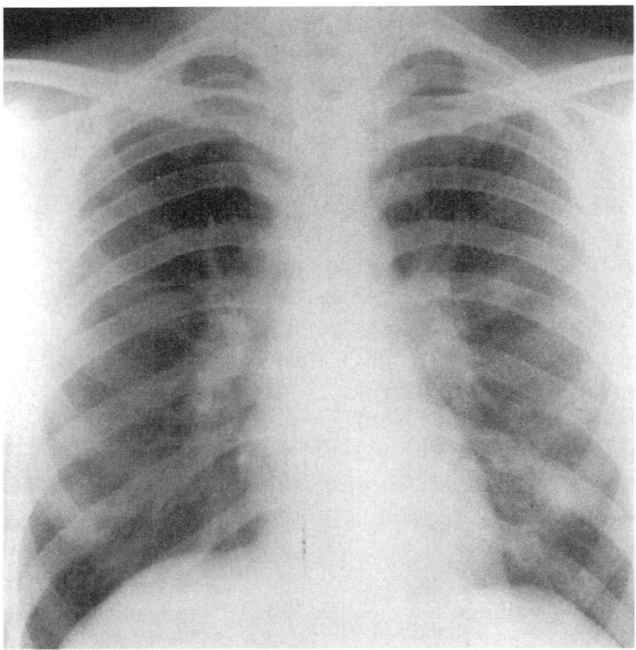

Figure 3 Sarcoidosis. Chest roentgenogram demonstrating bilateral hilar lymphadenopathy.

manifestations (106). Sarcoidosis is reported to account for 2% to 4% of all cases of uveitis. The uveitis may be anterior or posterior; anterior uveitis tends to be more common in black patients and posterior uveitis more common in white patients (206). The anterior uveitis is often of the granulomatous type, with "mutton fat" keratic precipitates and nodules, which may be in the iris, anterior chamber angle, and ciliary processes (Fig. 4) (170). Glaucoma can occur secondary to active disease, from posterior synechiae with iris bombe, or from angle damage with peripheral anterior synechiae. Posterior segment involvement is present in approximately one-quarter of patients with ocular disease. A vitreous cellular infiltrate with "snowball" opacities and a peripheral periphlebitis with "candle wax" exudates are almost pathognomonic (Fig. 5). Edema, of the macula and optic nerve head, chorioretinitis, and peripheral retinal neovascularization (secondary to ischemia and/or a direct effect of the inflammation) may also occur. Conjunctival granulomas and, less commonly, isolated choroidal, orbital, and lacrimal gland granulomas, also occur (110).

Histopathology

The characteristic tissue finding in sarcoidosis is noncaseating epitheliod cell granulomas, with giant cell formation and a surrounding rim of lymphocytes. There is a lack of necrosis, an intact reticulin pattern, and a failure to demonstrate any infective agent.

In the lung, the initial lesion is an alveolitis that proceeds to the formation of granulomas, which may proceed to resolution or become infiltrated by fibroblasts and transformed into hyalinized connective tissue. Sarcoidosis may be considered a "lymphoproliferative disorder" characterized by depressed delayed-type hypersensitivity imbalance of CD4/CD8 subsets, hyperactivity of B cells, and the circulation of immune complexes (105). T lymphocytes expressing helper/inducer phenotypes have been detected within the aggregates of epithelioid cells; suppressor/cytotoxic phenotypes are predominantly in the lymphocyte mantle surrounding each granuloma and are possibly attempting to restrict the immune response (161). The detection of the lymphokines, IFNγ and

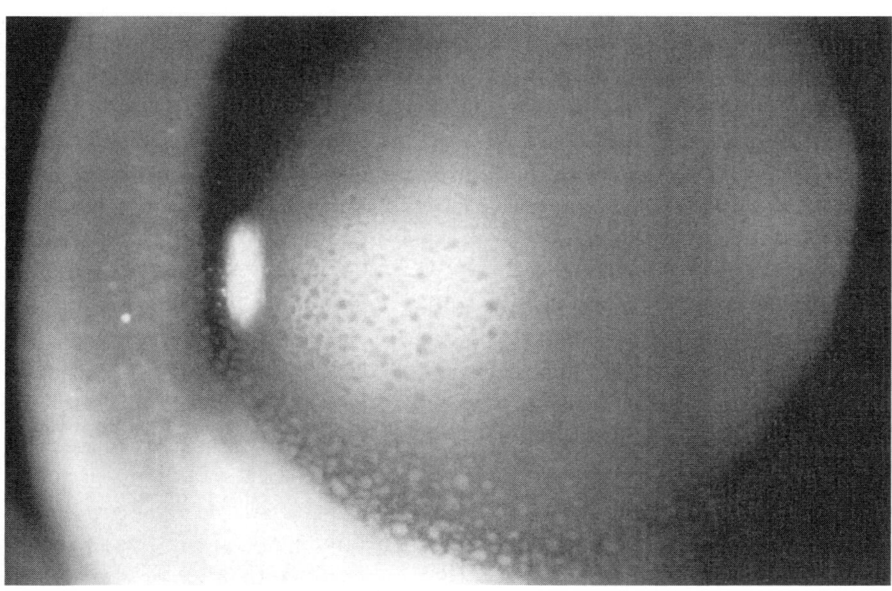

Figure 4 Sarcoidosis. Anterior uveitis with "mutton fat" keratic precipitates.

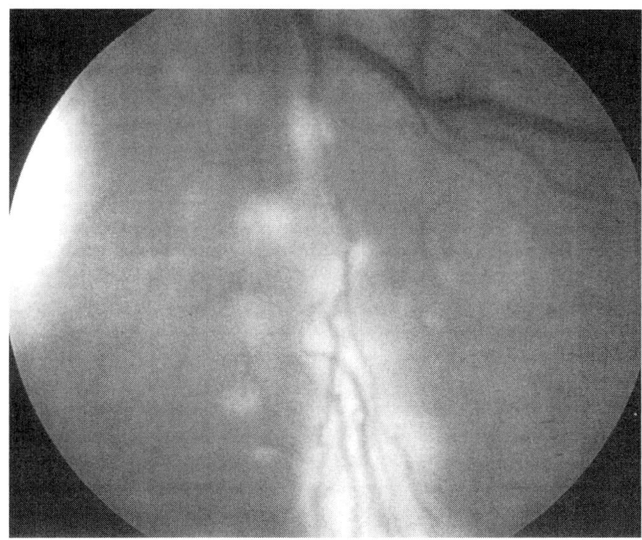

Figure 5 Sarcoidosis. Peripheral periphlebitis with "candle wax" exudates.

interleukin 2 (IL2) together with expression of IL2 receptors in T cells of patients with active sarcoidosis, further supports the role of T cells in the pathogenesis (95). The peripheral circulation may be lymphopenic with an absolute decrease in CD4 positive lymphocytes that have been consumed in the tissue granulomas. Such a redistribution of T lymphocytes may explain the cutaneous anergy seen to purified protein derivative in tuberculin testing in patients previously immunized with bacillus Calmette-Guérin (101). Circulating immune complexes have been found in patients with active sarcoidosis and may be associated with extrapulmonary involvement.

In a histopathological analysis, a widespread infiltrate of lymphocytes and plasma cells, epithelioid cells, and occasional multinucleate giant cells surrounded by a cuff of small and large lymphocytes was demonstrated (Fig. 6). The majority of lymphocytes were T cells (>90% CD4 cells, and <10% CD8 T cells). The suppressor/cytotoxic T cells were generally located in the lymphocyte cuff, and rarely within the granuloma. Class II MHC antigens were diffusely distributed over and within the granuloma. Cell membranes of T lymphocytes, macrophages, and epithelioid cells contained abundant IL2 receptors and IFNγ according to immunohistochemical analyses.

Etiology and Pathogenesis

That genetic factors are involved in sarcoidosis is suggested by the highly variable prevalence and incidence of the disease in individuals from different ethnic and racial groups, and by the existence of familial forms (65,251). As the sarcoid granulomatous process is mediated by activated macrophages and $CD4^+$ T cells, a genetic predisposition could be related to the regulation of the immunological response, to antigen presentation/processing, or to T-cell function. Numerous studies have emphasized associations between HLA class II alleles and sarcoidosis in patients of different racial or ethnic groups. Varying associations have been observed, depending on the populations studied. Whereas many alleles have been identified that confer susceptibility to the disease (including HLA-DR3, HLA-DR5, HLA-DR8, HLA-DR9, HLA-DR11, HLA-DR12, HLA-DR14, HLA-DR15, HLA-DR17, HLA-DPB1, HLA-DQB1), others seem to be protective (HLA-DR1, DR4). It may be that the influence of HLA class I alleles on sarcoidosis could be more pronounced than previously thought (93).

Other genes have been targeted because of their known expression in the course of the disease. It has

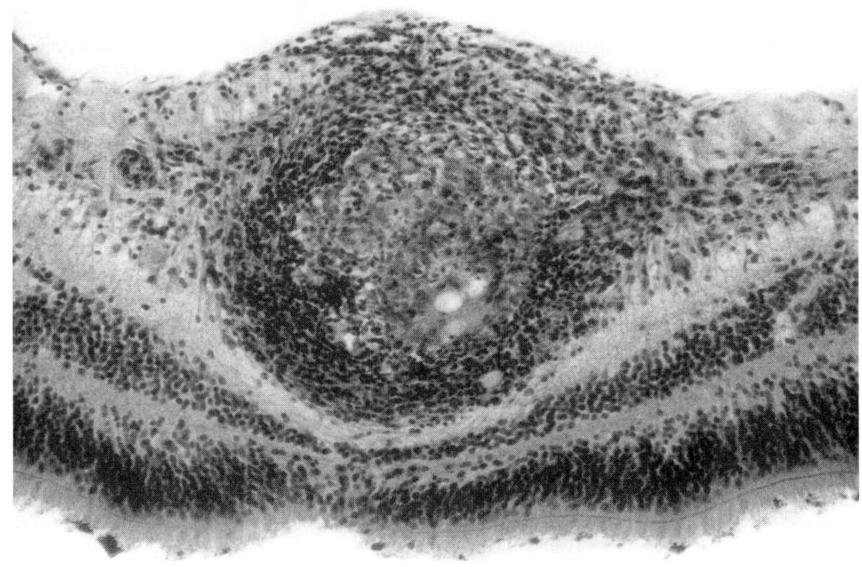

Figure 6 Sarcoidosis. A circumscribed aggregate of epithelioid macrophages, including multinucleated giant cells, is located in the inner retina. There is a surrounding mantle of lymphocytes and occasional plasma cells (hematoxylin and eosin, ×160). *Source*: Courtesy of Professor A. Garner.

been suggested that the SNPs in the *IL1A, TNF, CCR2, CCR5, ACE, VDR, NRAMP1, NRMP2* genes encoding IL1α, TNFα, CC chemokine receptor 2, CC chemokine receptor 5, angiotensin-converting enzyme (ACE), vitamin D receptor, natural resistance-associated macrophage protein 1, natural resistance-associated macrophage protein 1 and 2 (NRAMP1 and NRAMP2) or transporters associated with antigen processing (*TAP* genes) could play a role in sarcoidosis susceptibility. These studies suggest that different haplotypes may be associated with different forms of sarcoidosis. In this respect, a strong association between *CCR2* SNPs and Löfgren syndrome (a benign form of sarcoidosis associated with erythema nodosum and bilateral hilar lymphadenopathy) has been reported, suggesting a prominent role for this receptor in acute forms of sarcoidosis (230).

Genetic alterations such as microsatellite instability or loss of heterozygosity, which are known to be important in carcinogenesis, have been detected in some patients with sarcoidosis, suggesting an explanation for the higher risk of cancer following sarcoidosis.

SYSTEMIC LUPUS ERYTHEMATOSUS

General Remarks

SLE is a multisystemic chronic autoimmune disorder that can affect almost any organ system. The manifestations of SLE are protein and follow a relapsing and remitting course. It usually presents in women (90% of cases) and occurs much more frequently in the black population (72).

Clinical Features

Systemic

The course of SLE is highly variable, with some experiencing a mild, relatively benign disease and others an aggressive, rapidly progressive (and even fatal) course. Diagnosis frequently is based on of the presence of four or more qualifying criteria (serially or simultaneously over any time period) as defined by the American College of Rheumatology (ACR) (Table 2). These criteria originally were designed for classification in experimental studies but have been found to be 96% sensitive and specific for the diagnosis of SLE.

SLE usually presents with constitutional symptoms, such as fever, fatigue, weight loss, and symmetrical arthralgia, although a destructive arthritis seldom occurs. Skin lesions develop in 80% of cases, and the typical malar (butterfly) rash presents in about half the patients at diagnosis. A cutaneous vasculitis may produce nail fold hemorrhages, a punctate erythematosus rash, or livedo reticularis. Discoid lupus erythematosus is a variant of SLE in which well-demarcated erythematous papules occur, typically in the malar regions, in the absence of systemic manifestations. Alopecia may be present. Renal involvement is present in approximately 50% of cases and usually manifests as a nephrotic syndrome, although asymptomatic proteinuria, an acute nephritis, or chronic renal failure with hypertension can occur. Pleurisy, with effusion, pericarditis, Raynaud phenomenon, and nervous system involvement are other features of SLE.

Table 2 American College of Rheumatology Criteria for the Classification of Systemic Lupus Erythematosus

Malar rash
Discoid rash
Photosensitivity (skin)
Oral ulcers (oral or nasopharyngeal, usually painless)
Arthritis (nonerosive)
Serositis (pleurisy, pericarditis)
Renal involvement (proteinuria, cellular casts)
Neurologic disorder (seizures, psychosis)
Hematologic disease (leukopenia, thrombocytopenia, lymphopenia)
Immunologic disorder [lupus erythematosus (LE) cells; anti-DNA; anti-Smith (anti-Sm); biologic false-positive (BFP) serologic test for syphilis (STS); antiphospholipid antibodies]

Ocular

Retinal vascular disease is the most common ophthalmic manifestation of SLE, occurring in 3% to 29% of patients (96). It consists of diffuse arteriolar and capillary nonperfusion, manifest by cotton-wool spots, retinal hemorrhages, optic disc swelling, and serous retinal detachment. Sheathing of the retinal blood vessels is common, suggesting a vasculitis, but tissue examination has not confirmed inflammation in the vascular wall. Occlusion of the central retinal artery and vein can occur, and a widespread multifocal arterial occlusion with deposits in the arterial walls has been reported (44). Retinal neovascularization with subsequent tractional retinal detachment can occur secondary to the widespread retinal ischemia. A choroidopathy (168) manifest clinically by multifocal, serous elevations of the RPE has also been reported (125). Most (80–90%) cases of retinopathy in SLE are associated with active disease typically cerebral SLE, and its development is a poor prognostic indicator for survival (197). The presence of "lupus" anticoagulant (antibodies to cardiolipin, a phospholipid) is a risk factor for occlusovascular retinal disease and patients may present with retinal vascular occlusion, with new vessels and vitreous hemorrhage (176). After RA, SLE is the next most frequent cause of scleritis, which is typically diffuse or nodular. Other ocular manifestations of SLE include mucocutaneous disease and sSS.

Histopathology

The fundamental pathological change of SLE is inflammation of small arteries with fibrinoid necrosis of the vessel walls and of the connective tissue under the serous sacs (such as the pericardium and pleura), the synovium of joints, and the endocardium. There is usually only a mild inflammatory cellular reaction, but the presence of hematoxyphil bodies, the histological counterpart of the lupus erythematosus (LE) cell is virtually diagnostic. Examination of involved skin discloses atrophy of the epidermis, hydropic degeneration of the basal cells, and an infiltrate of mostly lymphocytes in the dermis. In the kidney, a characteristic wire-loop lesion is produced by thickening of the basement membrane of the capillaries in the glomerulus. Necrosis of endocardium can lead to valvular vegetations and subsequent Libman-Sacks endocarditis.

Ocular

Retinal SLE exhibits similar fibrinoid necrosis of the small arteries and arterioles, with multifocal occlusions and microinfarctions, but active vasculitis or foci of inflammatory cells have not been reported. Examination of the choroid, however, may show a mononuclear cell infiltration as well as fibrinoid necrosis of the arterioles (Fig. 7) (89).

Etiology and Pathogenesis

A genetic contribution to SLE susceptibility is supported by an increased sibling risk (as much as 20-fold) and by an increased disease concordance in monozygotic twins (255).

A whole genome linkage scan for SLE-associated genes has identified multiple loci (188,239). Among them a locus for SLE susceptibility named SLEB2 on chromosome 2 (2q37) contains the *PDCD1* gene which encodes for a cell surface receptor involved immune modulation. PDCD1 is known to regulate peripheral tolerance in T and B cells, and mice lacking the counterpart develop SLE-like phenotypes. The *PDCD1* gene was sequenced in family members, in whom the SLEB2 locus was detected and seven SNPs were identified. One of five haplotypes was transmitted more frequently in affected individuals and confirmed the positive linkage.

A susceptibility locus and allele has been identified for HLA-DR2, but not for HLA-DR3 (88). HLA-DR2 and HLA-DR3 have been consistently associated with SLE. An analysis of SNPs in and around the HLA locus of European–American SLE patients showed that the genetic association centered on HLA-DR2 effectively eliminating SNPs at the surrounding loci. SLE patients with HLA-DR3 had so little variation across a large extended haplotype, that SNPs at the surrounding genes could not be excluded from consideration. In the case of the HLA-DR3 haplotype, multiple interdependent alleles may be simultaneously required for SLE susceptibility. Candidates for such a contribution include the null alleles in genes encoding for complement components C2 and C4, the TNF receptor, and HLA-DQ, HLA-A, HLA-B, and HLA-C.

Autoantibody production is a hallmark of SLE pathogenesis. Over one hundred specific autoantibodies have been described in patients with SLE and several of them have been associated with disease activity (224). The development of autoantibodies reflects a loss of B- or T-cell tolerance, which is likely to result from a combination of a genetic predisposition, persistent inflammatory responses, abnormal handling of apoptotic material and immune complexes, abnormal presentation of self-antigens and other events (279). Antibodies directed against chromatin components (dsDNA, nucleosomes and histones) are of principal importance in SLE and anti-dsDNA serum levels are generally elevated in African-American and Mexican-Hispanic patients with higher disease activity having an enhanced predictive value for lupus nephritis (20). Several studies report conflicting data relating serum anti-dsDNA titers and disease activity. Other autoantibodies, including anti-Ro, anti-La, anti-Sm, anti-U1RNP, anti-extractable nuclear antigen (ENA) and anti-phospholipid (aPL), have not shown consistent clinical usefulness in

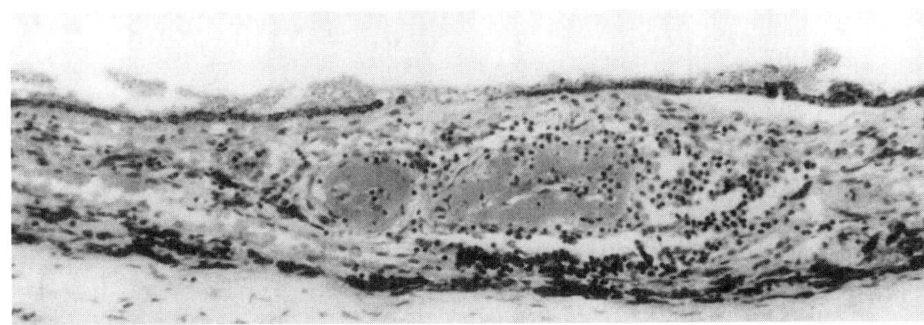

Figure 7 Systemic lupus erythematosus. Two blood vessels of arteriolar caliber are seen, showing fibrinoid necrosis and a mild surrounding lymphocytic infiltrate (hematoxylin and eosin, ×170). *Source*: Courtesy of Professor A. Garner.

identifying activity or predicting flares. Anti-Ro and anti-La are associated with the skin manifestations of SLE and with the syndrome of neonatal SLE (27). Autoantibodies against the q subfraction of the first component of complement (C1q) appear to correlate with renal involvement (149), whereas aPL antibodies are associated with the aPL syndrome of thrombocytopenia, recurrent thrombosis, and recurrent fetal loss (265). Studying peripheral blood leukocytes, several groups have identified a pattern of enhanced gene expression involving genes regulated by IFNs type I in patients with SLE. These findings have focused attention on both myeloid and plasmacytoid dendritic cells (DCs) as potential sources of IFNs. A crucial balance between activating and inhibitory receptors for immune complexes on DCs determines the net response to immune complexes and this balance is influenced by both the genome of the host and the cytokine milieu (32). Toll-like receptors (TLRs) are likely to have an important role in this response and this contribution might depend in part on the balance of DNA and RNA species in the complexes, which, in turn, will determine the types of TLR that are engaged. TLRs are type I transmembrane proteins that recognize pathogens and activate immune cell responses as a key part of the innate immune system. In vertebrates, they can help activate the adaptive immune system, linking innate and acquired immune responses. TLR are pattern recognition receptors, binding to pathogen-associated molecular patterns, small molecular sequences consistently found on pathogens.

The contributions of both B cells and T cells is well established in SLE and genetic associations with variants of PDCD1 and protein tyrosine phosphatase non-receptor type 22 (PTPN22). PDCD1 and PTPN22 are both putatively involved in lymphocyte activation, suggesting intrinsic differences in lymphocyte function may combine with variants in Ig receptors, in acute phase reactants, and possibly other molecules in the SLE diathesis (52). Overproduction of the B-cell–stimulating factor TNFSF13B (tumor necrosis factor ligand, member 13B; also known as zTNF4) and TALL1 (TNF and Apol-related leukocyte-expressed ligand 1) disrupts the architecture of lymphoid follicles, which may contribute to lymphocyte dysfunction and compromised immune tolerance in lupus-prone mice (92). Raised serum levels of TNFSF13B have been found in patients with autoantibodies but without other clinical SLE or signs of inflammatory disease. The implications of sustained elevations of TNFSF13B for the integrity of normal immune function are unclear.

High levels of circulating and tissue immune complexes are common in SLE. Although some authors have proposed that these immune complexes result from the high titers of antibodies combining with antigen (mainly DNA), this remains unproven. The presence of the antibodies in such complexes has been difficult to demonstrate and a consistent correlation of immune complex concentration to patterns or activity of disease has not been observed (5). Two hypotheses to explain the presence of serum antibodies and immune complexes are (*i*) a failure of the immune response, allowing overproduction of "forbidden" antibodies and (*ii*) failure of elimination of immune complexes produced as a normal response to the abnormal presentation of antigen (167). Studies of the anti-DNA antibodies have revealed public idiotype 16/6, which is present in the serum and kidney biopsies of many patients with SLE (214). Procainamide, which can induce clinical SLE, may induce an increased production of these idiotypes (215). Immunization of healthy mice with an antibody containing this idiotype leads to a SLE type of disease. PMNs that have ingested nuclear material within a large intracytoplasmic vacuole, LE cells, are present in approximately 80% of cases. The inclusion is characteristically amorphous, deeply staining, and less basophilic then the normal nucleus of this leukocyte.

RELAPSING POLYCHONDRITIS

General Remarks

Relapsing polychondritis (RP) is a rare, generally fatal systemic disease affecting primarily cartilage and proteoglycan-rich tissues (4). Ocular inflammation occurs in approximately 60% of cases with episcleritis and intractable scleritis being the most frequent manifestations. Approximately one-third of patients have circulating antibodies to native collagen type II, the titer correlating with the severity of inflammation. Since there is no cartilage or collagen type II in human sclera, an indirect mechanism has been invoked for the scleritis, namely, an immune complex vasculitis (see Chapter 3). Other ocular manifestations include uveitis, keratitis, retinopathy, ischemic neuropathy, keratoconjunctivitis sicca, proptosis and eye muscle palsy.

RP is an uncommon disorder of connective tissue characterized by recurrent inflammation and subsequent destruction of cartilage, typically the auricular, nasal, and laryngotracheal cartilages (Fig. 8).

Clinical Features

Systemic

Conductive hearing loss secondary to Eustachian tube involvement, serous otitis media, outer ear cartilage collapse, or sensory/hearing loss with accompanying vestibular symptoms due to internal auditory artery vasculitis is frequently present. The associated polyarthritis is typically non-deforming, RF negative, and nonerosive. Cardiovascular involvement takes the

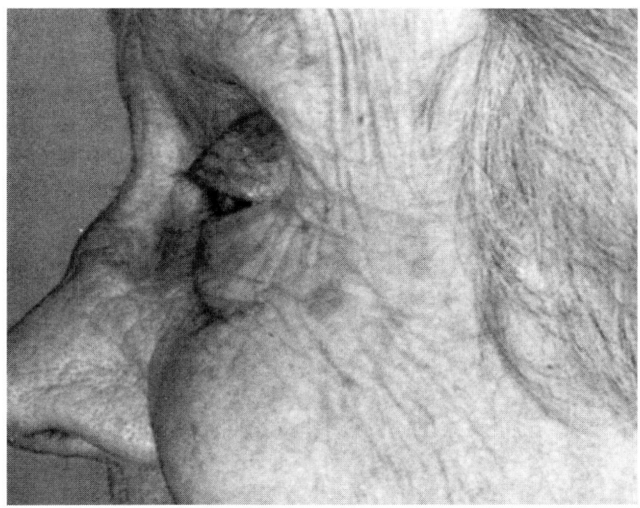

Figure 8 Relapsing polychondritis. Nasal cartilage collapse leading to "saddle nose" deformity.

form of a vasculitis of any sized blood vessel, aneurysms, and valvular heart disease (82).

The kidneys are uncommonly affected and usually manifest as focal proliferative glomerulonephritis with crescent formation, although IgA nephropathy has been identified. Males and females are equally affected, with a median age of 51 years at diagnosis. As many as 37% of patients with RP have an associated hematologic disorder, connective tissue disease, vasculitis, skin disorder, or other autoimmune disease (141).

Ocular

Over 50% of patients develop ocular manifestations; most commonly episcleritis. Scleritis and corneal guttering occur less frequently. Uveitis (119), retinal vasculitis and exudative retinal detachment (23), optic neuritis (30), and proptosis with extraocular muscle palsy also take place (179).

Histopathology

Microscopic examination of affected cartilage reveals a marked perichondritis characterized by degenerated disorganized chondrocytes and decreased basophilia of the ECM due to loss of proteoglycans. There is a cellular infiltration of lymphocytes, macrophages, plasma cells, and PMNs (83)

The first account of the ocular histopathology was reported by Verity et al. (250), who described a "minimal decrease of basophilia and fragmentation of elastic tissue in the scleroconjunctival angle," together with scattered mast cells, plasma cells, and lymphocytes around the episcleral blood vessels. Barth and Berson (18) reported an infiltration of the iris with lymphocytes and plasma cells, but no evidence of granuloma formation or vasculitis. Other studies have, however, disclosed vasculitis, with mononuclear cell infiltration and mast cell degeneration and granular deposits of Ig and the C3 (245), as well as CD4+ lymphocytes and plasma cells. Non-specific granulation tissue is common, however, if inflamed perichondral tissue is sampled, specimens may show more characteristic features (236). The vacuolated and necrotic chondrocytes are eventually replaced by fibrous tissue.

Evidence of cell-mediated changes has been found, including abnormal cellular responses to cartilage proteoglycans and imbalance of T-lymphocyte subsets. T cells directed against a peptide corresponding to residues 261–273 of collagen type II have been isolated from a patient with RP by Buckner et al. (36). The T-cell clones were restricted to either the DRB1*0101 or the DRB1*0401 allele. T-cell responses to collagen types IX and XI have also been reported in a patient with RP having severe tracheomalacia (10).

Etiology and Pathogenesis

The cause and pathogenesis of RP is poorly understood. Affected individuals have a significant increase in the frequency HLA-DR4, but there is no predominant HLA-DR4 subtype (134) and the disease is associated negatively with HLA-DR6 (275). HLA-DQ6/8 transgenic mice develop auricular chondritis after immunization with collagen type II (34). Antibodies to collagen types II, IX, and XI have been described, but they lack sensitivity and specificity. Cell-mediated immunity is important in the pathogenesis of RP. Levels of MIF are higher than in control subjects. Furthermore, one patient has been characterized with T-cell clones specific for a collagen type II epitope (37). Rarely, a mechanical insult to cartilage as in piercing the cartilaginous portion of the ear correlates temporarily with the onset of RP.

Nonspecific markers of an inflammatory state may be present with active RP. Antineutrophil cytoplasmic antibodies have been found in some patients with RP, but other serologic tests are nonspecific or suggest overlapping syndromes. The most frequent causes of death are infection, systemic vasculitis, and malignancy and 10% of deaths are attributable to airway disease. A saddle-shaped nose and systemic vasculitis indicate a poor prognosis, especially in younger patients (155).

RP was initially thought to be perpetuated by cellular immune mechanisms. In 1978, however, Foidart and collaborators demonstrated the presence of antibodies to collagen type II in 5 of 15 patients with RP that were detected at the onset of the disease and in titer that appeared to correlate with the severity of the disease. These antibodies were almost entirely restricted to RP and were found in only one of 92 patients with other arthritides, and in none of 75 normal volunteers. The presence of such antibodies has been confirmed and these antibodies may be the primary event in the pathogenesis of RP. Circulating immune complexes have been detected in the same patients; immunofluorescence studies reveal granular deposits of IgG, IgA, IgM, and C3 at the chondrofibrous junction, which also supports the presence of immune complexes, although their role in the disease is still unclear.

Autoantibodies are found in the sera of patients with RP. They have usually been generated against collagen types II, IX, and XI (271), which form the major fibrillar scaffold in cartilage and mediate the interaction of collagen fibrils and proteoglycans. Autoantibodies against cartilaginous collagen raise the possibility that they may play a crucial role in the pathogenesis of RP. Increased titers of antibodies to matrilin-1, a cartilage matrix protein, have been described in sera from 13 to 97 patients with RP, and positive titers correlated with respiratory symptoms in 69% of the cases (96). Significant responses to collagen type II and cartilage oligomeric matrix protein (COMP) were also detected. A cellular immune response to matrilin-1 was also demonstrated in an RP patient with respiratory symptoms (36).

WEGENER GRANULOMATOSIS

General Remarks

Wegener granulomatosis (WG) is a multisystem granulomatous inflammatory disorder of presumed autoimmune origin. It has a predilection for the upper and lower respiratory tracts and kidneys. The associated vasculitis preferentially affects small-caliber arteries, and to a lesser extent, veins. It usually presents in the fourth or fifth decade and in a male–female ratio of 3:2 (124).

Clinical Features

Systemic

The respiratory tract is most commonly involved in WG, the patient typically presenting with severe rhinorrhea, nasal mucosal ulceration, or paranasal sinus pain. Cough, hemoptysis, and pleuritic pain indicate involvement of the lower respiratory tract, and sometimes fever, which is not necessarily secondary to an infective focus. Purpura, ulceration, papules or vesicles may indicate a cutaneous vasculitis. Glomerulonephritis occurs in about 80% of cases and, once started, usually takes a fulminant course. Unlike polyarteritis nodosa it does not usually cause hypertension.

Ocular

Ocular involvement occurs in 28% to 50% of cases and may be the initial presentation of the disease. Orbital and extraocular manifestations are generally secondary to granulomatous paranasal sinus disease, and involvement of the globe usually results from a focal vasculitis. The most common ocular manifestation is proptosis, with pain and limited extraocular movement, which may begin suddenly. There may be accompanying visual loss, due to either compression or vasculitis of the optic nerve. Conjunctivitis, episcleritis, and necrotizing sclerokeratitis also occur and, less commonly, nasolacrimal duct obstruction, uveitis, and choroidal and retinal detachments.

Histopathology

WG is characterized by necrotizing granulomas in the upper or lower respiratory tract (Fig. 9), generalized focal necrotizing vasculitis, and glomerulonephritis. Necrosis, vasculitis, and granulomatous inflammation are the major histopathological changes found, although these features are not present in all biopsy material (148). A study of 126 head and neck biopsy specimens of 70 patients with WG found that samples from the paranasal sinuses had the highest diagnostic yield (61). The necrosis is often termed geographic and is typified by basophilic patches of tissue necrosis, usually with serpiginous borders and surrounded by varying amounts of granulomatous inflammation consisting of palisaded macrophages and sometimes multinucleated giant cells. Microabscesses consisting of nodular collections of PMNs mixed with fewer macrophages, lymphocytes, and plasma cells may also be found. These may represent an early form of necrosis. Multinucleate giant cells may be scattered, associated with areas of necrosis, or involved in poorly formed non-necrotizing granulomas (Fig. 10).

Examination of the blood vessels may reveal fibrinoid necrosis of the vessel wall or granulomatous vasculitis. Marked destruction of lymphocytes, plasma cells, and PMNs occurs. When present, the vasculitis is not necessarily related to foci of necrosis and granulomatous inflammation. WG can be differentiated from polyarteritis nodosa by the involvement of small arteries and veins and the presence of necrotizing granulomas frequently remote from the areas of vascular involvement.

Renal examination reveals proliferative focal glomerulonephritis with necrosis and thrombosis of individual loops or larger parts of the glomeruli. Sometimes almost all glomeruli are destroyed, accompanied by capsule adhesions and proliferations.

The precise connection between infections and pulmonary vasculitis remains poorly understood. Nasal colonization with *Staphylococcal aureus* is an independent risk factor for relapse of WG suggesting infectious pathogens as potential triggers of a cascade of events that result in vascular inflammation. Multiple laboratory studies have contributed to a

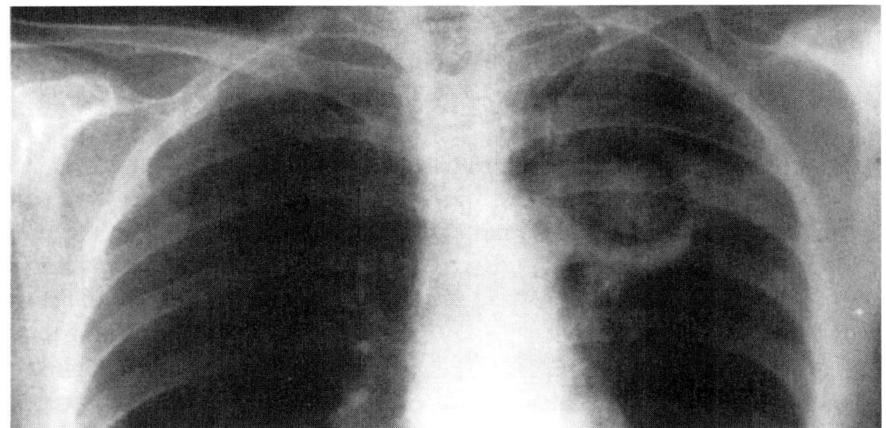

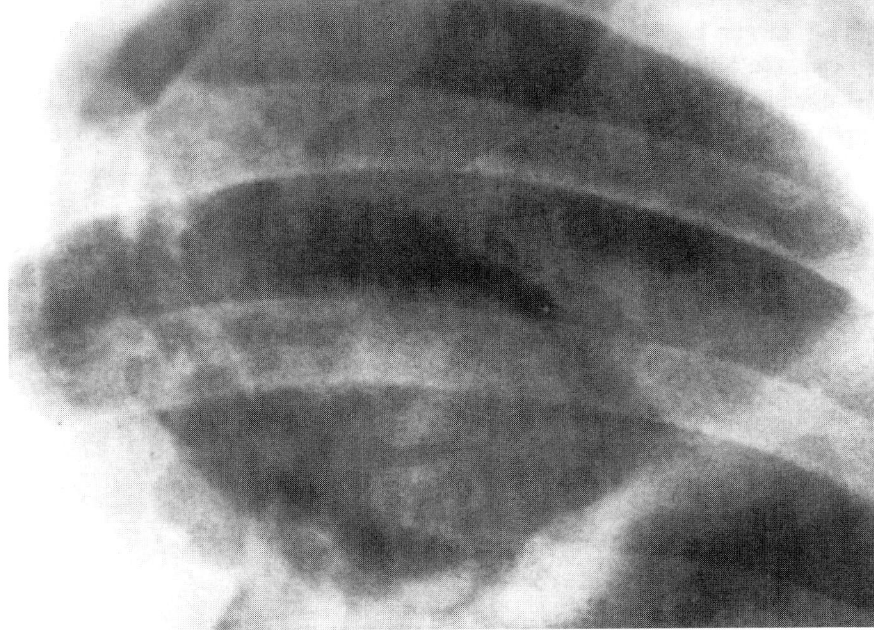

Figure 9 Wegener granulomatosis. Chest roentgenogram with cavitating lesion.

coherent and plausible theory about the pathogenesis of antineutrophil cytoplasmic antibody (ANCA)-associated vasculitis in which infection plays a critical role. In susceptible individuals immune tolerance may break down and ANCA production resulting from molecular mimicry ensues. In addition, bacterial superantigens may serve as potent stimulators of the immune system (41). Circulating immune complexes have been demonstrated, but deposits in the kidney or lung are rare. The vascular lymphoid infiltrates are composed predominantly of T cells and monocytes, suggesting that cellular rather than humoral immune mechanisms are responsible.

A major advance in diagnosing WG was made with the discovery of an IgG autoantibody against intracytoplasmic extranuclear components of granulocytes–ANCA. Testing for ANCA, by using either immunofluorescence and/or enzyme-linked immunospecific assay (ELISA), is of significant diagnostic value in the vasculitides named above. Using ELISA, the cANCA pattern is found to react with proteinase-3, whereas the pANCA pattern typically reacts with myeloperoxidase (MPO) (69).

A meta-analysis of cANCA testing in WG reported a pooled sensitivity of 91% and specificity of 99% for active WG (194). The sensitivity of pANCA/anti-MPO for WG is reported to be about 10% to 12% and hence not a reliable marker for WG. A combination of IF and ELISA is recommended for ANCA testing, because ELISA techniques are more specific, whereas IF has a greater sensitivity (145). An international consensus statement recommends that IF testing be performed on all serum samples of new patients, with positive patients undergoing ELISA testing for PR3-ANCA and MPO-ANCA (213).

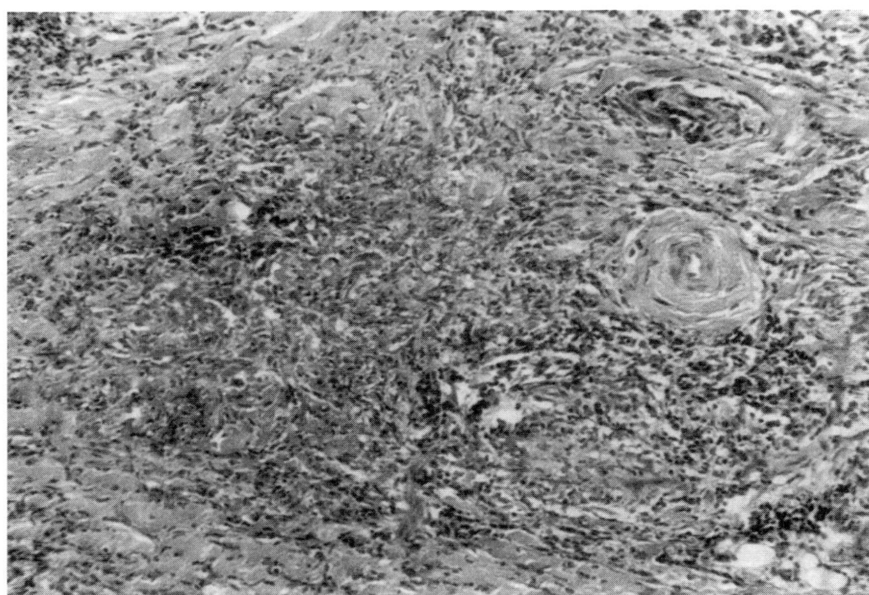

Figure 10 Wegener granulomatosis. Orbital connective tissue showing granulomatous inflammation and vascular occlusion (hematoxylin and eosin, ×170). *Source*: Courtesy of Professor A. Garner.

Etiology and Pathogenesis

Several findings suggest a genetic predisposition to WG. The membrane expression of the main ANCA target is proteinase 3 (previously designated myeloblastin, azurophil granulae protein 7 and PR3) encoded by the *PRTN3* gene is genetically determined (216). A SNP in promoter of *PRTN3* is associated with WG and affects a putative SP1-transcription factor-binding site (81). This SNP leads potentially to increased *PRTN3* expression which encodes a member of the serine proteinase family. PRTN3 is inhibited by the serine protease inhibitors (serpins), their genes clustering on chromosome 14 (14q32.1) in addition to further loci. Linkage disequilibrium of haplotypes in this gene cluster is associated with WG (29). PMN-derived proteins represent a source of innate immune defense playing a role in the recognition and neutralization of the proinflammatory surface components (e.g., endotoxins) of bacteria. Binding of ANCA to antigens on the surface of PMNs results in cellular activation as mediated by Fcγ receptors (FcγR) (129). Most analyses of these highly polymorphic genes have failed to detect significant differences in genotype distributions or allele frequencies between patients with WG and controls. Yet, a trend for increased homozygosity of the *FcγRIIIb-NA1* allele is evident which may have implications for disease susceptibility being significant in MPO-ANCA$^+$ patients (240). The adhesiveness of leukocytes to the endothelium is an important pathophysiological element of WG. Adhesion is augmented by expression of molecules like CD11, CD18, ICAM-1, and E-selectin. Whereas specific associations in the aforementioned genes as risk factors for WG have not been identified, linkage has been detected between given *CD18* alleles and myeloperoxidase-antinuclear cytoplasmic antibody vasculitides (MPO-ANCA vasculitides) (80). WG patients with a defined *TNF* 1/1 phenotype have a higher mean disease extension index than *TNF* 1/2 individuals (84). In part these results were confirmed in another study that excluded certain *IL2* and *IL5Rγ* alleles as predisposing genes. Furthermore, SNPs in the *ILIB* (encoding IL1β) and *IL1R* (encoding IL1Rγ) genes were examined concerning the clinical manifestation and outcome of ANCA-associated systemic vasculitides (AASV), such as WG, Churg-Strauss syndrome, and microscopic polyangiitis. A distinct combination of these SNPs leads to a pro-inflammatory genotype increased in PRTN3-ANCA$^+$ patients with end-stage-renal disease. In a Swedish WG population variations in the *IL4* and *IL10* genes were investigated. Whereas *IL4* variations were not associated with WG, a microsatellite polymorphism located in the promotor region of *IL10* was present in a higher percentage of patients heterozygous for two specific alleles (278). In addition, another study on Caucasians, a significant shift toward the homozygous AA genotype of an *IL10* polymorphism was observed in WG patients. Furthermore, the latter study excluded the SNPs in codon 25 of the *TGFB1* gene encoding transforming growth factor β_1 (TGFβ_1) as a genetic risk factor for WG (17). Major histocompatibility genes that encode cell surface molecules initiating acquired immune responses to invading pathogens (potentially also *S. aureus* for WG). SNPs in these genes were extensively studied to determine possible associations with WG. Different alleles including *HLA-B8, -B50, -DR9, -DR1, -DR2, -DQw7* and the haplotype HLA-DR4DQ7, were increased in frequency in WG patients, whereas a decrease of *HLA-DR3* alleles and *HLA-DR13DR6* heterozygotes among WG or systemic vasculitides (SV) patients has also been observed (268). In a systematic association screen with 202 microsatellites certain alleles within a region of chromosome 6 (6p21.3) were significantly associated with WG. *HLA-DPB1* genotyping of this comparatively large cohort of 150 patients revealed an increased frequency of the *DPB1*0401* allele. In contrast, the frequency of the **0301* allele was significantly decreased. These results were confirmed in an independent WG patient cohort. Furthermore, two additional genes (*CASP14* and *RIPK1*), which encode for caspase 14 and receptor-interacting serine/threonine kinase 1 represent good candidates for WG predisposition. SNPs in these genes may cause subtle shifts in the balance of apoptosis (104).

POLYARTERITIS NODOSA

General Remarks

Polyarteritis nodosa (PN) is characterized by focal, episodic, necrotic inflammation of the walls of medium-sized and small arteries and can involve any organ.

Clinical Features

Systemic

PA affects males more than females (2–3:1) and usually presents in the fifth and sixth decades, with fever, weight loss, and malaise. Abdominal pain reflects widespread gastrointestinal arteritis, which may produce infarction. Cutaneous features include ulcers, digital vasculitis, and gangrene. Renal disease develops in 70% to 80% and may cause hypertension. Peripheral neuropathy, arthritis, and myocardial infarction may also occur, but pulmonary involvement is uncommon (51). Causes of death include infection (usually pulmonary), renal failure, cardiomegaly, pericarditis, coronary artery involvement leading to ischemia and infarction, and gastrointestinal bleeding.

Ocular

The eye is estimated to be involved in at least 20% of cases. Most ocular tissues can be affected, but choroidal and posterior ciliary vessels are most often affected due to the arteritis and/or systemic hypertension. Choroidal vasculitis is the most common manifestation, but retinal vasculitis, anterior and posterior ischemic optic neuropathy, and vascular occlusions also occur (67). FA demonstrating retinal vasculitis with multiple areas of retinal and choroidal ischemia can aid diagnosis. Necrotizing scleritis, iritis, and conjunctival vasculitis have been reported (178), although involvement of the anterior segment is less common.

Histopathology

Systemic

Skeletal muscle is traditionally used for biopsy, but a positive result is obtained in <40% of cases. Renal biopsies are helpful but potentially hazardous because of the danger of rupturing an aneurysm or producing arteriovenous fistulas. Biopsies of skin lesions give the highest frequency of positive results, but correlation between biopsy and systemic disease may be poor (219).

The lesions consist of focal, panmural necrotizing inflammation in small and medium-sized arteries, with a predilection for involvement at the vascular bifurcation. Extensive denudation of the endothelium is associated with intimal and intraluminal fibrinoid necrosis, an inflammatory infiltrate of the intima and inner media, primarily with PMNs, and fewer lymphocytes and eosinophils. The normal architecture of the blood vessel wall is disrupted with a variable intramural deposition of fibrin. Thrombosis or aneurysmal dilatation may develop at the site of the lesion (53). Healed areas of arteritis contain proliferations of fibrous tissue and endothelial cells that can lead to vessel occlusion. The kidney is involved in up to 80% of cases and glomerulonephritis (usually segmental and proliferative) may be present in one-third of cases. The peripheral nerves are involved in 50% of patients, the vasculitis resulting in fascicular degeneration with loss of myelinated nerve fibers (228).

The blood vessels of the jejenum and liver are commonly affected. The presence of aneurysms can be demonstrated by angiography and they tend to be associated with severe hypertension, hepatitis B antigenemia, and clinically severe disease (68).

Ocular

Lesions similar to those in other parts of the body occur in the ocular tissues. A study of conjunctiva in PN showed severe vasculitis of the small and medium-sized arteries with fibrinoid necrosis and infiltration with PMNs (Fig. 11). Immunohistochemical studies disclosed extensive immune complex and complement deposition in the vessels (190).

Etiology and Pathogenesis

The cause of PN is unknown, although it may be triggered by viruses, notably the hepatitis B virus, or

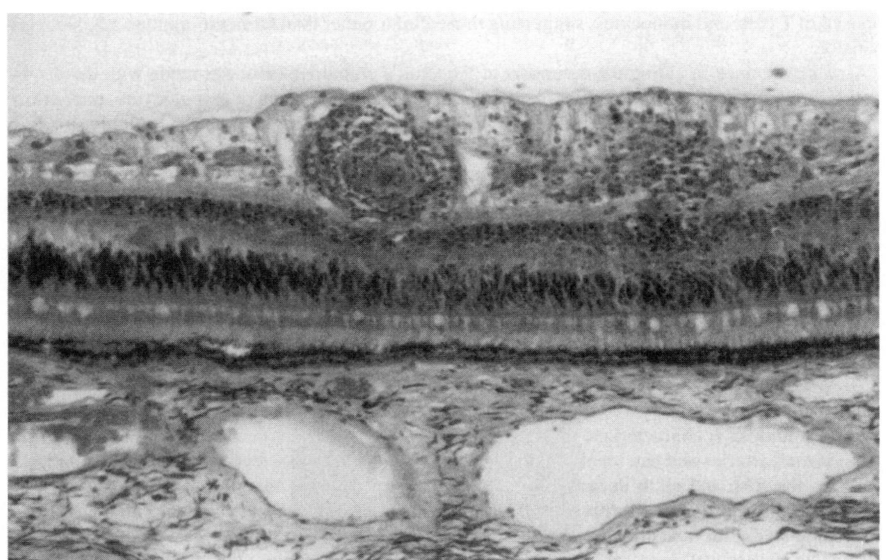

Figure 11 Polyateritis nodosa. Involvement of retinal arterioles with leukocytic infiltration of the entire thickness of the vessel wall (hematoxylin and eosin, ×170). *Source*: Courtesy of Professor A. Garner.

occasionally by drug abuse (175). PN is generally considered to involve an immune complex-mediated mechanism, but although circulating immune complexes may be detected. Deposits are found infrequently, suggesting either that there is a transient deposition or that immune complexes are not involved. Early studies of experimental immune complex vasculitis showed that complexes are sparse initially and are quickly lost from the tissue involved; biopsies must therefore be performed early if immune deposits are to be demonstrated (49).

ANCA and antiendothelial cell antibodies have been detected in microscopic polyarteritis and may be involved in this pathological process as well as PN (71).

ANKYLOSING SPONDYLITIS

General Remarks

Ankylosing spondylitis (AS) is an inflammatory arthritis of the spine and sacroiliac joints that usually develops in the late teens or early twenties. It affects 1–10 Caucasian adults per thousand (42), but a true frequency is difficult to determine because radiographic evidence of disease is much more common than clinical disease. Men are afflicted with AS approximately two to three times more frequently than women (280).

Clinical Features

Systemic

Early symptoms include episodic low back pain, which is worse on awaking and eases with exercise. The disease may present as an asymmetric peripheral arthritis, usually of the large weight-bearing joints. Spinal fusion and the radiological appearance of the "bamboo spine" are the result of longstanding disease (Fig. 12). Extraarticular manifestations include plantar fasciitis (causing heel pain), a nonspecific aortitis that can cause aortic valve regurgitation and aneurysmal dilatation, and compressive neuropathies. Although chest expansion can be severely restricted, this is compensated by increased diaphragmatic excursion. Secondary amyloidosis is a well-recognized cause of renal failure in these patients.

Ocular

The eye is involved in about 25% of patients, predominantly with intense, painful, acute anterior uveitis and conjunctivitis. Uveitis is more common in HLA-B27$^+$ patients and is the presenting feature in 10% of cases (162). The presence of HLA-A2 in B27$^+$ AS patients may further increase the risk of uveitis (46), which is frequently bilateral and recurrent. It is not related to the general activity but is associated with peripheral joint involvement.

Histopathology

In contrast to RA, in which the primary lesion is in the synovium, the primary site in AS is at the insertion of the ligaments and tendons into bone. At these sites, chondrified and calcified parts of the ligament and the bone to which they are attached become replaced by soft connective tissue containing variable numbers of lymphocytes and plasma cells, which tend to spread along blood vessels lying within the undamaged part of the ligaments (13). The erosion in the bone surface is repaired by the deposition of reactive (woven) bone,

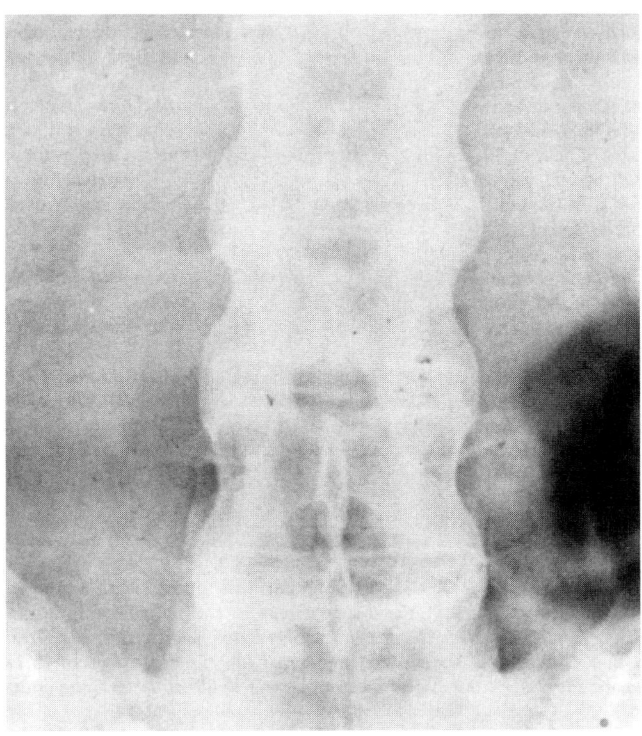

Figure 12 Ankylosing spondylitis. "Bamboo spine" in long-standing disease.

which fills in the defect, becomes attached to the eroded end of the ligament, and is later remodeled and replaced by lamellar bone. Similar changes occur at the attachment of the outer fibers of the annulus fibrosus of the vertebral body; the deposition of reactive bone results in a type of bone outgrowth known as a syndesmophyte, which can grow to form a bony bar. Synovial membranes are affected similarly to RA, with a diffuse lymphocyte and plasma cell infiltration and the formation of lymphoid follicles (198).

Immunohistochemical examinations of synovium have revealed equal numbers of $CD4^+$ T cells and $CD8^+$ T cells in AS, whereas in RA there are greater numbers of $CD4^+$ T cells, suggesting that there are disease-specific inflammatory responses within the synovial membranes. Examination of the synovial fluid, however, has disclosed a reduced CD4 T-cell/CD8 T-cell ratio in AS, with an increased number of T cells expressing class II MHC antigens. The bone marrow of the AS samples is edematous and contains cellular infiltrates. The density of all cell types in the bone marrow is higher in AS than in RA. There are also more $CD8^+$, $CD3^+$, $CD4^+$, and $CD20^+$ T cells in the AS group. In particular, the $CD3^+$ cell subset is increased five fold in the AS group compared with the RA group. Within the AS group, the predominant T cells are $CD8^+$ cells (26).

Etiology and Pathogenesis

The prevalence of HLA-B27 in the general population ranges from 4% to 8%, but HLA-B27 is found in >90% of patients with AS. A HLA-$B27^+$ first-degree relative of a HLA-B27+ proband with AS has a 16 times greater chance of developing the condition than HLA-$B27^+$ individuals in the population at large (225). Available evidence favors the belief that HLA-B27 itself, rather than any linked gene, is the major predisposing factor for AS (120). An increased frequency of HLA-DQW3 has also been reported, and HLA-BW60 may increase susceptibility to AS in HLA-$B27^+$ individuals (202). AS occurs infrequently in nonwhite populations, correlating with the rarity of HLA-B27 in these ethnic groups. HLA-B2705 is the dominant subtype and is associated with AS across broad ethnic and geographic boundaries. Of the subtypes studied to date, it appears that HLA-B2706 and HLA-B2709 do not confer susceptibility to AS. Although the HLA-B27 has remained a center of extensive research, the mechanism whereby HLA-B27 confers susceptibility to AS is not well defined. Molecular mimicry is proposed as a possible mechanism for HLA-B27-related disorders. This postulates that the antibodies against foreign antigens arising during a bacterial infection are cross-reactive with HLA-B27. In this regard Fiorillo et al. (73) recently showed an allele-dependent similarity between a "viral" antigen and a "self"-peptide derived from vasoactive intestinal peptide receptor (VIPR) presented by HLA-B27 subtypes carrying the B*2709 or B*2705 alleles. A crystallographic study sheds light on the possible structural basis of differential susceptibility to AS conferred by different B27 subtypes (103). HLA-*B2705, an AS-associated subtype, has the capacity to bind a candidate autoantigen in two different conformations, in a way that is not shared by HLA-*B2709, which is a non-AS-associated subtype. Abnormal forms of HLA-B27 may react with $CD4^+$ T cells or natural killer cells, rather than $CD8^+$ T cells. The HLA-B27 molecule appropriately loaded with peptide usually interacts with $CD8^+$ T cells. HLA-B27-restricted $CD8^+$ T cells are unlikely to serve as effector cells in the transgenic rat model of HLA-B27-associated disease, but $CD4^+$ T cells are capable of inducing arthritis (150).

Several studies have evaluated genes other than HLA-B27 in AS (276). Genes in regions outside the MHC, especially on chromosome 6 (6q) and chromosome 11 (11q), may be important in AS susceptibility. SNPs for the genes that encode HLA-B60, HLA-DR1, TNFα (*TNF*), the homologue of the mouse gene for progressive ankylosis (*Ank*) (*ANKH*), MMP-3 (*MMP3*), TGFβ (*TGFB*), IL1 (*IL1A, IL1B*), and IL1 receptor antagonist (*IL1RN*) have been examined as candidate genes for AS susceptibility, but these studies are inconclusive because of the positive and negative results.

REITER SYNDROME

General Remarks

Reiter syndrome (RS) comprises the association of an arthritis that is seronegative for RF with a nonspecific urethritis or cervicitis and conjunctivitis, although the diagnosis can be made confidently in the absence of conjunctivitis.

Clinical Features

Systemic

RS typically affects young males, who usually present 4 to 6 weeks after sexual exposure to *Chlamydia* or an attack of dysentery. There is an asymmetric oligoarthritis which predominantly affects the knees, ankles, feet, and wrists. Plantar fasciitis occurs in up to 20% of cases, and true ankylosing spondylitis can develop (140). Nonspecific urethritis is common to both genital and dysenteric forms of the disease and is generally responsive to antibiotic treatment, unlike the other manifestations of the condition. Mucocutaneous involvement resembles psoriasis. The typical skin lesion is keratoderma blennorrhagica, which affects up to 15% of cases. It is usually confined to the palms and soles and may be associated with circinate balanitis. Buccal and lingual ulcers and a psoriatic type of nail dystrophy also occur. The presence of such mucocutaneous changes helps distinguish RS from AS. Pericarditis, aortitis, pleurisy, amyloidosis, and deep vein thrombosis develop occasionally.

Ocular

The most common ophthalmic manifestation is conjunctivitis, which is papillary or follicular with a mucopurulent discharge. It occurs in about 60% of cases (136) and is generally self-limiting and requires no treatment. Keratitis starts as superficial epithelial and subepithelial punctate opacities and may develop in isolation or follow conjunctivitis. Pleomorphic anterior stromal infiltrates develop, typically in the mid-periphery, where they may underlie ragged epithelial erosions (147).

Anterior uveitis develops in a small proportion of cases and characteristically is accompanied by fine keratic precipitates, although it can be more severe with fibrin and a hypopyon. Posterior uveitis and scleritis may also occur (127).

Histopathology

Examination of the synovium in early disease reveals a hyperplastic synovial lining cells, with an infiltration of PMNs, increased surface fibrin, and vascular congestion with occlusion of blood vessels by platelets and fibrin (218). TEM has disclosed intra- and extracellular particles consistent with *Chlamydia* and staining with antichlamydial antibodies. However, initial reports of the isolation of this organism from the joints of patients with RS (123) have not been confirmed. Biopsies taken later in the disease discloses a tendency for a reduction in PMNs and an increased infiltration of lymphocytes and plasma cells, with moderate degrees of synovial lining hyperplasia (260). The deposition of IgM and C3 in blood vessel walls and interstitial tissue of the synovium supports an underlying immunological pathogenetic mechanism (14).

Ocular

Inflamed conjunctiva has a mononuclear cell infiltrate composed predominantly of lymphocytes in the submucosa. An extensive nonspecific deposition of fibrin is present in the epithelial basement membrane, regardless of the degree of current inflammation (190). Arteritis has been identified within the conjunctiva in one patient, perhaps reflecting a more widespread disorder than simple conjunctivitis. The deposition of IgM, C3, and IgG in the conjunctiva has also been reported (24).

Etiology and Pathogenesis

The cause is not known, but several microorganisms, such as *Campylobacter, Chlamydia, Salmonella, Shigella,* and *Yersinia,* have been implicated as triggering factors, *Chlamydia* is the commonest causative agent in RS. DNA, mRNA, and rRNA from *Chlamydia* and intact Chlamydia-like infected cells have been found in synovial tissues and peripheral blood (51). The treatment of such infections does not appear to affect the ensuing course of the disease (132) except in the case of *Chlamydia* infections (135).

Up to 75% of patients with RS are HLA-B27 positive, the presence of HLA-B27 correlating with the presence of uveitis, severe constitutional manifestations, and a chronic relapsing course. In one study, the haplotypes A2 and B27 appeared to be associated with a generalized increase in disease severity, whereas BW35 appeared to be protective (217).

RS is considered to be an autoimmune disorder despite the absence of immune complexes or autoantibodies. However, other autoimmune disorders such as RA, SLE, and AS, are found less frequently in patients with RS. An imbalance in the production of proinflammatory cytokines by peripheral blood mononuclear cells during acute arthritis (low production of TNF) has been observed (39). IL10.G12 microsatellite polymorphism is reported to be associated with a reduced risk for the development of RS, while IL10.G8 polymorphism is a marker of chronicity (116). After microbes invade the mucosa they persist either in the epithelium or within associated lymphoid tissues, liver, and spleen. Viable organisms or bacterial antigens disseminate to the joint, causing a local inflammatory response. A $CD4^+$ T-cell response to the invading microorganism drives, and probably supports, the arthritic process. An abnormal/poor T helper (Th)2 cytokine response may favor the persistence of the microbes/microbial antigens and contribute to the poor elimination of the antigens in the host.

Genetically engineered mice in which the *p55 tnf* gene is switched off [tumor necrosis factor receptor (TNFR) p55 knockout mice] develop more severe arthritis after Yersinia infection (278). Butrimiene et al. (39) showed that in chronic RS TNFα production was higher and TNFα positive and IFNγ positive $CD3^+$ cells were significantly higher, suggesting that the Th1 response in chronic ReA is more dominant than that in acute ReA. In ReA, both $CD8^+$ and $CD4^+$ cells exhibit a Th1 profile with higher production of TNFα and IFNγ, suggesting that T cells contribute to pathogenesis by inducing a Th1 type cytokine response (199).

GIANT CELL ARTERITIS

General Remarks

Giant cell arteritis (GCA) is a chronic systemic vasculitis that affects people over the age of 50 years (mean age 70 years). It occurs more frequently in females, relative risk 2.5- to 3-fold, commonly in Caucasians but rarely in blacks and Asians.

Clinical Features

Initial symptoms are usually fever, malaise, anorexia, and weight loss, accompanied by a severe temporal headache (60%). Extreme scalp tenderness on combing the hair, and jaw claudication, especially on eating, are common. A tender, thickened, nonpulsatile temporal artery is typically found on physical examination. Neurological findings are diverse and common (30% of cases), reflecting the widespread nature of the vasculitis (40). A considerable number of patients present with constitutional symptoms, and this can delay the diagnosis and treatment (45).

Ocular

Ocular complications occur in 40% of patients and the most common presentation is a sudden painless visual loss due to an anterior ischemic optic neuropathy, which is usually irreversible (98). One study suggested that such neuropathy due to arteritis occurs more frequently in eyes with normally sized optic discs and nonarteritic anterior ischemic optic neuropathy occurs more often in those with small optic discs. Central retinal artery occlusion occurs less commonly. The two eyes may be affected simultaneously, or the second eye may lose vision hours or days after the first. Amaurosis fugax, cortical blindness, internuclear ophthalmoplegia, and ptosis may also occur as the relevant arteries are affected (3).

A raised ESR is considered a hallmark of the disease and is commonly used as an indirect measure of disease activity (75). However, the ESR is influenced (inversely) by the hematocrit and may be normal despite active arteritis. Ocular pneumoplethysmography, by demonstrating a reduced ocular blood flow, may aid the clinical diagnosis but is rarely used in practice (31). Along with the local vasculitis, there is usually a prominent systemic inflammatory response. The peripheral circulation contains upregulated monocytes, which secrete cytokines, including IL6. This results in the raised acute phase response, including an elevated ESR and CRP. One study suggests that patients with severe systemic symptoms, and high levels of peripheral IL6 and CRP, have a lower rate of ischemic episodes (261), but this observation has not been confirmed.

Histopathology

Arteries with active arteritis typically have a thickened edematous intima with granulomatous inflammation concentrated in the region of the elastic lamina, which is focally or diffusely disrupted. The media and intima are infiltrated with multinucleate giant cells, macrophages, and lymphocytes, which may be present at all levels of the arterial wall (70). Examination of a "healed" artery shows thickening of the blood vessel walls, fragmentation and loss of the internal elastic lamina, intimal fibrosis, and organization of thrombus (Fig. 13). The intimal proliferation is dependent on several factors. The amount of arterial wall thickening is limited by the blood supply. Usually the intima and media are avascular, hence neovascularization is an important pathological process, without which lumen obliteration is less likely because neovascularization increases luminal thickening and in turn luminal obliteration (115). Vascular endothelial growth factor (VEGF) expression is associated with this process (264). In the arterial wall inflammation leads to myofibroblast hyperplasia, which is thought to be a response to platelet-derived growth factor (PDGF) (114). Affected arteries with significant intimal hyperplasia express higher levels of INFγ (secreted by T cells), IL1, and PDGF. They also have a higher chance of having multinucleated giant cells, which secrete VEGF, allowing intimal growth.

Unfortunately, false negative biopsies occur with a frequency varying from 9% to 61% (142). This may be partly because of focal involvement of the arteries, with intervening normal areas (35), inadequate processing of the specimen (8), or an inability to distinguish age-related vascular changes from "burned out" or treated arteritis (151). A biopsy should be performed before or within a few weeks of the initiation of corticosteroid therapy, because the

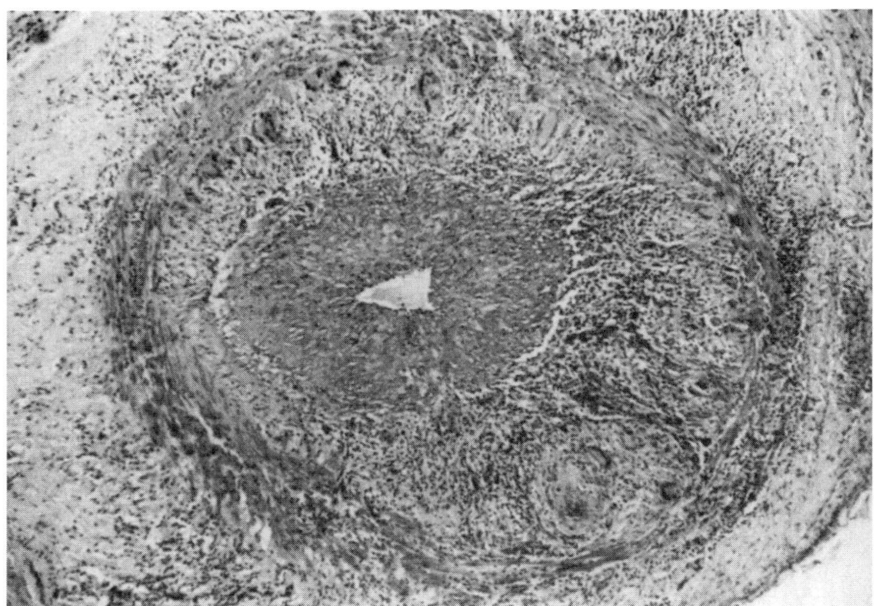

Figure 13 Giant cell arteritis. Mononuclear cell infiltration and numerous multinucleated giant cells in the wall of a temporal artery (hematoxylin and eosin, ×65). *Source*: Courtesy of Professor A. Garner.

typical histopathological features of active arteritis may be absent after 7 to 8 weeks of treatment. Bilateral temporal artery biopsies may reduce the false negative rate.

Etiology and Pathogenesis

Population and genetic studies suggest an inherited component to GCA, with disease more frequently encountered among people of Scandinavian and Northern European descent, irrespective of their place of residence (90). There are reports of concordance within monozygotic twins, and familial clustering. Most studies have shown an association of GCA and HLA-DR4 and HLA-DRB1*04 alleles. HLA-DRB classes may play a pathogenic role, with the HLA-DRB1*04 allele appearing to be both a strong risk factor for disease severity, and a marker of corticosteroid resistance in some populations (196). SNPs involving genes that are involved in the immunologic processes, such as TNFα (*TNF*), intracellular adhesion molecule-1 (ICAM-1), may influence GCA susceptibility independent of HLA class (86).

GCA and polymyalgia rheumatica (PMR) are associated conditions and some consider them to be different phases of the same disease. GCA presents with the symptoms of PMR in up to 50% of patients with GCA (86). However, more frequently PMR is an isolated condition unrelated to GCA. PMR has not been shown to have the strength of association with HLA class II genes as GCA and the susceptibility to isolated PMR varies from one population to another. Relapses of PMR, however, are found to be significantly more common in patients with the HLA-DRB1*04 allele.

It remains unclear whether GCA is an autoimmune disease. A variety of infectious agents have been implicated, including Parvovirus B19, *C. pneumoniae* (200), *Varicella-zoster* virus as well as other human herpes viruses (169), but these claims are balanced by others reporting negative findings for these organisms (204). The presence of infectious pathogens may represent a coincidental infection, to date the role of microbial pathogens in the pathogenesis of GCA remains uncertain.

Current theory on the pathogenesis of GCA described by Weyand and Goronzy suggests that an early event in GCA is the inappropriate activation of the adaptive immune system via immature dendritic cells, which normally reside within the adventitia–media border of the arterial wall (263). Immature dendritic cells normally inhibit T-cell activation in the perivascular space. Following activation, dendritic cells produce pro-inflammatory cytokines and express receptors required for dendritic cell T-cell interaction. Dendritic cells most likely represent the antigen-presenting cells in GCA (254) and when activated the cells release chemokines, which attract both T cells and macrophages. Macrophages and T cells then enter the arterial wall via the vasa vasorum.

Affected arteries contain predominantly T-cell aggregates of $CD4^+$ (T helper/inducer) cells in excess of $CD8^+$ (suppressor/cytotoxic) cells. Selective clonal expansion of T cells within the vessel wall then occurs suggesting an adaptive immune system-driven response (262). The antigens that incite clonal expansion of $CD4^+$ cell populations remain unknown.

SCLERODERMA

General Remarks

Scleroderma, also known as systemic sclerosis (SSc), is a complex autoimmune disease characterized by pathological remodeling of connective tissues. Although the earliest and most frequent manifestations include blood vessel and immunological abnormalities, the systemic and progressive lesions suggests that fundamental interactions between microvascular damage and inflammation are mechanistically linked to obliterative tissue fibrosis (1).

Clinical Features

Scleroderma is typically a disease of middle-aged women, initially presenting with Raynaud phenomenon and swelling of the hands and feet. As fibrosis develops, the skin becomes thickened and tethered, appearing smooth and tight, and ulceration and gangrene of the extremities can occur. Reduced esophageal motility occurs in 90% of patients, some of whom complain of dysphagia; and involvement of the upper small intestine can cause malabsorption. Lung involvement can cause pulmonary hypertension and interstitial fibrosis. An arthritis that is seronegative for RF and pericarditis can also occur. The major cause of death is renal failure from kidney involvement.

In cutaneous scleroderma, the skin disease is unaccompanied by systemic involvement. Some authors include the patients with the CREST syndrome (calcinosis, Raynaud phenomenon, esophageal hypomotility, sclerodactyly, and telangiectasia) in this group. Morphea is a localized benign indurated sclerodermatous lesion that rarely proceeds to systemic disease.

The American College of Rheumatology (former American Rheumatism Association – ARA) has defined criteria that are 97% sensitive and 98% specific for SSc as follows:

Major Criterion:

- Proximal diffuse (truncal) sclerosis (skin tightness, thickening, non-pitting induration)

Minor Criteria:

- Sclerodactyly (only fingers and/or toes)
- Digital pitting scars or loss of substance of the digital finger pads (pulp loss)
- Bibasilar pulmonary fibrosis

The patient should fulfill the major criterion or two of the three minor criteria (233).

Clinical examination of the nail fold capillaries discloses a distinctive pattern of grossly dilated and distorted capillary loops, alternating with avascular areas the severity of the abnormalities correlating well with the degree of multisystemic involvement (97).

Ocular

Ocular disorders that appear to be specifically related to scleroderma include telangiectasia and dermal fibrosis of the eyelid, deficient tear secretion, congestion as well as telangiectasis and sludging of the blood columns in conjunctival blood vessels, and shallow conjunctival fornices. Despite a normal fundal appearance on fundoscopy, FA may disclose patchy areas of nonperfusion of choroidal capillaries even in the absence of hypertension (91). A retinopathy comparable to that seen in accelerated hypertension may occur (13). The central corneal thickness may be thicker than normal in patients with morphea (223), indicating that the condition is not localized to the skin.

Histopathology

Biopsies of involved skin show a marked increase in collagen types I and III in the dermis, hyalinization and obliteration of the small blood vessels, and loss of normal dermal appendages and thinning of the epidermis. A mononuclear cell infiltrates, predominantly of activated T lymphocytes, the degree of infiltration correlating with the degree of subsequent fibrosis. Calcification from the deposition of calcium hydroxyapatite can occur, typically in the CREST syndrome.

The major vascular changes are in the small arteries and arterioles, where there is marked proliferation of endothelial cells and intimal thickening that can occlude the vascular lumen, which subsequently fibroses. The number of blood vessels may diminish considerably and the remaining vessels dilate and become visible in the skin as telangiectasia. Similar changes occur in other organs, notably the kidney, lungs, heart, and joints. The afferent arterioles of patients with renal failure manifest smooth muscle hyalinization and fibrinoid necrosis of the arteriolar wall, changes similar to those of malignant hypertension although the blood pressure may remain normal (174). The glomeruli may appear normal or frankly necrotic. Interstitial fibrosis and arteriolar thickening commonly occur in the lung and can be associated with pulmonary hypertension. Patients with generalized scleroderma are more likely to develop renal manifestations, and those with CREST syndrome are at a greater risk of developing pulmonary hypertension (238).

Mast cells may be involved in the disease process. The observation that many patients with scleroderma complain of itchy skin raises the possibility of histamine release and, indeed, the number of mast cells in the skin of "early scleroderma" is elevated. Moreover, such skin also has a greater number of mast cells than uninvolved skin of the same patient.

Fibrosis can be caused by profibrotic cytokines, such as TGFβ, IL4, PDGF, and CTGF. The vasculopathy may be caused by TGFβ, PDGF, while the paucity of blood vessels in skin lesions can be attributed to anti-endothelial cell autoantibodies. Activation of the immune system is important in the pathogenesis of SSc. T cells are activated by antigen, infiltrate early the skin lesions in SSc, and produce the profibrotic cytokine IL4. T cells are also required for autoantibody production. B cells may contribute to fibrosis, as a deficiency of CD19, a B cell transduction molecule, results in decreased fibrosis in animal models of fibrosis (210).

The most prominent clinical vascular dysfunction in SSc relates to dysregulation of the vascular tone leading to vascular spasm and a reduction in blood flow, best illustrated by the Raynaud phenomenon. It results from digital arterial closure after cold exposure (111). In SSc, an imbalance in endothelial signals (increased vasoconstrictory endothelin release), impaired vasodilatory mechanisms involving nitric oxide (NO), endothelial dependent relaxation factor (EDRF), enhanced platelet aggregation and deficient neuropeptide levels lead to the vasospastic propensity in the disease.

Increased endothelin expression in microvascular endothelial cells of the upper dermis in association with an increased number of endothelin-binding sites is also reported in SSc. There is a similar relationship in respect of lung fibrosis. Impaired NO production may contribute to platelet activation and to oxidative injury of endothelial cells, as well as promote inflammation and enhance the arteriolar internal proliferation in SSc (112). Endothelial cell apoptosis may also be a primary event in scleroderma. It may relate to infection by viruses, including cytomegalovirus (CMV). ACE levels inversely related to levels of von Willebrand factor have been proposed as markers of vascular endothelial cell (EC) injury. It is not clear yet if ACE plasma activity reflects a decreased synthesis or inhibition of enzyme activity. Further indicators of vascular injury include increased serotonin-induced platelet aggregation. In SSc, EC expressing increased numbers of ligands of 1-integrins as well as mucosal adressin cell adhesion molecule (MadCAM1), CD34, endothelial cell leukocyte adhesion molecule (ELAM-1), and ICAM-1 facilitate the interaction with lymphocytes, which express 1- and 2-integrins. In this way the transcapillary migration of inflammatory cells is mediated, leading to prominent T-cell infiltrates around blood vessels in early skin lesions. The anti-endothelial autoantibodies also induce leukocyte adhesion to EC. Circulating levels of endothelin-1, P-selectin, E-selectin, VCAM-1(vascular cell adhesion molecule-1 (VCAM-1) and ICAM-1 are useful markers of vascular and fibrotic change in SSc (94).

Several cytokines and growth factors, such as the interleukin 1 (IL1) interleukin 2 (IL2), interleukin 4 (IL4), interleukin 6 (IL6), interleukin 8 (IL8), interleukin 10 (IL10), interleukin 13 (IL13), TGFβ, PDGF, TNFα, IFNγ, and particularly the high-affinity IL2 receptor, can also be found elevated in the serum of patients with SSc (113). To some extent they correlate with the degree of organ involvement and disease activity.

One suspected mechanism behind the autoimmune phenomena is the existence of microchimerism, i.e., fetal cells circulating in maternal blood, triggering an immune reaction to what is perceived as "foreign" material (108).

Etiology and Pathogenesis

SSc is not inherited in a Mendelian fashion but genome-wide screening and candidate gene approaches have identified genetic associations between SSc and SNPs with SSc(6). To date, implicated SNPs include those in genes coding for vasomotor regulatory factors, such as ACE (*ACE*), endothelin (*EDN1, EDNRA, EDNRB*) and nitric oxide synthase (*NOS1*), B-cell markers [CD19 antigen (*CD19*)], chemokines and chemokine receptors [monocyte chemotactic protein-1 (MCP-1) and IL8 receptor beta [also known as chemokine (C-X-C) receptor 2] (*IL8RB* also known as *CXCR2*], cytokines [IL1α (*IL1A*), IL4 (*IL4*) and TNFα (*TNF*)], growth factors and their receptors [bone morphogenetic protein receptor type II (*BMPR2*), connective tissue growth factor (*CTGF*) and transforming growth factor-β (*TGFB1*)], an antioxidant glutathione S-transferase (*GSTP1*) and ECM proteins [fibronectin (*FN1*), fibrillin (*FBN1*) and secreted protein, acidic and rich in cysteine (*SPARC*) (109). The most significant genetic associations are between HLA types and the presence of defined autoantibody profiles, the latter of which are often present in specific scleroderma clinical subsets (212). This might suggest strong immunogenetic influences in SSc with aberrant activation of both the B-cell and T-cell compartments, providing potential mechanism (s) for autoimmunity. HLA is associated with scleroderma: Al, B8, and DR5 with generalized disease, DR1 with the CREST syndrome, and A3, B7, and DR2 with morphea.

BEHÇET DISEASE

General Remarks

Behçet disease (BD) is a chronic relapsing inflammatory disorder with multisystemic involvement. Its typical presentation is of iridocyclitis with hypopyon (Fig. 14), aphthous mouth ulceration, and genital ulceration. BD is relatively more frequent in countries around the Mediterranean Sea and in the Middle East

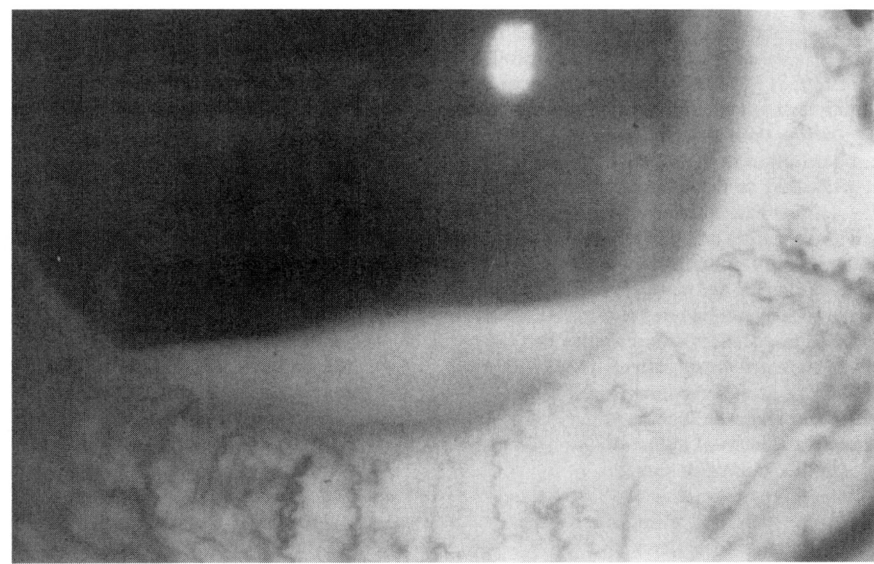

Figure 14 Behçet disease. Uveitis with sterile hypopyon.

and Far East, with a prevalence of approximately 1:10,000 in Japan. Males are affected more frequently than females.

An association exists between BD and HLA-B*51 has been well documented in a wide range of ethnic groups, with the HLA-B*5101 subtype being the most frequently expressed (up to 98%) (158,159). HLA B27 and B12 have been associated with predominantly arthritic and mucocutaneous manifestations, respectively (139).

Clinical Features

Systemic

The clinical diagnosis is made on the presence of major and minor criteria. The more frequent major findings are buccal and genital ulceration, skin lesions (typically erythema nodosum), and eye lesions (typically uveitis or occlusive retinal vasculitis). Minor findings are arthritis, gastrointestinal, cardiovascular, and renal disease, epididymitis, and thrombophlebitis (249). Painful ulceration, typically of the mucous membranes of the lips, gums, mouth, and tongue, and genitals (particularly around the scrotum and vulva), are the most frequent presenting complaints and the lesions heal with scarring. About two-thirds of patients have other skin lesions, such as erythema nodosum, folliculitis, and superficial thrombophlebitis. Approximately half of the cases develop joint involvement, typically a recurrent, asymmetric arthralgia, most frequently involving the knee and usually accompanied by fever and erythema nodosum. Superficial and deep thrombophlebitis with subsequent vein occlusion can occur and superior vena caval obstruction may cause death. CNS involvement may present with a generalized meningoencephalitis, benign intracranial hypertension, or more localizing features that may mimic multiple sclerosis. Nonspecific gastrointestinal symptoms frequently occur, but ulceration is uncommon. Epididymitis occurs in a small but significant proportion of men.

Ocular

The frequency of ocular manifestations is from 70% to 85% (173). The eye disease is typically a recurrent chorioretinitis with prominent occlusive retinal vasculitis. Patients may present with the pain and photophobia of anterior uveitis or blurring of vision from posterior uveitis and retinal vasculitis. The anterior uveitis is typically severe, with extensive posterior synechiae and hypopyon (but less than a third of patients with eye disease have hypopyon). Posterior segment involvement has a much worse prognosis than BD patients with anterior uveitis and vision is frequently lost (144). Sakamoto et al. (Fukuoka, Japan) (209) recorded an unfavorable visual outcome in 35 of 101 eyes (about 35%) in BD patients and another group from Tokyo reported a similar outcome (34%) (272). The essential feature is a progressive obliterative vasculitis, first detectable in the veins, progressing to arterial and capillary closure, with foci of retinitis and accompanying vitritis (102). Initially edema, hemorrhage, and exudates may present in the retina and this progresses to large areas of infarction with occluded blood vessels that are visible as thin white threads. Neovascularization and phthisis bulbi may occur.

Histopathology

All involved tissues manifest a systemic perivasculitis with an infiltration of lymphocytes and plasma cells and swollen hyperplastic EC, which leads to thrombosis and fibrinoid necrosis (171). In addition, these vascular abnormalities and early oral mucosal lesions contain an infiltration of lymphocytes and monocytes and at the base of the ulcers that infiltrates also contain PMNs (138). Findings in the skin include a perivascular infiltrate with fibrinoid deposition in the vascular walls, mainly affecting venules. In the brain, infarction may complicate thrombosis of the cerebral arteries.

The histopathologic trademark of ocular BD is usually a bilateral infiltration of leukocytes in and around blood vessels, occlusive retinal perivasculitis, and thrombosis that may be induced by antecedent microbial infection cross-reacting with putative autoantigens, being influenced by the genetic susceptibility of both HLA associations and SNPs in genes that encode cytokines (102). BD is characterized by periphlebitis, periarteritis, necrotizing arteriolitis, and tissue destruction with an infiltration of PMNs during active period of BD.

Biopsies of oral ulcers have disclosed numerous activated T cells and the expression of class II MHC antigens by keratinocytes. Biopsies of erythema nodosum-like skin lesions have shown an infiltrate predominantly of PMNs in early lesions and lymphocytes in chronic lesions (270). Most lymphocytes (60–80%) in all specimens have the $CD4^+$ phenotype, and a smaller number (20–40%) are $CD8^+$ with natural killer cells constituting only 5%. B cells are virtually absent. An immmunohistochemical analysis of five eyes enucleated from patients with BD disclosed a predominance of T cells in the inflammatory infiltrate (19). B-cell abnormalities have also been detected in active disease, and antibodies to oral mucosa and the outer retina have been found in patients with ocular BD.

Etiology and Pathogenesis

Huluci Behçet himself postulated a viral trigger for BD. Sixty-five years later, it remains unclear whether a virus or bacterium initiates and/or prolongs the characteristic mucosal and endothelial hyper-reactivity observed at the gastrointestinal and vascular endothelial surfaces, respectively. However, it has become increasingly apparent that these events, once triggered, may be influenced by numerous interdependent and independent genetic regions. The idea that BD may be initiated by a virus is supported by the finding of virus-like particles in the vitreous of affected individuals (63) and, the demonstration that at least part of the *Herpes simplex* genome is transcribed in mononuclear cells of some patients with BD and the observation of an impaired T-cell response specific to the *H. simplex* virus (HSV). An animal model for BD was described in 1997, in which 30% of *Herpes simplex* type 1 (HSV-1) innoculated mice were reported to exhibit BD-like manifestations, which included skin, tongue, gastrointestinal and genital ulcers, ocular inflammation and arthritis (229). Since HSV-1 immunity is common in the general population, it is possible that certain genetic haplotypes may influence the immune response of an individual to HSV-1 infection at the gastrointestinal mucosal surface. Streptococcal antigens have also been implicated in the induction of systemic symptoms of BD after skin testing with the streptococcal antigen and elevated antigen titers in some patients.

Studies have demonstrated that both *Streptococcus sanguis* and a human heat shock protein (HSP) (especially the 60/65 kDa HSP) activate gamma/delta T cells in patients with BD, but not in controls (62,137). However, BD is rare, *Streptococcus* sp. is common in oral fauna, and HSP is ubiquitously expressed by stressed cells. To be validated, this model would require an escape of T-cell clonal deletion (or positive selection) in the thymus in BD or, alternatively, irregular leukocyte behavior at the mucosal surface in patients, which may itself be influenced by certain HLA types (249).

Immune complexes may play a role in the pathogenesis of BD. They have been reported in the transition from focal oral ulceration to the systemic syndrome, are present in over 50% of patients, and appear to be associated with active fulminant disease, although Kasp et al. suggested that they may confer a beneficial role (120). Immunocomplex-mediated damage may be responsible for the increased PMN chemotaxis that is observed in BD. Serum levels of PMN priming cytokines, such as TNF, IL1β, and IL8 are known to be raised in BD patients (152), and myeloperoxidase levels generated by active PMNs are also raised (2).

An association between BD and alleles in the TNF promotor region was first reported in Japanese patients with BD (157). Two possible alleles may exist at the promotor site: TNFB*1 and TNFB*2. The latter is associated with higher TNF production by stimulated monocytes than the former and is not only more prevalent among patients with BD but is also weakly associated with a poor visual outcome. Although neither allele is rare, TNFB*2 has been associated with higher leukocyte TNF production, and might therefore lead to a more severe and prolonged inflammatory response. However, the TNFB*2 allele is also in linkage with HLA-B51, and these two alleles may therefore be co-inherited, each contributing both to disease risk and to severity of organ involvement.

A second gene in linkage with HLA-B51 is the MHC class I chain related (*MIC*) gene. An association between *MICA* genes and BD was first described in 1997, when it was shown that the prevalence of a certain "triplet repeat" polymorphism in the transmembrane region of the *MICA* gene (the MICA A6 allele) was raised in Japanese patients with BD (159).

BD confers up to a 14-fold risk of developing systemic venous thrombosis, and the risk in males is reported to be six times higher than in females (11). Factor V Leiden, a variant of the protein Factor V needed for blood clotting is a major risk factor for idiopathic systemic venous thrombosis and has also been associated with BD, in which systemic venous thrombosis occurs in up to 40% of all patients. The mutation has been associated with ocular disease, and in particular the development of ocular vaso-occlusion. This may indicate that genes outside the MHC may contribute independently to morbidity in BD.

ICAM molecules interact with their ligand molecules on leucocytes, enabling the movement of pro-inflammatory cells across the blood vessel wall into the tissues. Once released from the endothelial surface, the soluble form of ICAM-1 (sICAM-1) may be detected in the peripheral blood of patients with a variety of inflammatory disorders, including BD (248). Until the effect of the allelic variants on the function of ICAM-1 is known, the relevance of these findings to BD remains unclear. However, this association supports a multifactorial cause of BD.

Despite 20 years of intense efforts to identify other associated genetic regions in chromosome 6 and elsewhere, HLA-B51 remains foremost among candidate risk factors for disease. TNF and MICA alleles in the MHC are also implicated, but their close linkage with HLA-B51 has made their independent contribution to disease less easy to define. Newly characterized regions on different chromosomes may also contribute to disease, through their influence on the clotting cascade, on the events that underlie the leukocyte recruitment into the tissues, and on PMN activation. These discoveries have important implications for the management of patients with BD. Firstly, they provide a rationale for new forms of immunomodulation that are now under investigation such as TNF and ICAM blockade, and the use of IFNα2a and IFNα2b. In the case of factor V Leiden, anticoagulative measures, in addition to immunosuppression, may be valuable in managing patients with severe and recurrent ocular occlusive disease. Secondly, increasing knowledge of genetic disease severity markers may enable early identification of vulnerable patients before irreversible ocular complications ensue.

REFERENCES

1. Abrahama DJ, Varga J. Scleroderma: from cell and molecular mechanisms to disease models. Trends in Immunol November 2005; 26(11):587–95.
2. Accardo-Palumbro A, Triolo G, Carbone MC, et al. Polymorphonuclear leukocyte myeloperoxidase levels in Behçet's disease. Clin Exp Rheumatol 2000; 18:495–8.
3. Afshari NA, Afshari MA, Lessell S. Temporal arteritis. Int Ophthalmol Clin Winter 2001; 41(1):151–8.
4. Afshari NA, Afshari MA, Foster CS. Inflammatory conditions of the eye associated with rheumatic diseases. Curr Rheumatol Rep 2001; 3:453–8.
5. Agnello V, Koffler D, Kunkel HG. Immune complex systems in the nephritis of systemic lupus eryhthematosis. Kidney Int 1973; 3:90–9.
6. Ahmed SS, Tan FK. Identification of novel targets in SSc: update on population studies, cDNA arrays, SNP analysis, and mutations. Curr Opin Rheumatol 2003; 15:766–71.
7. Alarcon-Segovia, Alarcon-Riquelme. Etiopathogenesis of systemic lupus erythematosus. In: Lahita RG, ed. Systemic Lupus Erythematosus. 4th ed. Academic Press, 2004:93–107.
8. Allsop CJ, Gallagher PJ. Temporal artery biopsy in giant cell arteritis: a reappraisal. Am J Surg Pathol 1981; 5:317–23.
9. Alsaeid KM, Haider MZ, Al-Awadhi AM, et al. Role of human leukocyte antigen DRB1*0307 and DRB1*0308 in susceptibility to juvenile rheumatoid arthritis. Clin Exp Rheumatol 2003; 21:399–402.
10. Alsalameh J, Mollenhauer F, Scheuplein et al. Preferential cellular and humoral immune reactivities to native and denatured collagen types IX and XI in a patient with fatal relapsing polychondritis. J Rheum 1993; 20:1419–24.
11. Ames PR, Steuer A, Pap A, et al. Thrombosis in Behçet's disease: a retrospective survey from a single UK centre. Rheumatology 2001; 40:652–5.
12. Ashton N, Hobbs HE. Effect of cortisone on rheumatoid nodules of the sclera (scleromalacia perforans). Br J Ophthalmol 1952; 56:373–84.
13. Ashton N, Coomes EN, Garner A, Oliver DO. Retinopathy due to progressive systemic sclerosis. J Pathol Bacterial 1968; 96:259–68.
14. Baldassare AR, Weiss TD, Tsai CC, et al. Immunoprotein deposition in synovial tissue in Reiter's syndrome. Ann Rheum Dis 1981; 40:281–5.
15. Ball J. Articular pathology of ankylosing spondylitis. Clin Orthop 1979; 143:30–7.
16. Barron KS, DeCunto CL, Montalvo JE, et al. Abnormalities of immunoregulation in juvenile rheumatoid arthritis. J Rheumatol 1989; 76:940–8.
17. Bartfai Z, Gaede KI, Russell KA, et al. Different gender-associated genotype risks of Wegener's granulomatosis and microscopic polyangiitis, Clin Immunol 2003; 109:330–7.
18. Barth WE, Berson EL. Relapsing polychondritis, rheumatoid arthritis and blindness. Am J Ophthalmol 1968; 66: 890–96.
19. Barton K, Charteris D, McCartney A, Lightman S. Investigation of the inflammatory cellular infiltrates in ocular Behçet's disease. Invest Ophthalmol Vis Sci 1990; Suppl 31:67.
20. Bastian HM, Roseman J, McGwin G Jr, et al. Systemic lupus erythematosus in three ethnic groups: XII. Risk factors for lupus nephritis after diagnosis. Lupus 2002; 11:152–60.
21. Benson WE. Posterior scleritis. Surv Ophthalmol 1988; 52: 297–316.
22. Bertoni M, Niccoli L, Pociello G, et al. Pulmonary hypertension in primary Sjögren's syndrome: report of

a case and review of the literature. Clin Rheum 2005; 24 (4):431–4.
23. Bhagat N, Green RL, Feldon SE, Lim JI. Exudative retinal detachment in relapsing polychondritis: case report and literature review. Ophthalmology 2001; 108:1156–9.
24. Bialasiewic AA, Holbach L. Ocular findings in infection-linked immune phenomena and secondary disease (the so-called Reiter's syndrome). Klin Monatsbl Augenheilkd 1990; 796:196–201.
25. Binaghi M, Kamoun MM, Coscas KG. Fluorescein angiography in the diagnosis of polyarteritis nodosa. J Fr Ophthalmol 1984; 7:19–30.
26. Blanco P, Viallard JF, Pellegrin JL, Moreau JF. Cytotoxic T lymphocytes and autoimmunity. Curr Opin Rheumatol November 2005; 17:731–4.
27. Boh EE. Neonatal lupus erythematosus. Clin Dermatol 2004; 22:125–8.
28. Bonfioli AA, Orefice F. Sarcoidosis. Semin Ophthalmol 2005; 20:177–82.
29. Borgmann S, Endisch G, Urban S, et al. Linkage disequilibrium between genes at the serine protease inhibitor gene cluster on chromosome 14q32.1 is associated with Wegener's granulomatosis. Clin Immunol 2001; 98:244–8.
30. Borrout. Neuro-ophthalmologic manifestations of rheumatologic and associated disorders. Curr Opin Ophthalmol December 1996; 7(6):8–10 (Review).
31. Bosley TM, Savino PJ, Sergott RC, et al. Ocular pneumoplethysmography can help in the diagnosis of giant cell arteritis. Arch Ophthalmol 1989; 707:379–81.
32. Boule MW, Broughton C, Mackay F, et al. Toll-like receptor 9-dependent and -independent dendritic cell activation by chromatin-immunoglobulin G complexes. J Exp Med 2004; 199:1631–40.
33. Bowman SJ, Ibrahim GH, Holmes G, et al. Estimating the prevalence among caucasian women of primary Sjögren's syndrome in two general practices in Birmingham. Scand J Rheumatol 2004; 33:39–43.
34. Bradley DS, Das P, Griffiths MM, et al. HLA-DQ6/8 double transgenic mice develop auricular chondritis following type II collagen immunization: a model for human relapsing polychondritis. J Immunol 1998; 161:5046–53.
35. Brownstein S, Nicolle DA, Codere E. Bilateral blindness in temporal arteritis with skip areas. Arch Ophthalmol 1983; 101:388–91.
36. Buckner J, Van Landeghen M, Kwok WW, Tsarknaridis L. Identification of type II collagen peptide 261–273-specific T cell clones in a patient with relapsing polychondritis. Arthritis Rheum 2002; 46:238–44.
37. Buckner JH, Wu JJ, Reife RA, et al. Autoreactivity against matrilin-1 in a patient with relapsing polychondritis. Arthritis Rheum 2000; 43:939–43.
38. Burke CD. Science, medicine and the future treatment of rheumatoid arthritis. Brt Med J 1997; 315:236–8.
39. Butrimiene I, Jarmalaite S, Ranceva J, et al. Different cytokine profiles in patients with chronic and acute reactive arthritis. Rheumatology. Oxford, 2004; 43: 1300–4.
40. Calvo-Romero JM, Giant cell arteritis. Postgrad Med J 2003; 79:511–5.
41. Capizzi SA, Specks U. Does infection play a role in the pathogenesis of pulmonary vasculitis? Semin Respir Infect 2003; 18:17–22.
42. Carmona L, Villaverde V, Hernandez-Garcia C, et al. The prevalence of rheumatoid arthritis in the general population of Spain. Rheumatology. Oxford, 2002; 41: 88–95.
43. Carpenter AB, Eisenbeis CH Jr, Carrabis S, et al. Soluble interleukin-2 receptor: elevated levels in serum and synovial fluid of patients with rheumatoid arthritis. J Clin Lab Anal 1990; 4:130–4.
44. Carrero JL, Sanjurjo FJ. Bilateral cilioretinal artery occlusion in antiphospholipid syndrome. Retina. 2006; 26:104–6.
45. Chan CC, Paine M, O'Day J Predictors of recurrent ischemic optic neuropathy in giant cell arteritis. J Neuroophthalmol 2005; 25:14–7.
46. Chang JH, McCluskey PJ, Wakefield D. Acute anterior uveitis and HLA-B27. Surv Ophthalmol 2005; 50:364–88.
47. Chisholm DM, Mason DK. Labial salivary gland biopsy in Sjögren's syndrome. J Clin Pathol 1968; 21:656–60.
48. Cochrane CG. Mechanisms involved in the deposition of immune complexes in tissues. J Exp Med 1971; Suppl 134: 75–89.
49. Cochrane W, Davies DV, Dorling J. Ultramicroscopic structure of the rheumatoid nodule. Ann Rheum Dis 1964; 23:345–63.
50. Colmegna I, Cuchacovich R, Espinoza LR. HLA-B27-associated reactive arthritis: pathogenetic and clinical considerations. Clin Microbiol Rev 2004; 17:348–69.
51. Colmegna I, Maldonado-Cocco JA. Polyarteritis nodosa revisited. Curr Rheumatol Rep 2005; 7:288–96.
52. Croker JA, Kimberly R. Genetics of susceptibility and severity in SLE. Curr Opin Rheumatol 2005; 17: 529–37.
53. D'Agati V, Chander R, Nash M, Mancilla-Jimenez R. Idiopathic microscopic polyarteritis nodosa: ultrastructural observations on the renal and vascular and glomerular lesions. Am J Kidney Dis 1986; 7:95–110.
54. Daniels TE, Fox PC. Salivary and oral components of Sjögren's syndrome. Rheum Dis Clin North Am 1992; 18: 571–89.
55. Dawson LJ, Field EA, Harmer AR, Smith PM. Acetylcholine-evoked calcium mobilization and ion channel activation in human labial gland acinar cells from patients with primary Sjögren's syndrome. Clin Exp Immunol 2001; 124:480–5.
56. Dawson TM, Starkebaum G, Wood BlL, et al. Epstein – Barr virus, methotrexate and lymphoma in patients with rheumatoid arthritis and primary Sjögren's syndrome: case series. J Rheumatol 2001; 28:47–53.
57. DeBenedetti F, Meazza C, Vivarelli M, et al. Functional and prognostic relevance of the -173 polymorphism of the macrophage migration inhibitory factor gene in systemic-onset juvenile idiopathic arthritis. Arthritis Rheum 2003; 48:1398–1407.
58. DeBenedetti F, Vivarelli M, Pignatti P, et al. Circulating levels of soluble E-selectin, P-selectin and intracellular adhesion molecule-1 in patients with juvenile idiopathic arthritis. J Rheum 2000; 27:2246–50.
59. DeClerck LS, Struyf NJ, Bridts CH et al. Humoral immunity and composition of immune complexes in patients with rheumatoid arthritis, with special reference to IgE containing immune complexes. Clin Exp Rheumatol 1989; 7:485–92.
60. DeRycke L, Peene I, Hoffman IE et al. Rheumatoid factor and anticitrullinated protein antibodies in rheumatoid arthritis: diagnostic value, association with radiological progression rate and extra articular manifestations. Ann Rheum Dis 2004; 63:1587–93.
61. Devaney KO, Travis WD, Hoffman G, et al. Interpretation of head and neck biopsies in Wegener's granulomatosis: a pathological study of 126 biopsies in 70 patients. Am J Surg Pathol 1990; 14:555–64.

62. Direskeneli H, Eksioglu-Demiralp E, Yavuz S, et al. T cell responses to 60/65 kDa heat shock protein derived peptides in Turkish patients with Behcet's disease. J Rheumatol 2000; 27:708–13.
63. Direskeneli H. Behcet's disease: infectious aetiology, new autoantigens, and HLA-B51. Ann Rheum Dis 2001; 60: 996–1002.
64. Doita M, Maeda S, Kawai K, et al. Analysis of lymphocyte subsets of bone marrow in patients with rheumatoid arthritis by two colour immunofluorescence and flow cytometry. Ann Rheum Dis 1990; 49:168–71.
65. du Bois RM, Goh N, McGrath D, Cullinan P. Is there a role for microorganisms in the pathogenesis of sarcoidosis? J Intern Med 2003; 253:4–17.
66. El-Shabrawi Y, Livir-Rallatos C, Christen W, et al. High levels of interleukin-12 in the aqueous humor and vitreous of patients with uveitis. Ophthalmology 1998; 105:1659–63.
67. Emad Y, Basaffar S, Ragab Y, et al. A case of polyarteritis nodosa complicated by left central retinal artery occlusion, ischemic optic neuropathy, and retinal vasculitis. Clin Rheumatol 2006 Mar 31; Epub ahead of print. PMID: 16575492.
68. Ewald EA, Griffin D, McCune WJ. Correlation of angiographic abnormalities with disease manifestations and disease severity in polyarteritis nodosa. J Rheumatol 1987; 14:952–6.
69. Falk RJ, Jennette JC. Anti-neutrophil cytoplasmic anutoantibodies with specificity for myeloperoxidase in patients with systemic vasculitis and idiopathic necrotizing and crescentic glomerulonephritis. N Engl J Med 1988; 318:1651–7.
70. Fauchald P, Rygvold O, Oystese B. Temporal arteritis and polymyalgia rheumatica. Clinical and biopsy findings. Ann Intern Med 1972; 77:L845–52.
71. Ferraro G, Meroni PL, Tincani A, et al. Anti-endothelial cell antibodies in patients with Wegener's granulomatosis and micropolyarteritis. Clin Exp Immunol 1990; 79:47–53.
72. Fessel WJ. Systemic lupus erythematosis in the community. Arch Intern Med 1974; 134:1021–35.
73. Fiorillo MT, Ruckert C, Hulsmeyer M, et al. Allele-dependent similarity between viral and self-peptide presentation by HLA-B27 subtypes. J Biol Chem 2005; 280:2962–71.
74. Fong LP, Sainz de la Maza M, Rice BA, et al. Immunopathology of scleritis. Ophthalmology 1991; 98:472–9.
75. Foroozan R, Danesh-Meyer HV, Savino PJ et al. Thrombocytosis in patients with biopsy proven giant cell arteritis. Ophthalmology 2002; 109:1267–71.
76. Foster CS, Forstot SL, Wilson LA, et al. Mortality rate in rheumatoid arthritis patients developing necrotizing scleritis or peripheral ulcerative keratitis. Ophthalmology 1984; 91:1253–63.
77. Fox RI. Sjögren's syndrome. Lancet 2005; 366: 321–31.
78. Fraunfelder FT, Watson PG. Evaluation of eyes enucleated for scleritis. Br J Ophthalmol 1976; 60:227–30.
79. Gal I, Lakos G, Zeher M. Comparison of the anti-Ro/SSA autoantibody profile between patients with primary and secondary Sjögren's syndrome. Autoimmunity 2000; 32: 89–92.
80. Gencik M, Meller S, Borgmann S, Fricke H. Proteinase 3 gene polymorphisms and Wegener's granulomatosis. Kidney Int 2000; 58:2473–7.
81. Gencik M, Meller S, Borgmann S, et al. The association of CD18 alleles with anti-myeloperoxidase subtypes of ANCA-associated systemic vasculitides. Clin Immunol 2000; 94:9–12.
82. Gergely P Jr, Poor G. Relapsing polychondritis. Best Pract Res Clin Rheumatol 2004; 18:723–38.
83. Giroux L, Paquin F, Guerard-Desjardins MJ, Lefaivre A. Relapsing polychondritis: an autoimmune disease. Semin Arthritis Rheum 1983; 13:182–7.
84. Giscombe R, Wang X, Huang D, Lefvert AK. Coding sequence 1 and promoter single nucleotide polymorphisms in the CTLA-4 gene in Wegener's granulomatosis. J Rheumatol 2002; 29:950–3.
85. Godfrey WA, Lindsley CB, Cuppage FE. Localization of IgM in plasma cells in the iris of a patient with iridocyclitis and juvenile rheumatoid arthritis. Arthritis Rheum 1981; 24:1195–8.
86. Gonzalez-Gay MA, Garcia-Porrua C, Salvarani C, Hunder GG. Diagnostic approach in a patient presenting with polymyalgia. Clin Exp Rheumatol 1999; 17: 276–8.
87. Gonzalez-Gay MA. Genetic epidemiology in giant cell arteritis and polymyalgia rheumatica. Arthritis Res 2001; 3:154–7.
88. Graham RR, Ortmann WA, Langefeld CD, et al. Visualizing human leukocyte antigen class II risk haplotypes in human systemic lupus erythematosus. Am J Hum Genet 2002; 71:543–53.
89. Graham EM, Spalton DJ, Barnard RO, et al. Cerebral and retinal vascular changes in systemic lupus erythematosus. Ophthalmology 1985; 92:444–8.
90. Gran JT, Myklebust G. The incidence of polymyalgia rheumatica and temporal arteritis in the county of Aust Agder, south Norway: a prospective study 1987–94. J Rheumatol 1997; 24:1739–43.
91. Grennan DM, Forrester J. Involvement of the eye in SLE and scleroderma: a study using fluorescein angiography in addition to clinical ophthalmic assessment. Ann Rheum Dis 1977; 36:152–6.
92. Gross JA, Johnston J, Mudri S. et al. TACI and BCMA are receptors for a TNF homologue implicated in B-cell autoimmune disease. Nature 2000; 404:995–9.
93. Grunewald J, Eklund A, Olerup O. Human leukocyte antigen class I alleles and the disease course in sarcoidosis patients. Am J Respir Crit Care Med 2004; 169:696–702.
94. Gruschwitz MS, Hornstein OP, von den Driesch P. Correlation of soluble adhesion molecules in the peripheral blood of scleroderma patients with their in situ expression and with disease activity. Arthritis Rheum 1995; 18:184–9.
95. Hancock WW, Kobzik L, Colby AJ, et al. Detection of lymphokines and lymphokine receptors in pulmonary sarcoidosis. Am J Pathol 1986; 123:1–8.
96. Hansson, Heinegard D, Piette JC, et al. The occurrence of autoantibodies to matrilin 1 reflects a tissue-specific response to cartilage of the respiratory tract in patients with relapsing polychondritis. Arthritis Rheum 2001; 44:2402–12.
97. Haustein U-F, Systemic sclerosis – scleroderma. Dermatology Online Journal 8(1):3 http://dermatology.cdlib.org/DOJvol8num1/reviews/scleroderma/haustein.html)
98. Hayreh SS. Posterior ischaemic optic neuropathy: clinical features, pathogenesis, and management. Eye. 2004; 18: 1188–206.
99. Hazelton RA. Immunogenic insights into rheumatoid arthritis: a family study. Q J Med 1982; 51:336–40.
100. Henkind P, Gold D. Ocular manifestations of rheumatic disorders. Rheumatology 1973; 4:13–59.

101. Hudspith BN, Flint KC, Geraint-James D, et al. Lack of immune deficiency in sarcoidosis: compartmentalisation of the immune response. Thorax 1987; 42:250–5.
102. Hughes EH, Dick AD. The pathology and pathogenesis of retinal vasculitis. Neuropathol Appl Neurobiol 2003; 29: 325–40.
103. Hulsmeyer M, Fiorillo MT, Bettosini F, et al. Dual, HLA-B27 subtype-dependent conformation of a self-peptide. J Exp Med 2004; 119:271–81.
104. Jagiello PM, Gencik L, Arning S, et al. New genomic region for Wegener's granulomatosis as revealed by an extended association screen with 202 apoptosis-related genes. Hum Genet 2004; 114:468–77.
105. Jain SS, Rao P, Kothari K, et al. Posterior scleritis presenting as unilateral secondary angle-closure glaucoma. Indian J Ophthalmol 2004; 52:241–4.
106. James DG. The many faces of sarcoidosis. Sarcoidosis 1990; 7:1–8.
107. James DG, Neville E, Siltzbach LE. A worldwide review of sarcoidosis. Ann NY Acad Sci 1976; 278:321–4.
108. Jimenez SA, Derk CT. Following the molecular pathways toward an understanding of the pathogenesis of systemic sclerosis. Ann Intern Med 2004; 140:37–50.
109. Johnson RW, Tew MB, Arnett FC, et al. The genetics of systemic sclerosis. Curr Rheumatol Rep 2002; 4:99–107.
110. Jones NP, Sarcoidosis and uveitis. Ophthalmol Clin North Am 2002; 15:319–26.
111. Kahaleh B, Matucci-Cerinic M. Raynaud's phenomenon and scleroderma. Dysregulated neuroendothelial control of vascular tone. Arthritis Rheum 1995; 38:1–4.
112. Kahaleh MB, LeRoy EC. Autoimmunity and vascular involvement in systemic sclerosis. Autoimmunity 1999; 31:195–214.
113. Kahaleh MB, Yin T. Enhanced expression of high-affinity interleukin-2 receptors in scleroderma: possible role for IL-6. Clin Immunol Immunopathol 1992; 62:97–102.
114. Kaiser M, Weyand CM, Bjornsson J, et al. Platelet derived growth factor, intimal hyperplasia, and ischaemic complications in giant cell arteritis. Arthritis Rheum 1998; 41: 623–33.
115. Kaiser M, Younge B, Bjornsson J, et al. Formation of new vasa vasorum in vasculitis. Production of angiogenic cytokines by multinucleated giant cells. Am J Pathol 1999; 155:765–74.
116. Kaluza W, Leirisalo-Repo M, Marker-Hermann E, et al. IL10G microsatellites mark promoter haplotypes associated with protection against the development of reactive arthritis in Finnish patients. Arthritis Rheum 2001; 44:1209–14; Erratum in: Arthritis Rheum 2001; 44: 2212.
117. Kanski JJ. Juvenile arthritis and uveitis. Sum Ophthalmol 1990; 34:253–61.
118. Kanski JJ. Screening for uveitis in juvenile chronic arthritis. Br J Ophthalmol 1989; 73:225–8.
119. Karim A, Allali F, Tachfouti S. Bilateral uveitis in relapsing polychondritis. A case report. J Fr Ophthalmol 2005; 28:530–2.
120. Kasp E, Graham EM, Stanford MR, et al. Retinal autoimmunity and circulating immune complexes in ocular Behçet's disease. In: Lehner T, Barnes CG, eds. Recent Advances in Behçet's Disease. London: Royal Society of Medicine Services, 1982:67–71.
121. Katano K, Kawano M, Koni I, et al. Clinical and laboratory features of anticentromere antibody positive primary Sjögren's syndrome. J Rheumatol 2001; 28: 2238–44.
122. Kataria RK, Brent LH. Spondyloarthropathies. Am Fam Physician 2004; 69:2853–60.
123. Keat A, Thomas BJ, Taylor Robinson D. Chlamydial infection in the aetiology of arthritis. Br Med Bull 1983; 59:168–74.
124. Khan AM, Elahi F, Hashmi SR, et al. Wegener's granulomatosis: a rare, chronic and multisystem disease. Surgeon 2006; 4:45–52.
125. Khng CG, Yap EY, Au-Eong KG, et al. Central serous retinopathy complicating systemic lupus erythematosus: a case series. Clin Experiment Ophthalmol 2000; 28: 309–13.
126. Kilding R, Wilson AG. Mapping of a novel susceptibility gene for rheumatoid arthritis in the telomeric MHC region. Cytokine 2005; 32:71–5.
127. Kiss S, Letko E, Qamruddin S, et al. Long-term progression, prognosis, and treatment of patients with recurrent ocular manifestations of Reiter's syndrome. Ophthalmology 2003; 110:1764–9.
128. Kobayashi M, Kawano S, Hatachi S et al. Enhanced expression of programmed death -1 (PD-1)/PD-L1 in salivary glands of patients with Sjögren's syndrome. J Rheumatol 2005; 32:2156–63.
129. Kocher M, Siegel ME, Edberg JC, Kimberly RP. Cross-linking of Fc gamma receptor IIa and Fc gamma receptor IIIb induces different proadhesive phenotypes on human neutrophils. J Immunol 1997; 159:3940–8.
130. Konttinen YT, Bergroth V, Kunnamo I, Haapasaari J. The value of biopsy in patients with monoarticular juvenile rheumatoid arthritis of recent onset. Arthritis Rheum 1986; 29:47–53.
131. Koufakis DI, Karabatsas CH, Sakkas LI, et al. Conjunctival surface changes in patients with Sjögren's syndrome: a transmission electron microscopy study. Invest Ophthalmol Vis Sci 2006; 47:541–4.
132. Kvien TK, Gaston JS, Bardin T, et al. Three month treatment of reactive arthritis with azithromycin: a EULAR double blind, placebo controlled study. Ann Rheum Dis 2004; 63:1113–9.
133. Lacomba MS, Martin CM, Chamond RR, et al. Aqueous and serum interferon gamma, interleukin (IL) 2, IL-4, and IL-10 in patients with uveitis. Arch Ophthalmol 2000; 118: 768–72.
134. Lang B, Rothenfusser A, Lanchbury JS, et al. Susceptibility to relapsing polychondritis is associated with HLA-DR4. Arthritis Rheum 1993; 36:660–4.
135. Lauhio A, Leirisalo-Repo M, Lahdevirta J, et al. Double-blind, placebo-controlled study of three-month treatment with lymecycline in reactive arthritis, with special reference to Chlamydia arthritis. Arthritis Rheum 1991; 34:6–14.
136. Lee DA, Barker SM, Daniel Su, et al. The clinical diagnosis of Reiter's syndrome. Ophthalmic and non-ophthalmic aspects. Ophthalmology 1988; 95:350–6.
137. Lehner T. The role of heat shock protein, microbial and autoimmune agents in the aetiology of Behçet's disease. Int Rev Immunol 1997; 14:21–32.
138. Lehner T, Batchelor JR. Classification and an immunogenetic basis of Behçet's syndrome. In: Lehner T, Barnes CG, eds. Behçet's Syndrome. London: Academic Press, 1976: 13–32.
139. Lehner T. Pathology of recurrent oral ulceration in Behçet's syndrome: light, electron and fluorescence microscopy. J Pathol 1969; 97:481–94.
140. Leirisalo-Repo M. Reactive arthritis. Scand J Rheumatol 2005; 34:251–9.

141. Letko E, Zafirakis P, Baltatzis S, et al. Relapsing polychondritis: a clinical review. Semin Arthritis Rheum 2002; 31:384–95.
142. Lie JT. Temporal artery biopsy diagnosis of giant cell arteritis: lessons from 1109 biopsies. Anat Pathol 1996; 1: 69–97.
143. Ma-Krupa W, Kwan M, Goronzy JJ, Weyand CM. Toll-like receptors in giant cell arteritis. Clin Immunol 2005; 115: 38–46.
144. Mamo JG. The rate of visual loss in Behçet's disease. Arch Ophthalmol 1970; 84:451–2.
145. Mandl LA, Solomon DH, Smith EL, et al. Using antineutrophil cytoplasmic antibody testing to diagnose vasculitis: can test-ordering guidelines improve diagnostic accuracy. Arch Intern Med 2002; 162:1509–15.
146. Mariette X. Lymphomas in patients with Sjögren's syndrome: review of the literature and physiopathological hypothesis. Leukaemia and Lymphoma 1999; 33:93–9.
147. Mark DB, McCulley JB. Reiter's keratitis. Arch Ophthalmol 1982; 100:781–4.
148. Mark EJ, Matsubara O, Tan-Liu FR. The pulmonary biopsy in the early diagnosis of Wegener's (pathergic) granulomatosis. Hum Pathol 1988; 19:1065–71.
149. Marto N, Bertolaccini ML, Calabuig E, et al. Anti-C1q antibodies in nephritis: correlation between titres and renal disease activity and positive predictive value in systemic lupus erythematosus. Ann Rheum Dis 2005; 64: 444–8.
150. May E, Dorris ML, Satumtira N, et al. CD8 alpha beta T cells are not essential to the pathogenesis of arthritis or colitis in HLA-B27 transgenic rats. J Immunol 2003; 170: 1099–1105.
151. McDonnell PJ, Moore GW, Miller NR, et al. Temporal arteritis: a clinicopathological study. Ophthalmology 1986; 93:518–30.
152. Mege J-L, Dilsen N, Sanguedolce V, et al. Overproduction of monocyte derived TNF, Interleukin (IL) 6, IL 8 and increased neutrophil superoxide generation in Behçet's disease. A comparative study with familial Mediterranean fever and healthy subjects. J Rheumatol 1993; 20: 1544–9.
153. Merriam JC, Chylack LT, Albert DM. Early-onset pauciarticular juvenile rheumatoid arthritis: a histopathological study. Arch Ophthalmol 1983; 101:1085–92.
154. Messmer EMM, Foster CS. Destructive corneal and scleral disease associated with rheumatoid arthritis. Cornea 1995; 14:408–17.
155. Michet CJ, McKenna CH, Luthra HS, O'Fallon WM. Relapsing polychondritis: survival and predictive role of early disease manifestations. Ann Intern Med 1986; 104: 74–8.
156. Miller JJ, Osborne CL, Hsu Y. Clq binding in serum in juvenile rheumatoid arthritis. J Rheumatol 1980; 7:665–70.
157. Mizuki N, Inoko H, Ohno S. Molecular genetics (HLA) of Behcet's disease. Yonsei Med J 1997; 38:333–49.
158. Mizuki N, Inoko H, Sugimura K, et al. RFLP analysis in the TNFβ gene and susceptaibility to alloreactive NK cells in Behçet's disease. Invest Ophthalmol Vis Sci 1992; 33: 3084–90.
159. Mizuki N, Ohno S, Tanaka H, et al. Association of HLA-B51 and lack of association of class II alleles with Behcet's disease. Tissue Antigens 1992; 40:22–30.
160. Mizuki N, Ota M, Kimura S, et al. Triplet repeat polymorphism in the transmembrane region of the MICA gene: a strong association of six GCT repetitions with Behçet's disease. Proc Natl Acad Sci U S A 1997; 94: 1298–303.
161. Modlin RL, Hofman EM, Meyer PR, et al. In situ demonstration of T lymphocyte subsets in granulomatous inflammation: leprosy, rhinoscleroma, and sarcoidosis. Clin Exp Immunol 1983; 57:430–8.
162. Monnet D, Breban M, Hudry C, et al. Ophthalmic findings and frequency of extraocular manifestations in patients with HLA-B27 uveitis: a study of 175 cases. Ophthalmology. 2004; 111:802–9.
163. Moroldo MB, Donnelly P, Saunders J, et al. Transmission disequilibrium as a test of linkage and association between HLA alleles and pauciarticular-onset juvenile rheumatoid arthritis. Arthritis Rheum 1998, 41:1620–4.
164. Muller K, Herner EB, Stagg A, et al. Inflammatory cytokines and cytokine antagonists in whole blood cultures of patients with systemic JIA. Br J Rheum 1998; 37:562–9.
165. National Rheumatoid Arthritis Society, Maidenhead. Berkshire: Making a diagnosis of rheumatoid arthritis. BJN 2005.
166. Newkirk MM, Goldbach-Mansky R, Senior BW, et al. Elevated levels of IgM and IgA antibodies to *Proteus mirabilis* and IgM antibodies to Escherichia coli are associated with early rheumatoid factor (RF) positive rheumatoid arthritis. Rheumatology 2005; 44:1433–41.
167. Ng YC, Walport MJ. Immunogenetics of SLE and primary Sjögren's syndrome. Ballieres Clin Rheumatol 1988; 2: 623–47.
168. Nguyen QD, Uy HS, Akpek EK, et al. Choroidopathy of systemic lupus erythematosus. Lupus 2000; 9:288–98.
169. Nordborg C, Nordborg E, Petursdottir V, et al. Search for Varicella zoster virus in giant cell arteritis. Ann Neurol 1998; 44:413–4.
170. Obenauf CD, Shaw HE, Sydnor CE, Klintworth GK. Sarcoidosis and its ophthalmic manifestations. Am J Ophthalmol 1978; 86:648–55.
171. O'Duffy JD. Vasculitis in Behçet's disease. Rheum Dis Clin North Am 1990; 76:423–31.
172. Ogilvie EM, Fife MS, Thompson SD, et al. The -174G allele of the interleukin-6 gene confers susceptibility to systemic arthritis in children: a multicenter study using simplex and multiplex juvenile idiopathic arthritis families. Arthritis Rheum 2003; 48:3202–6.
173. Okada AA, Rao NA, Usui M. Behçet's disease. In: Yanoff M, Duker JS, eds. Ophthalmology. 2nd ed. Mosby Inc., 2004: Part 10, Section 6, Chapter 176.
174. Oliver JA, Cannon PJ. The kidney in scleroderma. Nephron 1977; 78:141–50.
175. Oyoo O, Espinoza LR. Infection-related vasculitis. Curr Rheumatol Rep 2005; 7:281–7.
176. Paccalin M, Manic H, Bouche G, et al. Antiphospholipid syndrome in patients with retinal venous occlusion. Thromb Res 2006; 117:365–9.
177. Parking B, Chew JB, White VA, et al. Lymphocyte infiltration and enlargement of the lacrimal glands new subtype of primary Sjögren's syndrome? Ophthalmology 2005; 112:2040–7.
178. Pecorella I, La Cava M, Mannino G, et al. Diffuse granulomatous necrotizing scleritis. Acta Ophthalmol Scand 2006; 84:263–5.
179. Peebo BB, Peebo M, Frennesson C. Relapsing polychondritis: a rare disease with varying symptoms. Acta Ophthalmol Scand 2004; 82:472–5.
180. Peponis V, Kyttaris VC, Tyradellis C, et al. Ocular manifestations of systemic lupus erythematosus: a clinical review. Lupus 2006; 15:3–12.
181. Perez P, Kwon YJ, Alliende C, et al. Increased acinar damage of salivary glands of patients with Sjögren's

syndrome is paralleled by simultaneous imbalance of matrix metalloproteinase 3/tissue inhibitor of metalloproteinases1 and matrix metalloproteinase 9/tissue inhibitor of metalloproteinase 1 ratios. Arthritis Rheum 2005; 52:2751–60.

182. Perrot S, Calvez V, Escande JP, et al. Prevalences of herpes viruses DNA sequences in salivary gland biopsies from primary and secondary Sjögren's syndrome using degenerated consensus PCR primers. J Clin Virol 2003; 28: 165–8.
183. Pertovaara M, Raitala, Uusitalo H, et al. Mechanisms dependent on tryptophan catabolism regulate immune responses in primary Sjögren's syndrome. Clin Exp Immunol 2005; 142:155–6.
184. Petty RE, Viruses and childhood arthritis. Ann Med 1997; 29:149–52.
185. Petty RE, Hunt DE, Rollins DE, et al. Immunity to soluble retinal antigen in patients with uveitis accompanying juvenile rheumatoid arthritis. Arthritis Rheum 1987; 30: 287–93.
186. Prahalad S, Ryan MH, Shear ES, et al. Juvenile rheumatoid arthritis: linkage to HLA demonstrated by allele sharing in affected sibpairs. Arthritis Rheum 2000; 43: 2335–8.
187. Prochorec-Sobieszek M, Wagner T, Loukas M, et al. Histopathological and immunohistochemical analysis of lymphoid follicles in labial salivary glands in primary and secondary Sjögren's syndrome. Medical Science Monitor 2004 Apr; 10(4):BR115–21.
188. Prokunina L, Alarcon-Riquelme M, The genetic basis of systemic lupus erythematosus—knowledge of today and thoughts for tomorrow. Hum Mol Genet 2004; 13:R143–8.
189. Purcell JJ, Birkenkamp R, Tsai CC. Conjunctival lesions in periarteritis nodosa: a clinical and immunopathological study. Arch Ophthalmol 1984; 702:736–8.
190. Purcell JJ, Tsai CC, Baldassare AR. Conjunctival immunopathologic and ultrastructural alterations: occurrence in Reiter's syndrome. Arch Ophthalmol 1982; 700:1618–21.
191. Quinlan MP, Hitchings RA. Angle closure glaucoma secondary to posterior scleritis. Br J Ophthalmol 1978; 62: 330–5.
192. Ramo-Casals M, Font J. Primary Sjögren's syndrome: current and emergent aetiopathogenic concepts. Rheumatology 2005; 44:1354–67.
193. Ramos-Casals M, Garcia-Carrasco M, Cervera R, et al. Hepatitis C virus infection mimiking primary Sjögren's syndrome. A clinical and immunologic description of 35 cases. Medicine 2001; 80:1–8.
194. Rao JK, Weinberger M, Oddone EZ, et al. The role of antineutrophil cytoplasmic antibody (c-ANCA) testing in the diagnosis of Wegener granulomatosis. A literature review and meta-analysis. Ann Intern Med 1995; 123: 925–32.
195. Rao NA, Marak GE, Hidayat AA. Necrotizing scleritis: a clinico-pathologic study of 41 cases. Ophthalmology 1985; 92:1542–9.
196. Rauzy O, Fort M, Nourhasemi F, et al. Relation between HLA-DRB1 alleles corticosteroid resistance in giant cell arteritis. Ann Rheum Dis 1998; 57:380–2.
197. Read RW, Clinical mini-review: systemic lupus erythematosus and the eye. Ocul Immunol Inflamm 2004; 12: 87–99.
198. Revell PA, Mayston V. Histopathology of the synovial membrane of peripheral joints in ankylosing spondylitis. Ann Rheum Dis 1982; 41:579–86.
199. Rihl M, Gu J, Baeten D, et al. Alpha beta but not gamma delta T cell clones in synovial fluids of patients with reactive arthritis show active transcription of tumour necrosis factor alpha and interferon gamma. Ann Rheum Dis 2004; 63:1673–6.
200. Rimeti G, Blasi F, Cosentini R, et al. Temporal arteritis associated with *Chlamydia pneumoniae* DNA detected in an arterial specimen. J Rheumatol 2001; 28:1738–9.
201. Riono WP, Hidayat AA, Rao NA. Scleritis: a clinicopathological study of 55 cases. Ophthalmology 1999; 106: 1328–33.
202. Robinson WP, van der Linden SM, Khan MA, et al. HLA-Bw60 increases susceptibility to ankylosing spondylitis in HLA B27 positive individuals. Arthritis Rheum 1989; 52: 1135–41.
203. Rochat GF. Scleritis necroticans. Ned Tijdschr Geneeskd 1934; 77:4935–8.
204. Rodriguez-Pla A, Bosch-Gil JA, Echevarria-Mayo JE, et al. No detection of parvovirus B19 or Herpesvirus DNA in giant cell arteritis. J Clin Virol 2004; 31:11–15.
205. Rosenberg AM. The clinical associations of antinuclear antibodies in juvenile rheumatoid arthritis. Clin Immunol Immunopathol 1988; 49:19–27.
206. Rothova A, Alberts C, Glasius E, et al. Risk factors for ocular sarcoidosis. Doc Ophthalmol 1989; 72:287–96.
207. Runstadler JA, Saila H, Savolainen A, et al. Analysis of MHC region genetics in Finnish patients with juvenile idiopathic arthritis: evidence for different locus-specific effects in polyarticular vs. pauciarticular subsets and a shared DRB1 epitope. Genes Immun 2003; 4: 326–35.
208. Sabates R, Smith T, Apple D. Ocular histopathology in juvenile rheumatoid arthritis. Ann Ophthalmol 1979; 11: 733–37.
209. Sakamoto M, Akazawa K, Nishioka Y, et al. Prognostic factors of vision in patients with Behcet disease. Ophthalmology 1995; 102:317–21.
210. Sakas LI. New developments in the pathogenesis of systemic sclerosis. Autoimmunity 2005; 38:113–6.
211. Santos Lacomba M, Marcos Martin C, Gallardo Galera JM, et al. Aqueous humor and serum tumor necrosis factor-alpha in clinical uveitis. Ophthalmic Res 2001; 33:251–5.
212. Sato H, Lagan AL, Alexopolou C., et al. The TNF-863A allele strongly associates with anticentromere antibody positivity in SSc. Arthritis Rheum 2004; 50:558–64.
213. Savige J, Gillis D, Benson E, et al., International consensus statement on testing and reporting of antineutrophil cytoplasmic antibodies (ANCA). Am J Clin Pathol 1999; 111:507–13.
214. Schoenfeld Y, Isenberg D. DNA antibody idiotype: a review of their genetic, clinical, and immunopathologic features. Semin Arthritis Rheum 1987; 76:245–52.
215. Schoenfeld Y, Vilner Y, Reshef T, et al. Increased presence of common systemic lupus erythematosis (SLE) anti-DNA idiotypes (16/6 Id, 32/15 Id) is induced by procainamide. J Clin Immunol 1987; 7:410–9.
216. Schreiber A, Busjahn A, Luft FC, Kettritz R. Membrane expression of proteinase 3 is genetically determined. J Am Soc Nephrol 2003; 14:68–75.
217. Schultz JS, Good AE, Sing CE, Kapur JJ. HLA profile and Reiter's syndrome. Clin Genet 1981; 19:159–67.
218. Schumacher HR, Magge S, Varghese Cherian P, et al. Light and electron microscopic studies on the synovial membrane in Reiter's syndrome. Arthritis Rheum 1988; 331:937–46.
219. Scott DG, Bacon PA, Elliott PJ, et al. Systemic vasculitis in a district general hospital 1972–80; clinical and laboratory features, classification of 80 cases. Q J Med 1982; 203: 292–311.

220. Sebbag M, Parry SL, Brennan FM et al. Cytokine stimulation of T lymphocytes regulates their capacity to induce monocyte production of tumour necrosis factor alpha, but not interleukin-10: possible relevance to pathophysiology of rheumatoid arthritis. European J Immunol 1997; 27:624–32.
221. Semenzato G, Bambara LM, Biasi D, et al. Increased serum levels of soluble interleukin-2 receptor in patients with systemic lupus erythematosis and rheumatoid arthritis. J Clin Immunol 1988; 8:447–52.
222. Senkpiehl I, Marget M, Wedler M, et al. HLA-DRB1 and anti-cyclic citrullinated peptide antibody production in rheumatoid arthritis. Int Arch Allergy Immunol 2005; 137:315–8.
223. Serup J, Serup L. Increased central cornea thickness in localized scleroderma (morphoea). Metab Pediatr Syst Ophthalmol 1985; 8:11–14.
224. Sherer Y, Gorstein A, Fritzler MJ, Shoenfeld Y. Autoantibody explosion in systemic lupus erythematosus: more than 100 different antibodies found in SLE patients. Semin Arthritis Rheum 2004; 34:501–37.
225. Sims AM, Wordsworth BP, Brown MA. Genetic susceptibility to ankylosing spondylitis. Curr Mol Med 2004; 4: 13–20.
226. Smerdel A, Lie BA, Finholt C, et al. An additional susceptibility gene for juvenile idiopathic arthritis in the HLA class I region on several DR-DQ haplotypes. Tissue Antigens 2003; 61:80–4.
227. Smerdel A, Lie BA, Ploski R, et al. A gene in the telomeric HLA complex distinct from HLA-A is involved in predisposition to juvenile idiopathic arthritis. Arthritis Rheum 2002, 46:1614–9.
228. Sobue G, Kachi T, Yamada T, Hashizume Y. Pathology of the peripheral nervous system in polyarteritis nodosa: a clinicopathological study of two autopsy cases. Rinsho Shinkeigaku 1989; 29:209–15.
229. Sohn S, Lee ES, Bang D, et al. Behcet's disease-like symptoms induced by the Herpes simplex virus in ICR mice. Eur J Dermatol 1998; 8:21–3.
230. Spagnolo P, Renzoni EA, Wells AU, et al. C-C chemokine receptor 2 and sarcoidosis: association with Löfgren's syndrome. Am J Respir Crit Care Med 2003; 168:1162–6.
231. Squirrell DM, Winfield J, Amos RS. Peripheral ulcerative keratitis 'corneal melt' and rheumatoid arthritis: a case series. Rheumatology (Oxford) 1999; 38:1245–8.
232. Strom H, Lindvall N, Hellstrom B, Rosenthal L. Clinical, HLA, roentgenological follow-up study of patients with juvenile arthritis: comparison between the long-term outcome of transient and persistent arthritis in children. Ann Rheum Dis 1989; 48:918–23.
233. Subcommittee for Scleroderma Criteria of the American Rheumatism Association Diagnostic and Therapeutic Criteria Committee. Preliminary criteria for the classification of systemic sclerosis (scleroderma). Arthritis Rheum 1980; 23:581–90.
234. Thoen J, Frre O. Phenotypes of peripheral blood T lymphocytes in rheumatoid arthritis and juvenile rheumatoid arthritis: Findings in patients with varying disease activity and clinical subgroups. Clin Rheumatol 1988; 7:188–96.
235. Toda Y, Aoki R, Ikeda Y, et al. Detection of ABCA7 positive cells in salivary glands from patients with Sjögren's syndrome. Pathology Int 2005; 55:639–43.
236. Trentham DE, Le CH, Relapsing polychondritis. Ann Intern Med 1998; 129:114–22.
237. Triantafyllopoulou A, Moutsopoulos HM. Autoimmunity and coxsackievirus infection in primary Sjögren's syndrome. Ann New York Acad Sci 2005; 1050:389–96.
238. Trostle DC, Bedetti CD, Steen VD, et al. Renal vascular histology and morphometry in systemic sclerosis. Arthritis Rheum 1988; 31:393–400.
239. Tse WY, Abadeh S, Jefferis R, et al. Neutrophil FcgammaRIIIb allelic polymorphism in anti-neutrophil cytoplasmic antibody (ANCA)-positive systemic vasculitis. Clin Exp Immunol 2000; 119:574–7.
240. Tse WY, Abadeh S, Jefferis R, et al. Neutrophil FcgammaRIIIb allelic polymorphism in anti-neutrophil cytoplasmic antibody (ANCA)-positive systemic vasculitis. Clin Exp Immunol 2000; 119:574–7.
241. Tsokos GC, Inghirami G, Pillemer SR, et al. Immunoregulatory aberrations in patients with polyarticular juvenile rheumatoid arthritis. Clin Immunol Immunopathol 1988; 47:62–74.
242. Tsokos GC, Mavridis A, Inghirami G, et al. Cellular immunity in patients with systemic juvenile rheumatoid arthritis. Clin Immunol Immunopathol 1987; 42:86–92.
243. Uchida K, Akita Y, Matsuo K, et al. Identification of specific autoantigens in Sjögren's syndrome by SEREX. Immunology 2005; 116:53–63.
244. Uchiyama RC, Osborn TG, Moore TL. Antibodies to iris and retina detected in sera from patients with juvenile rheumatoid arthritis with iridocyclitis by indirect immunofluorescence studies on human eye tissue. J Rheum 1989; 76:1074–8.
245. Valenzuela R, Cooperrider PA, Gogate P, et al. Relapsing polychondritis. Immunomicroscopic findings in cartilage of ear biopsy specimens. Human Pathology 1980; 11:19–22.
246. Valla DC, Benhamou JP. Hepatic granulomas and hepatic sarcoidosis. Clin Liver Dis 2000; 4:269–85.
247. Verhoeff FH, King MJ. Scleromalacia perforans: report of a case in which the eye was examined microscopically. Arch Ophthalmol 1938; 20:1013–5.
248. Verity DH, Wallace GR, Seed P, et al. Soluble adhesion molecules in Behçet's disease. Ocul Immunol Inflamm 1998; 6:81–92.
249. Verity DH, Wallace GR, Vaughan RW, Stanford MR. Behcet's disease: from Hippocrates to the third millennium. Br J Ophthalmol 2003; 87:1175–83.
250. Verity MA, Larson WM, Madden SC. Relapsing polychondritis: report of two necropsied cases with histochemical investigation of the cartilage lesion. Am J Pathol 1963; 42:251–69.
251. Verleden GM, du Bois RM, Bouros D, et al. Genetic predisposition and pathogenetic mechanisms of interstitial lung diseases of unknown origin. Eur Respir J 2001; 32:17s–29s.
252. Verma MJ, Lloyd A, Rager H, et al. Chemokines in acute anterior uveitis. Curr Eye Res 1997; 16:1202–8.
253. Vitali C, Bombardieri R, Jonsson HM, et al. Classification criteria for Sjögren's syndrome: a revised version of the European criteria proposed by the American–European Consensus Group. Ann Rheum Dis 2002; 61:554–8.
254. Wagner AD, Wittkop U, Prahst A, et al. Dendritic cells colocalize with activated CD4+ T cells in giant cell arteritis. Clin Exp Rheumatol 2003; 21:185–92.
255. Wakeland EK, Liu K, Graham RR, Behrens TW. Delineating the genetic basis of systemic lupus erythematosus. Immunity 2001; 15:397–408.
256. Walker SM, McCurdy DK, Shaham B, et al. High prevalence of IgA rheumatoid factor in severe polyarticular-onset juvenile rheumatoid arthritis, but not in

systemic-onset or pauciarticular-onset disease. Arthritis Rheum 1990; 33:199–204.

257. Watson PG. The diagnosis and management of scleritis. Ophthalmology 1980; 87:716–20.
258. Watson PG, Hayreh, SS. Scleritis and episcleritis Br. J. Ophthalmol. 1976; 60:163–191.
259. Watson PG, Young RD. Changes at the periphery of a lesion in necrotising scleritis: anterior segment fluorescein angiography correlated with electron microscopy. Br J Ophthalmol 1985; 69:656–63.
260. Weinberger WH, Ropes MW, Kulka JR, Bauer JW. Reiter's syndrome, clinical and pathological observations: a long term study of 16 cases. Medicine (Baltimore) 1962; 47: 5–91.
261. Weyand CM, Fulbright JW, Hunder GG, et al. Treatment of giant cell arteritis. Interleukin-6 as a biological marker of disease activity. Arthritis Rheum 2000; 43:1041–8.
262. Weyand CM, Goronzy JJ, Kurtin PJ. Lymphoma in rheumatoid arthritis: an immune system set up for failure. Arthritis Rheum 2006; 54:685–9.
263. Weyand CM, Goronzy JJ. Pathogenic principles in giant cell arteritis. Int J Cardiol 2000; 75:S9–15.
264. Weyand CM, Goronzy JJ. The pathogenesis of giant cell arteritis. Bull Rheum Dis 2002; 51:8–111.
265. Wilson WA, Gharavi EA, Koike T, et al. International consensus statement on preliminary classification criteria for definite antiphospholipid syndrome: report of an international workshop. Arthritis Rheum 1999; 42: 1309–11.
266. Witte T, Matthias T, Arnett FC, et al. IgA and IgG autoantibodies against alpha-fodrin as markers for Sjögren's syndrome. Systemic lupus erythematosus. J Rheum 2000; 27:2617–20.
267. Wood NC, Symons JA, Duff GW. Serum interleukin-2-receptor in rheumatoid arthritis: a prognostic indicator of disease activity? J Autoimmun 1988; 7:353–61.
268. Wucherpfennig KW. Insights into autoimmunity gained from structural analysis of MHC-peptide complexes. Curr Opin Immunol 2001; 13:650–6.
269. Wynne-Roberts CR, Anderson CH, Turano AM, Baron M. Light and electron-microscopic findings of juvenile rheumatoid arthritis snyovium: comparison with normal juvenile synovium. Semin Arthritis Rheum 1978; 7: 287–302.
270. Yamama S, Jones SL, Aoi K, Aoyama T. Lymphocyte subsets in erythema nodosum-like lesions from patients with Behçet's disease. In: Lehner T, Barnes CG. eds. Recent Advances in Behçet's Disease. London: Royal Society of Medicine Services, 1986:117–21.
271. Yang J, Brinckmann HF Rui, et al. Autoantibodies to cartilage collagens in relapsing polychondritis. Arch Dermatol Res 1993; 285:245–9.
272. Yoshida A, Kawashima H, Motoyama Y, et al. Comparison of patients with Behcet's disease in the 1980s and 1990s. Ophthalmology 2004; 111:810–15.
273. Young S. Ocular involvement in connective tissue disorders. Curr Allergy Asthma Rep 2005; 5:323–6.
274. Young RD, Watson PG. Microscopical studies of necrotising scleritis. I. Cellular aspects. Br J Ophthalmol 1984; 65: 770–80.
275. Zeuner M, Straub RH, Rauh G, et al. Relapsing polychondritis: clinical and immunogenetic analysis of 62 patients. J Rheumatol 1997; 24:96–101.
276. Zhang G, Luo J, Bruckel J, et al. Genetic studies in familial ankylosing spondylitis. Arthritis Rheum 2004; 50: 2246–54.
277. Zhao YX, Lajoie G, Zhang H, et al. Tumor necrosis factor receptor p55-deficient mice respond to acute Yersinia enterocolitica infection with less apoptosis and more effective host resistance. Infect Immun 2000; 68: 1243–51.
278. Zhou Y, Giscombe R, Huang D, Lefvert AK. Novel genetic association of Wegener's granulomatosis with the interleukin 10 gene. J Rheumatol 2002; 29:317–20.
279. Zieve, Khusial PR. The anti-Sm immune response in autoimmunity and cell biology. Autoimmun Rev 2003; 2:235–40.
280. Zink A, Braun J, Listing J, Wollenhaupt J. Disability and handicap in rheumatoid arthritis and ankylosing spondylitis—results from the German rheumatological database. J Rheumatol 2000; 27:613–22.
281. Zvaifler NJ. New perspectives on the pathogenesis of rheumatoid arthritis. Am J Med 1988; 55:12–7.

7

Tumor Immunology

Zita F. H. M. Boonman
Department of Ophthalmology, Leiden University Medical Center, Leiden, The Netherlands

René E. M. Toes
Department of Rheumatology, Leiden University Medical Center, Leiden, The Netherlands

Martine J. Jager
Department of Ophthalmology, Leiden University Medical Center, Leiden, The Netherlands

INTRODUCTION

Various factors regulate the balance between immunity and tolerance against intraocular tumors. Investigating these ongoing immune processes in animals with intraocular tumors teaches us about the basic strategies cancer uses to escape tumor elimination, since the eye, an immune-privileged site, is especially hostile to any form of aggressive antitumor immunity. Understanding these fundamental immunological processes will help us to better understand how to develop safe and efficient immune intervention strategies against uveal melanoma and its metastases.

IMMUNOLOGY OF INTRAOCULAR TUMORS

Intraocular Tumors and Immune Privilege

Hypothetically ocular immune privilege would favor the development of intraocular tumors; however, the contrary is true. Intraocular tumors do not appear more frequently than malignancies arising in conventional body sites. In experimental animal models, ocular immune privilege allows the growth of tumor cells that are not growing elsewhere in the body. In the following paragraphs some aspects of general tumor immunology together with their significance for intraocular tumor growth are discussed. Furthermore, findings in immune responses against intraocular tumors from human and experimental animal studies together with current and future immune intervention strategies against uveal melanoma and their metastases will be elucidated.

Basic Immunology

The defense against pathogens is regulated by innate and adaptive immune mechanisms which are interactive. The innate immune system acts as a first barrier against infection by recognizing common structures shared between pathogens. Important players in the innate immune system are the macrophage, the dendritic cell (DC) and granulocytes (eosinophils, basophils and neutrophils).

Granulocytes and macrophages are able to discern the presence of "danger" and attack immediately. If the danger cannot successfully be dealt with and removed, macrophages and DCs can pick up pieces of the invader and present these pieces to the adaptive immune system. This adaptive immune system comprises humoral (B cells and their antibodies) and cellular responses (T cells). They functionally complement each other to specifically recognize and destroy foreign invaders. Immunological memory is generated after the attack, characterized by a subsequent more rapid and vigorous response to a second invasion by the same pathogen.

The cellular arm (T cells) of the immune system is able to trace down and eradicate intracellular pathogens, such as viruses (see Chapter 8). These T cells are constantly scanning the pool of peptides within a cell which are being presented at the cell surface in the groove of major histocompatibility complex (MHC) molecules (75). Thus, cells with altered self-antigens, because of malignant transformation, should be recognized and killed with similar ease and efficiency as virus-infected cells.

The generation of optimal cell-mediated antitumor immune responses requires the activation of antigen-specific CD4+ and CD8+ T cells. Antigens are presented to T cells as peptide fragments of whole proteins by MHC class I molecules to CD8+ T cells and by MHC class II molecules to CD4+ T cells. The tumor can present antigens to T cells directly, or, more commonly, tumor antigens are presented by antigen-presenting cells (APC), such as DCs. This process is called cross-priming (44). The APC captures antigen and migrates through the lymphatic drainage pathway into the T-cell–rich areas of the draining lymph nodes (DLNs). Here, the APC presents peptide fragments of tumor antigens to CD4+ and CD8+ T cells (68). Optimal activation of a T cell requires both the interaction between the T-cell receptor (TCR) and the peptide–MHC complex (signal 1) and a second (costimulatory) signal, provided by a group of immuno-adjuvant molecules such as CD80 or CD86, Toll-like receptors (resembling the Toll transmembrane receptor of *Drosophila*), CD40 (67), and receptors for the constant fragment of immunoglobulin (Fc receptors) found on the professional APC. In the absence of the appropriate costimulus, a T cell exposed to a tumor antigen peptide/MHC complex becomes specifically tolerized rather than activated (44). Thus, systemic tolerance may develop instead of a clinically useful antitumor response.

Cancer Immune Surveillance

In 1909, Ehrlich (19) proposed that if the immune system did not survey the body for continuously arising malignant cells, the frequency of cancer would increase enormously. This theory did not get much attention until the late 1950s when at about the same time Burnet (8) and Thomas (65) suggested that distinctive features of tumor cells are recognized by the immune system. They proposed that the primary function of cellular immunity was the defense against altered self or neoplastic cells. The finding of "tumor-specific antigens" provided additional evidence that the immune system can recognize and destroy newly emerging transformed cells (31). In 1970, these promising discoveries were incorporated into the formal hypothesis of "cancer immunosurveillance," as proposed by Burnet and Thomas (9). In 1978, this hypothesis lost favor when T-cell–deficient nude mice failed to experience a higher incidence of malignancies (58). Now we know that nude mice are not completely immunocompromised. They contain detectable populations of $\alpha\beta$ T cells, $\gamma\delta$ T cells (see Chapter 3 for definition) and natural killer (NK) cells, all of which can mediate antitumor immunity. Almost 30 years later, around the mid-1990s, renewed interest in the immunosurveillance theory arose by the discovery that mice with complete immunodeficiency, which lack recombination activating gene 1 (*RAG1*) or recombination activating gene 2 (*RAG2*), have a higher incidence of tumors and a more rapid progression of malignancy following exposure to carcinogens (63). Furthermore, transplant patients who are immunosuppressed and people with primary immunodeficiencies carry a significantly higher relative risk of developing cancer (23). Additional studies not only support the importance of immune system control of tumor formation, but also suggest the involvement of both the innate and adaptive immune responses in cancer immunosurveillance. Thus, the unmanipulated immune system is capable of recognizing and eliminating primary tumors. Cancer immunosurveillance seems to apply to intraocular tumors as well, since such tumors are rare and occur with a frequency that is not higher than of malignancies arising in conventional body sites. Thus, ocular immune privilege does not appear to hinder cancer immunosurveillance.

Tumor Escape

Why do tumors occur in immunocompetent people given the existence of cancer immunosurveillance? And why does spontaneous clearance of established tumors by endogenous immune responses rarely take place? Indeed, tumor-specific antigens expressed by growing tumors are recognized by the immune system but are mostly not sufficiently immunogenic to induce an effective antitumor response (70). Hence most tumors are antigenic, though not immunogenic. Numerous factors contribute to the failure of the immune system to effectively control tumor outgrowth.

As tumors originate from nontransformed tissues, antigens expressed by tumor cells are often self-antigens and presented in a noninflammatory environment (21). Immune responses to self-antigens are strictly regulated. In the course of T-cell differentiation and maturation, elaborate positive and negative selection processes are in place in the thymus to eliminate self-antigen-specific T cells. This selection process, called central tolerance, is incomplete and potential pathogenic autoreactive T cells do escape into the periphery (40). Autoimmunity mediated by these escaping autoreactive T cells is regulated by several strategies, collectively referred to as peripheral tolerance, such as ignorance and the generation of regulatory T cells (TReg) (see Chapter 3). As already mentioned above, an effective antitumor immune response is not only determined by specific TCR–peptide–MHC complex interactions (signal 1) between immune cells, but also by the context in which these tumor antigens are presented to the immune system (41). This is mainly regulated by a network of professional APCs or DCs, since these cells not only detect the tumor, but also direct the ensuing immune response (tolerance vs. immunity). The DCs must be activated for proper T-cell activation. Differentiation of the DC into a potent APC is triggered by molecular stimuli that are released as a result of tissue disturbance and a local inflammatory response caused by the pathogen. The absence of these "danger signals" in tumors, which behave in many ways as "healthy" tissues, leads to inactivated DCs (21,41). These DCs are able to present tumor antigens to the T cells in the tumor-DLN without resulting in appropriate tumor immunity and eventually the T cells become tolerant of the tumor (45). Indeed, T cells recognizing self-antigens presented by tissue-resident DCs are inactivated and sometimes eliminated (1).

When some tumors activate DCs which are capable of generating proper antitumor responses, immunoediting might come into play to give the tumor another chance to escape (16,45,61). Immunoediting postulates that the immune system creates tumor cells that are superior in surviving immune attacks during tumor development. Immunoediting consists of three phases: elimination, equilibrium, and escape. Immunosurveillance occurs during the elimination process. During the equilibrium phase, a "survival-of-the-fittest" battle between the immune system and the escaped tumor cell variants can last for a prolonged period. During this process, many of the original escaped tumor cell types are destroyed, but new ones arise, carrying different mutations that provide them with increased resistance to immune attack. This leads to tumor escape, resulting in the appearance of clinically apparent tumors.

Another feature of developing malignancies, which is in harmony with the above-mentioned phenomena, is that tumors establish their own immunosuppressive environment (76). Cancer cells can be major producers of vascular endothelial growth factor, which suppresses DC differentiation and maturation (22). Additionally, tumor cells, tumor-associated macrophages, and TReg cells often produce interleukin-10 and transforming growth factor (TGFβ), which also suppress DC maturation and function (55). Abundant infiltrating TReg cells present in the tumor microenvironment favor tolerizing conditions (74). Thus, not only the tumor cells but also their microenvironment help tumor cells to escape effective antitumor immunity actively. From this perspective it seems that the eye and spontaneous tumors share common pathways to establish and maintain an immunosuppressive environment. Moreover, ocular immune privilege can be terminated (25), suggesting that there are methods of preventing immune privilege within the eye that may be useful in terminating immunosuppressive factors within other tumors.

UVEAL MELANOMA

General Remarks

Uveal melanoma is the most common primary intraocular neoplasm in adults, accounting for 70% of all primary eye tumors and an annual incidence of six to eight per million Caucasian individuals (18) (see Chapter 59). Uveal melanomas arise in the iris in approximately 3% of patients, in the ciliary body in 5% to 10%, and in the choroid in about 90% of cases (64). Melanomas occur in all age groups but nearly two-thirds of cases are seen in patients 50 to 70 years old. The five-year survival rate is around 65% to 81% but decreases to 50% for large tumors (15,42,62).

The incidence of obvious metastases at the time of presentation is around 2% to 3% (71) and, unfortunately, successful eradication of the primary tumor does not reduce the rate of subsequent tumor spread (12,42). Uveal melanoma disseminates hematogenously and in 19% to 35% of patients metastases appear within five years after treatment of the intraocular tumor, primarily in the liver. The prognosis of patients with metastases is poor, with a median survival time of only four to six months (64).

Once the "high-risk" patients are identified, additional treatment strategies capable of eradicating the micrometastases would be very useful to bring down the high mortality rate. An attractive method of dealing with micrometastases would be to use some form of adjuvant immunotherapy. To develop effective immune strategies, a thorough understanding of the basic immunological mechanisms behind intraocular tumor growth and uveal melanoma behavior is mandatory. An additional challenge is the eye itself, since the intraocular environment is an immune-privileged site in which different immunologic laws rule. All these features will be discussed below to understand the difficulties one faces when trying to apply immune intervention strategies.

Immune Responses Against Intraocular Tumors in Mice

Several experimental animal models have been studied in recent years to understand the influence of the immune system on intraocular tumor growth. Either syngeneic murine tumor cells or xenogeneic human uveal melanoma cells are inoculated into the eyes of inbred mice or immunocompromised mice. Unfortunately, most murine intraocular tumors do not arise in the uveal tract, so their direct relevance to human uveal melanoma is limited. However, they help us to find fundamental immunological principles regulating intraocular tumor growth which in the long run could be beneficial to patients with intraocular tumors. A selection of representative studies will be discussed showing the various elicited immune responses leading to different end results in tumor-bearing mice. The deviant intraocular immune responses allow the intraocular growth of tumor cells that are not growing elsewhere in the body, providing a model to understand the specific immunological characteristics of tumors in the eye.

Antigens on intraocular tumors, including melanoma-associated antigens expressed on syngeneic murine melanomas (52), elicit anterior chamber-associated immune deviation (ACAID) with suppression of delayed-type hypersensitivity (DTH) reactions in combination with normal antibody production and cytotoxic T lymphocyte (CTL) responses (51). The formation of ACAID in murine intraocular tumor models is linked to progressive tumor growth. Nonetheless, not all intraocular tumors induce ACAID. Tumors that fail to induce ACAID mostly express potent tumor-specific antigens and bring forth strong DTH and CTL reactions leading to intraocular tumor rejection (32,54). This shows that immune privilege of the eye can be aborted in some intraocular tumor models.

Immune-mediated rejection of intraocular tumors can follow two fundamental patterns (32), and a third model has recently come to light (60,72). The first type strongly resembles a DTH-mediated process and leads to extensive collateral damage of all structures of the eye, eventually leading to phthisis bulbi (53). The damage is CD4+ T-cell–dependent. However, infiltrating mononuclear cells characteristic of DTH (CD4+ T cells) were not found in these tumors, although histological features resembled a localized DTH reaction (53). In contrast, the second pattern of intraocular tumor eradication mainly involves tumor-specific CTL and leaves the eye morphologically intact (32). Analysis of tumor-infiltrating lymphocytes (TILs) revealed the presence of mainly CD8+ and CD4+ T cells. Depletion of these cells resulted in progressive intraocular tumor growth (3). The third pattern of intraocular tumor rejection is also CD4+ T-cell–dependent (60); however, the elimination is tumor-specific and thus leaves the eye intact, not leading to phthisis bulbi compared to the first DTH rejection pattern.

The model that Schurmans et al. (60) used was developed using intraocular tumors that express a highly immunogenic antigen derived from the early region 1 of human adenovirus type 5 (Ad5E1). When Ad5E1-modulated tumor cells are placed in the anterior chamber of an immunocompetent host, an intraocular tumor will develop. The development of natural immune responses against these intraocular tumors was studied in depth together with new intervention protocols that could activate an effective immune response. As already mentioned, in this syngeneic murine intraocular Ad5E1-expressing tumor model, the intraocular tumor disappears with the help of CD4+ T cells without causing collateral damage elsewhere in the eye. Tumor-necrosis-factor-related apoptosis-inducing ligand, interferon gamma (IFNγ), and macrophages play important roles in this specific CD4+ T-cell–dependent intraocular tumor clearance (7,60,72). Tumor growth depends on the type of tumor used. Using a slightly different model where the tumor cells express the early region 1A of human adenovirus type 5 (Ad5E1A) plus the oncogene EJ-ras, the intraocular tumor grows progressively. Some support the idea that intraocular tumor antigens from growing tumors in the anterior chamber of the eye drain directly into the spleen inducing systemic tolerance for this specific tumor antigen. The tumor antigen-draining pathways of the Ad5E1A-expressing anterior-chamber tumor were studied in detail, and surprisingly, intraocular E1A-tumor antigens were found to drain primarily to the local tumor-DLNs in the neck, specifically the submandibular LN, triggering tumor-specific CD8+ T cells. Unfortunately, the primed E1A-specific CTLs that were also present in the tumor-DLN did not disseminate systemically and were therefore unable to eradicate the intraocular tumor. Additional help from CD40 antibodies, which has been proven to be a successful antitumor treatment in other tumor models, was not powerful enough to induce an effective antitumor response, indicating the lasting effects of the immune-privileged intraocular environment (5). An additional finding was that intraocular tumor antigens are cross-presented by CD11c+ cells to tumor-specific CTLs in the tumor-DLN. These CD11c+ cells, most probably DCs, become activated in hosts in which the anatomical integrity of the tumor-bearing eye is lost (phthisis bulbi) (6). This activation of local APCs leads to the systemic distribution of tumor-specific CTLs that protects against secondary, otherwise lethal, subcutaneous Ad5E1-tumor challenges. Tumor-specific CTLs did not spread systemically in tumor-bearing hosts with an "intact" eye, despite the progressively growing intraocular tumor. Therefore, these animals are not protected against secondary lethal tumor deposits and also not against otherwise nonlethal tumor injections which will eventually kill the host.

Immune Responses Against Uveal Melanoma in Humans

Even though intraocular tumors are shielded in an immune-privileged environment, this does not prevent their detection by the immune system. However, intraocular tumors, just like tumors in other body sites, try to circumvent immune responses which endanger their survival. In this light, intraocular tumors have an advantage compared to other tumors because they are already situated in an immunosuppressive environment.

Clinical observations support the fact that the immune system is involved in taming intraocular tumor growth. Spontaneous eradication of uveal melanomas has been described in some patients (29,56). Serum antibodies against melanoma-associated antigens were detected in 16 out of 22 patients (11). Also, positive DTH reactions against melanoma-associated antigens were demonstrated in patients with uveal melanoma. Lymphocytes cytotoxic to uveal and skin melanoma cells were collected from the blood of ocular melanoma patients (30). Melanoma-specific CD8+ T cells from patients with choroidal melanoma were able to recognize autologous and allogeneic uveal melanoma cells, indicating that tumor-associated antigens are shared between the various uveal melanoma cell lines (26,35). Unfortunately, these immune cells are unable to reject the intraocular tumor, which is similar to the situation described earlier in this chapter regarding mice.

A variety of cutaneous melanoma antigens recognized by antimelanoma CTLs have been identified due to the pioneering work of van der Bruggen et al. (70). Apart from the melanoma tumor-specific antigens, members of the melanoma antigen gene (MAGE) family, the melanocytic lineage-specific tyrosinase, and the differentiation antigens GP100, Melan-A/MART-1, and gp75 have also been described. Similar to cutaneous melanomas, uveal melanomas have been shown to be antigenic. In one study, uveal melanoma cells did not express the MAGE genes, but they expressed higher-than-normal levels of tyrosinase, MART-1, and GP100 (50). In contrast to the previous study, other groups demonstrated the appearance of MAGE tumor antigens in primary and metastatic uveal melanoma that are recognized by tumor-specific T cells (10,36,37). It has been reported that uveal melanoma patients have precursor lymphocytes that can recognize and kill T cells presenting these peptides (59).

These tumor antigens can only be recognized by CD8+ T cells in an MHC class I-restricted manner. In humans, the MHC complex is referred to as human leukocyte antigen (HLA) system (see Chapter 3). Alterations of the HLA phenotype will have serious consequences for the hosts' defense against tumor growth. In many tumors, including cutaneous and uveal melanoma, expression of HLA class I is downregulated (4,14,27). Loss of HLA class I molecules may prevent recognition of the tumor cells by cytotoxic T cells. HLA class I loss is associated with a worse patient survival in cutaneous melanoma, in contrast with uveal melanoma where a low HLA class I expression is correlated with a better patient survival (4,20,34). In addition, downregulation of HLA class II is also correlated with better survival of patients with uveal melanoma (20,34). Lower expression of HLA class I on uveal melanoma causes the cells to become more susceptible to NK-cell–mediated lysis in vitro (37). TGFβ has been shown to decrease HLA expression (38). Although NK-cell–mediated lysis of uveal melanomas is inhibited in the eye by macrophage migration inhibitory factor, it is suggested that melanoma cells that disseminate from the eye into the liver are at risk for surveillance by NK cells (28,57). Progressive intraocular tumor growth and an increase in hepatic metastases were observed in experimental animal models deficient of NK cells (2,37).

Various TILs, such as CD8+ and CD4+ T cells and NK cells, can be detected in uveal melanomas (14,17). The prognostic relevance of these TILs in uveal melanoma is unclear. According to different studies, TILs are either favorable or unfavorable for the survival of patients (13,73). In addition, the presence of high numbers of tumor-infiltrating lymphocytes within the primary ocular melanoma is associated with an increased mortality in patients with uveal melanoma (Fig. 1) (39). These observations show that the immune system plays a role in uveal melanoma, although immune responses seem not to be related to decreased survival, not to a better prognosis. Perhaps the influence of the intraocular environment is such that immunosuppression instead of immune stimulation is achieved, and this may have important implications for prospective immunotherapy, as discussed below.

Immune Intervention Strategies Against Uveal Melanoma in Humans

Although many treatments are available for intraocular melanoma, no effective therapy is available for its distant metastases. Trials with small numbers of

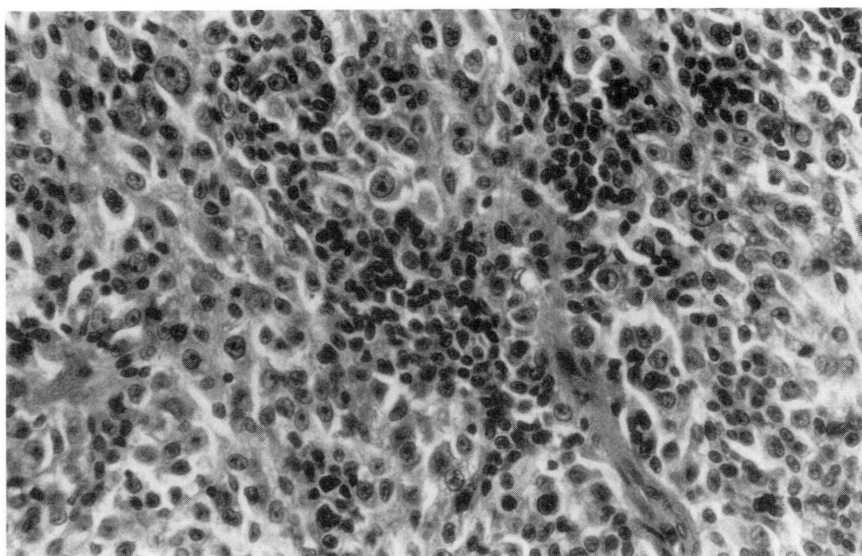

Figure 1 Choroidal malignant melanoma with patchy lymphocytic infiltration (hematoxylin and eosin, ×480).

"high-risk" patients prone to develop metastases, investigated nonspecific tumor vaccines, such as methanol-extracted residue of bacilli Calmette-Guérin and/or interferon 2α (IFN2α) (24,42). Both treatments were tolerated by the patients but did not result in a substantial prognostic benefit. The progress of therapeutic vaccines has been most evident in patients with cutaneous melanoma. Mitchell used cell lysates from allogeneic cutaneous melanoma cell lines in combination with adjuvants (Melacine®) (Corixa, Seattle, Washington, U.S.A.). This proved to be beneficial in phase I and II trials for patients with disseminated cutaneous melanoma in which 10% to 20% of patients cleared some metastases and another 10% to 20% of patients developed stable disease (46,69). Patients treated with Melacine compared to patients treated with chemotherapy did not show any difference in response rate or survival in a multicentered phase III study (48). The same cutaneous melanoma cell lysates resulted in primary tumor regression in an 81-year-old patient with uveal melanoma in whom surgery and radiation therapy were contraindicated (47). A similar vaccine preparation, Canvaxin™, showed a small increase in survival in vaccinated patients compared to patients treated with surgery and chemotherapy against dispersed cutaneous melanoma (49). Further evidence that therapeutic vaccines enhance antitumor immune responses was observed in melanoma patients treated with melanoma-specific antigen 3 (MAGE-3)-based vaccines. Tumor regression occurred in 20% of the treated patients and in about half of these patients tumor-specific CTL responses were found (66). The discovery of such tumor-specific antigens in uveal melanoma (10,36,50) initiated the current European multicenter phase I/II study in which patients with disseminated ocular melanoma are treated with a cocktail of tumor-specific and tumor differentiation peptides.

The results of tumor-antigen-based vaccines in patients with cutaneous melanoma are promising, although one would have expected more. A number of reasons can be given for these moderate outcomes: for example, all these trials have been performed in patients with advanced disease. The tumors in these patients have already overcome many obstacles and therefore created the best conditions for their own survival, leading to the presence of suppressive regulatory T cells, inactivated DCs, and the production of immunosuppressive cytokines (76). Better results may be expected by adding components into tumor treatments that subvert these immune-tolerizing conditions, together with substances that enhance natural immune effectors. New insights in these ruling processes in cancer are continuously provided by ongoing fundamental research in the field of tumor immunology and can eventually be expected to get us nearer the cure for cancer.

REFERENCES

1. Adler AJ, Marsh DW, Yochum GS, et al. CD4+ T cell tolerance to parenchymal self-antigens requires presentation by bone marrow-derived antigen-presenting cells. J Exp Med 1998; 187:1555–64.
2. Apte RS, Sinha D, Mayhew E, et al. Cutting edge: role of macrophage migration inhibitory factor in inhibiting NK cell activity and preserving immune privilege. J Immunol 1998; 160:5693–6.
3. Benson JL, Niederkorn JY. In situ suppression of delayed-type hypersensitivity: another mechanism for sustaining the immune privilege of the anterior chamber. Immunology 1991; 74:153–9.
4. Blom DJ, Luyten GP, Mooy C, et al. Human leukocyte antigen class I expression: marker of poor prognosis in

uveal melanoma. Invest Ophthalmol Vis Sci 1997; 38: 1865–72.

5. Boonman ZF, Van Mierlo GJ, Fransen MF, et al. Intraocular tumor antigen drains specifically to submandibular lymph nodes, resulting in an abortive cytotoxic T cell reaction. J Immunol 2004; 172:1567–74.
6. Boonman ZF, Van Mierlo GJ, Fransen MF, et al. Maintenance of immune tolerance depends on normal tissue homeostasis. J Immunol 2005; 175:4247–54.
7. Boonman ZF, Schurmans LR, Van Rooijen N, et al. Macrophages are vital in spontaneous intraocular tumor eradication. Invest Ophthalmol Vis Sci 2006; 47:2959–65.
8. Burnet FM. The biology of the cancer cell. Fed Proc 1958; 17:687–90.
9. Burnet FM. The concept of immunological surveillance. Prog Exp Tumor Res 1970; 13:1–27.
10. Chen PW, Murray TG, Uno T, et al. Expression of MAGE genes in ocular melanoma during progression from primary to metastatic disease. Clin Exp Metastasis 1997; 15:509–18.
11. Cochran AJ, Foulds WS, Damato BE, et al. Assessment of immunological techniques in the diagnosis and prognosis of ocular malignant melanoma. Br J Ophthalmol 1985; 69: 171–6.
12. Damato B. Developments in the management of uveal melanoma. Clin Experiment Ophthalmol 2004; 32: 639–47.
13. De la Cruz PO Jr, Specht CS, McLean IW. Lymphocytic infiltration in uveal malignant melanoma. Cancer 1990; 65: 112–5.
14. De Waard-Siebinga I, Hilders CG, Hansen BE, et al. HLA expression and tumor-infiltrating immune cells in uveal melanoma. Graefes Arch Clin Exp Ophthalmol 1996; 234: 34–42.
15. Diener-West M, Earle JD, Fine SL, et al. The COMS randomized trial of iodine 125 brachytherapy for choroidal melanoma, III: initial mortality findings. COMS Report No. 18. Arch Ophthalmol 2001; 119:969–82.
16. Dunn GP, Bruce AT, Ikeda H, et al. Cancer immunoediting: from immunosurveillance to tumor escape. Nat Immunol 2002; 3:991–8.
17. Durie FH, Campbell AM, Lee WR, Damato BE. Analysis of lymphocytic infiltration in uveal melanoma. Invest Ophthalmol Vis Sci 1990; 31:2106–10.
18. Egan KM, Seddon JM, Glynn RJ, et al. Epidemiologic aspects of uveal melanoma. Surv Ophthalmol 1988; 32: 239–51.
19. Ehrlich P. Ueber den jetzigenstand der Karzinomforschung. Ned Tijdschr Geneeskd 1909; 5:273–90.
20. Ericsson C, Seregard S, Bartolazzi E, et al. Association of HLA class I and class II antigen expression and mortality in uveal melanoma. Invest Ophthalmol Vis Sci 2001; 42: 2153–6.
21. Fuchs EJ, Matzinger P. Is cancer dangerous to the immune system? Semin Immunol 1996; 8:271–80.
22. Gabrilovich DI, Chen HL, Girgis KR, et al. Production of vascular endothelial growth factor by human tumors inhibits the functional maturation of dendritic cells. Nat Med 1996; 2:1096–103.
23. Gatti RA, Good RA. Occurrence of malignancy in immunodeficiency diseases: a literature review. Cancer 1971; 28:89–98.
24. Gragoudas ES, Egan KM, Seddon JM, et al. Survival of patients with metastases from uveal melanoma. Ophthalmology 1991; 98:383–9; discussion 390.
25. Gregory MS, Koh S, Huang E, et al. A novel treatment for ocular tumors using membrane FasL vesicles to activate innate immunity and terminate immune privilege. Invest Ophthalmol Vis Sci 2005; 46:2495–502.
26. Huang XQ, Mitchell MS, Liggett PE, et al. Non-fastidious, melanoma-specific CD8+ cytotoxic T lymphocytes from choroidal melanoma patients. Cancer Immunol Immunother 1994; 38:399–405.
27. Hurks HM, Metzelaar-Blok JA, Mulder A, et al. High frequency of allele-specific down-regulation of HLA class I expression in uveal melanoma cell lines. Int J Cancer 2000; 85:697–702.
28. Jager MJ, Hurks HM, Levitskaya J, Kiessling R. HLA expression in uveal melanoma: there is no rule without some exception. Hum Immunol 2002; 63:444–51.
29. Jensen OA, Andersen SR. Spontaneous regression of a malignant melanoma of the choroid. Acta Ophthalmol (Copenh) 1974; 52:173–82.
30. Kan-Mitchell J, Liggett PE, Harel W, et al. Lymphocytes cytotoxic to uveal and skin melanoma cells from peripheral blood of ocular melanoma patients. Cancer Immunol Immunother 1991; 33:333–40.
31. Klein G. Tumor antigens. Annu Rev Microbiol 1966; 20: 223–52.
32. Knisely TL, Luckenbach MW, Fischer BJ, Niederkorn JY. Destructive and nondestructive patterns of immune rejection of syngeneic intraocular tumors. J Immunol 1987; 138:4515–23.
33. Knisely TL, Niederkorn JY. Emergence of a dominant cytotoxic T lymphocyte antitumor effector from tumor-infiltrating cells in the anterior chamber of the eye. Cancer Immunol Immunother 1990; 30:323–30.
34. Krishnakumar S, Abhyankar D, Lakshmi SA, et al. HLA class II antigen expression in uveal melanoma: correlation with clinicopathological features. Exp Eye Res 2003; 77: 175–80.
35. Ksander BR, Geer DC, Chen PW, et al. Uveal melanomas contain antigenically specific and non-specific infiltrating lymphocytes. Curr Eye Res 1998; 17:165–73.
36. Luyten GP, van der Spek CW, Brand I, et al. Expression of MAGE, gp100 and tyrosinase genes in uveal melanoma cell lines. Melanoma Res 1998; 8:11–6.
37. Ma D, Luyten GP, Luider TM, Niederkorn JY. Relationship between natural killer cell susceptibility and metastasis of human uveal melanoma cells in a murine model. Invest Ophthalmol Vis Sci 1995; 36:435–41.
38. Ma D, Niederkorn JY. Transforming growth factor-beta down-regulates major histocompatibility complex class I antigen expression and increases the susceptibility of uveal melanoma cells to natural killer cell-mediated cytolysis. Immunology 1995; 86:263–9.
39. Makitie T, Summanen P, Tarkkanen A, Kivela T. Tumor-infiltrating macrophages (CD68(+) cells) and prognosis in malignant uveal melanoma. Invest Ophthalmol Vis Sci 2001; 42:1414–21.
40. Matzinger P. Why positive selection? Immunol Rev 1993; 135:81–117.
41. Matzinger P. Tolerance, danger, and the extended family. Annu Rev Immunol 1994; 12:991–1045.
42. McLean IW, Berd D, Mastrangelo MJ, et al. A randomized study of methanol-extraction residue of bacille Calmette-Guérin as postsurgical adjuvant therapy of uveal melanoma. Am J Ophthalmol 1990; 110:522–6.
43. McLean IW, Zimmerman LE, Foster WD. Survival rates after enucleation of eyes with malignant melanoma. Am J Ophthalmol 1979; 88:794–7.
44. Melief CJ. Mini-review: regulation of cytotoxic T lymphocyte responses by dendritic cells: peaceful coexistence of cross-priming and direct priming? Eur J Immunol 2003; 33:2645–54.

45. Melief CJ. Cancer immunology: cat and mouse games. Nature 2005; 437:41–2.
46. Mitchell MS, Kan-Mitchell J, Kempf RA, et al. Active specific immunotherapy for melanoma: phase I trial of allogeneic lysates and a novel adjuvant. Cancer Res 1988; 48:5883–93.
47. Mitchell MS, Liggett PE, Green RL, et al. Sustained regression of a primary choroidal melanoma under the influence of a therapeutic melanoma vaccine. J Clin Oncol 1994; 12:396–401.
48. Mitchell MS. Perspective on allogeneic melanoma lysates in active specific immunotherapy. Semin Oncol 1998; 25: 623–35.
49. Morton DL, Hsueh EC, Essner R, et al. Prolonged survival of patients receiving active immunotherapy with Canvaxin therapeutic polyvalent vaccine after complete resection of melanoma metastatic to regional lymph nodes. Ann Surg 2002; 236:438–48; discussion 448–9.
50. Mulcahy KA, Rimoldi D, Brasseur F, et al. Infrequent expression of the MAGE gene family in uveal melanomas. Int J Cancer 1996; 66:738–42.
51. Niederkorn JY, Streilein JW, Kripke ML. Promotion of syngeneic intraocular tumor growth in mice by anterior chamber-associated immune deviation. J Natl Cancer Inst 1983; 71:193–9.
52. Niederkorn JY. Suppressed cellular immunity in mice harboring intraocular melanomas. Invest Ophthalmol Vis Sci 1984; 25:447–54.
53. Niederkorn JY. The immunopathology of intraocular tumour rejection. Eye 1991; 5 (Pt 2):186–92.
54. Niederkorn JY. Immunoregulation of intraocular tumours. Eye 1997; 11 (Pt 2):249–54.
55. Qin Z, Noffz G, Mohaupt M, Blankenstein T. Interleukin-10 prevents dendritic cell accumulation and vaccination with granulocyte-macrophage colony-stimulating factor gene-modified tumor cells. J Immunol 1997; 159:770–6.
56. Reese AB, Archila EA, Jones IS, Cooper WC. Necrosis of malignant melanoma of the choroids. Am J Ophthalmol 1970; 69:91–104.
57. Repp AC, Mayhew ES, Apte S, Niederkorn JY. Human uveal melanoma cells produce macrophage migration-inhibitory factor to prevent lysis by NK cells. J Immunol 2000; 165:710–5.
58. Rygaard J, Povlsen CO. The mouse mutant nude does not develop spontaneous tumours: an argument against immunological surveillance. Acta Pathol Microbiol Scand [B] 1974; 82:99–106.
59. Saba J, McIntyre CA, Rees RC, Murray AK. Recognition of melanoma-associated peptides by peripheral blood mononuclear cells of ocular melanoma patients. Adv Exp Med Biol 1998; 451:241–4.
60. Schurmans LR, Diehl L, den Boer AT, et al. Rejection of intraocular tumors by CD4(+) T cells without induction of phthisis. J Immunol 2001; 167:5832–7.
61. Shankaran V, Ikeda H, Bruce AT, et al. IFN gamma and lymphocytes prevent primary tumour development and shape tumour immunogenicity. Nature 2001; 410: 1107–11.
62. Shields JA, Shields CL, De Potter P, Singh AD. Diagnosis and treatment of uveal melanoma. Semin Oncol 1996; 23: 763–7.
63. Shinkai YG, Rathbun KP, Lam EM, et al. RAG-2 deficient mice lack mature lymphocytes owing to inability to initiate V(D)J rearrangement. Cell 2002; 68:855–67.
64. Singh AD, Borden EC. Metastatic uveal melanoma. Ophthalmol Clin North Am 2005; 18:143–50, ix.
65. Thomas L. In: Lawrence H, ed.: Cellular and Humoral Aspects of the Hypersensitive States. New York: Hoeber-Harper, 1959:529–32.
66. Thurner B, Haende I, Roder C, et al. Vaccination with mage-3A1 peptide-pulsed mature, monocyte-derived dendritic cells expands specific cytotoxic T cells and induces regression of some metastases in advanced stage IV melanoma. J Exp Med 1999; 190:1669–78.
67. Toes RE, Schoenberger SP, van der Voort EI, et al. CD40–CD40 ligand interactions and their role in cytotoxic T lymphocyte priming and anti-tumor immunity. Semin Immunol 1998; 10:443–8.
68. Toes RE, Van der Voort EI, Schoenberger SP, et al. Enhancement of tumor outgrowth through CTL tolerization after peptide vaccination is avoided by peptide presentation on dendritic cells. J Immunol 1998; 160: 4449–56.
69. Vaishampayan U, Abrams J, Darrah D, et al. Active immunotherapy of metastatic melanoma with allogeneic melanoma lysates and interferon alpha. Clin Cancer Res 2002; 8:3696–701.
70. Van der Bruggen P, et al. Tumor-specific shared antigenic peptides recognized by human T cells. Immunol Rev 2002; 188:51–64.
71. Wagoner MD, Albert DM. The incidence of metastases from untreated ciliary body and choroidal melanoma. Arch Ophthalmol 1982; 100:939–40.
72. Wang S, Boonman ZF, Li HC, et al. Role of TRAIL and IFN-gamma in CD4+ T cell-dependent tumor rejection in the anterior chamber of the eye. J Immunol 2003; 171: 2789–96.
73. Whelchel JC, Farah SE, McLean IW, Burnier MN. Immunohistochemistry of infiltrating lymphocytes in uveal malignant melanoma. Invest Ophthalmol Vis Sci 1993; 34:2603–6.
74. Woo EY, Chu CS, Goletz TJ, et al. Regulatory CD4(+)CD25 (+) T cells in tumors from patients with early-stage non-small cell lung cancer and late-stage ovarian cancer. Cancer Res 2001; 61:4766–72.
75. Zinkernagel RM, Doherty PC. Restriction of in vitro T cell-mediated cytotoxicity in lymphocytic choriomeningitis within a syngeneic or semiallogeneic system. Nature 1974; 248:701–2.
76. Zou W. Immunosuppressive networks in the tumour environment and their therapeutic relevance. Nat Rev Cancer 2005; 5:263–74.

8

Viral Disease

Sara E. Miller
Department of Pathology, Duke University, Durham, North Carolina, U.S.A.

David N. Howell
Department of Pathology, Duke University and Durham Veterans Administration Medical Center, Durham, North Carolina, U.S.A.

Alan D. Proia
Department of Pathology, Duke University, Durham, North Carolina, U.S.A.

INTRODUCTION

Ocular viral infections are a particularly complex topic for diagnosticians and clinicians alike. The eye's component parts, though packed into a space measuring approximately one inch in diameter, are rich in diversity and varied in embryonic origin, inviting infection by viruses with a wide range of tissue tropisms. Some of the eye's compartments have evolved mechanisms of immune privilege; while offering potential protection against injurious effects of inflammation on the transparency of the eye's optical path, these mechanisms may alter the immune response to pathogens, including viruses. The anterior segment of the eye is separated from the external world by only a thin mucous membrane, providing ready access for a panoply of viral carriers, including airborne particulate matter, purposely introduced foreign bodies such as contact lenses, and the occasional errant finger. Blood vessels and the optic nerve provide alternative portals for virus entry.

Diagnosis of viral infections in the eye often requires a multidisciplinary approach, including both a growing battery of clinical imaging modalities and a broad armamentarium of pathology diagnostic techniques, the latter of which are reviewed in this chapter. In spite of limitations on the availability and size of biopsy specimens, light microscopic examination of tissue biopsies is important for the diagnosis of infections with many viruses. Where relevant for a given virus, light microscopic findings are included in the section entitled Histopathology. For viruses lacking this section, histologic findings are nonspecific, unknown, or of limited diagnostic value. Transmission electron microscopy (TEM) also has several appealing advantages for application to ocular viral pathology. It is ideally suited (indeed, constrained) to the analysis of small tissue samples. It can be applied to solid tissues and liquid specimens such as tears, the latter with great rapidity. Perhaps most important, it has the potential to detect virtually any viral pathogen without requiring pre-selection of analyte-specific reagents. Ultrastructural attributes of each viral pathogen are discussed. As appropriate, clinical laboratory tests, including culture, serology, and analysis of viral proteins and nucleic acids, are also reviewed.

VIROLOGY

Virus Classification

Viruses are very small (~20 nm to a few hundred nanometers in diameter) obligate intracellular parasites. They contain a genetic code but not all the necessary components for reproduction, and thus make use of their host's cellular metabolic machinery to provide the mechanisms for replication. Unlike other microorganisms, they have only one kind of nucleic acid, either DNA or RNA, but not both. Some are large enough to contain a few proteins that help to direct reproduction, but all rely on the host cells to produce necessary building blocks. The genome is packaged inside a protein coat called a capsid or nucleocapsid. Some viruses are further enclosed in a pliable membrane, usually derived by budding through cellular membranes into which some viral proteins have been inserted as part of the viral replicative program.

Historically, virus classification was based on host range, disease caused, organ tropism, or mode of transmission. Some viruses were simply named for their discoverers, without recourse to a specific taxonomic scheme. With the advent of molecular techniques, genetic properties have been used to determine relationships between the viruses. Today the International Committee on the Taxonomy of Viruses (29) uses an organization based on the type of nucleic acid present in the genome (DNA or RNA), the presence of single (unpaired) or double (paired) nucleic acid strands (ssDNA/RNA or dsDNA/RNA) and, for ssRNA viruses, the polarity (direction of reading) of the RNA (with RNA in the same polarity as cellular mRNA referred to as "sense" or "plus-stranded" and RNA in the complementary orientation called "antisense" or "minus-stranded") (Table 1). Additional characteristics that may be used for classification are whether the nucleic acid is linear or circular and whether it is one molecule that codes for several proteins or is segmented into two or more nucleic acid strands.

DNA viruses replicate their genomic material and produce mRNA using mechanisms similar to and, in some cases, borrowed from their cellular hosts. Replication of RNA viruses requires virus-encoded enzymes that produce either RNA or a DNA intermediate from the genomic RNA. The latter enzymes are referred to as reverse transcriptases. Hepatitis B virus (HBV), a dsDNA virus, also uses a reverse transcriptase to produce DNA from an RNA intermediate transcribed from the genome. In plus-stranded RNA viruses, the genome can be translated directly to produce viral proteins; in minus-stranded viruses, the genome must be used as a template to produce either plus-stranded RNA or DNA that is then transcribed into mRNA before protein synthesis can occur.

Table 1 Virus Classification

DNA
Group 1: double stranded DNA (dsDNA)
Group 2: single stranded DNA (ssDNA)
RNA
Group 3: double stranded RNA (dsRNA)
Group 4: plus sense single stranded RNA (+ssRNA) (like mRNA)
Group 5: negative sense single stranded RNA (−ssRNA)
RNA or DNA
Group 6: single stranded RNA-reverse transcriptase (ssRNA-RT)
Group 7: double stranded DNA-reverse transcriptase (dsDNA-RT)

Virus Identification

Properties used to identify viruses include the type of nucleic acid, morphology (e.g., size, shape, outer covering—as in naked or enveloped), tissue tropism (e.g., encephalitis viruses), and sometimes the mode of transmission [e.g., arboviruses (arthropod borne viruses)].

Atlases (23,103) segregate viruses into two broad categories: DNA or RNA viruses. Their location inside cells is a clue to the type of nucleic acid and, hence, to identification by TEM. Generally, DNA viruses are constructed in the nucleus and RNA viruses are assembled in the cytoplasm; there are exceptions. By light microscopy, the virus factories show up as inclusions (a smudgy or "ground glass" spot), and by TEM, actual virions can be seen. If there are particles/inclusions in the nucleus, the infection is almost always with a DNA virus. An exception is that in para- and orthomyxovirus (RNA viruses) infections, immunostaining can demonstrate some viral proteins, but not complete particles, in the nucleus. Occasionally, very late in enterovirus (RNA viruses) infection, empty nucleocapsids might be seen in the nucleus. Visualization of virus inclusions or particles in the cytoplasm, but not the nucleus, indicates an RNA virus, with the exception of poxviruses (DNA viruses). Observation of viral components in both the nucleus and cytoplasm may indicate a naked DNA virus that has gotten into the cytoplasm by lysing the nuclear membrane or an enveloped DNA virus that has arrived there by budding through the nuclear membrane into the cytoplasm.

In addition to direct visualization of virus particles or inclusions formed by aggregates of them, virus infection can sometimes be inferred by indirect effects on cell or tissue morphology. Some viruses cause cell membranes to fuse (e.g., herpesviruses, myxoviruses), producing multinucleated giant cells or syncytia. Cytomegalovirus (CMV) causes individual cells to enlarge with the increasing burden of viral particles. In this case, the cell has only one nucleus, and the nuclear pattern of clumped nucleocapsids surrounded by a clear space results in a diagnostic appearance resembling an "owl's eye". Aggregates of viral proteins such as HBV surface antigen can sometimes be detected in cell cytoplasm as areas with a cleared appearance. Several viruses also produce characteristic patterns of programmed cell death [e.g., the random hepatocyte apoptosis of hepatitis C virus (HCV) infection] or tissue necrosis (e.g., the geographic necrosis often seen in adenovirus infection).

Virus Morphology

Morphological features of classification include whether the virus is naked or enveloped. Naked human viruses are icosahedral, remain essentially spherical in TEM examinations, and range from 22 to 90 nm (e.g., parvovirus, papillomavirus, adenovirus). Enveloped viruses have an outer covering that, in most cases, is derived from cellular membranes as the virus buds through them. This pliable covering makes the virions pleomorphic. They may have a visible layer of spikes called peplomers on the surface (e.g., influenza virus with 8-nm projections, coronavirus with 20-nm projections) or appear relatively smooth by TEM (e.g., herpesvirus, rubellavirus)—although most enveloped viruses do have some membrane projections. They range in size from 40 nm (e.g., flaviviruses) to 300 nm (e.g., paramyxoviruses, poxviruses); some filamentous viruses are 80 nm by up to 1400 nm in length (e.g., Ebola virus). Many virus pictures are available online (www.ncbi.nlm.nih.gov/ICTVdb/index.htm).

MECHANISMS OF VIRAL DISEASE

Viral Entry and Replication

Virus entry into the host can be mediated through inoculation into the skin by vector bites, application to abrasions, or via mucosal surfaces. Viruses enter cells in different ways, depending on their outer covering, which has receptors for cell membranes. Many receptors are specific for certain target cells (e.g., poliovirus for motor neurons). Entry into cells can be by fusion of the virus envelope with the cellular membrane, allowing the nucleocapsid access to the inside, or by endocytosis and proteolysis within hydrolytic compartments.

The genetic information in viruses gets replicated in different ways. RNA viruses are unique, as they are the only organisms that use RNA as their genetic map. They replicate either by producing RNA from RNA or by producing DNA from RNA, followed by DNA replication and transcription (6). Both of these methods require enzymatic mechanisms not found in uninfected cells that must be encoded in the viral genome.

DNA viruses, except for poxviruses, have to transport their genome to the nucleus. They may use enhancers (regulatory nucleic acid sequences) to take over the cell transcription machinery or may take into the cell with them proteins (transcription factors) that aid replication of their DNA. Some can only replicate in cells that are themselves actively undergoing cell division. There are many different mechanisms for initiating the duplication of DNA, and some viruses (e.g., hepadnaviruses) use a hybrid procedure (6). Sometimes viral DNA becomes incorporated into the host cell genome and becomes latent (e.g., papillomaviruses). Viruses may have circular or linear DNA, and replication may proceed in a number of configurations (e.g., circular to circular, linear to circular to linear, hairpins to concatamers to hairpins).

Tissue Tropism

Some viruses were originally named because they home to specific tissues (e.g., hepatitis viruses). This tendency can also be used to identify viruses. However, in the case of immunosuppressed individuals, tissue and organ tropisms may broaden.

Viral Disease

In addition to acute disease (e.g., influenza), virus infection may result in silent or subclinical persistent infection whereby the virus is present but symptoms are mild or nonexistent (e.g., polyomavirus), or latent infection where the virus genome persists in tissue and occasionally causes symptoms (e.g., herpesviruses). Additionally, they may cause diseases that develop over a period of months to years [e.g., measles in subacute sclerosing panencephalitis (SSPE)] or potentiate oncogenesis by causing the normal growth-restriction mechanisms of the cell to fail (e.g., retroviruses). The size of the inoculum and the tissue of entry play roles in the type and severity of disease. Host factors modify the effects of viral infection; very young, very old, malnourished, and immunocompromised individuals usually have a more severe disease. In some cases, the detrimental effects of a viral illness are due to the host immunological response to it (e.g., some forms of hepatitis).

VIRAL DETECTION

Methods

Frequently, material from lesions is inoculated into tissue culture and sometimes into embryonated eggs or animals. Recognition of the infection may be from observation of the resulting cell or tissue changes, such as cytopathic effect (CPE) in tissue culture, and histology or appearance of diseased tissue (e.g., giant multinucleated cells), or detection of viral products produced. Tests detecting viruses and viral components include TEM, immunohistochemistry, enzyme-linked immunosorbent assay (ELISA), radioimmunoassay, polymerase chain reaction (PCR), hemagglutination inhibition (HI), enzyme immunoassay, immunofluorescent antibody (IFA), and complement fixation. The type of nucleic acid, the proteins, and morphological structure are all used in identification.

Detection of antibodies produced in the infected organism (serological tests) can be used once the body has had a chance to produce them. Some tests may be virus-specific. Some tests make use of complement fixation, neutralization, neutralization inhibition, or hemagglutination to detect virus group-specific or type-specific antibodies after an individual has produced a response. These tests confirm an exposure or infection but are not useful for rapid diagnosis of acute disease.

Advantages/Limitations of Detection Systems

Culture studies afford the advantage that they amplify viral numbers and make viruses easier to detect, but require that they be cultivable. Sometimes, viruses grow poorly or not at all in in vitro systems; if not transported under favourable conditions, they may not be viable when they reach the culture laboratory. Serological studies measure the body's response to a virus, yet early after infection, there may not be a recognizable immunological response. Serology is good for confirming an infection, detecting exposure to a pathogen, and detecting a chronic infection (e.g., hepatitis), but may not be useful if the infection is acute or if the patient is not immunocompetent. Histology and immunohistochemistry are extremely useful as rapid tests. They examine specimens directly from the patient if enough cellular material is available, but histological changes may be non-specific, and immunostaining requires an accurate choice of antibody reagents to match the infection present. PCR also can be rapid (several hours), and is extremely sensitive, but also requires the choice of appropriate primers to detect the infection. TEM provides an "open view" [term coined by Hans Gelderblom (41)] of whatever may be present, i.e., it does not require an a priori notion of what agent might be present for selection of the correct reagent. Additionally, TEM diagnosis of viruses in liquids by negative staining with heavy metal salt solutions is very rapid (a matter of minutes). However, viruses must be present in sufficient numbers in bodily fluids ($\sim10^5$ to 10^6/mL) for detection. Concentration procedures have been described for increasing the likelihood of seeing them (90). Visualization of viruses by TEM in tissues requires ultrathin sectioning, the preparation for which takes several hours to overnight. Focal infections may be missed by microscopical methods due to selection of tissue not containing the virus. Short term in vitro cultivation and TEM of the culture has been described to enhance viral numbers (89). Methods have been described for locating focal pathological tissue by light or confocal microscopy and then processing the exact area for TEM (14,44).

VIRAL EYE DISEASES

Infection

Viruses causing eye problems include those that directly infect the eye and surrounding tissues and those that cause immunosuppression and destruction by other organisms or metabolic events. Direct infection may occur from the outside through the conjunctiva and occasionally corneal transplants, where the external eye is mainly affected (e.g., adenovirus). Alternatively, infection may occur through hematogenous spread from a generalized infection (e.g., CMV) or neurologic spread through nerves [e.g., varicella zoster virus (VZV)]. Additionally, the mucous membranes of the eye can be an entryway for viruses to cause systemic infection [e.g., human immunodeficiency virus (HIV)]. The major human viral pathogens are listed in Table 2 and are discussed individually.

Virus Spread

Tissue to Tissue

Some viruses cause epithelial cell damage at the site where they attach and enter (e.g., respiratory and gastroenteric viruses). Others enter and become disseminated via the blood or lymphatics to produce a generalized illness (e.g., measles). The conjunctiva can be a site of viral entry, both for conjunctivitis (e.g., adenovirus, coxsackievirus, see below) and for systemic disease (e.g., enterovirus 70, HIV, Ebola virus).

Table 2 Viruses Associated with Ocular Disease

Virus family	Viruses	NA	NA symmetry	Coating	NC size (nm)	Virion size (nm)	Ocular disease
Adenoviridae	Adenovirus	DNA	Icosahedral	Naked	70–90	70–90	Pharyngeal conjunctival fever Epidemic keratoconjunctivitis Follicular conjunctivitis, keratoconjunctivitis
Bunyaviridae	Rift Valley fever virus	RNA	Helical	Enveloped	Variable × 9	80–120	Conjunctivitis, uveitis, retinitis
	Sandfly fever virus						Conjunctivitis
Flaviviridae	Dengue virus	RNA	Spherical	Enveloped	25–30	35–50	Retrobulbar pain, conjunctival congestion, eyelid swelling
	Powassan virus						Diplopia, ophthalmoplegia
	West Nile virus						Uveitis, vitritis, chorioretinitis, papilledema, occlusive retinal vasculitis
	Yellow fever virus						Conjunctivitis, conjunctival hemorrhage
Filoviridae	Ebola virus	RNA	Helical	Enveloped	50	Variable up to 1400 × 80	Hemorrhagic conjunctivitis, uveitis
	Marburg virus						Hemorrhagic conjunctivitis, uveitis
Hepadnaviridae	Hepatitis B virus	DNA	Icosahedral	Enveloped	28	42	Neuroretinitis, yellow skin or eyes, ocular circulation compromise, optic nerve dysfunction, cataract formation
Herpesviridae	Cytomegalovirus	DNA	Icosahedral	Enveloped	100	120–200	Uveitis, retinitis
	Epstein–Barr virus						Conjunctivitis
	Herpes simplex virus 1, 2						Conjunctivitis, keratitis, retinitis, uveitis
	Kaposi sarcoma herpes virus						Eyelid or conjunctival tumors
	Varicella zoster virus						Conjunctivitis, keratitis, scleritis, iridocyclitis, optic neuritis
Orthomyxoviridae	Influenza virus	RNA	Helical	Enveloped	Variable × 9–15	Variable × 80–120	Follicular conjunctivitis, iritis, interstitial keratitis, dacryoadenitis, macular hemorrhage, retinitis
Papillomaviridae	Papillomavirus	DNA	Icosahedral	Naked	55	55	Eyelid margin warts, verrucous keratitis, conjunctivitis, dysplastic or carcinomatous lesions in transition zone between cornea and conjunctiva
Paramyxoviridae	Measles (rubeola) virus (red measles)	RNA	Helical	Enveloped	Variable × 12–21	100–500	Mucopurulent conjunctivitis, punctate keratitis, corneal erosion, retinitis
	Mumps virus						Dacryoadenitis, conjunctivitis, uveitis, iritis, optic neuritis, neuroretinitis, posterior vitritis
	Newcastle disease virus						Follicular conjunctivitis, preauricular lymphadenopathy, keratitis
Picornaviridae	Bovine foot and mouth disease virus	RNA	Icosahedral	Naked	24–30	24–30	Mucopurulent conjunctivitis, punctate keratitis
	Coxsackievirus						Conjunctivitis, acute idiopathic maculopathy
	Enterovirus						Hemorrhagic follicular conjunctivitis
	Hepatitis A virus						Conjunctivitis, yellow eyes due to icterus from liver disease
Polyomaviridae	JC polyomavirus	RNA	Icosahedral	Naked	40–45	40–45	Visual loss from brain infection and demyelination

(Continued)

Table 2 Viruses Associated with Ocular Disease (*Continued*)

Virus family	Viruses	NA	NA symmetry	Coating	NC size (nm)	Virion size (nm)	Ocular disease
Poxviridae	Molluscum contagiosum virus	DNA	Complex	Enveloped	(Dumbell-shaped)	320 × 250 × 200	Blepharoconjunctivitis, keratoconjunctivitis
	Orf virus					220–300 × 140–170	Follicular and papillary conjunctivitis
	Vaccinia virus					250 × 200 × 200	Mucopurulent blepharoconjunctivitis, keratitis, iritis, choroiditis, optic neuritis
	Variola (smallpox) virus					250 × 200 × 200	Eyelid lesions, blepharoconjunctivitis, keratoconjunctivitis
Retroviridae	Human immunodeficiency virus	RNA	Isometric	Enveloped	(Cone-shaped)	80–140	Retinopathy, opportunistic ocular infections due to immunosuppression
Rhabdoviridae	Rabies virus	RNA	Helical	Enveloped	Coiled: 15–16 Uncoiled: 3–6	100–430 × 45–100	Ciliary body and choroid inflammation, retinal exudate, periphlebitis, retinal ganglion cell loss
Rubiviridae	Rubella virus (German measles)	RNA	Icosahedral	Enveloped	30–35	60–70	Acquired (post natal): conjunctivitis, iritis, superficial keratitis, bilateral exudative retinal detachments, veiling, poliosis, panuveitis; congenital: microphthalmia, cataracts, glaucoma, strabismus, nasolacrimal duct occlusion, corneal clouding, iris atrophy, iritis, chorioretinitis, optic atrophy

Abbreviations: Enveloped, has glycoprotein membrane (organic solvent-sensitive); NA, nucleic acid; Naked, without glycoprotein membrane (not organic solvent-sensitive); NC, nucleocapsid.

The opposite route, from systemic disease to eye, can also occur (e.g., measles, VZV). Herpes simplex virus (HSV) and VZV travel through nerves to re-infect surface locations. Reactivation of endogenous infection can occur during immunosuppression [e.g., JC polyomavirus in progressive multifocal leukoencephalopathy (PML)], during which the virus becomes productive and destructive again. Another tissue-to-tissue (or human to human) mode of transmission is through organ transplantation (e.g., as with herpesviruses). Transplanting an organ from a CMV seropositive individual to a seronegative patient can result in serious, sometimes life-threatening infections. Herpes viruses have been transmitted with corneal transplants.

Human to Human

Virus spread from person to person is modified by numerous host factors, including host pre-exposure (immunity), age, gender, and virus characteristics such as dosage, virulence, and entry portal. Some viruses almost always cause disease in the host (e.g., measles), while others may result in a subclinical infection (e.g., polyomavirus). Mother to fetus transmission occurs, and the effect on the unborn child is a function of its developmental stage (e.g., as in rubella infection). Viruses (e.g., CMV) have also been transmitted from mother to baby in milk. Sexual transmission results from mucous membrane contact with infected body fluids (e.g., HIV). Respiratory infection occurs from airborne viruses in droplets as well as from fomites to membranes (e.g., adenoviruses); some viruses are shed in saliva and can be transmitted by sharing food or utensils [e.g., Epstein–Barr Virus (EBV)]. Ease of viral transmission by contact of skin surfaces varies; poxviruses are easily transmissible in this fashion, while measles is not.

Zoonoses

Some animal virus diseases can be transmitted through bites (e.g., rabies), while others occur from skin contact with infected animals (e.g., orf). Many arenaviruses (e.g., Lassa fever) and hantaviruses (e.g., Hantaan) are shed in animal urine, and human infection may occur from inhaling dried waste.

Spread by Arthropods

In the early days of virology, the mechanism of spread was an important factor in naming viruses. Arboviruses are viruses that are transmitted by arthropod vectors, most commonly mosquitoes and ticks. Later, viral classification schemes placed them into several different groups, including bunyavirus (e.g., LaCross), flavivirus (e.g., dengue), alphavirus (eastern equine encephalitis), and reovirus (e.g., Colorado tick fever) families.

Antiviral Agents

Antiviral drugs are targeted to inhibit viral replication mechanisms while leaving the host metabolism intact. One way is to prevent virus attachment by supplying agents that mimic the viral receptor protein on the cell and occupy the sites on the membrane that attract viruses. Attachment can also be prevented by supplying agents that mimic the cell receptor on the virus and bind to the virions themselves. Another mechanism is to introduce a nucleoside or nucleotide analog that gets incorporated into the viral nucleic acid, but which the replicase enzyme cannot recognize, and thus acts as a chain terminator. A different mechanism is to prevent viral release from the cell; two new influenza antivirals block release of mature virions by inhibiting viral neuraminidase. Some drugs act by inhibiting viral enzymes such as reverse transcriptase or protease. Finally, some therapies operate by boosting the host immune system. Vaccines are available for many viruses, including influenza, measles, mumps, poliomyelitis, rabies, rubella, hepatitis A virus (HAV) and HBV, VZV, and yellow fever. Genetically engineered interferon can be used to protect uninfected cells from internalizing a virus released from nearby cells. Pooled gamma globulin is given for passive immune prophylaxis post-exposure (e.g., influenza in high risk cases, rabies).

VIRUSES

Viruses that affect the ocular structures are summarized in Table 2. For ease of finding information on specific viruses, the viruses are listed alpabetically in the text rather than in the order of their frequency.

Adenoviruses

Virology

Adenoviruses are dsDNA, naked icosahedral particles, ranging from 70 to 90 nm in diameter, depending on the strain (1). The family is subdivided into four genera; the Mastadenovirus genus contains the human and other mammalian adenoviruses. There are at least 19 designated species to date. Adenoviruses are constructed in the nuclei of infected cells, and may be seen as nuclear "ground glass" inclusions by light microscopy. However, other DNA viruses (e.g., polyomavirus) produce similar inclusions. By negative staining and TEM of fluids (e.g., stool, tears), the particles appear spherical with flat triangular facets made up of 8- to 10-nm bead-like capsomers (Fig. 1A). Depending on how they land on the plastic support film, the circumference may appear hexagonal. Viruses from culture, but rarely from clinical material, may have long (~55 nm) fibers (penton antigens)

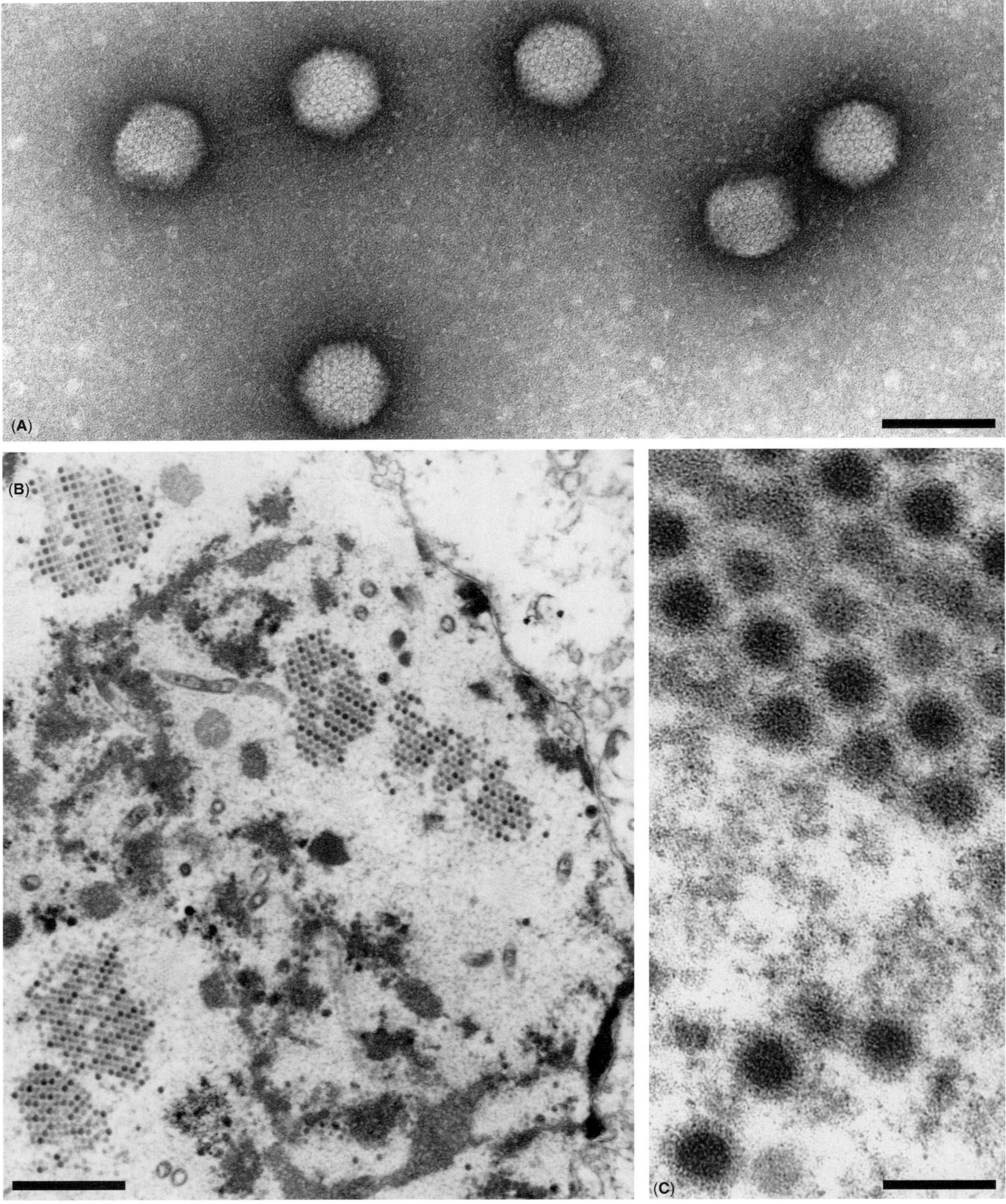

Figure 1 Adenovirus. (**A**) Negative stain; note naked icosahedral capsids with flat, triangular facets. Bar = 100 nm. (**B**) Thin section of virus-infected cell with paracrystalline arrays of virions in the nucleus. Bar = 1 μm. (**C**) High magnification of virus; note electron-dense core with less dense capsid coat. Bar = 100 nm.

protruding from the vertices of the triangles. In thin sections, viral factories may be seen in paracrystalline arrays in the nucleus (Figs. 1B and C). Late in the course of the infection when the cell membranes have started to break down, viruses can be seen dispersed in the cytoplasm as well.

Epidemiology

Adenoviruses have over 30 different serotypes that cause human disease, typically in the upper respiratory tract, gastrointestinal tract, and ocular mucosa. They can be spread by medical instruments, swimming pools, and fomites with hand to eye contact (142). Types 31 and 40 cause 30% to 80% of gastrointestinal infections; types 1–3, 5, 7, and 31 have also been isolated. The actual incidence of adenovirus in ocular disease is difficult to ascertain due to the variation in severity of the infection, but it may be the causative agent for around 20% of viral conjunctivitis. The serotypes associated with eye disease are 1–11, 14–17, 19–22, 26, 27, 29, and 37, the most frequent ones being 7, 8, 11, 19, and 37 (47). Adenovirus 1, 2, 4–6, and 19 are associated with acute follicular conjunctivitis, and 8 and 19 with epidemic keratoconjunctivitis (EKC). In the United States EKC is most often due to adenovirus type 19, but worldwide type 8 is the most common. Adenovirus types 3 and 7 frequently cause pharyngeal conjunctival fever (PCF) and are commonly seen in epidemics of swimming pool conjunctivitis; type 7 is one of the most commonly seen viruses in acute hemorrhagic conjunctivitis (AHC). Serotype 11 and Coxsackievirus A24, a picornavirus (see below), also cause AHC. Epidemics have been reported in Asia, India, and West Africa.

Clinical Presentation

Almost half of adenovirus infections are subclinical. Many serotypes cause respiratory infections resulting in pharyngitis, tonsillitis, laryngitis, and pneumonia; symptoms are similar to those caused by other respiratory viruses. Adenoviruses are the most common cause of febrile convulsion. In children, there may be fever (39.4°C) for several (2–13) days. Infection in newborns may result in disseminated disease that is often fatal. Enteric infection results in gastritis, with watery, but not bloody, stools. Diarrhea lasts between 3 and 11 days; fever and vomiting are common. Adenoviruses can cause hemorrhagic cystitis in bone marrow recipients and occasionally renal transplant recipients. The incidence of adenovirus infection in bone marrow transplant patients is high (>20%); infection in this setting may occur as a result of reactivation of latent virus or transmission via donor marrow or blood. It is also a serious problem in liver transplant patients and HIV-positive individuals. Uncommon manifestations include meningoencephalitis, myocarditis, celiac disease, urethritis, and vaginal and genital ulcers.

Adenovirus infection may result in conjunctivitis and sometimes uveitis. Serotypes 8, 19, and 37 most commonly affect the eye. Acute follicular conjunctivitis begins unilaterally and usually spreads to the other eye; it may last up to a month but resolves without sequelae. PCF is characterized by pharyngitis, headache, diarrhea, coryza, rash, and lymphadenopathy. After about 2 weeks, it resolves without sequelae. AHC is characterized by a sudden, painful follicular conjunctivitis. There may be regional lymphadenopathy and subepithelial corneal infiltrates. Rarely, nongranulomatous iritis may occur a week after infection; it resolves spontaneously with time.

Adenovirus can cause persistent infections by producing proteins that modulate the immune system. Persistent virus has been detected in intestine, tonsil, and adenoid tissue. Such infection may result in fecal shedding of virus for several years; the mucosa-associated lymphoid tissue is a potential source of excreted virus (40). Persistent infection with adenovirus may also contribute to reactivation of other viruses such as herpesviruses.

Histopathology

Histopathological examination of conjunctiva from patients with adenovirus infection discloses nonnecrotizing inflammation with the formation of lymphoid follicles, along with stromal edema and vascular dilation (130). Corneal epithelial scrapings from individuals with acute EKC exhibit swollen, edematous epithelial cells that may fuse to form syncytia (84). Maudgal observed intranuclear vacuolar inclusions with and without dense bodies (84). Adenovirus particles are detectable in the corneal and conjunctival epithelium by TEM in the acute disease (20,84).

Rare reports document the histopathology in intact corneas from patients with corneal opacities following adenovirus keratoconjunctivitis (82,138). In these, an inflammatory infiltrate was noted immediately beneath the Bowman layer or in areas where the Bowman layer was disrupted. In the case reported by Lund and Stefani (82), the inflammatory infiltrate consisted mostly of lymphocytes, while Tullo et al. reported the inflammatory infiltrate to be mostly macrophages (138). In two corneas examined histologically by the authors, the corneal inflammation consisted mostly of macrophages with lesser numbers of lymphocytes (Fig. 2).

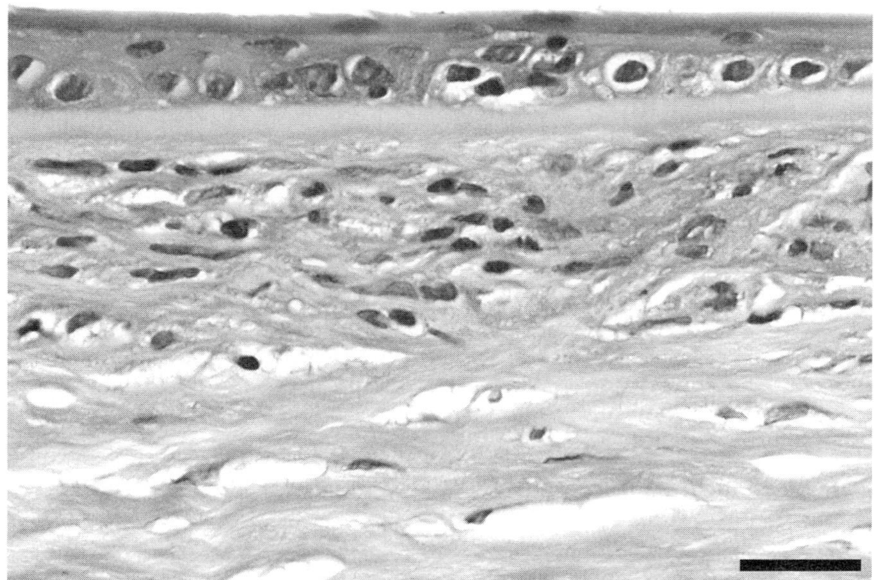

Figure 2 Adenoviral keratitis. Corneal opacities following adenoviral keratoconjunctivitis are the result of macrophages and lymphocytes accumulating in the superficial stroma beneath the Bowman layer. Hematoxylin and eosin; bar = 25 μm.

Diagnosis

In tissue culture, adenoviruses cause cells to become more globular in shape. Aggregation and lysis of chromatin and formation of basophilic or eosinophilic nuclear inclusions may also occur. CPE may be evident between 1 and 8 days after inoculation, if the specimen was taken within a week of symptom onset. A rapid ELISA is available that is 81% sensitive and 100% specific, compared to culture (67). PCR for adenovirus is highly sensitive, but is not widely used at present. TEM of fluids such as tears is rapid and can demonstrate the naked icosahedral particles; in thin sections of tissues, viruses are seen in the nucleus. Antibodies are available for immunostaining. Serological testing is useful in epidemiologic studies, but is not practical as a diagnostic procedure.

In the differential diagnosis, HSV and VZV, along with chlamydial infections (see Chapter 10) should be considered. Other less common agents include coxsackievirus and other picornaviruses, Newcastle disease virus, influenza virus, and bacteria.

Bunyaviruses

Rift Valley Fever Virus

Virology

Rift Valley fever virus (RVFV) is a bunyavirus, an enveloped segmented ssRNA particle with a coiled circular nucleocapsid (29). It is about 90 to 120 nm in diameter, and because of lack of surface detail, is impossible to identify in clinical specimens by negative staining (Fig. 3A). In thin sections, bunyaviruses can be seen budding into cytoplasmic vesicles (Figs. 3B and C).

Epidemiology

This virus is an animal disease in sub-Saharan Africa that is transmitted to humans by mosquitoes and sand flies. It can persist in mosquito eggs during drought and re-emerge during hatching after rainfall. It is amplified in cattle, sheep, and goats. RVFV can be transmitted by direct contact or aerosol spread from infected animals during necropsy or slaughter, or by aerosols produced in laboratory settings. Persistence of other bunyaviruses has been described (25), but attempts to identify persistent RVFV and its reservoir between outbreaks have been unsuccessful (19).

Clinical Presentation

The infection presents as an acute febrile illness (up to 104°F) with chills, headache, myalgia, and malaise between 2 and 7 days after inoculation. The acute phase resolves in 2 to 5 days, but a prolonged convalescence may follow. Gastrointestinal symptoms may occur later in the disease, and the fever may relapse. Conjunctivitis and uveitis may occur during the acute phase, and unilateral or bilateral retinitis may present with loss of central vision 1 to 3 weeks after onset (22). There may be macular exudates and hemorrhage; vasculitis and vascular occlusion may be evident by fluorescein angiography. The ocular symptoms usually resolve over months. A few patients may develop serious sequelae such as hepatitis, encephalitis, and visceral hemorrhage. In the serious form of the disease, half the patients have a permanent loss of central vision due to macular scar formation, retinal detachment, or ischemic maculopathy (125,126).

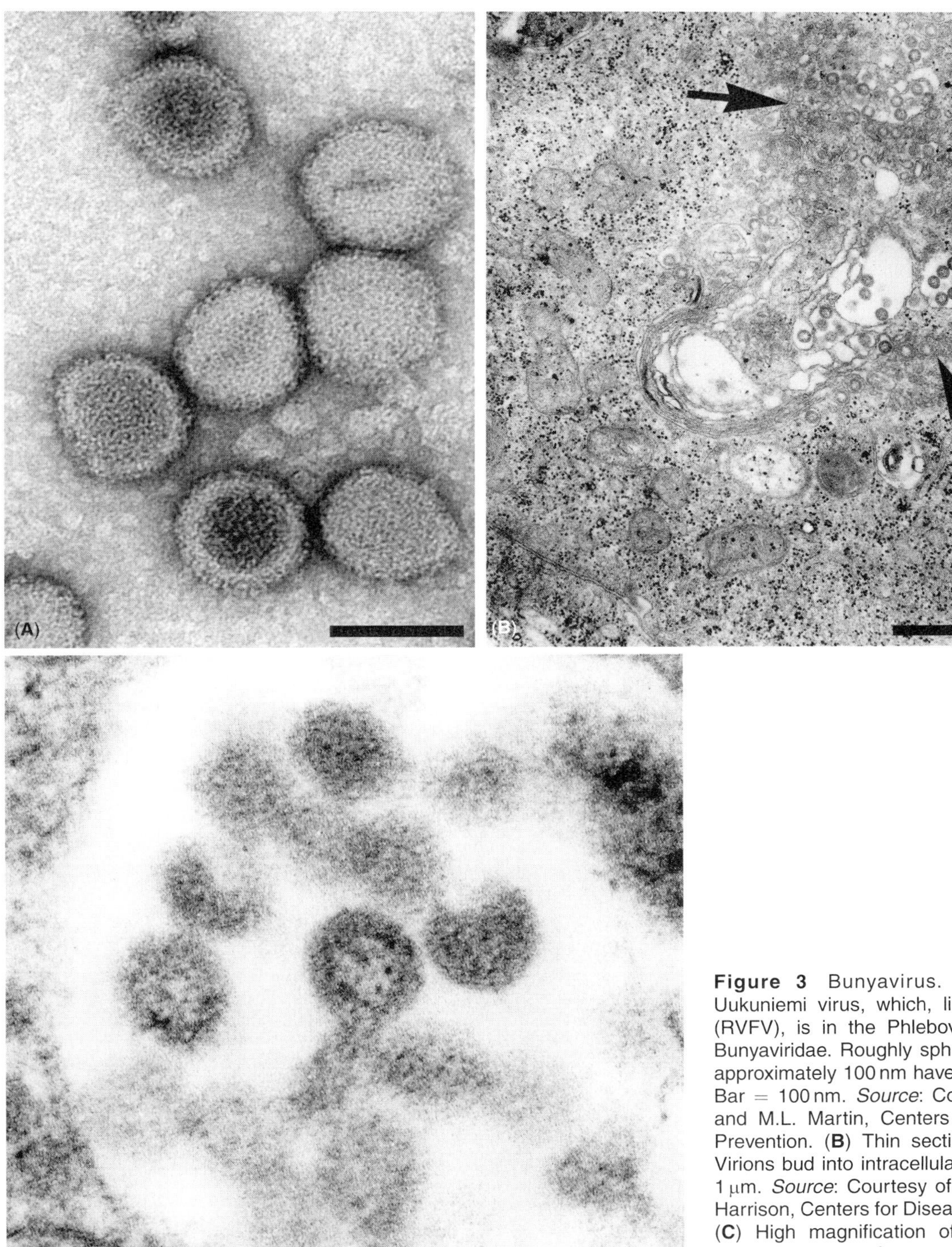

Figure 3 Bunyavirus. (**A**) Negative stain of Uukuniemi virus, which, like Rift Valley fever virus (RVFV), is in the Phlebovirus genus of the family Bunyaviridae. Roughly spherical enveloped virions of approximately 100 nm have short surface projections. Bar = 100 nm. *Source*: Courtesy of Dr. E.L. Palmer and M.L. Martin, Centers for Disease Control and Prevention. (**B**) Thin section of RVFV-infected cell. Virions bud into intracellular vesicles (*arrows*). Bar = 1 μm. *Source*: Courtesy of Dr. F.A. Murphy and A.K. Harrison, Centers for Disease Control and Prevention. (**C**) High magnification of RVFV showing surface projections as a fuzzy outer layer. Bar = 100 nm. *Source*: Courtesy of Dr. F.A. Murphy and A.K. Harrison, Centers for Disease Control and Prevention.

Diagnosis

RVFV should be suspected in patients with ocular signs living in or traveling through endemic areas. In the acute phase, the virus can be grown in tissue culture from blood and in mice or hamsters. HI, complement fixation (CF), IFA, and ELISA tests are available, but are less sensitive than culture (99). A four-fold rise in CF and HI antibodies from acute to convalescent phase helps to confirm infection. In the late stage with central nervous system (CNS) and ocular disease, serology is more helpful than both culture and molecular tests. Lyme disease and rickettsial diseases should be in the differential diagnosis.

Flaviviruses

Virology

The Flaviviridae family includes dengue, Japanese encephalitis, West Nile, Powassan, and yellow fever viruses. Flaviviruses are small (40–60 nm) enveloped plus-sense ssRNA viruses. The envelope has 10- to 12-nm ring-like subunits on the surface when negative stained preparations are viewed by TEM (Fig. 4A). The core is about 30 nm in diameter and appears round in thin sections (Figs. 4B and C). Cryoelectron microscopy has determined that the nucleocapsid has icosahedral symmetry (29).

Dengue Virus

Epidemiology

Dengue fever is endemic in the tropics. The principal carrier is the *Aedes aegypti* mosquito, and due to its increased spread, the disease has reached epidemic proportions in South America. It is estimated that over 100 million cases occur each year (85), which may be low due to inapparent infections. Between 100 and 200 cases per year are reported in travelers returning to the United States, Australia, and Europe; additionally, several cases are reported each year in the southern United States. Dengue fever is caused by four serotypes of virus. Infection with one serotype confers full immunity to future infections by that serotype, but predisposes patients to a more serious manifestation of disease after infection with a different serotype.

Clinical Presentation

After a 2- to 7-day incubation, an acute illness characterized by high fever, headache, retrobulbar pain, back pain, conjunctival congestion, eyelid swelling, and flushing occurs (117). Early in the infection, a rash may appear, often beginning on the trunk and spreading centripetally; desquamation sometimes occurs. The fever may last 6 to 7 days or subside and return, during which time, there is malaise, anorexia, and nausea. Cough, pharyngitis, and rhinitis may be present. The white blood cell and platelet counts are depressed, and occasionally, hemorrhagic phenomena are present. Neurologic disorders and Reye syndrome have been reported. Convalescence may be lengthy and may include weakness, cardiac arrhythmias, and depression.

Diagnosis

History of travel to endemic areas is a clue to diagnosis. Differential diagnoses include infections due to arboviruses, influenza, rubella, rubeola, typhus and malaria.

The virus can be isolated in mosquito tissue cultures, which then can be examined by immunofluorescence microscopy. Viral antigen can be detected in serum by immunohistochemical staining of peripheral blood mononuclear cells, reverse transcription-polymerase chain reaction (RT-PCR) with digoxigenin probes, countercurrent immunoelectrophoresis, or RIA with monoclonal antibody. Serological confirmation depends on at least a four-fold rise in antibody titer as demonstrated by HI, CF, or neutralization.

Due to the increased possibility of hemorrhagic dengue fever in secondary infections, it is necessary to differentiate primary from secondary exposure. In secondary infections, HI antibodies are present in the acute phase and high in the convalescent phase. The IgM:IgG antibody ratio in acute phase sera is >1.5, while in convalescence sera, the ratio is reversed, and ELISA for IgG and IgM is useful for determining primary versus secondary infection (18).

Powassan Virus

Epidemiology

Powassan virus is a rare arthropod-borne flavivirus that goes through a cycle in small animals such as squirrels and groundhogs. Encephalitis due to this agent has been reported in Russia, Canada, the United States, and Mexico, mostly in male patients under 20 years old, possibly due to outdoor exposure to ticks.

Clinical Presentation

Powassan virus causes encephalitis, and in the United States, it has been recognized with increasing frequency in New England. There is a febrile prodrome that may include a rash, followed by CNS symptoms in about a third of patients. Meningitis and encephalitis may be severe and may resemble HSV temporal lobe infection. Olfactory hallucinations, unilateral or bilateral facial paresis or paralysis, muscle tremors or rigidity may occur. In one case, in addition to general symptoms of nausea, vomiting, diarrhea, dizziness, uncoordination, arm weakness, urinary retention, fever, and delirium, there was diplopia and almost total ophthalmoplegia. After several months, most symptoms abated, but eye movements remained slow and did not improve (76).

Diagnosis

Diagnosis is by serology or, in fatal cases, by virus culture of brain. Herpesvirus should be in the differential diagnosis.

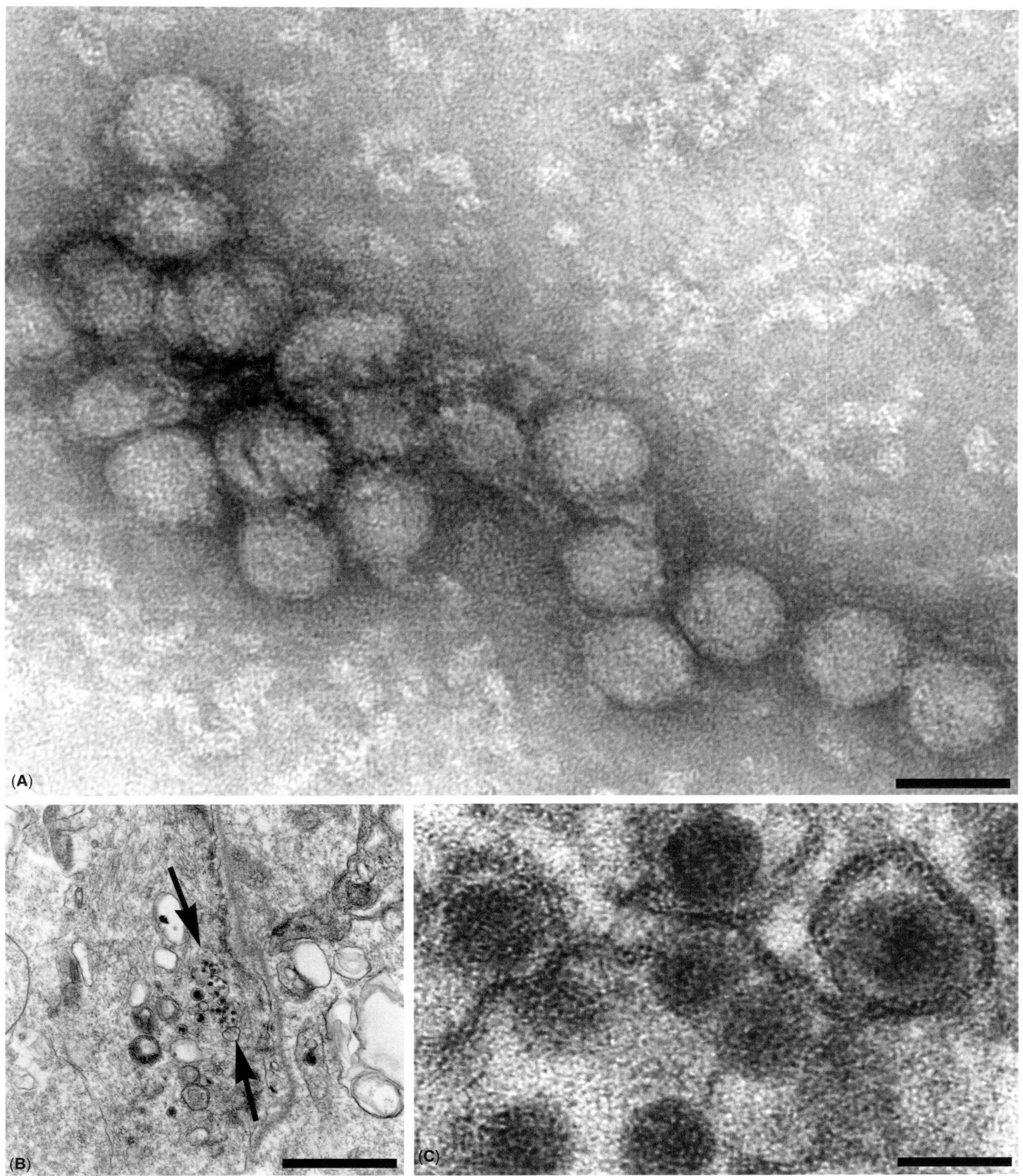

Figure 4 Flavivirus. (**A**) Negative stain of West Nile virus showing the 40- to 60-nm enveloped particles. Short projections are irregularly positioned on the surface. Bar = 100 nm. *Source*: Courtesy of C.S. Goldsmith and Dr. P.E. Rollin, Centers for Disease Control and Prevention. (**B**) Thin section of a brain biopsy from a patient who was serologically positive for St. Louis encephalitis virus. Small particles bud into the cisternae of endoplasmic reticulum (*arrows*). Note that they are, in general, smaller than neurosecretory vesicles. Bar = 1 μm. (**C**) High magnification of budding virus. Bar = 100 nm.

West Nile Virus

Epidemiology

West Nile virus causes fatal encephalitis in birds and can be transmitted to humans by mosquitoes. It has a wide distribution and has been seen increasingly in the United States, especially in crows and blue jays. West Nile virus has been reported in other animals, including horses, dogs and cats.

Clinical Presentation

West Nile virus infection causes fever and flu-like symptoms in humans. Uveitis, vitritis, chorioretinitis, papilledema, and occlusive retinal vasculitis can also occur during West Nile virus infection (11,39,64,94).

Histopathology

Though several recent articles document ocular manifestations of West Nile virus infection, histopathologic descriptions of human ocular lesions for this and other flaviviruses are scant. In great horned owls and goshawks, West Nile virus infection may result in lymphoplasmacytic endophthalmitis (147).

Diagnosis

West Nile virus can be isolated from blood in the early stages of infection following amplification in tissue culture, embryonated eggs, or mice inoculated intracranially. Serological tests are less useful because of cross-reaction with other flaviviruses, such as St. Louis encephalitis virus. PCR for the virus and ELISA for IgM antibody can be used.

Hepadnavirus

Virology

The Hepadnaviridae family includes two genuses: Orthohepadnavirus, which contains HBV that infects humans and other mammals, and Avihepadnavirus, which infects birds (29). HBV is an enveloped dsDNA/partially ssDNA virus. The complete virion of 40 to 45 nm, called a Dane particle, has a dense core of 32 to 36 nm. Empty particles, made up of HBV surface antigen (HBsAg), may be 16 to 25 nm or filaments 20 nm in diameter and of variable length (Fig. 5A). In thin sections, cores can be found both in the nucleus and the cytoplasm, but complete virions (the 42-nm Dane particles) are seen only in the cytoplasm (Fig. 5B). Frequently, the endoplasmic reticulum will contain large amounts of dense deposits composed of HBsAg (Fig. 5C).

Hepatitis B Virus

Epidemiology

Transmission is by blood and other body fluids, and can be by sexual contact; mother to fetus; fomites such as toys, toothbrushes, and needles (intravenous drug users); laboratory accidents; and health equipment, including ophthalmic instruments.

Clinical Presentation

The virus homes to the liver, where it can cause persistent infection and may cause cirrhosis and hepatocellular carcinoma. Neuroretinitis has been reported in association with HBV infection (28). It is usually a self-limiting disease and is thought to be an immune-mediated disorder. Hepatitis can cause jaundice, which may be manifested in yellow skin or eyes. Ocular circulation may be compromised, and autoimmune reactions may contribute to optic nerve dysfunction and cataract formation (17).

Histopathology

To our knowledge, no specific ocular histopathologic findings have been described in patients with hepatitis B infection. In eyes that we have examined at autopsy from patients with cirrhosis due to chronic HBV infection, we have not seen any changes that could be attributed to the hepatitis virus.

Diagnosis

Diagnosis of hepatitis due to HBV is usually based on serological markers, and algorithms for different causal agents have been designed (66). In cases of acute hepatitis, the presence of HBsAg with or without IgM anti-hepatitis B core antigen (HBcAg) indicates HBV infection. If IgM anti-HBcAg is present, the infection is recent; if not, the infection may be either a chronic infection or one resolved in the remote past. In cases of chronic hepatitis, the presence of HBsAg and IgG anti-HBcAg identifies chronic HBV infection. If HBeAg is detected, a highly replicative chronic HBV infection is indicated which can be substantiated by testing for HBV DNA in the serum. In the absence of HBV infection, HCV RNA should be tested.

There may also be superinfection with other hepatitis viruses, including hepatitis delta virus (HDV), hepatitis A virus (HAV), and hepatitis C virus (HCV). The differential diagnosis of hepatitis B includes hepatitis due to other viruses such as herpesviruses, paramyxoviruses, adenoviruses, enteroviruses, rubella virus, and yellow fever virus. Some exotic viruses, not commonly found in the United States, which can cause hepatitis, include the hemorrhagic fever viruses from several families (e.g., filovirus, bunyavirus). Aside from viruses, hepatitis can also be caused by some parasites (e.g., *Toxoplasma gondii* in neonates and immunocompromised individuals); some drugs (e.g., anesthetic agents, alcohol), and other conditions (e.g., cholecystitis, heart failure, and metastatic neoplasms).

necrosis. About one-third of AIDS patients with a CD4 count $<50/mm^3$ have CMV retinitis, and frequently, this is the presenting manifestation of HIV infection (107). Patients may complain of blurred vision, floaters, light flashes, scotoma, or central vision loss. Posterior lesions may resemble congenital toxoplasmosis or toxocariasis.

A complication of antiretroviral therapy is retinitis if the CD4 cell count can be raised to 100 to 150 per mm^3. When the CD4 count starts to recover after therapy, inflammatory cells can infiltrate the infected tissue, and may result in vitritis and macular edema.

Congenital infection may result in hearing loss and mental retardation. Ocular infection may be mild or may result in chorioretinitis or retinal necrosis. Resolution may result in a hyperplastic pigmented macular scar or multiple lesions with pigmented scars.

Histopathology

The most frequent ocular manifestation of CMV infection encountered histologically is CMV retinitis in immunocompromised individuals (45,93). CMV infection results in retinal necrosis with minimal inflammation. Infected neurosensory retinal cells exhibit a variable degree of cytomegaly with both nuclear and cytoplasmic enlargement. Nuclear and cytoplasmic inclusion bodies are often seen, and the infected retinal cells may fuse to form a large multinucleated syncytium (Fig. 7). The cytoplasmic inclusion bodies are amphophilic to deeply basophilic, and their presence can be highlighted using a colloidal iron stain for glycosaminoglycans (GAGs). Infected nuclei have a single inclusion body that is usually deeply basophilic, round to oval with a smooth border, and surrounded by a clear halo. CMV may also infect retinal pigment epithelium (RPE) cells resulting in cytomegaly and prominent nuclear and cytoplasmic inclusion bodies. A thin fibroglial scar is the usual residue of CMV-induced retinal necrosis.

CMV rarely infects the conjunctiva of immunocompromised individuals and is manifest histologically as cytomegalic cells within and around conjunctival blood vessels along with accompanying acute inflammation (10). CMV infection of the corneal epithelium has been reported in a man with AIDS (144) and as a rare cause of stromal keratitis following penetrating keratoplasty (143).

Diagnosis

A diagnosis is made on the characteristic clinical findings with confirmation by culture, especially of throat and urine. Rapid techniques that detect early viral proteins in culture can increase the detection.

In tissue biopsies, the typical "owl's eye" cell is strongly suggestive of CMV infection (Fig. 7). Immunostaining with anti-CMV antibody is particularly helpful when infection is early and focal. By negative staining and TEM of fluids (e.g. tears) icosahedral nucleocapsids (~100 nm in diameter) appear slightly larger than adenoviruses, but are indistinguishable from HSV. They may be seen unenveloped or within membranes if the stain has penetrated the envelope. Enveloped particles are ~150 nm or more in diameter and may contain one or several nucleocapsids (Fig. 6A).

A febrile illness with >10% atypical lymphocytes and a negative heterophile test may suggest primary CMV; a high IgM antibody against CMV is a good indicator of CMV mononucleosis. A serologic evaluation at presentation and 2 months later may demonstrate a rise in IgG antiviral titer and help to differentiate CMV from toxoplasmosis. However, tests for antibodies of the IgM type can be falsely positive if rheumatoid factor is present. Serological tests are not useful in immunosuppressed individuals such as AIDS patients. PCR and in situ hybridization are sensitive techniques for viral nucleic acid in tissue, including ocular specimens, but are less sensitive in bronchoalveolar lavage samples.

Epstein–Barr Virus

Virology

Like other herpesviruses, EBV (also known as human herpesvirus type 4) is a dsDNA virus (29). During an active infection it produces ~100-nm nucleocapsids and ~150- to 200-nm enveloped virions that are morphologically indistinguishable from CMV, HSV, and VZV.

Epidemiology

EBV is responsible for infectious mononucleosis, Burkitt lymphoma, nasopharyngeal carcinoma, and some cases of chronic fatigue syndrome. EBV serology demonstrates that close to 90% of Americans have been exposed to the virus by early adulthood, and it can be isolated from saliva in up to 25% of asymptomatic individuals (120). The virus enters the oropharynx and replicates in parotid epithelial cells and salivary gland ducts and then spreads to B cells. It is shed in the oropharynx of about a fifth of seropositive people in the absence of disease. The main mechanism of transmission is virus shedding into saliva, and infection has been called the "kissing disease".

Frequently, EBV DNA persists in B cells, but it may not produce complete virions recognizable by TEM. Some individuals become carriers. A small number of lymphocytes continue to produce virions that can be shed in up to 20% of infected people. Reactivation of latent virus causes recurrent eye disease, including epithelial keratitis, stromal keratitis, trabeculitis, keratouveitis, glaucoma, and rarely, acute retinal necrosis (ARN) (9). ARN is more often caused by HSV-1 and HSV-2, VZV, and CMV.

EBV may cause tumors in lymphoid tissues [e.g., Burkitt lymphoma, post transplant lymphoproliferative disease (PTLD) in transplant patients on immunosuppressive therapy]. Even though complete viruses may not be produced, some antigens are evident by immunostaining.

Clinical Presentation

EBV infection may be asymptomatic, but about 50% of infected individuals develop infectious mononucleosis, which may present with sore throat, respiratory tract symptoms, fever, lymphadenopathy, and hepatosplenomegaly. Up to a third of them may develop follicular conjunctivitis. Other potential ocular diseases include stromal keratitis, iritis, episcleritis, optic neuritis, and ophthalmoplegia (38).

Retinal involvement during mononucleosis is rare and usually mild, but macular edema, retinal hemorrhages, chorioretinitis, punctate outer retinitis, multifocal chorioretinitis, and the panuveitis syndrome have been reported (146). Conjunctivitis and keratitis are rare but can occur. Dacryoadenitis, episcleritis, uveitis and optic neuritis, papilledema, and vitritis have also been documented.

Histopathology

Polyclonal or monoclonal conjunctival lymphocytic infiltrates in EBV infection may be unilateral or bilateral (30). EBV antigen is demonstrable immunohistochemically in the infected lymphocytes (30). EBV infection may also induce PTLD in the iris (113) or elsewhere in the uveal tract (21). The PTLD is similar histologically to that seen in different parts of the body and may be composed of a monomorphic or polymorphic lymphocytic proliferation. Viral inclusions are not observed using light microscopy. A periocular T-cell lymphoma with EBV-infected lymphocytes has also been documented histologically (128), as has ARN (52). A patient with EBV-related ARN had X-linked lymphoproliferative disorder, which predisposes to EBV infection. A retinal biopsy in that patient disclosed retinal hemorrhage and necrosis with diffuse replacement of the photoreceptor layer by large multinucleated cells having enlarged hyperchromatic nuclei. A mixed population of B cells and T cells was present in the necrotic retina, and the lymphocytes exhibited cytological atypia compatible with their being infected by EBV. Viral inclusions were not evident, but EBV DNA was demonstrable using in situ hybridization (52).

Diagnosis

Serological tests for heterophile antibodies (antibodies directed against antigens on the surface of sheep erythrocytes or "Paul-Bunnell" antigens), IgM antibodies against the viral capsid antigen, or antibodies against early viral antigens are used in diagnosis. Due to the ubiquity of the virus, the presence of antibodies must be viewed with caution; a rising titer may indicate a primary infection. Viral DNA can also be demonstrated by PCR and Southern blot or in situ hybridization. Immunostaining of biopsied tissue sections can demonstrate infected cells.

Herpes Simplex Virus

Virology

Like other herpesviruses, HSV is a 150- to 200-nm dsDNA virus with a 100 nm icosahedral nucleocapsid (Fig. 6A) (29). Two major subtypes, HSV-1 (herpes labialis or human herpesvirus type 1) and HSV-2 (herpes genitalis or human herpesvirus type 2) are common causes of human infections. They have predilections for the perioral and genital regions, respectively, but are by no means restricted to these areas. Morphologically, single virions resemble those of other herpes viruses. However, HSV does not form the large cytoplasmic viral factories that develop in CMV infection; frequently, the virions are seen as single or double nucleocapsids inside cytoplasmic vesicles (Figs. 6D and E).

Epidemiology

Most cases of primary HSV infection are subclinical, and between 50 and 80% of individuals in the United States have antibodies to HSV by 30 years of age. Seroconversion is higher in lower socioeconomic groups, and occurs earlier in less developed countries (95). Establishment of latency in the trigeminal ganglia with one strain results in immunity to infection with another strain at that site. However, it is possible to be infected with different strains of HSV in different sites at the same time, particularly in AIDS patients. Patients infected with HSV-2 have some resistance to HSV-1, but the reverse is not true.

HSV-1 is responsible for most ocular HSV disease. Twenty percent of patients with ocular disease develop stromal disease, particularly after recurrent herpes keratitis, and more than half of these patients develop disciform keratitis (79). Most cases of HSV-2 ocular disease are genitally acquired, and mother to baby transmission may result in chorioretinitis, keratoconjunctivitis, optic atrophy, and/or encephalitis. Transmission usually occurs during birth, but transplacental infection can take place.

Clinical Presentation

Primary HSV infection may present as gingivostomatitis, pharyngitis, rhinitis, or tonsillitis, and the manifestations include fever, chills, myalgias, and lymphadenopathy. Vesicular eruptions may occur and resolve in about a week. Neonatal infection may result in disseminated disease, often affecting the liver, lungs, and CNS (140).

HSV DNA hides in the root ganglia of sensory nerves and can become reactivated during times of immune insufficiency (e.g., cancer patients on chemotherapy, HIV-infected individuals, and persons stressed from emotional trauma or sun exposure). During latency, most viral proteins are repressed; however, DNA remains active, and transcription produces RNA called the latency-associated transcripts whose function has not been clearly defined (35).

Primary ocular infection with HSV usually presents as acute follicular keratoconjunctivitis. It may be associated with lymphadenitis, ulcerative blepharitis, keratitis, or dacryoadenitis. In recurrent infections, epithelial ulcers, stromal interstitial keratitis, and iridocyclitis may be present. A postinfectious sterile ulceration may follow an impaired adhesion of the corneal epithelium to its underlying basal lamina.

Corneal ulceration is a common manifestation of HSV and is often associated with recurrences. The infection is thought to be via nerves rather than inoculation directly onto the cornea (136). Prognosis is poor due to delayed diagnosis and treatment and because of the rapid destruction of the cornea. Corneal disease is manifest in three ways. Lytic infection of the epithelium produces dendritic lesions, which may ulcerate if untreated. Under the ulcers, antigen-antibody-complement-mediated damage may produce white infiltrations that may progress to stromal vascularization of the cornea; they should be distinguished from secondary infections. Another form of corneal infection is disciform endotheliitis leading to stromal edema. This may result from a delayed hypersensitivity reaction in the cornea without necrosis or vascularization. In severe cases, there may be edema, folds in the Descemet membrane, and vascularization. This may progress to ulceration and stromal thinning with iritis. The other type of corneal disease is stromal keratitis, whereby the immune response causes inflammation, scarring, and eventually, corneal opacification (Fig. 9). The type of corneal disease may be a function of the strain of HSV as well as the genetic makeup of the host (137).

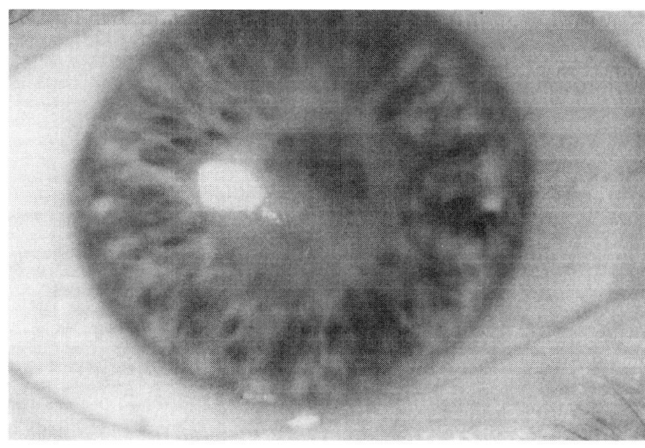

Figure 9 Severe herpes simplex virus-induced stromal keratitis.

HSV iritis may be granulomatous, with keratic precipitates in the corneal endothelium. Iridocyclitis and trabeculitis may lead to increased intraocular pressure (IOP). A nongranulomatous iridocyclitis can be present with or without skin lesions in immunosuppressed individuals. The eye may be red and painful with tearing, blurred vision, and miosis. Cells and a flare are present in the aqueous humor with glaucoma and sometimes hypopyon, thought to result from an immune reaction. The virus may directly invade the retina to cause a choroiditis and vitritis with retinal infiltrates, vascular sheathing and hemorrhage that results in permanent scarring and an atrophic retina.

HSV retinitis has a variable presentation that depends on the age and immune status of the patient. Documented intrauterine retinitis is rare and usually associated with CNS and skin infections. HSV retinitis may be contracted during delivery, and these cases are associated with infection of other tissues, such as the skin. Almost all reported cases of neonatal retinitis have been caused by HSV-2.

Adult HSV retinitis is usually bilateral, frequently associated with encephalitis, and caused by HSV-1. In immunosuppressed patients, retinitis is a rapidly progressive bilateral infection sometimes associated with a fatal encephalitis (127). Retinal whitening, vasculitis, papilledema, and nerve hemorrhage are characteristic and may result in early retinal detachment. Patients may present with blurred vision due to vitritis and pain from inflammation of the anterior segment. When the retina is visible through the inflammation, edema, hemorrhage, and vascular occlusion can be seen.

HSV retinitis in most documented reports has been in late stage disease, which does not shed light on its progression. In early disease, acute or chronic inflammation of the retina, RPE, and optic nerve may be present along with necrosis, hemorrhage, and/or vascular occlusion of the retina. Much of the tissue destruction is due to the immunological response.

The ARN syndrome can be caused by HSV-1 and HSV-2, as well as VZV, CMV, and rarely EBV. Symptoms may include floaters, decreased vision, ocular and periocular pain, and photophobia. Focal peripheral areas of necrotic retinitis rapidly become confluent. Vitritis, optic disc edema, retinal arteritis, vaso-occlusion, and granulomatous anterior uveitis may be present (124). The ARN syndrome caused by

HSV is associated with an exudative retinal detachment, while that resulting from VZV may not be.

Histopathology

HSV infection of the eyelid skin is manifest histologically in a fashion similar to that of skin elsewhere in the body, though eyelid lesions are uncommon. The earliest changes in HSV infection are seen in the epidermal cell nuclei, which enlarge, develop a homogenous "ground glass" appearance, and have peripherally clumped chromatin. Intraepidermal vesicles form secondary to ballooning and acantholysis of keratinocytes. Destruction of the basal layer of epidermis may result in subepidermal vesicles. Multinucleated keratinocytes are more conspicuous in lesions that have been present for several days. HSV infection causes eosinophilic nuclear inclusions, which are more common in the multinucleated cells (Fig. 10).

HSV infection of the conjunctiva results in follicular conjunctivitis (130), while corneal infection results in a complex array of histological manifestations (131). Corneas removed at penetrating keratoplasty often have edematous epithelium of irregular or interrupted thickness; fibrous or fibrovascular tissue between the epithelium and the residual Bowman layer (pannus); partial or complete absence of the Bowman layer due to anterior stromal scarring; stromal scarring, with or without stromal vascularization, in deeper layers of the stroma depending on the severity of the herpetic keratitis; a stromal infiltrate of chronic inflammatory cells of variable intensity; and folds or breaks in the Descemet membrane (131). All of these histological changes are nonspecific and may be seen in other forms of corneal injury, either traumatic or infectious (109). HSV keratitis may also result in granulomatous inflammation involving any layer of the stroma or in association with disrupted Descemet membrane (Fig. 11) (53,135). The presence of granulomatous inflammation together with stromal scarring is a useful, though not completely specific (109), marker for prior HSV keratitis. HSV antigens are detectable immunohistochemically in keratocytes, endothelial cells, and foci of epithelioid histiocytes and multinucleated giant cells around the Descemet membrane in some, but not all, corneas removed during graft surgery (53).

HSV retinitis exhibits retinal necrosis, chronic inflammation in the retina, and there may also be phlebitis, venous occlusion, arteritis, and chronic inflammation of the vitreous and choroid. Eosinophilic nuclear viral inclusions may be seen in retinal cells adjacent to the necrotic areas (Fig. 12) (45,55). Healed lesions are characterized by chorioretinal scarring.

Diagnosis

Skin lesions caused by HSV can be a clue to the causation of the associated ocular lesions. Diagnosis is usually made by viral culture or an immunofluorescent study of the abnormal tissue. ELISA on skin scrapings can detect antigen after treatment has been initiated when culture would be negative, and PCR can detect viral DNA. TEM of scrapings or fluid may disclose herpesvirus, but it would not be able to differentiate between different species. It can,

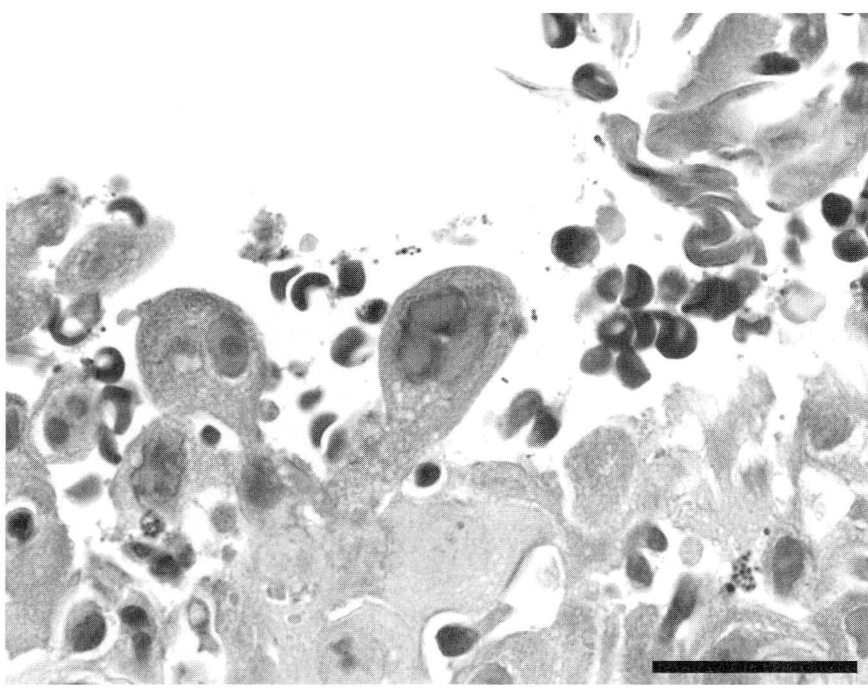

Figure 10 Herpes simplex virus (HSV) eyelid infection. HSV infection of the eyelid skin causes the epidermal cells to swell and lyse, resulting in intraepidermal vesicles. Epidermal cells may become multinucleated with eosinophilic nuclear inclusions, as exhibited by the cell in the center of this photomicrograph. Hematoxylin and eosin; bar = 25 μm.

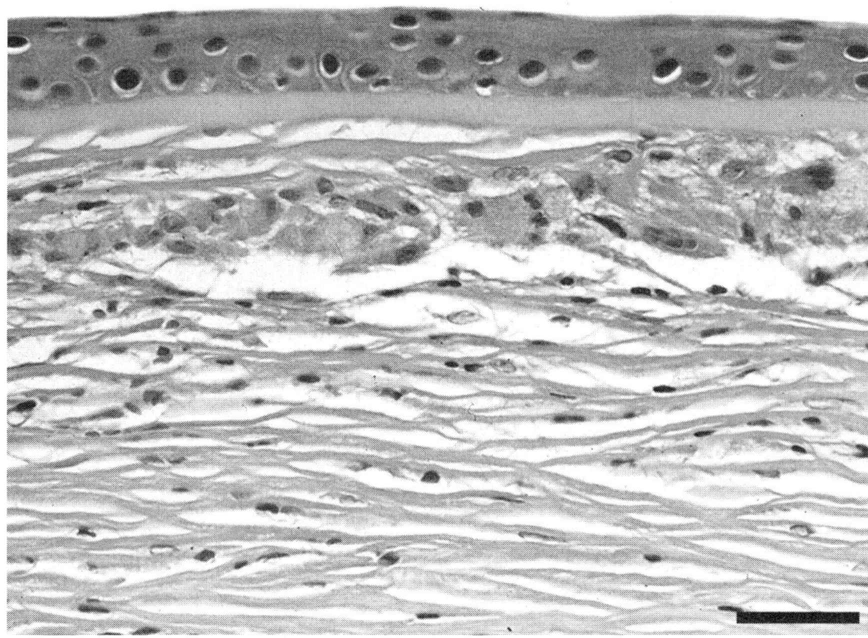

Figure 11 Herpes simplex virus (HSV) keratitis. HSV keratitis may lead to granulomatous inflammation involving any layer of the stroma. The presence of granulomatous inflammation together with stromal scarring is a useful, though not completely specific, marker for HSV keratitis. Hematoxylin and eosin; bar = 25 μm.

however, be useful in detecting virus initially and rapidly or in following a resolving infection after therapy when the virus does not grow in culture.

Herpes Virus B

Virology

Herpes virus B (HV-B) (also known as Cercopithecine herpesvirus 1, Herpesvirus simiae, monkey B virus, or B-virus) is morphologically and genetically similar to HSV as described above.

Epidemiology

HV-B is indigenous in macaque monkeys (*Macaca* sp.), which are 30% to 80% seropositive. It has also been isolated from other species of monkeys. The virus can be transmitted by bites, scratches, or punctures from contaminated instruments (133). Most human HV-B

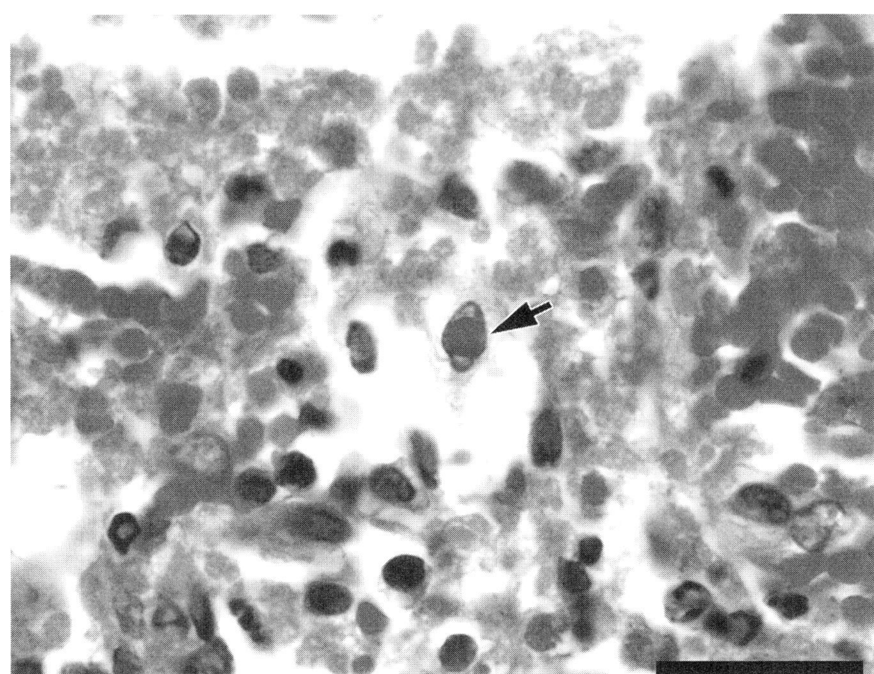

Figure 12 Herpes simplex virus (HSV) retinitis. HSV retinitis results in retinal necrosis, and there may be large, eosinophilic, nuclear inclusions in retinal cells (*arrow*). Hematoxylin and eosin; bar = 25 μm.

disease has been contracted from monkeys without apparent lesions; thus, anyone handling these animals should consider all potentially infective. Fortunately, human disease is rare because contact with these animals is uncommon, except in animal handlers like laboratory workers. The mortality rate is high despite treatment with antiviral drugs. Latency has not been documented in humans, perhaps because of the high lethality.

Clinical Presentation

The disease depends on the exposure site and the amount of inoculum and starts with general flu-like symptoms. There may be lymphadenitis, gastrointestinal upset, abdominal pain and hiccups. Spread to the CNS results in a rapid ascending meningitis and encephalitis. It can progress to necrotizing retinitis, retinal scarring, retinal detachment, optic nerve atrophy, and panuveitis, even in immunocompetent individuals. Once disease from HV-B spreads, deaths from respiratory failure due to ascending paralysis are frequent (58).

Histopathology

One report documented the ocular histopathologic findings in a fatal case of HV-B infection, which occurred after a cutaneous penetrating wound from a rhesus monkey. The man died 6 weeks after his injury, and examination of the patient's left eye revealed a multifocal necrotizing retinitis associated with a vitritis, optic neuritis, and prominent panuveitis. Herpes-type virus was identified in the involved retina by TEM, and postmortem vitreous cultures and retinal cultures were positive for HV-B. Thus, HV-B produces infection and destruction of retinal tissues similar to that seen in other herpesvirus infections (97).

Diagnosis

Since other herpesviruses can cause symptoms similar to HV-B infection, a history of a monkey bite is a significant diagnostic clue. A rising CF titer, a positive ELISA for anti HV-B antibodies, and virus culture may be used to confirm the diagnosis. In the absence of a monkey bite, Lyme disease, rickettsioses, and Behçet disease may be considered in the event of both CNS and retinal involvement.

Kaposi Sarcoma Herpes Virus

Virology

Kaposi sarcoma herpes virus (KSHV) (human herpesvirus type 8) is morphologically similar to other viruses in the herpes virus family. It belongs to the Rhadinovirus genus in the subfamily Gammaherpesvirinae and is the only human pathogenic rhadinovirus discovered to date. Like other herpesviruses, it can replicate in two ways: a lytic and a latent mode. In the former, the viral DNA is produced by a viral polymerase and packaged into infectious particles. In the latter, circular viral episomes replicate with host DNA using host enzymes. The reservoir during asymptomatic infection is CD19+ B cells (3).

Epidemiology

Kaposi sarcoma (KS) is a vascular tumor (see Chapter 62) seen in HIV-positive individuals and HIV-negative elderly men from certain areas including the Mediterranean, Africa, and Asia. KSHV infection is necessary, but not sufficient, for tumor formation; genetic and immunologic factors alter risk for KS (48). KSHV has been reported in a 20-year-old (non HIV-infected) treated with 0.1% Tacrolimus (FK-506) ointment for atopic blepharitis and dermatitis. The facial lesions resolved with intravenous acyclovir therapy (91).

Clinical Presentation

In AIDS patients, transplant recipients, and in young children, the infection is particularly aggressive and can disseminate to cause death. KSHV may cause three proliferative diseases, KS, body cavity-based or primary effusion lymphoma, and a plasma cell form of multicentric Castleman disease in AIDS patients. It can also result in acute failure of bone marrow transplants to engraft.

In AIDS patients, ~2% have ocular KS; of those, 10% to 20% have eyelid or conjunctival tumors (60).

Histopathology

KS involving the eyelid is similar histologically to that in the skin covering other body sites (87). Proliferations of irregular, often jagged, vascular channels within the dermis are features of the patch stage of KS. The vascular channels have thin walls lined by plump or inconspicuous endothelial cells. Some channels have perivascular lymphocytes and plasma cells, and there may be extravasated erythrocytes and hemosiderin deposits. The plaque and nodular stages of KS feature interlacing bundles of spindle cells and poorly defined, slit-like vessels within the dermis (Fig. 13). Chronic inflammatory cells are present focally, and there are extravasated erythrocytes and deposits of hemosiderin. There may be small, eosinophilic hyaline globules within the cell cytoplasm or extracellularly; these are positive using periodic acid-Schiff stain, and they are bright red with the Masson trichrome stain. KSs of the conjunctiva (130) and eyelid, but not in the deep orbit, which lacks lymphatic vessels (61), have an appearance similar to those in the plaque and nodular stages in the skin. Antibodies to KSHV stain the nuclei of infected cells (Fig. 14).

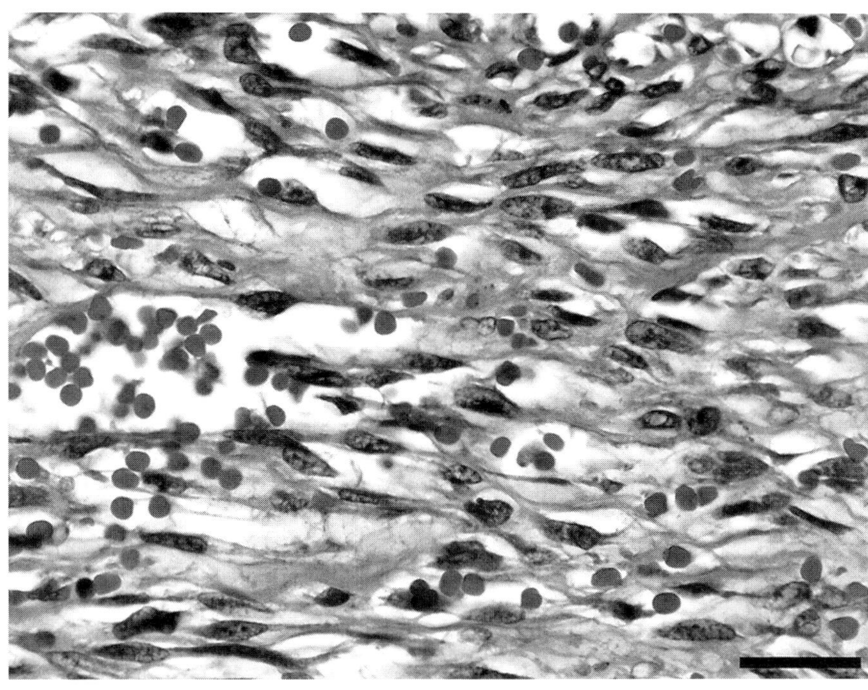

Figure 13 Kaposi sarcoma. Interlacing bundles of spindle cells and poorly defined vascular channels are histological features of Kaposi sarcoma. Hematoxylin and eosin; bar = 25 μm.

Diagnosis

Serological assays can detect KSHV in ~90% of infected individuals. Indirect fluorescence staining is used to detect antibodies in patient sera when incubated with infected cells. Various assays have different positive and negative attributes; detection of the latency-associated nuclear antigen is easy and results in low false positive results, but is subjective. Assays for the lytic antigen and an ELISA for the complete virion are more sensitive but have a risk of cross-reactivity with lymphocyte antigens. Tests using recombinant antigens have been described and are being refined, but a combination of tests provides the best opportunity for detection (70). PCR for viral DNA

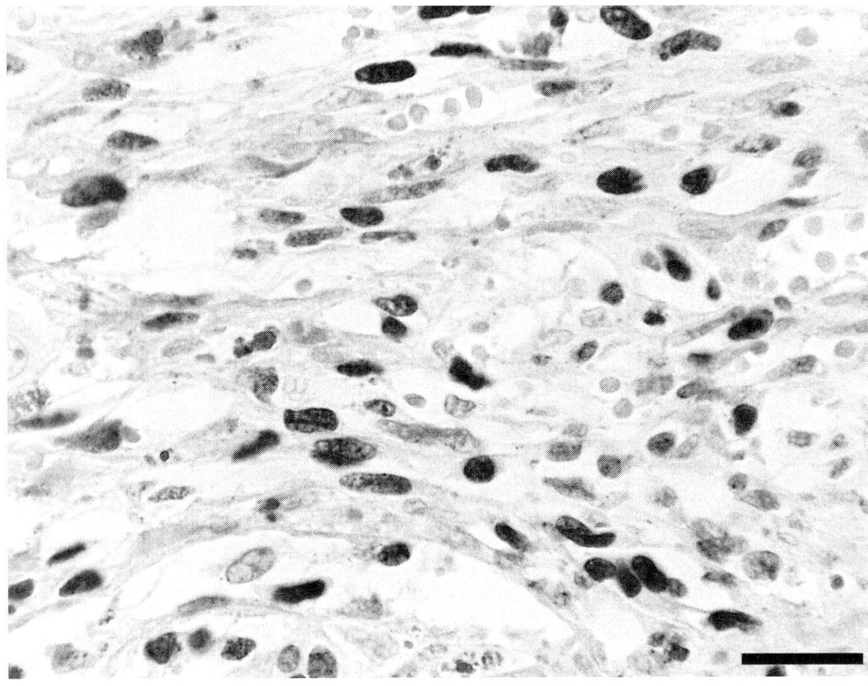

Figure 14 Antibodies to Kaposi sarcoma herpesvirus (KSHV) cause nuclear staining of the infected endothelial cells in Kaposi sarcoma. Immunohistochemical stain with anti-KSHV antibody; bar = 25 μm.

in serum is less sensitive, suggesting that viremia is not a significant feature of KS.

Varicella Zoster Virus

Virology

Varicella zoster virus (herpes zoster virus, varicella virus, human herpesvirus type 3) is morphologically similar to other members of the herpesvirus family (29).

Epidemiology

The virus is ubiquitous, but after a vaccine was developed in 1995, the prevalence of the infection and the sequelae of reactivation were dramatically reduced. Until a vaccine became available, close to 3 million cases of VZV infection were diagnosed in the United States per year, peaking in the spring. The infection is spread by contact with skin lesions or respiratory secretions. In infected individuals, VZV retinitis can occur in all ages from infancy to the elderly in either primary disease or reactivation. It may occur in both normal and immunocompromised individuals, though a genetic predisposition has been reported (54).

Clinical Presentation

VZV gains entry via infection of the upper respiratory tract. In non-vaccinated individuals, after local replication, the virus spreads through the lymphatic system in monocytes/macrophages, producing a viremia that may last 2 to 3 weeks, followed by a primary cutaneous vesicular eruption referred to as varicella or chickenpox. The cutaneous vesicles of varicella are of variable size and usually form scabs that heal without scarring. These are major distinguishing characteristics from poxvirus lesions: deep-seated vesicles that often leave scars and are generally all at the same stage at any given time.

Following primary cutaneous infection, VZV spreads through nerves to the dorsal root ganglia, where it establishes latency in almost all cases (80). It can subsequently become reactivated in the setting of immunosuppression due to a variety of causes, including stress, waning immunity in the elderly, cancer therapy, or AIDS. Upon reactivation, it travels from the dorsal root ganglia back to the skin surface, causing a painful condition called zoster or shingles. Zoster is frequently preceded by a flu-like prodrome with fever, malaise, and fatigue. Typical lesions begin with a burning sensation and then erupt into painful blisters, usually over a single dermatome, sometimes affecting the ophthalmic division of the trigeminal nerve and resulting in ocular involvement. The lesions appear initially as macules and then progress to papules and vesicles that eventually rupture and crust over.

Pneumonia and encephalitis have been diagnosed in very few cases of VZV infection, usually in immunocompromised hosts or in fetuses of non-immune mothers. In mothers who contract either varicella or zoster during pregnancy, congenital infection can occur with serious consequences, including skin or chorioretinal scars, optic nerve atrophy, retinopathy microphthalmia, cataracts, retardation, and limb hypoplasia (63).

Herpes zoster ophthalmicus results when VZV reactivates in the ophthalmic division of the trigeminal nerve (Fig. 15). It accounts for about 25% of cases of shingles. Conjunctivitis, episcleritis and scleritis are seen in half the cases and appear as hemorrhages and a regional lymphadenopathy. Ptosis and a secondary bacterial infection may occur.

Punctate epithelial keratitis consisting of multiple lesions may progress to a dendritic pattern resembling the corneal ulceration of herpes simplex or plaques of swollen epithelial cells. Finely granular infiltrates under the epithelium are thought to be antigen–antibody complexes. This may lead to anterior stromal keratitis about a week after the initial symptoms. Keratitis occurs in 40% of the patients and may appear with or without stromal edema or ulceration; it may be mistaken for HSV keratitis. Rarely, this may progress to a deep stromal keratitis with edema. Neovascularization with lipid infiltrates may occur, or there may be corneal melting and perforation. Severe corneal

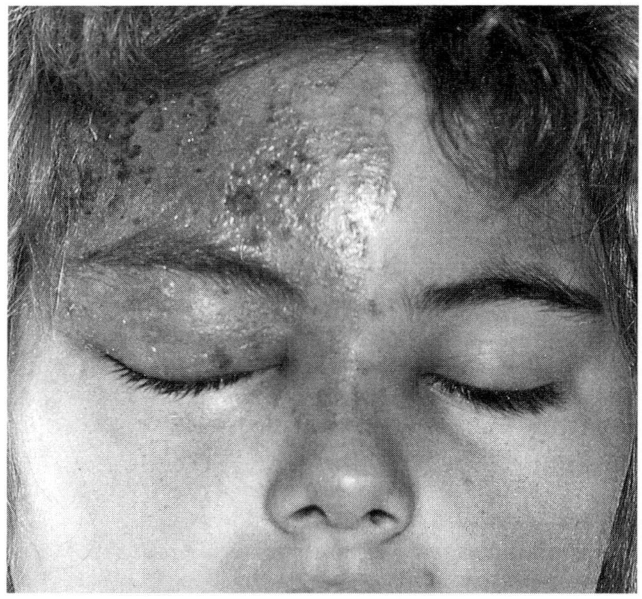

Figure 15 Herpes zoster ophthalmicus. A vesicular eruption of the skin involves the ophthalmic division of the trigeminal nerve. *Source*: Reproduced from Klintworth GK, Landers MB, III. The Eye. Baltimore, MD: Williams & Wilkins, 1976.

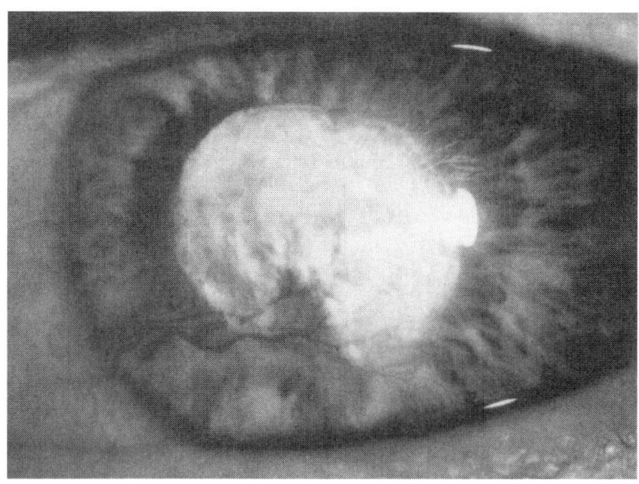

Figure 16 Severe corneal scarring with lipid deposition following herpes zoster ophthalmicus.

scarring and lipid deposition can occur as sequelae (Fig. 16).

Uveitis without corneal disease is rare, and when present, it may be misdiagnosed, or diagnosis may be delayed with a poor prognosis (118). There may be vascular occlusion, scleritis, and uveitis. Iris atrophy, hypopyon, anterior segment necrosis, and phthisis bulbi may be caused by vasculitis. Glaucoma may occur acutely or several months later. Other potential serious sequelae include chronic ocular inflammation, vision loss, and disabling pain (118,122).

Retinitis occasionally develops during the primary infection or more frequently during reactivation. It may present as ARN, which was originally described in otherwise healthy individuals; it has since been shown to occur more frequently in patients with specific histocompatibility types, including HLA-DQw7, Bw62, and DR4 (54). Initially, patients may experience pain, photophobia, and vitreous "floaters." Manifestations include focal areas of necrosis in the peripheral retina, which may progress rapidly in the absence of antiviral therapy; vasculopathy; and inflammation in the vitreous and anterior chamber. Optic atrophy, scleritis, and ocular pain may also occur. With treatment, many immunocompetent patients have a good visual prognosis.

AIDS patients with a low CD4 cell count (110) and others with immunodeficiencies (78) may experience a deep retinal opacification with minimal vitritis called progressive outer retinal necrosis (PORN). A painless reduction in central vision follows the progression of the retinal lesions to confluence without much inflammation and finally to complete retinal necrosis. Unlike CMV retinitis, PORN is multifocal, lacks granular borders and hemorrhage, and spreads rapidly (26). In contrast to ARN, both eyes are frequently affected, and retinal vasculitis and optic neuritis develop less often. The infection has a limited response to therapy, and the prognosis is poor, with most patients eventually losing the ability to perceive light.

Post-herpetic neuralgia occasionally occurs and may last months or years. Affected individuals may become depressed and even suicidal. Rarely, optic neuritis or cranial nerve palsies may occur.

Histopathology

Eyelid lesions of VZV infection are intraepidermal vesicles with swollen and multinucleated epidermal cells (Fig. 17). The swollen epidermal cells lose their attachment to adjacent cells and separate from them. If this process involves basal epidermal cells, then a subepidermal vesicle may result. Eosinophilic nuclear inclusions are found in some of the multinucleated keratinocytes, and polymorphonuclear leukocyes (PMNs) are present within vesicles and within the subjacent dermis. Follicular conjunctivitis often accompanies the eyelid infection (130), and there may be corneal involvement with chronic inflammation, scarring and stromal vascularization (109,131). Eyes removed from patients after herpes zoster ophthalmicus have histopathological findings that may include perineuritis, patchy or diffuse iris and ciliary body necrosis, retinal thrombophlebitis, and granulomatous choroiditis (45). Retinal infection in immunocompromised patients, such as those with AIDS, causes progressive necrosis of the outer retina (45), and eosinophilic nuclear viral inclusions are sometimes evident in the residual retinal cells (Fig. 18).

Diagnosis

Blister fluid, vitreous, or retinal biopsy sections can be examined on slides by immunofluorescence microscopy; this technique is faster than culture and is more likely to be positive if transportation of the specimen is delayed. VZV can be grown in culture from material obtained from active lesions, but it is labile and must be transported and planted onto cells soon after being harvested. Unlike HSV-1 and HSV-2, both of which can be isolated in culture from latent infections of nerve ganglia, culture of VZV from sites of latency has not been successful. Cultures of human fibroblast origin (amnion, human embryo lung fibroblasts, and human thyroid gland) support growth, but replication takes longer than HSV—up to a week. The use of shell vials and centrifugation can hasten growth to within 24 to 48 hours. Culture is more likely to be positive if specimens are taken during the acute phase of

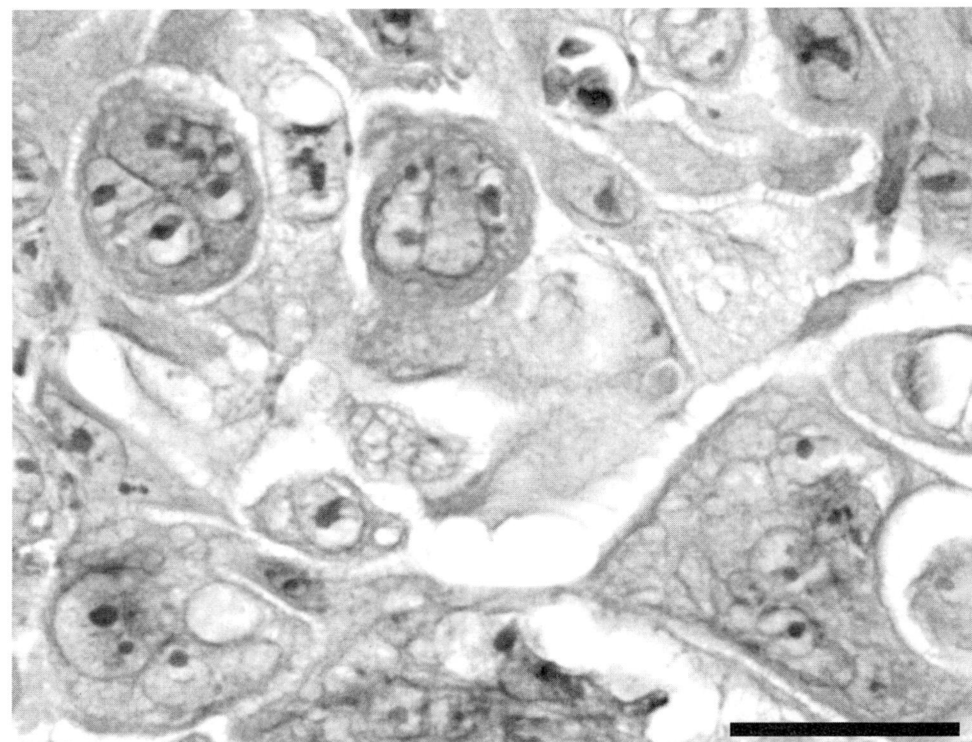

Figure 17 Herpes zoster eyelid infection. Swollen and multinucleated epidermal cells are a prominent feature in herpes zoster infection of the eyelid. Hematoxylin and eosin; bar = 25 μm.

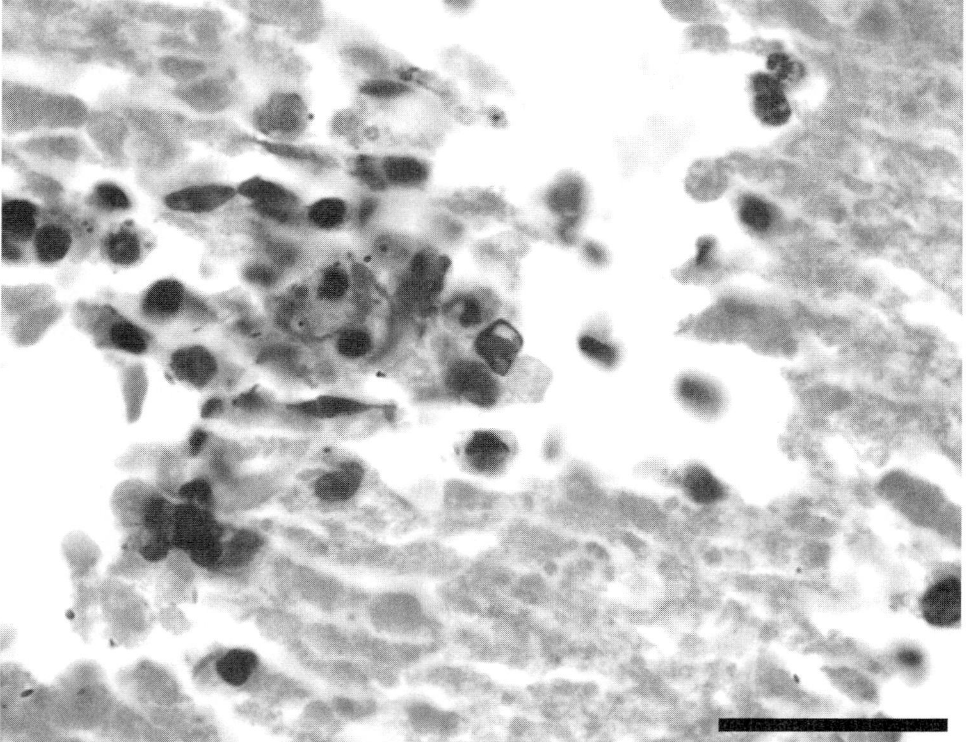

Figure 18 Herpes zoster retinitis in a patient with acute retinal necrosis. Most of the tissue is necrotic, but one of the residual cells (slightly left of center) displays a prominent intranuclear inclusion. Hematoxylin and eosin; bar = 25 μm.

infection. Antiviral drug therapy reduces the likelihood of virus isolation.

PCR is a sensitive method for detecting the VZV genome and can be performed within hours. Care must be taken to avoid cross-contamination to prevent false positive results.

Orthomyxoviruses

Virology

Orthomyxoviruses are ssRNA enveloped viruses that include influenza type A viruses, influenza type B viruses, influenza type C viruses, and two other genuses (*Thogotovirus* and *Isavirus*) with similar morphology. *Thogotovirus* is transmitted to vertebrates by ticks in central Africa, Egypt, and Sicily. *Isavirus* causes disease in fish. The spherical or ovoid particles are typically 80 to 120 nm in diameter (Fig. 19A), and some strains produce long filamentous particles of 80 by over 1000 nm. The surface is studded with "spikes" composed of hemagglutinin and neuraminidase proteins that are important in virus adherence to the cell surface and penetration into cells. The RNA is packaged into a helical nucleocapsid 9 to 15 nm in diameter. Influenza viruses are produced in the cell cytoplasm; the nucleocapsids migrate to the cell membrane into which viral proteins have been incorporated, and bud into the extracellular space through the plasma membrane (Figs. 19B and C).

Epidemiology

Influenza type A viruses (including avian influenza) are subtyped based on surface proteins (hemagglutinin and fusion proteins). Genome recombination is common when different strains are present in the same host and frequently occurs in Asia where human, avian, and swine species live in close proximity. Another form of alteration is antigenic shift, which is a sudden major mutation of the genes encoding surface proteins, recognized in influenza A, but not influenza B. Influenza viruses can also change by antigenic drift, small alterations that happen continually over time, eventually rendering a strain unrecognizable by the immune system.

Influenza epidemics occur in cycles about every 2 to 3 years, depending on the antigenic makeup of the surface antigens. These changes in surface proteins (recombination, shift, and drift) are responsible for the constant guesswork of world health care providers and vaccine producers in their attempt to produce flu vaccines that contain the strains most likely to be in the western community the following year.

Influenza B virus circulates widely in people, but not in animals. It does not undergo rapid change, and is not subtyped. Influenza C results in a mild illness and is not believed to cause epidemics.

Influenza viruses do not cause latency in the traditional sense, although some neurological diseases may follow infection. These may include optic neuritis, extraocular muscle palsy, accommodative abnormalities, mydriasis, and papilledema (124). Additionally, since more than one strain may be transmitted, it is possible for an individual to recover from the flu and then contract the infection again from a different strain during the same season.

Clinical Presentation

Patients with influenza present with fever, headache, and myalgia. The symptoms start acutely and progress rapidly, more so than the common cold. The disease is self-limiting and resolves after about a week; however, young, old, and debilitated individuals may suffer cardiopulmonary complications and sometimes death. Some strains of influenza virus, such as the 1918 strain and avian influenza, have caused high mortality even in normal individuals.

Conjunctivitis, iritis, interstitial keratitis, and dacryoadenitis may be present during the acute phase, but usually resolve after several weeks. Macular hemorrhage, a macular lipid star vasculopathy and/or retinitis may occur concomitant with influenza, suggesting the influenza virus may be responsible. Retinitis with hemorrhage and edema may resolve with time, returning the patient to normal vision but leaving microscopic residua (111).

Histopathology

We are unaware of any reports of ocular histopathology of human eyes after influenza virus infection. Injection of influenza virus into the anterior chamber of rabbits and guinea pigs causes corneal clouding due to endothelial damage (65). Iridocyclitis and uveitis are also reported following inoculation of human influenza virus into the anterior chamber of the guinea pig eye (114).

Diagnosis

A diagnosis of influenza can be established by an immunohistochemical evaluation of cells from a nasopharyngeal aspiration (Fig. 20). Serological confirmation can be done by detecting a four-fold rise in anti-influenza virus titers by ELISA, HI, or CF.

Papillomaviruses

The Papillomaviridae family contains 16 genuses, four of which cause disease in humans and are designated alpha-, beta-, gamma-, and nupapillomaviruses. *Pa*pillomaviruses used to be included together with

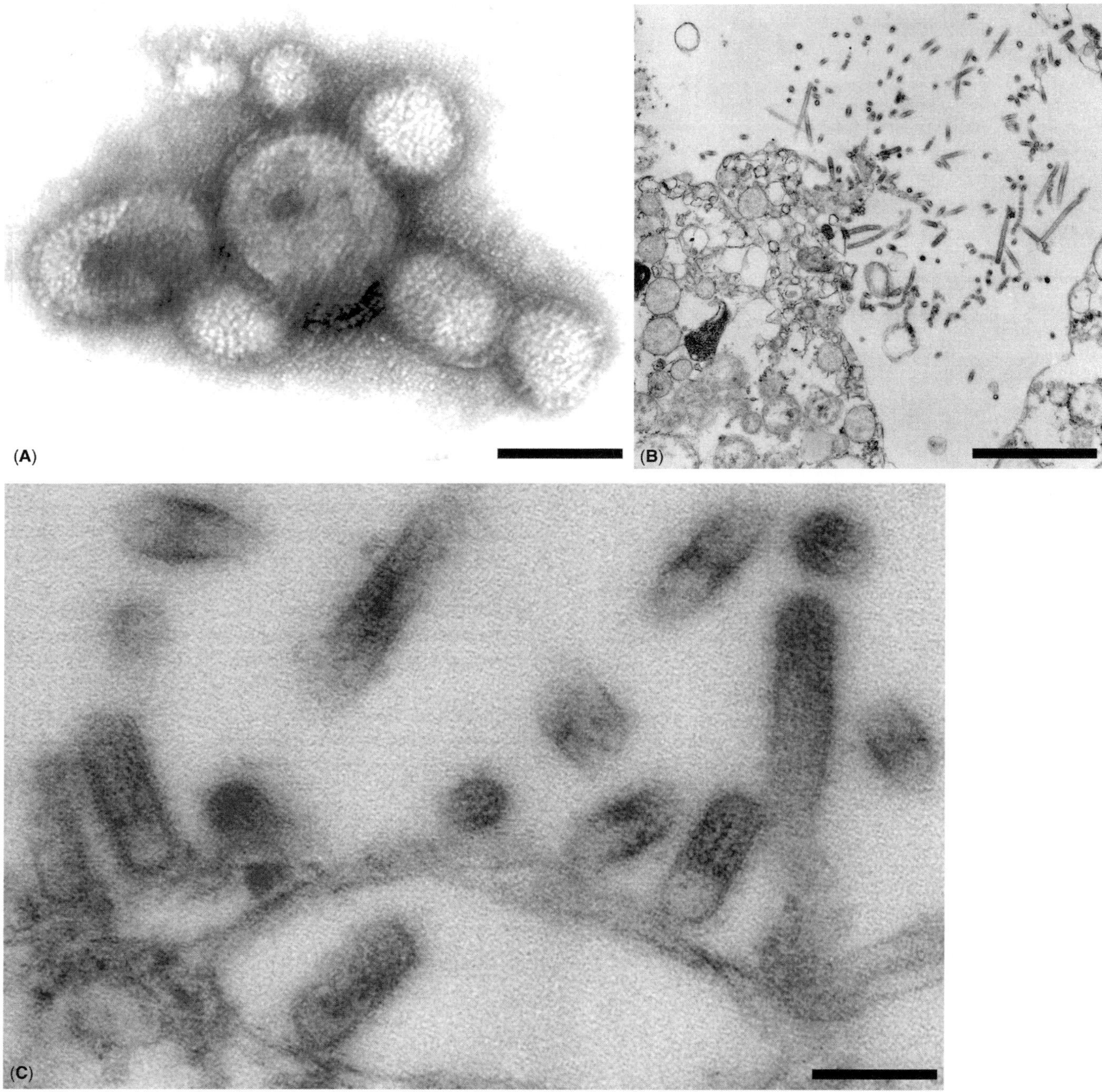

Figure 19 Orthomyxoviruses. (**A**) Negative stain of influenza A virus. Virus particles are enveloped with 8- to 9-nm spikes of hemagglutinin and fusion proteins on the surface. They may be round, ovoid, or long and filamentous (80 nm by up to 1000 nm). Bar = 100 nm. (**B**) Low magnification of thin section of influenza virus budding from the cytoplasmic membrane of an infected cell. Bar = 1 μm. *Source*: Courtesy of C.S. Goldsmith and Dr. E.L. Palmer, Centers for Disease Control and Prevention. (**C**) High magnification of budding particles. Bar = 100 nm. *Source*: Courtesy of C.S. Goldsmith and Dr. E.L. Palmer, Centers for Disease Control and Prevention.

*po*lyomaviruses and *va*cuolating agent (pa-po-va) in the Papovaviridae family, as they were all naked icosahedral viruses with similar morphology. The former papovaviruses all have now been categorized into separate families (29). Papillomaviruses are 55 nm in diameter, slightly larger than polyomaviruses, but otherwise indistinguishable in TEM of negative stains (see Fig. 23A). In TEM of thin sections, they appear in

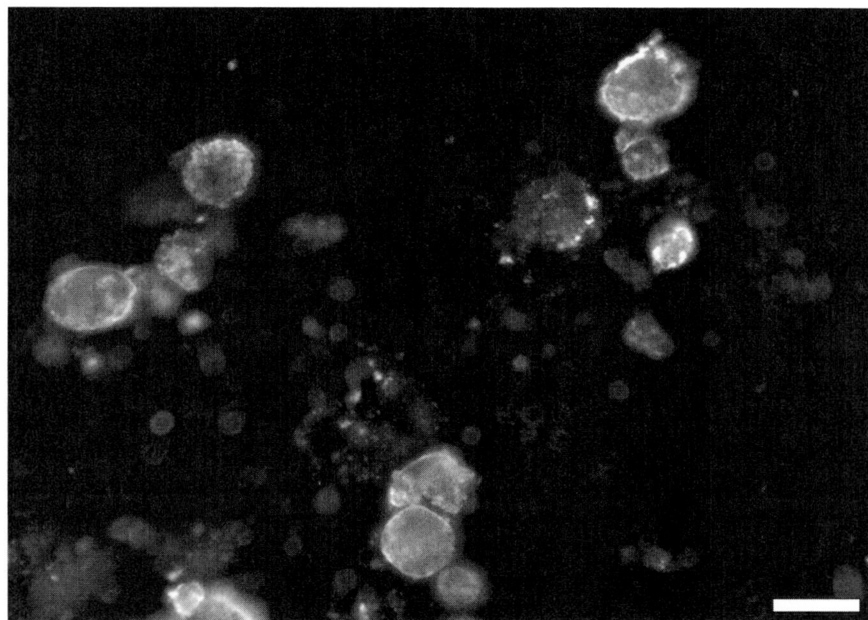

Figure 20 Fluorescence micrograph of influenza A-infected cells. Immunostaining is in a diffuse cytoplasmic pattern and frequently is denser at the edge where the virions bud out. Additionally, some nuclear proteins fluoresce; however, note that complete, enveloped virions are not found in the nucleus by transmission electron microscopy. *Source*: Courtesy of Dr. N.G. Henshaw, Duke University.

the nuclei of cells; sometimes in paracrystalline arrays (see polyomavirus thin sections).

Virology

The papillomavirus genome is circular dsDNA, and may exist in an integrated form in cells (e.g., in cervical cancers) or may be present in an episomal state (e.g., in skin carcinomas). All human papillomaviruses (HPV) require terminal differentiation of host cells for replication and virus production (29). They do not grow in routine diagnostic tissue culture, and can be propagated (inefficiently) only in specialized research conditions. There are over 60 serotypes, and they are very host-specific and tissue restricted.

Epidemiology

Several strains are found in ocular disease. Types 6 and 11 infect mucous membranes like conjunctiva and form papillomatous or condylomatous lesions, while types 5, 8, 16, and 18 cause epithelial dysplasia or carcinoma. Transmission is by close contact, and the rate of new infections with papillomavirus is increasing dramatically.

Viral DNA has been identified in the majority of conjunctival papillomata, dysplasias, and carcinomas (86). However, it has also been detected in the conjunctiva in the absence of ocular disease. Ultraviolet light (UV) had been thought to be responsible for conjunctival neoplasia in papillomavirus-infected tissue; however, this has not been verified. Smokers have an increased risk of conjunctival dysplasia as they do of cervical carcinoma. An immune deficiency is associated with an increased risk of HPV infections.

Unlike herpesvirus infections, papillomavirus infections do not undergo a latent phase in which the disease goes into remission and reappears at a later date. However, the DNA can be present in deep tissues that are not actively producing virions, and excision of visible wart tissue may not yield a cure due to persistence of viral nucleic acid in the tissue. Additionally, some strains (types 16 and 18) are oncogenic and cause cervical carcinomas well as conjunctival dysplasias and carcinomas (see Chapter 57).

Clinical Presentation

Papillomata on the conjunctiva are usually pedunculated fleshy growths that may be heavily vascularized. Inverted papillomata, though rare, are the most common manifestation in the lacrimal sac; they invaginate into the stroma as opposed to forming warty structures. Dysplastic and carcinomatous conjunctival lesions may result from solitary or multiple infections of the squamous epithelia on the cornea or conjunctiva. They may be white, gray, or yellow, and pedunculated or sessile lesions. Many involve the junction between corneal and conjunctival epithelium, a transition zone that may favor rapid cellular turnover conducive to cancer.

Histopathology

Conjunctival papillomas are most often pedunculated lesions with fibrovascular cores covered by epithelium having a variable proportion of non-keratinizing squamous epithelial cells and goblet cells (130). There may be a variable degree of acute inflammation in the papilloma, depending on how much irritation has resulted from its presence. Papillomas of the conjunctiva arising at the corneoscleral limbus tend to be sessile, flat, and with a broad base (130). The epithelium of sessile limbal papillomas is usually moderately to markedly thickened, and it often has only a few goblet cells among the non-keratinizing squamous epithelial cells. There are fibrovascular cores within the thick epithelium (130). Inverted papillomas of the conjunctiva are characterized by lobules of epithelium that appear to push into the substantia propria (130). The epithelium is composed of non-keratinizing squamous epithelial cells with a varying number of goblet cells.

Conjunctival intraepithelial neoplasia is a term used to encompass lesions varying from mild dysplasia through carcinoma in situ (27) (see Chapter 57). The dysplastic lesions have disorganized, cytologically atypical cells occupying a variable proportion of the epithelial thickness depending on whether the degree of dysplasia is mild, moderate, or severe (130). In situ carcinoma of the conjunctiva has epithelial cells with malignant cytological features occupying the full thickness of the epithelium but without invasion of the underlying substantia propria.

Histologically, verruca vulgaris has marked hyperkeratosis and acanthosis with prominent papillomatosis in the filiform variant. The papillomatous projections have parakeratosis, often arranged as vertical tiers. The granular cell layer is usually prominent, and the cells contain coarse clumps of basophilic keratohyaline granules. Cells infected with papillomavirus may be evident in the granular cell layer as vacuolated cells with deeply basophilic nuclei surrounded by a clear halo (32). Dilated capillary loops may be conspicuous in the core of the papillary projections.

Diagnosis

Aside from the tissue diagnosis by light microscopy, immunohistochemical methods are the usual routes of identifying papilloma viral antigens. Molecular diagnostic techniques include Southern blot and in situ hybridization. PCR is a highly sensitive procedure for identifying HPV DNA in small ocular specimens. TEM is not useful due to the fact that the diagnostic infected cells may not produce recognizable virions.

Paramyxoviruses

The Paramyxoviridae family is divided into two subfamilies: the Paramyxovirinae, with 7 genera (e.g., mumps, measles, hendra viruses, and others) and the Pneumovirinae, with 2 genera (e.g., respiratory syncytial virus and metapneumovirus) (29). They contain linear ssRNA within a helical (like a Slinky) nucleocapsid of 13- to 18-nm diameter and up to 1000 nm long. The complete enveloped virion is widely pleomorphic, ranging from 100 to 300 nm in diameter, with 8- to 9-nm hemagglutinin and/or neuraminidase "spikes" or "fuzz" on the surface (Fig. 21A). Some genera lack neuraminidase and others lack hemagglutination activity. The nucleocapsids are helical filaments 18 nm in diameter and may be up to 1000 nm long (Fig. 21B). In thin sections, nucleocapsids can be seen in the cytoplasm as "wormy" structures in virus factories. They migrate to the cytoplasmic membrane that has been programmed to contain viral proteins and bud out into the extracellular space, taking cell membrane as their outer covering. In thin sections, the budding virus has a thickened, darker-appearing membrane resulting from the viral hemagglutinin and neuraminidase spikes on the surface (Figs. 21C and D). Paramyxoviruses morphologically resemble orthomyxoviruses in that they are both enveloped particles with spikes on the outside. In general, the orthomyxoviruses are more ovoid (~100 nm) with long filamentous particles (100 × 1500 nm), while the paramyxoviruses are more pleomorphic, ranging up to ~300 nm in a globular shape, and do not usually form long filaments. However, this generalization is of populations as a whole, and individual particles in each family may be identical to those in the other.

Paramyxoviruses are mainly found in mammals and birds, although they have been reported rarely in fish and reptiles (29). They are eliminated by the immune system though long-term shedding can occur. Latent infection is unknown, although long-term infection with a defective strain can occur in subacute sclerosing panencephalitis (SSPE) and in canine distemper. Paramyxoviruses can be grown in cell culture where the infection is usually lytic, but can be

Figure 21 (*Shown on facing page*) Paramyxoviruses. (**A**) Negative stain of measles virus. Note the fuzz or fringe around the outside, similar to orthomyxoviruses. The enveloped particles are pleomorphic. Bar = 100 nm. (**B**) Negative stain of naked helical nucleocapsids. Bar = 100 nm. (**C**) Low magnification of measlesvirus-infected cell. Curvy helical nucleocapsids develop in the cytoplasm (*arrow*) and migrate to the cytoplasmic membrane where they bud out through areas containing some viral proteins. The dense areas of the cytoplasmic membrane contain virus-coded proteins, and the dark-rimmed vesicles to the right of the cell are complete virions. Bar = 1 μm. (**D**) High magnification of budding measles virus. Bar = 100 nm.

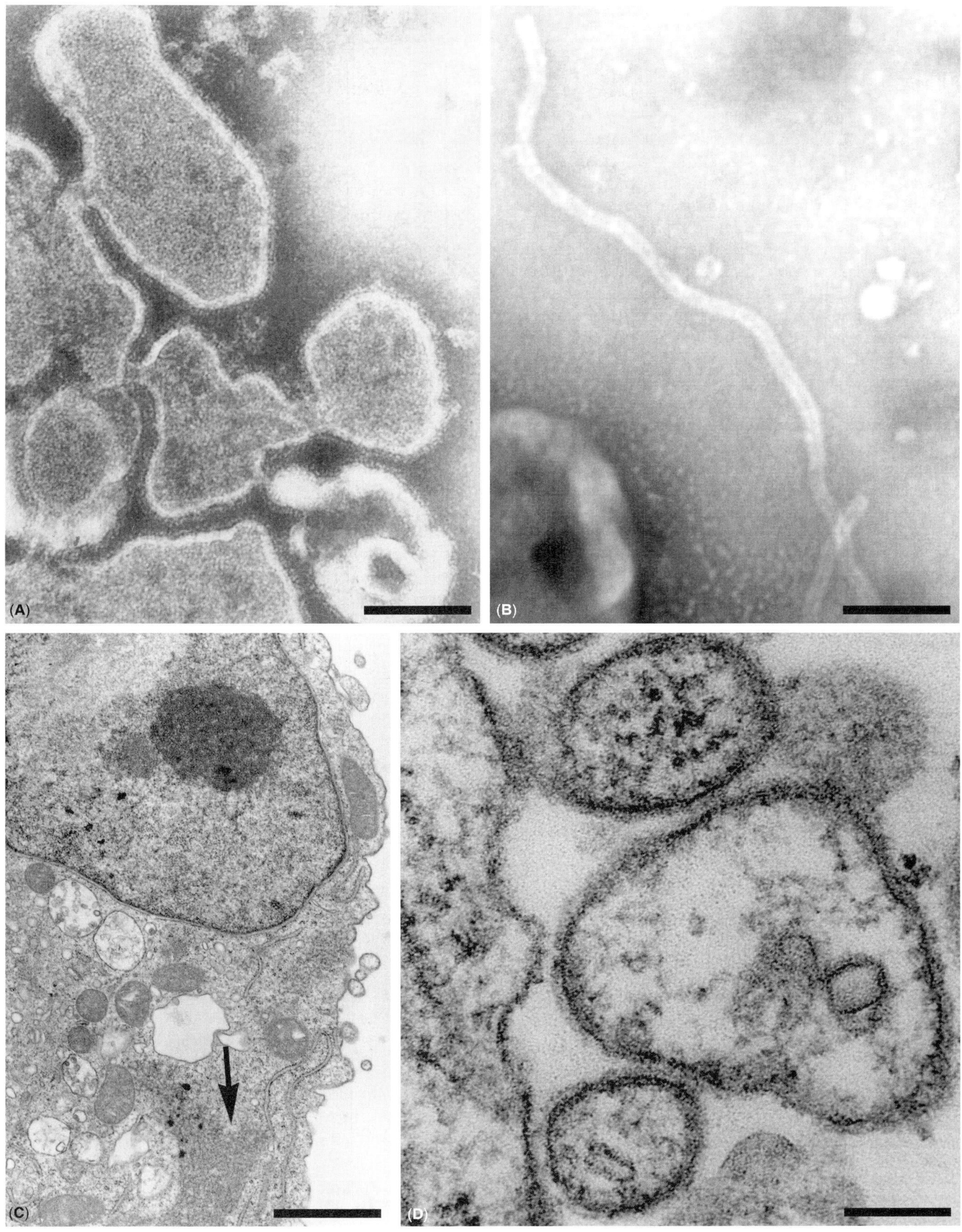
(A)
(B)
(C)
(D)

persistent. Syncytia (giant fused cells with multiple nuclei) are common.

Measles

Virology

Rubeola (measles) virus (Fig. 21A) is a paramyxovirus and lacks neuraminidase activity. A variant of the measles virus that causes SSPE is a slow virus, a term given to agents that take months to years to produce symptoms (see below). Wild type measles virus nucleocapsids are found in the cytoplasm of infected cells; however, in persistent measles virus infections (long-term infections that do not kill the cells) in tissue culture and in SSPE in vivo, nucleocapsids, but not the whole virus, can be seen in the nucleus.

Transmission is by aerosols, and vectors are not known. Measles is a rare disease in the United States today due to the introduction of a vaccine in 1963, but it still occurs in non-immunized children and occasionally in older children who received the vaccine at an early age. A booster is now being given, which has reduced the number of cases. However, in developing countries more than a million children per year die as a result of measles. There is a push by the World Health Organization (WHO) to provide vaccines to these countries.

Epidemiology

The measles virus is transmitted in nasopharyngeal secretions, either airborne or via contact with droplets on mucous membranes where it replicates. It is then spread through the mononuclear phagocytic system causing hyperplasia of infected epithelia and multinucleated giant cells. Viremia ensues.

Clinical Presentation

After an incubation period of a week and a half, mild fever, cough, coryza, and conjunctivitis begin. The temperature increases over the next week; Koplik spots (small red spots with a bluish white center) appear in the mouth, and a rash appears, first around the ears, forehead and neck, then spreading to the trunk. The Koplik spots grow and coalesce to cover the whole membranous surface with numerous whitish peaks. The erythema and rash diminish after a few days leaving a brownish skin tone. Three different forms of CNS disease may occur (100). Acute postinfectious encephalitis is due to an autoimmune reaction, whereas progressive infectious encephalitis is a direct infection of the brain by the virus, and SSPE results from a latent infection as described above.

Conjunctivitis and keratitis are very common in cases of measles, but usually resolve after 1 to 2 weeks. However, in third world countries, secondary bacterial disease frequently results in blindness. Corneal erosion can occur after the keratitis resolves, and this is a major cause of blindness in developing countries. Retinitis may include macular edema and star formation, attenuated arterioles, disc edema, or neuroretinitis (119). Blindness may result from optic neuritis, chorioretinitis, corneal ulceration, perforation, leukoma, and phthisis bulbi. Blindness following measles virus infection may also result from a simultaneous herpesvirus infection, folk remedies containing noxious compounds, and vitamin A deficiency (see Chapter 49) (34).

Histopathology

Measles retinitis (measles maculopathy) may occur alone as part of a measles infection or in the course of SSPE (45). The retina in measles maculopathy exhibits necrosis, lymphocytic infiltration, and multinucleated cells during active retinitis; intranuclear viral inclusions may be seen in retinal neurons. Atrophy and gliosis may develop after the retinitis resolves (45,98). Viral antigen is demonstrable in infected retinal cells immunohistochemically, while intranuclear and cytoplasmic viral nucleocapsids may be observed ultrastructurally (45). Injection of measles virus into the anterior chamber of guinea pigs causes iridocyclitis, keratoconjunctivitis, and follicular conjunctivitis (116).

Diagnosis

The diagnosis of measles is made clinically based on the pathognomonic presenting manifestations that include a characteristic rash and Koplik spots, cough, conjunctivitis, and coryza. Multinucleated giant cells with eosinophilic inclusions are present in infected tissue. Fluorescent antibody staining of nasopharyngeal fluids and isolation of the virus in tissue culture can be performed in cases when the diagnosis is uncertain. Detection of early anti-measles virus IgM can confirm infection. HI, ELISA, or CF tests can detect serum antibody concentration, and a four-fold rise after two to four weeks is confirmatory (42).

Subacute Sclerosing Panencephalitis

Virology

SSPE, also known as Dawson inclusion body encephalitis, is a rare disorder that has now been etiologically linked, with considerable confidence, to a defective form of measles virus lacking the viral M protein and other envelope proteins. Evidence for its pathogenesis includes ultrastructural detection of paramyxovirus-like particles in infected tissues, elevated circulating anti-measles antibodies in affected individuals, and detection of measles virus components in brain tissue and cerebrospinal fluid (CSF) by immunologic and nucleic-acid-based methods. Additional evidence has been provided by the development of encephalitis in experimental animals inoculated with brain tissue from patients with SSPE and recovery of virus particles and antigens from explanted brain tissue co-cultivated or fused with human or simian cells (see Chapter 70).

Epidemiology

SSPE occurs most frequently in individuals who have contracted measles at less than two years of age; its incidence has been estimated at 1 to 10 per million measles cases. The predilection of the disorder for individuals who contract measles infections in the first two years of life suggests that the virus may be incompletely cleared by the immature immune system of early childhood. SSPE is primarily a disease of childhood and adolescence, though occurrence in adults has been documented. Males are three to four times more susceptible than females. Like measles itself, SSPE has decreased in incidence with the advent of measles vaccination, but remains prevalent in developing countries where such vaccination is not routinely available.

Clinical Presentation

SSPE is a slowly progressive neurodegenerative disorder that resembles multiple sclerosis in some of its manifestations (7). SSPE typically presents with an insidious onset of progressive intellectual and personality deterioration, followed by development of myoclonic movements. These clinical symptoms are often accompanied by characteristic electroencephalographic (EEG) changes. The disease is generally progressive and fatal, though the course is sometimes prolonged and rare survivals have been reported. Ophthalmic abnormalities, including cortical blindness, nystagmus, and visual impairment due to involvement of the brain and/or focal chorioretinitis, have been reported in approximately 50% of affected individuals. The retinal changes have a predilection for the macular or perimacular area. More detailed information is provided elsewhere in this volume (see Chapter 70).

Histopathology

See measles virus.

Diagnosis

In subjects with SSPE the CSF usually contains a few lymphocytes and a normal glucose level; although the total protein is often normal or moderately raised, the gamma globulin is usually elevated. An elevated titer of measles antibodies is consistently present in the CSF. IgM and IgG antibodies to measles are both normally high in the serum and CSF in SSPE (15). Measles-specific IgD activity is also significantly increased in SSPE (104). A brain biopsy has been used to confirm the diagnosis, but is no longer indicated.

Mumps Virus

Virology

Mumps virus, an enveloped ssRNA virus (29) in the genus *Rubulavirus*, is morphologically indistinguishable from measles virus (see Fig. 21A) but does not share cross-neutralization with other paramyxoviruses. It has both hemagglutinin and neuraminidase activities. Other viruses in the genus include human parainfluenza viruses, simian viruses, and porcine and other animal viruses.

Epidemiology

Transmission is from person to person by contact with nasopharyngeal droplets. Mumps virus is endemic and may cause epidemics every 2 to 3 years except in countries where mumps vaccine is available. It has recently made a comeback in the United States, beginning in Kansas. Most infections occur in children, but when an unexposed adult contracts the virus, a more severe disease ensues.

Clinical Presentation

Mumps starts, after a two-and-a-half-week incubation, as an upper respiratory infection that includes fever, headache, malaise, and myalgia. The virus becomes disseminated, leading to swollen parotid and submandibular salivary glands. In addition to parotitis, infection of other systems may result in orchitis (25% of males infected after puberty), meningitis (10% of patients), encephalitis, and less commonly, pancreatitis, carditis, oophoritis, mastitis, and arthritis. Meningitis may develop in 10% of patients.

Dacryoadenitis and conjunctivitis are common in mumps (112). There may also be iritis, optic neuritis, neuroretinitis, or posterior vitritis. Documented corneal lesions include a punctate epitheliopathy, nummular anterior stromal keratitis, and unilateral central interstitial keratitis. These may cause a profound decrease in visual acuity about a week after parotitis, but the corneal lesions resolve with minimal scars without vascularization in about a month. Uveitis, changes in IOP, and, rarely, episcleritis and scleritis may be present. Cranial nerve palsies and opsoclonus-myoclonus with acute cerebellar ataxia have been seen as mumps complications. Mumps vaccination has reduced mumps infection and related ocular disease.

Histopathology

Injection of mumps virus into the anterior chamber of guinea pig eyes causes follicular conjunctivitis, corneal clouding due to keratitis, iridocyclitis, and dacryoadenitis (65,115). While these changes in animals recapitulate the ophthalmological changes observed clinically in humans, we are unaware of any histopathological observations conducted on human ocular tissues during infection with this virus.

Diagnosis

The disease is usually diagnosed clinically based on symptoms. Infection can be confirmed by culture of bodily fluids and serological tests (a four-fold rise in antibody titers detected in convalescent serum by HI, CF, neutralization, or ELISA).

Newcastle Disease Virus

Virology

Newcastle disease virus (NDV), a paramyxovirus in the *Avulavirus* genus, is morphologically similar to measles virus (29), and has both hemagglutinin and neuraminidase activities. There are many strains that cause infections of considerable morbidity and mortality in poultry. They can be transmitted to human eyes in individuals such as poultry workers and veterinarians.

Clinical Presentation

NDV infection may cause fever, headache, and malaise. After 24 to 48 hours, an acute follicular conjunctivitis with a tender preauricular lymphadenopathy and a mild keratitis are common. Conjunctival papillary and follicular hypertrophy is associated with chemosis and hyperemia. Systemic symptoms are mild and subside in a couple of days, while eye involvement resolves in about a week (49).

Histopathology

Naturally occurring Newcastle disease results in suppurative conjunctivitis in double-crested cormorants (69). Acute inflammation is present in the epithelium and substantia propria of the conjunctiva, though the degree of inflammation varies among birds (69). The substantia propria also has an infiltrate of lymphocytes and plasma cells (69). Other ocular histopathological findings in naturally infected cormorants include epidermal erosions in the eyelids, acute keratitis, corneal epithelial erosions, corneal ulceration with stromal neovascularization, and suppurative anterior uveitis (69). Inoculation of chickens with NDV results in conjunctivitis manifest histologically by variable degrees of focal hyperplasia of conjunctival epithelial cells with lymphocytic infiltration and edema of the substantia propria (96). More severely affected chickens also had vascular necrosis and conjunctival hemorrhage (96). Intraocular injection of chickens with NDV causes uveitis involving the iris, ciliary body, and choroid (101). We are unaware of any histopathological observations conducted on human ocular tissues during infection with this virus.

Diagnosis

The differential diagnosis includes acute keratoconjunctivitis due to adenovirus, which is usually more severe; chlamydia, which has a coarser punctate epithelial keratitis and prolonged course; and other bacteria, which is purulent and lacks conjunctival follicles and preauricular lymphadenopathy. Newcastle disease is usually diagnosed because of a history of contact with infected birds and can be confirmed by culturing NDV or detecting a rise in anti-NDV antibody.

Picornaviruses

Picornaviruses are small ssRNA naked icosahedral particles (29). There are nine genuses, including enterovirus, rhinovirus, cardiovirus, hepatovirus (hepatitis A virus), and others. By negative staining and TEM, they can be visualized as round, 27- to 30-nm particles without distinguishing marks to make them identifiable specifically (Fig. 22A). In thin sections of infected tissue or tissue culture, virions can be seen in the cytoplasm (Fig. 22B), and sometimes lined up along ribosomes associated with cytoplasmic membranes (Fig. 22C), or in paracrystalline arrays (Fig. 22D). Picornaviruses may be difficult to distinguish

Figure 22 (*Shown on facing page*) Picornaviruses. (**A**) Negative stain of hepatitis A virus (HAV). Bar = 100 nm. *Source*: Courtesy of Dr. C.D. Humphrey, Centers for Disease Control and Prevention. (**B**) Low magnification of a picorrnavirus (Nodamura) in mouse muscle showing paracrystalline arrays of virus in the cytoplasm. Bar = 1 μm. *Source*: Courtesy of Dr. F.A. Murphy and A.K. Harrison, Centers for Disease Control and Prevention. (**C**) Thin section of an enterovirus-infected tissue culture cell inoculated from a patient specimen. Virions are small, about the size of ribosomes, and frequently hard to see in clinical material. Often, they are aligned with ribosomes or seen associated with membranes; however, they are naked, not enveloped, icosahedral viruses. Bar = 100 nm. (**D**) High magnification of a picornavirus (Nodamura) in mouse muscle showing paracrystalline arrays of virus in the cytoplasm. Bar = 100 nm. *Source*: Courtesy of Dr. F.A. Murphy and A.K. Harrison, Centers for Disease Control and Prevention.

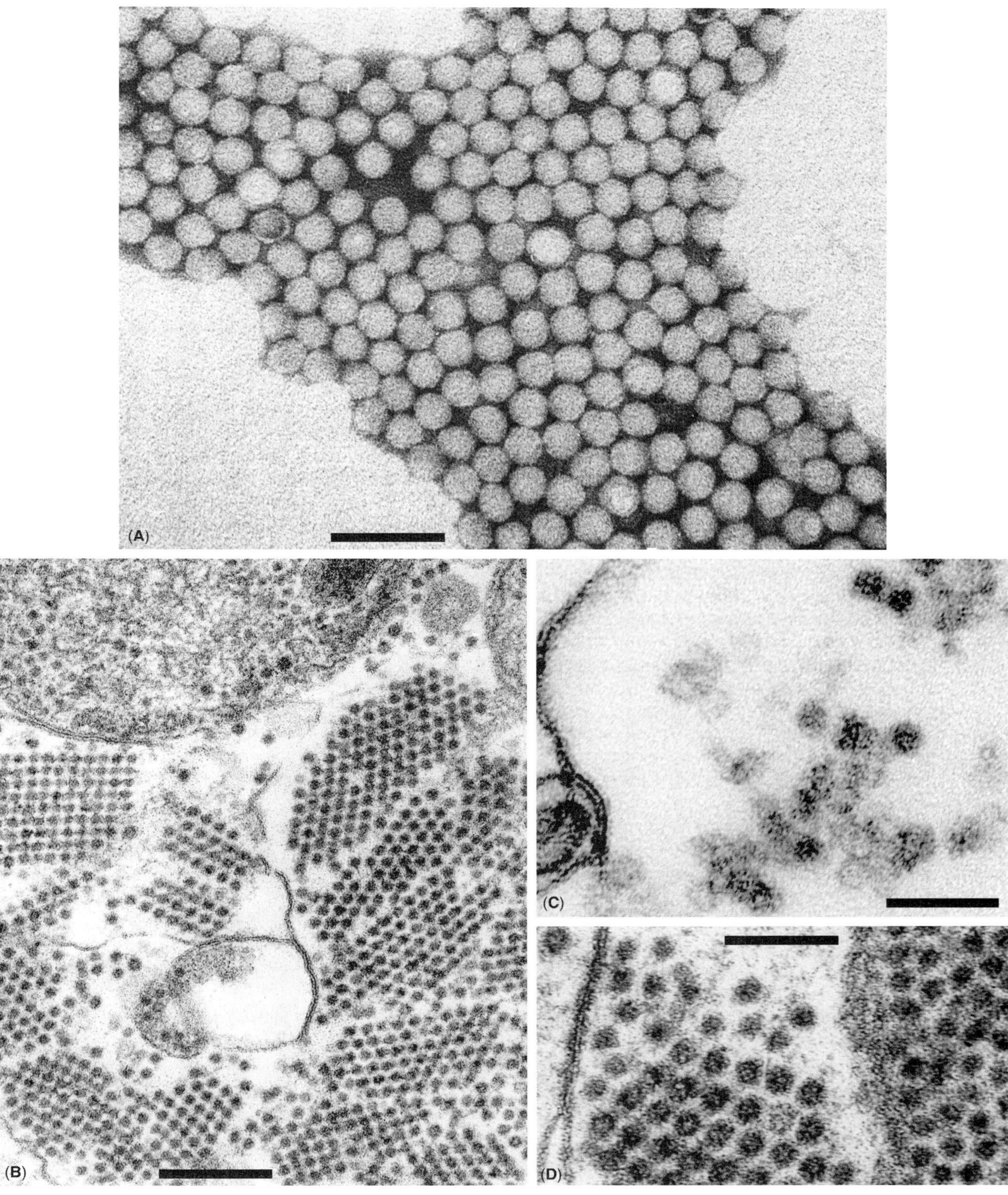
(A)
(B)
(C)
(D)

from ribosomes because of their similar size. Infected cells may contain large polyribosomes and cytoplasmic masses of smooth-membraned vesicles. Degenerated cells are vacuolated at their periphery. Infection is usually lytic, but some species can cause persistent infections.

Enteroviruses

Virology

The enterovirus genus includes coxsackieviruses, poliovirus, echoviruses, hepatitis A virus and others. They infect humans, apes, swine, and cattle and multiply primarily in the gastrointestinal tract but replicate in other organs such as respiratory and ocular mucosa, nerve, and muscle. Infections may be asymptomatic or may cause meningitis, encephalitis, myelitis, myocarditis, and conjunctivitis (29).

Epidemiology

Enteroviruses are very stable and resist acids, solvents, proteolytic enzymes, and many disinfectants. They can survive in the acidic gastric contents and in sewage for long periods of time. The fecal-oral route is the most common mechanism of transmission, but they can also be spread by respiratory droplets, insects, and ocular diagnostic instruments. Infections more commonly occur in the summer. Coxsackievirus A24 variant virus causes acute hemorrhagic conjunctivitis and has been responsible for epidemics in Asia, India, Egypt, Cuba, Puerto Rico, and Brazil. Coxsackieviruses are highly contagious and spread person-to-person. Virus is present in throat washings and stool specimens.

Clinical Presentation

Infection may be subclinical or may result in serious illnesses. The manifestations include a sore throat, gastroenteritis, meningitis, encephalitis, myocarditis, hepatitis, herpangina, hand-foot-and-mouth disease (HFMD), and pneumonia (92). When the eye is involved, it is most likely from direct inoculation.

Coxsackieviruses are usually cytolytic; however, viral RNA persistence is associated with rare chronic diseases (e.g., dilated cardiomyopathy, characterized by dilation and dysfunction of the ventricles; chronic myocarditis; congestive heart failure; insulin-dependent diabetes mellitus). Infection in quiescent cells (in phase G0 of the cell cycle) may lead to persistence, and virus reactivation during a change in the growth cycle may trigger chronic viral or immune-mediated disease (31). However, there does not appear to be any long-term ocular involvement.

Acute hemorrhagic conjunctivitis syndrome, a painful follicular conjunctivitis, can be caused by several enterovirus species (e.g., Coxsackievirus type A24, enterovirus 70, echovirus 7) as well as adenoviruses. Patients have excessive lacrimation, pain, swelling, photophobia, and conjunctival hemorrhage that develops over 24 to 48 hours and resolves without sequelae in 1 to 2 weeks (31). The onset is usually unilateral after an incubation period of 18 to 36 hours, followed by involvement of the other eye within a day. The infection is characterized by photophobia, eyelid swelling, and a seromucous conjunctival discharge that later becomes watery. Many patients have a regional lymphadenopathy. A follicular conjunctivitis may be present and rarely, radiculomyelitis. The characteristic sign is subconjunctival hemorrhage, which is exacerbated by manipulation. The cornea may have punctate epithelial keratitis without nummular opacities. Retinitis is rare and may be asymptomatic during the systemic infection, but an acute idiopathic maculopathy has been reported following HFMD. HFMD is usually seen in the preteen or early teen years and is most often caused by Coxsackievirus A16, but other coxsackieviruses have been reported (8).

A rare neurologic complication may occur in 0.01% of patients with enterovirus acute hemorrhagic conjunctivitis. After a latent period of 1 to 8 weeks following ocular symptoms, patients may experience prodromal symptoms (e.g., fever, malaise, myalgia, headache), followed by flaccid paralysis of the lower limbs, similar to that caused by polio (13).

Histopathology

Topical application of rabbit enterovirus 70 to the rabbit eye results in conjunctivitis with numerous punctate areas of epithelial absence in the superior palpebral conjunctiva and lymphoid follicles without germinal centers in the palpebral and tarsal conjunctiva (71). Injection of ophthalmotropic enterovirus into the anterior chamber of primate eyes results in uveitis (68) that mimics enterovirus uveitis of infants (72,73). Following injection of the primate eye, enteroviral antigen was detected mainly in the anterior segment of the infected eye during acute uveitis, while later the antigen was mostly in the posterior segment (68). Krichevskaia et al. speculate that the long persistence of enterovirus antigen in the eye may explain many of the late complications observed in children with enterovirus uveitis (68), which include cataract, glaucoma, and blindness (81). To our knowledge, there have been no reports yet of the histopathological findings in the eyes of children following enterovirus uveitis.

Diagnosis

Enteroviruses can be cultured from conjunctival swabs and occasionally from throat swabs and feces, and culture is the gold standard for diagnosis. However, specimens must be obtained early in the infection, and not all cell lines commonly maintained in diagnostic laboratories support growth of enteroviruses. Coxsackieviruses can also be grown in tissue culture, but suckling mice are the system of choice for the Coxsackievirus A group. Due to technical difficulty of inoculation and maintenance of mouse colonies, this modality is seldom used. Antigen detection is not widely used because viruses in this family do not share a common antigen, and antibody reagent preparation has been limited to Coxsackievirus group B. PCR and reverse transcription-PCR (RT-PCR) tests are highly successful and rapid, but are not routinely available in most diagnostic virology laboratories. Serological tests (IFA, HI, ELISA) can be used and are the only mechanism for confirming the cause of neurologic cases, but have a limited role because of the lack of common antigens between the different enteroviruses. Differentiation of serotypes is usually unnecessary because enteroviral diseases are not serotype specific. However, in pediatric patients, it may be necessary to differentiate pathogenic enteroviruses from the vaccine strain of poliovirus, which immunized children may shed for several weeks.

Interpretation of enteroviral detection must be considered in the light of the specimen source. Enteroviruses can be shed from the nasopharynx and gastrointestinal tract for weeks, and their detection may not signify the presence of disease. While patients with aseptic meningitis will shed enterovirus in stool, many individuals with stool enteroviruses are asymptomatic. Thus, a positive feces test may be less specific than a positive pharyngeal test. Detection of virus from the CNS, blood, genitourinary tract, or eye is usually significant in the diagnosis of disease.

Adenovirus infection, Lyme disease, Rocky Mountain spotted fever, and bacterial diseases should be in the differential diagnosis.

Hepatitis A

Virology

Hepatitis A (HAV, hepatovirus) is an enterovirus, but, while there are several strains, none have much genetic similarity with other picornaviruses. There are two biotypes with different preferred hosts; one infects all species of primate, and the other infects green and cynomolgus monkeys. HAV grows in epithelial cells of the small intestine and hepatocytes, causing an acute, usually self-limiting hepatitis (29). Transmission is by the fecal-oral route, and while the virus can be isolated from bodily fluids (e.g., saliva, urine), they are not a significant source of transmission. Uncooked or undercooked shellfish are common sources, and infected food handlers of uncooked foods can spread it. HAV can be spread by contaminated water, but waterborne disease is uncommon in developed countries.

Clinical Presentation

The incubation is between 2 and 7 weeks, depending on dosage. Clinical symptoms include fever, jaundice, light-colored stools, abdominal pain, and diarrhea. In children, the infection may be silent, and the severity of symptoms increases in teenagers and adults; however, the mortality rate is low (0.3%) (75). Extrahepatic disease is rare and may include cardiac, CNS, renal, and hematological manifestations. Conjunctivitis may be associated with systemic virus disease, and the icterus from liver disease can discolor the eye yellow.

Diagnosis

Hepatitis A is clinically indistinguishable from other types of hepatitis. It is usually diagnosed serologically by detecting IgM antibodies, which indicate a recent infection. RIA and ELISA tests measure total antibodies, which may persist for life, and thus, they are not useful in determining current infection.

Polyomavirus

Virology

Polyomaviruses are circular dsDNA viruses morphologically very similar to papillomaviruses, but slightly smaller in size (~40–45 nm) (29). By negative staining they appear to have "bumps" on the surface (Fig. 23A), but the pattern does not appear as regular as in larger icosahedral viruses (e.g., adenoviruses). Virions are constructed in the nucleus; spherical 40-nm particles can be seen singly and in paracrystalline arrays (Figs. 23B and C). Occasionally, aberrant filamentous forms are present. Two well-characterized pathogenic human species have been identified, BK and JC polyomaviruses, named with the initials of the patients in whom they were first discovered. Ten other species infect monkeys [e.g., simian virus 40 (SV40)], baboons, cattle, rabbits, mice, and hamsters. Each virus is very host- and cell-specific; however, cells that do not support replication can be transformed by early gene products (29).

Epidemiology

Polyomaviruses are very prevalent (~80% of adults worldwide are seropositive). The mode of transmission is not known, but respiratory infections have been seen, and other potential sources include

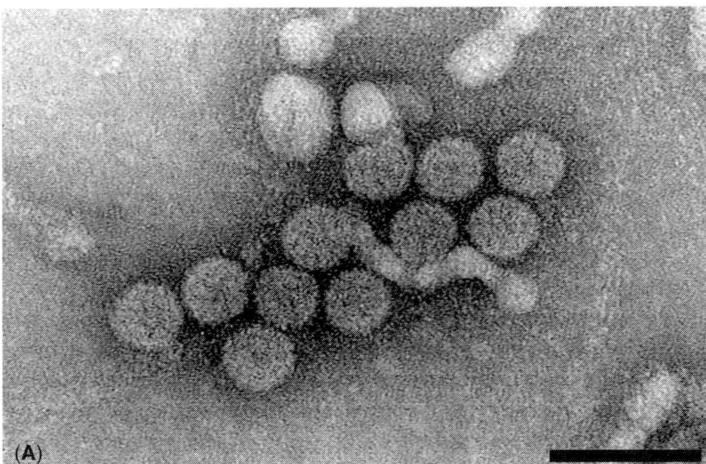

Figure 23 Polyomavirus: (A) Negative stain of polyomavirus in urine from a kidney transplant patient. Viruses are 40 nm. Bar = 100 nm. (B) Thin section of polyomavirus in the nucleus of a cell in skin from an immunosuppressed patient (*arrows*). Bar = 1 μm. (C) High magnification of naked virions. Bar = 100 nm.

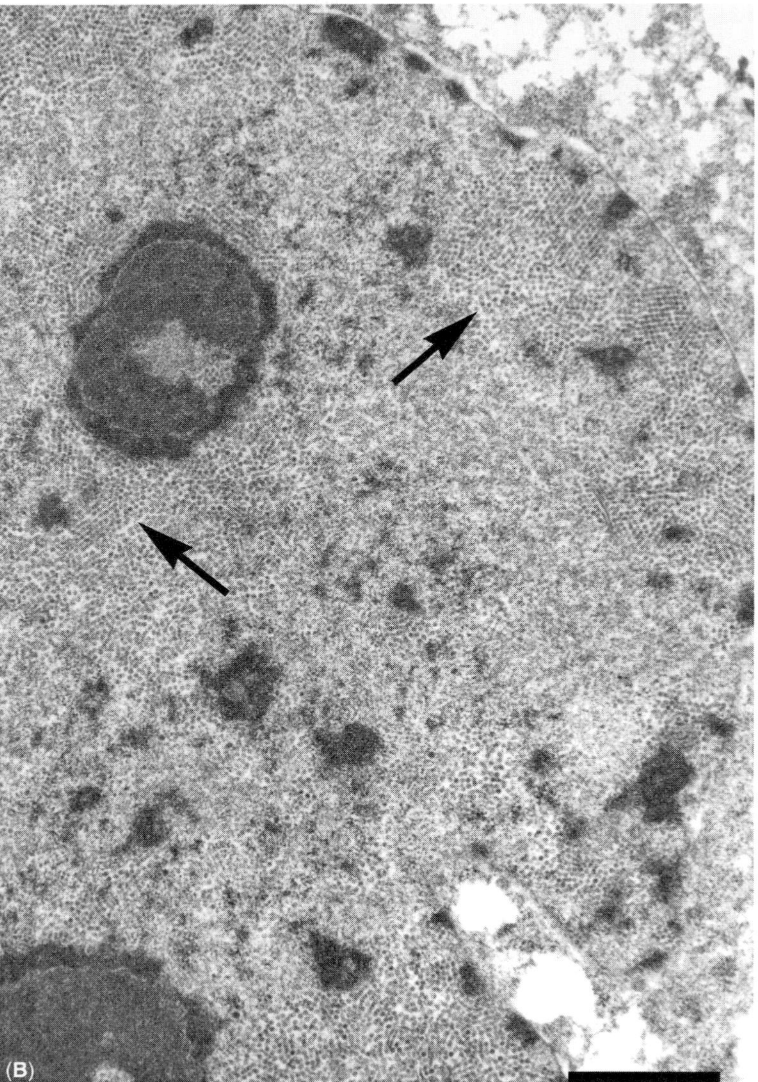

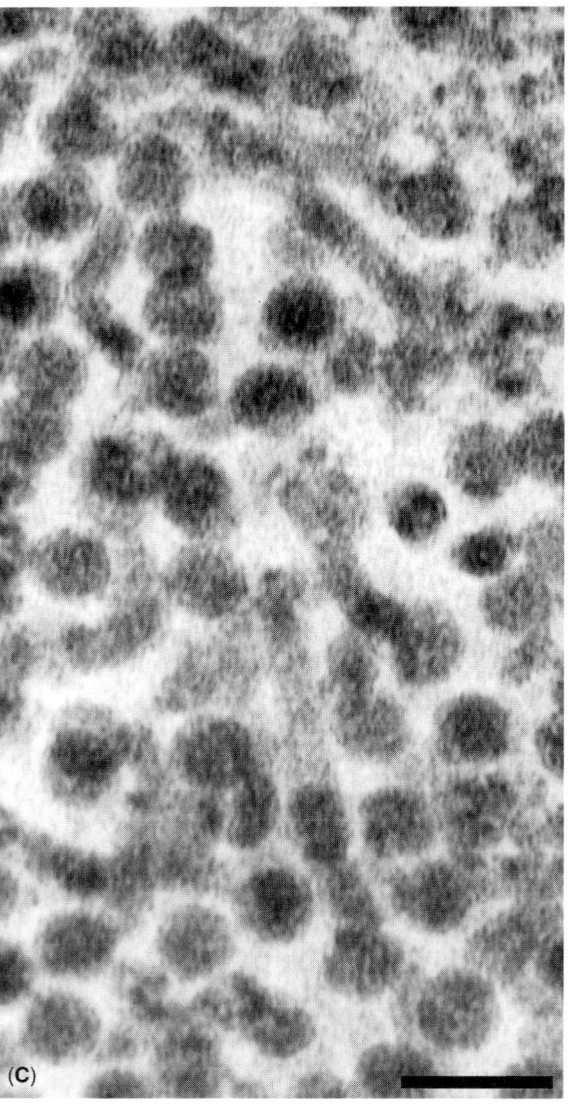

food and water. BK polyomavirus is seen in the urinary tract, particularly in bone marrow and kidney transplant patients, and has been demonstrated in the urine of normal pregnant women. JC polyomavirus is found in the brain in progressive multifocal leukoencephalopathy (PML) (see Chapter 70) and occasionally in the urinary tract.

Clinical Presentation

JC polyomavirus remains latent in the brain, but can cause PML in immunosuppressed hosts. This degenerative infection of oligodendroglia results in CNS symptoms, including motor dysfunction, disorientation, and seizures. Visual disturbances may also occur. Visual decrement in immunocompromised patients may be a signal of PML (102). PML needs to be differentiated from lymphoma and various CNS infections found in immunosuppresed individuals, such as cryptococcus meningitis and toxoplasmosis, as the therapies differ.

PML is an often-fatal subacute progressive demyelinating disease of the human CNS characterized by multiple foci of demyelination and abnormal oligodendrocytes that contain large numbers of intranuclear papovavirus virions (1,62). While PML can potentially involve the optic nerve, severe visual loss has followed involvement of the occipital lobe (5). Tumors of the CNS develop in some PML patients in whom cell-mediated immunity is suppressed. Most affected individuals are adults with lymphoproliferative disorders, but the disease also occurs in persons with AIDS and following immunosuppression for organ transplantation (141). It has also rarely been reported with sarcoidosis (59).

Other viruses (BKV and SV40) have been implicated in some cases of PML, but a recent analysis of affected tissue in two cases previously attributed to SV40 using biotinylated DNA probes and monoclonal antibodies casts serious doubt on the notion that SV40 can cause PML (132).

Histopathology

The eyes of a 29-year-old man with AIDS who developed BK virus retinitis showed several areas of full-thickness retinal necrosis without any viral inclusions evident by light microscopy (51). BK virus VP1 capsid protein was detected immunohistochemically in the retina only in and adjacent to the necrotic retina (51)

Diagnosis

Diagnosis of urinary tract infections can be made by negative staining of virus particles pelleted from urine, which is a rapid, sensitive, and non-invasive diagnostic modality (56).

Polyomaviruses can also be demonstrated in thin sections of cells sedimented from urine by low speed centrifugation, but this method requires embedment and thin sectioning, which take longer to accomplish than negative staining. Polyomavirus-infected cells can be demonstrated by cytology and immunofluorescence if the patient is shedding infected cells (decoy cells). PCR detection of polyomavirus in blood is likely significant, because the detection limit probably signifies active disease but, in most cases, requires the services of a referral laboratory. Unless quantitative methods are used, PCR detection of polyomavirus in urine is of limited value, as ~80% of individuals have been exposed to the virus and asymptomatic shedding detectable by PCR is common.

Diagnosis of CNS disease is done by biopsy and immunohistochemistry or TEM.

Poxviruses

Poxviruses are large brick-shaped viruses with a single linear dsDNA molecule (29). The orthopoxviruses (e.g., vaccinia) are about 250 × 200 × 200 nm, and molluscipoxes (e.g., molluscum contagiosum) are about 320 × 250 × 200 nm. Both genuses appear in TEM of negative stains to have furrows on the surface, like the gyri of brain (Fig. 24A). The parapoxviruses (e.g., orf) are longer and narrower, more like a medicine capsule, measuring 220 to 300 nm in length and 140 to 170 nm in diameter. Their surface appears to be wrapped with string-like striations in a crisscrossed pattern (Fig. 24B). In thin sections, poxviruses are found in the cytoplasm (Figs. 24C and D), sometimes in a matrix of dense material or inclusion body (e.g., cowpox). The genetic material is packaged together with nucleoproteins into a biconcave or cylindrical core. There may be one or two lateral bodies in the concave region between the core and the outer membrane.

Viruses synthesize their envelopes de novo in the cytoplasm, producing particles called intracellular mature virus (IMV). Some particles may become associated with cell membranes and acquire an additional membranous host-derived layer; such particles are referred to as intracellular enveloped virus (IEV). These particles have an antigenically different surface from the IMV. The IEV can be externalized and bound to the surface to form cell-associated virus (CEV) or released from the surface as extracellular enveloped virus (EEV).

CEV, EEV, and IMV are all infectious. CEV and EEV are primarily responsible for cell-to-cell spread of virus within an individual, while IMV appears to play a major role in infection of new hosts.

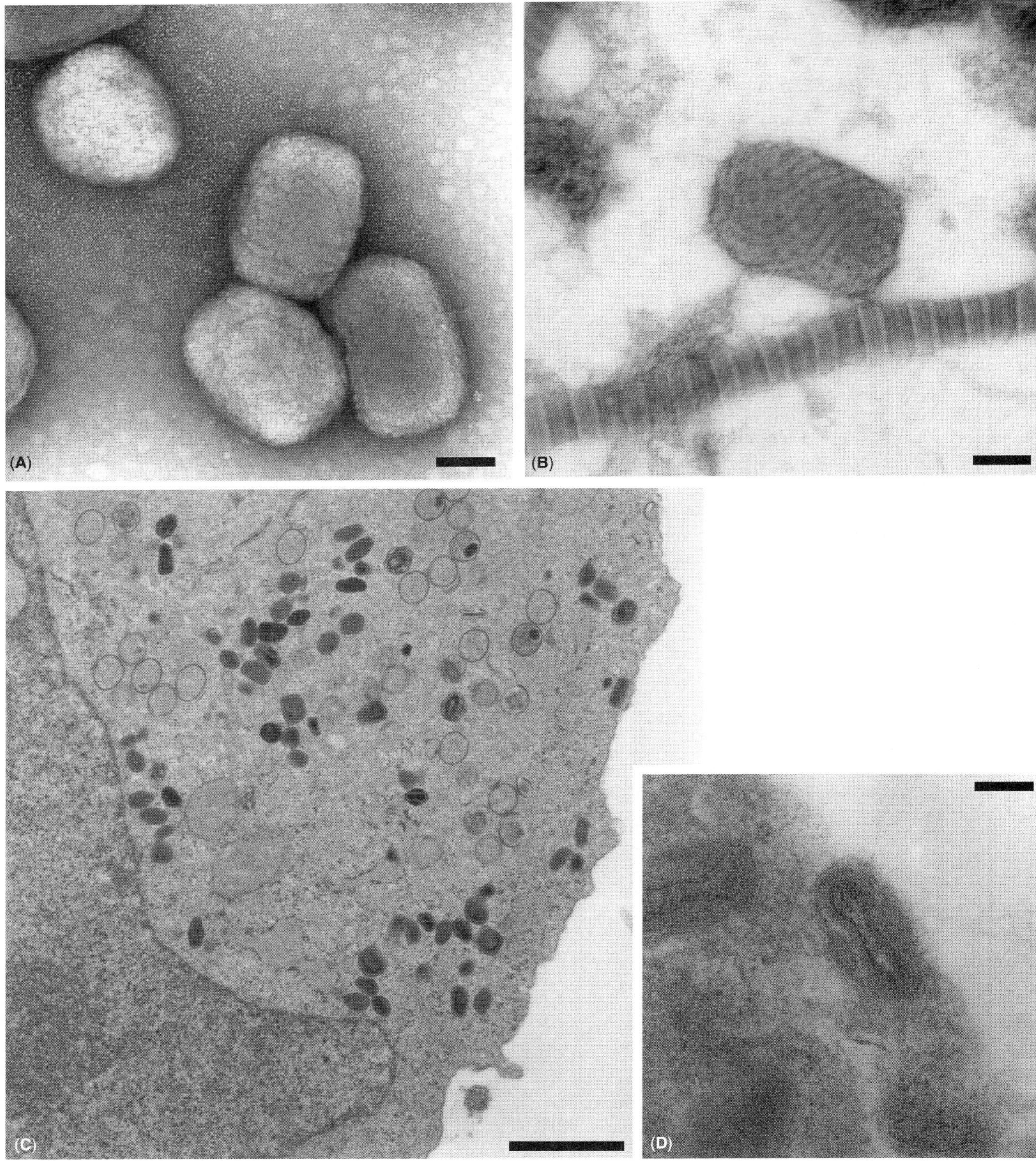

Figure 24 Poxviruses. (**A**) Negative stain of orthopoxvirus. Enveloped particles are brick shaped, and the surface is rough, like the gyri of brain. They are about 250 × 200 × 200 nm in size. The virion may have an envelope, in which case, the surface will appear fluffy; however, more commonly, there is no envelope, in which case, the appearance varies, depending on whether the stain penetrates the outer layer. The mulberry, or "M", form has a rough surface, while the stain-penetrated form may show a distention of the core. Bar = 100 nm. Note that due to large virus size, the magnification is shown at half that of other virus high magnification micrographs (×100,000, instead of ×200,000). (*Caption continues on facing page*)

Molluscum Contagiosum

Virology

Molluscum is a brick-shaped virion, ~320 × 250 × 200 nm, in the Molluscipoxvirus genus, and morphologically resembles the orthopoxviruses. There is only one species, but restriction mapping suggests that there are at least four strains.

Epidemiology

Molluscum is spread by direct contact. In children, the lesions have a predilection for the extremities and trunk, whereas in adults, they can be a sexually transmitted disease and affect other parts of the skin, including the genital region. Molluscum contagiosum can be spread by skin contact in sports such as wrestling. It can involve the eyelid from inoculation by scratching and is the most common poxvirus to infect the ocular tissues. The lesions in individuals with AIDS are larger than usual, multiple, and often widely disseminated. Such attributes have led to the diagnosis of AIDS in some cases (74).

Clinical Presentation

Molluscum contagiosum appears as 2- to 4-mm hard white or cream-colored, centrally umbilicated nodules; they are larger, more severe, and persistent in immunocompromised patients, including individuals infected with HIV, with congenital immunodeficiencies, with leukemia, or on immunosuppressive therapy. The lesions are painless and usually lack inflammation. They resolve, but may cause scarring if there is bacterial superinfection.

One or both eyelids can be affected, and the classic umbilicated appearance may be lacking. Rarely, there may be caruncular pinkish or yellowish lesions without follicular conjunctivitis; the lesions are discrete and can be easily excised. Follicular conjunctivitis and superficial keratitis may reflect an immunologic reaction to the virus. Secondary chronic follicular conjunctivitis or keratitis can develop with varied corneal involvement.

Nodules usually resolve spontaneously after several weeks, but may lead to a trachoma-like disease with loss of vision. In HIV-infected individuals, they do not resolve spontaneously.

Histopathology

Eyelid lesions of molluscum contagiosum have inverted lobules of hyperplastic epidermis that expand into the underlying dermis (32). Infected keratinocytes have eosinophilic inclusions that occupy almost the entire cell (Figs. 25A and B). The inclusion bodies (molluscum bodies) begin to form in keratinocytes just above the basal layer, and they progressively enlarge towards the epidermal surface. The inclusions may become basophilic near the skin surface. The viral inclusion bodies and keratinous debris are extruded into dilated ostia leading to the skin surface.

Shedding of viral particles into the conjunctiva from a molluscum lesion on the eyelid margin may result in follicular conjunctivitis (130) manifest histologically as lymphoid follicles in the substantia propria of the conjunctiva. Primary molluscum contagiosum lesions of the eyelid are rare and mainly reported in patients with the acquired immunodeficiency syndrome (12,130). In conjunctival lesions, the epithelium is thickened and molluscum bodies lie within the epithelial cells (12,130).

Diagnosis

Molluscum contagiosum lesions can frequently be identified by their appearance. The virus does not grow readily in tissue culture, although some CPE has been described. The clinical differential diagnosis of molluscum contagiosum includes numerous cutaneous infections that may be due to viruses (e.g., VZV, HSV, papillomavirus), fungi (e.g., *Cryptococcus neoformans*), bacteria (furuncles), as well as cysts and tumors (including keratosis and basal cell carcinoma). The easiest, fastest (10–15 min), and least traumatic method for detecting poxvirus is TEM of negatively stained lesion scrapings. This procedure can differentiate between poxvirus and herpesvirus and between orthopoxvirus and parapoxvirus. However, it cannot differentiate between the various strains of orthopoxvirus (e.g., vaccinia, smallpox) or molluscum

Figure 24 (*Continued*) (**B**) Negative stain of parapoxvirus. This genus has rounder ends, like a medicine capsule, and is generally longer and slimmer than orthopoxviruses (220–300 × 140–170 nm). It appears to be wrapped with string, and because of the upper and lower surface superimposition, appears to be wrapped in a criss-cross pattern. Bar = 100 nm. Note that due to large virus size, the magnification is shown at half that of other virus high magnification micrographs. (**C**) Thin section of poxviruses in an infected cell. Poxviruses are the exception to the general rule that DNA viruses are usually constructed in the nucleus. Oval and brick-shaped particles are seen here in the cytoplasm. Immature round to oval particles with less dense centers mature as the core condenses; they become more brick-shaped and contain a bone-shaped core. Lateral bodies may be visible in the concave portion of the bone. Bar = 1 μm. (**D**) High magnification of a mature poxvirus particle showing the dumbbell-shaped core. Bar = 100 nm. Note that due to large virus size, the magnification is shown at half that of other virus high magnification micrographs.

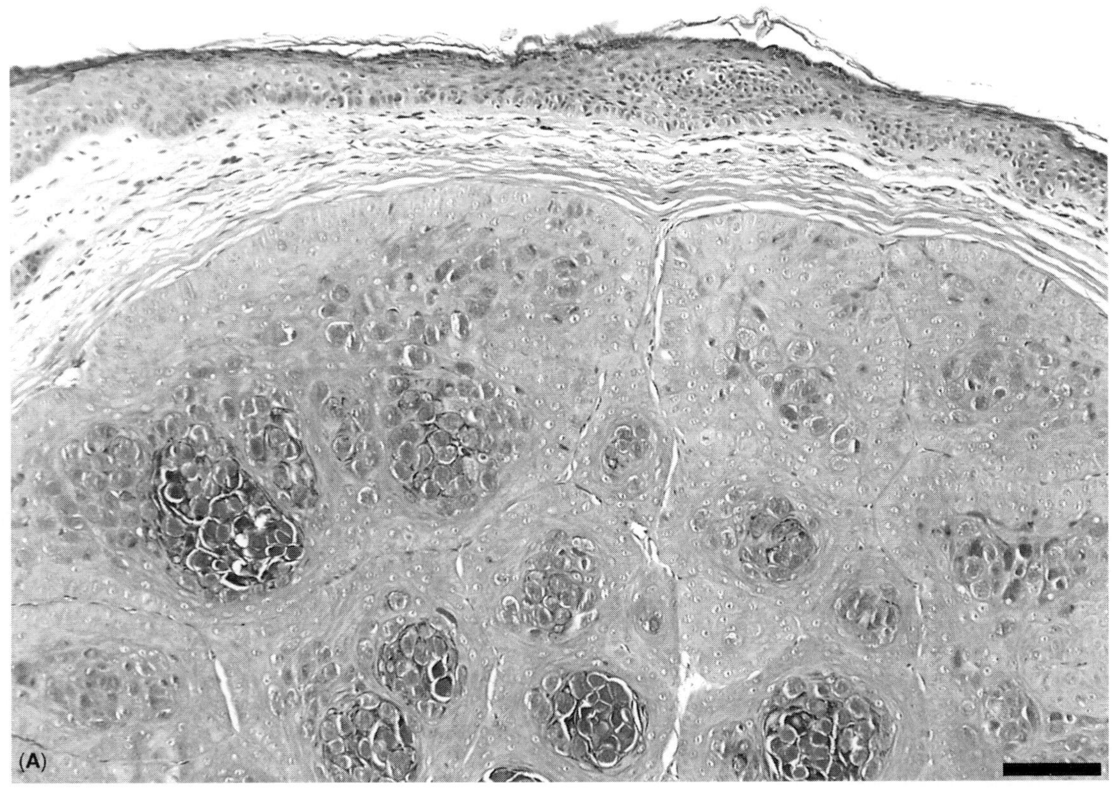

Figure 25 Molluscum contagiosum. (**A**) Lobules of infected epidermal cells are present in the dermis (hematoxylin and eosin; bar = 100 μm). (*Continued*)

contagiosum. Biopsies show eosinophilic hyaline inclusions in the cytoplasm; the virions are large (~0.2–0.3 μm) and can just be discerned by light microscopy of material spread from a lesion and stained with a supravital dye. Immunohistochemistry, PCR, and hybridization techniques can be used to differentiate further between poxviruses if necessary. The differential diagnosis includes basal cell carcinoma on the face or neck, or cutaneous cryptococcosis in AIDS patients.

Orf

Virology

Parapoxviruses are ovoid, resembling a medicine capsule, and are clearly distinguishable from the brick-shaped orthopoxviruses. They are 220 to 300 nm in length and 140 to 170 nm in diameter, with a surface that appears to be wrapped diagonally around the diameter with string, first in one direction, followed by wrapping in the other direction in a criss-crossed pattern (Fig. 24B). There are five species plus four tentative species in the parapoxvirus genus (29).

Epidemiology

Parapoxviruses normally cause diseases of ungulates and domesticated livestock, and occasionally can be transmitted to humans by contact with the lesions or fomites.

Most human infections occur in animal handlers such as veterinarians and ranchers. Person to person transmission has not been documented.

Clinical Presentation

The lesions involve the skin and appear as maculopapules that progress to a bull's eye appearance (red center, white halo, red outer halo), and then to an umbilicated ulcer. Those of orf are larger than lesions of another parapoxvirus, pseudocowpox (milker nodule), and molluscum contagiosum. Finally, an eschar develops, and the epidermis regenerates. Usually there is no fever or other symptoms, but a regional lymphadenopathy is common, and the lesions may itch. Ocular disease is rare, but a follicular and papillary conjunctivitis and involvement of the canthus have been reported. A case of blindness resulting from bacterial superinfection has been described.

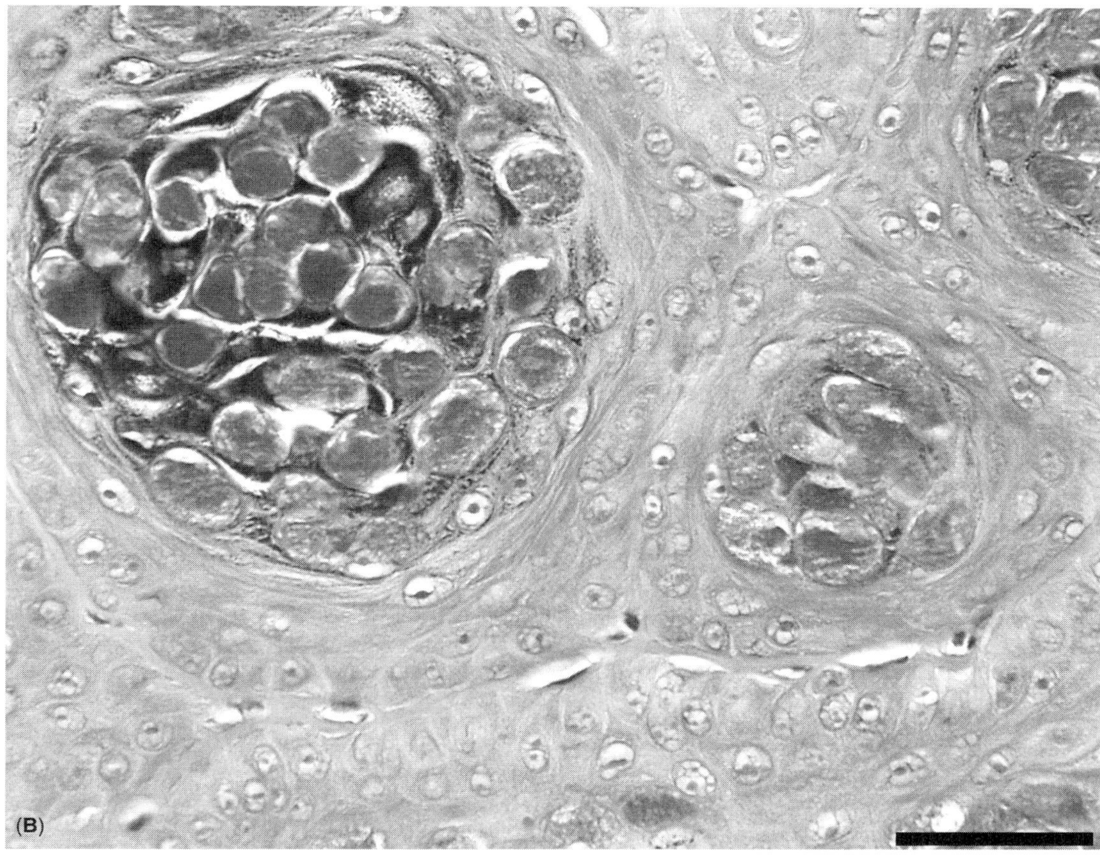

Figure 25 (*Continued*) Molluscum contagiosum. (**B**) Numerous cytoplasmic inclusions are readily apparent under higher magnification (hematoxylin and eosin; bar = 50 μm).

Diagnosis

Orf is usually diagnosed on the basis of the clinical appearance of the lesions and a history of contact with an infected animal. The diagnosis can be easily confirmed by performing TEM on scrapings from affected skin. By light microscopy, eosinophilic cytoplasmic inclusions are seen in epidermal cells, and inflammatory cells are present. The orf virus can be isolated in primary sheep or goat cells and can then be passaged into human embryonic fibroblasts or monkey kidney cells. The virus in culture can be further identified by immunological staining. The differential diagnosis of orf includes molluscum contagiosum, anthrax, keratoacanthoma, and pyogenic granuloma.

Vaccinia

Virology

Vaccinia is a poxvirus very similar to the cowpox virus that Jenner used to vaccinate against smallpox. It is a laboratory virus, and several strains exist with different levels of virulence; laboratory-acquired infections may occur. The vaccinia virus does not cause latent infections but will re-infect an area locally if reinoculated. The degree of re-infection depends on the individual's immune status; more recent vaccination may lead to a greatly reduced "take" (size, induration of lesion). The live vaccine strain, which is used to offer protection against smallpox, can cause morbidity, including eye disease.

Epidemiology

The most common ocular poxvirus infection in the recent past has been vaccinia spread from the local vaccination site. During the middle of the 20th century when the WHO was in the midst of eradicating smallpox from the world, vaccinia was occasionally and accidentally transmitted from the vaccination lesion to the eye by rubbing the lesion and then touching the eye. Because of the fear of smallpox following bioterrorism, some military and health care personnel have been vaccinated with vaccinia virus (57,123).

Clinical Presentation

The cutaneous lesion begins a few days following inoculation, with papules progressing to vesicles, and it itches extensively. After a couple of weeks, it forms a scab that eventually falls off in another couple of weeks, leaving a scar. Adverse reactions from vaccination include fever, headache, fatigue, myalgia, chills, local skin reactions, rashes, erythema multiforme, lymphadenopathy, and pain at the site of vaccination. Serious reactions requiring treatment may include generalized vaccinia, eczema vaccinatum, progressive vaccinia, CNS disease, or fetal vaccinia (16).

Transfer of infection from a vaccination site to the eye of a previously vaccinated individual causes mucopurulent blepharoconjunctivitis. Vesicles form, followed by white pustules that umbilicate and indurate. Scarring, madarosis, and symblepharon or ankyloblepharon formation occur, but usually, the infection is confined to the eyelid and conjunctiva. Rarely, there may be corneal involvement (ranging from superficial keratitis to necrotic keratitis), iritis, choroiditis, or optic neuritis. The preauricular nodes may be enlarged and infected.

Severe eye disease occurs during primary accidental inoculation or in immunosuppressed individuals. Keratitis more frequently complicates primary vaccinations than revaccinations.

Histopathology

After immunization against smallpox, accidental autoinoculation may result in vaccinia infection of the eyelids, conjunctiva, or cornea (106,121). Skin infection by vaccinia leads to intracellular edema of keratinocytes with resulting ballooning degeneration, cell rupture, and formation of multilocular vesicles with acute inflammation (87). Extensive epidermal necrosis may be present. Intracytoplasmic viral inclusion bodies may be seen in epidermal keratinocytes; they are small, eosinophilic, surrounded by a clear halo, and located near the nucleus (87).

Diagnosis

A diagnosis of a vaccinia infection is usually based on clinical observations after a recent vaccination, but the lesions need to be differentiated from infections due to HSV, VZV, adenovirus, enterovirus, and protozoa (acanthamoebic keratitis). Smears of the lesions disclose PMNs and eosinophilic cytoplasmic inclusion bodies (Guarnieri bodies). Poxviruses can be easily and rapidly differentiated from other viruses by TEM. Vaccinia grows in tissue cultures normally maintained by diagnostic virology laboratories, including HeLa and primary monkey kidney cells. Confirmatory tests include immunohistochemistry, PCR, and a restriction endonuclease analysis (88).

Variola

Virology

Variola is an orthopox virus, a brick-shaped particle of $250–300 \times 200 \times 200$ nm. Two forms have been identified. Variola major, the casual agent of smallpox, is a highly contagious, highly virulent form. Variola minor is a mild disease caused by a less virulent form of variola with a mortality rate of ~1%. Other synonyms include alastrim, Cuban itch, Kaffir pox, milk pox, pseudosmallpox, pseudovariola, West Indian smallpox, and white pox smallpox.

Epidemiology

Smallpox had considerable ocular consequence prior to immunization, accounting for one third of blindness in Europe (121). The mortality rate for smallpox was 30%, and survivors had multiple deep nonpigmented scars. Smallpox was eradicated in the wild throughout the world in the late 1970s, and does not occur today. Its current significance lies in the fact that variola virus is feared as a potential bioterrorism agent (2).

Clinical Presentation

Variola is contracted through the respiratory tract, where it multiplies and moves to the regional lymph nodes and then disseminates to a systemic disease. There is a febrile prodrome (fever of 101°F or more) occurring 1 to 4 days before the onset of the rash, and the patient is toxic or moribund, with prostration, headache, backache, chills, vomiting, and/or severe abdominal pain. Skin lesions begin in the oral mucosa and on the extremities, including the face, palms, and soles, and move centripetally toward the trunk. They begin as macules and develop slowly to papules, then to pustules, over several days. The mature lesions are deep-seated, hard, round, and well-circumscribed vesicles or pustules. Some may become umbilicated or confluent. In any one area on the body, the lesions are all in the same stage of development (similar in size and appearance). In survivors, they eventually fall off, leaving pitted scars (www.cdc.gov/nip/smallpox).

Histopathology

The eyelid lesions in smallpox are similar to those elsewhere on the body and are similar histologically to vaccinia infection. Infection leads to intracellular edema of keratinocytes with subsequent ballooning degeneration, cell rupture, and formation of multilocular vesicles with acute inflammation (87). There may be extensive epidermal necrosis. Intracytoplasmic viral inclusions, termed Guarnieri bodies, may be seen in epidermal keratinocytes; they are small, eosinophilic, surrounded by a clear halo, and located near the nucleus (87).

Diagnosis

A rapid method for detecting a poxvirus infection is TEM, and thus TEM laboratories are included in the Laboratory Response Network (LRN), an organization of laboratories in the United States designed to identify and manage emerging disease and potential release of organisms by bioterrorists. TEM can rapidly distinguish between poxviruses and herpesviruses (e.g., varicella zoster), and can distinguish between orthopoxviruses (e.g., smallpox and vaccinia) and parapoxviruses (e.g., orf virus). However, it cannot differentiate between the various orthopoxviruses. PCR tests are now available through the LRN and the Centers for Disease Control and Prevention (CDC) for specific smallpox diagnosis but are not readily available in local diagnostic virology laboratories. Once smallpox cases have been identified in an area, the diagnosis can be suggested by symptomatology (see above) and confirmed by PCR or TEM.

Retroviruses

Retrovirus virions are roughly spherical enveloped particles of 80 to 140 nm, containing a nucleoid that is spherical and may be eccentric, concentric, or cone-shaped, depending on the virus. The envelope has 8-nm glycoprotein surface projections.

There are five genuses in the subfamily Orthoretrovirinae, which contains the pathogenic retroviruses. The genome of orthoretroviruses is a dimer of linear, positive sense ssRNA.

Members of the Spumaretrovirinae subfamily cause a "foamy" cytopathology in cell culture, but no diseases have been associated with these viruses. The genome of spumaretroviruses is a dsDNA, and reverse transcription is a late step in the life cycle.

Human T-lymphotropic virus types 1 and 2 are in the Deltaretrovirus genus, and HIV types 1 and 2 are in the Lentivirus genus. Species delineation is based on genome sequence, gene product sequences, host range, and oncogenes incorporated.

Retroviruses have an enzyme, reverse transcriptase, that allows them to produce DNA from the viral RNA that can become integrated into the host DNA, causing persistent infections. While some retroviruses cause neoplasms (e.g., human T-cell leukemia virus), others cause a depletion of certain immune cells and their precursors (e.g., HIV). This, in turn, results in a profound immunodeficiency that may result in the individual's demise from opportunistic infections.

Human Immunodeficiency Virus (HIV)

Virology

HIV is an enveloped ssRNA virus of 80 to 140 nm (29). It has a cone-shaped core that can be visualized by a special negative staining technique using detergent (Fig. 26A), and short spikes on the surface that may be difficult to see. Construction occurs in the cell cytoplasm, and the nucleocapsid buds through the plasma membrane to the extracellular space (Fig. 26B and C) and occasionally into intracellular cytoplasmic vesicles. The presence of both HIV and CMV in the same retinal cell has been shown, and it has been suggested that the two viruses may enhance each other when present in the same cell (129).

Epidemiology

HIV in the United States was first identified in the homosexual community in the early 1980s. It is transmitted by bodily fluids, including blood in intravenous drug users. Not restricted to homosexuals, it is primarily a heterosexual disease in Africa and other third world countries.

Clinical Presentation

In HIV infection, almost every organ and system can be involved, either directly by the virus or as a result of opportunistic infections due to the profound immunodeficiency created by the destruction of T-lymphocytes. Infection of lymphocytes by HIV causes lymphadenopathy, with early disease resulting in follicular hyperplasia, followed by late lymphoid depletion. Other direct systemic manifestations of HIV infection include cardiac disorders (myocarditis, pericarditis, endocarditis), renal disease (HIV-associated nephropathy), and infections of the CNS (e.g., vacuolar myelopathy).

Ocular complications of HIV infection are many and varied. The immunosuppression engendered by HIV potentiates the development of ocular opportunistic infections with a wide range of organisms, including, CMV, HSV, VZV, fungi (*Candida* sp., *Cryptococcus neoformans*, *Pneumocystis carinii*) (see Chapter 11), *Toxoplasma gondii* (see Chapter 12), and mycobacteria (36). Opportunists are not the only culprits in HIV-associated eye disease; HIV can affect the eye through direct infection of ocular tissues or via indirect effects of CNS infections or tumors. KS, a neoplasm common in patients with AIDS (discussed earlier), can also be seen occasionally on the conjunctiva or eyelids.

Retinal lesions in AIDS patients usually result from opportunistic infections by other organisms such as CMV, HSV, mycobacteria, cryptococcus, and *Toxoplasma gondii*; however, HIV itself can be found in the retina and can cause or contribute to the damage. The most common direct manifestation HIV in the eye is HIV retinopathy. As in CMV retinopathy, focal ischemia disrupts axonal transport, and the axons swell, causing the white opaque spots (cotton wool spots) visible ophthalmoscopically in the nerve fiber layer (139). Intraretinal hemorrhages may be seen in up to 20% of patients. In one study, a high plasma viral load was the most predictive factor of the presence of retinal angiopathy. The prevalence of angiopathy

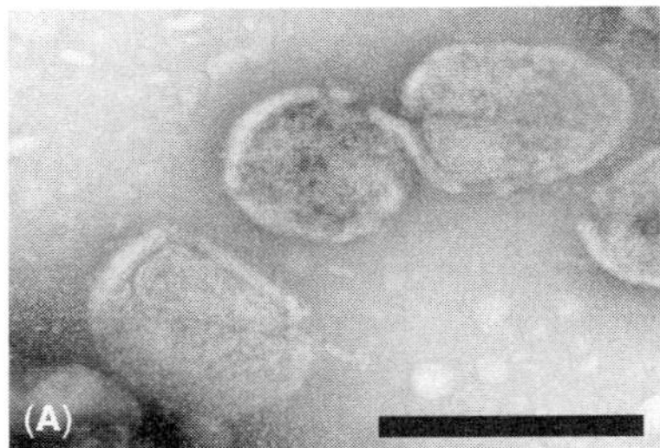

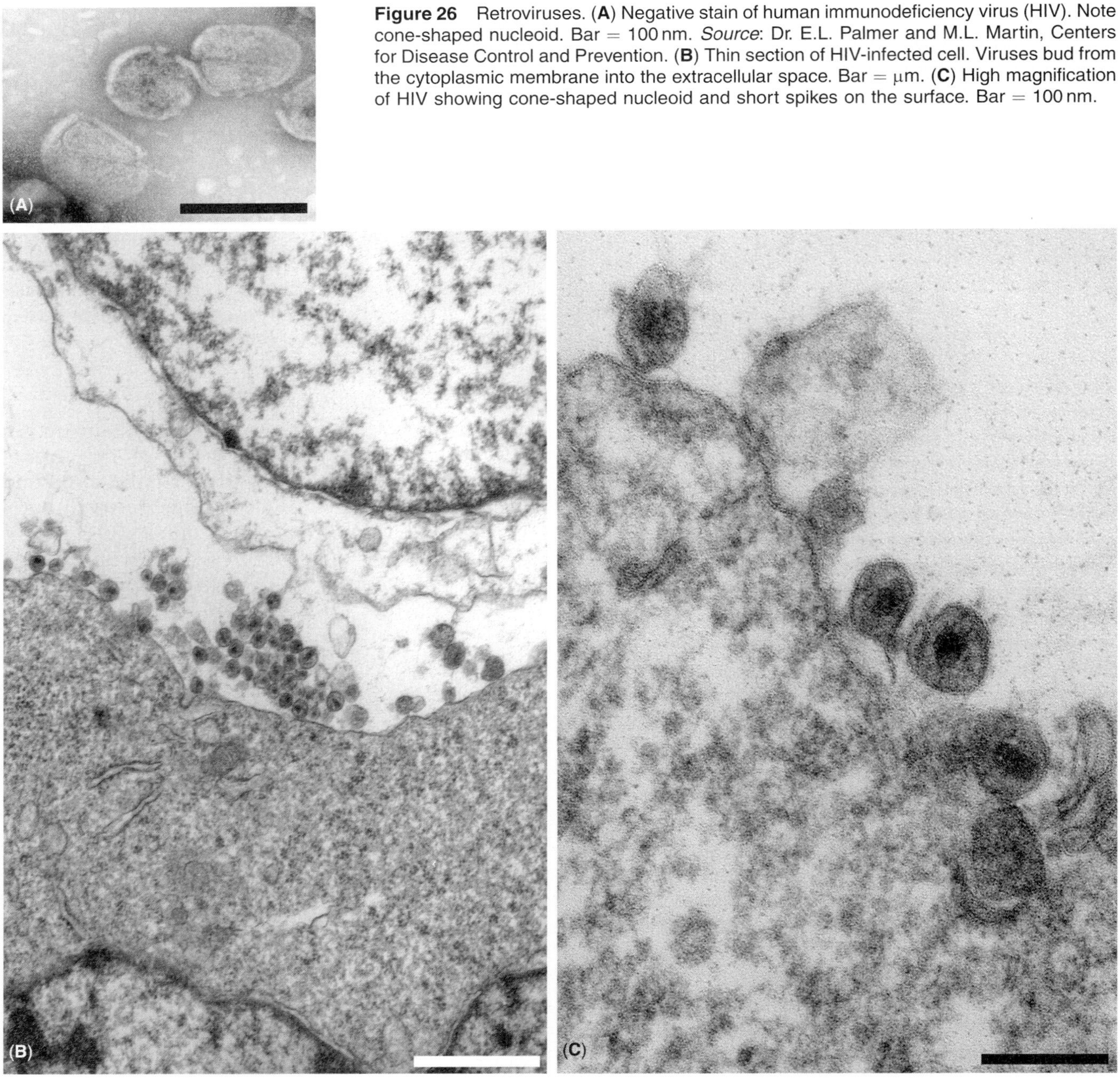

Figure 26 Retroviruses. (**A**) Negative stain of human immunodeficiency virus (HIV). Note cone-shaped nucleoid. Bar = 100 nm. *Source*: Dr. E.L. Palmer and M.L. Martin, Centers for Disease Control and Prevention. (**B**) Thin section of HIV-infected cell. Viruses bud from the cytoplasmic membrane into the extracellular space. Bar = μm. (**C**) High magnification of HIV showing cone-shaped nucleoid and short spikes on the surface. Bar = 100 nm.

correlates with the HIV viral load of the patient, and to some extent with lowered CD4+ T-cell count (37).

Ulcerative keratitis due to HIV may mimic that caused by herpesviruses. Other manifestations that may be caused directly by HIV include follicular conjunctivitis, iritis, glaucoma, vasculitis, hemorrhages, microaneurysms, Roth spots (round white spots surrounded by hemorrhage), ischemic maculopathy, retinal periphlebitis, and papilledema (105). HIV infection of neural tissues leads to neuronal atrophy and demyelination. Optic nerve damage may result from opportunistic infection or from papilledema due to increased intracranial pressure from an intracerebral lymphoma (145). Brain infections may involve different parts of the gray and white matter. Impaired ocular motility with muscle paralyses may occur (77).

Histopathology

Histopathological studies of eyes from individuals dying of AIDS have confirmed the clinical ocular manifestations that occur in this disease (45). Many of the ocular changes are due to opportunistic infections by viruses discussed elsewhere in this chapter. Other retinal manifestations include retinal hemorrhages and distended hypereosinophilic axons in the retinal nerve fiber layer (cotton-wool spots). HIV itself has been isolated from retina, and its presence has been inferred by immunohistochemical studies on sections of the retina including the vascular endothelium (108).

Diagnosis

A diagnosis of HIV infection is made by ELISA and Western blot for HIV antibody and by a determination of the ratio of T-helper cells to T-suppressor cells. The virus can be grown from bodily fluids early in infection, but diagnosis is not usually made by culture. Later, infected cells are few, and virus isolation in culture is reduced. Microscopical techniques are not routinely used in diagnosis; however, tubuloreticular inclusions (not pathognomonic and observed also in other diseases such as systemic lupus erythematosus) may be suggestive of HIV infection.

Rhabdoviruses

Rabies Virus

Virology

The Rhabdovirus family consists of minus-stranded ssRNA viruses in six genuses, two of which infect animals (29). The *Lyssavirus* genus contains rabies virus, bat lyssavirus, and others, which are neurotropic. The *Vesiculovirus* genus contains vesicular stomatitis virus (VSV) and seven others that occasionally infect humans, plus numerous others that infect other species (29).

By negative staining, rhabdoviruses appear as bullet-shaped particles 45 to 100 nm in diameter and 100 to 430 nm long (Fig. 27A). The end that buds from the cell cytoplasmic membrane is rounded, and the back end is flat where it breaks off from the infected cell. Sometimes the nucleocapsid spills out of the back opening that has not sealed. The 30- to 70-nm nucleocapsid is helical with 30 to 35 coils and is contained in a lipoprotein envelope. The surface is studded with glycoprotein spikes (G protein), which are responsible for cell membrane recognition and entry. The G protein is responsible for different serotypes and induces virus-neutralizing antibodies.

By thin sectioning, bullet-shaped virions can be seen budding from the cytoplasmic membrane, or cut in cross-section, they appear round (Figs. 27B and C). Collections of nucleocapsids can be seen in the cytoplasm within a dense matrix and appear circular or filamentous, depending on the plane of section. Some strains of rabies acquire an envelope de novo in

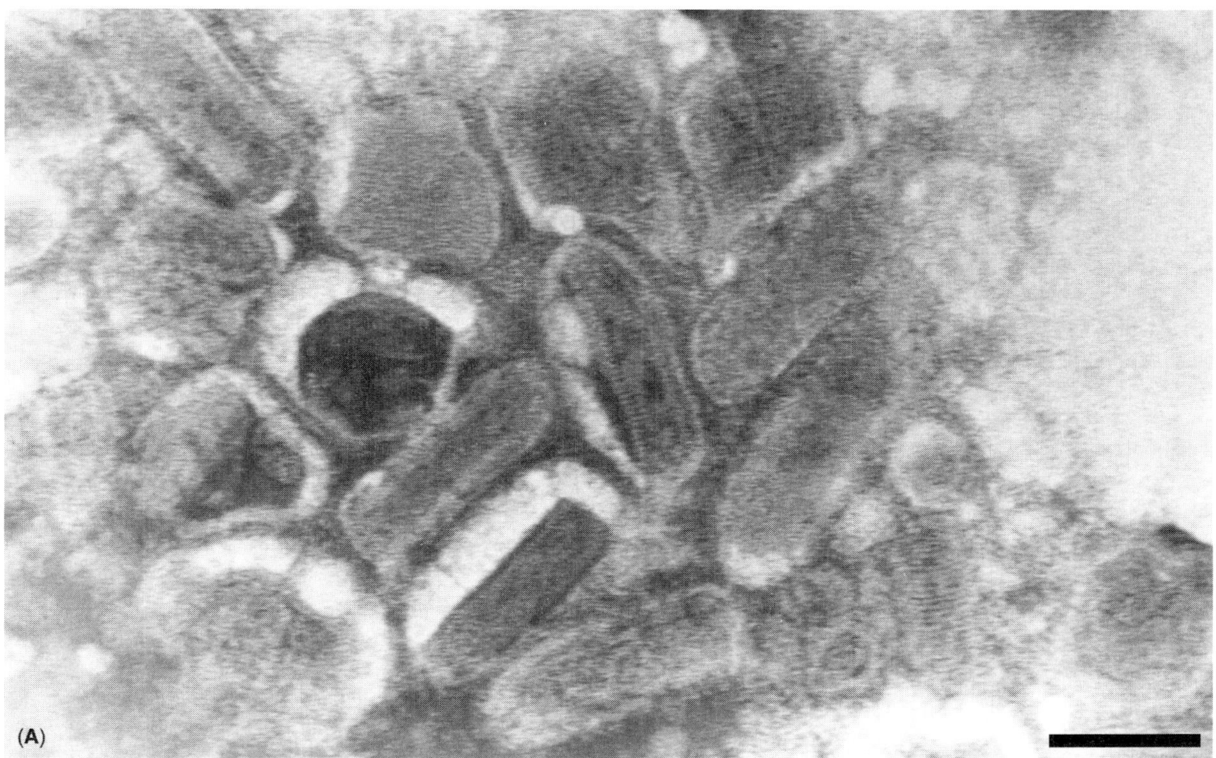

Figure 27 Rhabdovirus. (**A**) Negative stain of vesicular stomatitis virus, a bullet-shaped virus, identical in morphology to rabies virus. Bar = 100 nm. (*Continued*)

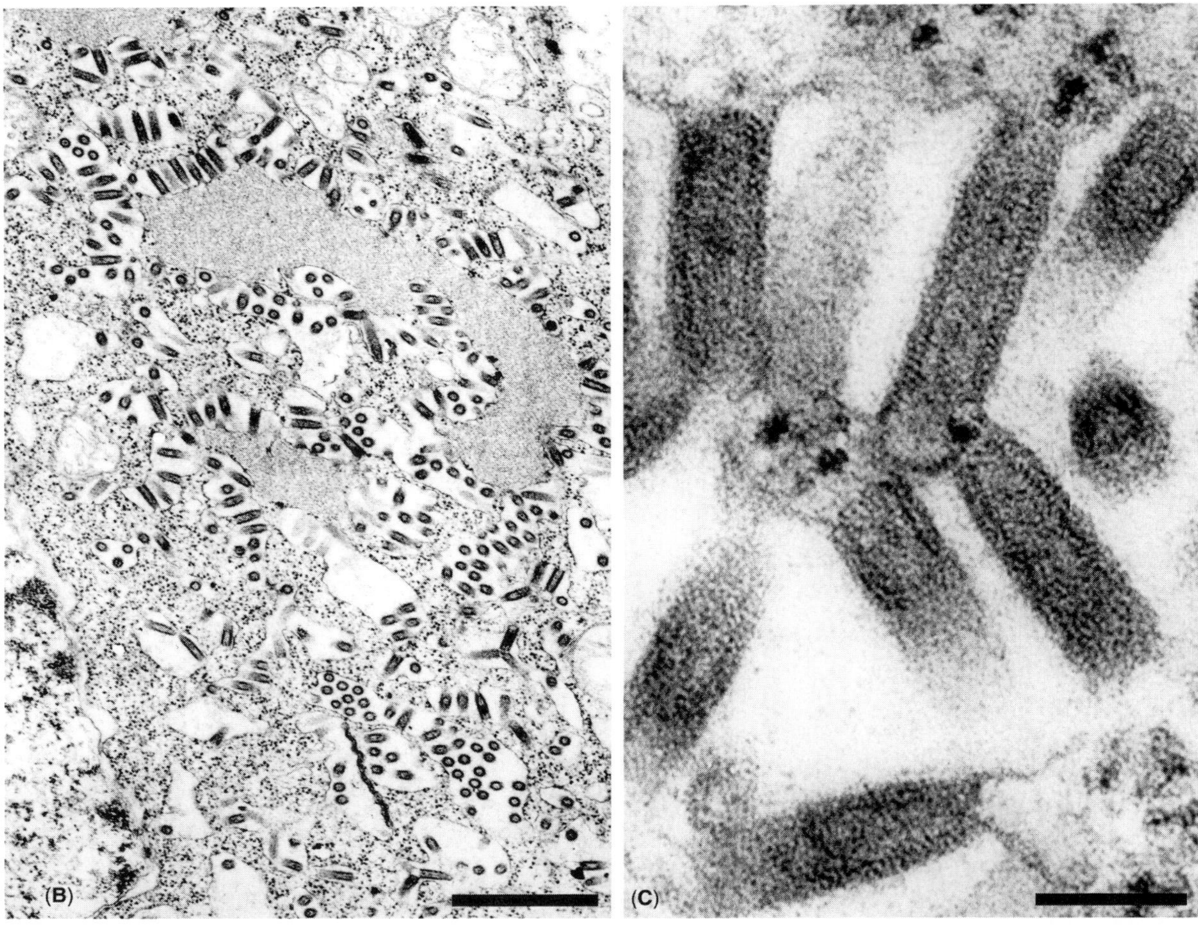

Figure 27 (*Continued*) (**B**) Thin section of a rabies virus-infected cell. Virions bud out from the cytoplasmic membrane. Bar = 1 μm. (**C**) High magnification of rabies virus. The rounded end protrudes from the cell, and the flat end breaks off from the cell membrane. Bar = 100 nm. *Source*: (**B** and **C**) Courtesy of Dr. F.A. Murphy and A.K. Harrison.

the matrix, but most rhabdoviruses mature by budding out of the cell.

VSV is somewhat smaller (~170 × 70 nm) than rabies virus, which is longer and varies more in diameter (200–300 nm × 50–80 nm).

Epidemiology

Rabies transmission is usually through saliva in bites from infected animals, but aerosols and corneal and other organ transplants have been known to spread the disease (4,43). A reported case of sudden onset of bilateral vision decrement resulted from corneal endotheliitis. Aqueous humor was cultured, and a rhabdovirus was identified by TEM (83), but not further identified.

Clinical Presentation

There is an incubation period of a few days to months, shorter if the bite is on the head or in children. In a longer incubation and with a lack of history of a bite, the disease may go unnoticed until too late. The prodrome may last 2 to 7 days and is characterized by nonspecific flu-like symptoms that may include headache, agitation, and irritability.

There are two potential manifestations of the disease, a hyperactive or "furious rabies" and a paralytic or "dumb rabies" form. In the former, patients have severe agitation, hallucinations, and anxiety. Laryngeal spasms may be triggered by drinking, seeing, or thinking of liquids, hence the designation "hydrophobia". In ~20% of cases, the paralytic form prevails with progressive weakness and flaccid paralysis that may resemble Landry-Guillain-Barré syndrome.

Rabies is almost always fatal once disease symptoms have appeared; only a small handful of cases have been reported where the patient survived. Usually death ensues within ~7 days without support or within 2 weeks with intensive support and assisted ventilation. Up to 50,000 deaths per year occur in developing countries due to rabies. The only defense is vaccination prior to exposure with a booster after a bite, or a series of passive and active vaccinations of a non-immune host following exposure.

Histopathology

In CNS tissue, the hallmark lesion of rabies infection is the Negri body, a cytoplasmic inclusion seen in neurons, particularly in the spinal cord, upper brainstem, and thalamus. By TEM, viral particles in a dense matrix have been demonstrated in these inclusions, which are sometimes accompanied by perivascular inflammation and focal microglial nodules. Haltia et al. reported the ocular pathological findings in a 30-year-old bat scientist who died 7 weeks after a bat bite (50). There was chronic inflammation of the ciliary body and choroid, proteinaceous exudate in the outer plexiform layer of the retina and subretinally, periphlebitis, and loss of retinal ganglion cells (50). Rabies-related viral antigen was detected in retinal ganglion cells, but viral particles could not be identified by TEM (50).

Diagnosis

The diagnosis in an infected animal is made by direct immunofluorescence staining of a touch preparation of brain (Fig. 28), after which a positive result warrants vaccination of the bitten person or animal. Diagnosis in humans can be confirmed by fluorescence staining, but is unnecessary after death following a bite and typical disease. A corneal impression test has been used for diagnosing rabies virus encephalitis; it was positive for virus by fluorescence before CSF, serum, saliva and culture tests showed evidence of the infection (148). Other tests include inoculating mice or tissue cultures and staining with fluorescent antibody, or detecting neutralizing antibody in serum of a person who has not been prevaccinated.

Rubiviruses

Rubella Virus

Virology

Rubella virus (German measles) is a small (50–70 nm) enveloped ssRNA virus (29). The non-structural proteins share some sequence homology with the non-structural proteins of alphaviruses and Hepevirus (hepatitis E virus). Although the nucleocapsid is icosahedral, by TEM it is non-distinct. The outer surface has a hemagglutinin protein, but it is not evident as spikes by TEM as those in the paramyxo- and orthomyxoviruses are, and the surface appears morphologically smooth. Thus, in negative stains of clinical material, it cannot be distinguished from cellular debris because both the outer surface detail and the nucleocapsid are not distinctive (Fig. 29A). In thin sections of infected cells, particles with a dense, nondescript 30 to 35 nm core can be seen budding from the cytoplasmic membrane (Figs. 29B and C).

Epidemiology

Prior to widespread vaccination, epidemics of rubella occurred in 6- to 9-year cycles, typically in children. Rubella virus replicates in the respiratory tract and is

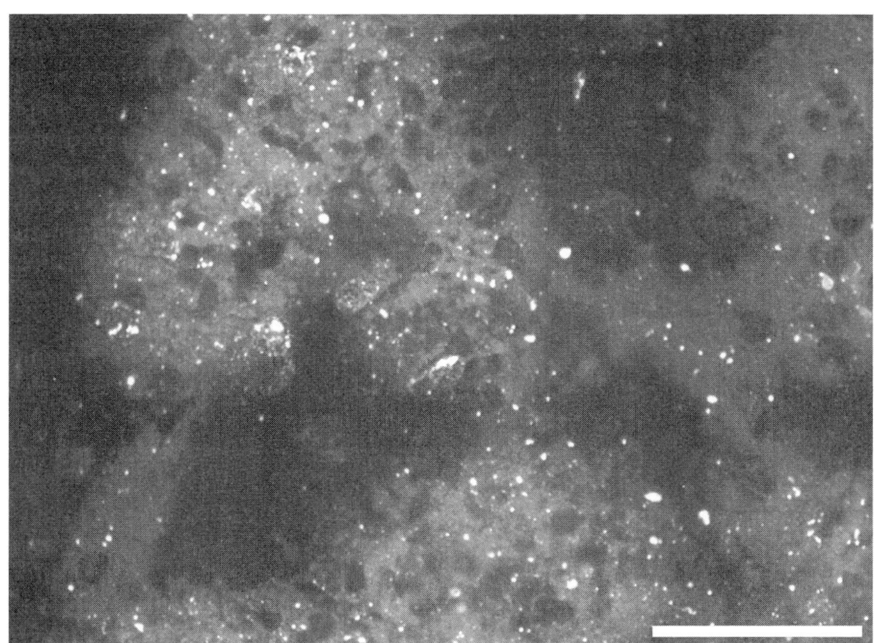

Figure 28 Fluorescence micrograph of a touch preparation of a rabies virus-infected brain. *Source*: Courtesy of M. Brinson, North Carolina State Laboratory of Public Health. Bar = 25 μm.

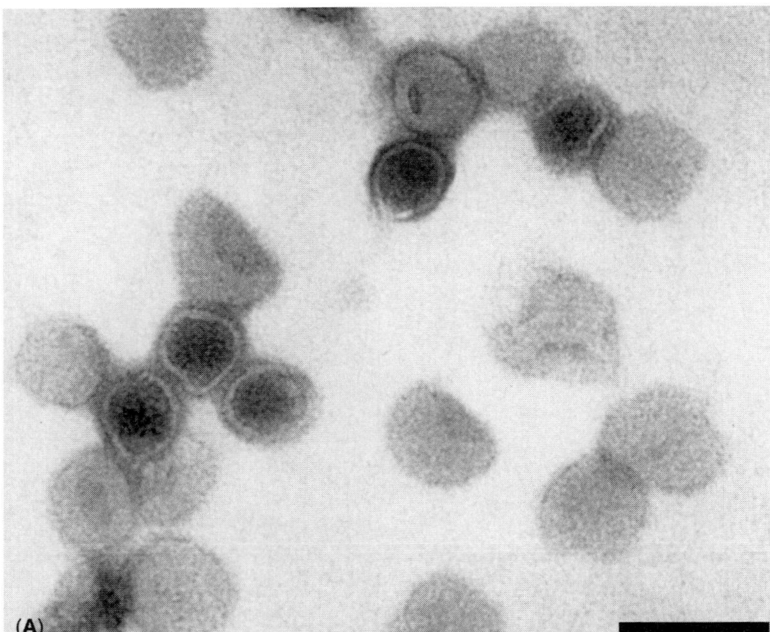

Figure 29 Rubivirus. (**A**) Negative stain of rubella virus. Particles are ~60 nm and are relatively smooth on the surface. They would be indistinguishable from cell debris in a clinical specimen. Bar = 100 nm. *Source*: Courtesy of Dr. R.B. Simmons, Georgia State University. (**B**) Low magnification of rubella virus in the extracellular space between cells (*center*). Bar = 1 μm. *Source*: Courtesy of Dr. F.A. Murphy and A.K. Harrison, Centers for Disease Control and Prevention. (**C**) High magnification of thin section of rubella virus in tissue culture. Virions bud from the cytoplasmic membrane to the extracellular space. Bar = 100 nm. *Source*: Courtesy of Dr. F.A. Murphy and A.K. Harrison, Centers for Disease Control and Prevention.

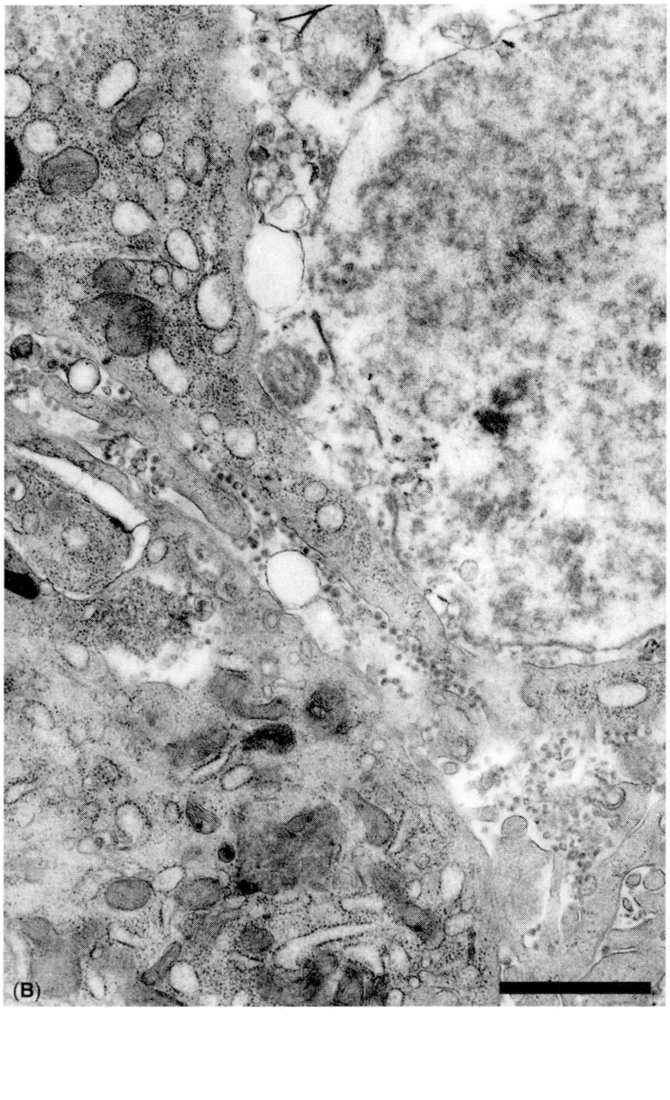

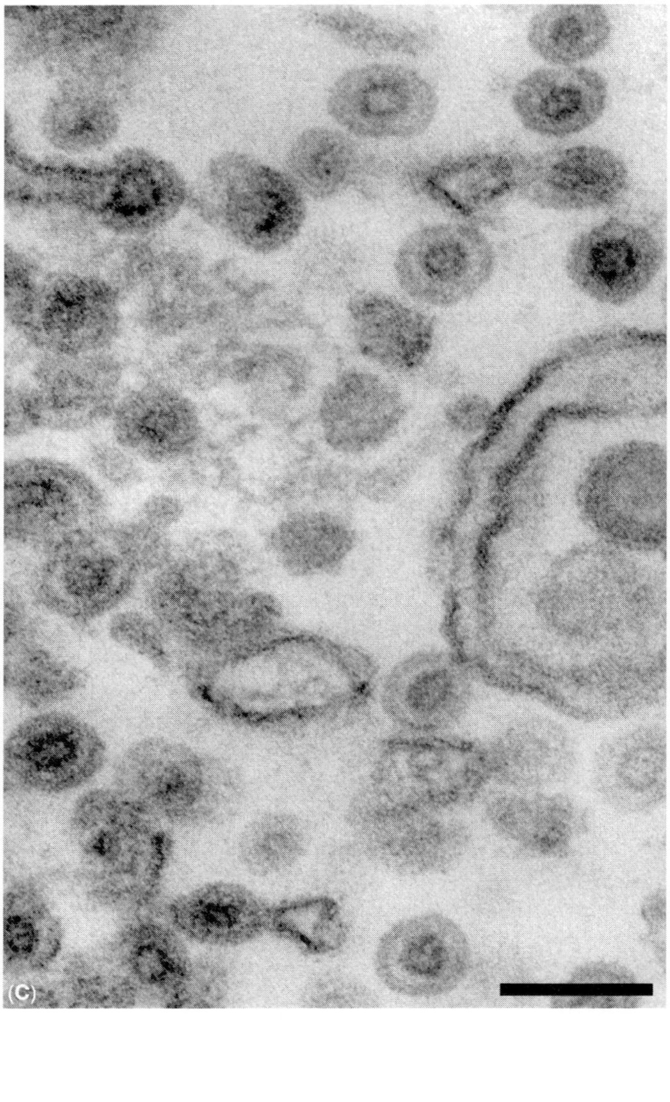

spread via droplets from the nasopharyngeal area. Up to ~25% of pregnant women do not have immunity, and fetal infection results in direct consequences. Persistent infections may be established whereby the virus can be isolated several years after the disease (42). Rubella is pandemic; however, vaccination controls it in the developed world.

Clinical Presentation

An infection acquired after birth results in fever, headache, and malaise. A maculopapular rash on the trunk spreads centrifugally to the extremities. It progresses to a systemic infection where antibodies are formed and rash occurs. When severe, there may be thrombocytopenic purpura, lymphadenopathy, or splenomegaly. Other manifestations that may occur include encephalitis, arthritis, hemorrhage, carditis, hearing loss, and genitourinary disorders (33). If the eye is affected, there may be conjunctivitis, iritis, superficial keratitis, bilateral exudative retinal detachments, veiling, peliosis, and panuveitis.

Serious consequences of rubella occur from intrauterine transmission to a fetus during the first trimester of pregnancy. Fetal manifestations of congenital rubella depend on the gestational age at the time of virus exposure. Infection early in pregnancy may result in abortion. Later first-trimester infection may result in a congenital rubella syndrome (CRS) with numerous birth defects, including deafness, blindness, and heart malformation. CRS patients, and occasionally patients who contract the disease later in life, may develop autoimmune and psychiatric problems years later, including progressive rubella panencephalitis, a fatal neurodegenerative disease.

Ocular features may include microphthalmia, cataracts, glaucoma, strabismus, nasolacrimal duct occlusion, corneal clouding, iris atrophy, iritis, chorioretinitis, and optic atrophy. A fundus photograph of a patient with congenital rubella may show alternating hypopigmented and hyperpigmented areas of the RPE with a diminished foveal light reflex that have been termed "salt and pepper fundus". The salt and pepper appearance of the retina may occur in acquired as well as congenital disease. This picture remains throughout life, even though vision can be close to normal. Second and third trimester infection may not harm the fetus.

Histopathology

The lens in children with congenital rubella cataract is more spherical than usual and has nuclear sclerosis with retained nuclei in the nuclear lens fibers (24). There may be an abrupt transition from normal cortex to the sclerotic central nucleus, or there may be lateral displacement of the sclerotic nucleus if the cortex has liquefactive degeneration (24). The degree of cortical degeneration varies widely, and the amount of spherophakia is generally directly proportional to the amount of cortical degeneration (24). Rarely, the cataractous lens may be spontaneously absorbed leaving behind only the transparent capsule (24). Congenital rubella retinopathy is manifest as areas of increased pigmentation of the RPE with other areas having loss of RPE cells or decreased pigment within the cells (45).

Diagnosis

Congenital rubella can be diagnosed clinically with characteristic fetal abnormalities and a history of maternal infection during the pregnancy. Rubella virus can be cultured from oropharyngeal fluids of the infected newborn and identified with fluorescent staining. In acquired disease, IgM antibodies may be present, and a four-fold rise in hemagglutination inhibition or complement fixation of ELISA antibodies may support the diagnosis.

REFERENCES

1. Aksamit AJ, Major EO, Ghatak NR, et al. Diagnosis of progressive multifocal leukoencephalopathy by brain biopsy with biotin labeled DNA:DNA in situ hybridization. J Neuropathol Exp Neurol 1987; 46:556–66.
2. Alibek K, Handelman S, Biohazard. The Chilling Story of the Largest Covert Biological Weapons Program in the World–Told from Inside by the Man Who Ran It. New York: Dell, 1999.
3. Ambroziak JA, Blackbourn DJ, Herndier BG, et al. Herpes-like sequences in HIV-infected and uninfected Kaposi's sarcoma patients. Science 1995; 268:582–3.
4. Anderson LJ, Williams LP Jr, Layde JB, et al. Nosocomial rabies: investigation of contacts of human rabies cases associated with a corneal transplant. Am J Public Health 1984; 74:370–2.
5. Appen RE, Roth H, ZuRhein GM, Varakis JN. Progressive multifocal leukoencephalopathy. A cause of visual loss. Arch Ophthalmol 1977; 95:656–9.
6. Ball LA. Replication strategies of RNA viruses. In: Knipe DM, Howley PM, Griffin DE, Lamb RA, Martin MA, Roizman B, Straus SE, eds. Fields Virology. 4th ed. New York: Lippincott Williams & Wilkins, 2001:105–18.
7. Barrero PR, Grippo J, Viegas M, Mistchenko AS. Wild-type measles virus in brain tissue of children with subacute sclerosing panencephalitis, Argentina. Emerg Infect Dis 2003; 9:1333–6.
8. Beck AP, Glasser DA, Pollack JS. Is Coxsackievirus the cause of unilateral acute idiopathic maculopathy? Arch Ophthalmol 2004; 122:121–3.
9. Bonfioli AA, Eller AW. Acute retinal necrosis. Semin Ophthalmol 2005; 20:155–60.
10. Brown HH, Glasgow BJ, Holland GN, Foos RY. Cytomegalovirus infection of the conjunctiva in AIDS. Am J Ophthalmol 1988; 106:102–4.
11. Chan CK, Limstrom SA, Tarasewicz DG, Lin SG. Ocular features of west Nile virus infection in North America: a study of 14 eyes. Ophthalmology 2006; 113:1539–46.
12. Charles NC, Friedberg DN. Epibulbar molluscum contagiosum in acquired immune deficiency syndrome. Case

report and review of the literature. Ophthalmology 1992; 99:1123–6.
13. Chopra JS, Sawhney IM, Dhand UK, Prabhakar S, Nalk S, Sehgal S. Neurological complications of acute haemorrhagic conjunctivitis. J Neurol Sci 1986; 73:177–91.
14. Chu CT, Howell DN, Morgenlander JC, et al. Electron microscopic diagnosis of human flavivirus encephalitis: use of confocal microscopy as an aid. Am J Surg Pathol 1999; 23:1217–26.
15. Connolly JH, Haire M, Hadden DS. Measles immunoglobulins in subacute sclerosing panencephalitis Br Med J 1971; 1:23–5.
16. Cono J, Casey CG, Bell DM. Smallpox vaccination and adverse reactions. Guidance for clinicians. MMWR Recomm Rep 2003; 52:1–28.
17. Cusnir V, Slepova O, Dumbrava V, et al. Ocular manifestations of hepatitis B. Oftalmologia 1997; 41: 25–7.
18. Cuzzubbo AJ, Vaughn DW, Nisalak A, et al. Comparison of PanBio Dengue Duo IgM and IgG capture ELISA and venture technologies dengue IgM and IgG dot blot. J Clin Virol 2000; 16:135–44.
19. Davies FG. Observations on the epidemiology of Rift Valley fever in Kenya. J Hyg (Lond) 1975; 75:219–30.
20. Dawson CR, Hanna L, Togni B. Adenovirus type 8 infections in the United States. IV. Observations on the pathogenesis of lesions in severe eye disease. Arch Ophthalmol 1972; 87:258–68.
21. Demols PF, Cochaux PM, Velu T, Caspers-Velu L. Chorioretinal post-transplant lymphoproliferative disorder induced by the Epstein–Barr virus. Br J Ophthalmol 2001; 85:93–5.
22. Deutman AF, Klomp HJ. Rift Valley fever retinitis. Am J Ophthalmol- 1981; 92:38–42.
23. Doane FW, Anderson N. Electron Microscopy in Diagnostic Virology. A Practical Guide and Atlas. New York: Cambridge University Press, 1987.
24. Eagle RC Jr, Spencer WH. Lens. In: Spencer WH, ed. Ophthalmic Pathology An Atlas and Textbook. 4th edn. Philadelphia: W.B. Saunders Co., 1996:372–437.
25. Elliott RM, Wilkie ML. Persistent infection of Aedes albopictus C6/36 cells by Bunyamwera virus. Virology 1986; 150:21–32.
26. Engstrom RE Jr, Holland GN, Margolis TP, et al. The progressive outer retinal necrosis syndrome. A variant of necrotizing herpetic retinopathy in patients with AIDS. Ophthalmology 1994; 101:1488–502.
27. Erie JC, Campbell RJ, Liesegang TJ. Conjunctival and corneal intraepithelial and invasive neoplasia. Ophthalmology 1986; 93:176–83.
28. Farthing CG, Howard RS, Thin RN. Papillitis and hepatitis B. Br Med J 1986; 292:1712.
29. Fauquet CM, Mayo MA, Maniloff J, et al. eds. Virus Taxonomy. Classification and Nomenclature of Viruses. Eighth Report of the International Committee on the Taxonomy of Viruses. New York: Elsevier Academic Press, 2005.
30. Feinberg AS, Spraul CW, Holden JT, Grossniklaus HE. Conjunctival lymphocytic infiltrates associated with Epstein–Barr virus. Ophthalmology 2000; 107:159–63.
31. Feuer R, Mena I, Pagarigan R, et al. Cell cycle status affects coxsackievirus replication, persistence, and reactivation in vitro. J Virol 2002; 76:4430–40.
32. Font RL. Eyelids and lacrimal drainage system. In: Spencer WH, ed. Ophthalmic Pathology: An Atlas and Textbook. 4th ed. Philadelphia: W.B. Saunders Co., 1996: 2218–437.
33. Forrest JM, Turnbull FM, Sholler GF, et al. Gregg's congenital rubella patients 60 years later. Med J Australia 2002; 177:664–7.
34. Foster A, Sommer A. Corneal ulceration, measles, and childhood blindness in Tanzania. Br J Ophthalmol 1987; 71:331–43.
35. Fraser NW, Block TM, Spivack JG. The latency associated transcripts of herpes simplex virus: RNA in search of function. Virology 1992; 191:1–8.
36. Furrer H, Fux C. Opportunistic infections: an update. J HIV Ther 2002; 7:2–7.
37. Furrer H, Barloggio A, Egger M, Garweg JG. Retinal microangiopathy in human immunodeficiency virus infection is related to higher human immunodeficiency virus-1 load in plasma. Ophthalmology 2003; 110:432–6.
38. Gardner BP, Margolis TP, Mondino BJ. Conjunctival lymphocytic nodule associated with Epstein–Barr virus. Am J Ophthalmol 1991; 112:567–71.
39. Garg S, Jampol LM. Systemic and intraocular manifestations of West Nile virus infection. Surv Ophthalmol 2005; 50:3–13.
40. Garnett CT, Erdman D, Xu W, Gooding LR. Prevalence and quantitation of species C adenovirus DNA in human mucosal lymphocytes. J Virol 2002; 76: 10608–16.
41. Gentile M, Gelderblom HR. Rapid viral diagnosis: role of electron microscopy. New Microbiol 2005; 28:1–12.
42. Gershon AA. Rubella virus (German measles). In: Mandell GL, Douglas GG, Bennett JE, eds. Principles and Practice of Infectious Diseases. 3rd ed. New York: Churchill Livingstone, 1990:1242–7.
43. Gode GR, Bhide NK. Two rabies deaths after corneal grafts from one donor. Lancet 1988; 2:791.
44. Grant K, Jerome WG. Laser captures microdissection as an aid to ultrastructural analysis. Microsc Microanal 2002; 8:170–5.
45. Green WR. Retina. In: Spencer WH, ed. Ophthalmic Pathology An Atlas and Textbook. 4th ed. Philadelphia: W.B. Saunders Co., 1996:667–1331.
46. Griffiths PD, Baboonian C. A prospective study of primary cytomegalovirus infection during pregnancy: final report. Br J Obstet Gynaecol 1984; 91:307–15.
47. Guo DF, Shibata R, Shinagawa M, et al. Genomic comparison of adenovirus type 3 isolates from patients with acute conjunctivitis in Japan, Australia, and the Philippines. Microbiol Immunol 1988; 32:833–42.
48. Guttman-Yassky E, Dubnov J, Kra-Oz A, et al. Classic Kaposi sarcoma. Cancer 2005; On-line.
49. Hales RH, Ostler HB. Newcastle disease conjunctivitis with subepithelial infiltrates. Br J Ophthalmol 1973; 57: 694–7.
50. Haltia M, Tarkkanen A, Kivela T. Rabies: ocular pathology. Br J Ophthalmol 1989; 73:61–7.
51. Hedquist BG, Bratt G, Hammarin AL, et al. Identification of BK virus in a patient with acquired immune deficiency syndrome and bilateral atypical retinitis. Ophthalmology 1999; 106:129–32.
52. Hershberger VS, Hutchins RK, Witte DP, et al. Epstein–Barr virus-related bilateral acute retinal necrosis in a patient with X-linked lymphoproliferative disorder. Arch Ophthalmol 2003; 121:1047–9.
53. Holbach LM, Font RL, Naumann GO. Herpes simplex stromal and endothelial keratitis. Granulomatous cell reactions at the level of Descemet's membrane, the stroma, and Bowman's layer. Ophthalmology 1990; 97:722–8.
54. Holland GN, Cornell PJ, Park MS, et al. An association between acute retinal necrosis syndrome and HLA-

DQw7 and phenotype Bw62, DR4. Am J Ophthalmol 1989; 108:370–4.

55. Holland GN. Executive committee of the American Uveitis Society. Standard diagnostic criteria for the acute retinal necrosis syndrome. Am J Ophthalmol. 1994; 117:663–7.
56. Howell DN, Smith SR, Butterly DW, et al. Diagnosis and management of BK polyomavirus interstitial nephritis in renal transplant recipients. Transplantation 1999; 68: 1279–88.
57. Hu G, Wang MJ, Miller MJ, et al. Ocular vaccinia following exposure to a smallpox vaccinee. Am J Ophthalmol 2004; 137:554–6.
58. Huff JL, Barry PA. B-virus (Cercopithecine herpesvirus 1) infection in humans and macaques: potential for zoonotic disease. Emerg Infect Dis 2003; 9:246–50.
59. Iannarella G, Makdassi R, Schmit JL, et al. Association of progressive multifocal leukoencephalitis and sarcoidosis. Ann Med Interne (Paris). 1992; 143:71–4.
60. Jabs DA, Green WR, Fox R, et al. Ocular manifestations of acquired immune deficiency syndrome. Ophthalmology 1989; 96:1092–9.
61. Jakobiec FA, Bilyk JR, Font RL. Orbit. In: Spencer WH, ed. Ophthalmic Pathology an Atlas and Textbook. 4th ed. Philadelphia: W.B. Saunders Co., 1996:2438–933.
62. Johnson RT. Evidence for polyomaviruses in human neurological diseases. In: Sever JL, Maddend DL, eds. Polyomaviruses and Neurological Disease. New York: Alan R. Liss 1983:183–90.
63. Jones KL, Johnson KA, Chambers CD. Offspring of women infected with varicella during pregnancy: a prospective study. Teratology 1994; 49:29–32.
64. Kaiser PK, Lee MS, Martin DA. Occlusive vasculitis in a patient with concomitant West Nile virus infection. Am J Ophthalmol 2003; 136:928–30.
65. Kirber MW, Kirber HP. Effect of ultraviolet-irradiated homologous virus on experimental mumps and influenza infections in animal eyes. J Bacteriol 1966; 92:1570–5.
66. Korenblat KM, Dienstag JL. Viral Hepatitis. In: Richman DD, Whitley RJ, Hayden FG, eds. Clinical Virology. 2nd ed. Washingnton, D.C.: ASM Press, 2002:59–77.
67. Kowalski RP, Gordon YJ. Comparison of direct rapid tests for the detection of adenovirus antigen in routine conjunctival specimens. Ophthalmology 1989; 96: 1106–9.
68. Krichevskaia GI, Katargina LA, Andzhelov VO, et al. [Persistence of ophthalmotropic enteroviruses in ocular tissues after enterovirus uveitis]. Vestn Oftalmol 1997; 113:26–9.
69. Kuiken T, Wobeser G, Leighton FA, et al. Pathology of Newcastle disease in double-crested cormorants from Saskatchewan, with comparison of diagnostic methods. J Wildl Dis 1999; 35:8–23.
70. Lang D, Hinderer W, Rothe M, et al. Comparison of the immunoglobulin-G-specific seroreactivity of different recombinant antigens of the human herpesvirus 8. Virology 1999; 260:47–54.
71. Langford MP, Yin-Murphy M, Barber JC, et al. Conjunctivitis in rabbits caused by enterovirus type 70 (EV70). Invest Ophthalmol Vis Sci 1986; 27:915–20.
72. Lashkevich VA, Koroleva GA, Lukashev AN, et al. Enterovirus uveitis. Rev Med Virol 2004; 14:241–54.
73. Lashkevich VA, Koroleva GA, Lukashev AN, et al. (Acute enterovirus uveitis in infants). Vopr Virusol 2005; 50: 36–45.
74. Leahey AB, Shane JJ, Listhaus A, Trachtman M. Molluscum contagiosum eyelid lesions as the initial manifestation of acquired immunodeficiency syndrome. Am J Ophthalmol 1997; 124:240–1.
75. Lemon SM, Shapiro CN. The value of immunization against hepatitis A. Infectious Agents and Disease—CK this title. 1994; 3:38–49.
76. Lessell S, Collins TE. Ophthalmoplegia in Powassan encephalitis. American Academon of Neurology. 2003; 60: 1726–7.
77. Levy RM, Bredesen DE, Rosenblum ML. Neurological manifestations of the acquired immunodeficiency syndrome (AIDS): experience at UCSF and review of the literature. J Neurosurg 1985; 62:475–95.
78. Lewis JM, Nagae Y, Tano Y. Progressive outer retinal necrosis after bone marrow transplantation. Am J Ophthalmol 1996; 122:892–5.
79. Liesegang TJ. Epidemiology of ocular herpes simplex. Natural history in Rochester, Minn, 1950 through 1982. Arch Ophthalmol 1989; 107:1160–5.
80. Liesegang TJ. Biology and molecular aspects of herpes simplex and varicella-zoster virus infections. Ophthalmology 1992; 99:781–99.
81. Lukashev AN, Lashkevich VA, Koroleva GA, et al. Molecular epidemiology of enteroviruses causing uveitis and multisystem hemorrhagic disease of infants. Virology 2003; 307:45–53.
82. Lund OE, Stefani FH. Corneal histology after epidemic keratoconjunctivitis. Arch Ophthalmol 1978; 96: 2085–8.
83. Madhavan HN, Goldsmith CS, Rao SK, et al. Isolation of a vesicular virus belonging to the family rhabdoviridae from the aqueous humor of a patient with bilateral corneal endotheliitis. Cornea 2002; 21:333–5.
84. Maudgal PC. Cytopathology of adenovirus keratitis by replica technique. Br J Ophthalmol 1990; 74:670–5.
85. McBride WJ, Bielefeldt-Ohmann H. Dengue viral infections; pathogenesis and epidemiology. Microbes Infect 2000; 2:1041–50.
86. McDonnell JM, McDonnell PJ, Sun YY. Human papillomavirus DNA in tissues and ocular surface swabs of patients with conjunctival epithelial neoplasia. Invest Ophthalmol Vis Sci 1992; 33:184–9.
87. McKee PH, Calonje E, Granter SR. Pathology of the Skin with Clinical Correlations. 3rd ed. Philadelphia: Elsevier Mosby, 2005.
88. Meyer H, Damon IK, Esposito JJ. Orthopoxvirus diagnostics. In: Isaacs SN, ed. Methods in Molecular Biology: Vacinnia Virus and Poxvirology Methods and Protocols. Totowa NJ: Humana Press, 2004:119–31.
89. Miller SE, Lang DJ. Rapid diagnosis of herpes simplex infection: amplification for electron-microscopy by short-term in vitro replication. J Infect. 1982; 4:37–41.
90. Miller SE. Detection and identification of viruses by electron microscopy. J Electron Microscopy Tech 1986; 4: 265–301.
91. Miyake-Kashima M, Fukagawa K, Tanaka M, et al. Kaposi varicelliform eruption associated with 0.1% Tacrolimus ointment treatment in atopic blepharitis. Cornea 2004; 23:190–3.
92. Modlin JF. Coxsackieviruses, echovirus, and new enteroviruses. In: Mandell GL, Douglas FG, Bennett JE, eds. Principles and Practice of Infectious Diseases. New York: Churchill Livingston, 1990.
93. Murray HW, Knox DL, Green WR, Susel RM. Cytomegalovirus retinitis in adults. A manifestation of disseminated viral infection. Am J Med. 1977; 63: 574–84.

94. Myers JP, Leveque TK, Johnson MW. Extensive chorioretinitis and severe vision loss associated with west Nile virus meningoencephalitis. Arch Ophthalmol. 2005; 123: 1754–6.
95. Nahmias AJ, Lee FK, Beckman-Namias S. Sero-epidemiological and -sociological patterns of herpes simplex virus infection in the world. Scand J Infectious Disease 1990; 69:19–36.
96. Nakamura K, Ohta Y, Abe Y, et al. Pathogenesis of conjunctivitis caused by Newcastle disease viruses in specific-pathogen-free chickens. Avian Pathol 2004; 33: 371–6.
97. Nanda M, Curtin VT, Hilliard JK, et al. Ocular histopathologic findings in a case of human herpes B virus infection. Arch Ophthalmol 1990; 108:713–6.
98. Nelson DA, Weiner A, Yanoff M, DePeralta J. Retinal lesions in subacute sclerosing panencephalitis. Arch Ophthalmol 1970; 84:613–21.
99. Niklasson B, Grandien M, Peters CJ, Gargan TP II. Detection of Rift Valley fever virus antigen by enzyme-linked immunosorbent assay. J Clin Microbiol 1983; 17: 1026–31.
100. Norrby E, Kristensson K. Measles virus in the brain. Brain Res Bull 1997; 44:213–20.
101. Obaldia N III, Hanson RP. Effect of Newcastle disease virus on ocular and paraocular tissues in experimentally inoculated chickens. Avian Dis 1989; 33:285–90.
102. Ouwens JP, Haaxma-Reiche H, Verschuuren EA, et al. Visual symptoms after lung transplantation: a case of progressive multifocal leukoencephalopathy. Transpl Infect Dis 2000; 2:29–32.
103. Palmer EL, Martin ML. Electron Microscopy in Viral Diagnosis. Boca Raton: CRC Press, 1988.
104. Patrick BA, Mehta PD, Sobczyk W, et al. Measles virus-specific immunoglobulin D antibody in cerebrospinal fluid and serum from patients with subacute sclerosing panencephalitis and multiple sclerosis. J Neuroimmunol 1990; 26:69–74.
105. Pavan-Langston D. Manual of Ocular Diagnosis and Therapy. 4th ed. New York: Little, Brown and Company, 1996.
106. Pepose JS, Margolis TP, LaRussa P, Pavan-Langston D. Ocular complications of smallpox vaccination. Am J Ophthalmol 2003; 136:343–52.
107. Pertel P, Hirschtick R, Phair J, et al. Risk of developing cytomegalovirus retinitis in persons infected with the human immunodeficiency virus. J Acquir Immune Defic Syndr 1992; 5:1069–74.
108. Pomerantz RJ, Kuritzkes DR, de la Monte SM, et al. Infection of the retina by human immunodeficiency virus type I. N Engl J Med 1987; 317:1643–7.
109. Proia AD. Cornea and sclera. In: Sassani JW, ed. Ophthalmic Pathology with Clinical Correlations. Philadelphia: Lippincott-Raven Publishers, 1997:125–44.
110. Purdy KW, Heckenlively JR, Church JA, Keller MAMD. Progressive outer retinal necrosis caused by varicella-zoster virus in children with acquired immunodeficiency syndrome. Pediatric Infections Disease 2003; 22:382–286.
111. Rabon RJ, Louis GJ, Zegarra H, Gutman FA. Acute bilateral posterior angiopathy with influenza A viral infection. Am J Ophthalmol 1987; 103:289–93.
112. Riffenburgh RS. Ocular manifestations of mumps. Arch Ophthalmol 1961; 66:739–43.
113. Rohrbach JM, Krober SM, Teufel T, et al. EBV-induced polymorphic lymphoproliferative disorder of the iris after heart transplantation. Graefes Arch Clin Exp Ophthalmol 2004; 242:44–50.
114. Rozina EE, Khudaverdyan OE, Ghendon Yu Z. Clinical and morphologic studies on the guinea pig eye infected with human influenza virus strains of different virulence. Acta Virol 1987; 31:340–5.
115. Rozina EE, khudaverdian OE, Shteinberg L. Comparative clinico-morphological research on measles and mumps infections in an experiment on guinea pigs. Vopr Virusol 1988; 33:342–7.
116. Rozina EE, Khudaverdyan OE, Brudno IA, et al. Comparative clinico-morphological investigations of the CNS of monkeys and of the eye teguments of guinea pigs infected with different measles virus strains. Acta Virol 1988; 32:123–8.
117. Sabin AB. Research on dengue during World War II. Am J Tropical Med Hygiene 1952; 1:30–50.
118. Santos C. Herpes simplex uveitis. Bol Asoc Med P R. 2004; 96:71–4, 77–83.
119. Scheie HG, Morse PH. Rubeola retinopathy. Arch Ophthalmol 1972; 88:341–4.
120. Schooley RT, R.D. Epstein–Barr virus (infectious mononucleosis). In: Mandell GL, Douglas RG, Bennett JE, eds. Principles and practice of infectious diseases. 3rd ed. New York: Churchill Livingstone, 1990:1172–85.
121. Semba RD. The ocular complications of smallpox and smallpox immunization. Arch Ophthalmol 2003; 121: 715–9.
122. Shaikh S, Ta CN. Evaluation and management of herpes zoster ophthalmicus. Am Fam Physician. 2002; 66:1723–30.
123. Shalala DE. Bioterrorism: how prepared are we? Emerg Infect Dis 1999; 5:492–3.
124. Shuttleworth G, Shimeld C, Easty D. Viral disease of the eye. In: Richman DD, Whitley FJ, Hayden FG, eds. Clinical Virology. 2nd ed. Washington, DC: ASM Press, 2002:145–69.
125. Siam AL, Meegan JM. Ocular diseases resulting from infection with Rift Valley fever virus. Trans R Soc Trop Med Hyg 1980; 74:539–41.
126. Siam AL, Meegan JM, Gharbawi KF. Ritf Valley fever ocular manifestations: observations during the 1977 epidemic in Egypt. Br J Ophthalmol 1980; 64:366–74.
127. Sidikaro Y, Silver L, Holland GN, Kreiger AE. Rhegmatogenous retinal detachments in patients with AIDS and necrotizing retinal infections. Ophthalmology 1991; 98:129–35.
128. Sjo LD, Juhl BR, Buchwald C, et al. Epstein–Barr positive T-cell lymphoma in the ocular region. Eur J Ophthalmol 2006; 16:181–5.
129. Skolnik PR, Pomerantz RJ, de la Monte SM, et al. Dual infection of retina with human immunodeficiency virus type 1 and cytomegalovirus. Am J Ophthalmol 1989; 107: 361–72.
130. Spencer WH. Conjunctiva. In: Spencer WH, ed. Ophthalmic Pathology An Atlas and Textbook. 4th ed. Philadelphia: W.B. Saunders Co., 1996:38–155.
131. Spencer WH. Cornea. In: Spencer WH, ed. Ophthalmic Pathology an Atlas and Textbook. 4th ed. Philadelphia: W. B. Saunders Co., 1996:157–333.
132. Stoner GL, Ryschkewitsch CF. Evidence for JC virus in two progressive multifocal leukoencephalopathy (PML) brains previously reported to be infected with SV 40. J Neuropathol Exp Neurol 1991; 50:342.
133. Straus SE. Introduction to herpesviridae. In: Mandell GL, Douglas RG, Bennett JE, eds. Principles and Practice of infectious Diseases. 3rd ed. New York: Churchill Livingstone, 1990:1139–44.
134. Taylor GH. Cytomegalovirus. Am Fam Physician 2003; 67:519–24.

135. Teitelbaum CS, Streeten BW, Dawson CR. Histopathology of herpes simplex virus keratouveitis. Curr Eye Res 1987; 6:189–94.
136. Tullo AB, Shimeld C, Blyth WA, et al. Latent infection following ocular herpes simplex in non-immune and immune mice. J Gen Virol 1982; 63:95–101.
137. Tullo AB, Coupes D, Klapper P, et al. Analysis of glycoproteins expressed by isolates of herpes simplex virus causing different forms of keratitis in man. Curr Eye Res 1987; 6:33–8.
138. Tullo AB, Ridgway AE, Lucas DR, Richmond S. Histopathology of adenovirus type 8 keratitis. Cornea 1987; 6:234.
139. Verougstraete C. White spots syndromes. Bull Soc Belge Ophtalmol 2001:67–78.
140. Waggoner-Fountain LA, Grossman LB. Herpes simplex virus. Am Acad Pediat 2004; 25:86–93.
141. Walker DL. Progressive multifocal leukoencephalopathy. In: Vinken PJ, Bruyn GW, eds. Handbook of Clinical Neurology. Amsterdam: North Holland, 1985: 503–24.
142. Wegman DH, Guinee VF, Milliani SF. Epidemic keratoconjunctivitis. Am J Public Health 1970; 60:1230–7.
143. Wehrly SR, Manning FJ, Proia AD, et al. Cytomegalovirus keratitis after penetrating keratoplasty. Cornea 1995; 14: 628–33.
144. Wilhelmus KR, Font RL, Lehmann RP, Cernoch PL. Cytomegalovirus keratitis in acquired immunodeficiency syndrome. Arch Ophthalmol 1996; 114:869–72.
145. Winward KE, Hamed LM, Glaser JS. The spectrum of optic nerve disease in human immunodeficiency virus infection. Am J Ophthalmol 1989; 107:373–80.
146. Wong KW, D'Amico DJ, Hedges TR III, et al. Ocular involvement associated with chronic Epstein–Barr virus disease. Arch Ophthalmol 1987; 105:788–92.
147. Wunschmann A, Shivers J, Bender J, et al. Pathologic and immunohistochemical findings in goshawks (Accipiter gentilis) and great horned owls (Bubo virginianus) naturally infected with West Nile virus. Avian Dis 2005; 49:252–9.
148. Zaidman GW, Billingsley A. Corneal impression test for the diagnosis of acute rabies encephalitis. Ophthalmology. 1998; 105:249–51.

9

Bacterial Infections

Curtis E. Margo
University of South Florida, Tampa, Florida, U.S.A.

INTRODUCTION

Knowledge concerning human diseases caused by bacteria has been accumulating at an extraordinary rate since bacteria were first discovered nearly 175 years ago. This, however, is a minuscule fraction of the 3.5 billion years that bacteria have inhabited the earth and learned to adapt to their environment. The prokaryotic genome with its ability to acquire new DNA and rearrange existing genes gives bacteria an effective mechanism by which to colonize the vast number of ecological niches that exist on earth. The eye, like other body surfaces, is constantly exposed to bacteria, yet only a small proportion ever causes disease. In an idealized setting, bacteria and the human host would co-exist in a symbiotic relationship. In reality, however, co-existence is limited by either increased bacterial virulence or lapses in host defenses that result in infection.

Infectious disease can be conceptualized as a state of diminished health caused by an imbalance between microbial virulence factors and human defense mechanisms. When it comes to ocular infections, there are a variety of physical, cellular and molecular strategies used to avert, limit, or discourage the adherence, penetration and growth of bacteria on the surface of the globe and to maintain the sterility of the interior of the eye. This chapter reviews the different clinical patterns of ocular infection in context of the interaction between bacterial virulence factors and host defense mechanisms.

OCULAR DEFENSES

Tear Film

The mucosal surface of the eye is lined by a relatively thin epithelial layer (compared to skin), which in turn is coated by the tear film. The tear film is the first line of anti-bacterial defense. It has been traditionally viewed as a trilaminar film composed of mucin, aqueous, and lipid. Recent studies suggest that mucin may be more evenly distributed throughout the tear film than the trilaminar model would indicate (105). Tears are kept at near neutral pH, supplied constantly with glucose and maintained at an osmolarity just below the physiologic averuse. This nutrient-rich, moist environment would be ideal for bacterial growth if not for a variety of antibacterial substances that are also present.

Mucin, a complex meshwork of proteins and polysaccharides, helps to mechanically trap bacteria and prevent them from gaining access to the mucosal epithelia. The aqueous layer contains a variety of substances such as lactoferrin that inhibit bacterial proliferation. Most pathogenic bacteria require free iron for growth, which in the human body is kept at low concentration by binding to ferritin, transferritin, hemoglobin, and lactoferritin. To survive in low iron environments, bacteria use low molecular weight chelators of iron, known as siderophores, to trap this essential growth factor. Lactoferrin, present in human tears in a concentration of 1.5 gm/L (none detectable in serum), competes with bacterial siderophores for free iron. Lactoferrin may have other secondary roles in host defense. It appears to augment bacterial killing by polymophonuclear leukocytes (PMNs) and also serves a protective function by binding potentially toxic iron released from dying cells (19).

Antibacterial proteins such as lysozyme are found in relatively high concentrations in the tears. Lysozyme makes up to 40% of the total protein content of the tears (118). In the gut, lysozyme has been shown to digest the walls of Gram-positive bacteria and it can inflict similar damage to Gram-negative organisms, but only after their outer membrane has been injured by bile salts. Tear lysozyme probably acts against Gram-positive bacteria in the conjunctiva in a similar manner. Its concentration decreases with age, dry eye syndrome (see Chapter 30) and certain types of infections.

Beta-lysin has antibacterial actions that parallel those of lysozyme, but it may act against bacterial cell membranes rather than cell walls. It is more concentrated in serum than tears and probably originates from non-conjunctival sources.

Conjunctiva

The conjunctiva is guarded by a reservoir of subepithelial lymphoid tissues that acts as a processing center for foreign antigens and an immunological repository for antigen-specific antibodies (57). The resident conjunctival lymphoid tissue is considered as a part of the mucosa-associated lymphoid tissue (MALT) system used to protect the respiratory, alimentary, and genitourinary tracts from bacterial infection. Among the most important functions of MALT is the production of antigen-specific antibodies of the immunoglobulin A (IgA), immunoglobulin G (IgG), and immunoglobulin E (IgE) types (5,21,118).

IgA is the predominant immunoglobulin in tears as it is in other seromucous secretions. The mechanism of IgA secretion has been more thoroughly studied in non-conjunctival mucosal tissues. The IgA dimer is synthesized by plasma cells and bound to epithelial cell receptors soon after its release. The dimer, which is vulnerable to proteolytic digestion, is endocytosed by epithelium for transport across the epithelial cell. When the IgA molecule is released onto the mucosal surface, it has a secretory component derived from the cleavage of the receptor (107). This secretory component appears to provide the IgA molecule with added protection from proteolytic enzymes present in the tear film. The main role of secretory IgA is to coat bacteria and toxins in the tear film and prevent them from adhering to cell surfaces (22).

IgG is not found in any appreciable concentration in normal tears. Under certain conditions IgG is called into action where it functions as a second line of defense. IgG binds bacteria, fixes complement and enhances phagocytosis. IgG antibodies bind to the surface of bacteria where they interact with complement proteins. Opsonization of bacteria by activated complement enhances the uptake of bacteria by phagocytes. The classical complement pathway (see Chapter 3) can also be activated by mannose-binding lectins that bind mannose residues on bacteria. The alternative pathway is activated by binding of certain bacterial surface molecules to complement components. Components of the complement cascade result in histamine release from mast cells, act as chemoattractants for phagocytic cells, and can directly injure or kill bacteria.

The immune response to bacteria involves multiple steps starting with bacterial antigens being processed by an antigen-processing cell. The processed fragment of the antigen is displayed on its surface and presents it in a highly immunogenic form to T helper cells and B cells. The T cell recognizes separate determinants on the antigen to those recognized by the B cell. B-cell activation depends on the antigen interacting with B-cell immunoglobulin receptors and a second factor from the T helper cell to prompt optimal growth and differentiation. Acquired humoral immunity, although not a primary conjunctival defense, serves an important role in preventing bacterial infection.

Polymorphonuclear Leukocytes and Phagocytosis

PMNs (see Chapter 1) contain substances with antibacterial actions including hydrolyses, cationic proteins, and myeloperoxidases (25). Ingestion of bacteria triggers degranulation and the production of hydrogen peroxide or superoxide. Bacteria are killed intracellularly by a variety of mechanisms. Most but not all bacteria can be destroyed by the detergent-like action of cationic proteins, low intracellular pH, lysozyme, and other antibacterial enzymes found in PMNs.

Phagocytosis of bacteria by PMNs involves attachment, engulfment, and ingestion. Ingestion is often mediated by surface protein receptors and the coating of bacteria with opsin enhances attachment and ingestion. As mentioned earlier, antigen-specific IgG and complement are the two major opsonic substances. Antibodies neutralize antiphagocytic molecules on the surface of bacteria. A cooperative interaction of receptors involved in phagocytosis exists when organisms are coated with both IgG and the third component of complement (C3). Nonspecific serum factors such as fibronectin and laminin also promote phagocytosis by less well understood mechanisms. Once the foreign bacteria have been ingested, there is a burst of oxidative activity and cytoplasmic degranulation coordinated to deliver the toxic products of degranulation to the phagocytic vacuoles. Unfortunately, the process of degranulation is not limited to contact between foreign microorganisms and PMNs. When the toxic components of phagocytic digestion are exposed to host tissue, they cause collateral damage.

Cytokines play important stimulatory and regulator roles in the cellular defense system (see Chapter 3). Various cytokines direct the exit of PMNs from blood vessels and their movement in interstitial tissue. Tumor necrosis factor and interleukin-1, for example, induce monocytes and PMNs to leave the bloodstream via endothelial transmigration. Once outside the vascular space, inflammatory cells depend on various chemical signals (chemotaxis) to migrate to the site of infection. PMNs, for instance, are able to follow the changing gradient of the fifth component of complement (C5) to an infection site.

Cell Mediated Immunity

Cell mediated immunity (see Chapter 3) operates in concert with humoral immunity and has a particularly important role in defense against obligate intracellular pathogens. The cellular immune response is initiated on the surface of the eye by Langerhans cells, which are concentrated at the sclerocorneal limbus and are scattered throughout the bulbar conjunctiva (43). The concentration of Langerhans cells is lowest in the center of the cornea (23). The surface of the Langerhans cell contains human leukocyte antigen, -DR antigens (class II histocompatibility antigens), receptors for complement, and the crystallizable (Fc) portion of immunoglobulin (43,57). The Langerhans cell may have other functions beyond that of an antigen processing cell, (there being evidence that the cell serves to stimulate local inflammatory reaction through nonspecific mechanisms).

The usual histopathologic manifestation of the cell mediated immune response is granulomatous inflammation. Bacteria that typically elicit such a reaction include, but are not limited to, mycobacteria, *Listeria monocytogenes*, spirochetes, *Salmonella* sp. and *Brucella*, and *Franciscella tularensis* (137). As pointed out in Chapter 3, the T cells in granulomas are composed of $CD4^+$ T cells centrally and $CD8^+$ T cells towards the periphery (107).

Mechanical Barriers

The vast majority of bacteria in the tear film has a limited life expectancy and does not cause invasive disease. Intraocular sterility is maintained in large part by the mechanical barriers created by the cornea, conjunctiva and sclera. The effectiveness of epithelium in preventing bacterial infection is due in part, to the fact that skin surfaces are a recent evolutionary development of complex, multicellular organisms. Bacteria have not had enough time to develop strategies to by-pass this type of barrier short of waiting for an accidental or surgical injury. However, one should not under estimate the creative potential of these unicellular organisms. Bacteria are making some progress. Take, for example, the strategy used by *Borrelia burgdorferi* that gains entrance into the sterile confines of the body by colonizing the digestive tracts of biting insects.

Bacterial Flora of the Conjunctiva

It is generally believed, although not fully proven, that the normal commensal flora of the conjunctiva has a role in protecting the host from invasive bacteria by competing for nutrients and receptor sites on host cells. Commensal flora may also produce substances that are toxic to pathogenic bacteria or stimulate the host's immune system to cross-react with potentially invasive organisms. The flora of the conjunctiva and eyelid margin is similar and consists of a dynamic population of organisms. Despite their similarity, quantitative studies have disclosed higher colony counts in the eyelid margins (4,63,87). The most frequently encountered bacteria in the conjunctiva are coagulase-negative staphylococci, *Staphylococcus aureus*, corynebacteria, *Propionibacterium* species, and anaerobic Gram-positive cocci (18,76,98).

The ocular flora changes with environmental factors. There is increased representation of more virulent bacteria, such as Gram-negative rods, in hospitalized patients, patients admitted to burn units, and in persons on immunosuppressive drugs or infected with human immunodeficiency virus (HIV) (40,79,103) (see Chapter 8).

DETERMINANTS OF BACTERIAL PATHOGENICITY

The effectiveness of a bacterium to cause disease is a function of its virulence and attributable to properties of mobility, adhesiveness, invasiveness, and replicability. How much damage a bacterium causes depends upon a variety of molecular interactions between the organism and host. Success of a pathogen is measured by its ability to multiply maximally and secure its biological niche without killing the host.

The origins of pathogenicity are beginning to be unraveled by molecular genetics. The bacterial chromosome is a highly integrated and stable entity that tends to resist rearrangement despite an ability to transfer its genetic material. Analyses of natural populations of pathogenic bacteria have shown a prominent representation of relatively few clones of pathogenic subtypes (117). Virulence factors are conserved. Of the 182 distinct *Hemophilus influenzae* type b clonal types, as few as 9 contribute to 80% of all invasive disease worldwide (81). If horizontal transfer of genetic material through recombination were a frequent occurrence, homogenization of the bacterial chromosome would be expected. In fact, bacterial species have remained distinct taxonomic entities and serious disease is caused by a small proportion of the total number of clones within a bacterial species (106).

Changes in the environment can affect the expression of the determinants of virulence. Bacteria have the ability to regulate their virulence factors according to changes in temperature, ionic concentration, oxygen concentration, calcium concentration, pH, and trace metal concentration (106). Many of the genes that control these regulatory functions have been identified in pathogenic bacteria including *B. pertussis, V. cholerae, S. aureus*, and *E. coli* (106).

Bacterial Adherence

The initial contact between a microorganism and its host is termed adherence. This process of simply sticking together is mediated by molecules on the surface of bacteria called adhesins and host receptor molecules known as ligands. There are several classes of bacterial adhesins, the most common of which are fimbrial and nonfimbrial. Bacteria with fimbrial adhesins include *Escherichia coli, Neisseria gonorrhea, Salmonella* (type 1), and *Vibrio cholerae*. Nonfimbrial adhesins are found on *B. pertussis, M. pneumoniae, Treponema pallidum*, and *Yersinia* (99). Lipoteichoic acid is an adhesin for *Streptococcus pyogenes*. A single adhesin may interact with one or multiple receptor molecules. Cellular receptors vary considerably in their structure and include immunoglobulins, integrins, transport proteins, complement receptors, and growth factors (99). The activity of adhesins may be conformationally controlled or it may involve proteolytic processing.

Bacterial Capsule and Cell Wall

The bacterial cell wall and capsule are common determinants of virulence. Most bacteria have a rigid cell envelope and a cytoplasmic membrane surrounding a single chromosome of double-stranded DNA. Four different types of cell walls are found: Gram-negative, Gram-positive, mycobacterial, and spirochaetal.

The cell walls of Gram-negative bacteria are characterized by lamellar inner and outer phospholipid layers. Sandwiched between these layers are a cross linked peptidoglycan, which gives bacteria their rigid shape. A variety of other molecules have been found in the outer phospholipid layer including lipopolysaccharide (LPS) in Gram-negative organisms and various types of proteins. LPS is a major biological effector molecule that triggers host responses to bacterial infection (as in endotoxic shock and other conditions). Gram-positive bacteria differ by the greater thickness of the peptidoglycan layer. Outward radiating organelles such as flagella and pili originate from the inner membrane of both Gram-negative and Gram-positive bacteria. Surface antigens have functional roles in establishing virulence and are useful markers for the classification of bacteria.

The walls of mycobacteria contain prominent amounts of long chain fatty acids and mycolic acids covalently linked to different carbohydrates (16). The hydrocarbon chains of these lipids form an exceptionally thick bilayer making it relatively impermeable (17). Hydrophilic nutrients traverse the cell wall through special channels. Mycobacteria glycolipids are highly antigenic, and are also highly resistant to enzymatic digestion. The cell wall stimulates both a strong cell-mediated and humoral immune response. This immunogenic property of mycobacteria has been known for a considerable time and lead to the development of a commercial universal antigenic stimulant using mycobacterial cell wall preparations (Freud adjuvant).

Bacterial capsules are relatively unstructured polymer coatings. These polymers consist of pure and combined forms of peptides, protein-carbohydrates and polysaccharides. The most commonly studied group is the polysaccharides. The first protective roles ascribed to capsules were those of neutralizing complement activation and impeding phagocyte function. Some capsules rich in sialic acid, such as those in the K1 strain of *E. coli*, prevent the assembly of C3 (via the complement alternative pathway) on the bacterial surface thus reducing the likelihood of opsonization. Most polysaccharide capsules are hydrophobic and can inhibit phagocytosis by this nonspecific physicochemical property.

The most thoroughly studied antiphagocytic bacterial capsules are those from *N. meningitides*, *S. pneumoniae*, and *H. influenzae*. The only defense that checks the intravascular proliferation of these microorganisms is a capsular-specific antibody response. Without this response, PMNs are not able to ingest capsulated bacteria. In the case of *H. influenza* type b, normal antibody production to colonized bacteria in the throat does not occur for several years after birth. Historically, children have been at risk of serious *H. influenza* infection until they reach the age of 4 or 5 years when protective antibody titers are obtained. With the widespread use of *H. influenza* type b vaccine, the incidence of serious infection has significantly declined in recent years.

Bacteria have found methods to counter the effect of capsular-specific antibodies. Some subvert the host antibody response by producing capsules that resemble the polysaccharides in host's cells. *S. pyogenes* and some strains of *N. meningitides*, for instance, use this method of mimicry to diminish their immunogenicity (109).

Bacterial Toxins

Bacterial toxins were the first type of virulence factor discovered and studied in any detail. As the activities of these substances became elucidated, they provided strong support for the molecular theory of infectious disease. Bacterial toxins consist of heterogeneous groups of substances that have been divided traditionally into two broad groups: exotoxins and endotoxins (49). The term "exotoxins" was first used to describe toxins that were excreted from cells rather than being embedded in the cell surface (an endotoxin). More recently, the use of the word "exotoxins" has fallen out of favor because some toxins are not truly excreted but rather accumulate inside the cell until the time of cell death when they are released.

Toxin nomenclature is haphazard. Some toxins are named after the organism from which they are derived, such as diphtheria toxin, tetanus toxin, *Shiga* toxin, and cholera toxin. Other bacterial toxins are named according to the cell type they attack; examples include neurotoxin, leukotoxin, cardiotoxin and hepatotoxin. Yet other toxin names are based on their enzymatic activity. They include lecithinase (toxin produced by *C. perfringens*) and adenylate cyclase (toxin produced by *B. pertussis*). A more systematic approach to naming toxins is by mechanism of action. A three-category system has been proposed based on how toxins bind and interact with cell membranes (110).

Botulism is the prototype of an exotoxin disease: an acute form of bacterial poisoning caused by the ingestion of a preformed toxin in food. *Clostridium botulinum* is a spore forming, Gram-positive rod that normally grows in soil. Botulism occurs when spores germinate in foods leading to a bacterial proliferation and the production of toxin. Bacteria produce three toxins: botulinum toxin (botox), C2 toxin and C3 toxin. Botulinum toxin is the most lethal of the three and it has seven different serotypes (A through G). Types A and B are the ones most often implicated in human disease. Botulinum toxin binds to glycoproteins on the surface of neurons and when internalized it inhibits the release of acetylcholine. Clinically, the toxin interferes with neuromuscular transmission in cholinergic fibers causing ophthalmoplegia, ptosis, and mydriasis (127). Symptoms usually begin within 12 hours after ingestion of contaminated food. Visual symptoms can be the first manifestation of poisoning.

The toxin produced by *Clostridium diphtheria* is probably the most thoroughly studied of all naturally occurring toxins. *C. diphtheria* is a Gram-positive nonsporulating rod. A pathogen of the upper respiratory tract that occasionally infects the skin and conjunctiva, it causes a localized infection characterized by epithelial ulceration and severe exudation. The toxin is cleaved by proteolytic nicking after secretion, forming two small chains (A and B). Once the toxin is bound to a human cell, the host takes up the toxin in endocytic vesicles where a single molecule of the A chain can kill a eukaryotic cell (110). The gene encoding the diphtheria toxin is carried by a lysogenic bacteriophage. Only strains infected with the phages produce the toxin. Localized complications of ocular infection include symblepharon formation, corneal scaring, and dry eye. In untreated cases, the toxin can cause myocarditis and peripheral neuropathy. Ocular infections, however, do not tend to cause the severe, often life-threatening complications as diphtheria pharyngitis.

Endotoxin cell injury, on the other hand, is triggered by specific components of the bacterial cell walls. Tissue destruction is mediated by lysosomal enzymes from leukocytes and by activation of the complement cascade (115). LPS is the component of the Gram-negative outer membrane responsible for the toxic reaction. Most bacteria causing endotoxin injury are Gram-negative; many are normal commensals of the gastrointestinal tract. The typical setting in which bacterial endotoxic injury occurs is in chronically ill patients who have an underlying disease that predisposes them to sepsis. The role of endotoxins in the pathogenesis of ocular injury from infection is less clear than it is in systemic disease. The destructive effects of *Pseudomonas* keratitis are probably mediated by both exotoxins and endotoxins (53).

Biofilm

Biofilms are sessile communities of bacteria in which individual microorganisms live in close proximity to one another and within a hydrated polymeric matrix (27). This mode of individual and communal growth is just beginning to be understood. Biofilm formation has existed for at least 3 billion years based on findings from early fossil records. These structures allow bacteria to survive in environments that would normally be too hostile for individual organisms to exist in (46). Individual microorganisms that make up the community of bacterium display differences from their free-living counterparts both morphologically and physiologically. Biofilms have an important role in the pathogenesis of a variety of diseases from cystic fibrosis to dental caries and chronic gingivitis. Biofilms also serve as reservoirs for pathogens in the environment (95). Antibiotic resistance of bacteria living in biofilms likely contributes to the chronicity of certain infections. Resistance to antibiotics usually involves alterations of genetic information through plasmids, transposons, or mutations (126). Antibiotic resistance in biofilms takes advantage of the slimy hydrated matrix of polysaccharides and proteins in which the bacteria grow. This matrix can simply inhibit antibiotic penetration on a physicochemical basis.

The structure of biofilms is characterized by numerous mushroom-shaped assemblages of bacteria. These small units are separated by channels that are used to transport nutrients throughout the biofilm community. Biofilms create unique adaptive properties that give bacteria growth and proliferative advantage (29). *P. aeruginosa*, for instance, produces an acetylated form of the polysaccharide alginate, a polymer of mannuronic and glucuronic acid (100). This form of alginate forms a viscous gel that imparts a glistening appearance to colonies. The gel allows bacteria to better survive in moist environments like the respiratory tract. The acetylated alginate may also serve as an adhesin which increases resistance to phagocytosis.

Bacterial biofilms are suspected of playing roles in the pathogenesis of several ocular infection including contact lens-associated keratitis, pseudophakic endophthalmitis, and crystalline keratopathy (92,94). Endotoxins released from Gram-negative biofilms growing in sterilizers have been implicated in the development of diffuse lamellar keratitis after laser in situ keratomileusis (LASIK) (51).

Other Virulence Factors

Plasmids are self-replicating, nonchromosomal units of DNA. A class of plasmids known as R-plasmids has an important role in determining antimicrobial resistance. Most of the individual drug resistance determinants in R-plasmids contain transposons (111). Transposons possess both the gene for drug resistance and the genetic machinery to relocate itself on other plasmids (and even insert itself in bacterial chromosomes). R-plasmids in some cases can transfer this genetic information via conjugal transfer to other bacterial strains and occasionally to other species. Certain individual virulence factors like hemolysin and enterotoxin can exist in plasmids. Indiscriminate use of antibiotics helps to select for R-plasmids antibiotic resistant factors. Multiple resistance factors can exist on a single R-plasmid.

PATTERNS OF OCULAR INFECTION

Patterns of ocular infection refer to the intuitive classification of infection based on anatomic location. The natural anatomic barriers of the eye represent the simplest form of host defense. They are primarily responsible for keeping superficial infections localized and the internal contents of the eye sterile.

Bacterial Conjunctivitis

Essentially all bacterial infections of the conjunctiva are contracted from external sources, with the rare exceptions of endogenously spread spirochetes in secondary syphilis and perhaps in Lyme disease (caused by *Borrelia burgorferi*) (125). The classification of bacterial conjunctivitis is imperfect and can be based on duration of symptoms (acute vs. chronic), type of inflammation (non-granulomatous vs. granulomatous), predominant clinical feature (such as purulent, catarrhal, membranous, and pseudomembranous), or by the etiologic agent.

Endogenous Bacterial Conjunctivitis

Syphilitic conjunctivitis is the result of hematogenous dissemination of treponemal spirochetes during the secondary stage of the disease. During this stage of syphilis, lesions of the skin and mucous membrane are potentially infectious (71). The conjunctiva is usually mildly inflamed, but the condition can be easily overlooked when more prominent signs of intraocular infection co-exist. Histologically, the conjunctiva contains lymphocytes and plasma cells with either a granulomatous or non-granulomatous pattern of inflammation. Necrosis is seldom found. Spirochetes are present in large numbers, but require special stains (such as the Warthin-Starry stain) for visualization. Although the clinical manifestations of secondary syphilis are self limited in the non-immunocompromised host, the disease is transmittable during this stage through direct contract with lesions of the skin or mucous membrane.

Acute Bacterial Conjunctivitis

The distinction between acute and chronic conjunctivitis is clinical and has been arbitrarily based on the duration of inflammation. An often quoted dividing point is 3 or 4 weeks (15). A subset of acute conjunctivitis is referred to as "hyperacute" and is characterized by the sudden onset of intensely inflamed tissues with a purulent discharge. The organisms most often associated with this clinical picture are *N. gonorrhoae, Neisseria meningitides,* and *Hemophilus influenza* biotype II.

The clinical findings in *N. gonorrhoae* conjunctivitis are severe hyperemia and a thick purulent discharge (Fig. 1). The tarsal conjunctiva has a diffuse papillary reaction. If left untreated, the infection can result in a corneal infiltration, ulceration, and, in some situations, perforation. Gonorrheal conjunctivitis can be acquired by newborns as they pass through an infected birth canal or by adults through direct contact with a companion who has a genital infection.

Because *N. gonorrhoae* is a human-specific pathogen, research efforts have been slowed by the lack of an animal model. The Chang conjunctival cell line is one of the most popular and practical means of studying the bacterium in the laboratory. In cervical or urethral infections, *N. gonorrhoae* are ingested by epithelial cells and transported to the basolateral cell surface where they bind to cell surface receptors and stimulate an intense inflammatory reaction. A component of the outer membrane known as lipo-oligosaccharide is responsible for the resistance of *N. gonorrhoae* to membrane attack complex of complement (82). The organism also appears to stimulate certain host antibodies that block the action of other anti-bacterial antibodies (135). Once considered a strictly extracellular pathogen, *N. gonorrhoae* may derive some of its virulence from activity inside human cells. The hypervariability of gonococcal surface proteins has prevented the successful development of a vaccine.

Acute Catarrhal Conjunctivitis

Acute catarrhal conjunctivitis is characterized by moderate conjunctival hyperemia and a mucopurulent discharge. Symptoms usually begin abruptly. The tarsal inflammatory changes consist of small papillae; follicles are not seen in typical cases. A variety of bacteria can cause acute catarrhal conjunctivitis, with *S. pneumoniae* and *H. influenzae* being the two most common.

Membranous Conjunctivitis

In membranous conjunctivitis an inflammatory membrane forms over the conjunctiva during the acute phase of the infection. The membrane is composed of fibroblasts, small blood vessels, fibrin, and inflammatory cells. The causative organism that incites this process does so by seriously damaging the host's conjunctival epithelium. The membrane is interwoven with the underlying substantia propria of the conjunctiva and when peeled causes vigorous bleeding.

Clostridium diphtheria is the prototypical cause of pseudomembranous conjunctivitis, though rarely seen today. This Gram-positive, non-spore forming, aerobic rod usually is a pathogen of childhood. The infection is infrequently encountered in developed countries because of the widespread use of diphtheria toxoid vaccine. The diphtheria toxin is one of the most thoroughly studied of all bacterial metabolites and serves as a model of toxic injury. Diphtheria toxin has both local and systemic effects, including potent cardiac toxicity. In the past, diphtheria pharyngitis was a major cause of childhood morbidity. The gene encoding diphtheria toxin is carried on a group of

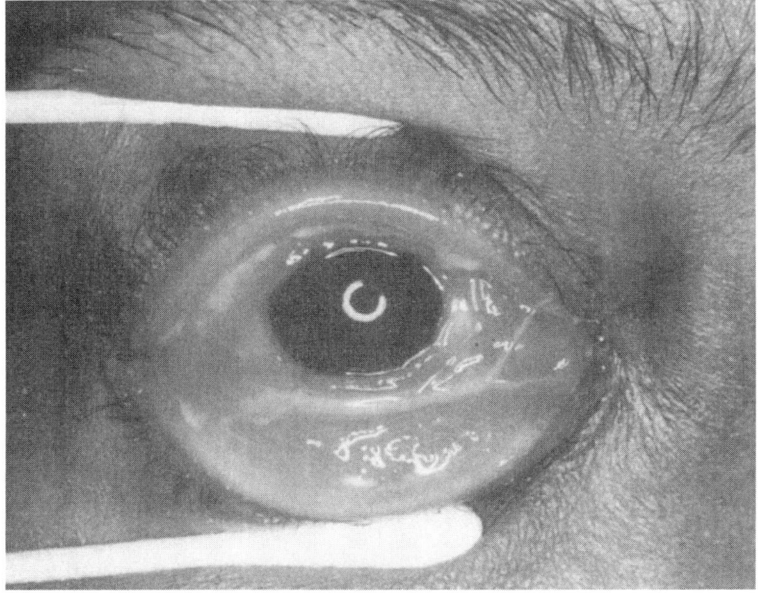

Figure 1 Hyperacute conjunctivitis due to *Neisseria gonorrheae*, showing beefy red mucosa and thick purulent discharge in the lower cul-de-sac and at the interface of the upper lid, and edematous conjunctiva. Photograph was taken 15 hours after topical and systemic antibiotic therapy was started.

related lysogenic bacteriophages. Only strains infected with these phages are able to produce the toxin.

Chronic Conjunctivitis

After prolonged exposure to a bacterial pathogen the conjunctiva adapts to some extent and displays nonspecific changes. Goblet cells increase in number, the epithelium becomes hyperplastic, vascular congestion increases and edema of the substantia propria creates overlying folds. The proliferation of lymphocytes leads to lymphoid follicles with germinal centers. Certain organisms, like staphylococci, produce toxins that result in marginal corneal infiltrates (Fig. 2) (132). These superficial infiltrates, which occur most often between 4 and 8 o'clock positions of the conjunctiva, are separated from the corneoscleral limbus by a thin clear area. Severe cases can lead to peripheral corneal ulceration. Chronic infection of the eyelid margin and conjunctiva by *Moraxella* gives rise to superficial excoriated skin lesion typically at the medial and lateral canthi (angular blephritis) (135).

Bacterial Keratitis and Corneal Ulceration

Highly virulent bacteria in the conjunctiva such as *N. gonorrhoeae* can cause ulcerative keratitis de novo. The vast majority of corneal ulcers, however, follow injury to the corneal epithelium. Common predisposing factors include contact lens use, accidental corneal abrasion, trichiasis, and bullous keratopathy. Alterations in the ocular surface from dry eyes, poor blink reflex, chronic blepharitis, diabetes mellitus, or alcoholism play important roles in the initiation and propagation of bacterial keratitis. Visual prognosis depends on several important variables including bacterial virulence, location of the primary ulcer, effectiveness of treatment, and host defense mechanisms. Bacterial keratitis that results in the permanent loss of vision or in enucleation is usually due to virulent organisms (68).

The histopathologic findings depend on when in the course of the corneal infection the tissue is examined. Most corneal tissue is studied when the condition is advanced, as when a perforated ulcer or secondary endophthalmitis is associated, or when the ulcer has healed and the corneal scar is removed by penetrating keratoplasty.

During the early stage of infection, the corneal epithelium is absent and the stroma is thin. The base of the ulcer shows degenerating collagen and a dense accumulation of PMNs. The density of the inflammatory infiltrate decreases the greater the distance from the epicenter of the ulcer. Full thickness stromal necrosis will lead to corneal perforation (Fig. 3). Because Descemet membrane is relatively resistant to enzymatic digestion, it can remain intact after the stromal collagen has been destroyed (Fig. 4). Infections causing a moderately severe degree of tissue destruction are usually associated with an anterior chamber reaction, trabeculitis, iritis, inflammatory deposits on the lens capsule and possibly an anterior vitritis. Uncontrolled infection can lead to endophthalmitis (68).

Atypical presentations of bacterial keratitis are becoming more common. This could be due to the more liberal and inappropriate use of antibiotics and immunosuppressive drugs (including topical corticosteroids), or because greater clinical awareness of these conditions exist. For example, *Capnocytophaga*, an anaerobic Gram-negative rod found normally in the oral cavity causes an indolent keratitis that is often unresponsive to

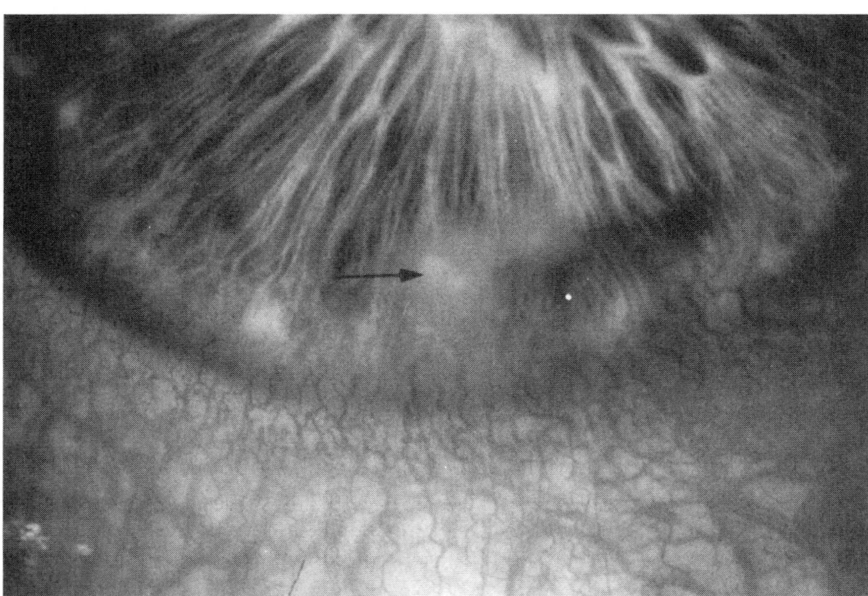

Figure 2 Staphylococcal blepharoconjunctivitis showing marginal infiltrates separated from the corneoscleral limbus by a narrow gap of less inflamed cornea.

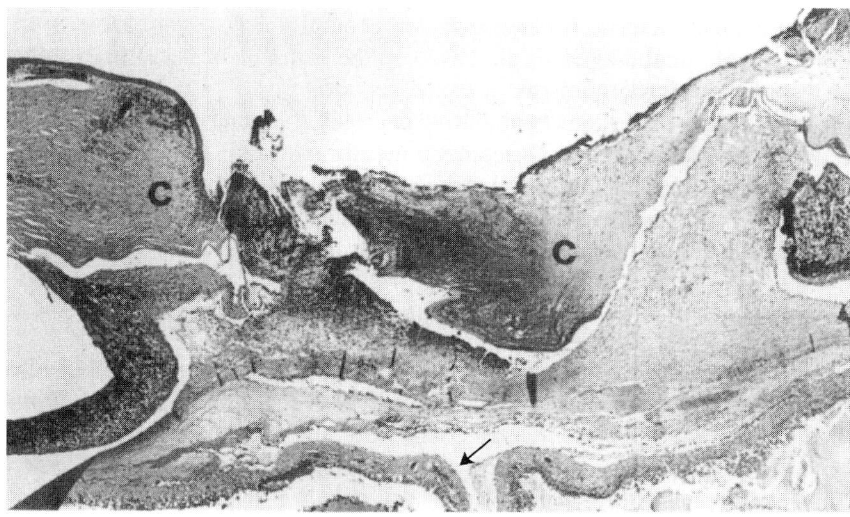

Figure 3 Perforated bacterial corneal ulcer showing edges of cornea (C) through which inflammatory debris and portions of intraocular tissue are being extruded. The neurosensory retina is present near the wound (*arrow*) (hematoxylin and eosin, ×53).

antimicrobial therapy (90,97,108). Clinically, patients with corneal infections due to *Capnocytophaga* present with a non-healing ulcer. A ring infiltrate, endothelial plaques, stromal necrosis and hypopyon may also be present (3). Risk factors for *Capnocytophaga* keratitis include recent surgical or accidental trauma, or systemic immunosuppression from HIV (129). *Capnocytophaga* has a predilection for the deep stroma just anterior to Descemet membrane (35).

Nontuberculous Mycobacterium Keratitis

The prevalence of nontuberculous mycobacterial infection is increasing. This may be due to increased awareness of this type of infection, better methods of detection, or the greater proportion of susceptible persons who are either elderly or immunosuppressed. Atypical mycobacteria are ubiquitous in the environment and are found worldwide in human water supplies and soil (34). Mycobacteria are remarkably hardy and can withstand high levels of environmental stress. Although most atypical mycobacteria have low human pathogenicity, their cell wall architecture, like mycobacteria in general, confers relative antibiotic resistance (16,17). The hydrophobicity of the cell wall makes for efficient nutrient uptake (104).

The cornea is the most common site of ocular infection with atypical mycobacteria, but external infections of the conjunctiva and sclera can also occur (73). Nontuberculous keratitis almost always follows accidental or surgical trauma (36). The histological

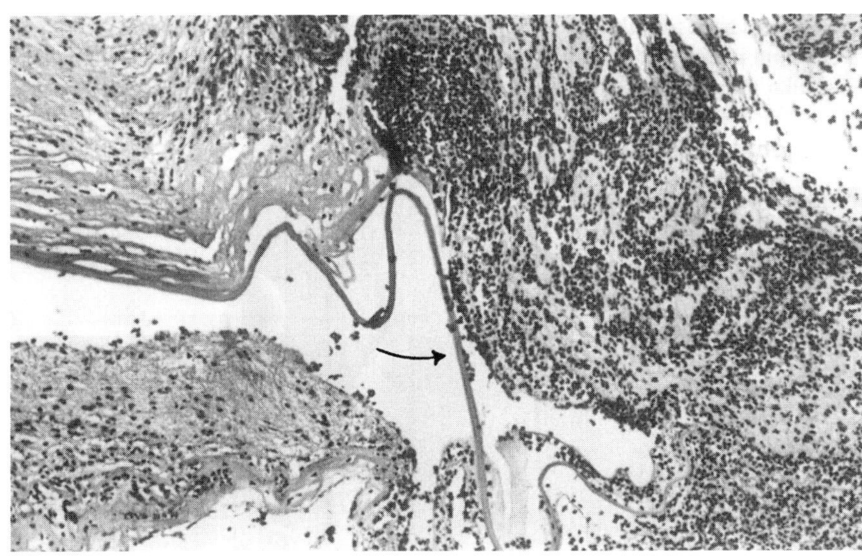

Figure 4 Perforated bacterial corneal ulcer under high magnification showing the edge of Descemet membrane (*arrow*). Descemet membrane is relatively resistant to enzymatic digestion by neurotrophils compared to the stroma (hematoxylin and eosin, ×187).

appearance of nontuberculous keratitis is indistinguishable from other types of severe infectious keratitis. There is widespread necrosis of keratocytes with acute and chronic inflammation. Many of the cell nuclei are in various stages of disintegration giving the stroma a peppered look (Fig. 5). Outbreaks of atypical myobacterial keratitis have been traced to surgical procedures such as laser assisted in situ keratomileusis (LASIK) (41,84). Disseminated infection is rare in persons who are not immunocompromised.

Crystalline Keratopathy

Crystalline keratopathy is a relatively recently reported clinical entity describing a condition in which a myriad of bacteria propagate in the corneal stroma without a significant inflammatory response (92). The bacteria are sequestered between collagen lamellae which gives them a crystal-like appearance on clinical examination (Fig. 6.). The lack of inflammation in invading bacteria is probably due to the use of topical corticosteroids. Because corticosteroids mediate their antiinflammatory effects in a variety of ways, it is unclear what part of the inflammatory pathway is most critically neutralized in this situation. Crystalline keratopathy is usually caused by low virulence bacteria such as *Streptococcus viridans* and almost always follows surgical or accidental trauma (94).

Intraocular Bacterial Infections

Bacterial Endophthalmitis

Bacterial endophthalmitis is an infection involving the internal contents of the globe. It is a type of endoththalmitis based on the broad category of infecting organisms. Other classifications of endothalmitis are based on the clinical setting (such as post-traumatic, or postoperative), route of infection (exogenous or endogenous), or according to the specific infectious agent. The term panophthalmitis usually denotes a more serious or widespread infection involving the outer sclerocorneal tunic, but this designation has been used inconsistently in the literature.

Postoperative Endophthalmitis

Postoperative bacterial endophthalmitis is one of the most serious complications of any type of intraocular surgery. A risk of endophthalmitis exists with all types of intraocular surgery, but because of space restraints this discussion will be limited to cataract extraction and glaucoma surgery. Visual prognosis with endophthalmitis is poor even with appropriate treatment.

Postoperative endophthalmitis following cataract surgery results in severe visual loss in a third of patients and blindness in nearly a fifth (88). The risk of endophthalmitis after cataract surgery in developed countries over the last two decades has ranged from 0.05% to 0.3% (26,58–60,80,116,119,124,134). The most common source of infection is the patient's conjunctiva and eyelids. Results from the Endophthalmitis Vitrectomy Study showed that 70% of culture-positive cases were due to coagulase-negative, Gram-positive micrococci, with *Staphylococcus epidermidis* being the single most frequent organism recovered (47).

Epidemics of pseudophakic bacterial endophthalmitis have occurred from contaminated lens implants. An example of such an epidemic was

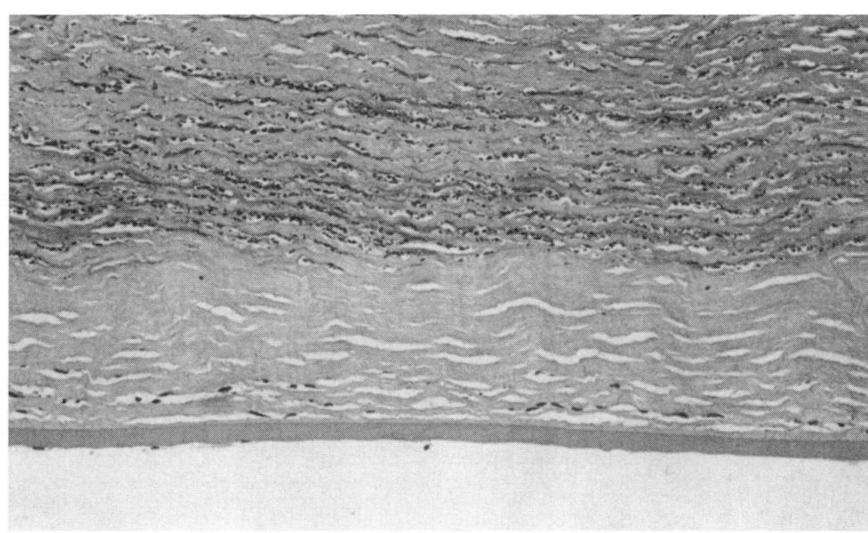

Figure 5 Necrotizing keratitis due to atypical mycobacterial infection. The anterior stroma has a peppered appearance due to the disintegration of cellular nuclei, while the posterior stroma is necrotic and nearly acellular. Acid-fast bacteria were demonstrated in large numbers with special stains (hematoxylin and eosin, ×208).

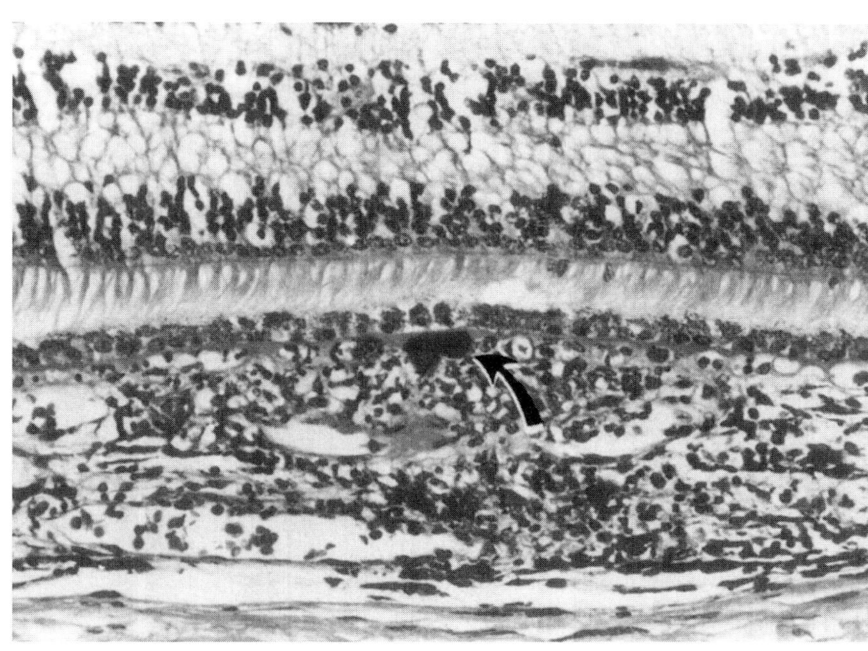

Figure 11 Early metastatic bacterial endophthalmitis showing an intravascular nidus of organisms in the choriocapillaris (*arrow*). A few polymorphonuclear leukocytes are present. The eye was obtained at autopsy (hematoxylin and eosin, ×415).

state within the human host. The pathogenic spirochetes cannot be routinely cultivated in the laboratory. The entire *T. pallidum* genome has been cloned and sequenced (39,85). A possible explanation for the organism's fastidious behavior is that many essential structural and enzyme cofactor genes are not found in its genome (39). Thus astidious behavior the clinical diagnosis of syphilis is presumptive based on clinical findings and the results of serological tests. The bacterium has a surface hyaluronidase which may play a role in tissue penetration along with periplasmic flagella (52). *T. pallidum* has developed some unique survival features including its ability to optimize metabolic activity when the oxygen concentration falls 10% to 20% (8).

The immunologic response to *T. pallidum* has been thoroughly studied. Humoral antibodies and cell-mediated immunity follow primary infection, but are not completely protective (65). Host defenses, however, cannot prevent early hematogenous dissemination or the development of the secondary stage. The outer coat of *T. pallidum* is rich in phospholipids and contains as many as 14 surface antigens (48). Measurable immune parameters to infection tend to correlate poorly with the waxing and waning of the clinical course of the disease (71). Both reagin and anti-treponema antibodies are predominately IgG, but appreciable concentrations of IgM are also present after the initial infection (6,89). The microorganisms reach a maximum number during the secondary stage of syphilis. The spirochetes then become less numerous as the host response suppresses the infection. The rate of spontaneous cure is unknown. *T. pallidum* can enter a stage of clinical latency for months or years and later manifest as neurosyphilis (general paresis, tabes dorsalis) or as cardiovascular disease (130).

T. pallidum is one of the few bacteria capable of penetrating normal mucous membranes. Within hours after entering the skin or a mucous membrane spirochetes gain access to the blood stream and disseminate throughout the body. The incubation period is followed by four stages of the disease: primary, secondary, latent and late. Successive stages do not necessarily occur in all patients even if left untreated (130). The ocular manifestations are broad and the infection can involve every part of the eye (71). The most common ocular findings are due to involvement of the uveal tract and retina during the secondary stage (Fig. 14). Late syphilis can present with signs of anterior neuro-visual pathway disease. Serious ocular complications are seen in infants and children who acquire transplacental infection. The ocular manifestations of congenital syphilis include corneal opacification, uveitis, cataract, secondary glaucoma, pigmentary retinopathy, and optic neuropathy (71,86).

The organism's outer membrane contains relatively few proteins, which may help it elude host immune-mediated defenses. The damage caused by *T. pallidum* in many organ systems is due to the inflammatory response and to circulating immune complexes bound to treponema proteins, fibronectin, and host antibodies (112).

The most common pathologic finding in all stages of the disease is an obliterative endarteritis. In

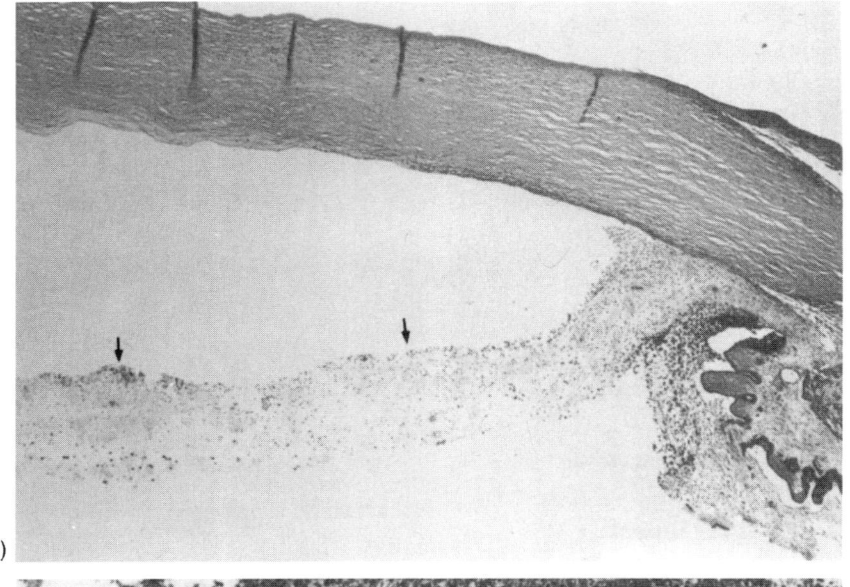

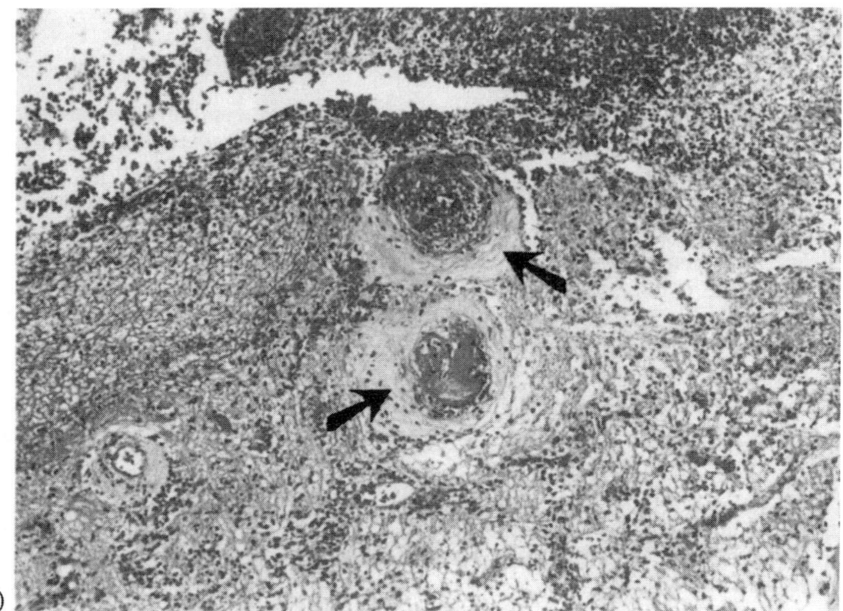

Figure 12 (**A**) Metastatic endophthalmitis due to *Clostridium perfingens* demonstrating ischemic necrosis of the anterior segment. The iris (*arrows*) has few visible cell nuclei. Inflammatory cells and peripheral anterior synechiae have closed the angle (hematoxylin and eosin, ×47). (**B**) Thrombosed choroidal vessels (*arrows*) are associated with widespread and severe ischemic necrosis of the posterior segment of the eye (hematoxylin and eosin, ×189).

the eye, various patterns of inflammation and repair are found. The conjunctiva can display a granulomatous inflammation indistinguishable from sarcoidosis (125). Syphilitic interstitial keratitis is associated with congenital syphilis, but can also occur as an acquired complication (49,75,86)

Cat-Scratch Disease

Cat-scratch disease is caused by a small pleomorphic, Gram-negative bacillus that requires special silver impregnation stains for visualization in tissue section. It is the most common single cause of Parinaud ocular glandular syndrome. Two unrelated but morphologically similar bacteria have been cultured from patients with this syndrome: *Bartonella henselae* (previously designated *Rochalimaea henselae*) and *Afipia felis* (12,67,97). Based on serological evidence, most cases of cat-scratch disease are due to *B. henselae* infection, but the clinical manifestations are probably broader than previously suspected (142).

Histologically, the conjunctiva contains a dense accumulation of lymphocytes and histiocytes (70). Small areas of necrosis may be present and some degree of granulomatous inflammation can be observed. The responsible small bacillus is identified with a modified Warthin-Starry stain (136). A palisading granuloma with necrosis is often found in clinically involved regional lymph nodes.

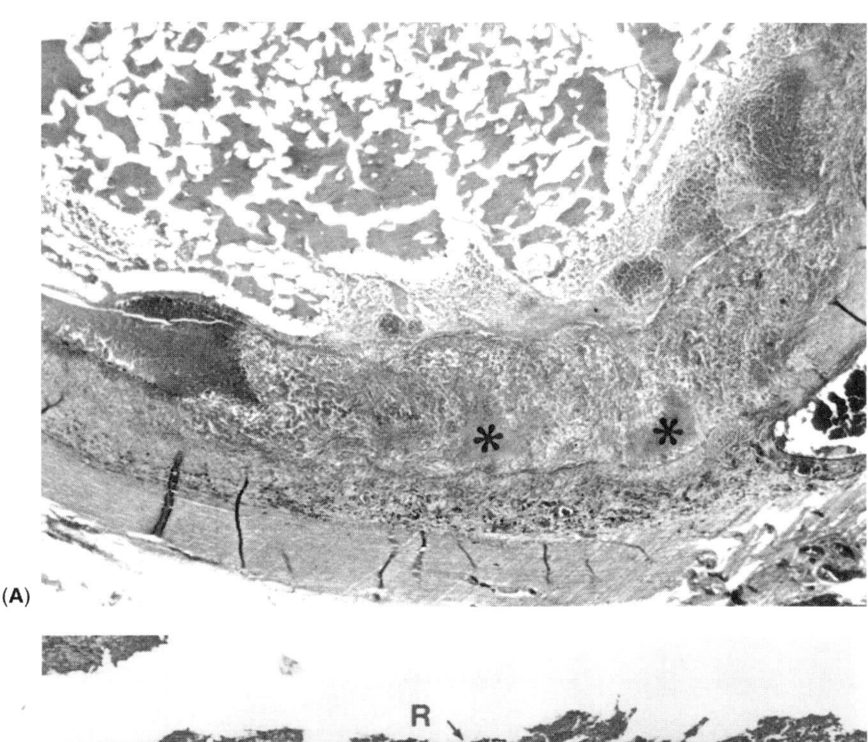

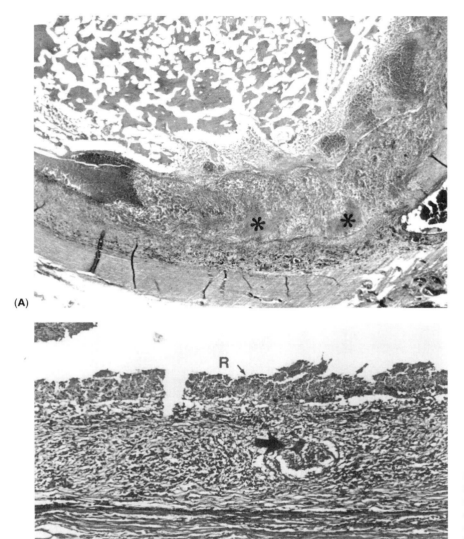

Figure 13 (**A**) The eye from a patient with miliary tuberculosis shows intense focal necrosis (*) and widespread inflammation of the posterior segment (hematoxylin and eosin, ×30). (**B**) High magnification reveals the retina (R) is totally necrotic. The choroid has been replaced by chronic granulomatous inflammation with multinucleated giant cells (*arrow*) (hematoxylin and eosin, ×120).

Lyme Disease

In 1975, an epidemiologic investigation of 12 cases of juvenile arthritis in Lyme, Connecticut led to the discovery of Lyme disease and the identification of *B. burgdorferi*, its causative bacterium (11). The disease has three stages starting with a cutaneous rash that begins at the site of a blood meal taken by the tick vector, *Ixodes*. This arthropod leaves spirochetes in the lower layers of the skin where the bacteria migrate for days creating a centrifugal inflammatory reaction (erythema migrans). The immunologic response to infection consists initially of *Borrelia*-specific IgM. *Borrelia* eventually gains access to the blood and disseminates throughout the body, but is effectively removed from the blood. Were it not for the bacterium's ability to invade and survive in a variety of tissues, including the heart, joints, and nervous system, the disease would be self limited. During stage 2 of the disease a *Borrelia*-specific IgG response develops and the neurological manifestations include cranial mononeuropathies and lymphocytic meningitis (64).

B. burgdorferi can lower its metabolic activity and exist in a quiescent phase for prolonged periods. The different sites of infection plus the latency between time of infection and clinical manifestations make Lyme disease notoriously difficult to diagnose. Like syphilis, the diagnosis is based on clinical findings and supportive laboratory studies rather than on culture results.

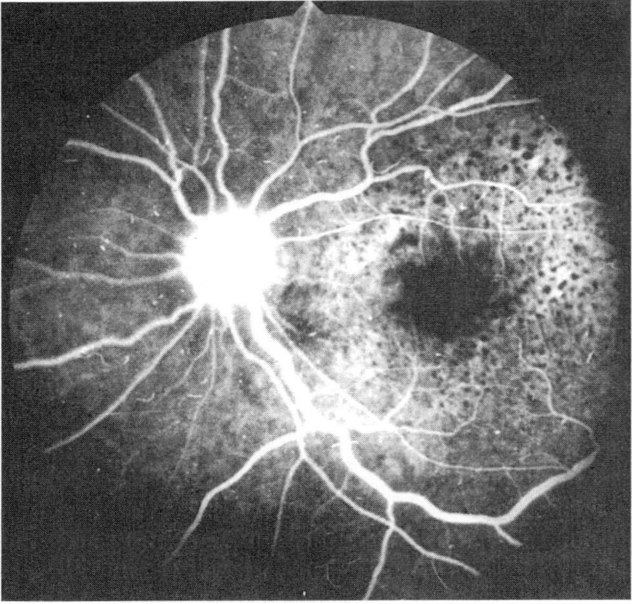

Figure 14 Fluorescein angiogram from a patient with secondary syphilis. On fundoscopy the left macula was thick and had a slightly yellow color. The plaquoid lesion has a "leopard spot" appearance in the midphase fluorescien angiogram. The disc stains intensely. *Source*: Courtesy of Dr. Scott Pautler.

The 25 μm long spiral-shaped bacterium has a Gram-negative cell wall composed of two membranes surrounding a central peptidoglycan layer. *B. burgdorferi* has 4 to 20 coils and is so thin (0.2 μm in diameter) that it cannot be seen by phase-contrast microscopy. The spirochete can be visualized by light microcopy using fluorescent labeled antibodies using immunohistochemistry. *Borrelia* was the first organism discovered with linear plasmids (it also has circular plasmids). For reasons that are not yet clear, *Borrelia* has considerably more of these autonomously replicating extrachromosomal DNA segments than other types of bacteria. The genome of *B. burgdorferi* has been completely sequenced (112). None of the genes appear to encode for an iron-requiring protein, which means that enzyme functions are dependent on other metals such as manganese.

The diagnosis of Lyme disease depends on correlating clinical findings with positive serological studies (20). In regions where Lyme disease is endemic, the seroprevalence of *B. burgdorferi* can be high and makes the interpretation of causal relationships challenging. Immunofluorescent and enzyme-linked immunosorbent assays are the two most commonly used tests (20), but they have established ranges of false-positive and false-negative rates. False-positive results can occur because of cross reactivity to other antigens such as flagellins of *T. pallidum*.

The ocular manifestations of Lyme disease are broad and include numerous patterns of ocular inflammation such as conjunctivitis, keratitis, uveitis, and vitritis. A variety of ophthalmic abnormalities have also been described, including optic neuropathy, defects of pupillary function, ocular motor nerve palsies, and supranuclear disorders of ocular motility (55,61,122,123,138,140). While discussion of these findings is beyond the scope of this chapter, the approach to diagnosing Lyme disease involves the exclusion of disorders that can present with similar clinical findings and obtaining supportive results from serological assays (56).

Chlamydial Infections

Chlamydia is a small bacteria and contains the second smallest bacterial genomes known next to Mycoplasma. Infections due to *Chlamydia* are covered in Chapter 10.

BACTERIAL INFECTIONS OF THE EYE IN ACQUIRED IMMUNODEFICIENCY SYNDROME

The eyes of patients with the acquired immunodeficiency syndrome (AIDS) are at risk for several types of bacterial infections, including *T. pallidum*, *Mycobacterium avium intracellulare*, and *Mycobacterium tuberculosis* (13,30,62,96). A variety of pathogenic and saprophytic bacteria have been reported to cause endogenous bacterial endophthalmitis and bacterial keratitis (121,141).

REFERENCES

1. Abrahams IW. *Propionibacterium acnes* endophthalmitis: an unusual manner of presentation. J Cataract Refract Surg 1989; 15:698–701.
2. Adamis AP, Schein OD. *Chlamydia* and *Acanthoamoeba* infections of the eye. In: Albert DM, Jakobeic FA, eds. Principles and Practice of Ophthalmology. Philadelphia: WB Saunders Company, 1994:179–89, Chapter 9.
3. Alexandrakis G, Palma LA, Miller D, Alfonso EC. *Capnocytophaga* keratitis Ophthalmology 2000; 107: 1503–6.
4. Allansmith MR, Ostler HB, Butterworth M. Concomitance of bacteria in various areas of the eye. Arch Ophthalmol 1969; 82:37–42.
5. Allansmith MR. Defense of the ocular surface. Int Ophthalmol Clin 1979; 19(2):93–100.
6. Baker-Zander SA, Hook EW 3rd, Bonin P, Handsfield HH, Lukehart SA. Antigens of *Treponema pallidum* recognized by IgG and IgM antibodies during syphilis in humans. J Infect Dis 1985; 151:264–72.
7. Barr CC, Prognostic factors in corneoscleral lacerations. Arch Ophthalmol 1983; 101:919–24.
8. Baseman JB, Nichols JC, Hayes NC. Virulent *Treponema pallidum*: aerobe or anaerobe? Infect Immun 1976; 13:704–11.
9. Beck AD, Grossniklaus HE, Hubbard B, Saperstein D, Haupert CL, Margo CE. Pathologic findings in late

endophthalmitis after glaucoma filtering surgery. Ophthalmology 2000; 107:2111–4.
10. Beer PM, Ludwig IH, Packer AJ. Complete visual recovery after Bacillus cereus endophthalmitis in a child. Am J Ophthalmol 1990; 110:212–3.
11. Berger BW, Johnson RC, Kodner C, Coleman L. Cultivation of *Borrelia burgdorferi* from erythema migrans lesions and perilesional skin. J Clin Microbiol 1992; 30:359–61.
12. Birkness KA, George VG, White EH, et al. Intracellular growth of *Afipia felis*: a putative etiologic agent of cat scratch disease. Infect Immun 1992; 60:2281–7.
13. Blodi BA, Johnson MW, McLeish WM, Gass JD. Presumed choroidal tuberculosis in a human immunodeficiency virus infected host. Am J Ophthalmol 1989; 108:605–7.
14. Bouza E, Cobo-Soriano R, Rodriguez-Creixems M, et al. A prospective search for ocular lesions in hospitalized patients with significant bacteremia. Clin Infect Dis 2000; 30:306–12.
15. Bozkir N, Stern GA. Chronic conjunctivitis. In: Margo CE, Hamed LM, Mames RN, eds. Diagnostic Problems in Clinical Ophthalmology, Philadelphia: WB Saunders Company, 1994:Chapter 18, 139–50.
16. Brennan PJ. Structure of mycobacteria: recent developments in defining cell wall carbohydrates and proteins. Rev Inf Dis 1989; 11(suppl 2):S420–30.
17. Brennan PJ, Nikaido H. The envelope of mycobacteria. Annu Rev Biochem 1995; 64:29–63.
18. Brinser JH, Burd EM: Principles of diagnostic ocular microbiology. In: Tabbara KF, Hyndiuk FA eds. Infection of the Eye. Boston: Little, Brown, 1986: Chapter 7, 73–92.
19. Brock J. Lactoferrin: a multifunctional immunoregulatory protein? Immunol Today 1995; 16:417–9.
20. Brown SL, Hansen SL, Lagone JJ. The role of serology in the diagnosis of Lyme disease. J Am Med Assoc 1999; 282: 62–66.
21. Chandler JW. Immunology of the ocular surface. Int Ophthalmol Clinc 1985; 25(2):13–23.
22. Chandler JW, Gillette TE. Immunologic defense mechanisms of the ocular surface. Ophthalmol 1983; 90: 585–91.
23. Chandler JW, Cummings M, Gillette TE. Presence of Langerhans cells in the central corneas of normal human infants. Invest Ophthalmol Vis Sci 1985; 26:113–116.
24. Chien AM, Raber IM, Fischer DH, et al. *Propionibacterium acnes* endophthalmitis after intracapsular cataract extraction. Ophthalmology 1992; 99:487–90.
25. Cohn ZA, Hirsch JG. The isolation and properties of specific cytoplasmic granules of rabbit polymorphornuclear leukocytes. J Exp Med 1960; 112:983–1004.
26. Colleaux KM, Hamilton WK. Effect of prophylactic antibiotics and incision type on the incidence of endophthalmitis after cataract surgery. Can J Ophthalmol 2000; 35:373–8.
27. Costerton JW, Stewart PS, Greenberg EP. Bacterial biofilms: a common cause of persistent infections. Science 1999; 21:284:1318–22.
28. Davey RT Jr, Tauber WB. Posttraumatic endophthalmitis: the emerging role of *Bacillus cereus* infection. Rev Infect Dis 1987; 9:110–23.
29. Davies DG, Parsek MR, Pearson JP, et al. The involvement of cell-to-cell signals in the development of a bacterial biofilm. Science 1998; 10:280:295–8.
30. Davis JL, Nussenblatt RB, Bachman DM, et al. Endogenous bacterial retinitis in AIDS. Am J Ophthalmol 1989; 107:613–23.
31. Dawson CR. Immunology of ocular chlamydial infections. Int Ophthalmol Clin 1985; 25:95–106.
32. Dawson CR, Whitcher JP, Horshiwara I, et al. Chlamydial infections of the eye: trachoma and inclusion conjunctivitis. Contact Lens 1980; 6:218–24.
33. Driebe WT, Mandelbaum S, Forster RK, et al. Pseudophakic endophthalmitis: diagnosis and management. Ophthalmology 1986; 93:442–8.
34. Falkinham JO III. Nontuberculous mycobacteria in the environment. Clin Chest Med 2002; 23:529–51.
35. Font RL, Jay V, Misra RP, Jones DB, Wilhelmus KR. *Capnocytophaga* keratitis. A clinicopathologic study of three patients, including electon microscopic observations. Ophthalmology 1994; 101:1929–34.
36. Ford JG, Huang AJ, Plugfelder SC, et al. Nontuberculous mycobacterial keratitis in south Florida. Ophthalmology 1998; 105:1652–8.
37. Forster RK. Endophthalmitis. In: Tasman W, Jaeger EA, eds. Duane's Clinical Ophthalmology. JB Lippincott, 1989; 4:Chapter 24, 1–29.
38. Fox GM, Joondeph BC, Flynn HW Jr, et al. Delayed-onset pseudophakic endophthalmitis. Am J Ophthalology 1991; 11:163–73.
39. Fraser CM, Norris SJ, Weinstock GM, et al. Complete genome sequence of Treponema pallidum, the sphyilis spirochete. Science 1998; 281:375–88.
40. Friedlaender MH, Masi RJ, Osumoto M, et al. Ocular microbial flora in immunodeficient patients. Arch Ophthalmol 1980; 98:1211–13.
41. Freitas D, Alvarenga L, Sampaio J, et al. An outbreak of *Mycobacterium chelonae* infection after LASIK. Ophthalmology 2003; 110:276–85.
42. Gerding DN, Poley BJ, Hall WH, et al. Treatment of *Pseudomonas* endophthalmitis associated with prosthetic intraocular lens implantation. Am J Ophthalmol 1979; 88: 902–8.
43. Gillette TE, Chandler JW, Greiner JV. Langerhans cells of the ocular surface. Ophthalmology 1982; 89:700–11.
44. Greenfield DS, Suner IJ, Miller MP, et al. Endophthalmitis after filtering surgery with mitomycin. Arch Ophthalmol 1996; 114:943–9.
45. Greenwald MJ, Wohl LG, Sell CH. Metastatic bacterial endophthalmitis. A contemporary reappraisal. Surv Ophthalmol 1986; 31:81–101.
46. Hall-Stoodley L, Costerton JW, Stoodley P. Bacterial biofilms: from the natural environment to infectious diseases. Nat Rev Microbiol 2004; 2:95–108.
47. Han DP, Wisniewski SR, Wilson LA, et al. Spectrum and susceptibilities of microbiologic isolates in the Endophthalmitis Vitrectomy Study. Am J Ophthalmol 1996; 122:1–17 [Erratum in Am J Ophthalmol 1996; 122:920].
48. Hanff PA, Miller JN, Lovett MA. Molecular characterization of common treponemal antigens. Infect Immun 1983; 40:825–8.
49. Hewlett EL. Toxins. In: GL Mandell, JE Bennett, Dolin R eds. Principles and Practice of Infectious Disease. 4th edn. New York: Churchill Livingston, 1995: Chapter 1, 21–30.
50. Hill JC, Maske R, Bowen RM. Secondary localized amyloidosis of the cornea associated with tertiary syphilis. Cornea 1990; 9:98–101.
51. Holland SP, Mathias RG, Morck DW, et al. Diffuse lamellar keratitis related to endotoxins released from sterilizer reservoir biofilms. Ophthalmology 2000; 107:1227–33.
52. Hovind Hougen K: Morphology. In: Schell RF, Musher DM eds. Pathogenesis and Immunology of Treponemal Infection. New York: Marcel Dekker, 1983:3–28, Ch 1.

53. Iglewski BH, Burns RP, Gipson IK. Pathogenesis of corneal damage from *Pseudomonas* exotoxin. Invest Ophthalmol Vis Sci 1977; 16:73–6.
54. Jackson TL, Eykyn SJ, Graham EM, Stanford MR. Endogenous bacterial endophthalmitis: a 17-year prospective series and review of 267 reported cases. Surv Ophthalmol 2003; 48:403–23.
55. Jacobson DM, Marx JJ, Dlesk A. Frequency and clinical significance of Lyme seropositivity in patients with isolated optic neuritis. Neurology 1991; 41:706–11.
56. Jacobson DM. Neuro-ophthalmic manifestations of Lyme disease. Ophthalmol Clin N Amer 1991; 4:463–778.
57. Jakobiec FA, Lefkowitch J, Knowles DM 2nd. B- and T-lymphocytes in ocular disease. Ophthalmology 1984; 91: 635–54.
58. Javitt JC, Street DA, Tielsch JM, et al. National outcomes of cataract extraction and endophthalmitis after outpatient cataract surgery. Cataract patient outcomes research team. Ophthalmology 1994; 101:100–5.
59. John T, Sims M, Hoffmann C. Intraocular bacterial contamination during sutureless, small incision, single-port phacoemulsification. J Cataract Refract Surg 2000; 26:1786–91.
60. Kattan HM, Flynn HW Jr, Pflugfelder SC, et al. Nosocomial endophthalmitis survey. Current incidence of infection after intraocular surgery. Ophthalmology 1991; 98:227–38.
61. Lesser RL, Kornmehl EW, Pachner AR, et al. Neuro-ophthalmologic manifestations of Lyme disease. Ophthalmology 1990; 97:699–706.
62. Levy JH, Liss RA, Maguire AM. Neurosyphilis and ocular syphilis in patients with concurrent human immunodeficiency virus infection. Retina 1989; 9:175–180.
63. Locatcher-Khorazo D, Seegal BC. Microbiology of the Eye. St Louis: Mosby, 1972.
64. Logigian EL, Kaplan RF, Steere AC. Chronic neurologic manifestations of Lyme disease. N Engl J Med 1990; 323: 1438–44.
65. Magnuson JH, Thomas EW, Olasnsky S, et al. Innoculation syphilis in human volunteers. Medicine (Baltimore) 1956; 35:33–82.
66. Mandelbaum S, Forster RK, Gelender H, Culbertson W. Late onset endophthalmitis associated with filtering blebs. Ophthalmology 1985; 92:964–74.
67. Margileth AM, Hayden GF. Cat scratch disease: from feline affection of human infection. N Engl J Med 1993; 329:53–54.
68. Margo CE. Eyes removed for primary ulcerative keratitis with endophthalmitis: Microbial and histologic findings. Ophthalmic Surg Laser 1999; 30:535–9.
69. Margo CE, Cole EL III. Postoperative endophthalmitis and asymptomatic bacteriuria due to group G *Streptococcus*. Am J Ophthalmol 1989; 107:430–1.
70. Margo CE, Grossniklaus HE. Ocular Histopathology. A Guide to Differential Diagnosis. Philadelphia: WB Saunders Company, 1991.
71. Margo CE, Hamed LM. Ocular syphilis. Surv Ophthalmol 1992; 37:203–20.
72. Margo CE, Mames RN, Guy JR. Endogenous *Klebsiella* endophthalmitis. Report of two cases and review of the literature. Ophthalmology 1994; 101:1298–1301.
73. Margo CE, Pavan PR. *Myocbacterium chelonae* conjunctivitis and scleritis following vitrectomy. Arch Ophthalmol 2000; 118:1125–8.
74. Margo CE, Pavan PR, Groden LR. Chronic vitritis with macrophagic inclusions. A sequelae of treated endophthalmitis due to a coryneform bacterium. Ophthalmology 1988; 95:156–61.
75. Martinez JA, Sutphin JE. Syphilitic interstitial keratitis masquerading as staphylococcal marginal keratitis. Am J Ophthalmol 1989; 107:431–3.
76. McNatt J, Allen SD, Wilson LA, Dowell VR Jr. Anaerobic flora of the normal human conjunctival sac. Arch Ophthalmol 1978; 96:1448–50.
77. Meisler DM, Mandelbaum S. *Propionibacterium*-associated endophthalmitis after extracapsular cataract extraction: review of reported cases. Ophthalmology 1989; 96:54–61.
78. Meisler DM, Palestine AG, Vastine DW, et al. Chronic *Proprionibacterium* endophthalmitis after extracapsular cataract extraction and intraocular lens implantation. Am J Ophthalmol 1986; 102:733–9.
79. Miller B, Ellis PP. Conjunctival flora in patients receiving immunosuppressive drugs. Arch Ophthalmol 1977; 95: 2012–14.
80. Morlet N, Li J, Semmens J, Ng J, Team EPSWA. The endophthalmitis population study of western Australia (EPSWA). First report. Br J Ophthalmol 2003; 87:574–6.
81. Musser JM, Kroll JS, Granoff DM, et al. Global genetic structure and molecular epidemiology of encapsulated Haemophilus influenza. Rev Infect Dis 1990; 12: 75–111.
82. Nassif X, Pujol C, Morand P, Eugene E. Interactions of pathogenic Neisseria with host cells. Is it possible to assemble the puzzle? Mol Microbiol 1999; 32:1124–32.
83. Neudorfer M, Barnea Y, Geyer O, Siegman-Igra Y. Retinal lesions in septicemia. Am J Ophthalmol 1993; 116:728–34.
84. Newman PE, Goodman RA, Waring GO III, et al. A cluster of cases of Mycobacterium chelonei keratitis associated with outpatient office procedures. Am J Ophthalmol 1984; 97:344–8.
85. Norgard MV, Miller JN. Cloning and expression of *Treponema pallidum* (Nichols) antigen genes in Escherichia coli. Infect Immun 1983; 42:435–45.
86. Oksala A. Studies on interstitial keratitis associated with congenital syphilis occurring in Finland. Acta Ophthalmol 1952; 30(suppl):5–109.
87. Okumoto M. Normal flora in the defense of the conjunctiva against infection. In: O'Connor GR (ed), Immunologic Disease of the Mucous Membranes: pathology, Diagnosis and Treatment. New York: Masson, 1980:33–9.
88. Olson RJ. Reducing the risk of postoperative endophthalmitis. Surv Ophthalmol 2004; 49(Suppl 2):S55–61.
89. O'Neill P, Nicol CS. IgM class anti-treponemal antibody in treated and untreated syphilis. Br J Vener Dis 1972; 48:460–3.
90. Ormerod LD, Foster CS, Paton BG, et al. Ocular *Capnocytophaga* infection in an edentulous, immunocompetent host. Cornea 1988; 7:218–22.
91. Ormerod LD, Ho DD, Becker LE, et al. Endophthalmitis caused by the coagulase-negative staphylococci, I: Disease spectrum and outcome. Ophthalmology 1993; 100:715–23.
92. Ormerod LD, Margo CE. Changing patterns of ocular infectious disease. Ophthalmol Clin N Amer 1995; 8:109–24.
93. Ormerod LD, Paton BG, Haaf J, et al. Anaerobic bacterial endophthalmitis. Ophthalmology 1987; 94:799–808.
94. Ormerod LD, Ruoff KL, Meisler DM, et al. Infectious crystalline keratopathy: role of nutrionally variant streptococci and other bacterial factors. Ophthalmology 1991; 98:159–69.
95. Parsek MR, Singh PK. Bacterial biofilms: an emerging link to disease pathogenesis. Ann Rev Microbiol 2003; 57: 677–701.
96. Passo MS, Rosenbaum JT. Ocular syphilis in patients with human immunodeficiency virus infection. Am J Ophthamol 1988; 106:1–6.

97. Paton BG, Ormedod LD, Peppe J, Kenyen KR. Evidence for a feline reservoir for dysgonic fermenter 2 keratitis. J Clin Microbiol 1988; 26:2439–40.
98. Perkins RE, Kundsin RB, Pratt MV, et al. Bacteriology of normal and infected conjunctiva. J Clin Microbiol 1975; 1: 147–9.
99. Petri WA Jr, Mann BJ. Microbial adherence. In: Mandell GL, Bennett JE, Dolin R eds. Principles and Practice of Infectious Disease. 4th edn. New York: Churchill Livingston, 1995:Chapter 2,11–18.
100. Pier GB. Peptides, *Pseudomonas aeruginosa*, polysaccharides and lippolysaccharides-players in the predicament of cytstic fibrosis patients. Trends Microbiol 2000; 8:247–51.
101. Piest KL, Kincaid MC, Tetz RM, et al. Localized endophthalmitis: a newly described cause of the so-called toxic lens syndrome. J Cataract Refract Surg 1987; 13:498–510.
102. Posenauer B, Funk J. Chronic postoperative endophthalmitis caused by *Proprionibacterium acnes*. Eur J Ophthalmol 1992; 2:94–7.
103. Pramhus C, Runyan TE, Lindberg RB. Ocular flora in the severely burned patient. Arch Ophthalmol 1978; 96:1421–24.
104. Primm TP, Lucero CA, Falkinham JO III. Health impacts of environmental mycobacteria. Clin Microbiol Rev 2004; 17:98–106.
105. Prydal JI, Campbell FW. Study of precorneal tear film thickness and structure by interferometry and confocal microscopy. Invest Ophthalmol Vis Sci 1992; 33:1996–2005.
106. Relman DA, Falkow S. A molecular perspective of microbial pathogenicity. In: Mandell GL, Bennett JE, Dolin R eds. Principles and Practice of Infectious Diseases. 4th edn. 1995:Chapter 3, 19–29.
107. Roitt I, Brostoff J, Male D. Immunology St Louis, CV Mosby, 1989: chapter 9, 9.2–9.12.
108. Roussel TJ, Osata MA, Wilhelmus KR: *Capnocytophaga* keratitis. Br J Ophthalmol 1985; 69:187–8.
109. Salyers AA, Whitt DD. Bacterial strategies for evading or surviving the defense systems of the human body. In Bacterial Pathogenesis. A Molecular Approach. Washington DC, ASM Press, 2nd edn. 2002:Chapter 8, 115–130.
110. Salyers AA, Whitt DD, Bacterial exotoxins: Important but still a mystery. In: Bacterial Pathogenesis. A Molecular Approach. 2nd edn. Washington DC: ASM Press, 2002: Chapter 9, 131–49.
111. Salyers AA, Whitt DD. How bacteria become resistant to antibiotics. In: Bacterial Pathogenesis. A Molecular Approach. 2nd ed. Washington DC: ASM Press, 2002: Chapter 11, 168–84.
112. Salyers AA, Whitt DD. The Spirochetes: *Borrelia burgdorferi* and *Treponema pallidum*.
113. Schachter J. Chlamydial infections. Parts 1–3. N Engl J Med 1978; 298:428–35, 490–5, 540–9.
114. Schiedler V, Scott IU, Flynn HW Jr, et al. Culture-proven endogenous endophthalmitis: clinical features and visual acuity outcomes. Am J Ophthalmol 2004; 137:725–31.
115. Schmitt CK, Meysick KC, O'Brien AD. Bacterial toxins: friends or foes? Emerg Infect Dis 1999; 5:224–34.
116. Schmitz S, Dick HB, Krummenauer F, Pfeiffer N. Endophthalmitis in cataract surgery: results of a German survey. Ophthalmology 1999; 106:1869–77.
117. Selander RK, Musser JM, Caugant DA, et al. Population genetics of pathogenic bacteria. Microbial Pathog 1987; 3:1–7.
118. Selinger DS, Selinger RC, Reed WP. Resistance to infection of the external eye. The role of tears Surv Ophthalmol 1979; 24:33–8.
119. Semmens JB, Li J, Morlet N, Ng J, Team EPSWA. Trends in cataract surgery and postoperative endophthalmitis in Western Australia (1980–1998): the endophthalmitis population study of western Australia. Clin Exp Ophthalmol 2003; 31:312–9.
120. Shammas HF. Endogenous *E. coli* endophthalmitis. Surv Ophthalmol 1977; 21:429–35.
121. Shuler JD, Engstrom RE Jr, Holland GN. External ocular disease and anterior segment disorders associated with AIDS. Int Ophthalmol Clin 1989; 29:98–104.
122. Smith JL. Ocular Lyme borreliosis- 1991. Int Ophthalmol Clin 1991; 31:17–38.
123. Smith JL. Neuro-ocular Lyme borreliosis. Neurol Clin 1991; 9:35–53.
124. Somani S, Grinbaum A, Slomovic AR. Postoperative endophthalmitis: incidence, predisposing surgery, clinical course and outcome. Can J Ophthalmol 1997; 32: 303–10.
125. Spektor FE, Eagle RC Jr, Nichols CW. Granulomatous conjunctivitis secondary to *Treponema pallidum*. Ophthalmology 1981; 88:863–65.
126. Stewart PS, Costerton JW. Antibiotic resistance of bacteria in biofilms. Lancet 2001; 358:135–138.
127. Terranova W, Palumbo J, Breman J. Ocular findings in botulism type B. JAMA 1979; 241:475–9.
128. Thompson NE, Ketterhagen MJ, Bergdoll MS, Schantz EJ. Isolation and some properties of an enterotoxin produced by *Bacillus cereus*. Infect Immun 1984; 43: 887–94.
129. Ticho BH, Urban RC Jr, Safran MJ, Saggau DD. *Capnocytophaga* keratitis associated with poor dentition and human immunodeficiency virus infection. Am J Ophthalmol 1990; 109:352–3.
130. Tramont EC. *Treponema pallidum* (syphilis). In: Mandell GL, Douglas RG Jr, Bennett JE eds. Principles and Practice of Infectious Diseases. 3rd ed. New York: Churchill Livingstone, 1990:1794–1808, Chapter 215.
131. Turnbull PC. *Bacillius cereus* toxin. Pharmacol Ther 1981; 13:453–505.
132. Valenton M, Okumoto M. Toxin producing strains of Staphylococcus epidermidis (albus): isolates from patients with staphylococcic blepharoconjunctivitis. Arch Ophthalmol 1973; 89:186–9.
133. Van Bijsterveld OP. Host-parasite relationship and toxonomic position of *Moraxella* and morphologically related organisms. Am J Ophthalmol 1973; 76:545–54.
134. Versteegh MF, Van Rij G. Incidence of endophthalmitis after cataract surgery in the Netherlands: several surgical techniques compared. Doc Ophthalmol 2000; 100:1–6.
135. Vogel U, Frosch M. Mechanisms of neisserial serum resistance. Mol Microbiol 1999; 32:1133–9.
136. Wear OJ, Malaty RH, Zimmerman LE, et al. Cat-scratch disease bacilli in the conjunctiva of patients with Parinaud's oculoglandular syndrome. Ophthalmology 1985; 92:1282–7.
137. Wing EJ, Remington JS. Cell-mediated immunity and its role in resistance to infection. In, Hook EW, Mandell JL, Gwaltney JM Jr, Sande MA (eds). Current Concepts of Infection Disease, New York: Wiley & Sons, 1977, Part Three, 89–116.
138. Winterkorn JM. Lyme disease: neurologic and ophthalmic manifestations. Surv Ophthalmol 1990; 35:191–204.
139. Wong JS, Chan TK, Lee HM, Chee SP. Endogenous bacterial endophthalmitis: an east Asian experience and a reappraisal of a severe ocular afflication. Ophthalmology 2000; 107:1483–91.
140. Zaidman GW. The ocular manifestions of Lyme disease. Int Ophthalmol Clin 1993; 33:9–22.
141. Zaidman GW. Neurosyphilis and retrobulbar neuritis in a patient with AIDS. Ann Ophthalmol 1986; 18:260–1.
142. Zangwill KM, Hamilton DH, Perkins BA, et al. Cat scratch disease in Connecticut: epidemiology, risk factors, and evaluation of a new diagnostic test. N Engl J Med 1993; 329:8–13.

10

Chlamydial Infections

Matthew J. Burton
International Centre for Eye Health, London School of Hygiene and Tropical Medicine, London, U.K.

INTRODUCTION

Chlamydia trachomatis causes trachoma, the most common infectious cause of blindness worldwide (98). It is one of nine species that comprise the family Chlamydiaceae, three of which cause disease in humans: *C. trachomatis, C. psittaci,* and *C. pneumoniae.* There has been a move to reclassify *Chlamydiaceae.* However, this has not been widely accepted, so the above nomenclature will be used here (42,84). Chlamydiae are obligate intracellular bacteria, which infect many species of mammals and birds causing diverse disease. *C. trachomatis* causes ocular, genital, and systemic infections that affect millions of people. As *C. trachomatis* is responsible for most ocular disease in humans it will be the principal focus of this chapter. *C. pneumoniae* is associated with acute respiratory infection and is implicated in a number of chronic conditions including ischemic heart disease. *C. psittaci* causes a variety of infections in animals, where it is responsible for major economic losses, and occasionally it may be transmitted to humans causing atypical pneumonia.

CHLAMYDIAL BIOLOGY

Chlamydial Structure

Chlamydiae exist in two principal forms during their developmental cycle: reticulate bodies (RBs) and elementary bodies (EBs). The RB is the metabolically active, intracellular form of the organism. It is larger (1 μm) than the EB and its nuclear material is in an open state. EBs are the small (0.3 μm), hardy, metabolically inactive extracellular form of the organism (63). It is in this form that Chlamydiae are transferred between host cells and organisms. Nuclear material is tightly packed with histone-like proteins into an electron-dense structure called a nucleoid (103). The cellular envelope of the EB is very similar to that of Gram-negative bacteria, having both an inner and an outer membrane with a periplasmic layer in-between, and is specialized to protect them in the extracellular environment (43), ensuring osmotic stability and limited permeability. All members of the *Chlamydia* genus share a common, heat-stable, lipopolysaccharide antigen, which has a molecular weight of approximately 10 kDa, and although it is readily demonstrated on the RB surface, it does not appear to be accessible on the surface of the EBs.

The major outer membrane protein (MOMP) accounts for 60% of the surface protein of *C. trachomatis* and it contains epitopes that exhibit genus, species, and serovar specificity. *C. trachomatis* can be separated into 19 different serovars. These are grouped into two biovars: the trachoma biovar, which consists of serovars A to K, and the lymphogranuloma venereum (LGV) biovar, which consists of serovars L1, L2, L2a and L3. Studies from trachoma endemic countries indicate that this disease is usually caused by serovars A, B, Ba, and C of *C. trachomatis* (100). A number of studies, however, have demonstrated that the conjunctiva can be infected by other serotypes of *C. trachomatis* (60). Genital chlamydial infection, which is a leading cause of pelvic inflammatory disease and infertility, is usually associated by serovars D to K. MOMP is encoded by *omp1*, a single copy gene on the chlamydial chromosome. It consists of four variable segments (VS) flanked by five conserved regions. The *omp1* gene is one of the most polymorphic regions of the chlamydial chromosome (17). The serovar specificity of *C. trachomatis* is determined by variations in the VS regions, which are exposed on the surface (31). MOMP appears to be an important target for the immune response to *Chlamydia*.

The *C. trachomatis* genome consists of a chromosome (1,042,519 bp) and a plasmid (7493 bp) (91). Each organism has a single copy of the chromosome and usually several copies of the plasmid. The complete genome sequence of *C. trachomatis* has been published (91). It is estimated that there are about 875 genes on the chromosome. This has lead to some important insights into chlamydial biology. *C. trachomatis* was originally believed to lack the ability to produce the vital energy-rich compounds adenosine triphosphate (ATP) and guanine triphosphate, functioning primarily as an "energy parasite" within eukaryotic cells (65). With the completion of the chlamydial genome project, a surprising number of genes related to energy metabolism have been found, suggesting that the organism might be less dependent on its host than previously thought and may be able to perform some limited ATP synthesis for at least part of its life cycle (91). Other molecules such as nucleotides, which are necessary for the completion of the chlamydial lifecycle, need to be obtained from the host cell.

Chlamydial Developmental Cycle

Attachment and Endocytosis

The chlamydial developmental cycle commences with the attachment of the EB to the surface of epithelial or other host cells. It appears that no single binding mechanism dominates but rather that a number of relatively weak interactions can occur. This may explain in part why the organism is able to infect a wide range of host cells (104). A heparan sulfate-like proteoglycan on the surface of *C. trachomatis* seems to contribute to the initial attachment and may be critical for endocytosis (27,28,90). The MOMP has been demonstrated to play a part in the attachment of EB to the host cell through a range of nonspecific hydrophobic and electrostatic interactions and also through an interaction with the host cell heparan sulfate receptor (92). Other structures that may play a role in the attachment step include HSP-70 (75) and a 38 kDa surface protein (57). Entry of *C. trachomatis* into the host cell is a highly efficient process (25). The attachment of the organism to the host surface triggers an intracellular signal that results in endocytosis. A number of signaling mechanisms are thought to be involved including cyclic guanosine monophosphate, calcium influx, and the tyrosine phosphorylation of a number of cytoskeleton proteins (44,105). Endocytosis can occur by means of either a classical clathrin-coated phagocytic vesicle or pinocytic mechanisms (52,77).

Intracellular Survival, Replication, and Release

Cells infected with *Chlamydia* are characterized by the presence of a chlamydial inclusion in the perinuclear region of the host cell. *Chlamydia* have developed mechanisms to evade intracellular destruction by preventing the attachment of lysosomes (59). As inclusion bodies mature they take on the surface properties of sphingomyelin-containing secretory vesicles of the Golgi system; masquerading as secretory vesicles they avoid the destructive attention of lysosomes (48–50). On entering the host cell the EB form transforms into the RB form, a process that takes six to nine hours in vitro. MOMP appears to function as a transmembrane porin-like structure (12). In the extracellular environment the EB MOMP is closed by the presence of extensive cross-linking of cysteine residues. On encountering the reducing environment of the intracellular space MOMP changes to an open, noncross-linked form permitting the entry of ATP and other molecules needed for active metabolism. The expression of genes by *C. trachomatis* at different stages in the development cycle has recently been investigated using gene microarray technology (14). One hour after the entry of the organism into a host cell the transcription of 29 genes increased, many of which are involved with the formation of the inclusion body and the translocation of metabolites into the organism. Between 3 and 24 hours a further 200 genes are transcribed, corresponding to the period when RBs are actively replicating. By the end of the developmental cycle, 40 hours after the initial infection, only 26 genes are expressed, including those for histone proteins. The RBs replicate by binary fission. Eventually the newly formed RBs transform into EBs, with condensation of nuclear material and an overall reduction in size (104). In vitro the chlamydial development cycle takes between 36 and 70 hours to complete. It is not known how long it takes in vivo. The newly formed EBs are released either by lysis of the host cell or by the fusion of the inclusion body with the plasma membrane (99).

Detection of *C. trachomatis*

A number of different diagnostic tests have been used over the years for the detection of conjunctival *C. trachomatis* infection. These have included Giemsa staining, direct immunofluorescence (DIF), tissue culture, enzyme-liked immunoassays, and most recently nucleic acid amplification tests. The methodologies vary widely as do the targets for detection, whole organisms, chlamydial antigens, or specific DNA sequences. Not surprisingly, when compared directly these various tests often give discordant results. There is no absolute "Gold Standard" test for *C. trachomatis*. Although previously culture was regarded as the standard for diagnosis it lacks sensitivity. Currently the polymerase chain reaction (PCR)-based tests tend to be favored for research purposes.

Cytology

Smears of conjunctival cells can be stained for chlamydial inclusion bodies, although rarely used now for diagnosis. The Giemsa preparation stains the inclusion a reddish-purple color. It is a highly specific test but lacks sensitivity (83). It has the advantage of allowing the adequacy of the specimen to be assessed and provides information about the presence of inflammatory cells and bacteria, but requires a skilled microscopist. To improve the sensitivity of cytology DIF uses fluorescein-labeled monoclonal antibodies to identify *C. trachomatis* antigens, such as MOMP (83). DIF is about as sensitive as tissue culture, but the specimens are more stable and offer a more practical option for collection of samples under field conditions.

Culture

For many years the reference technique for the detection of *C. trachomatis* was isolation in cell culture. It is the only method that can assess the viability of the organism. Several systems have been developed using different cell lines (DEAE-dextran-treated HeLa cells, cyclohexamidine-treated McCoy cells and BHK-21 cells), which are inoculated with EBs and cultured for three to six days. Following culture, the cells are stained with either Giemsa or a specific fluorescein-labeled monoclonal antibody to aid the identification of infected cells. Although tissue culture is very specific it lacks sensitivity (83,93,96). In addition, samples have to be handled very carefully; they are collected into 2-SP medium, snap frozen in liquid nitrogen and stored at −80°C; it is expensive, requires sophisticated laboratory equipment and a high degree of expertise.

Antigen Detection Tests

Enzyme-linked immunosorbant assays (ELISAs) detect the presence of a heat-stable glycolipid antigen on the surface of *C. trachomatis* by the binding of a specific antibody. The antibody is linked to an enzyme, which catalyzes a reaction that reports the presence of the antigen. ELISAs were first used for the detection of genital chlamydial infections and found to be both sensitive and specific (70). They have been used in a number of studies of conjunctival *C. trachomatis* infection (83). In high-risk populations, chlamydial enzyme immunoassays have been shown to have similar sensitivity and specificity compared to isolation of the organism in cell culture. Like DIF tests, enzyme immunoassays have a low positive predictive accuracy in populations with a low prevalence of chlamydial infection. However, the test is prone to false-positives due to cross-reaction with other bacteria such as *S. aureus* (78,83). In addition the detection of chlamydial antigen does not necessarily mean that there is active infection.

Serological Tests for *Chlamydia*

Antibodies to chlamydial antigens can be detected in both the serum and tears at the time and following an infection. These tests are of limited value in the diagnosis of a chlamydial infection as they are relatively insensitive and are not routinely used in the diagnosis of ocular chlamydial infection. Chlamydial immunoglobulin G (IgG) antibody may persist at low levels in the serum for many months after the organisms have been eradicated, hence its value as a diagnostic indicator of current disease has a low predictive accuracy. It was suggested that the measurement of both IgG and immunoglobulin M antichlamydial antibodies may give some indication about how recent the infection is and whether the individual has previously had an infection when all other tests are negative. The measurement of subclasses of tear immunoglobulin has been used in studies of the immune response to the infection.

Nucleic Acid Probes

Nucleic acid hybridization techniques offer the prospect of very high diagnostic specificity compared with immunodiagnostic tests (DIF and ELISA), which are based on antibody detection probes. The detection of *C. trachomatis* using in situ hybridization has generally shown a low degree of sensitivity, especially using probes based on chlamydial plasmid DNA. The reason for the poor sensitivity is probably that not all *Chlamydia* contain extra-chromosomal DNA.

Nucleic Acid Amplification Tests

More recently a number of nucleic acid amplification tests have become available for the diagnosis of *C. trachomatis* infections, the most commonly used are those based on PCR technology. A number of commercial tests are available, which are used in the diagnosis of both genital and ocular *C. trachomatis* infections. In trachoma research studies PCR is currently the preferred diagnostic method, but it is not suitable for routine use by control programs in endemic countries because of the cost and complexity (15,88). These tests are an improvement over the tests described above, as they are both highly specific and sensitive. In a PCR reaction a segment of target DNA is selectively amplified, through repeated cycles of the reaction, even from very low levels in the original sample. Various targets have been used including the chlamydial plasmid, the gene for MOMP (*omp1*), and chlamydial 16S rRNA (20,21). As the plasmid is usually present in multiple copies in the organism, assays using this target are probably more sensitive (88). As PCR is so sensitive, there is a risk of false-positive results through contamination. Additionally, the reaction can be inhibited leading to possible false-negative results. Both these problems can generally be overcome with careful laboratory practice. Recently quantitative real-time PCR has been used to measure the load of *C. trachomatis* infections in members of trachoma endemic communities to better define the major reservoirs of infection and monitor response to treatment (20,22,86,87). This method allows the accurate estimation of the number of copies a particular DNA sequence of interest in a sample.

CLINICAL FEATURES AND EPIDEMIOLOGY

From the epidemiological viewpoint, ocular infections caused by *C. trachomatis* are divided into two groups: (*i*) trachoma caused by eye-to-eye transmission of *C. trachomatis* serovars A, B, Ba, and C, and (*ii*) paratrachoma of sexually transmitted origin caused by *C. trachomatis* serovars D to K (56). Other species of *Chlamydia* have also rarely been reported to cause conjunctival infection.

Trachoma

Trachoma is the leading infectious cause of blindness worldwide (98). The disease was endemic in Ancient Egypt (6). The *Ebers Papyrus*, dating from the sixteenth century B.C., describes the condition and its treatment, and epilation forceps have been found in ancient Egyptian tombs (62). Hippocrates wrote about trachoma and trichiasis in Greece in the fifth century B.C. The name *trachoma* (from the Greek: *trachus* meaning rough) seems to have first been recorded by Discordes in *Materia Medica* dating from 60 A.D. (38).

The clinical manifestations of trachoma can be subdivided into active (early) and cicatricial (late-stage) disease, and are classified using the World Health Organization (WHO) grading system (35,97). Active disease is more commonly found in children. Infection of the ocular surface by *C. trachomatis* results in a chronic, recurrent follicular conjunctivitis. There may be minimal symptoms of ocular irritation and a slight watery discharge. In more severe cases there may be photophobia and copious watering. Active disease is characterized by lymphoid follicles and papillary hypertrophy, which are both most obvious in the upper tarsal conjunctiva (Figs. 1 and 2). Follicles are collections of lymphoid tissue subjacent to the tarsal conjunctival epithelium. Intense cases of active trachoma are characterized by the presence of papillary hypertrophy. When mild there is engorgement of the small vessels that appear as small red dots within the tarsal conjunctiva. More severe cases have a pronounced inflammatory thickening of the conjunctiva that obscures the normal deep tarsal blood vessels. During an episode of active disease the cornea can be affected: punctate epithelial keratopathy, superficial infiltrates, superficial vascular pannus, and limbal follicles, which as they resolve leave small depressions called Herbert pits.

The cicatricial or scarring sequelae of trachoma develop later in life, usually from around the third decade, but can present earlier in regions with more severe disease. Recurrent episodes of chronic inflammation lead to conjunctival scarring. This can range from a few linear or stellate scars to thick distorting bands of fibrosis with shortening of the fornices and symblepharon. The scarring causes entropion and trichiasis. Ultimately, blinding corneal opacification can develop. Women are more frequently affected by the blinding complications than men. About 75% of trichiasis and corneal blindness cases are in women, probably due to their greater lifetime exposure to *C. trachomatis* infection through contact with children (30).

The WHO estimates that 6 million people are blind from trachoma and a further 10 million people are in need of trichiasis surgery to prevent blindness (98). Six hundred million people are estimated to live in regions of the world where trachoma is endemic and about 146 million people are believed to have active trachoma at any given time. During the last

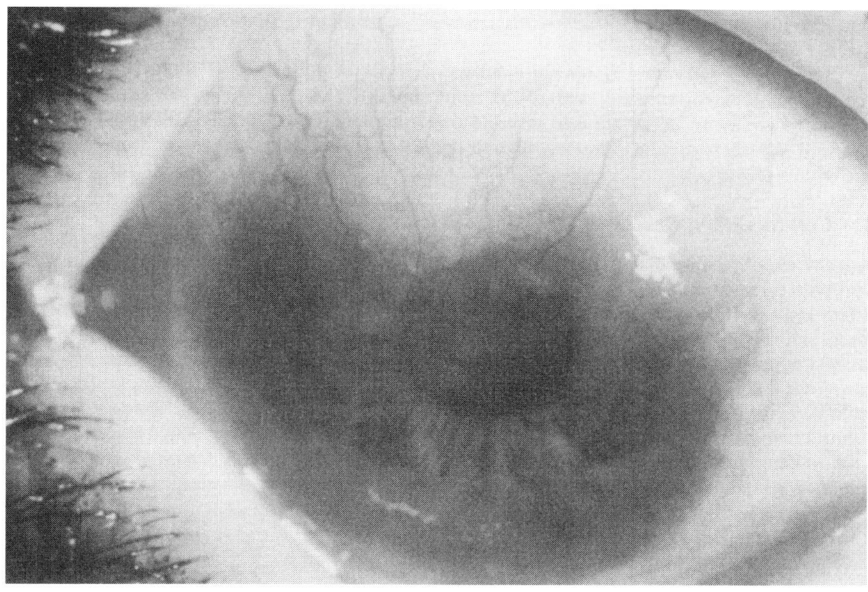

Figure 1 Severe trachoma, showing extensive pannus.

century trachoma retreated from some formerly endemic regions, such as Europe and North America. This reduction in prevalence is attributed to general improvements in the standard of living, as it occurred in the absence of any specific interventions against the disease (56). Today, trachoma is prevalent in large parts of Africa and in some regions of the Middle East, the Indian Subcontinent, Southeast Asia, and South America (69). Hyperendemic countries such as Ethiopia and Tanzania report rates of active trachoma in children in excess of 50% in many regions, with little or no reduction in disease being observed. For many trachoma endemic countries the general socioeconomic developments that might promote the disappearance of the disease are likely to be very slow in arriving, which in the light demographic trends and in the absence of effective control programs could lead to an increase in the amount of trachoma blindness (81).

C. trachomatis is probably transmitted from infected to uninfected individuals within a trachoma endemic community by a combination of mechanisms, such as direct spread from eye to eye during close contact, spread on fingers, indirect spread on fomites (such as face cloths), and transmission by eye-seeking flies (56). Individual and environmental risk factors, which promote the introduction and transmission of *C. trachomatis* in endemic communities, have

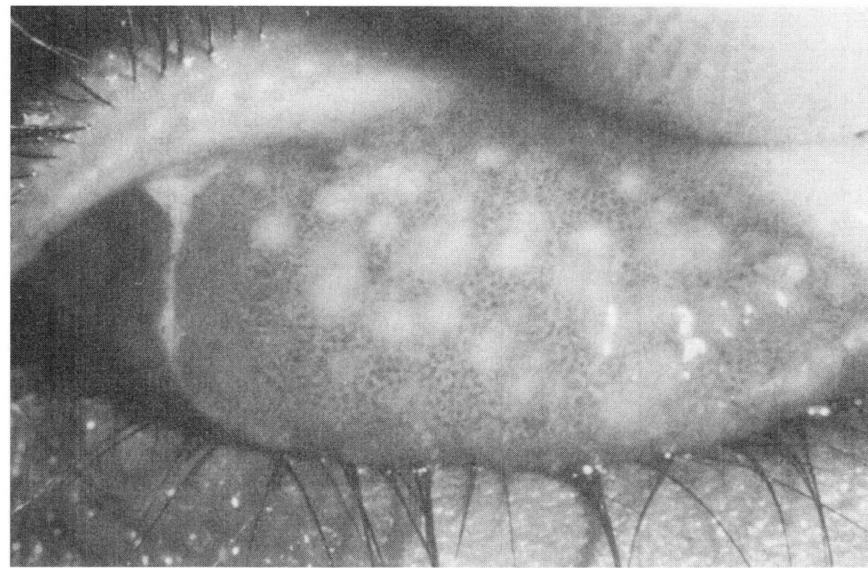

Figure 2 Everted upper tarsal conjunctiva of trachomatous eye, showing follicular and papillary hyperplasia.

been identified. Trachoma tends to cluster within communities and transmission is probably promoted by crowding (8). Limited water supply for face and hand cleaning is a risk factor for trachoma, probably by prolonging the presence of infected secretions on the face of children, so facilitating transmission (40,106). Eye-seeking flies probably act as vectors for *C. trachomatis* transmission in some environments (41). Poor sanitation such as a lack of latrines has often been associated with increased risk of trachoma (20). Controlling the fly population either through insecticide spraying or the provision of latrines is associated with reduced prevalence of active disease (41). No animal reservoir for *C. trachomatis* has been found in trachoma endemic environments, although there is an association with cattle, which may result in an abundance of flies (37). Migration of people between communities is probably important for maintaining trachoma endemicity through the introduction of new strains of *C. trachomatis* (22).

Paratrachoma

C. trachomatis infection of the urogenital tract, usually with serovars D to K, can sometimes cause conjunctival infection, which is referred to as paratrachoma. Because of the increasing incidence of chlamydial genital infections, ocular infection is likely to become more common. Paratrachoma comprises various clinical entities: chlamydial ophthalmia neonatorum, adult inclusion conjunctivitis, and chlamydial punctate keratoconjunctivitis.

Adult Inclusion Conjunctivitis

Adult inclusion conjunctivitis and chlamydial punctate keratoconjunctivitis are believed to be caused by transmission of *C. trachomatis* from the genital tract to the eye, either from the same individual or an infected partner. It accounts for about 2% of conjunctivitis cases seen in developed countries (46). Around 50% to 70% of individuals with adult inclusion conjunctivitis have simultaneous infection of the genital tract (89). Conversely, only around one in 300 cases of genital chlamydial infection have adult inclusion conjunctivitis. The infection is commonly unilateral and mainly affects young adults. Symptoms include a moderate watery discharge, eyelid swelling, redness, photophobia, and a foreign body sensation. There is thought to be an incubation period of one to three weeks. The clinical signs consist of moderate hyperemia, diffuse thickening, the development of papillae, and the formation of lymphoid follicles in the tarsal conjunctiva (102). The cornea is not usually involved, but may show a mild to moderate degree of punctate epithelial keratitis. In patients with chlamydial punctate keratoconjunctivitis the cornea may develop punctate subepithelial opacities resembling those in keratoconjunctivitis due to adenovirus. Occasionally, pannus or scarring of the conjunctiva may develop resembling the clinical picture of hyperendemic trachoma. However, it is usually a self-limiting condition as repeated ocular chlamydial infection does not usually occur to the same extent as it does in trachoma endemic regions. *C. trachomatis* is an increasingly common sexually transmitted infection worldwide, with about 90 million cases (47). Chlamydial urethritis is associated with discharge, dysuria, or frequency of urination. Most patients with chlamydial cervicitis are asymptomatic, although clinical signs consisting of mucopurulent discharge, hyperemia, hypertrophic erosions, follicles, and occasionally scars may be present. *C. trachomatis* may cause pelvic inflammatory disease in women leading to scarring of the fallopian tubes and infertility.

Ophthalmia Neonatorum

O. neonatorum due to *C. trachomatis* is acquired by the newborn during passage through the infected cervix of the mother. About 18% of babies born to infected mothers develop culture positive conjunctivitis (82). The incubation period is usually 5 to 14 days. The infection is acute, may affect both eyes, and is associated with excessive tearing, profuse mucopurulent discharge, and swelling and erythema of the eyelids. The bulbar conjunctiva is generally hyperemic, with mild to moderate chemosis but the cornea may remain normal. The tarsal conjunctiva is hyperemic, with a diffuse infiltration by lymphocytes and plasma cells and the formation of papillae related to the down growth of the surface epithelium. Untreated, the disease may last for months or years and may become associated with persistent lymphoid follicles, corneal pannus, and scarring identical to that in hyperendemic trachoma. Babies infected with *C. trachomatis* at birth are at risk of neonatal pneumonia, affecting 16% of those born to infected mothers (82).

Lymphogranuloma Venereum

LGV is a sexually transmitted disease caused by *C. trachomatis* serovars LI, L2, and L3. These organisms are more invasive than *C. trachomatis* serovars A to K. The characteristic feature of the disease is enlargement of and suppuration from the inguinal lymph nodes. Persistent infection may cause destructive lesions in the genital tract and rectal region. LGV is still common in Central and Southern Africa, Southeast Asia, and Central and South America. In the eye it has been rarely associated with Parinaud ocular glandular syndrome (24).

C. psittaci Infections

Psittacosis, caused by *C. psittaci*, is generally an infection of birds, but humans may contract the infection by inhalation of dried excreta or discharges from infected birds. In birds the infection often causes conjunctivitis or keratoconjunctivitis. Psittacosis is a serious occupational hazard of people in the poultry industry, in which the human infection may present as either respiratory or systemic disease. The organism has been incriminated in a case of interstitial keratitis and uveitis associated with the middle ear and cardiovascular lesions suggestive of Cogan syndrome (33). It has been suggested that there is an association between *C. psittaci* and adnexal lymphomas, although this finding is disputed (45). *Chlamidophila* felis, which was originally classified under *C. psittaci*, causes infections in domestic animals, particularly cats, and has been rarely found to produce conjunctivitis in humans (51).

C. pneumoniae Infections

C. pneumoniae is implicated in a number of human diseases. It probably causes 5% to 10% of acute community acquired pneumonia and may contribute to chronic pulmonary disease such as asthma. There is some evidence of an association with coronary artery disease, Alzheimer disease and multiple sclerosis. *C. pneumoniae* was first isolated from a Taiwanese girl with clinical signs of trachoma and has been identified as a cause of conjunctivitis occasionally since then.

RELATIONSHIP BETWEEN CLINICAL SIGNS AND DETECTION OF *CHLAMYDIA*

The relationship between the detection of *C. trachomatis* in the conjunctiva and the clinical signs of trachoma observed on examination is complex. Studies have consistently found a mismatch between the signs of disease and detection of the organism; people with signs of active trachoma without detectable *C. trachomatis* and conversely individuals with detectable *C. trachomatis* who are clinically normal (109). This is a significant problem for trachoma control programs, which rely on signs to guide antibiotic treatment. It also indicates the importance of the host response in the disease process. There are several contributory reasons for this mismatch. First, there may be an "incubation period" during which infection is present but disease has not yet developed. Secondly, the resolution of signs of disease lags behind the resolution of infection, often by many weeks (7). The duration of both disease and infection episodes are modified by age, lasting longer in children. Thirdly, it is possible that a subclinical persistent form of infection may develop under certain conditions in which the organism is not replicating but lies dormant and may not provoke the disease phenotype (83). Fourthly, the signs of conjunctival inflammation are not exclusive to trachoma and could be initiated by other pathogens. Finally, the presence of detectable chlamydial antigen or DNA does not necessarily equate to an established, replicating infection. Tests may be positive as a result of a transient inoculation of the conjunctiva with *C. trachomatis* following close contact with a heavily infected individual or the activities of eye seeking flies.

Quantitative PCR for *omp1* (a single copy gene on the *C. trachomatis* chromosome) has been used to determine the relative load of infection in members of trachoma endemic communities (20,22,86,87). The distribution of infection load is skewed; the majority of individuals have relatively low infection loads, whilst a smaller number have high loads. The highest infection loads are generally found in children, especially those with intense conjunctival inflammation. Clinically normal individuals with detectable *C. trachomatis* tend to have lower infection loads and do not have detectable expression of chlamydial 16S rRNA, a marker for a metabolically active replicating infection (21). In contrast, the presence of 16S rRNA expression was associated with high infection loads and clinical disease.

PATHOPHYSIOLOGY

The Stimulus for Inflammation

Clinically active trachoma is characterized by episodes of follicular conjunctivitis. Individuals who develop persistent, severe conjunctival inflammation in childhood are at greatest risk of developing scarring and trichiasis in later life (36,107). An inflammatory reaction is generated by the host immune system in response to *C. trachomatis* infection (18,21). It is believed that serial reinfection of the conjunctiva by *C. trachomatis* is the major stimulant to the development of the cicatricial complications. In primate models conjunctival scarring only developed after many episodes of *C. trachomatis* reinfection (94). However, the inflammatory signs often persist for many weeks or months after resolution of infection, suggesting that a proinflammatory immune response persists for reasons beyond a productive, replicating chlamydial infection (7). There is evidence that some individuals may have difficulty in resolving infections, with the same genotype of *C. trachomatis* being found on separate occasions several years apart (85). In vitro studies suggest that the organism may transform into a persistent nonreplicating form when stressed; however, this has not been confirmed in vivo. Bacterial conjunctival infection is a common finding in individuals with trichiasis and may provoke additional inflammation which could promote scarring (19,23). Corneal opacification and blindness probably result from trauma by the trichiasis and secondary bacterial infection (16,19,23).

Evidence from a monkey model for trachoma indicates that active disease develops in response to chlamydial heat shock protein 60 (HSP60) which is found within live whole organisms (95). Killed chlamydial EBs or surface antigens such as MOMP did not provoke an inflammatory response in previously infected animals. Heat shock proteins are found in both eukaryotic and prokaryotic cells and have extensive sequence homology. They are induced when a cell is under stress. It has been suggested that the chronic inflammatory reaction in trachoma could be partly an autoimmune reaction to the human equivalent of HSP60, however, the evidence for this is limited. Individuals with trachomatous scarring are more likely to have serum antibodies to HSP60 than controls (67).

Histopathology of Trachoma

Histological studies of conjunctival biopsy tissue from children with active trachoma have shown a marked inflammatory cell infiltrate (1,4,39). The conjunctival epithelium is hyperplastic, and chlamydial intracellular inclusion bodies can be seen within epithelial cells. In the subepithelial stroma there is a widespread inflammatory infiltrate. In places this is organized into follicles, with a surrounding lymphocytic mantle. Follicles are largely composed of B-lymphocytes. Between the follicles there is a diffuse mixed infiltrate of T- and B-lymphocytes, macrophages, plasma cells and neutrophils. Both CD4+ T cells and CD8+ T cells are found in the infiltrate (4). Staining for subtypes of collagen demonstrated a generalized increase in the amounts of collagen types I, III, and IV (normally found in the stroma) and deposition of collagen type V, which is not normally found at this site (3).

In trachomatous scarring the conjunctival epithelium is atrophic, often only one cell thick with a loss of goblet cells (5). The loose subepithelial stroma (normally collagen types I and III) is replaced with a thick scar containing collagen type V and with deposition of collagen type IV along the conjunctival basement membrane (2). These new fibers are orientated vertically and are firmly attached to the posterior surface of the tarsal plate causing its distortion (5). Biopsies from some scarred individuals have an inflammatory infiltrate dominated by T cells, corresponding to clinical conjunctival inflammation, which is frequently observed in people with established trichiasis (76). The tarsal plate is usually of normal thickness, but there is often atrophy of the meibomian glands and a chronic inflammatory infiltrate (5).

Immunity and Immunopathology in Trachoma

The human immune response to *C. trachomatis* is poorly understood. The resolution of infection is probably dependent on a cell-mediated response which, conversely, may also play a major role in the pathogenesis of trachomatous scarring. It appears that some degree of strain-specific immunity can develop. When previously uninfected human volunteers were challenged with *C. trachomatis* almost all develop infection whereas only half of those who had prior infections became infected (55). When rechallenged with the same strain of *C. trachomatis*, infection did not develop. However, if a different strain was used, infection developed. The finding that duration of *C. trachomatis* infection decreases with increasing age is consistent with an acquired immune response (7). It is likely that the scarring and blinding complications of trachoma arise from persistent or repeated severe inflammatory reactions to the infection (36). Chlamydial infection is usually confined to a minority of epithelial cells, whereas the inflammatory cell infiltrate extends deep into the substantia propria.

Innate Immune Response

The initial response to infection of the epithelial surface by *C. trachomatis* is probably made by the innate immune system. In vitro studies indicate that *C. trachomatis* infection triggers production of proinflammatory cytokines by epithelial cells: interleukin 1 (IL1), interleukin 6 (IL6) interleukin 8 (IL8) and tumor necrosis factor-α (TNFα) (74). Although these may have a limited direct antichlamydial action, their main effect is to promote rapid influx of neutrophils and macrophages, which may help to limit the initial infection through phagocytosis, but probably cause some direct tissue damage (11,34). Conjunctival biopsies from children with active trachoma reveal increased numbers of macrophages, which produce IL1β and TNFα (4). Ongoing activation of these cells even after infection has resolved probably plays an important part in the development of scarring.

Adaptive Immune Response

The initial innate immune response to *C. trachomatis* infection is followed by the development of adaptive immune responses with both antibody-meditated (humoral) and cell-mediated components. Current evidence indicates that a predominately T_H1 response is associated with a more favorable outcome in chlamydial infections.

Humoral Immunity

Antichlamydial antibodies have been found in the tears and serum of patients with clinically active trachoma (29,64,101). In a longitudinal study of a trachoma endemic community antichlamydial IgG in the tears of clinically normal individuals was associated with an increased incidence of developing clinically active trachoma (10). An opposite trend was found for antichlamydial immunoglobulin A (IgA).

Individuals with conjunctival scarring had significantly higher plasma titers of antichlamydial IgG and lower titers of IgA compared to normal controls (53). This suggests that antichlamydial IgG may enhance the entry of the organism into the host cell and may reflect a T_H2 helper T-cell–weighted response. Conversely, IgA may provide a defence against the initial stages of infection by interfering with attachment to host cells.

Cell-Mediated Immunity

Animal models of chlamydial infections suggest that effective cell-mediated immune responses are necessary for the resolution of chlamydial infection. Athymic mice are unable to clear genital infection with *C. trachomatis* (73), but this ability can be restored by the adoptive transfer of *Chlamydia*-specific T cells (71). Studies of patients with conjunctival *C. trachomatis* infection have demonstrated peripheral blood lymphocyte proliferation responses to chlamydial antigens (61). In a trachoma endemic community, individuals with clinically resolved active disease had greater lymphoproliferative responses to chlamydial antigens compared with individuals who had persistent clinical disease (9). In contrast, individuals with trachomatous conjunctival scarring had weaker peripheral blood lymphocyte proliferation responses with lower interferon γ (IFNγ) production compared with normal controls (53).

IFNγ appears to be the pivotal cytokine in the resolution of infection. IFNγ is primarily released by T_H1 cells. In vitro studies have demonstrated that IFNγ can inhibit the growth and differentiation of *Chlamydia* (13). Athymic mice can resolve *C. trachomatis* infection when given IFNγ, although other mechanisms probably contribute (72). Individuals with *C. trachomatis* infection have increased expression of IFNγ, IL2, and interleukin 12 (IL12) within the conjunctiva, consistent with a T_H1 helper T-cell–response (18). IFNγ has several antichlamydial actions (80). First, indoleamine 2,3-dioxygenase (IDO) is induced by IFNγ. IDO metabolizes L-tryptophan to *N*-formylkynurenine, depriving *C. trachomatis* of an essential amino acid. Polymorphisms in the *C. trachomatis* tryptophan synthase genes have been found, which indicate that genital, but not ocular, strains of the organism have maintained the ability to generate tryptophan. However, the significance of this finding is not currently known (26). Secondly, IFNγ increases inducible nitric oxide synthase, generating nitric oxide, which is active against *Chlamydia*. Thirdly, IFNγ appears to control chlamydial infection through the depletion of intracellular iron reducing the infectivity of EB and altering the morphology in chlamydial inclusions and the expression of various proteins.

The role of CD8+ cytotoxic lymphocytes (CTLs) in trachoma is uncertain. They may have an effect through triggering the apoptosis of infected cells or through IFNγ-mediated pathways. Studies in a genetically engineered murine model in which the MHC class I antigens are not expressed demonstrated that CTL responses are not essential for immunity to *Chlamydia* (108). However, this does not preclude some significant function in humans. Histological studies have found increased numbers of CD8+ T cells in conjunctival biopsies from individuals with active trachoma (4). A minority of individuals from a trachoma-endemic area were found to have peripheral blood CTL responses to chlamydial antigens (54). These responses were only found in children with resolved active disease episodes and in adults without conjunctival scarring. It appears that in mice CTL control of chlamydial infections is primarily through the production of IFNγ rather than by cell lysis mechanisms (58,68). However, the expression of perforin, which is mainly produced by CTL, was found to be elevated in the conjunctiva of individuals with *C. trachomatis* infection from a trachoma-endemic community (18).

Inflammation and Immunopathology

Clinically active trachoma often persists long after the infection becomes undetectable. Chronic severe conjunctival inflammation is associated with progression to scarring complications probably through the activation of fibrogenic pathways. Active disease, irrespective of the presence of infection, is associated with increased expression of the proinflammatory cytokines IL1β and TNFα, particularly in macrophages (4,18). The production of these cytokines may be triggered by various chlamydial antigens, but may not require the presence of a live replicating infection to be sustained (79). TNFα has been found more frequently in the tears of individuals with trachomatous scarring compared with controls, especially when chlamydial infection was present (32). A single base polymorphism of the TNFα promoter region, TNFA-308A, was associated with trachomatous scarring, although the functional significance of this polymorphism in trachoma is unclear (32). The principal antiinflammatory cytokine IL10 may have a significant role in the outcome of trachoma. It is expressed at increased levels in the conjunctiva of individuals with active trachoma (18). IL10 is produced by a number of cells including regulatory T cells (T_R) and type helper T cells (T_H2). It dampens the response to IL1β and TNFα, helping to limit the inflammation and therefore presumably the scarring complications (110). However, IL10 also opposes the action of the T_H1 response mediated through IFNγ, so may impede the resolution of infection. Polymorphisms have been identified in the IL10 gene, which are associated with increased risk of trachomatous scarring, although their functional significance remains to be elucidated (66).

Little is known about the fibrogenic processes leading to trachomatous scarring. As with many fibrotic diseases it is likely that TGFβ has a major role; however, it is difficult to measure its activity in vivo as it is posttranscriptionally regulated. Other fibrogenic cytokines associated with a T_H2 response, such as IL13, may also be important (110). Matrix metalloproteinases (MMPs) are a family of proteolytic enzymes central to the regulation of the extracellular matrix (ECM) that have been implicated in many scarring disorders. They can degrade the ECM and facilitate contraction of scar tissue. The expression of MMP-9 is elevated in the conjunctiva with active trachoma, becoming more marked with increasing severity of disease (18). MMP-9 has many ECM substrates, but also activates pro-IL1β and TGFβ, possibly helping to perpetuate the disease process.

REFERENCES

1. Abrahams C, Ballard RC, Sutter EE. The pathology of trachoma in a black South African population: light microscopical, histochemical and electron microscopical findings. S Afr Med J 1979; 55:1115–8.
2. Abu el-Asrar AM, Geboes K, Al Kharashi SA, et al. An immunohistochemical study of collagens in trachoma and vernal keratoconjunctivitis. Eye 1998; 12(Pt 6):1001–6.
3. Abu el-Asrar AM, Geboes K, Al Kharashi SA, et al. Collagen content and types in trachomatous conjunctivitis. Eye 1998; 12(Pt 4):735–9.
4. Abu el-Asrar AM, Geboes K, Tabbara KF, et al. Immunopathogenesis of conjunctival scarring in trachoma. Eye 1998; 12(Pt 3a):453–60.
5. Al Rajhi AA, Hidayat A, Nasr A, al Faran M. The histopathology and the mechanism of entropion in patients with trachoma. Ophthalmology 1993; 100:1293–6.
6. al Rifai KM. Trachoma through history. Int Ophthalmol 1988; 12:9–14.
7. Bailey R, Duong T, Carpenter R, et al. The duration of human ocular *Chlamydia trachomatis* infection is age dependent. Epidemiol Infect 1999; 123:479–86.
8. Bailey R, Osmond C, Mabey DC, et al. Analysis of the household distribution of trachoma in a Gambian village using a Monte Carlo simulation procedure. Int J Epidemiol 1989; 18:944–51.
9. Bailey RL, Holland MJ, Whittle HC, Mabey DC. Subjects recovering from human ocular chlamydial infection have enhanced lymphoproliferative responses to chlamydial antigens compared with those of persistently diseased controls. Infect Immun 1995; 63:389–92.
10. Bailey RL, Kajbaf M, Whittle HC, et al. The influence of local antichlamydial antibody on the acquisition and persistence of human ocular chlamydial infection: IgG antibodies are not protective. Epidemiol Infect 1993; 111: 315–24.
11. Barteneva N, Theodor I, Peterson EM, de la Maza LM. Role of neutrophils in controlling early stages of a *Chlamydia trachomatis* infection. Infect Immun 1996; 64: 4830–3.
12. Bavoil P, Ohlin A, Schachter J. Role of disulfide bonding in outer membrane structure and permeability in *Chlamydia trachomatis*. Infect Immun 1984; 44: 479–85.
13. Beatty WL, Byrne GI, Morrison RP. Morphologic and antigenic characterization of interferon gamma-mediated persistent *Chlamydia trachomatis* infection in vitro. Proc Natl Acad Sci USA 1993; 90:3998–4002.
14. Belland RJ, Zhong G, Crane DD, et al. Genomic transcriptional profiling of the developmental cycle of *Chlamydia trachomatis*. Proc Natl Acad Sci USA 2003; 100: 8478–83.
15. Bobo L, Munoz B, Viscidi R, et al. Diagnosis of *Chlamydia trachomatis* eye infection in Tanzania by polymerase chain reaction/enzyme immunoassay. Lancet 1991; 338: 847–50.
16. Bowman RJ, Faal H, Myatt M, et al. Longitudinal study of trachomatous trichiasis in the Gambia. Br J Ophthalmol 2002; 86:339–43.
17. Brunelle BW, Nicholson TL, Stephens RS. Microarray-based genomic surveying of gene polymorphisms in *Chlamydia trachomatis*. Genome Biol 2004; 5:R42.
18. Burton MJ, Bailey RL, Jeffries D, et al. Cytokine and fibrogenic gene expression in the conjunctivas of subjects from a Gambian community where trachoma is endemic. Infect Immun 2004; 72:7352–6.
19. Burton MJ, Bowman RJ, Faal H, et al. The long-term natural history of trachomatous trichiasis in the Gambia. Invest Ophthalmol Vis Sci 2006; 47:847–52.
20. Burton MJ, Holland MJ, Faal N, et al. Which members of a community need antibiotics to control trachoma? Conjunctival *Chlamydia trachomatis* infection load in Gambian villages. Invest Ophthalmol Vis Sci 2003; 44: 4215–22.
21. Burton MJ, Holland MJ, Jeffries D, et al. Conjunctival chlamydial 16S ribosomal RNA expression in trachoma: is chlamydial metabolic activity required for disease to develop? Clin Infect Dis 2006; 42:463–70.
22. Burton MJ, Holland MJ, Makalo P, et al. Reemergence of *Chlamydia trachomatis* infection after mass antibiotic treatment of a trachoma-endemic Gambian community: a longitudinal study. Lancet 2005; 365:1321–8.
23. Burton MJ, Kinteh F, Jallow O, et al. A randomised controlled trial of azithromycin following surgery for trachomatous trichiasis in the Gambia. Br J Ophthalmol 2005; 89:1282–8.
24. Buus DR, Pflugfelder SC, Schachter J, et al. *Lymphogranuloma venereum* conjunctivitis with a marginal corneal perforation. Ophthalmology 1988; 95:799–802.
25. Byrne GI, Moulder JW. Parasite-specified phagocytosis of *Chlamydia psittaci* and *Chlamydia trachomatis* by L and HeLa cells. Infect Immun 1978; 19:598–606.
26. Caldwell HD, Wood H, Crane D, et al. Polymorphisms in *Chlamydia trachomatis* tryptophan synthase genes differentiate between genital and ocular isolates. J Clin Invest 2003; 111:1757–69.
27. Chen JC, Stephens RS. *Chlamydia trachomatis* glycosaminoglycan-dependent and independent attachment to eukaryotic cells. Microb Pathog 1997; 22:23–30.
28. Chen JC, Stephens RS. Trachoma and LGV biovars of *Chlamydia trachomatis* share the same glycosaminoglycan-dependent mechanism for infection of eukaryotic cells. Mol Microbiol 1994; 11:501–7.
29. Collier LH, Sowa J, Sowa S. The serum and conjunctival antibody response to trachoma in Gambian children. J Hyg (Lond) 1972; 70:727–40.

30. Congdon N, West S, Vitale S, et al. Exposure to children and risk of active trachoma in Tanzanian women. Am J Epidemiol 1993; 137:366–72.
31. Conlan JW, Clarke IN, Ward ME. Epitope mapping with solid-phase peptides: identification of type-, subspecies-, species- and genus-reactive antibody binding domains on the major outer membrane protein of *Chlamydia trachomatis*. Mol Microbiol 1988; 2:673–9.
32. Conway DJ, Holland MJ, Bailey RL, et al. Scarring trachoma is associated with polymorphism in the tumor necrosis factor alpha (TNF-alpha) gene promoter and with elevated TNF-alpha levels in tear fluid. Infect Immun 1997; 65:1003–6.
33. Darougar S, John AC, Viswalingam M, et al. Isolation of *Chlamydia psittaci* from a patient with interstitial keratitis and uveitis associated with otological and cardiovascular lesions. Br J Ophthalmol 1978; 62:709–14.
34. Darville T, Andrews CW CW, Laffoon KK, et al. Mouse strain-dependent variation in the course and outcome of chlamydial genital tract infection is associated with differences in host response. Infect Immun 1997; 65: 3065–73.
35. Dawson CR, Jones BR, Tarizzo ML. Guide to Trachoma Control. Geneva: World Health Organization, 1981.
36. Dawson CR, Marx R, Daghfous T, et al. What clinical signs are critical in evaluating the intervention in trachoma? In: Bowein WR, ed. Chlamydial Infection. New York: Cambridge University, Press, 1990; 271–278.
37. De Sole G. Impact of cattle on the prevalence and severity of trachoma. Br J Ophthalmol 1987; 71:873–6.
38. Duke-Elder WS. Diseases of the outer eye, Part 1. London: Henry Kimpton, 1977:249–307.
39. El Asrar AM, Van den Oord JJ, Geboes K, et al. Immunopathology of trachomatous conjunctivitis. Br J Ophthalmol 1989; 73:276–82.
40. Emerson PM, Cairncross S, Bailey RL, Mabey DC. Review of the evidence base for the 'F' and 'E' components of the SAFE strategy for trachoma control. Trop Med Int Health 2000; 5:515–27.
41. Emerson PM, Lindsay SW, Alexander N, et al. Role of flies and provision of latrines in trachoma control: cluster-randomised controlled trial. Lancet 2004; 363: 1093–8.
42. Everett KD, Bush RM, Andersen AA. Emended description of the order Chlamydiales, proposal of Parachlamydiaceae fam. nov. and Simkaniaceae fam. nov., each containing one monotypic genus, revised taxonomy of the family Chlamydiaceae, including a new genus and five new species, and standards for the identification of organisms. Int J Syst Bacteriol 1999; 49(Pt 2):415–40.
43. Everett KD, Hatch TP. Architecture of the cell envelope of *Chlamydia psittaci* 6BC. J Bacteriol 1995; 177:877–82.
44. Fawaz FS, van Ooij C, Homola E, et al. Infection with *Chlamydia trachomatis* alters the tyrosine phosphorylation and/or localization of several host cell proteins including cortactin. Infect Immun 1997; 65:5301–8.
45. Ferreri AJ, Guidoboni M, Ponzoni M, et al. Evidence for an association between *Chlamydia psittaci* and ocular adnexal lymphomas. J Natl Cancer Inst 2004; 96:586–94.
46. Garland SM, Malatt A, Tabrizi S, et al. *Chlamydia trachomatis* conjunctivitis: prevalence and association with genital tract infection. Med J Aust 1995; 162:363–6.
47. Gerbase AC, Rowley JT, Heymann DH, et al. Global prevalence and incidence estimates of selected curable STDs. Sex Transm Infect 1998; 74(Suppl 1):S12–6.
48. Hackstadt T. Redirection of host vesicle trafficking pathways by intracellular parasites. Traffic 2000; 1:93–9.
49. Hackstadt T, Rockey DD, Heinzen RA, Scidmore MA. *Chlamydia trachomatis* interrupts an exocytic pathway to acquire endogenously synthesized sphingomyelin in transit from the Golgi apparatus to the plasma membrane. EMBO J 1996; 15:964–77.
50. Hackstadt T, Scidmore MA, Rockey DD. Lipid metabolism in *Chlamydia trachomatis*-infected cells: directed trafficking of Golgi-derived sphingolipids to the chlamydial inclusion. Proc Natl Acad Sci USA 1995; 92:4877–81.
51. Hartley JC, Stevenson S, Robinson AJ, et al. Conjunctivitis due to *Chlamydophila felis* (*Chlamydia psittaci* feline pneumonitis agent) acquired from a cat: case report with molecular characterization of isolates from the patient and cat. J Infect 2001; 43:7–11.
52. Hodinka RL, Davis CH, Choong J, Wyrick PB. Ultrastructural study of endocytosis of *Chlamydia trachomatis* by McCoy cells. Infect Immun 1988; 56:1456–63.
53. Holland MJ, Bailey RL, Hayes LJ, et al. Conjunctival scarring in trachoma is associated with depressed cell-mediated immune responses to chlamydial antigens. J Infect Dis 1993; 168:1528–31.
54. Holland MJ, Conway DJ, Blanchard TJ, et al. Synthetic peptides based on *Chlamydia trachomatis* antigens identify cytotoxic T lymphocyte responses in subjects from a trachoma-endemic population. Clin Exp Immunol 1997; 107:44–9.
55. Jawetz E, Rose L, Hanna L, Thygeson P. Experimental inclusion conjunctivitis in man: measurements of infectivity and resistance. JAMA 1965; 194:620–32.
56. Jones BR. The prevention of blindness from trachoma. Trans Ophthalmol Soc UK 1975; 95:16–33.
57. Joseph TD, Bose SK. A heat-labile protein of *Chlamydia trachomatis* binds to HeLa cells and inhibits the adherence of chlamydiae. Proc Natl Acad Sci USA 1991; 88:4054–8.
58. Lampe MF, Wilson CB, Bevan MJ, Starnbach MN. Gamma interferon production by cytotoxic T lymphocytes is required for resolution of *Chlamydia trachomatis* infection. Infect Immun 1998; 66:5457–61.
59. Levy NJ, Moulder JW. Attachment of cell walls of *Chlamydia psittaci* to mouse fibroblasts (L cells). Infect Immun 1982; 37:1059–65.
60. Mabey DC, Forsey T, Treharne JD. Serotypes of *Chlamydia trachomatis* in The Gambia [Letter]. Lancet 1987; 2:452.
61. Mabey DC, Holland MJ, Viswalingam ND, et al. Lymphocyte proliferative responses to chlamydial antigens in human chlamydial eye infections. Clin Exp Immunol 1991; 86:37–42.
62. MacCallan AF. The epidemiology of trachoma. Br J Ophthalmol 1931; 15:369–411.
63. Matsumoto A. Structural characteristics of chlamydial bodies. In: Barron AL, ed. Microbiology of Chlamydia. Boca Raton, FL: CRC Press, 1988:21–45.
64. McComb DE, Nichols RL. Antibodies to trachoma in eye secretions of Saudi Arab children. Am J Epidemiol 1969; 90:278–84.
65. Moulder JW. Interaction of chlamydiae and host cells in vitro. Microbiol Rev 1991; 55:143–90.
66. Natividad A, Wilson J, Koch O, et al. Risk of trachomatous scarring and trichiasis in Gambians varies with SNP haplotypes at the interferon-gamma and interleukin-10 loci. Genes Immun 2005; 6:332–40.
67. Peeling RW, Bailey RL, Conway DJ, et al. Antibody response to the 60-kDa chlamydial heat-shock protein is associated with scarring trachoma. J Infect Dis 1998; 177: 256–9.
68. Perry LL, Feilzer K, Hughes S, Caldwell HD. Clearance of *Chlamydia trachomatis* from the murine genital mucosa

does not require perforin-mediated cytolysis or Fas-mediated apoptosis. Infect Immun 1999; 67:1379–85.
69. Polack S, Brooker S, Kuper H, et al. Mapping the global distribution of trachoma. Bull World Health Organ 2005; 83:913–9.
70. Pugh SF, Slack RC, Caul EO, et al. Enzyme amplified immunoassay: a novel technique applied to direct detection of *Chlamydia trachomatis* in clinical specimens. J Clin Pathol 1985; 38:1139–41.
71. Ramsey KH, Rank RG. Resolution of chlamydial genital infection with antigen-specific T-lymphocyte lines. Infect Immun 1991; 59:925–31.
72. Rank RG, Ramsey KH, Pack EA, Williams DM. Effect of gamma interferon on resolution of murine chlamydial genital infection. Infect Immun 1992; 60:4427–9.
73. Rank RG, Soderberg LS, Barron AL. Chronic chlamydial genital infection in congenitally athymic nude mice. Infect Immun 1985; 48:847–9.
74. Rasmussen SJ, Eckmann L, Quayle AJ, et al. Secretion of proinflammatory cytokines by epithelial cells in response to Chlamydia infection suggests a central role for epithelial cells in chlamydial pathogenesis. J Clin Invest 1997; 99:77–87.
75. Raulston JE, Paul TR, Knight ST, Wyrick PB. Localization of *Chlamydia trachomatis* heat shock proteins 60 and 70 during infection of a human endometrial epithelial cell line in vitro. Infect Immun 1998; 66:2323–9.
76. Reacher MH, Pe'er J, Rapoza PA, et al. T cells and trachoma: their role in cicatricial disease. Ophthalmology 1991; 98:334–41.
77. Reynolds DJ, Pearce JH. Characterization of the cytochalasin D-resistant (pinocytic) mechanisms of endocytosis utilized by chlamydiae. Infect Immun 1990; 58:3208–16.
78. Rothburn M, Mallinson H, Mutton K. False-positive ELISA for *Chlamydia trachomatis* recognised by atypical morphology on fluorescent staining. Lancet 1986; 8513: 982–3.
79. Rothermel CD, Schachter J, Lavrich P, et al. *Chlamydia trachomatis*-induced production of interleukin-1 by human monocytes. Infect Immun 1989; 57:2705–11.
80. Rottenberg ME, Gigliotti-Rothfuchs A, Wigzell H. The role of IFN-gamma in the outcome of chlamydial infection. Curr Opin Immunol 2002; 14:444–51.
81. Schachter J, Dawson CR. The epidemiology of trachoma predicts more blindness in the future. Scand J Infect Dis Suppl 1990; 69:55–62.
82. Schachter J, Grossman M, Sweet RL, et al. Prospective study of perinatal transmission of *Chlamydia trachomatis*. JAMA 1986; 255:3374–7.
83. Schachter J, Moncada J, Dawson CR, et al. Nonculture methods for diagnosing chlamydial infection in patients with trachoma: a clue to the pathogenesis of the disease? J Infect Dis 1988; 158:1347–52.
84. Schachter J, Stephens RS, Timms P, et al. Radical changes to chlamydial taxonomy are not necessary just yet (Letter). Int J Syst Evol Microbiol 2001; 51:249.
85. Smith A, Munoz B, Hsieh YH, et al. OmpA genotypic evidence for persistent ocular *Chlamydia trachomatis* infection in Tanzanian village women. Ophthal Epidemiol 2001; 8:127–35.
86. Solomon AW, Holland MJ, Alexander ND, et al. Mass treatment with single-dose azithromycin for trachoma. N Engl J Med 2004; 351:1962–71.
87. Solomon AW, Holland MJ, Burton MJ, et al. Strategies for control of trachoma: observational study with quantitative PCR. Lancet 2003; 362:198–204.
88. Solomon AW, Peeling RW, Foster A, Mabey DC. Diagnosis and assessment of trachoma. Clin Microbiol Rev 2004; 17:982–1011.
89. Stenberg K, Mardh PA. Genital infection with *Chlamydia trachomatis* in patients with chlamydial conjunctivitis: unexplained results. Sex Transm Dis 1991; 18:1–4.
90. Stephens RS. Molecular mimicry and *Chlamydia trachomatis* infection of eukaryotic cells. Trends Microbiol 1994; 2:99–101.
91. Stephens RS, Kalman S, Lammel C, et al. Genome sequence of an obligate intracellular pathogen of humans: *Chlamydia trachomatis*. Science 1998; 282:754–9.
92. Su H, Raymond L, Rockey DD, et al. A recombinant *Chlamydia trachomatis* major outer membrane protein binds to heparan sulfate receptors on epithelial cells. Proc Natl Acad Sci USA 1996; 93:11143–8.
93. Taylor HR, Agarwala N, Johnson SL. Detection of experimental *Chlamydia trachomatis* eye infection in conjunctival smears and in tissue culture by use of fluorescein-conjugated monoclonal antibody. J Clin Microbiol 1984; 20:391–5.
94. Taylor HR, Johnson SL, Prendergast RA, et al. An animal model of trachoma. II. The importance of repeated reinfection. Invest Ophthalmol Vis Sci 1982; 23: 507–15.
95. Taylor HR, Johnson SL, Schachter J, et al. Pathogenesis of trachoma: the stimulus for inflammation. J Immunol 1987; 138:3023–7.
96. Taylor HR, Rapoza PA, West S, et al. The epidemiology of infection in trachoma. Invest Ophthalmol Vis Sci 1989; 30: 1823–33.
97. Thylefors B, Dawson CR, Jones BR, et al. A simple system for the assessment of trachoma and its complications. Bull World Health Organ 1987; 65:477–83.
98. Thylefors B, Negrel AD, Pararajasegaram R, Dadzie KY. Global data on blindness. Bull World Health Organ 1995; 73:115–21.
99. Todd WJ, Caldwell HD. The interaction of *Chlamydia trachomatis* with host cells: ultrastructural studies of the mechanism of release of a biovar II strain from HeLa 229 cells. J Infect Dis 1985; 151:1037–44.
100. Treharne JD. The microbial epidemiology of trachoma. Int Ophthalmol 1988; 12:25–9.
101. Treharne JD, Dwyer RS, Darougar S, et al. Antichlamydial antibody in tears and sera, and serotypes of *Chlamydia trachomatis* isolated from schoolchildren in Southern Tunisia. Br J Ophthalmol 1978; 62: 509–15.
102. Viswalingam ND, Wishart MS, Woodland RM. Adult chlamydial ophthalmia (paratrachoma). Br Med Bull 1983; 39:123–7.
103. Wagar EA, Stephens RS. Developmental-form-specific DNA-binding proteins in *Chlamydia* spp. Infect Immun 1988; 56:1678–84.
104. Ward ME. The immunobiology and immunopathology of chlamydial infections. APMIS 1995; 103:769–96.
105. Ward ME, Salari H. Control mechanisms governing the infectivity of *Chlamydia trachomatis* for HeLa cells: modulation by cyclic nucleotides, prostaglandins and calcium. J Gen Microbiol 1982; 128:639–50.
106. West S, Munoz B, Lynch M, et al. Impact of face-washing on trachoma in Kongwa, Tanzania [see comments]. Lancet 1995; 345:155–8.
107. West SK, Munoz B, Mkocha H, et al. Progression of active trachoma to scarring in a cohort of Tanzanian children. Ophthal Epidemiol 2001; 8:137–44.

108. Williams DM, Grubbs BG, Pack E, et al. Humoral and cellular immunity in secondary infection due to murine *Chlamydia trachomatis*. Infect Immun 1997; 65:2876–82.
109. Wright HR, Taylor HR. Clinical examination and laboratory tests for estimation of trachoma prevalence in a remote setting: what are they really telling us? Lancet Infect Dis 2005; 5:313–20.
110. Wynn TA. Fibrotic disease and the T(H)1/T(H)2 paradigm. Nat Rev Immunol 2004; 4:583–94.

11

Fungal Infections

William Robert Bell
Wilmer Eye Institute, Johns Hopkins University, Baltimore, Maryland, U.S.A.

Terrence P. O'Brien
Bascom Palmer Eye Institute of the Palm Beaches, Palm Beach Gardens, Florida, U.S.A.

W. Richard Green
Wilmer Eye Institute, Johns Hopkins University, Baltimore, Maryland, U.S.A.

INTRODUCTION

General Remarks

The systemic and ocular mycoses of humans are caused by fungi that are pathogenic and incite disease in the healthy host and other opportunistic fungi that produce disease in patients whose immune defenses are impaired. With an expanding population of individuals with acquired immunodeficiencies, fungi play an increasingly common role as causative agents of systemic and ocular infections. The increased detection of fungal infections is partly due to heightened clinical awareness and to improved laboratory diagnostic techniques with better reporting. Other factors cited as partially responsible for an increased involvement of fungi in ocular infections include the widespread use of antibiotics, immunosuppressive therapy, chemotherapeutic agents, and a variety of ocular prosthetic devices, including, contact lenses, punctal occlusive plugs, aqueous humor, shunt tubing, intraocular lenses, and scleral buckling materials.

Nature of Fungi

Fungi are eukaryotic organisms, differing from bacteria in cell wall composition, nuclear structure, ribosome structure, and size. They may be divided into yeasts and molds. They lack chlorophyll, are nonmotile (except for certain spore forms), and may grow as single cells (yeasts) or as long, branched, filamentous structures (mycelia). Virtually all fungi reproduce by forming spores through mitosis.

Cells of fungi pathogenic for humans have a rigid cell wall containing chitin and polysaccharides. This cell wall is readily stained by Gomori-methenamine silver. While the fungus remains viable, the periodic acid Schiff reagent also stains the cell wall. Most fungi, except *Candida*, are too faintly Gram positive to be seen well with the Gram stain.

A polysaccharide capsule around the cell wall is characteristic of the human pathogen *Cryptococcus neoformans*.

Inside the fungal cell wall is the sterol-containing cytoplasmic membrane that is the site of action of polyene macrolide antibiotics, such as amphotericin B and pimaricin (natamycin). Triazole antifungal agents inhibit the demethylation necessary in the formation of ergosterol, the major sterol in the fungal cytoplasmic membrane.

Diagnosis of Fungal Disease

Diagnosis is confirmed unequivocally by culturing the fungus from patient specimens on appropriate media and by specific laboratory methods (208), including the finding of fungi on direct microscopic examination of specially stained tissue sections. Histological features can be more rapidly diagnostic than culture when mycoses. Most pathogenic fungi grow readily within 48 to 72 hours (165), but some may take as long as 7 days to grow and some as long as 2 weeks (205). It is usually recommended that cultures be maintained for a period of no less than 21 days. Most fungal pathogens grow readily on blood agar at 35°C, but Sabouraud agar with gentamicin and without cycloheximide at room temperature is considered the most sensitive medium for the isolation of fungi.

Biopsy may also provide proof that the fungus is invading tissue, not merely a contaminant or saprophyte. Histological examination and culture ideally are performed together. Serological methods formerly received considerable emphasis in diagnosing systemic mycoses. These techniques include antigen detection (cryptococcosis) and antibody detection (coccidioidomycosis) in serum or identification of fungal forms in tissue using fluorescent antibody (histoplasmosis and North American blastomycosis). Widespread use of such methods has been hampered by poor standardization of reagents, cross-reaction with other fungal antigens, and frequent false positive and false negative results.

Skin testing is a useful means of measuring rates of infectivity for geographical and epidemiological studies but is not generally useful in clinical diagnosis of fungal infections. Many healthy inhabitants in an endemic area have a positive skin test (histoplasmosis and coccidiomycoses are examples) but experience no clinical manifestations.

Pathogenesis of Fungal Infections

The pathogenesis of ocular fungal infections varies with the site of involvement. Certain predisposing factors play an important role in most instances. Trauma, especially when plant or vegetable matter is involved, the use of topical antibiotics and corticosteroids, and local corneal diseases are important in initiating mycotic keratitis. Fungi can be recovered from the conjunctival sac in up to 25% of normal persons, and the prevalence increases with local disease and therapy.

Fungi are not known to produce endotoxins. Some exotoxins, such as aflatoxin, may be produced in vitro, but their precise roles in vivo are incompletely understood.

Fungal Infections of Ocular Tissues

Although fungi are less common causes of ocular infection than bacteria and viruses, they are worldwide pathogens in conjunctivitis, keratitis, endophthalmitis, and infections of the eyelids, lacrimal apparatus, and orbit (15,147,275).

Most fungi that cause ocular and orbital infection are ubiquitous. However, some have characteristic geographical distributions. For example, *Coccidioides immitis* is endemic in the southwestern United States, northwestern and central Mexico, Venezuela, and the Gran Chaco Plain of South America. *Blastomyces dermatitidis* (*Ajellomyces dermatitidis*), the causative agent of North American blastomycosis, occurs most frequently in the southeastern United States, but also occurs in other areas of the United States, Canada, and Africa. *Histoplasma capsulatum* (*Emmonsiella capsulata*) is a fungus endemic to the Ohio and Mississippi River valleys and the Appalachian Mountains in the United States. *Histoplasma duboisii* is found in Nigeria.

Exogenous mycotic endophthalmitis may occur with the introduction of organisms following accidental penetrating trauma, usually by a foreign body (especially wood). Intraocular extension of infection from the cornea may occur. Cataract extraction with excessive instrumentation and/or subsequent aspiration into the surgical incision of eyelid flora or flora of the conjunctival sac, a contaminated irrigating solution or a faulty or absent operating room air control system, and a keratoplasty with contaminated donor storage media may also introduce fungi into the eye. Local disease of the eyelid margin, conjunctiva, and lacrimal drainage system is also an important predisposing factor.

Endogenous mycotic endophthalmitis is an infrequent but important complication of systemic mycoses. The most frequently encountered fungus in this type of infection is *Candida*. The many factors that may play a role in the susceptibility to infection include systemic (usually debilitating) diseases, such as the acquired immunodeficiency syndrome (AIDS) (49,58), chemotherapy, antibiotics, immunosuppressive agents, therapy with corticosteroids, intravenous catheterization, and illicit intravenous drug abuse.

The principal orbital fungal infections, phycomycosis and aspergillosis, extend into the orbit from one of the paranasal sinuses. Diabetic acidosis predisposes to phycomycosis, whereas allergic diathesis with nasal polyps and/or deviated nasal septum commonly precedes orbital aspergillosis.

The principal predisposing factor in mycotic infections of the lacrimal drainage apparatus is partial or complete blockage of that system.

This chapter addresses chiefly ocular and periocular fungal infections. For information on systemic fungal infections, the reader is referred to several excellent sources (12,48,74,30,157,160,229,317).

SPECIFIC FUNGAL INFECTIONS

Aspergillosis

Aspergillus is widespread in nature and commonly resides in the nose (215), oropharynx, and paranasal sinuses (177,182,283). Infections of the periocular tissue by this fungus usually occur in persons from 40 to 60 years of age who have an allergic diathesis, deviated nasal septum, and nasal polyps. Aspergillosis also occurs in patients with debilitating disease (Figs. 1–3) (121). A geographical predisposition appears to exist in that the disease occurs more commonly in a hot and humid climate (217).

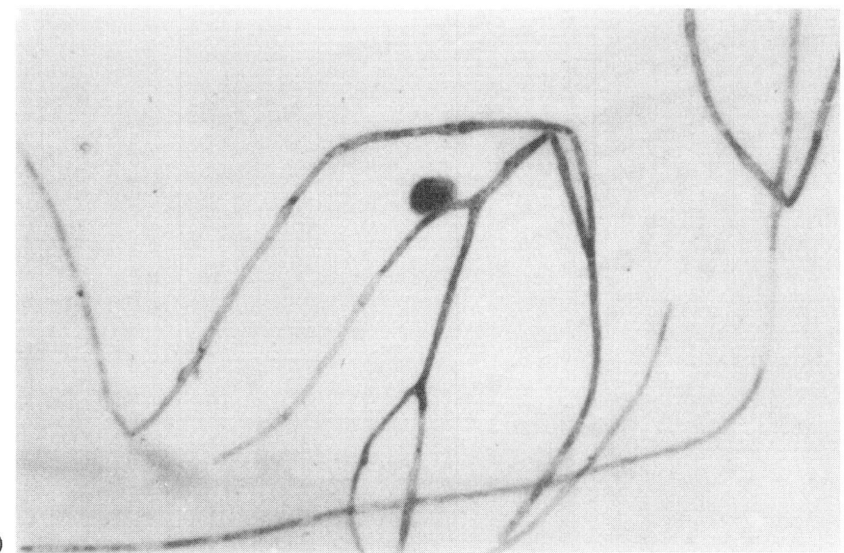

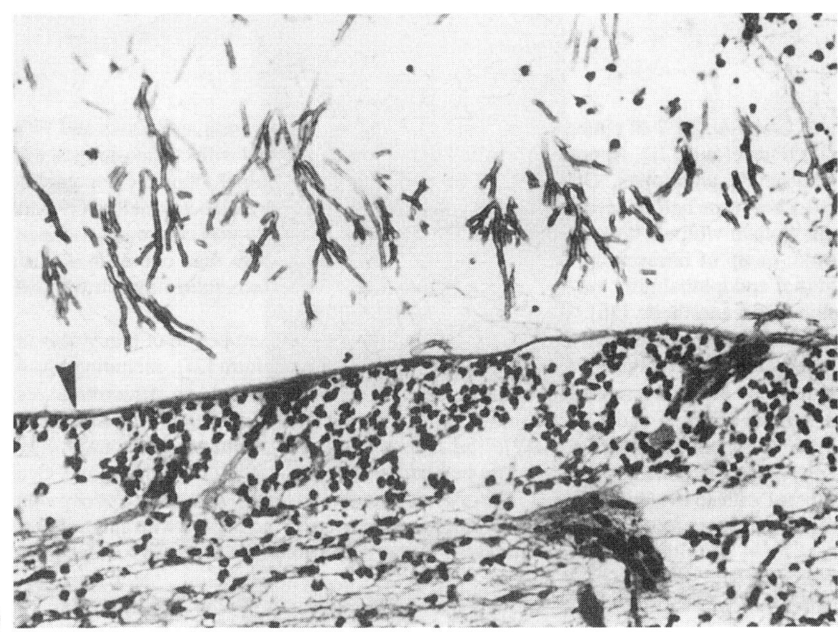

Figure 1 (**A**) Vitreous aspirate, showing branching septated hyphae from an eye with endophthalmitis of a 26-year-old man with known pulmonary aspergillosis who was on immunosuppressive therapy following renal transplantation (periodic acid Schiff, ×442). (**B**) Portion of enucleated eye, showing organisms in the vitreous and an inflammatory infiltrate, including giant cells in the subjacent retina (periodic acid Schiff, ×442). *Source*: Naidoff MA, Green WR. Endogenous *Aspergillus* endophthalmitis occurring after kidney transplant. Am J Ophthalmol 1975; 79:502–9.

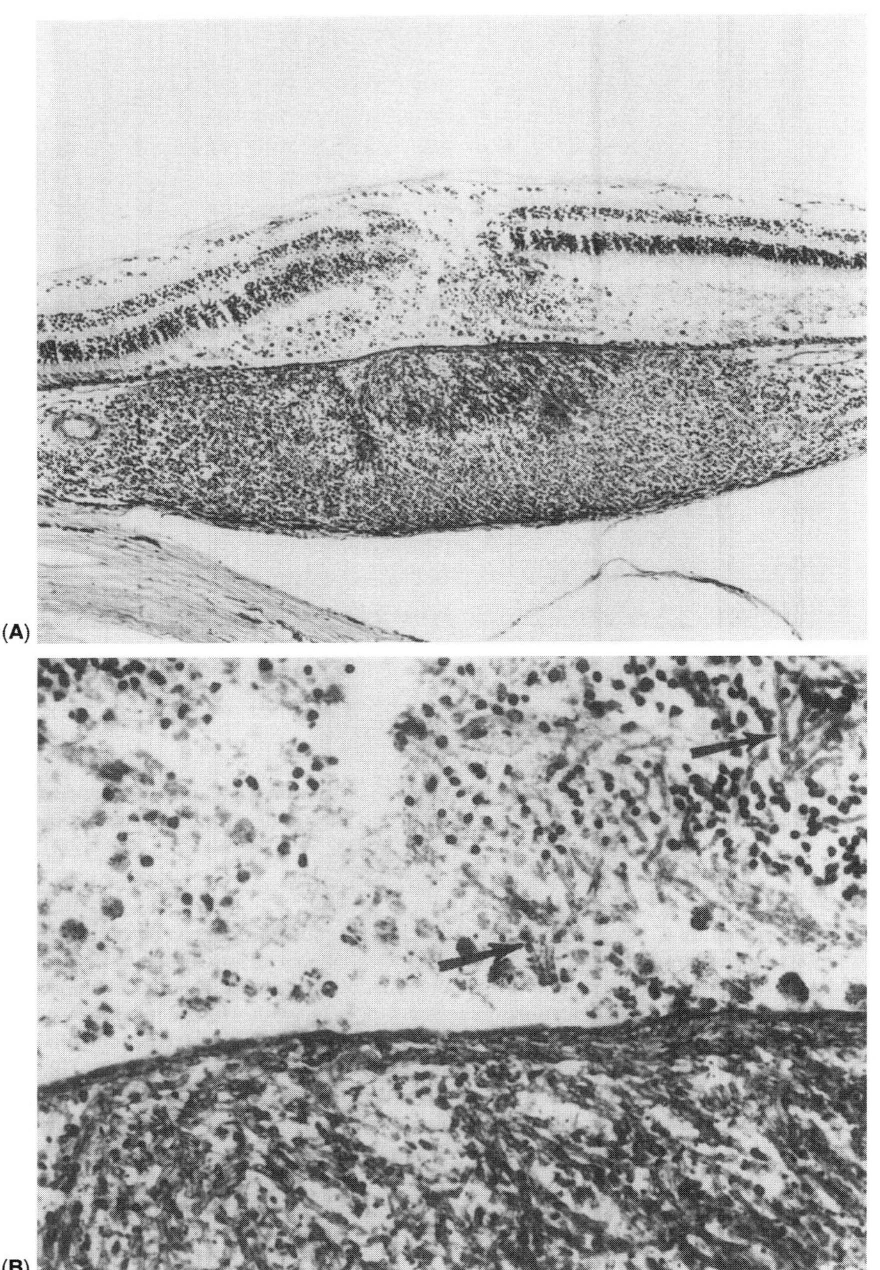

Figure 2 (**A**) Localized *Aspergillus* choroiditis with overlying retinal involvement in a 29-year-old woman on immunosuppressive therapy following renal transplantation (periodic acid Schiff, ×76). (**B**) Higher power, showing numerous organisms in the choroid and some extending into the subretinal space (*arrows*) (periodic acid Schiff, ×476). *Source*: Naidoff MA, Green WR. Endogenous *Aspergillus* endophthalmitis occurring after kidney transplant. Am J Ophthalmol 1975; 79:502–9.

Candidiasis

Because *Candida* is a ubiquitous fungus and common contaminant of culture media, caution and clinical judgment are needed to interpret the significance of positive cultures. The mouth is the most common site of infection (oral thrush), and the disease may be carried to the eyelids and conjunctiva. It primarily affects old, debilitated individuals or young children and may occur as an acute respiratory infection. The clinical diagnosis of candidiasis is also made difficult by the recovery of some patients with candidemia without antifungal agents (71,278). Indirect ophthalmoscopic examination is a useful adjunct to the clinical diagnosis of systemic candidiasis, since the discovery of one or more inflammatory foci in the retina is highly suggestive of candidemia with widespread candidiasis. In a postmortem series of 15 cases with documented ocular lesions, 13 had microabscesses containing *Candida* in at least one other organ, most commonly the kidney or heart (109).

Microscopic examination of the lesions in candidiasis usually discloses yeast forms or pseudomycelial elements in the presence of a suppurative inflammatory response (Figs. 4–7). In the eye, the primary focus is usually found in the inner choroid,

(A) 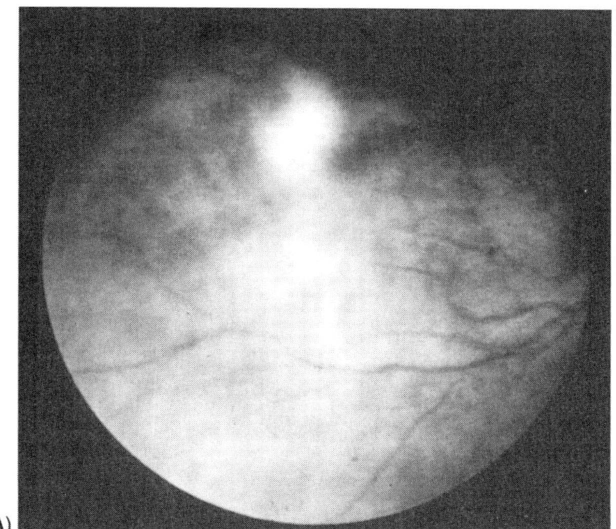

(B) 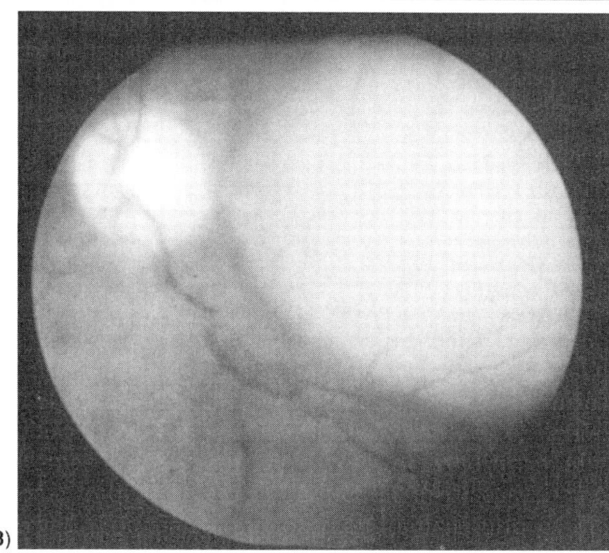

Figure 9 Cryptococcal retinitis of right (**A**) and left (**B**) eyes of a 36-year-old woman with a history of pulmonary tuberculosis, syphilis, and corticosteroid therapy for systemic lupus erythematosus. *Source*: From Ref. 141.

Ocular Histoplasmosis Syndrome

Histoplasmosis is associated with a characteristic syndrome (ocular histoplasmosis syndrome) in which *Histoplasma* organisms are probably first taken up by vascular endothelium in the choroid (243) during a transient fungemia that accompanies the initial pulmonary infection. This is thought to result in an asymptomatic, multifocal, usually bilateral choroiditis that heals spontaneously, leaving round, yellowish, atrophic choroidal scars with a punched-out appearance in the midperiphery of the fundus (Fig. 12) and, to a lesser degree, around the optic disc and macular area (Fig. 13). Typically, the anterior segment and vitreous are uninvolved. A scar in the macular area may become symptomatic 5 to 15 years later because of RPE neovascularization (Fig. 13) and hemorrhage. Disciform macular lesions can occur as late complications at sites of atrophic macular scars (92,239,241, 255,298), and their occurrence without a previous atrophic scar is rare (239,298). These atrophic scars seem to give rise to disciform lesions 10 to 30 years after a presumed initial histoplasmic choroiditis (88). The posterior pole has a predilection for neovascularization beneath the RPE, perhaps because of the high volume and pressure inflow from the short posterior ciliary arteries (91). The reason an old macular lesion becomes symptomatic remains unknown. A smoldering active choroiditis due to *H. capsulatum*, hypersensitivity phenomena, and vascular decompression at the margin of an atrophic choroidal scar have been postulated (92,313). The Macular Photocoagulation Study Group (1) determined that laser photocoagulation of the submacular choroidal neovascularization reduces the incidence of severe visual loss.

In the ocular histoplasmosis syndrome, the incidence of positive histoplasmin skin tests is much higher (93%) than in patients with other ocular varieties of uveitis (25%) (280,313). Positive histoplasmin skin tests were found in 59% of 842 persons in the general population of in Walkersville, Maryland, whereas each of 22 subjects with the ocular histoplasmosis syndrome had positive skin tests (254). It is noteworthy that a high percentage of patients with macular and peripapillary lesions of the ocular histoplasmosis syndrome have the histocompatibility antigen HLA-B27 (27,96,187).

Histopathological studies of eyes obtained postmortem from patients with ocular histoplasmosis syndrome have disclosed a fairly uniform picture (139,186). Asymptomatic mid-peripheral (Fig. 14) macular and peripapillary lesions are characterized by variable amounts of chorioretinal scarring and, in some instances, a mild to moderate lymphocytic infiltrate. Most scars show a discontinuity of Bruch membrane, and the RPE, usually absent centrally in the scar, may show varying degrees of hyperplasia and hypertrophy. Symptomatic macular scars invariably have a break in Bruch membrane, with choroidal neovascularization extending into a disciform lesion (Figs. 13 and 15). Irvine et al. (125) reported a case showing an unusually prominent choroidal inflammatory infiltrate in which indirect immunofluorescent microscopy revealed *Histoplasma* antigens but no organisms were identified.

The pathogenesis of late-onset macular lesions in the ocular histoplasmosis syndrome remains unknown. When Woods and Wahlen (313) first drew attention to the clinical picture, they suggested an immunological mechanism in the pathogenesis of the lesions. Gass (91) postulated that the disciform lesions

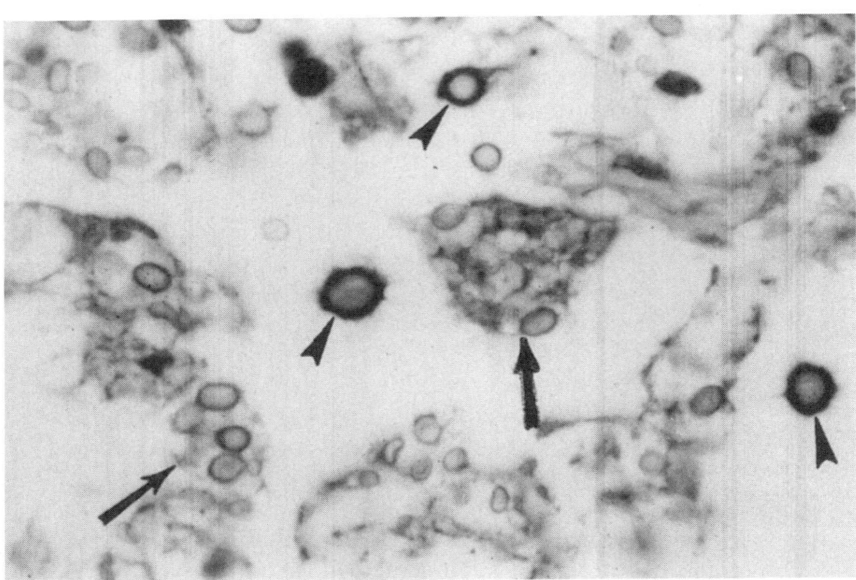

Figure 10 Area of retinitis in an eye with encapsulated and extracellular (*arrowheads*) and proliferative intracellular (*arrows*) cryptococcal organisms. The capsule stains positively for glycosaminoglycans and has a slight stellate configuration (*arrowheads*) (mucicarmine, ×653).

form in the posterior pole because of an inherent vascular instability in this portion of the eye. An active infective choroiditis is possible since the organism may be present for long periods of time (101,140), but organisms have not been cultured from an eye with the syndrome and amphotericin B has had no consistent therapeutic effect (94).

The macular lesion could result from a mechanical or immunological mechanism. Weber and Schlaegel (291) observed alterations in the pattern of skin test reactivity to a variety of antigens in patients with the ocular histoplasmosis syndrome. Lymphocyte transfer studies tend to manifest increased responsiveness of the cellular immune system in patients with macular scarring (87), who have a much higher incidence of peripapillary scarring (88). The macular lesions may bleed shortly after skin sensitivity tests with histoplasmin (151,242); this phenomenon has been observed in as many as 7% of the patients tested (242). Skin testing, a booster of cellular immunity to histoplasmin (89), has been postulated to cause the hemorrhage by immunological mechanisms. Reports document effective therapy for the macular disciform lesions with the immunosuppressive agent imuran (204) or desensitization (174). Edema with visual complaints often precedes occasional bleeding in the macular lesions. However, patients likely to be given the histoplasmin skin test are a select group who are very prone to develop associated hemorrhages in the normal course of the disease.

Choroidal lymphocytes, sensitized to antigens in *H. capsulatum*, are presumed to play an important role in activating the lesions (51,87). A hemorrhagic detachment of the RPE has been postulated to result from a hypersensitivity reaction to an excessive antigenic stimulation, as would occur, for example, after hematogenous dissemination, reinfection by the fungus, or the release of antigens from lesions.

Lymphocytes within the choroidal lesions do not necessarily play an active role in the pathogenesis of the disciform macular scar, especially since they are sometimes observed in AMD (see Chapter 18) and angioid streaks. Indeed, if lymphocytes are important in the genesis of the disciform lesions in the ocular histoplasmosis syndrome, their presence does not explain the predilection of the posterior pole for disciform scarring, since lymphocytes are also observed in some peripheral lesions. With the exception of elderly patients, disciform scarring has not been observed in the midperiphery or peripapillary area in the ocular histoplasmosis syndrome.

However, several other observations are also difficult to explain on a hypersensitivity basis: (*i*) Although bilateral involvement is common in the ocular histoplasmosis syndrome, it rarely presents bilaterally. (*ii*) If skin testing caused a flare in the posterior pole scars, why does it not occur at multiple sites, when numerous scars are present both at the posterior pole and in the midperiphery? (*iii*) A significant percentage of patients with the ocular histoplasmosis syndrome develop hemorrhages in the macular area even without a positive histoplasmin skin test.

Blood vessels invade the space beneath the RPE in a number of diseases, such as AMD, angioid streaks, and "lacquer cracks" in myopia (91). In these conditions, the common denominator appears to be a

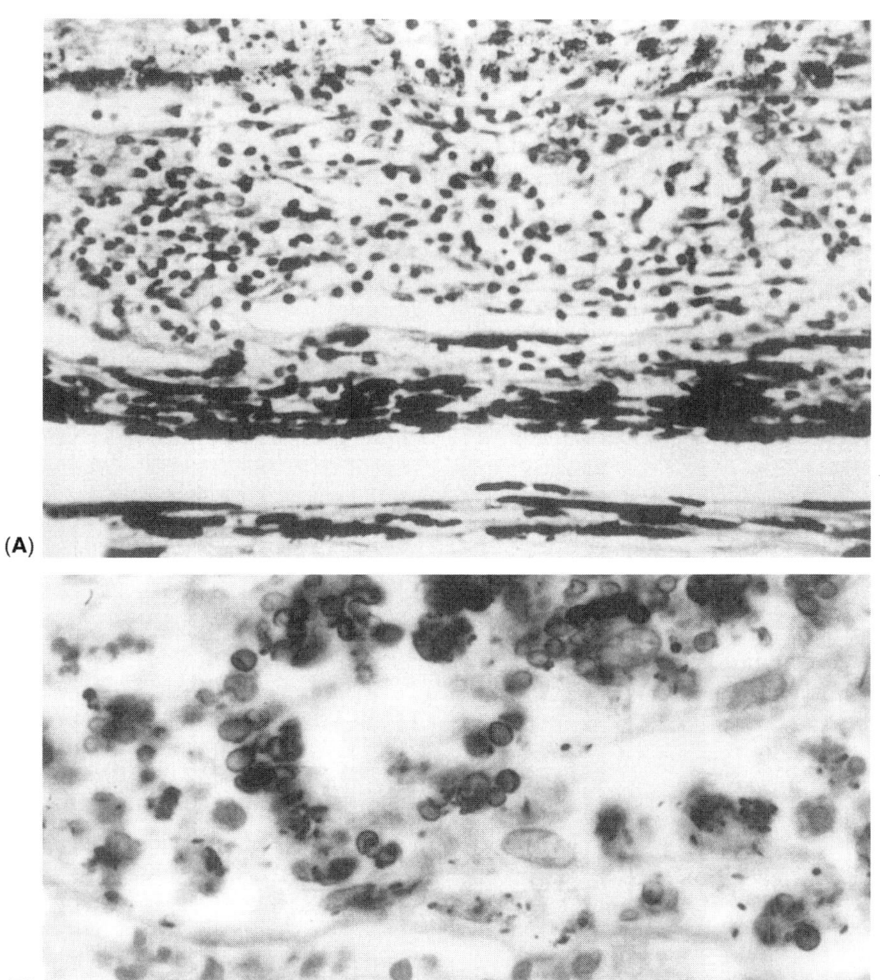

Figure 11 (**A**) Choroidal granuloma due to *Histoplasma capsulatum* in a 14-year-old immunologically deficient boy. There is disruption of the overlying retinal pigment epithelium, and the granuloma extends into the subretinal space (Grocott-Gomori-methanamine silver, ×262). (**B**) Higher power, showing the typical organisms of *Histoplasma capsulatum* (Grocott-Gomori-methanamine silver, ×660). *Source*: From Ref. 146.

breakdown of Bruch membrane, an abnormality documented in the macular, peripapillary, and midperipheral lesions of the ocular histoplasmosis syndrome (139,186). Rarely, persons with the peripapillary and midperipheral lesions of the ocular histoplasmosis syndrome develop macular subretinal neovascularization without prior abnormalities detected by ophthalmoscopy or fluorescein angiography (152,185,298). Although such lesions have been interpreted as indicating an active immunologic process, it is possible that a small pre-existing lesion was not clinically detectable or that the RPE healed, giving a normal ophthalmoscopic appearance.

The resolution of these questions awaits the introduction of a suitable animal model of the disciform macular lesion in histoplasmosis; this has already been accomplished for the peripheral lesions (206,256,310,312). Bilateral, multiple, whitish gray foci of choroiditis have been produced in animals by the intracarotid and intravenous injection of *H. capsulatum* (256,257,310). In the acute lesions organisms are easily demonstrated in the areas of granulomatous choroiditis. Such ocular lesions begin to resolve within 2 to 6 weeks; larger foci of choroiditis evolve into chorioretinal scars. About 6 to 9 weeks after the onset of clinical ocular activity, *H. capsulatum* is no longer demonstrable in sites of previous choroidal lesions. These observations support the hypothesis that the atrophic scars in the ocular histoplasmosis syndrome result from a focal, self-limited infection of the choroid during primary systemic histoplasmosis.

There are other unanswered questions. (*i*) Why does the posterior pole have a predilection for subretinal neovascularization? (*ii*) Why is there a latent period of 10–30 years between the initial exposure to *Histoplasma* and the development of the posterior pole lesions, and does it relate to degenerative changes in Bruch membrane? (*iii*) What, if any, is the role of the lymphocyte? (*iv*) Why are patients

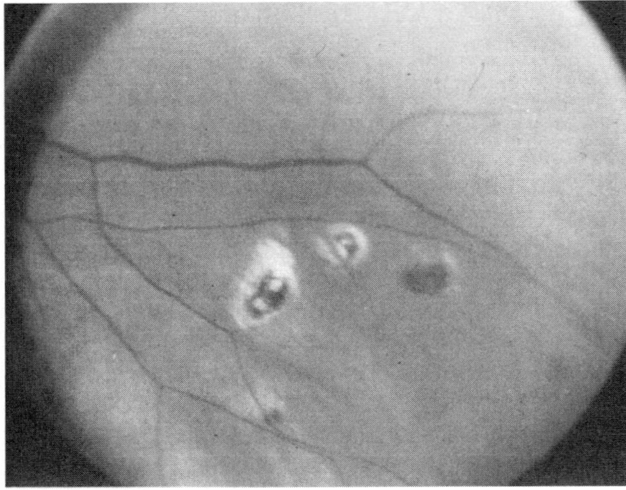

Figure 12 Midperipheral chorioretinal scars, "punched-out" lesions, in a patient with the ocular histoplasmosis syndrome.

with disciform macular lesions immunologically different from those with only peripapillary and peripheral lesions? (*v*) Why do so few patients with systemic histoplasmosis have ocular lesions, and does this relate to their different immunological reactivity? (*vi*) Does residual antigen in choroidal lesions contribute to the pathogenesis of the lesions?

North American Blastomycosis

The portal of entry for *B. dermatitidis* appears to be the lung. Thus, manifestations of disease at other body sites result from dissemination from a primary pulmonary infection, even if not clinically recognized. Intraocular involvement in North American blastomycosis is uncommon but manifests as an anterior uveitis often accompanied by secondary glaucoma (79). Yellow or yellowish white nodules may develop in the iris (40) or posterior fundus (249). Of eight cases of intraocular blastomycosis reported, endophthalmitis was observed in four, iritis or iridocyclitis in two, and choroidal lesions in four (24,79,124,164,240). A mixed acute and chronic granulomatous inflammatory respose is characteristic of North American blastomycosis.

Pneumocystosis

P. carinii is a eukaryotic microorganism that can infect numerous mammalian hosts with a life cycle superficially resembling that of both protozoa and fungi. Comparative analyses of small subunit ribosomal RNA from *P. carinii* have disclosed that this infectious agent is phylogenetically related to fungi (67,217, 265,288,289).

P. carinii pneumonia is a common opportunistic infection in AIDS, accounting for considerable

(A)

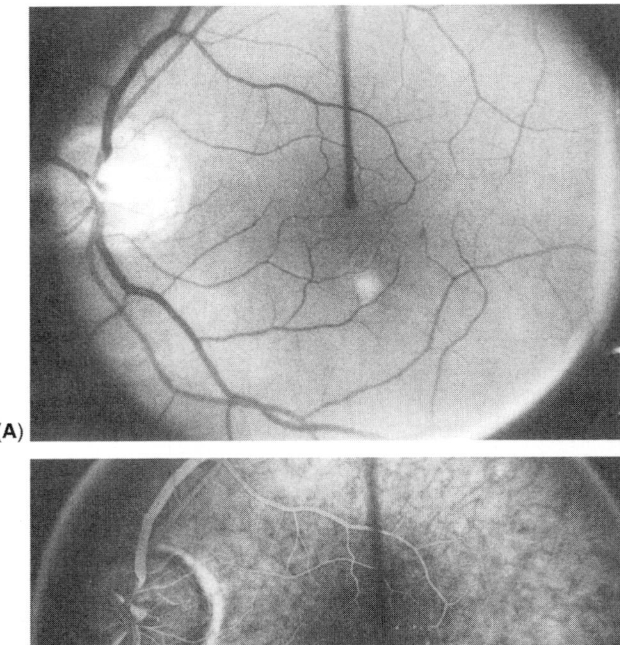

(B)

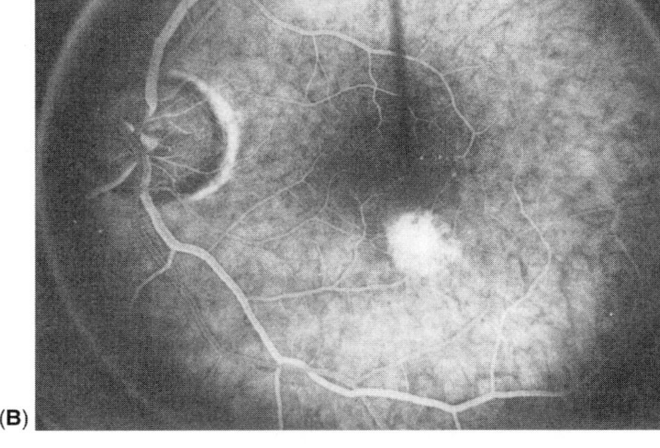

Figure 13 (**A**) Macular and peripapillary scars in the ocular histoplasmosis syndrome. (**B**) Fluorescein angiogram in early venous phase of the macular lesion seen in (**A**). The lesion fluoresces early and stains late.

morbidity and mortality in these and other immunocompromized patients. *P. carinii* causes choroiditis in patients with AIDS (64,82,86,170,221). A case with optic nerve involvement in a patient with acute lymphocytic leukemia has been reported (148). Clinically, the choroidal lesions are pale and oval, with minimal evidence of inflammation, and choroidal pneumocystosis should be suspected in immunocompromised patients with this fundoscopic appearance (86). *Cryptococcus* may produce similar lesions, but these are usually accompanied by an inflammatory reaction in the vitreous. Histopathological studies of the lesions in choroidal pneumocystosis have disclosed many eosinophilic, acellular, vacuolated, and frothy infiltrates within the affected tissue, including the choriocapillaris and other choroidal blood vessels (170,221). The cystic and crescentric organisms are readily demonstrated with Gomori-methenamine silver stain, and the thick-walled cystic organisms and trophozoites can also be identified using TEM (221).

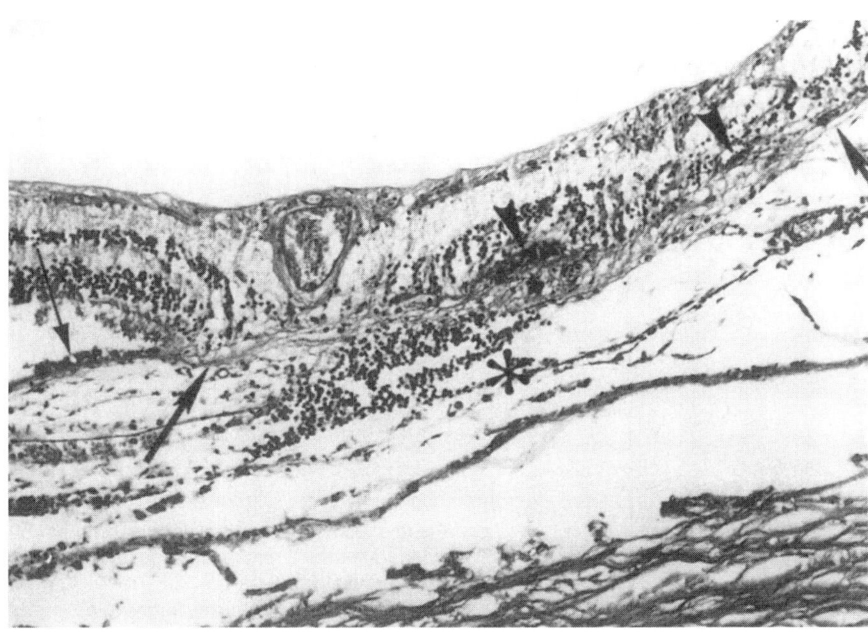

Figure 14 Midperipheral chorioretinal scar in patient with the ocular histoplasmosis syndrome. There is a discontinuity of the Bruch membrane (between *large arrows*) and loss of retinal pigment epithelium, except in two areas (*arrowheads*). The retinal pigment epithelium at the margin of the lesions is hypertrophic (*small arrow*). A small focus of lymphocytes is present in the subjacent choroid (*asterisk*). No choroidal neovascularization is present (periodic acid Schiff, ×130).

Rhinopsporidiosis

Rhinosporidiosis, a disease caused by *Rhinosporidium seeberi,* most often affects the nasal mucosa but may involve the conjunctiva (7,9,108). The conjunctival lesion was first described in India by Elliot and Ingram (70), and other reports quickly followed from that country (65,127,143,156,198,214,222,248,269). Elles (69) reviewed 22 cases of conjunctival rhinosporidiosis as well as three in which the lacrimal sac was affected. Conjunctival infection is relatively uncommon. The incidence of rhinosporidiosis in the ocular adnexa was reported by Kuriakose (154) in India as affecting the conjunctiva in 64%, the lacrimal sac in 24%, the canaliculi in 4%, the eyelids in 4%, and the sclera in 4%. The lesion is characterized by a polypoid or flattened mass that appears pinkish red, solid, and irregularly lobulated, sometimes protruding between the eyelids, preventing their closure. The mode of

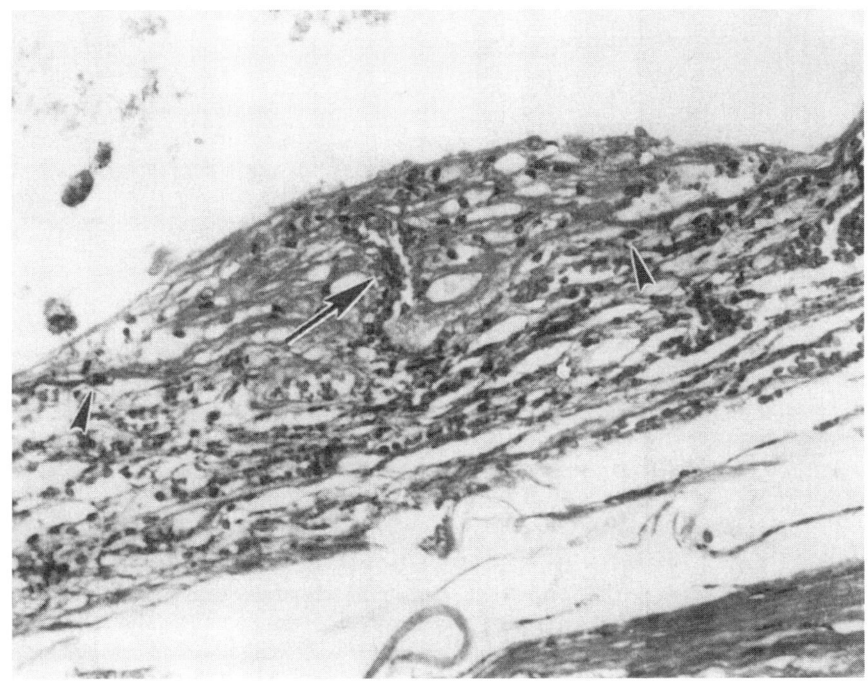

Figure 15 Small chorioretinal scar with choroidal neovascularization in the macular area of the eye illustrated in Figure 14. The *arrow* marks a vessel extending from the scar within the choroid through a break in Bruch membrane (between *arrowheads*) to the scar internal to the choroid (Van de Grift, ×233).

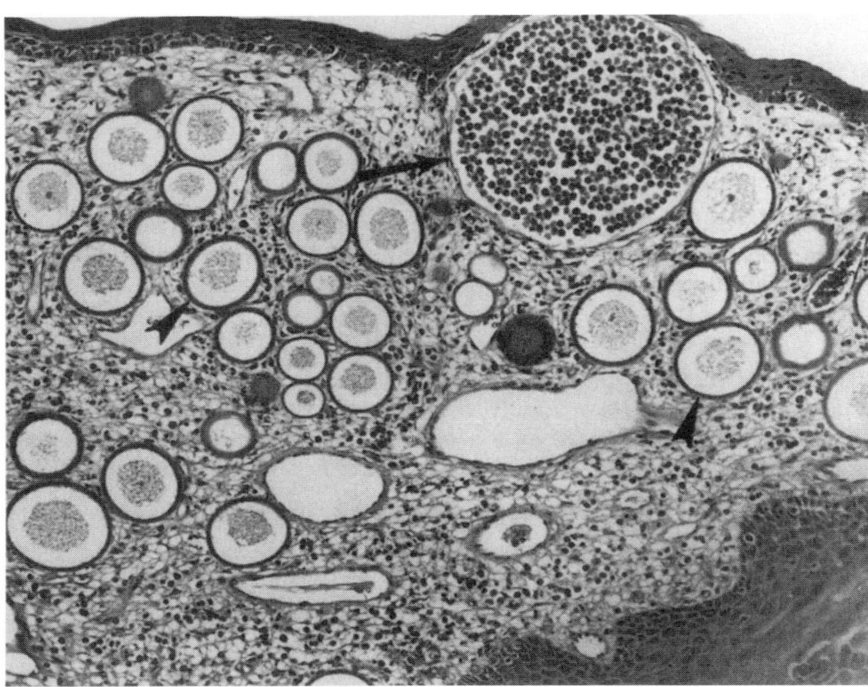

Figure 16 Conjunctival lesion due to rhinosporidiosis. There are numerous sporangia in various stages of development (*arrowheads*). A mature sporangium near the surface (*arrow*) has many spores (periodic acid Schiff, ×131). *Source*: Courtesy of Dr. Frank Winter.

infection is uncertain, but transmission by dust or water into a previously traumatized area seems probable. Transmission through handling of infected horses, cattle, pets, and other animals has also been suggested (7). The lesions of rhinosporidiosis contain numerous sporangia in various stages of development (Fig. 16). Mature sporangia near the surface have many spores (Fig. 17). Vukovic et al. (286) reported an outbreak of rhinospiridiosis associated with Silver Lake, a stagnant man-made body of water in eastern Serbia.

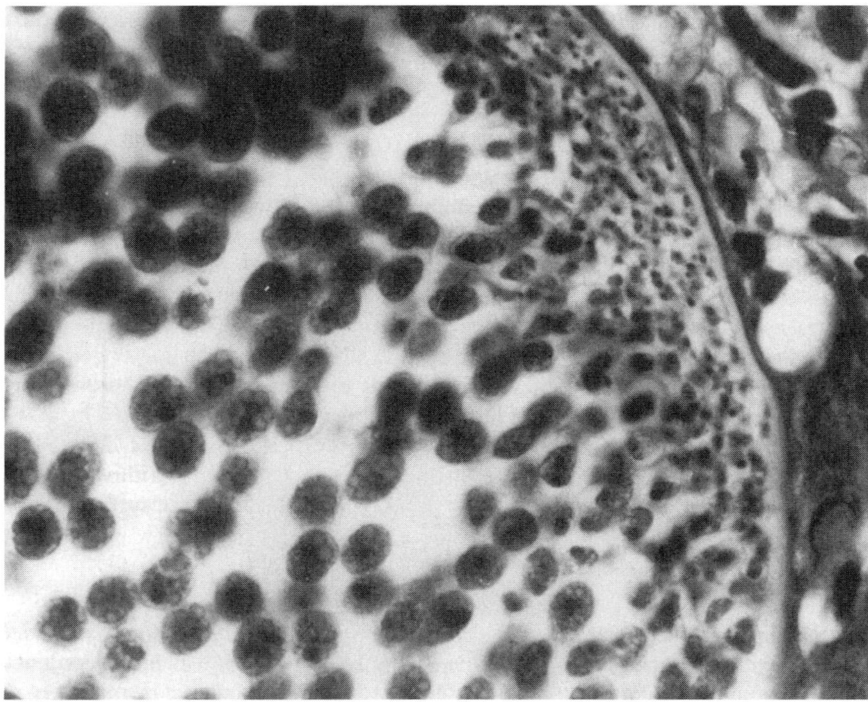

Figure 17 Rhinosporidiosis mature sporangium with mature spores developing from the germinative area in the periphery (periodic acid Schiff, ×1,213).

Sporotrichosis

Sporothrix schenckii, a saprophyte found on plants, green vegetables, and grass, enters the body at a site of injury and rarely causes systemic disease. After inoculation of the organism, a small nodule, which often ulcerates, develops at the site of injury, usually in the subcutaneous tissue. New nodules typically form along the draining lymphatic channels. Hematogenous seeding to extracutaneous sites is rare. Wilson et al. (301) observed ocular involvement in 5 (17%) of 30 patients with cutaneous sporotrichosis. Ocular sporotrichosis has generally been a localized infection, not the result of hematogenous spread.

Very rarely, *S. schenckii* lodges in the eyes of persons lacking overt lesions elsewhere but is perhaps the result of hematogenous dissemination from a small asymptomatic pulmonary infection (169). Anterior uveitis is the most common presenting sign in intraocular sporotrichosis (28). The organisms have a typical small cigar-shaped configuration in tissue sections (Fig. 18). The tissue response may be composed of typical granulomas with multinucleated giant cells and epithelioid cells or a suppurative granulomatous reaction with clusters of neutrophils. Fungi may be surrounded by a large, periodic acid Schiff–staining body, forming the so-called asteroid. Diagnosis is best accomplished by culture of the infected tissue. Cultures of blood or urine are rarely positive.

Zygomycosis

The Zygomycetes (Phycomycetes) are ubiquitous in soil and vegetable matter and, although ordinarily nonpathogenic, cause disease under certain conditions. The airborne spores of the organisms usually gain entry into the body through the respiratory tract, particularly the nose and paranasal sinuses, where the fungus proliferates, penetrates blood vessels, and spreads by vascular and direct extension to the orbit (Fig. 19) (263,226). The organisms proliferate within the blood vessels, producing a thrombosing vasculitis and thus infarction of the surrounding tissue (90). Several Zygomycetes, most commonly *Rhizopus*, cause the clinical syndrome of cerebrorhinoorbital phycomycosis. There is no age, sex, or geographical predilection in phycomycosis, and it is a lethal disease in the absence of treatment.

In adults, the infection occurs primarily in patients with diabetic ketoacidosis (90). Although about 50% of patients with zygomycosis are known to be diabetic, the infection can occur in patients with mild or unrecognized diabetes mellitus (14) and occasionally in healthy persons (314). Also, alcoholic cirrhosis, ulcerative colitis, multiple myeloma, lymphomas, carcinoma, extensive burns and deferoxamine therapy (50) have been associated with zygomycosis. Therapy with antimetabolites, corticosteroids and immunosuppression in bone marrow transplant patients (197) may predispose to infection with the Zygomycetes.

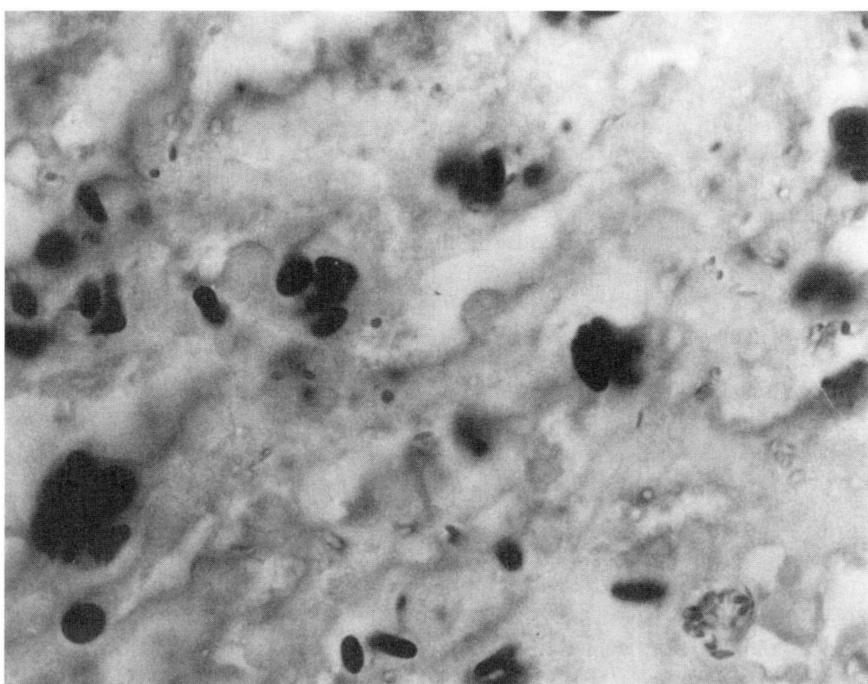

Figure 18 Small cigar-shaped organisms in the vitreous of a patient with endogenous sporotrichosis endophthalmitis (periodic acid Schiff, ×1,522).

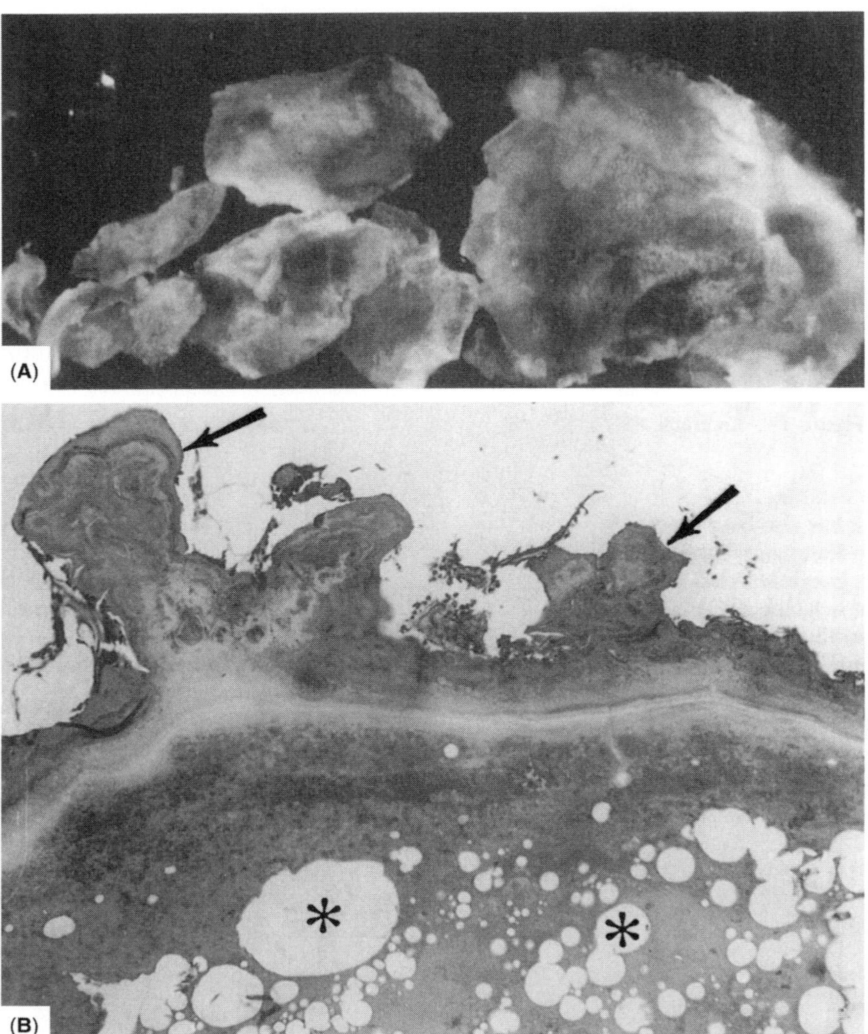

Figure 19 (**A**) Gross appearance of dacryoliths from the lacrimal sac of a 37-year-old with a history of recurrent dacryocystitis. (**B**) Dacryolith, showing an outer zone of lamination, central empty spaces (*asterisks*) from dissolved lipid, and irregular projections (*arrows*), which presumably represent sites of minor diverticula of the lacrimal sac.

In children, the infection is often a sequel to severe diarrhea with dehydration and metabolic acidosis (111), but it has also been reported in an otherwise healthy child (21). The fungus in some of these cases may be a species of Entomophthorales, not a member of the Phycomycetes.

Dark, gangrenous lesions occur in the periorbital skin, nasal mucosa, or palate. These characteristic areas of ischemic necrosis are virtually pathognomonic of cerebrorhinoorbital phycomycosis. The nasal septum, turbinates, and palate may undergo necrosis and perforate, and within the orbit the extraocular muscles may become infarcted. The fungal elements can invade the globe, and thrombosis of the ophthalmic and/or central retinal artery may result in extensive infarction of intraocular structures. Orbital cellulitis, sometimes with involvement of the optic nerve and the nerves that pass through the sphenoidal fissure (orbital apex syndrome) (116), commonly accompanies an associated, and usually fatal, cerebral involvement. Rare intraocular involvement has been noted (260).

In zygomycosis the organisms are located deep in the lesions, necessitating diagnosis by histological examination of excised tissue or scrapings from necrotic areas. In tissue sections, 30–50 μm wide nonseptate branching hyphae are found. A unique feature of this class of fungi, is their affinity for hematoxylin, which enables them to be easily identified in hematoxylin and eosin–stained tissue sections. The predominant lesion is infarcted tissue with a minimal cellular response to the fungi. Rarely, a granulomatous response is present at the sites of thrombosis and in surrounding necrotic tissue. A comprehensive review of ocular and orbital phycomycosis has been written by Schwartz and colleagues (245).

FUNGAL INFECTIONS IN SPECIFIC SITES

Conjunctivitis

Conjunctivitis is common but is infrequently caused by fungi (179). Mycotic conjunctivitis is rare and is pleomorphic in character. The lesions may be superficial or deep and granulomatous. Many species of fungi can be isolated from the conjunctival sac of a normal eye, most being usual inhabitants of soil and vegetable matter (202,302). The recovery rate of fungi from healthy eyes is variable and depends in part on geographical location. With increasing age, fungi can be isolated from healthy eyes with greater frequency (300), Younger individuals up to 30 years of age residing in rural agricultural areas are the most affected, possibly due to exposure from bathing in stagnant water or working in rice fields (275).

The use of topical antibiotics and corticosteroids increases the number of fungi isolated from healthy eyes. There is some evidence that after use of these drugs, nonpathogenic forms may assume pathogenic characteristics. Moreover, many may be saprophytic in the conjunctival sac, but when inadvertently introduced into the eye during ocular surgery or with trauma, become virulent pathogens (112). The predominant fungal genera isolated after use of topical antibiotics and corticosteroids are *Aspergillus*, *Candida*, and *Penicillium* (190).

Other rare fungal infections of the conjunctiva are aspergillosis, histoplasmosis, rhinosporidiosis, and sporotrichosis (106). Sporotrichosis of the conjunctiva is rare, but was first described by Debeurmann and Gougerot (55) in a patient with severe systemic involvement. After incubation from 11 to 17 days, small, yellow, soft nodules appear on the conjunctiva and eventually ulcerate, with associated purulent discharge. Schubach et al. (244) observed conjunctival sporotrichosis in two women. Rarely, intraocular complications and perforation of the sclera have been reported (42,274).

Knox et al. (149) observed a solitary granuloma in the conjunctiva due to *Histoplasma* in a 76-year-old female with no systemic disease.

Aspergillus is also a rare cause of conjunctival infection (25). Sehgal et al. (247) recovered *Aspergillus* sp. in 80 (16%) of 500 conjunctival swabs of normal individuals. *Aspergillus niger* was found in a case reported by Donahue (59), in whom a brownish black swelling involved the inferior canaliculus and conjunctiva. *Aspergillus* corneal infections and orbital infections are more common.

North American Blastomycosis

Blastomycosis due to the yeast-like fungus *B. dermatitidis* as a primary infection of the conjunctiva is rare. Conjunctival infection by this fungus is usually secondary to a primary lesion of the skin of the face and eyelids (252). An ulcerative lesion surrounded by a granulomatous reaction may appear in the conjunctival fornix. The bulbar conjunctiva is rarely affected, in which case the lesions are more superficial, resembling Bitot spots (128,273).

Coccidioidomycosis

Coccidioidomycosis may involve the conjunctiva in some 4% of systemic cases (173,251,253,299). The usual lesions are primarily cutaneous, including the eyelids, and affect the pulmonary system. Coccidioidal infection may resemble phlyctenular conjunctivitis.

Candidiasis

Infection of the conjunctiva by *Candida* sp. is relatively rare. Conjunctival and corneal involvement by *Candida* may be seen in patients who are anergic in delayed hypersensitivity reactions (309) and in the autoimmune, polyendocrinopathy, candidiasis, and ectodermal dystrophy syndrome (APECED) (MIM #240300) (2). The yeast organism may elaborate a heat-stable toxin capable of producing a follicular conjunctivitis (113). Conjunctival candidiasis with scarring and keloid formation has followed strabismus surgery (66).

Keratitis

More than 35 genera of fungi have been associated with corneal infection (56,134) throughout the world (276). Previously considered rare, fungal keratitis has increased in incidence and is usually caused by saprophytic organisms in the setting of trauma (99,262,276,309), ocular surgery (276), and altered host resistance at all ages, including children (213). Surgical procedures (276) include radial keratotomy (RK) (117,178,277); laser assisted in situ keratomileusis (LASIK) (223,230,261), and lamellar keratoplasty (212). The causative agents of mycotic keratitis vary remarkably with geographical locale. *Candida*, *Fusarium*, *Cephalosporium*, and *Aspergillus* are the most common genera in the United States and also vary in incidence within geographical areas (62,135,136,267). Rarely keratitis has been attributed to *Beauveria* sp. (144) and *Absidia corymbifea* (176). In a large series of suspected infectious keratitis from south Florida, fungi were recovered from 35% of patients from corneal scrapings (165,176). *Fusarium solani* was isolated in 57% of cases, nonpigmented fungi in 21%, pigmented fungi in 15%, and yeasts in 10%. In contrast, from a large series from New York City, fungi were recovered from only 1% of cases of suspected microbial keratitis and were principally *Candida* sp. with infrequent examples of *Fusarium* and 1 isolate of *Cryptococcus* (10). In a series of 19 cases from a 10 year period in Minnesota, *Candida* sp. were isolated in six, *Aspergillus* in six, *Alternaria* in four, and *Fusarium* in three (62). The relative infrequency of filamentous organisms as causative agents in fungal keratitis in northern latitudes probably relates to a lack of exposure in outdoor trauma. *Fusarium* sp. are ubiquitous in air, soil, and organic waste, the major fungal corneal pathogen in the southern United States (136,235). *F. solani* is the single most common isolate and has been reported throughout the world (161). *F. solani* produces several complex toxins and destructive enzymes that may result in severe, suppurative keratitis. An epidemic spanning 33 U.S. states and one U.S. territory of *Fusarium* sp. keratitis was reported with 164 confirmed cases from June 1, 2005 to June 30, 2006 and was associated with the use of a specific contact lens solution (44).

Aspergillus also produces various toxins and it may be the most common cause of fungal keratitis worldwide (131).

Corneal ulceration may also be caused by the action of proteolytic enzymes from *Cephalosporium* sp. This fungus is one of several pathogens causing suppurative skin lesions. *Cephalosporium* has been implicated in cases of postsurgical fungal endophthalmitis.

In one study *Curvularia* was the third most prevalent filamentous fungus among corneal isolates and the most common dematiaceous mold (296). One case of blastomycotic keratitis has been reported (233).

Candida is a ubiquitous yeast not directly linked to environmental factors for ocular infections, unlike the filamentous fungi. It is an extreme opportunist, causing keratitis in eyes with predisposing alterations in host defenses, including keratitis sicca, exposure keratitis, keratoplasty, viral keratitis, and chronic corticosteroid usage (193). Trauma or environmental and agricultural exposures are not necessary factors in the pathogenesis of candidal keratitis. *Candida* is the most common ocular fungal pathogen, also causing diseases of the eyelids, conjunctiva, lacrimal drainage system, and retina (277).

Filamentous organisms usually infect normal eyes of healthy individuals who have sustained mild abrasions to the corneal epithelium, typically with plant or vegetable matter. No other predisposing ocular or systemic immunological diseases or exogenous immunosuppressive therapy is required to establish filamentous fungal infections. In contrast, *Candida* and other yeasts cause opportunistic keratitis in the compromised corneas of immunologically incompetent individuals.

Pathogenesis of Fungal Keratitis

Multiple factors are involved in the pathogenesis of the tissue reaction in fungal infections including replicating and nonreplicating organisms, mycotoxins, proteolytic enzymes, and soluble fungal antigens. Although many mycotoxins have been isolated from numerous fungi and yeasts, their precise role in corneal disease has not been fully elucidated (304). The severity of fungal keratitis varies with the destructive potential of specific fungi. *Fusarium* causes a rapidly destructive keratitis; the less virulent *Cephalosporium*, *Allescheria*, *Aspergillus*, *Penicillium*, and *Phialophora* cause a more indolent keratitis. *Fusarium* has the ability to replicate at 35°C and releases a potent mycotoxin. The large hyphae escape phagocytic ingestion by polymorphonuclear leukocytes (PMNs). *Fusarium* may penetrate the stromal lamellae, as well as extend through Descemet membrane into the anterior chamber. A study of mycotic keratitis in 167 corneal buttons reported identifying risk factors for perforation were fungal load, depth of infiltration, and *Fusarium* species (282).

The adverse effects of *Candida* and other yeasts may result from release of a proteolytic enzyme causing lysis of host cells (122). Yeasts may also transform from blastospores to pseudohyphae and prevent effective phagocytosis by PMNs.

The use of topical corticosteroids or other immunosuppressive agents potentiates the invasive properties and virulence of fungi.

The salient clinical features of fungal keratitis are well described (135). The corneal surface typically appears gray or dirty white, with a dry, rough texture. Although such an appearance in the cornea is highly suggestive of a fungal infection, the specific pathogen cannot be predicted. The margins are delicately irregular, with feathery extensions beneath the intact epithelium into adjacent stroma. Focal areas of stromal infiltration or "satellite lesions" may exist apart from the central area corresponding to microabscesses. A crystalline pattern has been observed in a patient with *Candida guilliermondii* (3,297).

Additional clinical features of fungal keratitis include conjunctival hyperemia, endothelial plaque formation (138) with deposition of fibrinous material, and PMNs that may accumulate into hypopyon (Fig. 4). The inflammatory reaction within the cornea may be less marked than in bacterial keratitis. Fungi tend to invade the corneal stroma (Fig. 4) and sometimes align parallel to the lamellae of the collagen (201). The infection may produce extensive necrosis of the infected tissue, as with certain strains of *Fusarium* (63) and *Cephalosporium* (35), as a result of the elaboration of proteolytic enzymes. The ability of hyphae to penetrate the deeper layers of the corneal stroma accounts for the frequent failure of lamellar keratectomy in the treatment of fungal keratitis.

Less commonly, an immune ring may be the principal clinical feature and mimic *Herpes simplex* keratitis (80) or *Acanthamoeba* keratitis. Yeast keratitis, typically occurring in the setting of a compromised cornea, more closely resembles bacterial keratitis. In chronic cases there may be considerable necrosis with suppurative stromal inflammation and features indistinguishable from those of bacterial keratitis.

Superficial diagnostic corneal scrapings may fail to disclose organisms on microscopic examination in advanced fungal keratitis because hyphae are often absent in the superficial stroma. In deep fungal keratitis, a superficial keratectomy with deep corneal biopsy may be necessary to obtain diagnostic material (162,218). If neither scrapings nor keratectomy reveals the causative organisms, anterior chamber paracentesis for diagnostic smear and fungal culture have been suggested for deep mycotic keratitis (132,133). Gram and Giemsa stains may be ineffective in revealing fungal elements on diagnostic corneal scrapings. In addition to the periodic acid Schiff stain and the more specific Gomori-methenamine silver stain, fluorescent dyes (calcofluor white and acridine orange) and an ink-potassium hydroxide preparation may be effective in distinguishing fungal elements on corneal smears (8).

Fungal culture with specific media should be performed in all cases of suspected mycotic keratitis.

Scleritis

Fungal scleritis is infrequent and typically associated with trauma by vegetable matter or with surgery. In most cases of mycotic scleritis, the onset of symptoms occurs approximately two months after the initial traumatic event (290). A review of 426 pathological specimens of scleral disorders included 28 (6.5%) that were attributed to infectious causes and five were attributed to fungi (290).

Reported fungal infections affecting the sclera include *Aspergillus* sp., *Fusarium*, *Rhizopus* sp. *Sporothrix*, *Acremonium*, *Ovadendron*, *Pseudallescheria*, and *Scedosporium prolificans* (234).

Fungal scleritis has been observed following various ocular surgical procedures including cataract extraction (19,37,167), pterygium excision (175,195,268), and after trabeculectomy (19).

Intraocular Fungal Infections

Saprophytic fungi can cause endophthalmitis in a susceptible host, and about 20 different genera have been isolated from different cases of intraocular mycoses (66,137). Fungal endophthalmitis may originate from exogenous sources, such as extension of a fungal keratitis through Descemet membrane, or from surgical or nonsurgical trauma (58) that penetrates the globe and carries fungal elements into the eye. Fungi may also spread into the globe from local lesions or via a hematogenous route from distant sites. In individuals addicted to drugs, fungal endophthalmitis may follow intravenous injections with contaminated needles (142,266). Immunosuppresion from AIDS and other diseases predispose to fungal endophthalmitis. Studies of patients with AIDS have disclosed an infectious choroiditis due to a diverse group of microrgamisms including fungi, such as *Cryptococcus neoformans*, *Pneumocystis carini*, *Mycobacterium tuberculosis*, *Histoplasma capsulatum*, *Candida*, and *Aspergillus fumigatus* (126,181,196).

The main clinical difference between exogenously derived bacterial and fungal endophthalmitis is the time of onset of symptoms and signs, which are typically delayed when fungi are the causal agent. After intraocular surgery, a lapse of several weeks may precede the onset of ocular pain and hyperemia. Slit-lamp biomicroscopy may disclose a localized gray-white area in the vitreous. A transient hypopyon and additional satellite lesions may occur in the anterior vitreous. Rarely, the infection begins in the anterior chamber, usually near the chamber angle.

Since in cases of fungal endophthalmitis following intraocular surgery the anterior vitreous and other adjacent anterior segment structures are usually involved first, the posterior vitreous and retina are spared until later in the course of the infection. Patients may therefore maintain good light projection (70,270), a clinical sign of a reasonably intact functioning retina. Light projection may be preserved for a remarkably long period after the inflammatory process appears in the anterior segment and is a useful clinical feature in distinguishing fungal from bacterial endophthalmitis. The latter tends to be more rapidly progressive and destructive, involving posterior vitreous and retina at an early stage.

The incidence of postsurgical fungal endophthalmitis is very low. One series of 36,000 cataract extractions included only two cases (6). Fungal endophthalmitis may follow other surgical procedures (166), including intraocular lens implantation (199,207), penetrating keratoplasty (3,17,297), glaucoma filtering procedures (164), and retinal reattachment surgery (159,192). Approximately 20 different species of fungi have been cultured from eyes with postsurgical mycotic endophthalmitis (271), These include *Volutella* sp. (80), *Neurospora sitophilia* (272), *Monosporium apiospermum* (95), *Candida parakrusei* (236), and *Cephalosporium* sp. (103), *Exophilia* (17), and others (81,180).

With endogenous fungal endophthalmitis, the ocular involvement may be the first or only clinical manifestation. In such cases, reduced vision is the usual initial symptom, at which time only a slight preretinal vitreous haze may be detected on ocular examination. Within a few days, fluffy white balls accumulate in the vitreous adjacent to the retina. The degree of inflammation varies from a localized abscess to involvement of all intraocular structures. Chorio- or vitreoretinal scarring severely reduces vision and may necessitate enucleation of the eye.

In eyes with fungal endophthalmitis, vitreous (93,258) and/or anterior chamber aspiration (231) is useful for obtaining material for diagnostic staining and culture.

Aspergillosis

At least 37 patients with endophthalmitis due to *Aspergillus* have been reported (28,294), and most of these were associated with underlying systemic debilitating conditions. Antibiotics, corticosteroids, and immunosuppressive therapy, alone or in combination, are frequently used before the onset of septicemia. The onset of endophthalmitis due to *Aspergillus* is accompanied by blurred vision, conjunctival hyperemia, and ocular pain. The most common ocular presenting signs are iridocyclitis or vitritis with associated yellow-white retinal or choroidal lesions (Figs. 3 and 5). Scleritis, hypopyon, retinal hemorrhages, and panoph-thalmitis occur in some cases. Because endophthalmitides due to *Aspergillus*, and other fungi are indistinguishable (62), the diagnosis cannot be made solely by light microscopy and the pathogen requires identification by culture.

Candidiasis

Candida albicans is the most frequently reported cause of endogenous fungal endophthalmitis (23,68,77,109, 184,189,191,220,279,293), and intraocular infection by this organism has increased impressively over the past four decades, partly accounted for by increased clinical suspicion and improved culture techniques. Whereas 26 cases of intraocular candidiasis were documented from 1943 to 1969, 74 examples were reported from 1970 to 1975 (28).

Candida is a common saprophyte of the gastrointestinal tract, and the fungus can gain access to the body from this site when certain factors permit it to become pathogenic. These include gastrointestinal trauma and surgery (231) and underlying diseases treated with antibiotics and corticosteroids (231). Indwelling venous catheters (103,191) and hyperalimentation lines (54), as well as diabetes mellitus, malignancy, and other debilitating conditions (20), also predispose to candidiasis. In a review of 100 cases of endophthalmitis due to *Candida*, 85% of patients previously received broad-spectrum antibiotics and 17% received systemic corticosteroids (28). Approximately half of the patients treated with corticosteroids were concurrently on systemic antibiotics. Other associations included abdominal, thoracic, or cardiac surgery performed a short time before development of candidiasis (53 patients), diabetes mellitus (nine patients), and chronic alcoholism with cirrhosis (six patients). In this series, *Candida* was commonly isolated from the blood, urine, or tip of intravenous catheters and sometimes from more than one of these sites. *Candida* chorioretinitis was observed in 9% of patients with candidemia in a prospective multicenter study (60). Candidal endophthalmitis may occur in otherwise healthy persons following an intravenous injection of a contaminated anesthetic (36).

The ocular symptoms generally become manifest following a latent period of many days (average 18 days) after the diagnosis of systemic candidiasis is established by culture (28), and include blurred vision, pain, and redness of the eyes. Fluffy yellow-white retinal, chorioretinal, or vitreoretinal lesions with indistinct borders (Figs. 5–7) are usually seen, with small foci of retinal involvement sometimes simulating cotton-wool spots (105,123,287). The lesions are usually bilateral, and a hazy vitreous often overlies small retinal hemorrhages, which may be surrounded by a white halo (Roth spots). Occasionally, patients present with an iris abscess (188). The onset of suppuration in the vitreous is a poor prognostic sign (77,105,109). *Candida* retinitis and vitritis may resolve spontaneously in a patient with anterior chamber flare and cells, cells in the vitreous, and lesions deep in the retina surrounded by serous detachment of the sensory retina (54).

Cryptococcosis

At least 32 cases of cryptococcal endophthalmitis have been reported (5,28). The organisms are generally located in the retina and may excite little inflammatory response (Fig. 10). Both eyes are often involved (36,119,141), and cryptococcal meningitis may precede or succeed the ocular involvement (36,107,119,141).

Weiss and colleagues (295) were the first to isolate *Cryptococcus* from subretinal fluid in an eye with retinal detachment and uveitis.

Pseudoallescheriasis

There have been reports of 17 cases of ophthalmic infections by *P. boydii*, of which seven were endophthalmitis (183). Predisposing factors in these cases were trauma (three cases) and immunosuppression (three cases), but in one patient there were no predisposing factors. McGuire et al. (183) observed no difference between the ability of *Aspergillus fumigatus* and *P. boydii* to cause endophthalmitis in an exogenous experimental model in immunocompetent and immunosuppressed rabbits.

Sporotrichosis

At least 20 cases of *S. schenckii* endophthalmitis have been reported (28,38,155,303), including two patients with AIDS (38,155). Direct extension from lesions of the eyelids and conjunctiva may erode the eye or orbit. Of these cases, 12 resulted from widespread systemic disease and six patients were healthy without apparent systemic involvement (28,39,78,100).

Endophthalmitis may be a manifestation of coccidioidomycosis, histoplasmosis, and North America blastomycisis as discussed earlier.

Fungal Infections of Eyelids

The eyelid may be involved in North American blastomycosis, coccidioidomycosis, sporotrichosis, candidiasis, *Malassezia* (11), and, rarely, *Aspergillus niger* infection (200). Lesions of the eyelids are the most common ocular manifestations of North American blastomycosis, occurring in 25% of patients with systemic disease (83). The most frequent site of sporotrichosis of importance to ophthalmologists is the eyelid (75). A solitary eyelid nodule due to cryptococcus was observed in a 37-year-old man with AIDS (46). Slack et al. (252) observed blastomyces in the eyelid and conjunctiva in a 37 year old male who presented with a recurrent papillary lesion. Vieira-Dias et al. (285) reported ocular involvement in a 12-year-old girl with cutaneous sporotrichosis.

Rarely, granulomas due to *C. immitis* have been observed on the eyelids (73,124,313). In some instances the conjunctiva is principally involved and Parinaud oculoglandular syndrome develops (305). Bartley (13) observed involvement of the eyelids in only 1 of 79 patients with systemic blastomycosis.

Chronic infection of eyelid and conjunctiva by *Candida* sp. may accompany widespread superficial candidiasis and has been documented in patients with diminished delayed hypersensitivity (anergy), hypoparathyroidism, and adrenal insufficiency (2,31,311). The cell-mediated immune response to *Candida* can be reconstituted by allogeneic lymphocyte transfusion and the administration of transfer factor (311),

Fungal Infections of Lacrimal Drainage Apparatus

Fungal growth with or without inflammation may occur in lacrimal canaliculus, lacrimal sac (275), or lacrimal duct. The fungal overgrowth alone or with associated dacryoliths sometimes obstructs the lacrimal sac or lacrimal duct partially or completely (Figs. 19 and 20).

C. albicans is the most frequently encountered fungus in the lacrimal sac (66,76,281,307,308). Other fungal infections in this location include sporotrichosis, cryptococcosis, aspergillosis, cephalosporiosis, trichophytosis, pityrosporiosis (66,306), and rhinosporidiosis (16).

Lacrimal canaliculitis typically occurs in women with unilateral chronic conjunctivitis and is characterized clinically by epiphora and a mass in the upper or lower canalicular area (Fig. 20). It is sometimes caused by fungi, such as *Candida* (205) and *Aspergillus* (29,84,153,224), but *Actinomyces* (34,227) (previously streptothrix) has most commonly been isolated. *Arachnia (Actinomyces) proprionica* is now considered the major cause of lacrimal canaliculitis with typical concretions (246). This organism is now regarded as a bacterium. An undetected lacrimal canaliculitis can cause a unilateral recalcitrant conjunctivitis, and such persons have an increased risk of developing postsurgical endophthalmitis.

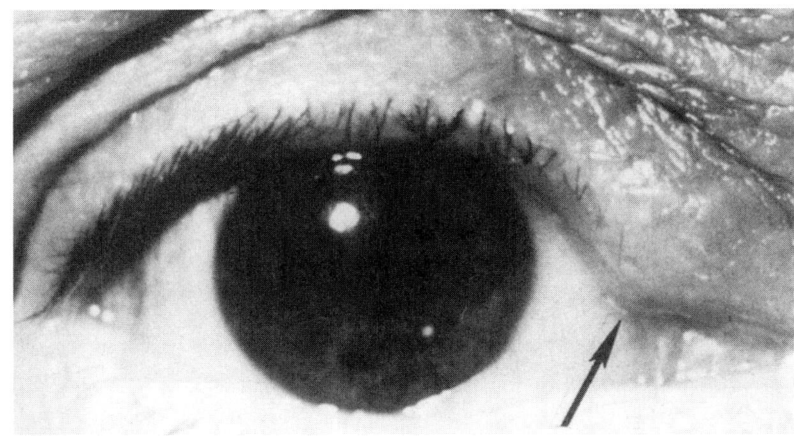

Figure 20 Lacrimal canaliculitis in right upper eyelid (*arrow*) of a 56-year-old woman.

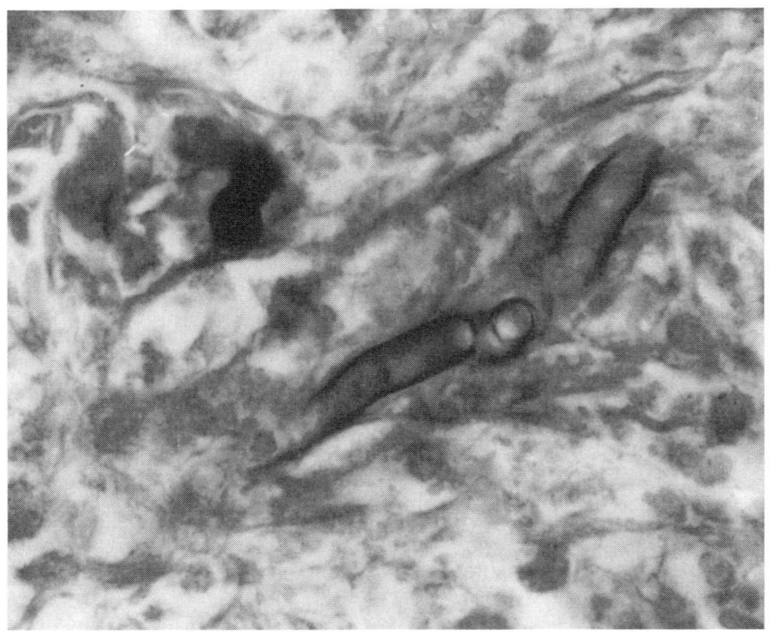

Figure 21 Broad hyphae of orbital phycomycosis in a nonacidotic child (Grocott-Gomori-methanamine silver, ×1,400).

Fungal Infections of Orbit

Fungal infections of the lacrimal gland are uncommon, but there are documented cases due to *B. dermatitidis*, *H., duboisii*, and *S. schenkii*. The most common fungi causing orbital infections (85) belong to the class Zygomycetes (Phycomycetes) (Fig. 21) (90,245) and the genus *Aspergillus* (104) that reach the orbit from the paranasal sinuses (147).

Aspergillosis

Aspergillus infection may develop and spread to the orbit on rare occasions (52,104,283,163). Orbital infection with *Aspergillus* results in a slowly progressive, granulomatous, fibrosing disease (Fig. 3). Thus, patients, may be asymptomatic for extended periods of time, and the duration of symptoms may range from several months to as long as 16 years. The chief clinical manifestations are ocular pain, decreased vision, and unilateral proptosis. The fibrosing nature of the granulomatous inflammation in the orbit may strangle the optic nerve, causing edema of the optic nerve head, venous engorgement, and central retinal artery occlusion. Other signs of inflammation, such as edema of the eyelids and conjunctiva, fever, and leukocytosis, are usually absent. In some instances, the fungus is highly invasive and in others may have a prominent allergic component with eosinophils (53,145). Sivak-Collcott et al. (250) reported four cases and 17 previously reported cases of invasive sino-orbital aspergillosis.

An extremely important fungal infection of the orbit is zygomycosis, which was discussed earlier.

Orbital Involvement by Other Fungi

Penicillium, the ubiquitous producer of penicillin, is rarely pathogenic even in debilitated hosts. A questionable case of orbital involvement by extension from a primary infection in the maxillary and ethmoid sinuses has been reported (194). Orbital infection with *H. capsulatum* has not been documented; however, the related species *H. duboisii* may cause a dacryoadenitis with secondary orbital rim osteomyelitis (211). Orbital infections by *B. dermatitidis* (284), *S. schenckii* (264), and *Cryptococcus* (61) have been recognized.

REFERENCES

1. Anonymous. Argon laser photocoagulation for ocular histoplasmosis. Results of a randomized clinical trial. Arch Ophthalmol 1983; 101:1347–57.
2. Ahonen, P, Myllarniemi, S, Sipila, I and Perheentupa, J. Clinical variation of autoimmune polyendocrinopathy-candidiasis-ectodermal dystrophy (APECED) in a series of 68 patients. N Engl J Med 1990; 322:1829–36.
3. Ainbinder DJ, Parmley VC, Mader TH, Nelson ML Infectious crystalline keratopathy caused by Candida guilliermondii. Am J Ophthalmol 1998; 125:723–5.
4. Ajello L and Arizona State Departmentt of Health. Coccidioidomycosis; papers. In: Ajello L ed. Tucson: Publication arrangements under the direction of Arizona State Department of Health University of Arizona Press, 1967.
5. Alexander PB, Coodley EL. Disseminated coccidioidomycosis with intraocular involvement. Am J Ophthalmol 1967; 64:283–9.
6. Allen HF. Amphotericin B and exogenous mycotic endophthalmitis after cataract extraction. Arch Ophthalmol 1972; 88:640–4.
7. Anderson WB, Byrnes TH. A case of Rhinosporidium of the conjunctiva. Am J Ophthalmol 1939; 22:1383–8.

8. Arffa RC, Avni I, Ishibashi Y, Robin J, Kaufman HE. Calcofluor and ink-potassium hydroxide preparations for identifying fungi. Am J Ophthalmol 1985; 100: 719–23.
9. Arnold R, WJ. Rhinosporidiosis of the conjunctiva. Am J Ophthalmol 1942; 25:1227–30.
10. Asbell P, Stenson S. Ulcerative keratitis. Survey of 30 years' laboratory experience. Arch Ophthalmol 1982; 100:77–80.
11. Ashbee HR, Evans EG. Immunology of diseases associated with Malassezia species. Clin Microbiol Rev 2002; 15:21–57.
12. Baker RD. Human Infection with Fungi, Actinomycetes and Algae. New York: Springer-Verlag, Berlin, 1971.
13. Bartley GB. Blastomycosis of the eyelid. Ophthalmology 1995; 102:2020–3.
14. Baum JL. Rhino-orbital mucormycosis occurring in an otherwise apparently healthy individual. Am J Ophthalmol 1967; 63:335–9.
15. Behrens-Baumann W, Rèuchel R. Mycosis of the Eye and Its Adnexa. New York: Karger, Basel, 1999.
16. Bell R, Font RL. Granulomatous anterior uveitis caused by Coccidioides immitis. Am J Ophthalmol 1972; 74: 93–8.
17. Benaoudia F, Assouline M, Pouliquen Y, Bouvet A, Gueho E. Exophiala (Wangiella) dermatitidis keratitis after keratoplasty. Med Mycol 1999; 37:53–6.
18. Bennington JL, Haber SL, Morgenstern NL. Increased Susceptibility To Cryptococcosis Following Steroid Therapy. Dis Chest 1964; 45:262–3.
19. Bernauer W, Allan BD, Dart JK. Successful management of Aspergillus scleritis by medical and surgical treatment. Eye 1998; 12(Pt 2):311–6.
20. Bernhardt HE, Orlando JC, Benfield JR, Hirose FM, Foos RY. Disseminated candidiasis in surgical patients. Surg Gynecol Obstet 1972; 134:819–25.
21. Blodi FC, Hannah FT, Wadsworth JA. Lethal orbitocerebral phycomycosis in otherwise healthy children. Am J Ophthalmol 1969; 67:698–705.
22. Blumenkranz MS, Stevens DA. Endogenous coccidioidal endophthalmitis. Ophthalmology 1980; 87:974–84.
23. Bonatti WD, Jaeger EA, Frayer WC. Endogenous Fungal Endophthalmitis. Clinical Course In A Successfully Treated Case. Arch Ophthalmol 1963; 70:772–4.
24. Bond WI, Sanders CV, Joffe L, Franklin RM. Presumed blastomycosis endophthalmitis. Ann Ophthalmol 1982; 14:1183–8.
25. Boralkar AN, Dindore PR, Fule RP, Bangde BN, Albel MV, Saoji AM. Microbiological studies in conjunctivitis. Indian J Ophthalmol 1989; 37:94–5.
26. Boyden BS, Yee DS. Bilateral coccidioidal choroiditis. A clinicopathologic case report. Trans Am Acad Ophthalmol Otolaryngol 1971; 75:1006–10.
27. Braley RE, Meredith TA, Aaberg TM, Koethe SM, Witkowski JA. The prevalence of HLA-B7 in presumed ocular histoplasmosis. Am J Ophthalmol 1978; 85: 859–61.
28. Brightbill FS, Fraser LK. Unilateral keratoconjunctivitis with canalicular obstruction by Aspergillus fumigatus. Arch Ophthalmol 1974; 91:421–2.
29. Brod RD, Clarkson JG, Flynn HWJ, Green WR. Endogenous fungal endophthalmitis. In: Duane's Clinical Ophthalmology. Philadelphia: W.B. Saunders, 1990.
30. Bronnimann DA, Adam RD, Galgiani JN, Habib MP, Petersen EA, Porter B, Bloom JW. Coccidioidomycosis in the acquired immunodeficiency syndrome. Ann Intern Med 1987; 106:372–9.
31. Bronsky D, Kushner DS, Dubin A, Snapper I. Idiopathic hypoparathyroidism and pseudohypoparathyroidism: case reports and review of the literature. Medicine 1958; 37:317–52.
32. Brown WC, Hudson KE, Nisbet AA. Pulmonary coccidioidomycosis associated with Jensen's disease. Am J Ophthalmol 1957; 43:965–7.
33. Brown WC, Kellenberger RE, Hudson KE. Granulomatous uveitis associated with disseminated coccidioidomycosis. Am J Ophthalmol 1958; 45:102–4.
34. Bruce GM, Locatcher-Khorazo D. Actinomyces: Recovery of the streptothrix in a case of superficial punctate keratitis. Arch Ophthalmol 1942; 27:294–8.
35. Burda CD, Fisher E Jr. Corneal destruction by extracts of Cephalosporium mycelium. Am J Ophthalmol 1960; 50:926–37.
36. Cameron ME, Harrison A. Ocular cryptococcosis in Australia, with a report of two further cases. Med J Aust 1970; 1:935–8.
37. Carlson AN, Foulks GN, Perfect JR, Kim JH. Fungal scleritis after cataract surgery. Successful outcome using itraconazole. Cornea 1992; 11:151–4.
38. Cartwright MJ, Promersberger M, Stevens GA. Sporothrix schenckii endophthalmitis presenting as granulomatous uveitis. Br J Ophthalmol 1993; 77:61–2.
39. Cassady JR, Foerster HC. Sporotrichum schenckii endophthalmitis. Arch Ophthalmol 1971; 85:71–4.
40. Cassady JV. Uveal Blastomycosis. Arch Ophthalmol 1946; 35:84–97.
41. Catanzaro A. Suppressor cells in coccidioidomycosis. Cell Immunol 1981; 4:235–45.
42. Chaillous MJ. Sporotrichose gommeuse disseminee, gomme intra-oculaire, perforation de la sclerotique (1). Ann Oculist Paris 1912; 745:321–8.
43. Chandler JW, Kalina RE, Milam DF. Coccidioidal choroiditis following renal transplantation. Am J Ophthalmol 1972; 74:1080–5.
44. Chang DC, Grant GB, O'Donnell K, Wannemuehler KA, Noble-Wang J, Rao CY, Jacobson LM, Crowell CS, Sneed RS, Lewis FM, Schaffzin JK, Kainer MA, Genese CA, Alfonso EC, Jones DB, Srinivasan A, Fridkin SK, Park BJ. Multistate outbreak of Fusarium keratitis associated with use of a contact lens solution. Jama 2006; 296:953–63.
45. Chapman-Smith JS. Cryptococcal chorioretinitis: a case report. Br J Ophthalmol 1977; 61:411–3.
46. Coccia L, Calista D, Boschini A. Eyelid nodule: a sentinel lesion of disseminated cryptococcosis in a patient with acquired immunodeficiency syndrome. Arch Ophthalmol 1999; 117:271–2.
47. Cohen DB, Glasgow BJ. Bilateral optic nerve cryptococcosis in sudden blindness in patients with acquired immune deficiency syndrome. Ophthalmology 1993; 100:1689–94.
48. Conant NF. Manual of Clinical Mycology. Philadelphia: Saunders, 1971.
49. Coskuncan NM, Jabs DA, Dunn JP, Haller JA, Green WR, Vogelsang GB, Santos GW. The eye in bone marrow transplantation. VI. Retinal complications. Arch Ophthalmol 1994; 112:372–9.
50. Daly AL, Velazquez LA, Bradley SF, Kauffman CA. Mucormycosis: association with deferoxamine therapy. Am J Med 1989; 87:468–71.
51. Davidorf FR. The role of T-lymphocytes in the reactivation of presumed ocular histoplasmosis scars. Int Ophthalmol Clin 1975; 15:111–24.

52. De Buen S, Duran S. Aspergillosis orbitaria. An Soc Mex Oftalmol 1969; 42:17–32.
53. de Juan E Jr, Green WR, Iliff NT. Allergic periorbital mucopyocele in children. Am J Ophthalmol 1983; 96:299–303.
54. Dellon AL, Stark WJ, Chretien PB. Spontaneous resolution of endogenous Candida endophthalmitis complicating intravenous hyperalimentation. Am J Ophthalmol 1975; 79:648–54.
55. Deubeurmann M, Gougerot M. Sporotricuose cachectisante mortelle. Bull Soc Med Hasp Paris 1909; 26:1046–50.
56. DeVoe AG, Silva-Hutner M. Fungal infections of the eye. In: Microbiology of the Eye. St. Louis: C.V. Mosby, 1972.
57. Diamond RD. Effects of stimulation and suppression of cell-mediated immunity on experimental cryptococcosis. Infect Immun 1977; 17:187–94.
58. Diamond RD. The growing problem of mycoses in patients infected with the human immunodeficiency virus. Rev Infect Dis 1991; 13:480–6.
59. Donahue HC. Unusual mycotic infection of the lacrimal canaliculi and conjunctiva. Am J Ophthalmol 1949; 32: 207–10.
60. Donahue SP, Greven CM, Zuravleff JJ, Eller AW, Nguyen MH, Peacock JE Jr, Wagener MW, Yu VL. Intraocular candidiasis in patients with candidemia. Clinical implications derived from a prospective multicenter study. Ophthalmology 1994; 101:1302–9.
61. Doorenbos-Bot AC, Hooymans JM, Blanksma LJ. Periorbital necrotising fasciitis due to Cryptococcus neoformans in a healthy young man. Doc Ophthalmol 1990; 75:315–20.
62. Doughman DJ, Leavenworth NM, Campbell RC, Lindstrom RL. Fungal keratitis at the University of Minnesota: 1971–1981. Trans Am Ophthalmol Soc 1982; 80:235–47.
63. Dudley MA, Chick EW. Corneal lesions produced in rabbits by an extract of fusarium moniliforme. Arch Ophthalmol 1964; 72:346–50.
64. Dugel PU, Rao NA, Forster DJ, Chong LP, Frangieh GT, Sattler F. Pneumocystis carinii choroiditis after long-term aerosolized pentamidine therapy. Am J Ophthalmol 1990; 110:113–7.
65. Duggan JN. A case of Rhinosporidium kinealyi. Br J Ophthalmol 1928; 72:526–30.
66. Duke-Elder S, Leigh AG. Diseases of the outer eye, Parts 1 and 2. In: System of Ophthalmology. St. Louis: C.V. Mosby, 1974:385–98, 793–801.
67. Edman JC, Kovacs JA, Masur H, Santi DV, Elwood HJ, Sogin ML Ribosomal RNA sequence shows Pneumocystis carinii to be a member of the fungi. Nature 1988; 334:519–22.
68. Edwards JE Jr, Foos RY, Montgomerie JZ, Guze LB. Ocular manifestations of Candida septicemia: review of seventy-six cases of hematogenous Candida endophthalmitis. Medicine (Baltimore) 1974; 53:47–75.
69. Elles NB. Rhinosporidium seeberi infection in the eye. Arch Ophthalmol 1941; 25:969–91.
70. Elliot RH, Ingram AC. A case of Rhinosporidium kinealyi of the conjunctiva. Ophthalmoscope 1912; 70:428–32.
71. Ellis CA, Spivack ML. The significance of candidemia. Ann Intern Med 1967; 67:511–22.
72. Eng RH, Bishburg E, Smith SM, Kapila R. Cryptococcal infections in patients with acquired immune deficiency syndrome. Am J Med 1986; 81:19–23.
73. Faulkner RF. Ocular coccidioidomycosis. Report of a case of coccidioidal granuloma of the conjunctiva associated with cutaneous coccidioidomycosis. Am J Ophthalmol 1962; 53:822–7.
74. Fetter BF, Klintworth GK, Hendry WS. Mycoses of the central nervous system. Baltimore: Williams & Wilkins, 1967.
75. Fine BS, Zimmerman LE, Exogenous intraocular fungus infections with particular reference to complications of intraocular surgery. Am J Ophthalmol 1959; 48:151–65.
76. Fine M, Waring WS. Mycotic obstruction of nasolacrimal duct (Candida albicans). Arch Ophthalmol 1947; 39:39–42.
77. Fishman LS, Griffin JR, Sapico FL, Hecht R. 1972. Hematogenous Candida endophthalmitis–a complication of candidemia. N Engl J Med 1972; 286:675–81.
78. Font RL, Jakobiec FA. Granulomatous necrotizing retinochoroiditis caused by Sporotrichum schenkii. Report of a case including immunofluorescence and electron microscopical studies. Arch Ophthalmol 1976; 94:1513–9.
79. Font RL, Spaulding AG, Green WR. Endogenous mycotic panophthalmitis caused by blastomyces dermatitidis. Report of a case and a review of the literature. Arch Ophthalmol 1967; 77:217–22.
80. Forster RK, Rebell G. The diagnosis and management of keratomycoses. I. Cause and diagnosis. Arch Ophthalmol 1975; 93:975–8.
81. Foster JB, Almeda E, Littman ML, Wilson ME. Some intraocular & conjunctival effects of amphotericin B in man and in the rabbit. AMA Arch Ophthalmol 1958; 60:555–64.
82. Foster RE, Lowder CY, Meisler DM, Huang SS, Longworth DL. Presumed Pneumocystis carinii choroiditis. Unifocal presentation, regression with intravenous pentamidine, and choroiditis recurrence. Ophthalmology 1991; 98:1360–5.
83. François J, Rysselaere M. Oculomycoses. Springfield, Ill: Thomas, 1972.
84. François J, Rysselaere M, Société belge d'ophtalmologie. Les mycoses oculaires. Imprimerie Medicale et Scientifique, Brussels, 1968.
85. Freeman LN, Green WR. Periocular infections. In: Principles and Practice of Infectious Diseases. New York: Churchill Livingstone, 1990.
86. Freeman WR, Gross JG, Labelle J, Oteken K, Katz B, Wiley CA. Pneumocystis carinii choroidopathy. A new clinical entity. Arch Ophthalmol 1989; 107:863–7.
87. Ganley JP. The role of the cellular immune system in patients with macular disciform histoplasmosis. Int Ophthalmol Clin 1975; 15:83–91.
88. Ganley JP, Smith RE, Knox DL, Comstock GW. Presumed ocular histoplasmosis. 3. Epidemiologic characteristics of people with peripheral atrophic scars. Arch Ophthalmol 1973; 89:116–9.
89. Ganley JP, Smith RE, Thomas DB, Comstock GW, Sartwell PE. Booster effect of histoplasmin skin testing in an elderly population. Am J Epidemiol 1972; 95:104–10.
90. Gass JD. Ocular manifestations of acute mucormycosis. Arch Ophthalmol 1961; 65:226–37.
91. Gass JD. Pathogenesis of disciform detachment of the neuroepithelium. Am J Ophthalmol 1967; 63(Suppl): 1–139.
92. Gass JD, Wilkinson CP. Follow-up study of presumed ocular histoplasmosis. Trans Am Acad Ophthalmol Otolaryngol 1972; 76:672–94.
93. Getnick RA, Rodrigues MM. Endogenous fungal endophthalmitis in a drug addict. Am J Ophthalmol 1974; 77:680–3.
94. Giles CL, Falls HF. Amphotericin B therapy in the treatment of presumed Histoplasma chorioretinitis: a further appraisal. Trans Am Ophthalmol Soc 1967; :136–45.

95. Glassman MI, Henkind P, Alture-Werber E. Monosporium apiospermum endophthalmitis. Am J Ophthalmol 1973; 76:821–4.
96. Godfrey WA, Sabates R, Cross DE. Association of presumed ocular histoplasmosis with HLA-B7. Am J Ophthalmol 1978; 85:854–8.
97. Goldstein E, Rambo ON. Cryptococcal infection following steroid therapy. Ann Intern Med 1962; 56:114–20.
98. Gonzales CA, Scott IU, Chaudhry NA, Luu KM, Miller D, Murray TG, Davis JL. Endogenous endophthalmitis caused by Histoplasma capsulatum var. capsulatum: a case report and literature review. Ophthalmology 2000; 107:725–9.
99. Gopinathan U, Garg P, Fernandes M, Sharma S, Athmanathan S, Rao GN. The epidemiological features and laboratory results of fungal keratitis: a 10-year review at a referral eye care center in South India. Cornea 2002; 21:555–9.
100. Gordon DM. Ocular sporotrichosis: Report of a case. Arch Ophthalmol 1947; 37:56–72.
101. Green WR. Uvea. In: Ophthalmic Pathology. An Atlas and Textbook. Philadelphia: W.B. Saunders, 1986.
102. Green WR, Bennett JE. Coccidioidomycosis. Report of a case with clinical evidence of ocular involvement. Arch Ophthalmol 1967; 77:337–40.
103. Green WR, Bennett JE, Goos RD. Ocular penetration of amphotericin B: a report of laboratory studies and a case report of postsurgical cephalosporium endophthalmitis. Arch Ophthalmol 1965; 73:769–75.
104. Green WR, Font RL, Zimmerman LE. Asperillosis of the orbit. Report of ten cases and review of the literature. Arch Ophthalmol 1969; 82:302–13.
105. Greene WH, Wiernik PH. Candida endophthalmitis. Successful treatment in a patient with acute leukemia. Am J Ophthalmol 1972; 74:1100–4.
106. Greeves RA. Streptothrix conjunctivitis. Br J Ophthalmol 1952; 36:653.
107. Grieco MH, Freilich DB, Louria DB. Diagnosis of cryptococcal uveitis with hypertonic media. Am J Ophthalmol 1971; 72:171–4.
108. Griffey EW. Rhinosporidiosis: A case report. Am J Ophthalmol 1939; 22:1389–90.
109. Griffin JR, Pettit TH, Fishman LS, Foos RY. Blood-borne Candida endophthalmitis. A clinical and pathologic study of 21 cases. Arch Ophthalmol 1973; 89: 450–6.
110. Grosse G, Mishra SK, Staib F. Selective involvement of the brain in experimental murine cryptococcosis. II. Histopathological observations. Zentralbl Bakteriol (Orig A) 1975; 233:106–22.
111. Hale LM. Orbital-cerebral phycomycosis. Report of a case and a review of the disease in infants. Arch Ophthalmol 1971; 86:39–43.
112. Hammeke JC, Ellis PP. Mycotic flora of the conjunctiva. Am J Ophthalmol 1960; 49:1174–8.
113. Hanabusa J. Toxin of Candida albicans. Ada Soc Ophthalmol Jpn 1953; 57:158–60.
114. Hart PD, Russell E Jr, Remington JS. The compromised host and infection. II. Deep fungal infection. J Infect Dis 1969; 120:169–91.
115. Harvey RP, Stevens DA. In vitro assays of cellular immunity in progressive coccidioidomycosis: evaluation of suppression with parasitic-phase antigen. Am Rev Respir Dis 1981; 123:665–9.
116. Hedges, TR, Leung, LS. Parasellar and orbital apex syndrome caused by aspergillosis. Neurology 1976; 26:117–20.
117. Heidemann DG, Dunn SP, Watts JC. Aspergillus keratitis after radial keratotomy. Am J Ophthalmol 1995; 120:254–6.
118. Hicks HR, Northey WT. Studies on responsive thymectomized mice to infection with Coccidioide immitis. In: Coccidioidomycosis. Tucson: University of Arizona Press, 1967.
119. Hiles DA, Font RL. Bilateral intraocular cryptococcosis with unilateral spontaneous regression. Report of a case and review of the literature. Am J Ophthalmol 1968; 65:98–108.
120. Hoefnagels KL, Pijpers PM. Histoplasma capsulatum in a human eye. Ophthalmologica 1968; 156:90.
121. Houle TV, Ellis PP. Aspergillosis of the orbit with immunosuppressive therapy. Surv Ophthalmol 1975; 20:35–42.
122. Howlett JA, Squier CA. Candida albicans ultrastructure: colonization and invasion of oral epithelium. Infect Immun 1980; 29:252–60.
123. Hvidberg-Hansen A. Endogenous mycotic retinopathy. Report of a case. Acta Ophthalmol (Copenh) 1972; 50:515–9.
124. Irvine AR Jr. Coccidioidal granuloma of lid. Trans Am Acad Ophthalmol Otolaryngol 1968; 72:751–4.
125. Irvine AR, Spencer WH, Hogan MJ, Meyers RL, Irvine SR. Presumed chronic ocular histoplasmosis syndrome: a clinical-pathologic case report. Trans Am Ophthalmol Soc 1976; 74:91–106.
126. Jabs DA, Green WR, Fox R, Polk BF, Bartlett JG. Ocular manifestations of acquired immune deficiency syndrome. Ophthalmology 1989; 96:1092–9.
127. Jimenez JF, Young DE, Hough AJ Jr. Rhinosporidiosis. A report of two cases from Arkansas. Am J Clin Pathol 1984; 82:611–5.
128. Joannides T. A case of blastomycosis of the conjunctiva. Bull Soc Hellen Ophthalmol 1952; 20:13.
129. Johnson JE, Fekety FR, Cluff LE, Kadull PJ, Perry JE. Laboratory-acquired coccidioidomycosis: A report of 210 cases. Ann Intern Med 1964; 60:941–56.
130. Joklik WK, Willett HP, Amos DB, Zinsser H. Zinsser Microbiology. New York: Appleton-Century-Crofts, 1980.
131. Jones BR. Principles in the management of oculomycosis. XXXI Edward Jackson memorial lecture. Am J Ophthalmol 1975; 79:719–51.
132. Jones BR, Jones DB, Lim AS, Bron AJ, Morgan G, Clayton YM. Corneal and intra-ocular infection due to Fusarium solani. Trans Ophthalmol Soc UK 1970; 89:757–79.
133. Jones BR, Jones DB, Richards AB. Surgery in the management of keratomycosis. Trans Ophthalmol Soc UK 1970; 89:887–97.
134. Jones BR, Richards AB, Morgan G. Direct fungal infection of the eye in Britain. Trans Ophthalmol Soc UK 1970; 89:727–41.
135. Jones DB. Fungal keratitis. In: Duane's Clinical Ophthalmology. Philadelphia: J.B. Lippincott, 1990.
136. Jones DB, Forster FK, Rebell G. Fusarium solani keratitis treated with natamycin (pimaricin): eighteen consecutive cases. Arch Ophthalmol 1972; 88:147–54.
137. Katz BJ, Scott WE, Folk JC. Acute histoplasmosis choroiditis in 2 immunocompetent brothers. Arch Ophthalmol 1997; 115:1470–2.
138. Kaufman HE, Wood RM. Mycotic Keratitis. Am J Ophthalmol 1965; 59:993–1000.
139. Key SN, Green WR, Maumenee AE. Pathology of macular lesion of ocular histoplasmosis: its pathogenic and therapeutic implication. In: Controversy in Ophthalmology. Philadelphia: W.B. Saunders, 1977.

140. Khalil MK. Histopathology of presumed ocular histoplasmosis. Am J Ophthalmol 1982; 94:369–76.
141. Khodadoust AA, Payne JW. Cryptococcal (torular) retinitis. A clinicopathologic case report. Am J Ophthalmol 1969; 67: 745–50.
142. Kim RW, Juzych MS, Eliott D. Ocular manifestations of injection drug use. Infect Dis Clin North Am 2002; 16: 607–22.
143. Kirkpatrick H. Rhinosporidium of the lacrimal sac. Ophthalmoscope 1916; 14:411–19.
144. Kisla TA, Cu-Unjieng A, Sigler L, Sugar J. Medical management of Beauveria bassiana keratitis. Cornea 2000; 19:405–6.
145. Klapper SR, Lee AG, Patrinely JR, Stewart M, Alford EL. Orbital involvement in allergic fungal sinusitis. Ophthalmology 1997; 104:2094–100.
146. Klintworth GK, Hollingsworth AS, Lusman PA, Bradford WD. Granulomatous choroiditis in a case of disseminated histoplasmosis. Histologic demonstration of Histoplasma capsulatum in choroidal lesions. Arch Ophthalmol 197390:45–8.
147. Klotz SA, Penn CC, Negvesky GJ, Butrus SI. Fungal and parasitic infections of the eye. Clin Microbiol Rev 2000; 13:662–85.
148. Knox DL, Green WR. Pneumocystis carinii granuloma of the optic nerve: a histopathologic case report. J Neuroophthalmol 2001; 21:274–5.
149. Knox DL, O'Brien TP, Green WR. Histoplasma granuloma of the conjunctiva. Ophthalmology 2003; 110:2051–3.
150. Kovacs JA, Kovacs AA, Polis M, Wright WC, Gill VJ, Tuazon CU, Gelmann EP, Lane HC, Longfield R, Overturf G, et al. Cryptococcosis in the acquired immunodeficiency syndrome. Ann Intern Med 1985; 103:533–8.
151. Krause AC, Hopkins WG. Ocular manifestation of histoplasmosis. Am J Ophthalmol 1951; 34:564–6.
152. Krill AE, Archer D. Choroidal neovascularization in multifocal (presumed histoplasmin) choroiditis. Arch Ophthalmol 1970; 84:595–604.
153. Kumstat Z, Pospisil L. Aspergillose der Bindehaut und der Tranenkanalchen. Cesk Oftalmol 1963; 9:127–29.
154. Kuriakose ET. Oculosporidiosis: Rhinosporidiosis Of The Eye. Br J Ophthalmol 1963; 47:346–9.
155. Kurosawa A, Pollock SC, Collins MP, Kraff CR, Tso MO. Sporothrix schenckii endophthalmitis in a patient with human immunodeficiency virus infection. Arch Ophthalmol 1988; 106:376–80.
156. Kurup PK. Rhinosporidal affections of the human eye and its appendages. Proc All-India Ophthalmol Soc 1931; 2:104–8.
157. Kwon-Chung KJ, Bennett JE. Medical Mycology. Philadelphia: Lea & Febiger, 1992.
158. Kwon-Chung KJ, Rhodes JC. Encapsulation and melanin formation as indicators of virulence in Cryptococcus neoformans. Infect Immun 1986; 51:218–23.
159. Landolt E, Zuccoli A. Mykotische Panophthalmitis nach Netzhautoperation. Ophthalmologica 1970; 161:237–42.
160. Larone DH. Medically Important Fungi: A Guide to Identification. Hagerstown, Md.: Medical Dept. Harper and Row, 1976.
161. Leck AK, Thomas PA, Hagan M, Kaliamurthy J, Ackuaku E, John M, Newman MJ, Codjoe FS, Opintan JA, Kalavathy CM, Essuman V, Jesudasan CA, Johnson GJ. Aetiology of suppurative corneal ulcers in Ghana and south India, and epidemiology of fungal keratitis. Br J Ophthalmol 2002; 86:1211–5.
162. Lee P, Green WR. Corneal biopsy. Indications, techniques, and a report of a series of 87 cases. Ophthalmology 1990; 97:718–21.
163. Levin LA, Avery R, Shore JW, Woog JJ, Baker AS. The spectrum of orbital aspergillosis: a clinicopathological review. Surv Ophthalmol 1996; 41:142–54.
164. Lewis H, Aaberg TM, Fary DR, Stevens TS. Latent disseminated blastomycosis with choroidal involvement. Arch Ophthalmol 1988; 106:527–30.
165. Liesegang TJ, Forster RK. Spectrum of microbial keratitis in South Florida. Am J Ophthalmol 1980; 90:38–47.
166. Litricin O, Parunovic A. Mycose Intra-Oculaire Post-Operatoire. Ann Ocul (Paris) 1964; 197:164–71.
167. Locher DH, Adesina A, Wolf TC, Imes CB, Chodosh J. Postoperative Rhizopus scleritis in a diabetic man. J Cataract Refract Surg 1998; 24:562–5.
168. Lovekin LG. Coccidioidomycosis. Report of a case with intraocular involvement. Am J Ophthalmol 1951; 34:621–3.
169. Lynch PJ, Voorhees JJ, Harrell ER. Systemic sporotrichosis. Ann Intern Med 1970; 73:23–30.
170. Macher A, Rodrigues MM, Kaplan W, Pistole MC, McKittrick A, Lawrinson WE, Reichert CM. Disseminated bilateral chorioretinitis due to Histoplasma capsulatum in a patient with the acquired immunodeficiency syndrome. Ophthalmology 1985; 92:1159–64.
171. Macher AM, Bardenstein DS, Zimmerman LE, Steigman CK, Pastore L, Poretz DM, Eron LJ. Pneumocystis carinii choroiditis in a male homosexual with AIDS and disseminated pulmonary and extrapulmonary P. carinii infection. N Engl J Med 1987; 316:1092.
172. Macher AM, Bennett JE, Gadek JE, Frank MM. Complement depletion in cryptococcal sepsis. J Immunol 1978; 120:1686–90.
173. Maguire LJ, Campbell RJ, Edson RS. Coccidioidomycosis with necrotizing granulomatous conjunctivitis. Cornea 1994; 13:539–42.
174. Makley TA, Long JW, Suie X, Stephan JD. Presumed histoplasmic chorioretinitis with special emphasis on present modes of therapy. Trans Am Acad Ophthalmol 1965; 69:443–55.
175. Margo CE, Polack FM, Hood CI. Aspergillus panophthalmitis complicating treatment of pterygium. Cornea 1988; 7:285–9.
176. Marshall DH, Brownstein S, Jackson WB, Mintsioulis G, Gilberg SM, al-Zeerah BF. Post-traumatic corneal mucormycosis caused by Absidia corymbifera. Ophthalmology 1997; 104:1107–11.
177. Martinson FD, Alli AF, Clark BM. Aspergilloma of the ethmoid. J Laryngol Otol 1970; 84:857–61.
178. Maskin SL, Alfonso E. Fungal keratitis after radial keratotomy. Am J Ophthalmol 1992; 114:369–70.
179. McDonnell PJ, Green WR. Conjunctivitis. In: Principles and Practice of Infectious Diseases. New York: Churchill Livingstone, 1990.
180. McDonnell PJ, Green WR. Endophthalmitis. In: Principles and Practice of Infectious Diseases. New York: Churchill Livingstone, 1990.
181. McDonnell PJ, McDonnell JM, Brown RH, Green WR. Ocular involvement in patients with fungal infections. Ophthalmology 1985; 92:706–9.
182. McGinnis MR, Buck DL Jr, Katz B. Paranasal aspergilloma caused by an albino variant of Aspergillus fumigatus. South Med J 1977; 70:886–8.
183. McGuire TW, Bullock JD, Bullock JD Jr, Elder BL, Funkhouser JW. Fungal endophthalmitis. An experimental study with a review of 17 human ocular cases. Arch Ophthalmol 1991; 109:1289–96.
184. McLean JM. Oculomycosis. Am J Ophthalmol 1963; 56: 537–49.

185. Meredith TA, Aaberg TM. Hemorrhagic peripapillary lesions in presumed ocular histoplasmosis. Am J Ophthalmol 1977; 84:160–8.
186. Meredith TA, Green WR, Key SN, Dolin GS, Maumenee AE. Ocular histoplasmosis: clinicopathologic correlation of 3 cases. Surv Ophthalmol 1977; 22: 189–205.
187. Meredith TA, Smith RE, Braley RE, Witkowski JA, Koethe SM. The prevalence of HLA-B7 in presumed ocular histoplasmosis in patients with peripheral atrophic scars. Am J Ophthalmol 1978; 86:325–8.
188. Meyers BR, Lieberman TW, Ferry AP. Candida endophthalmitis complicating candidemia. Ann Intern Med 1973; 79:647–53.
189. Miale JB. Candida albicans infection confused with tuberculosis. Arch Pathol 1943; 35:421–31.
190. Michelson PE, Stark W, Reeser F, Green WR. Endogenous Candida endophthalmitis. Report of 13 cases and 16 from the literature. Int Ophthalmol Clin 1971; 11:125–47.
191. Miguelez S, Obrador P, Vila J. Infeccion Conjuntival Por Penicillium. Arch Soc Esp Oftalmol 2003; 78:55–7.
192. Milauskas AT, Duke JR. Mycotic scleral abscess. Report of a case following a scleral buckling operation for retinal detachment. Am J Ophthalmol 1967; 63:951–4.
193. Mitsui Y, Hanabusa J. Corneal infections after cortisone therapy. Br J Ophthalmol 1955; 39:244–50.
194. Moriarty AP, Crawford GJ, McAllister IL, Constable IJ. Severe corneoscleral infection. A complication of beta irradiation scleral necrosis following pterygium excision. Arch Ophthalmol 1993; 111:947–51.
195. Morinelli EN, Dugel PU, Riffenburgh R, Rao NA. Infectious multifocal choroiditis in patients with acquired immune deficiency syndrome. Ophthalmology 1993; 100: 1014–21.
196. Morrison VA, McGlave PB. Mucormycosis in the BMT population. Bone Marrow Transplant 1993; 11:383–8.
197. Morriss FH Jr, Spock A. Intracranial aneurysm secondary to mycotic orbital and sinus infection. Report of a case implicating penicillium as an opportunistic fungus. Am J Dis Child 1970; 119:357–62.
198. Moses JS, Balachandran C, Sandhanam S, Ratnasamy N, Thanappan S, Rajaswar J, Moses D. Ocular rhinosporidiosis in Tamil Nadu, India. Mycopathologia 1990; 11: 5–8.
199. Mosier MA, Lusk B, Pettit TH, Howard DH, Rhodes J. Fungal endophthalmitis following intraocular lens implantation. Am J Ophthalmol 1977; 83:1–8.
200. Mostafa MS. Aspergillus niger infection of the eye. Am J Ophthalmol 1966; 62:1204–5.
201. Naumann G, Green WR, Zimmerman LE. A histopathologic study of 73 cases. Am J Ophthalmol 1967; 64:668–82.
202. Nema HV, Ahuja OP, Mohapatra LN. Mycotic flora of the conjunctiva. Am J Ophthalmol 1966; 62:968–70.
203. Newcomer VD, Wright ET, Tarbet JE, Winer LH, Sternberg TH. The effects of cortisone on experimental coccidioidomycosis. J Invest Dermatol 1953; 20:315–27.
204. Newell FW, Krill AE. Treatment of uveitis with azathioprine (Imuran). Trans Ophthalmol Soc UK 1967; 87:499–511.
205. Newton JC, Tulevech CB. Lacrimal canaliculitis due to Candida albicans. Report of a case and a discussion of its significance. Am J Ophthalmol 1962; 53:933–6.
206. O'Connor GR. Experimental ocular histoplasmosis. In: Ocular Histoplasmosis. Boston: Little, Brown, 1975.
207. O'Day DM. Fungal endophthalmitis caused by Paecilomyces lilacinus after intraocular lens implantation. Am J Ophthalmol 1977; 83:130–1.
208. O'Day DM, Akrabawi PL, Head WS, Ratner HB. Laboratory isolation techniques in human and experimental fungal infections. Am J Ophthalmol 1979; 87:688–93.
209. Okun E, Butler WT. Ophthalmologic Complications Of Cryptococcal Meningitis. Arch Ophthalmol 1964; 71: 52–7.
210. Olavarria R, Fajardo LF. Ophthalmic coccidioidomycosis. Case report and review. Arch Pathol 1971; 92:191–5.
211. Olurin O, Lucas AO, Oyediran AB. Orbital histoplasmosis due to Histoplasma duboisii. Am J Ophthalmol 1969; 68:14–8.
212. Panda A, Pushker N, Nainiwal S, Satpathy G, Nayak N. Rhodotorula sp. infection in corneal interface following lamellar keratoplasty–a case report. Acta Ophthalmol Scand 1999; 77:227–8.
213. Panda A, Sharma N, Das G, Kumar N, Satpathy G. Mycotic keratitis in children: epidemiologic and microbiologic evaluation. Cornea 1997; 16:295–9.
214. Pe'er J, Gnessin H, Levinger S, Averbukh E, Levy Y, Polacheck I. Conjunctival oculosporidiosis in east Africa caused by Rhinosporidium seeberi. Arch Pathol Lab Med 1996; 120:854–8.
215. Pena CE. Aspergillus intranasal fungus ball. Report of a case. Am J Clin Pathol 1975; 64:343–4.
216. Pettit TH, Learn RN, Foos RY. Intraocular coccidioidomycosis. Arch Ophthalmol 1967; 77:655–61.
217. Pixley FJ, Wakefield AE, Banerji S, Hopkin JM. Mitochondrial gene sequences show fungal homology for Pneumocystis carinii. Mol Microbiol 1991; 5:1347–51.
218. Polack FM, Kaufman HE, Newmark E. Keratomycosis. Medical and surgical treatment. Arch Ophthalmol 1971; 85:410–6.
219. Rainin EA, Little HL. Ocular coccidioidomycosis. A clinicopathologic case report. Trans Am Acad Ophthalmol Otolaryngol 1972; 76:645–51.
220. Ramsey MS, Willis NR. Endogenous Candida endophthalmitis. Can J Ophthalmol 1972; 7:126–31.
221. Rao NA, Zimmerman PL, Boyer D, Biswas J, Causey D, Beniz J, Nichols PW. A clinical, histopathologic, and electron microscopic study of Pneumocystis carinii choroiditis. Am J Ophthalmol 1989; 107:218–28.
222. Rao NBK, Rao VBA. A case of Rhinosporidium of the eye and nose. Proc All-India Ophthalmol Soc 1931; 2:109–10.
223. Read RW, Chuck RS, Rao NA, Smith RE. Traumatic Acremonium atrogriseum keratitis following laser-assisted in situ keratomileusis. Arch Ophthalmol 2000; 118:418–21.
224. Reboucas JA. Micoses Oculares. Rev Bras Oftalmol 1953; 12:107–15.
225. Reid D, Scherer JH, Herbut PA, Irving H. Systemic histoplasmosis - Systemic histoplasmosis diagnosed before death and produced experimentally in guinea pigs. J Lab Clin Med 1942; 27:419–34.
226. Ribes JA, Vanover-Sams CL, Baker DJ. Zygomycetes in human disease. Clin Microbiol Rev 2000; 13:236–301.
227. Richards WW. Actinomycotic lacrimal canaliculitis. Am J Ophthalmol 1973; 75:155–7.
228. Rifkind D, Marchioro TL, Schneck SA, Hill RB Jr. Systemic fungal infections complicating renal transplantation and immunosuppressive therapy. Clinical, microbiologic, neurologic and pathologic features. Am J Med 1967; 43:28–38.
229. Rippon JW. Medical mycology; the pathogenic fungi and the pathogenic actinomycetes. Philadelphia: Saunders, 1974.
230. Ritterband D, Kelly J, McNamara T, Kresloff M, Koplin R, Seedor J. Delayed-onset multifocal polymicrobial keratitis

after laser in situ keratomileusis. J Cataract Refract Surg 2002; 28:898–9.
231. Robertson DM, Riley FC, Hermans PE. Endogenous Candida oculomycosis. Report of two patients treated with flucytosine. Arch Ophthalmol 1974; 91:33–8.
232. Rodenbiker HT, Ganley JP. Ocular coccidioidomycosis. Surv Ophthalmol 1980; 24:263–90.
233. Rodrigues M, Laibson P. Exogenous mycotic keratitis caused by blastomyces dermatitidis. Am J Ophthalmol 1973; 75:782–9.
234. Rodriguez-Ares MT, De Rojas Silva MV, Pereiro M, Fente Sampayo B, Gallegos Chamas G, Sanchez-Salorio M. Aspergillus fumigatus scleritis. Acta Ophthalmol Scand 1995; 73:467–9.
235. Rosa RH Jr, Miller D, Alfonso EC. The changing spectrum of fungal keratitis in south Florida. Ophthalmology 1994; 101:1005–13.
236. Rosen R, Friedman AH. Successfully treated postoperative Candida parakrusei endophthalmitis. Am J Ophthalmol 1973; 76:574–7.
237. Roth AM. Histoplasma capsulatum in the presumed ocular histoplasmosis syndrome. Am J Ophthalmol 1977; 84:293–8.
238. Ryan SJ. Histopathological correlates of presumed ocular histoplasmosis. Int Ophthalmol Clin 1975; 15: 125–37.
239. Ryan SJ Jr. De novo subretinal neovascularization in the histoplasmosis syndrome. Arch Ophthalmol 1976; 94: 321–7.
240. Safneck JR, Hogg GR, Napier LB. Endophthalmitis due to Blastomyces dermatitidis. Case report and review of the literature. Ophthalmology 1990; 97:212–6.
241. Sawelson H, Goldberg RE, Annesley WH Jr, Tomer TL. Presumed ocular histoplasmosis syndrome. The fellow eye. Arch Ophthalmol 1976; 94:221–4.
242. Schlaegel TF Jr, Weber JC, Helveston E, Kenney D. Presumed histoplasmic choroiditis. Am J Ophthalmol 1967; 63:919–25.
243. Scholz R, Green WR, Kutys R, Sutherland J, Richards RD. Histoplasma capsulatum in the eye. Ophthalmology 1984; 91:1100–4.
244. Schubach A, de Lima Barros MB, Schubach TM, Francesconi-do-Valle AC, Gutierrez-Galhardo MC, Sued M, de Matos Salgueiro M, Fialho-Monteiro PC, Reis RS, Marzochi KB, Wanke B, Conceicao-Silva F. Primary conjunctival sporotrichosis: two cases from a zoonotic epidemic in Rio de Janeiro, Brazil. Cornea 2005; 24:491–3.
245. Schwartz JN, Donnelly EH, Klintworth GK. Ocular and orbital phycomycosis. Surv Ophthalmol 1977; 22:3–28.
246. Seal DV, McGill J, Flanagan D, Purrier B. Lacrimal canaliculitis due to Arachnia (Actinomyces) propionica. Br J Ophthalmol 1981; 65:10–3.
247. Sehgal SC, Dhawan S, Chhiber S, Sharma M, Talwar P. Frequency and significance of fungal isolations from conjunctival sac and their role in ocular infections. Mycopathologia 1981; 73:17–9.
248. Shrestha SP, Hennig A, Parija SC. Prevalence of rhinosporidiosis of the eye and its adnexa in Nepal. Am J Trop Med Hyg 1998; 59:231–4.
249. Sinskey RM., Anderson WB. Miliary blastomycosis with metastatic spread to posterior uvea of both eyes. AMA Arch Ophthalmol 1955; 54:602–4.
250. Sivak-Callcott JA, Livesley N, Nugent RA, Rasmussen SL, Saeed P, Rootman J. Localised invasive sino-orbital aspergillosis: characteristic features. Br J Ophthalmol 2004; 88:681–7.
251. Skipworth GB, Bergin JJ, Williams RM. Coccidioidal granulomas of skin and conjunctiva treated with intravenous amphotericin B: Report of a case. Arch Dermatol 1960; 86:605–8.
252. Slack JW, Hyndiuk RA, Harris GJ, Simons KB. Blastomycosis of the eyelid and conjunctiva. Ophthal Plast Reconstr Surg 1992; 8:143–9.
253. Smith CE. Epidemiology of acute coccidiodomycosis with erythema nodosum ("San Joaquin" or "valley fever"). Am J Public Health 1940; 50:600–11.
254. Smith RE, Ganley JP. Presumed ocular histoplasmosis. I. Histoplasmin skin test sensitivity in cases identified during a community survey. Arch Ophthalmol 1972; 87:245–50.
255. Smith RE, Knox DL, Jensen AD. Ocular histoplasmosis. Significance of asymptomatic macular scars. Arch Ophthalmol 1973; 89:296–300.
256. Smith RE, Macy JI, Parrett C, Irvine J. Variations in acute multifocal histoplasmic choroiditis in the primate. Invest Ophthalmol Vis Sci 1978; 17:1005–18.
257. Smith RE, O'Connor GR, Halde CJ, Scalarone MA, Easterbrook WM. Clinical course in rabbits after experimental induction of ocular histoplasmosis. Am J Ophthalmol 1973; 76:284–93.
258. Snip RC, Michels RG. Pars plana vitrectomy in the management of endogenous Candida endophthalmitis. Am J Ophthalmol 1976; 82:699–704.
259. Spaeth GL. Absence of so-called histoplasma uveitis in 134 cases of proven histoplasmosis. Arch Ophthalmol 1967; 77:41–4.
260. Sponsler TA, Sassani JW, Johnson LN, Towfighi J. Ocular invasion in mucormycosis. Surv Ophthalmol 1992; 36:345–50.
261. Sridhar MS, Garg P, Bansal AK, Sharma S. Fungal keratitis after laser in situ keratomileusis. J Cataract Refract Surg 2000; 26:613–5.
262. Srinivasan M, Gonzales CA, George C, Cevallos V, Mascarenhas JM, Asokan B, Wilkins J, Smolin G, Whitcher JP. Epidemiology and aetiological diagnosis of corneal ulceration in Madurai, south India. Br J Ophthalmol 1997; 81:965–71.
263. Straatsma BR, Zimmerman LE, Gass JD. Phycomycosis. A clinicopathologic study of fifty-one cases. Lab Invest 1962; 11:963–85.
264. Streeten BW, Rabuzzi DD, Jones DB. Sporotrichosis of the orbital margin. Am J Ophthalmol 1974; 77:750–5.
265. Stringer SL, Hudson K, Blase MA, Walzer PD, Cushion MT, Stringer JR. Sequence from ribosomal RNA of Pneumocystis carinii compared to those of four fungi suggests an ascomycetous affinity. J Protozool 1989; 36: 14S–16S.
266. Sugar HS, Mandell GH, Shalev J. Metastatic endophthalmitis associated with injection of addictive drugs. Am J Ophthalmol 1971; 71:1055–8.
267. Tanure MA, Cohen EJ, Sudesh S, Rapuano CJ, Laibson PR. Spectrum of fungal keratitis at Wills Eye Hospital, Philadelphia, Pennsylvania. Cornea 2000; 19:307–12.
268. Taravella MJ, Johnson DW, Petty JG, Keyser RB, Foster CS, Lundberg BE. Infectious posterior scleritis caused by Pseudallescheria boydii. Clinicopathologic findings. Ophthalmology 1997; 104:1312–6.
269. Thakur SK, Sah SP, Badhu BP. Oculosporidiosis in eastern Nepal: a report of five cases. Southeast Asian J Trop Med Public Health 2002; 33:362–4.
270. Theodore FH. Etiology and diagnosis of fungal postoperative endophthalmitis. Ophthalmology 1978; 85:327–40.

271. Theodore FH. Mycotic Endophthalimitis After Cataract Surgery. Int Ophthalmol Clin 1964; 32:861–81.
272. Theodore FH, Littman ML, Almeda E. Endophthalmitis following catarct extraction due to Neurospora sitophila, a so-called nonpathogenic fungus. Am J Ophthalmol 1962; 53:35–9.
273. Theodorides E, Coutrolikos D. Two cases of blastomycosis of the conjunctiva. Trans Greek Ophthalmol Soc 1947; 74145–80.
274. Thibierge G, Chaillous J. Sporotrichose gommense disseminee avec lesions oculaires: Iritis et retinite. Clin Ophtalmol Paris 1914; 6:126–28.
275. Thomas PA. Current perspectives on ophthalmic mycoses. Clin Microbiol Rev (2003; 16:730–97.
276. Thomas PA. Fungal infections of the cornea. Eye 2003; 17:852–62.
277. Thygeson P, Okumoto M. Keratomycosis: a preventable disease. Trans Am Acad Ophthalmol Otolaryngol 1974; 78:OP433–9.
278. Toala P, Schroeder SA, Daly AK, Finland M. Candida at Boston City Hospital. Clinical and epidemiological characteristics and susceptibility to eight antimicrobial agents. Arch Intern Med 1970; 126:983–9.
279. Van Buren JM. Septic retinitis due to Candida albicans. AMA Arch Pathol 1958; 65:137–46.
280. Van Metre TE Jr, Maumenee AE. Specific Ocular Uveal Lesions In Patients With Evidence Of Histoplasmosis. Arch Ophthalmol 1964; 71:314–24.
281. Veirs ER. Lacrimal Disorders. St. Louis: C.V. Mosby, 1976.
282. Vemuganti GK, Garg P, Gopinathan U, Naduvilath TJ, John RK, Buddi R, Rao GN. Evaluation of agent and host factors in progression of mycotic keratitis: A histologic and microbiologic study of 167 corneal buttons. Ophthalmology 2002; 109:1538–46.
283. Veress B, Malik OA, el-Tayeb AA, el-Daoud S, Mahgoub ES, el-Hassan AM. Further observations on the primary paranasal aspergillus granuloma in the Sudan: a morphological study of 46 cases. Am J Trop Med Hyg 1973; 22:765–72.
284. Vida L, Moel SA. Systemic North American blastomycosis with orbital involvement. Am J Ophthalmol 1974; 77:240–2.
285. Vieira-Dias D, Sena CM, Orefice F, Tanure MA, Hamdan JS. Ocular and concomitant cutaneous sporotrichosis. Mycoses 1997; 40:197–201.
286. Vukovic Z, Bobic-Radovanovic A, Latkovic Z, Radovanovic Z. An epidemiological investigation of the first outbreak of rhinosporidiosis in Europe. J Trop Med Hyg 1995; 98:333–7.
287. Walinder PE, Kock E. Endogenous fungus endophthalmitis. Acta Ophthalmol (Copenh) 1971; 49:263–72.
288. Watanabe J, Hori H, Tanabe K, Nakamura Y. Phylogenetic association of Pneumocystis carinii with the 'Rhizopoda/Myxomycota/Zygomycota group' indicated by comparison of 5S ribosomal RNA sequences. Mol Biochem Parasitol 1989; 32:163–7.
289. Watanabe J, Nakata K, Nashimoto H, Ikeda H. Cloning and characterization of a repetitive sequence from Pneumocystis carinii. Parasitol Res 1992; 78:23–7.
290. Watson PG. The sclera and systemic disorders. Edinburgh, New York: Butterworth-Heinemann, 2004.
291. Weber JC, Schlaegel TF Jr. Delayed skin-test reactivity of uveitis patients. Influence of age and diagnosis. Am J Ophthalmol 1969; 67:732–7.
292. Weingeist TA, Font RL, Phelps CD, Zimmerman LE. Ocular involvement by Histoplasma capsulatum. Invest Ophthalmol Vis Sci 1979; 18(Suppl):192.
293. Weinstein AJ, Johnson EH, Moellering RC Jr. Candida endophthalmitis. A complication of candidemia. Arch Intern Med 1973; 132:749–52.
294. Weishaar PD, Flynn HW Jr, Murray TG, Davis JL, Barr CC, Gross JG, Mein CE, McLean WC Jr, Killian JH. Endogenous Aspergillus endophthalmitis. Clinical features and treatment outcomes. Ophthalmology 1998; 105:57–65.
295. Weiss C, Perry IH, Shevky MC. Infection of the human eye with Cryptococcus neoformans (Torula histolytica: Cryptococcus hominis) – A Clinical and Experimental Study with a New Diagnostic Method. Arch Ophthamol 1948; 39:739–51.
296. Wilhelmus KR, Jones DB. Curvularia keratitis. Trans Am Ophthalmol Soc (2001; 99:111–30; discussion 130–2.
297. Wilhelmus KR, Robinson NM. Infectious crystalline keratopathy caused by Candida albicans. Am J Ophthalmol 1991; 112:322–5.
298. Wilkinson CP. Presumed ocular histoplasmosis. Am J Ophthalmol 1976; 82:140–2.
299. Willett FM, Weiss A. Coccidiodomycosis in Southern California: Report of a new endemic area with a review of 100 cases. Ann Intern Med 1945; 23:349.
300. Williamson J, Gordon AM, Wood R, Dyer AM, Yahya OA. Fungal flora of the conjunctival sac in health and disease. Influence of topical and systemic steroids. Br J Ophthalmol 1968; 52:127–37.
301. Wilson DE, Mann JJ, Bennett JE, Utz JP. Clinical features of extracutaneous sporotrichosis. Medicine (Baltimore) 1967; 46:265–79.
302. Wilson LA, Ahearn DG, Jones DB, Sexton RR. Fungi from the normal outer eye. Am J Ophthalmol 1969; 67:52–6.
303. Witherspoon CD, Kuhn F, Owens SD, White MF, Kimble JA. Endophthalmitis due to Sporothrix schenckii after penetrating ocular injury. Ann Ophthalmol 1990; 22:385–8.
304. Wogan GN. Mycotoxins. Annu Rev Pharmacol 1975; 15: 437–51.
305. Wolter JR. Endogenous fungus endophthalmitis caused by Candida albicans. Arch Ophthalmol 1962; 68:337–40.
306. Wolter JR. Pityrosporum species associated with dacryoliths: in obstructive dacryocystitis. Trans Am Ophthalmol Soc 1977; 75:428–35.
307. Wolter JR, Deitz MR. Candidiasis of the lacrimal sac. Am J Ophthalmol 1963; 55:153–5.
308. Wolter JR, Stratford T, Harrell ER. Cast-like fungus obstruction of the nasolacrimal duct; report of a case. AMA Arch Ophthalmol 1956; 55:320–2.
309. Wong TY, Ng TP, Fong KS, Tan DT. Risk factors and clinical outcomes between fungal and bacterial keratitis: a comparative study. Clao J 1997; 23:275–81.
310. Wong VG. Focal choroidopathy in experimental ocular histoplasmosis. Trans Am Ophthalmol Soc 1972; 70:615–30.
311. Wong VG, Kirkpatrick CH. Immune reconstitution in keratoconjunctivitis and superficial candidiasis. The role of immunocompetent lymphocyte transfusion and transfer factor. Arch Ophthalmol 1974; 92:335–9.
312. Wood TR. Ocular coccidioidomycosis. Report of a case presenting as Parinaud's oculoglandular syndrome. Am J Ophthalmol 1967; 64(Suppl):587–90.
313. Woods AC, Wahlen HE. The probable role of benign histoplasmosis in the etiology of granulomatous uveitis. Am J Ophthalmol 1960; 49:205–20.
314. Yohai RA, Bullock JD, Aziz AA, Markert RJ. Survival factors in rhino-orbital-cerebral mucormycosis. Surv Ophthalmol 1994; 39:3–22.

315. Zakka KA, Foos RY, Brown WJ. Intraocular coccidioidomycosis. Surv Ophthalmol 1978; 22:313–21.
316. Zimmerman LE, Rappaport H. Occurrence of Cryptococcosis in patients with malignant disease of reticuloendothelial system. Am J Clin Pathol 1954; 24:1050–72.
317. Zinsser H, Joklik WK. Zinsser Microbiology. Norwalk, CT: Appleton & Lange, 1992.
318. Zuger A, Louie E, Holzman RS, Simberkoff MS, Rahal JJ. Cryptococcal disease in patients with the acquired immunodeficiency syndrome. Diagnostic features and outcome of treatment. Ann Intern Med 1986; 104:234–40.

12

Protozoal Infections

Mary K. Klassen-Fischer and Ronald C. Neafie
Armed Forces Institute of Pathology, Washington, D.C., U.S.A.

INTRODUCTION

Protozoa are single-celled eukaryotic microorganisms. Certain species cause disease of the eye or periocular tissues either by direct infection or by the indirect effect of vascular complications.

TOXOPLASMOSIS

General Remarks

Toxoplasmosis is a common and usually asymptomatic infection caused by the protozoan *Toxoplasma gondii.* In 1923, Janku described a retinal macular coloboma of a 11-month-old child, but it was not until the late-1930s when *T. gondii* organisms were isolated from a child with congenital toxoplasmosis and similar retinal lesions (47,82). *Toxoplasma* was transmitted to laboratory animals, and toxoplasmosis was recognized as a widespread disease affecting humans (82). In 1952, Wilder described organisms indistinguishable from *T. gondii* in 53 eyes from adults, who had been previously diagnosed histopathologically as having tuberculous choroiditis or syphilis (82). Subsequently, 21 of these patients were found to have positive serology for *T. gondii* (46). These findings led to the recognition that focal retinochoroidal scarring in adults is most likely due to toxoplasmosis.

Parasite Morphology

T. gondii occurs in human tissue in two stages, tachyzoites and bradyzoites. Tachyzoites are round, ovoid, or crescent-shaped, up to 5 μm in length, and lie free in the tissue or occur in groups. Tachyzoites have a well-defined nucleus and stain well with hematoxylin and eosin (H&E) (Fig. 1). Bradyzoites are nearly identical to tachyzoites, but are always within cysts. They also stain well with H&E (Fig. 2).

Epidemiology, Life Cycle, and Transmission

T. gondii infection occurs worldwide. Approximately 10% of children born to mothers infected by *T. gondii* during pregnancy (as evidenced by seroconversion) become infected. Cats are the preferred primary host of *T. gondii*. They have a brief illness, but shed large numbers of oocysts in feces (35). The extra intestinal cycle occurs in over 300 species of warm-blooded animals, including humans, who are infected by ingesting food contaminated with oocysts or undercooked meat containing bradyzoites. Tachyzoites are released in the lumen of the gastrointestinal tract, pass through the intestinal wall, and become disseminated. *T. gondii* actively crosses nonpermissive biological barriers such as the intestine, the blood–brain barrier, and the placenta, thereby gaining access to tissues where it invades cells and replicates to cause severe disease (3). In acute infection, tachyzoites multiply rapidly to form intracellular groups. Cell lysis may occur with release of organisms to parasitize other cells. In chronic infection, bradyzoites multiply slowly to form an intracellular "cyst" that may contain hundreds of parasites. The nucleus of the host cell may be marginalized or destroyed.

Clinical Features

Acute infection may be asymptomatic, may cause a febrile illness associated with lymphadenopathy, or may cause encephalitis in an immunocompromised host (35). Retinochoroiditis is an unusual sequel of acute infection. In contrast to traditional teaching, evidence suggests that most individuals with ocular toxoplasmosis were infected postnatally (43). Most infants with congenital toxoplasmosis have no symptoms at birth, but many will have retinal disease or neurological abnormalities later in life (40,49). Among untreated patients with congenital toxoplasmosis, up to 85% develop retinochoroiditis during childhood and up to 100% by adulthood (40,71).

Clinical symptoms of retinochoroiditis include blurred vision, floaters, pain, and discomfort. Examination may show one or more foci of active retinal inflammation. Involvement of tissues adjacent to the optic disc may cause inflammation of the optic

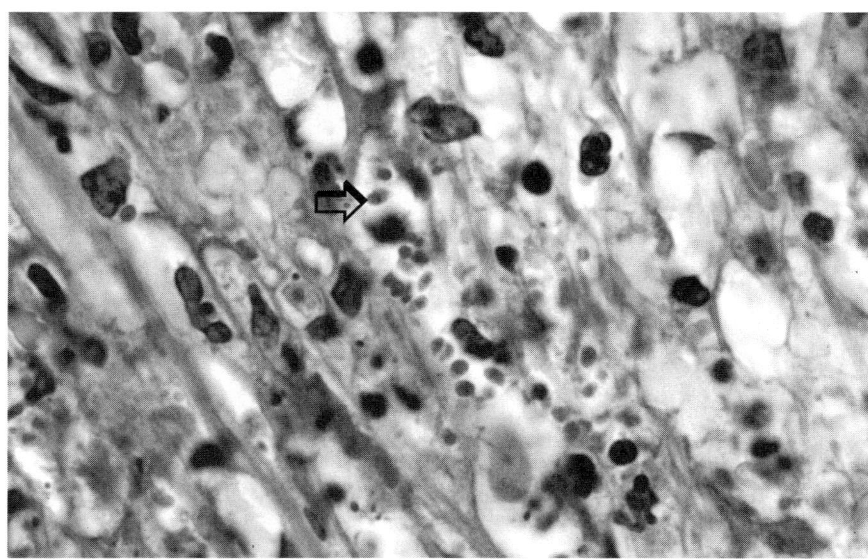

Figure 1 *Toxoplasma gondii* tachyzoites (*arrow*) lie free in inflamed choroid. Most are ovoid and have a prominent nucleus (hematoxylin and eosin, ×1,035).

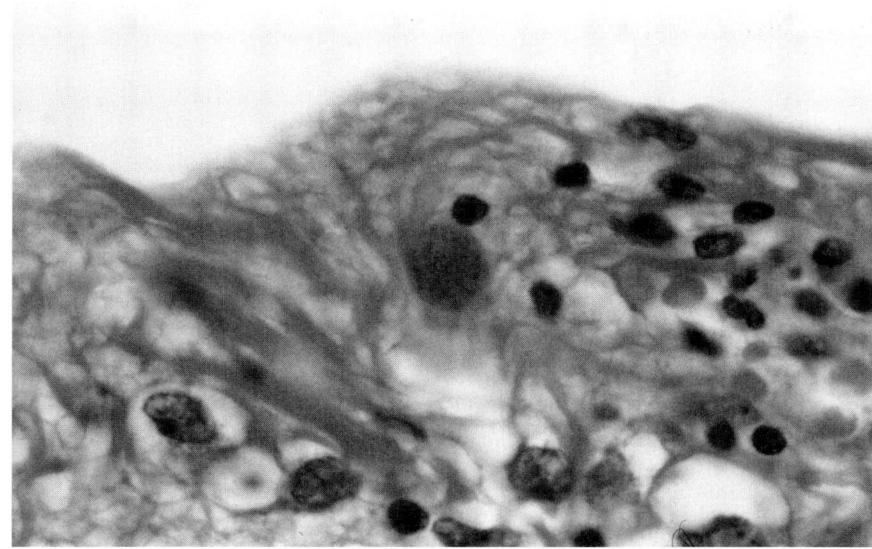

Figure 2 *Toxoplasma gondii* cyst filled with bradyzoites within retina. Individual bradyzoite cell boundaries are indistinct (hematoxylin and eosin, ×1,035).

nerve head. A lesion at the macula causes loss of central vision (75). In most cases inflammation gradually resolves, leaving a quiescent scar (57). A focus of active retinal inflammation may sometimes be present adjacent to an area of retinochoroidal scarring. The scars from which recurrent toxoplasmic retinochoroiditis arise may result from remote, acquired infections in many cases, rather than the residua of congenital infections as is commonly assumed (43). Deep punctate retinitis is a rare variant that may occur in association with a clear vitreous, which may later develop into the typical clinical picture (24). Retinal detachment and retinal hemorrhage are unusual complications (7).

Toxoplasmosis is a rare cause of neuroretinitis, a distinct clinical entity consisting of moderate to severe visual loss, optic nerve head edema, macular exudate in a stellate pattern, and variable vitreous inflammation (32). Recurrent episodes of neuroretinitis distinguish toxoplasmosis from idiopathic neuroretinitis, which is usually a monophasic illness. The differential diagnosis includes postviral, idiopathic, or other acute infectious causes.

Signs of inflammation may also be observed in the vitreous (where precipitates may be deposited upon the posterior vitreous face) or in the anterior chamber. Intravitreal fibrosis may cause retinal tears and retinal detachment. Other clinical signs that may develop include segmental periarteritis, retinal and vitreous hemorrhage, choroidal neovascularization, retinal branch artery occlusion, retinochoroidal anastomoses, and scleritis (23,31,50,74,81). Secondary cataract and glaucoma may also occur.

Congenital ocular toxoplasmosis presenting in childhood may interfere with the development of the eye and result in a different spectrum of clinical signs including optic atrophy, microphthalmia, and cataract. The differential diagnosis includes other infections (tuberculous or syphilitic choroiditis, candidiasis, cytomegalic inclusion disease, neonatal *Herpes simplex*, nocardiosis, cryptococcosis, and toxocariasis), Coats disease, retinal pigment epithelium (RPE) hypertrophy, retinoblastoma, traumatic choroidoretinal scarring, vitelliruptive macular dystrophy, familial macular coloboma, and Aicardi syndrome.

Diagnosis

The clinical characteristics, positive anti-*Toxoplasma* serology, and response to treatment are the usual bases for the diagnosis of toxoplasmic retinochoroiditis. A significantly higher antibody level in the aqueous humor than in the serum indicates a local immune response and is diagnostic (37). Increased anti-*Toxoplasma* IgM antibodies are indicative of recent acquired infection and provide evidence that focal retinochoroiditis occurring de novo is a sequel to recent acute toxoplasmosis. One may also make the diagnosis by histologic identification of the organism in enucleation specimens. Newer diagnostic techniques use detection of parasite DNA (44).

Histopathology

The histopathologic changes are similar in the enucleated eyes of adults with immunodeficiency and in the eyes of infants who have succumbed to congenital toxoplasmosis. The most common finding is retinochoroidal necrosis and necrotizing vasculitis that may be posterior, equatorial, or peripheral. The only recognizable retinal elements within the central necrotic area are karyolytic retinal cells. The surrounding inflammatory cell infiltrate is comprised of lymphocytes, plasma cells, epithelioid cells, multinucleated giant cells, and occasional eosinophils. Intraretinal dystrophic calcification may occasionally develop. *T. gondii* organisms may be seen on sections stained with H&E, mostly in the necrotic areas, but also sometimes in adjacent intact areas. Parasites are rarely present in ocular tissues other than the retina and choroid. The subjacent choroid is usually necrotic and surrounded by an infiltration of lymphocytes and plasma cells. A zone of relatively uninflamed sclera may separate the retinochoroidal lesion from a more superficial focus of scleral inflammatory change (74). The adjacent intact retina may show nonspecific chronic inflammatory changes including perivascular lymphocytic infiltration, clusters of mononuclear cells on the internal limiting membrane, edema, gliosis, and neuronal degeneration. The anterior segment may show nonspecific uveitis.

Pathogenesis

The pathogenesis and clinical presentation of toxoplasmosis vary depending on whether the infection is acquired congenitally or later in life, with the function of the host's immune system and the virulence of the strain. The outcome of congenital toxoplasmosis depends on gestational age at the time of maternal infection. If maternal infection occurs early in pregnancy, the rate of transmission to the fetus is low, but the disease is more severe. If maternal infection occurs during the last month of pregnancy, the rate of transmission is high, but the infection is subclinical in infancy. In most cases, pre- or postnatal parasitemia results in parasites in the retina where they may then remain dormant (26,56). Parasites may also remain dormant in brain, heart, or skeletal muscle (68), attributable to the CNS barrier to diffusion of antibodies (35) or to the low cell turnover rate. Later in life, parasitemia may occur following release of organisms from various tissues (70,71).

In persons with normal immune function, released bradyzoites are inactivated. The most common theory to explain the tissue destruction in the retina caused by *T. gondii* is that it is due to the host inflammatory response to the release of free parasites (35).

There are a number of *T. gondii* surface protein antigens, some of which engender humoral immune responses and some of which participate in antibody-dependent complement-mediated cell lysis and cell-mediated immune responses. Individual variations in immune responses to surface antigens may dictate the severity and frequency of recurrent ocular inflammation. There is a positive correlation between the size of the ocular lesions and serum level of immunoglobulin A (IgA) specific for tachyzoite-derived glycoinositolphospholipids (65).

Toxoplasma gondii strain variation in virulence is also likely to be a significant factor in predicting disease severity. Enhanced migration is associated with virulent strains of *Toxoplasma*, suggesting that this phenotype contributes to pathogenesis (3).

Macrophages and T lymphocytes are responsible for killing or halting the reproduction of *T. gondii* parasites in tissue because of lymphokine production by T lymphocytes stimulated by *T. gondii* antigen (6). Although macrophages from a host whose lymphocytes have not been exposed to *T. gondii* are able to engulf the parasites, they are not able to kill them because the resulting parasitophorous vacuole fails to fuse with lysosomes in the cytoplasm. By contrast, if the parasites are damaged, killed, or coated with antibody, phagolysosomes form in the macrophage and are then rapidly broken down and excreted. Active phagocytosis and killing of organisms by macrophages is accompanied by a release of acid hydrolases and other enzymes that may destroy adjacent normal cells and contribute to tissue damage. The T cells that infiltrate the eyes of patients with recurrent ocular toxoplasmosis are specific for *T. gondii*, a finding that supports their involvement in the local inflammatory response (29).

Cyst rupture in the retina may cause a hypersensitivity reaction to *T. gondii* antigen, which gives rise to the characteristic granulomatous inflammatory response (35). Subcutaneous inoculation of *T. gondii* antigen causes a delayed hypersensitivity reaction in severely infected patients. However, systemic immunity to *T. gondii* abrogates the acute severe inflammatory response in the retina that otherwise occurs following direct retinal inoculation by *T. gondii*. Indices of both humoral and cell-mediated immunity against retinal antigens are increased in a proportion of individuals with active toxoplasmic retinochoroiditis (61). It is therefore possible that in certain cases autoimmune mechanisms will contribute to the pathogenesis of the retinal inflammatory change.

Retinal damage may be due to replicating *T. gondii* organisms, the accompanying inflammatory response by a range of different mechanisms, or both. In persons who are immunodeficient due to human immunodeficiency virus (HIV) infection or other causes of impaired T-cell function, replication of tachyzoites is unchecked and leads to retinal damage directly in the absence of a significant inflammatory response (42). In such cases, the retinal damage may result from cytolytic and necrotizing actions of the parasite. Recurrent toxoplasmosis in patients receiving systemic corticosteroid therapy is uncommon (58).

AFRICAN TRYPANOSOMIASIS

General Remarks

Trypanosomes are flagellate, motile protozoa transmitted to a range of mammals through arthropod vectors. African trypanosomiasis, or African sleeping sickness, is caused by *Trypanosoma brucei gambiense* and *Trypanosoma brucei rhodesiense*, and they are transmitted by the bite of tsetse flies. Several mammals serve as reservoir hosts for *T. b. gambiense* and are of great significance in transmission to humans.

Parasite Morphology

T. b. gambiense and *T. b. rhodesiense* are morphologically indistinguishable. These trypanosomes are in the flagellate stage in blood and CSF. The flagellate form is polymorphic and 14–33 μm by 1.5–3.5 μm. They have a small, spherical, subterminal kinetoplast, large centrally placed nucleus, an undulating membrane, and at the anterior end a long free flagellum (Fig. 3).

Epidemiology, Life Cycle, and Transmission

T. b. gambiense infections occur in west and central Africa and Angola; *T. b. rhodesiense* infections occur in eastern and southern Africa with 300,000–500,000 people estimated to be infected per year. In some areas, the prevalence is as high as 20% to 50%. African trypanosomiasis is transmitted by species of *Glossina*, the tsetse fly. After the fly takes a blood meal from an infected mammal, parasites multiply, go through several developmental stages and migrate to the salivary glands. When the fly bites another mammal, infective trypanomastigotes are inoculated. The parasites multiply at the site of the bite for 1 to 2 days, before spreading to the host's blood and extracellular fluids such as CSF. Some enter the interstitium of tissues, especially lymph nodes and brain, where they multiply rapidly. Trypanosomes are rarely transmitted by laboratory accident, blood transfusion or organ transplantation.

Clinical Features

The clinical features of African trypanosomiasis are similar for both species, but are more acute in *T. b. rhodesiense* infections. African trypanosomiasis begins with inflammation at the site of the bite that may develop into a chancre, followed by headache, malaise, fever and lymphadenopathy. Eventually there is invasion of the CNS, with increasing somnolence, coma, and death. The prevailing view is that the disease is invariably fatal without anti-trypanosomal drug treatment. However, there have also been intriguing reports of wide variations in disease severity as well as evidence of asymptomatic carriers of trypanosomes (76).

The principal ocular finding is urticarial swelling of the eyelids, often with enlarged preauricular lymph nodes. Stromal keratitis, iritis or choroiditis may also develop (69).

Diagnosis

Diagnostic techniques include serologic screening and microscopic identification of the parasite in blood, CSF, chancre fluid or lymph node aspirate (14,17). Trypanosomes can sometimes be present in the aqueous humor.

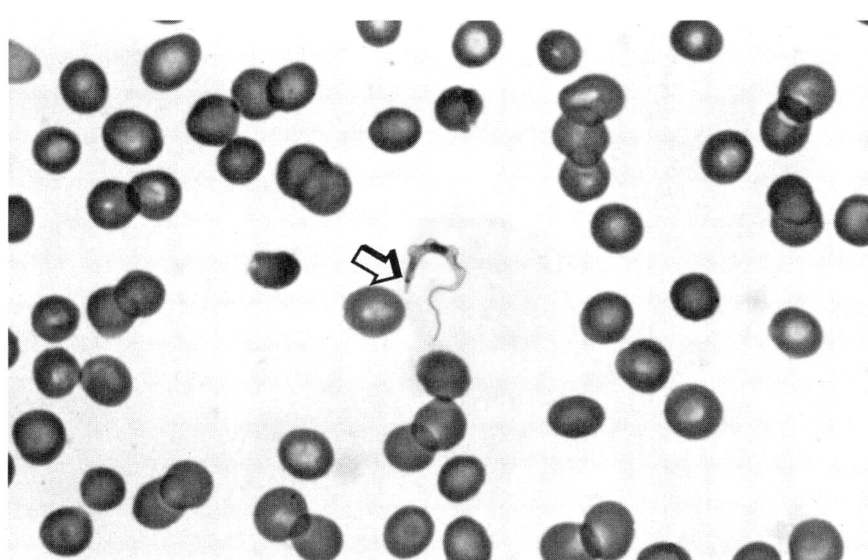

Figure 3 *Trypansoma brucei rhodesiense* flagellate in thin blood film. The flagellate has a small, spherical, subterminal kinetoplast (*arrow*), large centrally placed nucleus, an undulating membrane, and a long free flagellum at the anterior end (Giemsa, ×1,035).

Histopathology

In animal models, histologic sections of the eye and other tissues show vasculitis, thrombosis, acute or chronic inflammation, focal necrosis, or edema (59).

Pathogenesis

Trypanosomes are able to resist the host's immune response through rapid and repeated surface antigenic variation (25,76). In animal models, intravenous inoculation of parasites results in chronic panophthalmitis and eyelid swelling due to vasculitis and inflammatory edema (59).

AMERICAN TRYPANOSOMIASIS

General Remarks

Central and South American trypanosomiasis, also known as Chagas disease, is predominantly a disease of childhood caused by *Trypanosoma cruzi.* The organism is usually transmitted through defecation of biting reduvid bugs, but may also be transmitted by blood transfusion (27).

Parasite Morphology

In peripheral blood, the organism is in the trypomastigote stage, which is frequently C or U shaped. It is 16 to 22 μm in length and has a large central nucleus, a narrow undulating membrane, a large, spherical kinetoplast at the posterior end and a long free flagellum at the anterior end (Fig. 4). When the parasites invade cells, they transform into the amastigote stage. Amastigotes stain readily in histologic sections of brain or muscle, are 3 to 5 μm in diameter and have a nucleus and a rod-shaped kinteoplast (Fig. 5).

Epidemiology, Life Cycle, and Transmission

Chagas disease occurs exclusively in the Americas, from the southern United States to southern Argentina. It is one of the most significant endemic disease in Latin America where approximately 11 million people are infected. Triatomid bugs, or "kissing bugs," live in thatch and in the cracks of trees and houses and feed on sleeping humans at night. When the bug feeds on the blood of infected mammals, including humans and the numerous domestic and wild mammals that serve as reservoir hosts, it ingests trypomastigotes, which develop in the bug's gut. When the bug takes a blood meal, infective forms excreted in its feces are introduced into the bite or nearby mucosal tissue, such as conjunctiva. Infective trypomastigotes enter histiocytes, transform into amastigotes, and multiply. Within several days, parasitized cells rupture and release amastigotes, which then invade other cells. Some amastigotes transform into trypomastigotes that can circulate through blood or lymph channels to other cells, particularly myocardial, neuroglial, microglial, and reticuloendothelial cells, and to adipose tissue, where they can transform back into amastigotes. *T. cruzi* can also be transmitted congenitally, or through blood and blood-product transfusions, needle sharing, organ transplantation, and laboratory accidents.

Clinical Features

American trypanosomiasis starts with a reduvid bug bite. If the bite occurs in the periorbital region, it may lead to intense unilateral eyelid swelling, periorbital edema spreading onto the face, and conjunctivitis, constituting the diagnostic Romaña sign (Fig. 6) (77). Submandibular lymphadenopathy

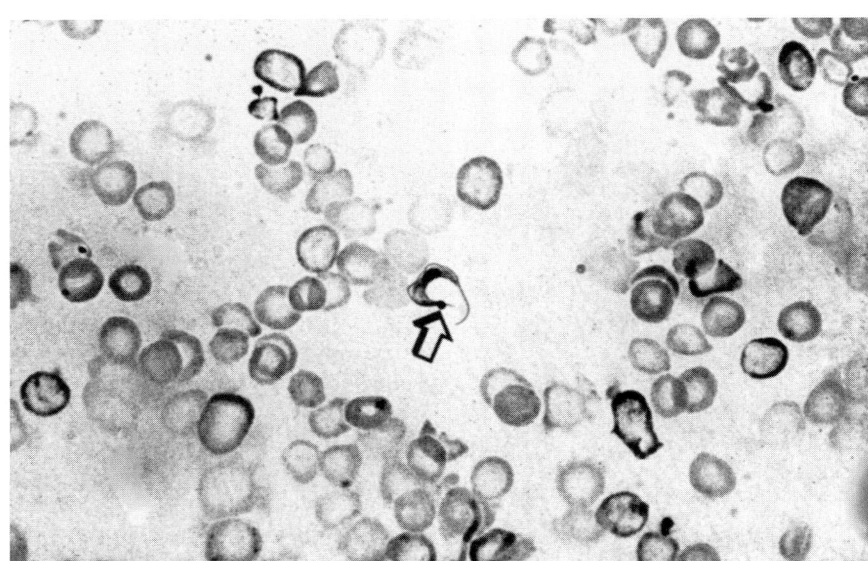

Figure 4 *Trypanosoma cruzi* C-shaped trypomastigote in thin blood film. It has a large nucleus, a narrow undulating membrane, a large spherical kinetoplast (*arrow*) at the posterior end, and a long free flagellum at the anterior end (Giemsa, ×1,035).

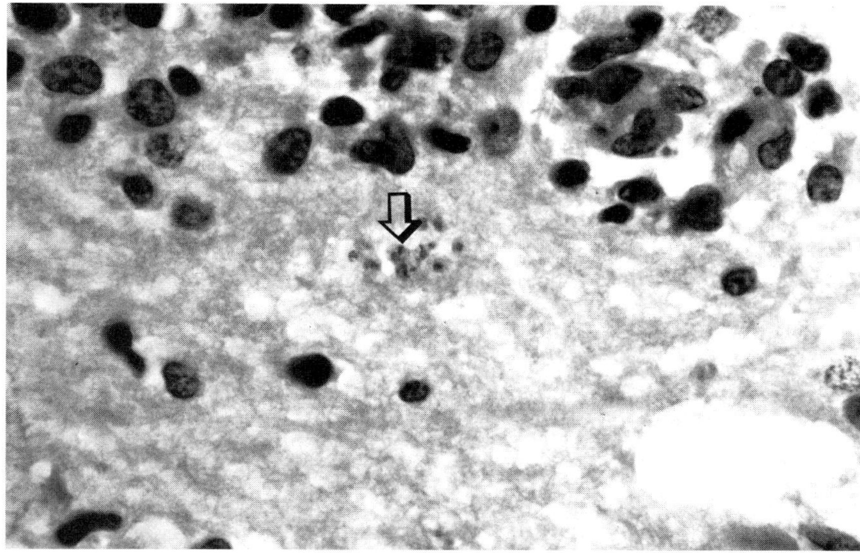

Figure 5 *Trypanosoma cruzi* amastigotes in brain. Each organism has a spherical nucleus and a rod-shaped kinetoplast (*arrow*), although frequently both are not observed in the same plane (hematoxylin and eosin, ×1,035).

often accompanies eyelid swelling. Intraocular lesions have not been reported (69). Patients with chronic Chagas disease may have alterations in the autonomic system that result in ocular findings, such as greater pupil diameter, irregularity of the pupil border, and altered response to dilating agents (66). Another reported autonomic disturbance is decreased ability to maintain intraocular pressure (IOP) with postural changes (55). Systemic disease ensues, often leading to a fatal cardiomyopathy if untreated. Exacerbations of *T. cruzi* infection may occur in patients receiving immunosuppressive therapy and for those with AIDS (77).

Diagnosis

Diagnostic techniques for Chagas disease include microscopic identification of the parasite in peripheral blood smears and serologic detection of specific antibodies (27). New serological and molecular biological techniques have improved the diagnosis of chronic infection (77).

Histopathology

Ocular lesions are seldom biopsied, but trypomastigotes may be found in wet mount preparations of chagomas. Histologic sections of skin typically show infiltration of the dermis and subcutaneous tissue

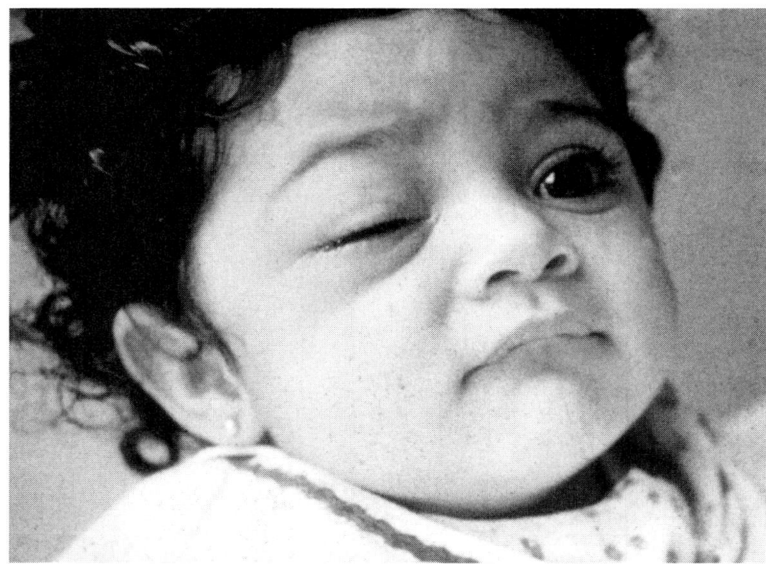

Figure 6 Romaña sign in child with Chagas disease. There is unilateral conjunctivitis, palpebral and periorbital edema, and preauricular lymphadenopathy.

by polymorphonuclear leukocytes (PMNs) monocytes, and lymphocytes.

Pathogenesis

Like African trypanosomes, *T. cruzi* parasites evade the immune response by variation of surface antigens (25). Two clinical forms of the disease are recognized, acute and chronic. During the acute stage, tissue damage is caused by the presence of the parasite. In the chronic stage parasites are few, and TNF, IFNγ, and the interleukins have roles in the pathogenesis. Autoimmune, neurogenic, and microvascular factors may be important in the pathogenesis (77).

LEISHMANIASIS

General Remarks

There are two principal forms of leishmaniasis, cutaneous and visceral. *Leishmania tropica* complex causes cutaneous leishmaniasis, known as oriental sore, in the Old World; and *Leishmania mexicana* complex and *Leishmania brasiliensis* complex cause cutaneous leishmaniasis in the New World. *Leishmania donovani* complex causes visceral leishmaniasis, known as kala-azar. In recent years, however, it has been determined that there is much overlapping among the leishmanial complexes and clinical disease and, for example, any species can cause cutaneous leishmaniasis. Various domestic and wild animals, such as canines and rodents, serve as potential reservoirs for human infection. *Leishmania* protozoa are in the flagellated form while within the sandfly vector (usually *Phlebotomus* sp.) and in the immotile amastigote form in the mammalian host.

Parasite Morphology

Leishmanial amastigotes are morphologically indistinguishable regardless of the species. They are generally ovoid, 2 to 4 μm in diameter, and have a prominent nucleus and a rod-shaped kinetoplast (Fig. 7) (18).

Epidemiology, Life Cycle, and Transmission

Cutaneous leishmaniasis occurs in the Americas from southern Texas to northern Argentina, parts of Africa, India, the Middle East, and the Mediterranean. There are approximately 300,000 cases of cutaneous leishmaniasis per year. Female sandflies (*Phlebotomus* in the East; *Lutzomyia* and *Pyschodogus* in the West) transmit metacyclic promastigotes to a host during a blood meal. Promastigotes transform into amastigotes, which replicate within a parasitophorous vacuole, leading to lysis and cell death. Released daughter amastigotes attach to and penetrate other cells where they continue to multiply. Rarely, transmission is congenital, sexual, occupational, or blood-borne through transfusion or intravenous drug use.

Clinical Features

Cutaneous leishmaniasis occurs at the sites of sandfly bites and thus predominates on exposed skin surfaces. Ocular involvement is rare, and reported cases have mostly affected the eyelids in the form of ulcers or nodules (62). Conjunctival and corneal lesions have also been reported (1,9).

Visceral leishmaniasis is a severe, chronic infection presenting with fever, weight loss, anemia, and

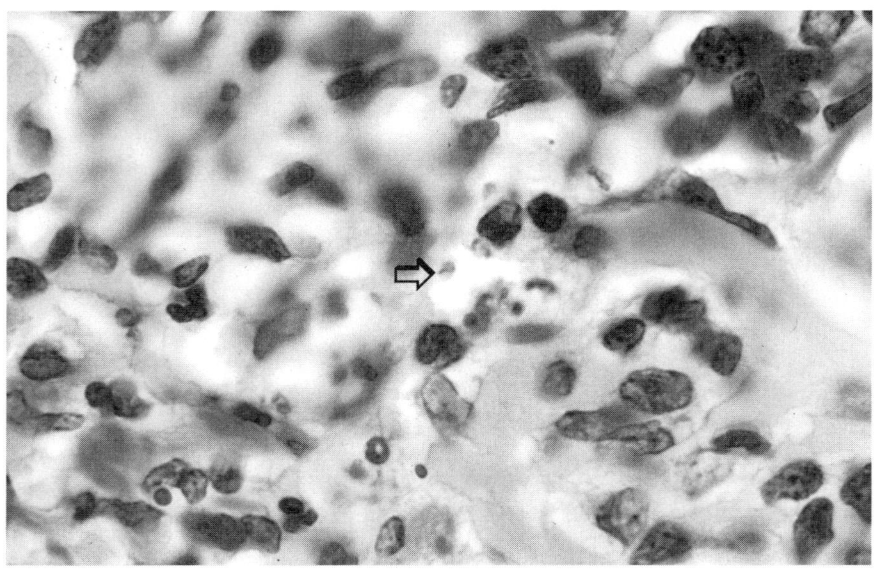

Figure 7 Leishmanial amastigote in skin demonstrating cytoplasm, spherical nucleus, and rod-shaped kinetoplast (*arrow*) (Brown and Hopps, ×1,140).

splenomegaly. Post-kala-azar ocular complications are not usual, but include anterior uveitis that may be complicated by angle-closure glaucoma, conjunctivitis, and blepharitis (22,28).

Diagnosis

The gold standard for the diagnosis of leishmaniasis is microscopic identification of amastigotes in cytologic or histologic preparations. Molecular testing and culture techniques may also be used.

Histopathology

Cutaneous leishmaniasis involving the eyelid is similar to that occurring on any skin surface. At first there are epidermal changes including pseudoepitheliomatous hyperplasia, parakeratosis, epidermal atrophy, and intraepidermal abscesses. In the dermis, there may be many amastigotes and an inflammatory infiltrate of histiocytes, lymphocytes, and plasma cells. The epidermis becomes increasingly hyperplastic and ulcerates. The dermis becomes necrotic and infiltrated by increasing numbers of vacuolated or epithelioid histiocytes, lymphocytes, plasma cells, and giant cells. There may be PMNs in the ulcer bed. As necrotizing or nonnecrotizing granulomas develop, amastigotes decline in number and may be almost impossible to find. As healing takes place, granulation tissue and fibrosis fill the ulcer crater.

Pathogenesis

Amastigotes are often within macrophages, where they multiply by binary fission. Survival within macrophages is attributable to the presence of an anionic lipophosphoglycan on the surface of the parasite that is able to both inactivate superoxide radicals and inhibit lysosomal hydrolases (13,79). Eventual elimination of the amastigotes is due at least in part by the intracellular production of nitric oxide boosted by immunologically determined IFNα and TNFα formation (38,51). The chronic and granulomatous inflammatory response to the amastigotes results in ulceration and cutaneous nodule formation. An allergic response may be the cause of post-kala-azar anterior uveitis (22).

ACANTHAMOEBA INFECTION

General Remarks

Members of the genus *Acanthamoeba* have the capacity to exist either as free-living organisms or as facultative parasites. Species reported to cause corneal infections include *Acanthamoeba castellani*, *Acanthamoeba polyphaga*, *Acanthamoeba culbertson*, *Acanthamoeba rhysodes*, and *Acanthamoeba hatchetti* (80). In spite of the parasite's prevalence, descriptions of *Acanthamoeba* keratitis were rare prior to the first published report in 1974 (60).

Parasite Morphology

Acanthamoeba trophozoites range in size from 10 to 45 μm and are usually uninucleate. The nucleus is distinctive and has a large dense karyosome, a thin, sharply outlined nuclear membrane and sometimes a clear space between the karyosome and the nuclear membrane (Fig. 8). The cytoplasm is foamy and has no specific diagnostic features (21). *Acanthamoeba* cysts are 7 to 15 μm in diameter, and have a foamy cytoplasm. The nucleus is essentially the same as in the trophozoite. Cysts can be identified by the presence of an outer usually wrinkled membrane (Fig. 9). The species of *Acanthamoeba* that infect humans are morphologically indistinguishable and cannot be determined by light microscopy.

Epidemiology, Life Cycle, and Transmission

Whereas earlier infections were associated with trauma, far more are now linked with contact lens use. The infection is more common among men and in those who fail to disinfect the lenses frequently, swim while wearing lenses, or use homemade saline solution. Adoption of disposable contact lenses has not decreased the risk of *Acanthamoeba* keratitis, and concerns remain regarding the effectiveness of some contact-lens disinfectants. The annual incidence during 1985 through 1987 was approximately 1.65 to 2.01 cases per million contact-lens wearers (73). Currently *Acanthamoeba* keratitis is estimated to affect one in every 30,000 contact lens wearers per year.

Acanthamoeba species are ubiquitous, occurring chiefly in stagnant water all over the world. They can withstand a wide range of temperatures, from the heat of a hot tub to nearly freezing swimming water (8,72). The life cycle involves trophozoite and cyst stages, the latter contributing to resistance to pharmacotherapy (60). Humans acquire the parasite by ingestion, inhalation, or contact with mucous membranes. The parasites may cross the nasopharyngeal or pulmonary mucosa then spread by direct extension or hematogenous dissemination to other sites.

Clinical Features

Apart from very few exceptional cases of uveitis that have accompanied CNS disease, the ocular manifestations of *Acanthamoeba* infection are corneal (Fig. 10) and represent direct invasion by exogenous organisms. Infection usually starts with a foreign body sensation. Over a period of weeks, there is cyclical loss and replacement of the corneal epithelium, stromal thinning and inflammation. The inflammatory cell infiltrate often has a characteristically annular configuration because of increased density at the periphery. If untreated, tissue destruction can culminate in corneal perforation and an increased risk for the development of fatal granulomatous amebic

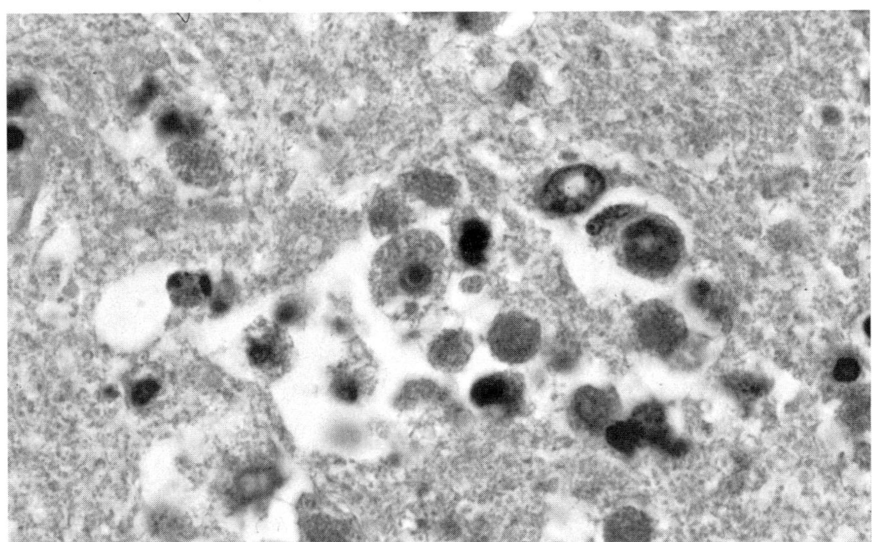

Figure 8 *Acanthamoeba* trophozoite in the brain. It has a foamy cytoplasm and a nucleus with a large spherical karyosome surrounded by a narrow halo (hematoxylin and eosin, ×1,140).

encephalitis. Diagnosis tends to be made later in patients in whom infection is not associated with contact lens wearing than in whom it is, resulting in a worse visual outcome. All patients with unresponsive microbial keratitis, even those without contact lens use, should be evaluated for *Acanthamoeba* (15).

Diagnosis

Laboratory diagnosis of *Acanthamoeba* corneal infection can be difficult. Smears are virtually useless, and scrapes need to reach as deep as is convenient because the viable organisms are mostly underneath the frankly necrotic zones. Diagnosis may require microscopic examination of histopathologic specimens from penetrating keratoplasty (16). When sections are examined by an experienced observer, H&E is the most useful stain for the detection of acanthamoeba keratitis (39). Special stains such as the periodic acid Schiff (PAS) and Gomori methenamine silver may be helpful. False-positive diagnoses may be made with calcofluor white and acridine orange stained slide because of staining of extracellular debris and other material. Some laboratories perform in vitro culture using media supplemented with *Escherichia coli*.

Histopathology

Histopathologic examination of affected corneas generally shows extensive loss of epithelium with absence of the underlying Bowman layer. There may be partial reepithelialization. Stromal necrosis is conspicuous and associated with a marked leukocytic infiltrate. PMNs tend to predominate and, when the

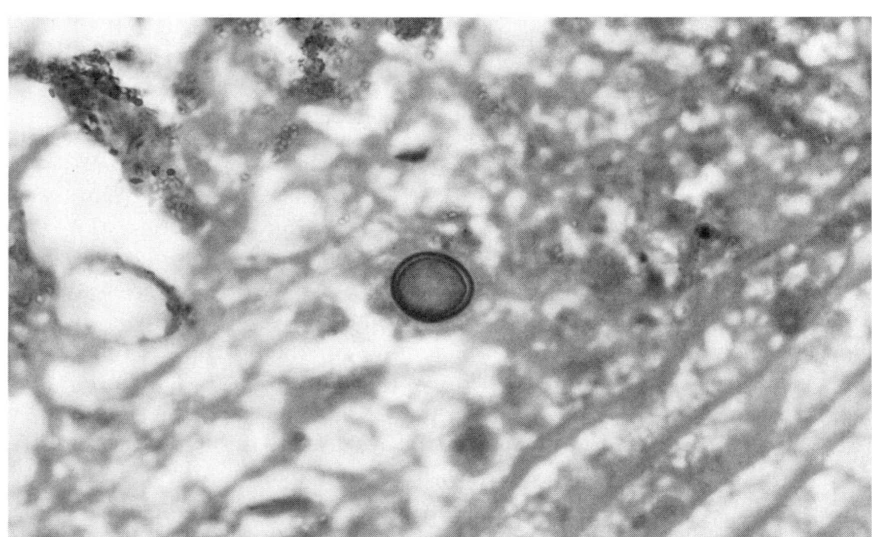

Figure 9 *Acanthamoeba* cyst in necrotic choroid in a case of endophthalmitis. Cysts have an inner membrane (endocyst) and an outer membrane (ectocyst) (Gomori methenamine silver, ×860).

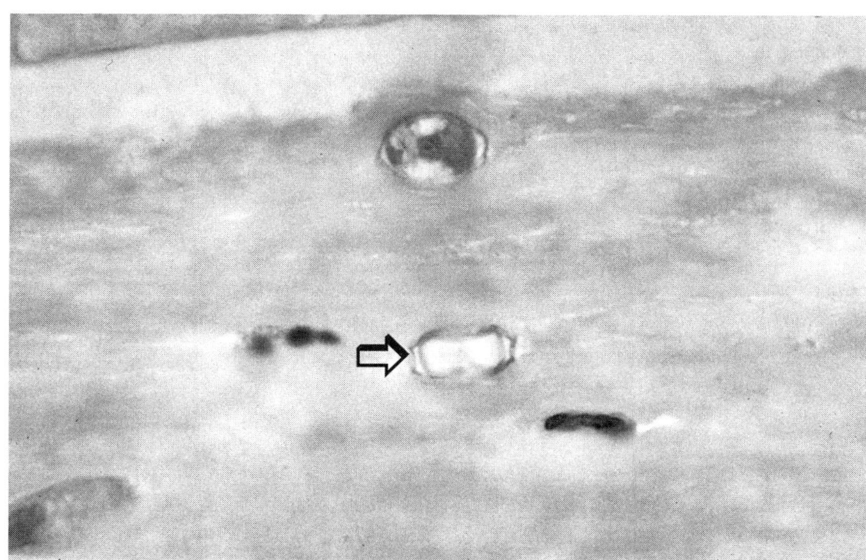

Figure 10 Two *Acanthamoeba* cysts in corneal stroma. Note the large karyosome in the top cyst and the outer wrinkled membrane in the bottom cyst (*arrow*) (hematoxylin and eosin, ×1,140).

infection reaches Descemet membrane, multinucleated giant cells may be seen with precipitates of PMNs and fibrin. Cases requiring enucleation of the globe usually show severe iridocyclitis, which can be granulomatous.

Pathogenesis

Physical trauma may be necessary for trophozoites to penetrate surface epithelium. It may be that contact lens-associated infection is attributable to microtrauma. Activation of the alternative complement pathway may engender the early acute inflammatory response to infection (30). Stromal necrosis is conspicuous and associated with a marked leukocytic infiltrate and it may be caused by ingestion of keratocytes by parasites or release of collagenolytic enzymes by either the parasites themselves or the leukocytic infiltrate (45). Extensive parasitic invasion can occur in the absence of stromal changes. The damage incurred by the inflammatory reaction is perhaps the predominant factor (36). Parasite-related toxic effects on keratocytes may be contributory.

Pathogenicity is a distinct property of certain strains of free-living amoebae and is independent of the circumstances giving rise to infection. Accurate species determination is problematic. Attempts to identify specific strains have thus far been unsuccessful. Clinically relevant isolates differ markedly from nonpathogenic isolates with respect to their physiological properties. In one study of 18 cases of amoeba-associated keratitis in contact lens wearers, 20 strains of free-living amoebae were discriminated based on 18S rDNA sequence similarities, only three of which were shown to be the cause of the keratitis: The virulent strains were identified as *Acanthamoeba polyphaga* and two strains of *Acanthamoeba hatchetti* (80).

ENTAMOEBA INFECTION

General Remarks

A variety of *Entamoeba* species are commensals in the human intestine. Among them *Entamoeba histolytica* can cause enteric disease.

Parasite Morphology

The parasite has a characteristic appearance in stool and tissue. Trophozoites are usually 15 to 25 μm in diameter and have a single nucleus with a tiny central karyosome and fine, beaded peripheral chromatin (Fig. 11). The cytoplasm contains vacuoles and may contain erythrocytes. Cysts are found only in stool specimens and are 10 to 20 μm in diameter and have a thick wall. Mature cysts contain four nuclei each with a central karysome and frequently cigar-shaped bodies in the cytoplasm (20).

Epidemiology, Life Cycle, and Transmission

A host ingests the parasite in contaminated water or food. The parasite is in the cyst form that allows it to escape gastric digestion. In the intestinal mucosa, the cyst walls dissolve and trophozoite forms develop, some of which invade the wall of the intestine. Parasites passed in the feces may contaminate water or food and perpetuate the life cycle.

Clinical Features

The prime disease manifestation is dysentery, the likelihood of which depends on parasite virulence and host debilitation. The parasite can spread to the liver and rarely its adjacent tissues. Peritonitis is the main cause of mortality.

Ocular involvement is extremely rare and includes a single case report of anterior uveitis (41) and exceptional reports of a maculopathy in which retinal hemorrhage and pigment disturbance surround a transparent cyst-like structure in the region of the posterior pole (48). There is also a case report of cutaneous amebiasis of the eyelid extending into the orbit of a 4-month-old with a history of trauma (5).

Diagnosis

A combination of serologic tests with detection of the parasite offers the best approach to diagnosis (78). Detection of serum markers is still only a research tool. The parasite is detected by microscopic examination or stool antigen detection. Culture of the parasite is not a routine clinical laboratory process. Molecular biology-based diagnosis, such as PCR assays that distinguish *Entamoeba* species, may become the technique of choice, but is not practical in many developing countries.

Histopathology

In cutaneous amebiasis, the dermis is hyperemic and infiltrated by lymphocytes, plasma cells, histiocytes, PMNs and sometimes eosinophils. Trophozoites are concentrated over the points of ulceration in adjacent epidermis and in the superficial layers of the ulcer.

Pathogenesis

Studies by TEM reveal degenerated epithelial cells as trophozoites approach, supporting the theory that trophozoites elaborate cytolytic substances. Pore-forming peptides and proteinases that cleave immunoglobulin and complement components secreted by the parasite may contribute to colonic cell lysis. Invasion by trophozoites causes the secretion of cytokines from host cells, leading to an acute inflammatory response.

MICROSPORIDIOSIS

General Remarks

Microspora is a large phylum of over 900 species of obligate intercellular spore-forming protozoa. They were once included in the phylum Sporozoa but research has shown that the microsporidia have no known relationship to other protists. Microsporidial infections are emerging in the HIV/AIDS epidemic. In HIV-infected patients, all three *Encephalitozoon* sp. [*E. hellem*, *E. cuniculi*, and *E.* (formerly *Septata*) *intestinalis*] may cause keratoconjunctivitis (33,34,54). Other microsporidia identified as pathogens in the corneal stroma of AIDS patients include *Nosema ocularum*, *Nosema algerae*, and *Vittaforma corneae* (formerly *Nosema corneum*) (67). *Brachiola* sp., *Brachiola vesicularum*, and *Brachiola* (formerly *Nosema*) *algerae* have been identified in the corneal stroma of patients without HIV infection. There is a case report of a patient with AIDS with disseminated infection due to *Encephalitozoon cuniculi* that involved the conjunctiva (33). There is one case report of keratitis due to *Trachipleistophora anthropopthera* in a man with HIV and one due to *Trachipleistophora hominis* in an immunocompetent patient (63,67).

The first reported cases of ocular microsporidiosis were an 11-year-old Sri Lankan boy and a

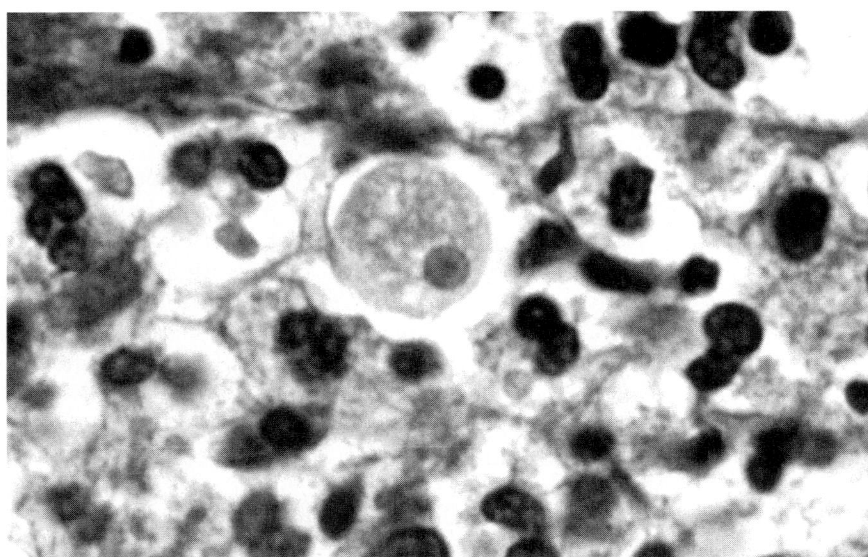

Figure 11 *Entamoeba histolytica* trophozoite in the colon. It has a foamy cytoplasm and a single nucleus with fine beaded chromatin inside the nuclear membrane and with a tiny central karyosome (hematoxylin and eosin, × 2,070).

26-year-old Botswanan woman. The boy presented with necrotizing stromal keratitis after a goat had gored him 6 years earlier (Fig. 12) (2). The woman had a perforated corneal ulcer (64). Both patients were otherwise healthy. The genera could not be determined, and the organisms were named *Microsporidium ceylonensis* and *Microsporidium africanum*, respectively (12).

Parasite Morphology

Histopathologic examination of *M. ceylonensis* shows $3.5 \times 1.5\,\mu m$ refractile ovoid bodies close to Descemet membrane both within macrophages and lying free (Fig. 12) (2). Most microsporidans that cause disease in humans can usually be identified by a dark staining band variously situated in the spore (Fig. 13). By TEM, the coiled tubular cytoplasmic filament and polar vacuole can be identified, confirming the diagnosis.

Clinical Features

Ocular microsporidiosis is second only to gastrointestinal infection as the most common manifestation of microsporidiosis in humans (34). Two types of ocular infection attributed to microsporidia have been observed (11). One type involves the corneal stroma leading to corneal ulceration and suppurative keratitis whereas the other type involves the conjunctival and corneal epithelium and occurs in HIV-positive individuals. Most HIV-infected patients with keratoconjunctivitis due to *Encephalitozoon* sp. present with bilateral conjunctivitis and exhibit a bilateral punctate epithelial keratopathy, leading to decreased visual acuity. The keratoconjunctivitis is often asymptomatic or moderate but can be severe; it rarely leads to corneal ulcers (53).

Diagnosis

Microsporidia should be considered in cases of culture-negative stromal keratitis refractory to medical therapy. Diagnosis of microsporidiosis is established by identification of spores. Originally, diagnosis required TEM, and an ultrastructural examination of corneal tissue may still be useful for determining the species (67). Now microsporidiosis is often diagnosed by light microscopic examination of corneal tissue. Immunofluorescent staining techniques for species differentiation are available only at research laboratories. Cell culture systems are not suitable for routine use. Serological tests detect antibodies to microsporidia, but their sensitivity and specificity are unknown, and they are not suitable for diagnosing microsporidial infections in immunocompromised persons. Recent success in nucleotide sequencing of various microsporidia has now led to the application of new molecular techniques (34).

Histopathology

The histopathologic changes in the cornea include acute and chronic inflammation (53). Stromal vascularization and reparative scarring may be seen. Spores may be seen within epithelial cells, within macrophages or free in the stroma (11).

Pathogenesis

Spores have a polar filament that is discharged through the anterior end and penetrates a suitable host cell. The sporoplasm is injected into the host cell where it undergoes repeated divisions by binary or multiple fissions (10). Disease occurs when a host cell dies and evokes an inflammatory response.

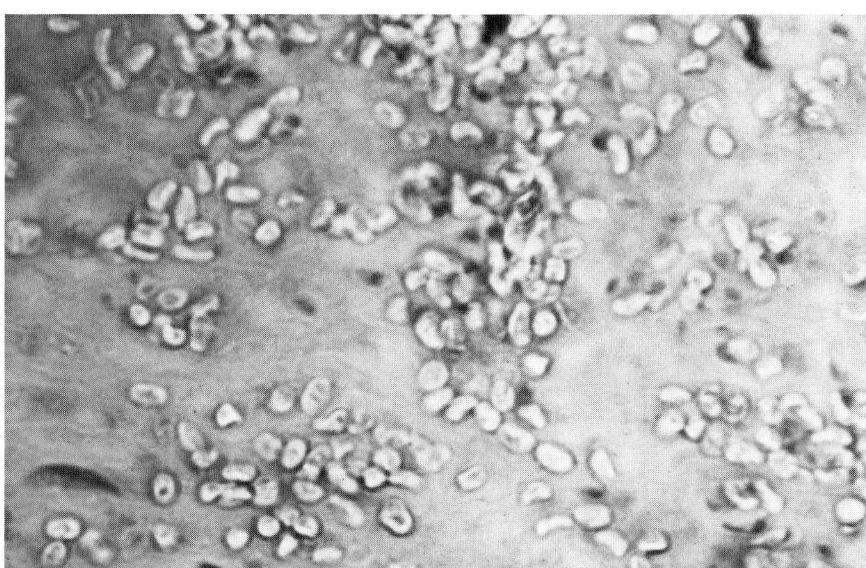

Figure 12 Necrotizing stromal keratitis in 11-year-old Sri Lankan boy. Numerous highly refractile $3.5 \times 1.5\,\mu m$ spores of *Microsporidium ceylonensis* just above Descemet membrane are shown (hematoxylin and eosin, ×2,180).

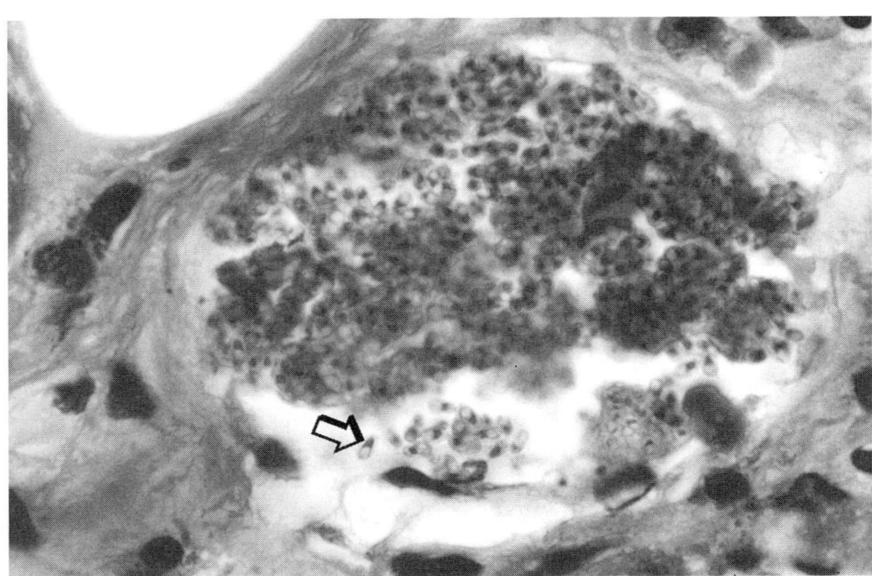

Figure 13 *Pleistophora ronneafiei* spores in muscle of deltoid. Note dark staining band (*arrow*) variously situated in the spore (Giemsa, ×1,005).

MALARIA

General Remarks

Malaria is one of the most prevalent infectious diseases. It threatens more than 40% of the world's population and causes a million deaths per year. *Plasmodium falciparum* causes the most serious form of malaria.

Parasite Morphology

When observed in thin peripheral blood films, erythrocytes infected with *P. falciparum* are of normal size (Fig. 14). Multiple infected erythrocytes are usually frequent, especially in heavy infections. Usually only trophozoites are observed in *P. falciparum* infection. Young ring trophozoites of *P. falciparum* are small (about one-fifth the diameter of an erythrocyte) and may have double chromatin dots. They have a delicate, threadlike line of cytoplasm and may be of various shapes: round, rectangular, flame-shaped or narrow band-shaped. Flattened marginal forms and bridge forms are more common than in other species. Older ring trophozoites contain traces of tiny grains of pigment, which give a yellowish tinge to the cytoplasm. Mature trophozoites have a characteristic small, dense, almost black clump of pigment. Mature schizonts usually contain 8 to 24 very small merozoites. Mature gametocytes are usually crescent or sausage shaped. Schizonts and gametocytes are not usually present in thin blood films.

Epidemiology, Life Cycle, and Transmission

Anopheles mosquitoes transmit malarial parasites to humans in the form of sporozoites, which invade the liver. Infected hepatocytes rupture, releasing merozoites into the blood stream where they invade erythrocytes and become trophozoites. As the trophozoite grows within the erythrocyte, it metabolizes hemoglobin and forms pigment granules. Trophozoites may undergo asexual or sexual division, resulting in schizonts (containing merozoites) or gametocytes, respectively. Merozoites are released into the bloodstream and invade other erythrocytes to begin another round of asexual reproduction. Gametocytes start the sexual reproductive cycle if they are taken up by the bite of an *Anopheles* mosquito.

Clinical Features

Patients with cerebral malaria often have retinal hemorrhages, which may provide visible evidence of vascular lesions involved in the pathogenesis of this condition (52). Subconjunctival hemorrhage develops in a minority of patients. The findings of one study of children with severe malaria supports the hypothesis that retinal signs were related to the cerebral pathophysiology (4). Retinopathy was present in most of those who had cerebral malaria and in many of those who had malarial anemia. In cerebral malaria, retinopathy and papilledema were risk factors for prolonged coma and death. Patients with malaria without brain involvement had better outcomes and less severe retinopathy than those with cerebral malaria. Cranial nerve palsies resulting in disturbed ocular movements have been attributed to vascular occlusion by parasitized erythrocytes; however, there is no histopathological evidence that they are direct manifestations of malaria.

Diagnosis

The gold standard for diagnosing malaria in a living patient is identification of malarial parasites in thick or thin peripheral blood films. Other methods include identifying malarial parasites by fluorescent dyes in a

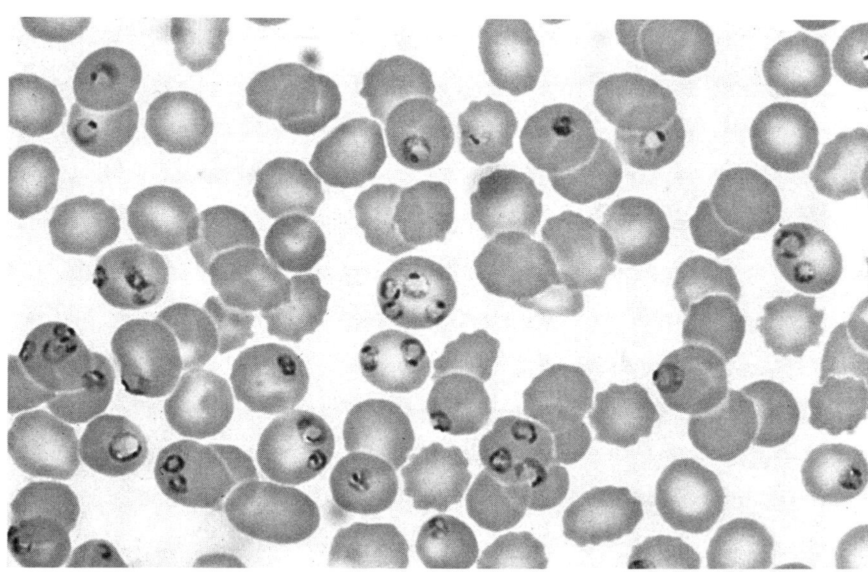

Figure 14 *Plasmodium falciparum* ring trophozoites in normal-sized erythrocytes in thin blood film. Many erythrocytes have multiple parasites, a common feature of *P. falciparum* infection (Giemsa, ×1,140).

capillary centrifuge tube by methods for detecting malarial antigens [enzyme-linked immunosorbent assay, radioimmunoassay and rapid dipstick tests for malarial antigens] and DNA hybridization and PCR tests for parasitic nucleic acid.

Histopathology

Microscopically, masses of erythrocytes fill the lumina of small and medium-sized blood vessels, distending them. Parasitized erythrocytes tend to lie against the endothelial surface (Fig. 15). Anoxia may result in non-specific congestion, edema, microinfarcts, and focal hemorrhage.

Pathogenesis

In *P. falciparum* infection there is a tendency for parasitized erythrocytes to sequestrate within such organs as liver, heart, and brain, where they attach to vascular endothelium leading to hypoxia of cerebral and other tissues, with eventual coma and death (19). This process probably accounts for the ocular complications of *P. falciparum* malaria.

ACKNOWLEDGMENT

The authors acknowledge Jose F. Rodriguez for his technical assistance with the images.

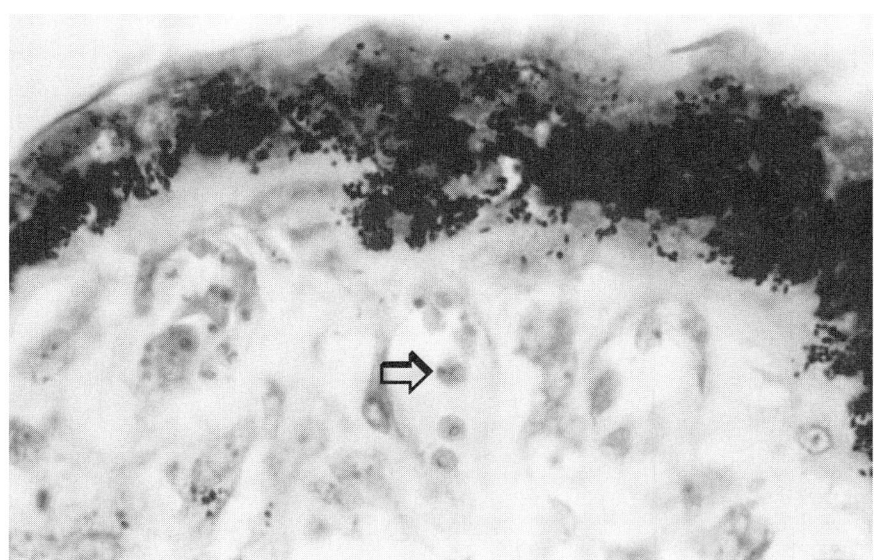

Figure 15 Ocular malaria caused by *Plasmodium falciparum.* Note parasitized erythrocytes (*arrow*) within blood vessels of ciliary process (Giemsa, ×860).

REFERENCES

1. Abrishami M, Soheilian M, Farahi A, Dowlati Y. Successful treatment of ocular leishmaniasis. Eur J Dermatol 2002; 12: 88–9.
2. Ashton N, Wirasinha PA. Encephalitozoonosis (nosematosis) of the cornea. Br J Ophthalmol 1973; 57:669–74.
3. Barragan A, Sibley LD. Migration of *Toxoplasma gondii* across biological barriers. Trends Microbiol 2003; 11: 426–30.
4. Beare NA, Southern C, Chalira C, et al. Prognostic significance and course of retinopathy in children with severe malaria. Arch Ophthalmol 2004; 122:1141–7.
5. Beaver PC, Villegas AL, Cuello C, D'Alessandro A. Cutaneous amebiasis of the eyelid with extension into the orbit. Am J Trop Med Hyg 1978; 27:1133–6.
6. Borges JS, Johnson WD Jr. Inhibition of multiplication of *Toxoplasma gondii* by human monocytes exposed to T-lymphocyte products. J Exp Med 1975; 141:483–96.
7. Bosch-Driessen LH, Karimi S, Stilma JS, Rothova A. Retinal detachment in ocular toxoplasmosis. Ophthalmology 2000; 107:36–40.
8. Brown TJ, Cursons RT. Pathogenic free-living amebae (PFLA) from frozen swimming areas in Oslo, Norway. Scand J Infect Dis 1977; 9:237–40.
9. Cairns JE. Cutaneous leishmaniasis (oriental sore): a case with corneal involvement. Br J Ophthalmol 1968; 52:481–3.
10. Cali A. General microsporidian features and recent findings on AIDS isolates. J Protozool 1991; 38:625–30.
11. Cali A, Meisler DM, Lowder CY, et al. Corneal microsporidioses: characterization and identification. J Protozool 1991; 38:215S–7S.
12. Canning EU, Curry A, Vavra J, Bonshek RE. Some ultrastructural data on *Microsporidium ceylonensis*, a cause of corneal microsporidiosis. Parasite 1998; 5:247–54.
13. Chakraborty P, Das PK. Suppression of macrophage lysosomal enzymes after *L. donovani* infection. Biochem Med Metab Biol 1989; 41:46–55.
14. Chappuis F, Stivanello E, Adams K, et al. Card agglutination test for trypanosomiasis (CATT) end-dilution titer and cerebrospinal fluid cell count as predictors of human African Trypanosomiasis (*Trypanosoma brucei gambiense*) among serologically suspected individuals in southern Sudan. Am J Trop Med Hyg 2004; 71:313–7.
15. Chynn EW, Lopez MA, Pavan-Langston D, Talamo JH. *Acanthamoeba* keratitis. Contact lens and noncontact lens characteristics. Ophthalmology 1995; 102:1369–73.
16. Cohen EJ, Buchanan HW, Laughrea PA, et al. Diagnosis and management of *Acanthamoeba* keratitis. Am J Ophthalmol 1985; 100:389–95.
17. Connor DH, Neafie RC, Dooley JR. African trypanosomiasis. In:Binford CH, Connor DH, eds. *Pathology of Tropical and Extraordinary Diseases: An Atlas*, Vol. 1. Washington D.C.: Armed Forces Institute of Pathology, 1976:252–7.
18. Connor DH, Neafie RC, Cutaneous leishmaniasis. In: Binford CH, Connor DH, eds. *Pathology of Tropical and Extraordinary Diseases: An Atlas*, Vol. 1. Washington D.C.: Armed Forces Institute of Pathology, 1976:258–64.
19. Connor DH, Neafie RC, Hockmeyer WT. Malaria. In: Binford CH, Connor DH, eds. *Pathology of Tropical and Extraordinary Diseases: An Atlas*, Vol. 1. Washington D.C.: Armed Forces Institute of Pathology, 1976:273–83.
20. Connor DH, Neafie RC, Meyers WM. Amebiasis. In: Binford CH, Connor DH, eds. *Pathology of Tropical and Extraordinary Diseases: An Atlas*, Vol. 1. Washington D.C.: Armed Forces Institute of Pathology, 1976:308–16.
21. Culbertson CG. Amebic meningoencephalitides. In: Binford CH, Connor DH, eds. *Pathology of Tropical and Extraordinary Diseases: An Atlas*, Vol. 1. Washington D.C.: Armed Forces Institute of Pathology, 1976:317–24.
22. Dechant W, Rees PH, Kager PA, et al. Post kala-azar. Br. J. Ophthalmol. 1980; 64:680–3.
23. Doft BH. Choroidoretinal vascular anastomosis. Arch Ophthalmol 1983; 101:1053–4.
24. Doft BH, Gass JDM. Punctate outer retinal toxoplasmosis. Arch Ophthalmol 1985; 103:1332–6.
25. Dubois ME, Demick KP, Mansfield JM. Trypanosomes expressing a mosaic variant surface glycoprotein coat escape early detection by the immune system. Infect. Immun. 2005; 73:2690–9.
26. Dutton GN. Toxoplasmic retinochoroiditis–a historical review and current concepts. Ann Acad Med Singapore 1989; 18:214–21.
27. Edgcomb JH, Johnson CM. American trypanosomiasis (Chagas' disease). In: Binford CH, Connor DH, eds. *Pathology of Tropical and Extraordinary Diseases: An Atlas*, Vol. 1. Washington D.C.: Armed Forces Institute of Pathology, 1976:244–51.
28. el Hassan AM, Khalil EA, el Sheikh EA, et al. Post kala-azar ocular leishmaniasis. Trans R Soc Trop Med Hyg 1998; 92:177–9.
29. Feron EJ, Klaren VN, Wierenga EA, et al. Characterization of *Toxoplasma gondii*-specific T cells recovered from vitreous fluid of patients with ocular toxoplasmosis. Invest Ophthalmol Vis Sci 2001; 42:3228–32.
30. Ferrante A, Rowan-Kelly B. Activation of the alternative pathway of complement by *Acanthamoeba culbertsoni*. Clin Exp Immunol 1983; 54:477–85.
31. Fine SL, Owens SL, Haller JA, et al. Choroidal neovascularization as a late complication of ocular toxoplasmosis. Am J Ophthalmol 1981; 91:318–22.
32. Fish RH, Hoskins JC, Kline LB. Toxoplasmosis neuroretinitis. Ophthalmology 1993; 100:1177–82.
33. Fournier S, Liguory O, Sarfati C, et al. Disseminated infection due to *Encephalitozoon cuniculi* in a patient with AIDS: case report and review. HIV Med 2000; 1: 155–61.
34. Franzen C, Muller A. Molecular techniques for detection, species differentiation, and phylogeneti analysis of microsporidia. Clin Microbiol Rev 1999; 12:243–85.
35. Frenkel JK. Toxoplasmosis. In: Binford CH, Connor DH, eds. *Pathology of Tropical and Extraordinary Diseases: An Atlas*, Vol. 1. Washington D.C.: Armed Forces Institute of Pathology, 1976:284–300.
36. Garner A. Pathogenesis of acanthamoebic keratitis: Hypothesis based on an histological analysis of 30 cases. Br J Ophthalmol 1993; 77:366–70.
37. Garweg JG. Determinants of immunodiagnostic success in human ocular toxoplasmosis. Parasite Immunol 2005; 27: 61–8.
38. Green SJ, Meltzer MS, Hibbs JB Jr, Nacy CA. Activated macrophages destroy intracellular *Leishmania major* amastigotes by an L-arginine dependent healing mechanism. J Immunol 1990; 144:278–83.
39. Grossniklaus HE, Waring GO IV, Akor C, et al. Evaluation of hematoxylin and eosin and special stains for the detection of acanthamoeba keratitis in penetrating keratoplasties. Am J Ophthalmol 2003; 136:520–6.
40. Guerina NG, Hsu HW, Meissner HC, et al. Neonatal serologic screening and early treatment for congenital *Toxoplasma gondii* infection. The New England Regional *Toxoplasma* Working Group. N Engl J Med 1994; 330: 1858–63.

41. Harris D, Birch CL. Bilateral uveitis associated with gastrointestinal *Endamoeba histolytica* infection: a case report. Am J Ophthalmol 1960; 50:496–500.
42. Holland GN, Engstrom RE Jr, Glasgow BJ, et al. Ocular toxoplasmosis in patients with the acquired immunodeficiency syndrome. Am J Ophthalmol 1988; 106:653–67.
43. Holland GN. Reconsidering the pathogenesis of ocular toxoplasmosis. Am J Ophthalmol 1999; 128:502–5.
44. Hovakimyan A, Cunningham ET Jr. Ocular toxoplasmosis. Ophthalmol Clin North Am 2002; 15:327–32.
45. Hurt M, Neelam S, Niederkorn J, Alizadeh H. Pathogenic *Acanthamoeba* spp secrete a mannose-induced cytolytic protein that correlates with the ability to cause disease. Infect Immun 2003; 71:6243–55.
46. Jacobs L, Cook MK, Wilder HC. Serologic data on adults with histologically diagnosed toxoplasmic chorioretinitis. Trans Am Acad Ophthalmol 1954; 55:193–200.
47. Janků J. Pathogenes a Pathologická Anatomic Tak Nazvaného Vrozeneho Kolobomu Zluté Skvyrny v Oku Nomalne Velikém a Mikrophthalmickem s Nalexem Parazitu v Sitnici. Cas. Lek. Ces. 1923; 62:1021–7, 1054–9, 1081–5, 1111–5, 1138–44.
48. King RE, Praeger DL, Hallett JW. Amebic choroidosis. Arch Ophthalmol 1964; 72:16–22.
49. Koppe JG, Loewer-Sieger DH, Roever Bonnett, H. Results of a 20-year follow-up of congenital toxoplasmosis. Lancet 1986; 1:254–6.
50. Kucukerdonmez C, Yilmaz G, Akova YA. Branch retinal arterial occlusion associated with toxoplasmic chorioretinitis. Ocul Immunol Inflamm 2004; 12:227–31.
51. Liew FY, Li Y, Millott S. Tumor necrosis factor-alpha synergizes with IFN-gamma in mediating killing of *Leishmania* major through the induction of nitric oxide. J Immunol 1990; 145:4306–10.
52. Looareesuwan S, Warrell DA, White NJ, et al. Retinal hemorrhage: A common sign of prognostic significance in cerebral malaria. Am J Trop Med Hyg 1983; 32:911–5.
53. Lowder CY. Ocular microsporidiosis. Int Ophthalmol Clin 1993; 33:145–51.
54. Lowder CY, McMahon JT, Meisler DM, et al. Microsporidial keratoconjunctivitis caused by *Septata intestinalis* in a patient with acquired immunodeficiency syndrome. Am J Ophthalmol 1996; 121:715–7.
55. Luna JD, Sonzini EE, Diaz HD, et al. Anomalous intraocular pressure changes in Chagas' disease elicited by postural test. Int Ophthalmol 1996–1997; 20:329–32.
56. McMenamin PG, Dutton GN, Hay J, Cameron S. The ultrastructural pathology of congenital murine toxoplasmic retinochoroiditis. Part I. The localization and morphology of *Toxoplasma* cysts in the retina. Exp Eye Res 1986; 43:529–43.
57. Mets MB, Holfels E, Boyer KM, et al. Eye manifestations of congenital toxoplasmosis. Am J Ophthalmol 1997; 123:1–16.
58. Morhun PJ, Weisz JM, Elias SJ, Holland GN. Recurrent ocular toxoplasmosis in patients treated with systemic corticosteroids. Retina 1996; 16:383–7.
59. Mortelmans J, Neetens A. Ocular lesions in experimental *Trypanosoma brucei* infection in cats. Acta Zool Pathol Antverp 1975; 62:149–72.
60. Naginton J, Watson PG, Playfair TJ, et al. Amoebic infection of the eye. Lancet 1974; 2:1537–40.
61. Nussenblatt RB, Mittal KK, Fuhrman S, et al. Lymphocyte proliferative responses of patients with ocular toxoplasmosis to parasite and retinal antigens. Am J Ophthalmol 1989; 107:632–41.
62. Oliveira-Neto MP, Martins VJ, Mattos MS, et al. South American cutaneous leishmaniasis of the eyelids: report of five cases in Rio de Janeiro State, Brazil. Ophthalmology 2000; 107:169–72.
63. Pariyakanok L, Jongwutiwes S. Keratitis caused by *Trachipleistophora anthropopthera*. J Infect 2005; 51:325–8.
64. Pinnolis M, Egbert PR, Font RL, Winter FC. Nosematosis of the cornea. Arch Ophthalmol 1981; 99:1044–7.
65. Portela RW, Bethony J, Costa MI, et al. A multihousehold study reveals a positive correlation between age, severity of ocular toxoplasmosis, and levels of glycoinositolphospholipid-specific immunoglobulin A. J Infect Dis 2004; 190:175–83.
66. Prata JA, Prata JA Jr, de Castro CN, et al. The pupil in the chronic phase of Chagas disease and the reaction to pilocarpine and phenylephrine. Rev Soc Bras Med Trop 1996; 29:567–70.
67. Rauz S, Tuft S, Dart JK, et al. Ultrastructural examination of two cases of stromal microsporidial keratitis. J Med Microbiol 2004; 53:775–81.
68. Remington JS, Cavanaugh EN. Isolation of the encysted form of *Toxoplasma gondii* from human skeletal muscle and brain. N Engl J Med 1965; 273:1308–10.
69. Rodger FC. Eye diseases. In: Manson-Bahr PEC, Bell DR (eds) *Manson's Tropical Diseases*, 19th ed., London: Bailliere Tindall; 1987, pp. 1133–82.
70. Rothova A, Van Knapen E, Baarsma GS, et al. Serology in ocular toxoplasmosis. Br J Ophthalmol 1986; 70:615–22.
71. Rothova A. Ocular manifestations of toxoplasmosis. Curr Opin Ophthalmol 2003; 14:384–8.
72. Samples JR, Binder PS, Luibel FJ, et al. *Acanlhamoeba* possibly acquired from a hot tub. Arch Ophthalmol 1984; 102:707–10.
73. Schaumberg DA, Snow KK, Dana MR. The epidemic of *Acanthamoeba* keratitis: where do we stand? Cornea 1998; 17:3–10.
74. Schuman JS, Weinberg RS, Ferry AR, Guerry RK. Toxoplasmic scleritis. Ophthalmology 1988; 95: 1399–403.
75. Stanford MR, Tomlin EA, Comyn O, et al. The visual field in toxoplasmic retinochoroiditis. Br J Ophthalmol 2005; 89:812–4.
76. Sternberg JM. Human African trypanosomiasis: clinical presentation and immune response. Parasite Immunol 2004; 26:469–76.
77. Tanowitz HB, Kirchhoff LV, Simon D, et al. Chagas' disease. Clin Microbiol Rev 1992; 5:400–19.
78. Tanyuksel M, Petri WA Jr. Laboratory diagnosis of amebiasis. Clin Microbiol Rev 2003; 16:713–29.
79. Turco SJ. The *Leishmania* lipophosphoglycan: a multifunctional molecule. Exp Parasitol 1990; 70:241–5.
80. Walochnik J, Haller-Schober E, Kolli H, et al. Discrimination between clinically relevant and nonrelevant *Acanthamoeba* strains isolated from contact lens-wearing keratitis patients in Austria. J Clin Microbiol 2000; 38:3932–6.
81. Wilder HC. Toxoplasma chorioretinitis in adults. Arch Ophthalmol 1952; 45:127–36.
82. Wolf A, Cowen D, Paige BH. Human toxoplasmosis. Occurrence in infants as an encephalomyelitis. Verification by transmission to animals. Science 1939; 89: 226–7.

13

Ocular Diseases Due to Helminths

J. Oscar Croxatto
Departments of Teaching and Research and Laboratory of Ophthalmic Pathology, Fundación Oftalmológica Argentina Jorge Malbran, Buenos Aires, Argentina

Alec Garner
Institute of Ophthalmology, Moorfields Eye Hospital, London, U.K.

INTRODUCTION

A variety of worms generally designated as helminths are associated with disease of the eye and its adnexae, some frequently, others rarely. Parasitism, which describes the relationship between the worm and its host, is defined as a state of symbiosis in which the symbiont benefits from the association and the host is harmed in some way. This is in contrast to commensalism, which refers to a symbiotic state wherein one symbiont, the commensal, benefits without detriment to the host, and to mutualism, in which both host and symbiont benefit from the association. A number of helminths responsible for human disease are obligate parasites in that humans are essential if the worm is to complete its life cycle (11). In other instances, however, human infection is accidental, the usual or elective hosts belonging to other species of the animal kingdom.

Helminth classification is based on the external and internal morphology of the egg, as well as the larval and adult stages. They include three large classes: trematodes (flukes), cestodes (tapeworms), and nematodes (roundworms). The trematodes and cestodes are grouped within the phylum Platyhelminthes. Nematodes inhabit intestinal and extraintestinal sites in adult and larval forms.

Disease attributable to parasitic helminths can arise in several ways, but in an ocular context the most important is a mechanical disturbance, such as an interference with retinal function by a worm in the vitreous or subretinal space, and immune-mediated inflammation (allergic phenomena). The inflammatory responses of the ocular tissue are determined by size, number, and location of the organism within the eye, whether the parasite is dead or alive and host immune response capabilities. It varies from no reaction or mild inflammation to localized granulomas and an extensive intraocular inflammatory reaction.

IMMUNOLOGIC ASPECTS OF HELMINTHIC DISEASE

The ability of eukaryotic parasites to survive in any mammal and wander throughout the body for a month or up to several years causing disease in several organs is accomplished by acquiring a unique mechanism for evading the host immune response (14). Composed of proteins that are foreign to the host, all helminths can be expected to be antigenic and to elicit an immunological response, but as a measure of their success as parasites, they are often little affected by it. In some instances this is because the parasite has developed a defense mechanism, but in others, particularly filarial infections, antigens attributable to the parasite can actively and specifically suppress the immune system (120). Furthermore individuals in endemic areas for a given helminth may acquire immune tolerance as a result of prenatal sensitization. Many antigens are common to worms of the same genus or family; a few are even more widely spread and this can produce difficulty when serological tests are used in diagnosis.

Protective Immunity

Some antibodies engendered by helminth infection appear to be irrelevant from a protective standpoint, and the production of antibodies at meaningful levels seems to depend on repeated infection over a prolonged period. Protective immunity is most readily achieved in unnatural hosts, and antibodies that protect against worm infection have been demonstrated by passive transfer experiments. This suggests that survival in the natural host is due to adaptive tolerance, a process that might develop in various ways:

1. *Acquisition of host antigens to provide an immunological screen.* This type of adaptation is well demonstrated in *Schistosoma mansoni* infection, adult worms being able to resist immunological attack even though incoming schistosomula are destroyed (143).
2. Antigenic modulation such that immune responses are less readily evoked (e.g., *Nippostrongylus brasiliensis* infection) (95).
3. Active immunosuppression of the host (e.g., *Trichinella spiralis*).
4. Accelerated sexual maturation such that larvae can be produced before the host's immune defenses are mobilized (e.g., *T. spiralis*).
5. Trickle infection: the level of infection may be insufficient to stimulate protective levels of antibodies and T cells.
6. Blocking antibodies, specifically of the IgG_4 isotype, may be formed, particularly with respect to filarial infections (116).

Even so, there is evidence that, despite the emergence of adaptive tolerance on the part of the established parasite, the immune process can be effective in preventing reinfection. Such concomitant immunity is directed against antigens unique to the as yet unestablished larvae, which are shed and replaced as the parasite matures (98). Protective immunity can also occur in other situations, when it acts against alternative stages in the helminth life cycle. Immunity to some filariae, especially *Onchocerca*, is maximal against the microfilarial stage, whereas in some worms there is prevention of larval maturation (e.g., *Toxocara canis* and several ascarid infections in animals other than humans). Significantly, in the interests of the parasite, this suppression is reduced during pregnancy of the host so that transplacental transmission of larvae occurs and survival of the helminth species is assured.

Immunoglobulin E (IgE) responses are the hallmark of parasitic infections, although much of the antibody is nonspecific, and are mediated by T-cell-derived interleukins (ILs), specifically IL4, with gamma interferon (IFNγ) serving to restrict the process (51). It is further suggested that patients with filariasis, who commonly have large numbers of microfilariae in their tissues but paradoxically low antibody levels, are exhibiting disproportionate IFNγ secretion (83). The frequent eosinophil response is also under T-cell control, this time mediated by IL5 (170,171). In evolutionary terms it is conceivable that the capacity for IgE and possibly other antibody-initiated cellular responses (antibody-dependent cell-mediated cytotoxicity) was originally promoted by the need to combat helminth infection (25).

Although most studies have concentrated on the role of antibodies, cell-mediated mechanisms may also be important in providing immunity. Precisely how this is affected is not entirely clear, but experiments in mice suggest that IL2 and IFNγ secretion by helper T cells may be important in addition to the recognized regulation of the IgE-eosinophil-mast cell axis (51).

Again, protection of a kind may be provided by the formation of a fibrous capsule around the parasite, a tissue response that is not necessarily immunologic-mediated.

Hypersensitivity-Based Response

Ironically, the most obvious results of the immune response to helminth infection are often deleterious to the host. This is nowhere more truly than in the eye and its adnexae, where the associated inflammatory reaction is almost always undesirable. Allergic reactions are usually, perhaps invariably, provoked by parasite death or the escape of antigenic material from larval cysts. The reaction can result in generalized anaphylaxis when large amounts of antigen are released into the circulating body fluids or a localized inflammatory lesion develops around the degenerating worms or a leaking cyst. These allergic manifestations are associated with a marked IgE production, and this is likely to be a major factor in both the blood eosinophilia and the heavy eosinophil infiltration of the focal inflammatory reaction. Besides giving rise to specific antibodies, which usually include immunoglobulin G (IgG) and immunoglobulin M (IgM) as well as IgE, helminth infection is said to have a nonspecific stimulatory effect on IgE formation.

At the tissue level, dying parasites provoke an inflammatory reaction characterized by an infiltrate of lymphocytes, plasma cells, and eosinophils. Macrophages, including multinucleated giant cells, collect somewhat later to constitute a granulomatous inflammation. Study of the earliest stages often shows that polymorphonuclear leukocytes (PMNs) predominate, possibly indicative of an Arthus-like reaction: lesions at this stage are most readily seen in experimental situations (45). In the more usual established lesions seen in human material, the parasite displays a variable degree of necrosis and the surrounding necrotic zone may contain remnants of degenerate eosinophils, with Charcot–Leyden crystals, and other leukocytes. Deposits of eosinophil major basic protein appear to be especially significant since they are directly helminthotoxic (82). This type of eosinophilic granuloma known as the Splendore–Hoeppli phenomenon (Fig. 1) is produced by several helminths as well as some fungi. Occasionally, such granulomas present in the conjunctiva as an isolated lesion in patients showing no other evidence of worm infection, and although parasite remnants can be demonstrated in some cases, in others they cannot (4). The morphology of the Splendore–Hoeppli lesions is so distinctive, however that even in these latter cases occult helminth infection is a strong possibility, provided the presence of fungi can be excluded (4). The pathogenesis of the Splendore–Hoeppli phenomenon includes antigen–antibody precipitates and eosinophilic basic proteins. Immunohistochemical studies revealed two staining patterns, one predominately of immunoglobulin deposition, the other primarily eosinophilic major basic protein (127). Experimental studies involving the injection of serum from *Ascaris*-infected patients and *Toxocara* larvae into the vitreous of rabbits indicate that eosinophils are able to exert a direct cytotoxic effect on these parasites (130).

HELMINTHIC DISEASES OF OPHTHALMIC IMPORTANCE

A detailed account of helminth taxonomy is out of place in a text dealing with ocular pathology, but a classification of worms of ocular importance is given in Table 1.

Diseases Due to Trematodes

Trematodes, or flukes, are flatworms that attach to the host by means of suckers and undergo a complicated life cycle entailing larval development in an intermediate host. The asexual phase of development takes place in snails, which are the intermediate host.

Depending on the habitat in the infected host, flukes can be classified as blood flukes, liver flukes, lung flukes, and intestinal flukes. The flukes that cause most human infections are *Schistosoma* species (blood fluke), *Paragonimus westermani* (lung fluke), and *Clonorchis sinensis* (liver fluke). The only flukes of ocular importance to humans are the *Schistosomes*,

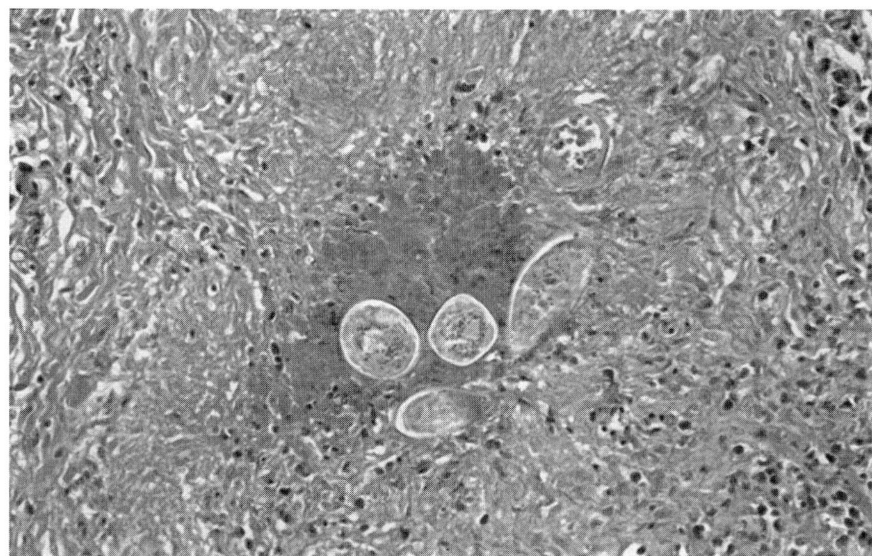

Figure 1 Splendore–Hoeppli phenomenon. Granulomatous inflammation with eosinophilic deposits adjacent to schistoma eggs (hematoxylin and eosin, $\times$ 60).

Table 1 Classification of Helminths of Ocular Importance to Humans

Phylum	Class	Subclass	Order	Superfamily	Family	Genus	Species
Nematoda	Adenophorea		Trichurida	Trichuroidea	Trichinellidae	Trichinella	*T. spiralis*
	Secernentea		Ascaridia		Ascarididae	Ascaris	*A. lumbricoides*
					Uncertain	Baylisascaris	*B. procyonis*
					Toxocaridae	Toxocara	*T. canis*
							T. cati
			Camallanida	Dracunculoidea	Dracunculidae	Dracunculus	*D. medinensis*
		Spiruria	Spirurida	Filarioidea	Filariidae	Brugia	*B. malayi*
						Dirofilaria	*D. immitis*
						Loa	*L. loa*
						Onchocerca	*O. volvulus*
						Wuchereria	*W. bancrofti*
				Gnathostomatoidea	Gnathostomatidae	Gnathostoma	*G. spinigerum*
				Thelazoidea	Thelaziidae	Thelazia	*T. callipaeda*
							T. californiensis
Platyhelminthes	Trematoda	Digenea	Strigeiderida		Schistomatidae	Schistosoma	*S. haematobium*
							S. japonicum
							S. mansoni
	Cestoda	Eucestoda	Pseudophyllidea		Diphyllobothriidae	Spirometra	*S. erinacei*
							S. erinaceieuropaei
							S. mansoni
							S. mansonoides
			Cyclophyllidea		Taeniidae	Taenia	*T. brauni*
							T. crassiceps
							T. multiceps
							T. saginata
							T. serialis
							T. solium
							T. taeniformis
						Echinoccocus	*E. granulosus*
							E. multilocularis
							E. oligoarthus
							E. vogeli

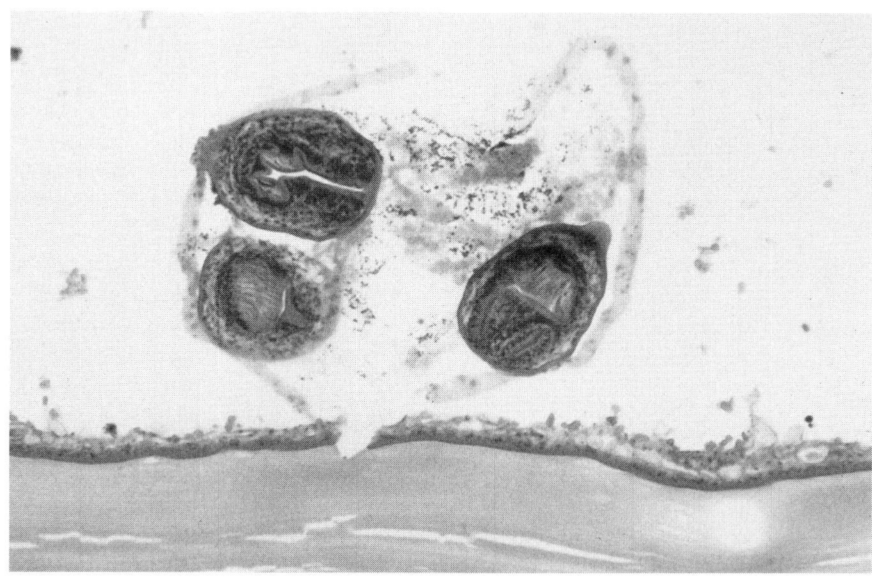

Figure 8 Echinococcosis. The wall of the cyst has a laminated membrane and an internal germinal layer containing a brood capsule with protoscolex (hematoxylin and eosin, ×120).

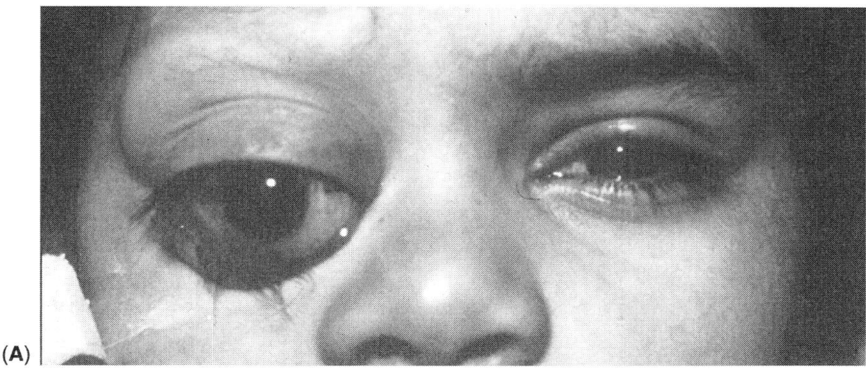

(**A**)

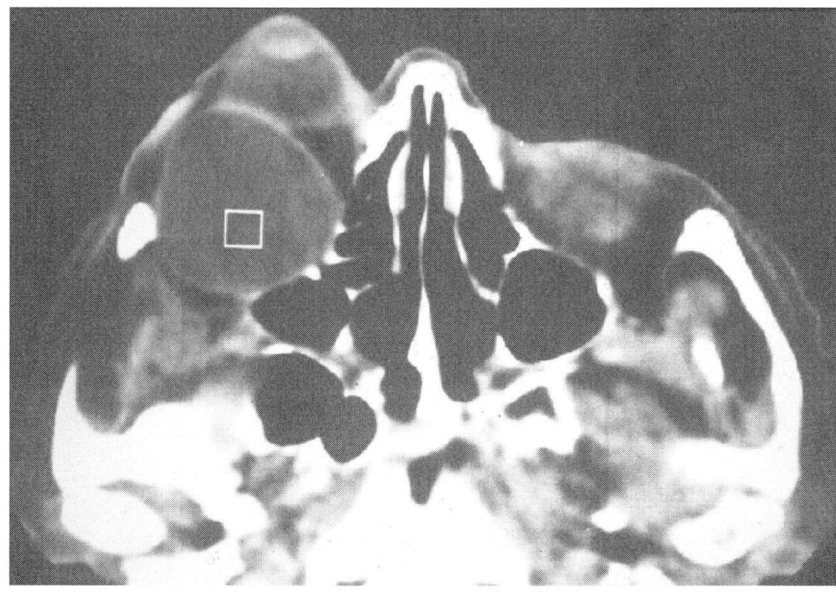

(**B**)

Figure 9 Echinococcosis. (**A**) Photograph of a child with prominent axial proptosis due to a cyst within the orbit. (**B**) Computed tomography scan revealing a large cyst filling the orbit with forward displacement of the eye.

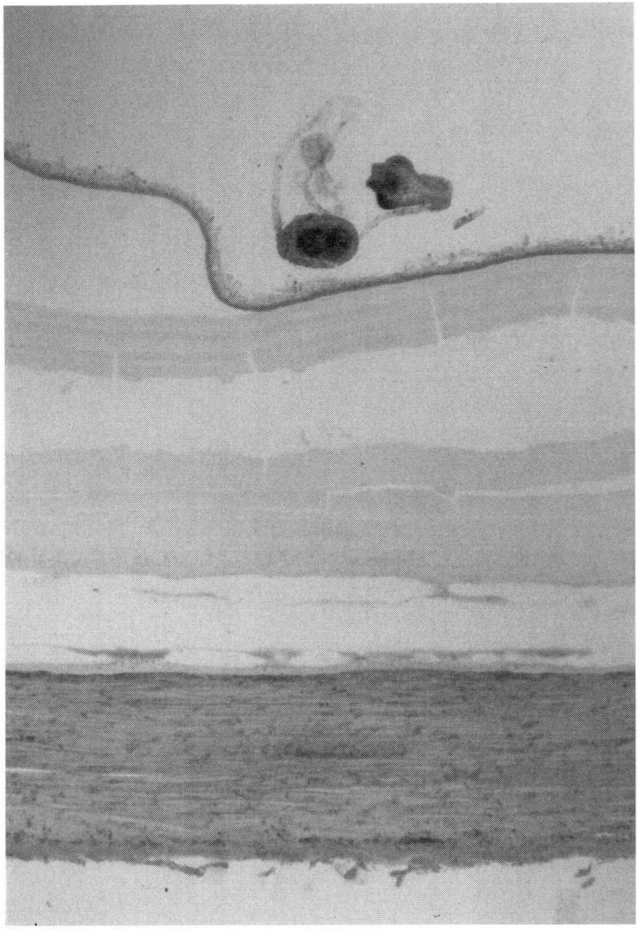

Figure 10 Intraocular echinococcosis. The laminated membrane, germinal layer, and a few protoscolices are seen lying inside the slcera (*bottom*) (hematoxylin and eosin, ×25).

Coenurosis

Adult worm of other species of *Taenia* are found in carnivorous animals (dog, wolf, and fox) with sheep, goat, and cattle acting as the intermediate hosts. Their larval stage or coenurus sometimes infects humans causing a disease named coenurosis. The developing larvae form cysts about 3 cm in diameter in the brain as a rule, but occasionally under the skin and elsewhere. Each cyst is known as a coenurus and, as a result of asexual multiplication, may contain up to 100 invaginated protoscolices. Three species of *Taenia* (formerly Multiceps) of which their larvae infect man are: *T. multiceps*, *T. serialis*, and *T. brauni*.

Ocular lesions: Ocular coenurosis, although not common, has been reported occasionally, with cysts developing in the conjunctiva or within the globe (13,50,69,166). In a case with subretinal involvement described by Manschot (97), there was a marked panophthalmitis characterized by lymphocytic, plasma cell, macrophage, and eosinophil infiltration of the retina, choroid, and sclera. The best treatment of intravitreal cestodes is its removal through vitrectomy before death of the parasite to prevent the release of toxins and severe intraocular inflammation. Orbital involvement is also reported (97,166), the cyst developing a fibrous capsule and an intervening collar of PMNs (97).

Sparganosis

Sparganosis in humans is caused by several species of diphyllobothrid tapeworms of the genus *Spirometra*. The second-stage larva of such parasites is known as a plerocercoid, in which there is a single invaginated anterior scolex within the solid elongated body. Carnivores represent the primary host, and freshwater crustaceans of the genus *Cyclops* and a variety of amphibians, reptiles, and mammals behave as successive intermediate hosts. Humans can also act as an intermediate host, infection being regarded as accidental and incurred in various ways: (*i*) ingestion of contaminated water, (*ii*) application of flesh from infected frogs to open sores and inflamed eyes as a poultice in parts of Southeast Asia, and (*iii*) ingestion of meat from infected animals.

In warm-blooded animals, maturation is arrested. Instead, each plerocercoid may simply increase in size (up to 8–10 cm in length) to constitute a sparganum. The developing sparganum tends to invade the deep tissues and initiates an intense irritation as the result of an associated inflammatory reaction. Ultimately, a surrounding capsule of fibrous tissue forms.

Ocular lesions: Involvement of the eyelids, especially the upper palpebral conjunctivae and orbit, is recorded (46,103) and is chiefly related to the direct application of infected tissue to the eyes. After an initial chemosis, a nodule up to 3 cm in diameter form, that may superficially resemble a fibroma (150). The presence of a live sparganum in the anterior chamber with attendant inflammation has been reported (89,141).

Diseases Due to Nematodes

Nematodes are unsegmented roundworms. Apart from members of the genus *Ascaris*, which follow a direct life cycle within a single host, most nematodes responsible for human disease require an intermediate host. Filarial worms constitute the largest group, all of them being tissue-dwelling parasites transmitted by the bite of a blood-sucking arthropod.

Ascaridiasis

Ascariasis

The adult form of *Ascaris lumbricoides* is the most common human helminthic infection. This fully developed largest nematode infecting man inhabits the small intestine. Here the fertilized female lays around 200,000 eggs each day, with many of them passing with the feces to the exterior, where they contaminate the drinking water and land and develop into second-stage infective larvae. Ingestion of eggs containing such larvae by other individuals allows the parasite to emerge from the surrounding shell and penetrate the intestinal mucosa. Once within the intestinal lymphatics and blood vessels, they proceed to the lungs, where a further stage of development takes place. They then break through the lining of the alveoli and ascend the bronchi and trachea, only to enter the esophagus and pass into the intestine for a second time before maturing into adult worms. The cycle from ingestion of infective eggs to oviposition by the adult female in the intestine lasts two to three months. High levels of IgE and IgG homocytotropic antibody are a characteristic of ascarid infections, and acute anaphylactic reactions with moderate eosinophilia are well documented. Larvae within the circulating blood may pass to tissues other than the lungs and provoke a localized eosinophilic granuloma.

Ocular lesions: Relative to the prevalence of ascariasis, estimated at around 700 million infected persons (103), ocular involvement is exceedingly rare and must be regarded as essentially an accident of aberrant larval migration. The experimental injection of larvae into the anterior chamber of rabbit eyes was attended within two hours by an acute eosinophilic iridocyclitis that later became granulomatous as the larvae began to degenerate (29). Other work suggests that the eosinophils may contribute directly to the larval degeneration (130). Allergic phenomena in the form of iridocyclitis (73) and chorioretinitis (40) have been observed in human eyes in the apparent absence of any direct infiltration. The uveal response in such cases has been attributed to the presence of toxic products derived from degenerating larvae, but tissue damage engendered by eosinophil-derived factors may also be involved (74). There is evidence implicating *A. lumbricoides* and *Ancylostoma* in the causation of bilateral Mooren ulceration of the cornea, possibly through antigen–antibody reactions to toxins derived from helminths that deposit in the peripheral cornea (see Chapter 5).

Baylisascariasis

The several species of *Baylisascaris,* nematodes of the Ascaridida order, are well-recognized intestinal parasites of lower carnivores. The raccoon roundworm, *Baylisascaris procyonis*, is the most common and widespread cause of clinical larva migrans in animals (60). In addition, it is increasingly recognized as a cause of devastating or fatal neural larva migrans in infants and young children and ocular larva migrans (OLM) in adults. Humans become infected by accidentally ingesting infective *B. procyonis* eggs from raccoon latrines or articles contaminated with their feces. Two features distinguish *B. procyonis* from other helminths that cause larva migrans: aggressive somatic migration and invasion of the central nervous system (CNS) and the continued growth of larvae to a large size (1500–2000 μm in length) within the CNS. Fatal infections in children have been reported as a result of visceral larva migrans (VLM) and acute fulminant eosinophilic meningoencephalitis (53,60).

Ocular lesions: In 1978, Gass and Scelfo (59) described a uniocular posterior segment disorder in children and young adults characterized by vitritis, papillitis, and recurrent crops of grayish lesions in the outer retina and RPE. The patients presented with early loss of central vision, but in time the visual fields were further reduced as optic nerve and RPE atrophy developed. Gass labeled the condition "diffuse unilateral subacute neuroretinitis" and suggested that a nematode could be responsible (59). A subsequent study revealed the presence of a motile nematode in each of 18 affected patients (58), chiefly located beneath or within the retina. Because of their size and negative serological tests, the larvae were not thought to represent *T. canis*: rather, in view of the observed capacity of the larvae to remain within the eye in a viable state for at least three years, Gass speculated that they might be ascarid worms (58). Goldberg et al. (65) presented morphometric, serologic, and epidemiologic support for *B. procyonis* as the causative agent. Although most cases occur in the southeastern United States and the Caribbean, cases from upper Midwestern United States, Europe, and South America have been reported (30,87,107).

Gass and Braunstein (58) believed that the retinal damage incurred by the larvae in their cases was caused by toxic products and secondary inflammation, there being no immediate tissue response to viable parasites. Experiments in which ova of *B. procyonis* were inoculated into monkeys support this interpretation, the observed tissue damage and inflammatory response developing in the wake as opposed to the close vicinity of the hatched larvae (80). As with the presumed human cases, most larvae entering the eye migrated to the retina and subretinal region, producing extensive changes in the outer retina and choroidal granulomas. Eosinophils were a notable feature of the inflammation developing in relation to the tracks of the larvae (80). Loss of vision due to atrophy of photoreceptors and RPE develops in the late stages resulting in abnormal electroretinograms. Bilateral eye involvement is extremely rare.

Toxocariasis

Two species of *Toxocara* (*T. canis* and *T. cati*), are implicated in human infection, but *T. cati* has not been identified histopathologically in human disease. The natural hosts of these nematodes of the ascarid group are dogs and cats, respectively. Human infection is accidental and is not obligatory for completion of the life cycle, since this can occur in the primary host alone. Humans do not develop adult worms or excrete eggs in their feces. Other species of *Toxocara* affecting domestic animals have been identified (*T. malayasiensis*, *T. lyncus*) (63,93). Although it is not known whether these species may cause human clinical disease, it may be likely that some unusual infections have resulted from exposure to their migrating larvae. Infestation of dogs by *T. canis* is throughout the world, the proportion affected varying widely, with estimates of 12% in the United Kingdom (128) and an average of 15% in the United States (64). Infection of puppies is usually acquired in utero by transplacental migration of larvae from the pregnant bitch, and it has been claimed that mature egg-laying worms may be present in 100% of puppies by three weeks after birth. In addition, following ingestion by younger dogs elder than five weeks, the infective eggs hatch and larvae penetrate the gut wall and migrate through the lungs, bronchial tree, and esophagus; adult worms develop and deposit ova in the small intestine. Immune mechanisms may inhibit the maturation of ova in the adult dog (112), which would explain the association of human toxocariasis with puppies and lactating bitches as opposed to mature animals.

There are relatively few data concerning the prevalence of *T. cati*, but figures of 8% (113) and 45% (41) have been cited in studies of cats in London; levels between 24% and 75% are reported in the United States (137).

Human infection is widespread and mostly confined to young children (19,79). It usually results from the ingestion of ova present in contaminated play areas, on toys, or on the coats of infected pets (99). Alternatively, transmission can follow licking of the face by affected puppies. Study of an adult sample population in the United Kingdom revealed positive serum antibodies in 2.8% of persons (170), which is indicative of a high level of transmission. A survey in rural areas of North Carolina in the United States showed positive antibody titers in 32% of kindergarten children (49). In another study from the Caribbean, the soil contamination rate was 46% and 80% of children had serologic evidence of *T. canis* infection (153). Human infection occurs in two forms, VLM, which encompasses diseases associated with major organs, and ocular toxocariasis (OLM) which is mainly restricted to the eye and optic nerve (34). Some asymptomatic patients may present with positive serologic titers (106). VLM following ingestion, ova develop to form first-stage larvae and then second-stage larvae, the latter emerging from the outer shell of the ova and penetrating the gut mucosa to enter the portal circulation and intestinal lymphatic channels. Many larvae lodge in the liver, but others ultimately may reach the lungs, brain, or eyes. During the acute phase of larval dissemination, fever is common and hepatosplenomegaly may develop; laboratory tests usually reveal leukocytosis with persistent eosinophilia. The affected child, most commonly of preschool age, may be gravely ill, but a benign course is more usual.

Ocular lesions: Rarely, larvae may reach the eye via the ophthalmic artery and enter the retinal or, less certainly, the uveal circulation (154). In most instances systemic involvement is subclinical, so that ocular involvement is ostensibly an isolated event, with blood eosinophilia either absent or slight. When an initial systemic episode can be documented, however, an interval as short as three months (96) or as long as 10 years (9) may elapse before the eye is affected. Ocular disease is most common in school-age children. Involvement is almost always unilateral (165). Reported cases have all implicated *T. canis*; the extent to which *T. cati* is responsible for ocular disease is unknown, although it may be relevant that Burren (24) found that larvae of *T. canis* entered the brain in all cases and the eye in 5% of experimentally infected mice, whereas only 8% of mice infected with *T. cati* developed lesions in the brain and in none were the eyes involved. Visual prognosis depends on the location of the lesions and the degree of inflammation. The coexistence of ocular toxocariasis and VLM is extremely rare (92). It is possible that ocular disease is caused by a strain of *Toxocara* with specific tropisms. Another hypothesis suggests that VLM is the result of several waves of migrating larvae and OLM occurs in children who have not been previously sensitized (79). Three main types of ocular involvement have been described.

1. *Peripheral retinitis and vitritis*. Currently, peripheral retinal and vitreous involvement is the most common form of presentation (70) and is one cause of unilateral peripheral uveitis in children. A study of 150 children with uveitis by Perkins (119) demonstrated positive skin tests for *Toxocara* in 10%. It is likely that the larva enters the eye via the ciliary circulation in such cases and/or that migration to this location reflects local retinal and choroidal microvascular anatomic arrangements. The inflammation stimulates the formation of vitreoretinal membranes that produces traction on the retina with a typical fold (Fig. 11). The presence of more than one peripheral focus of inflammation, most likely related to more than one larva is extremely rare.
2. *Posterior retinal granuloma*. The lesion in these patients is similar to that of chronic endophthalmitis,

(A)

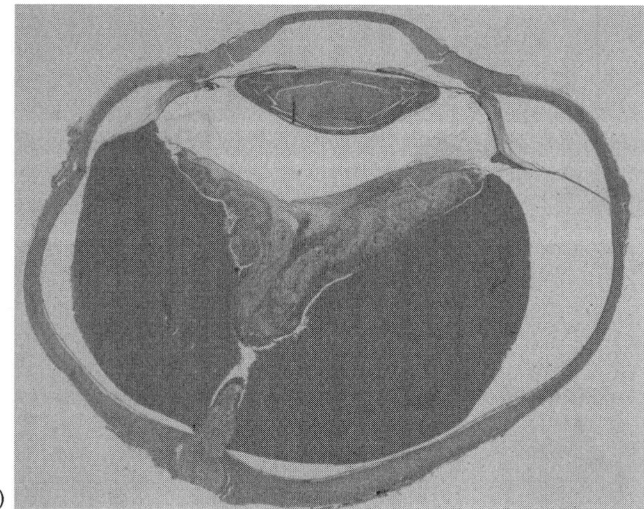

(B)

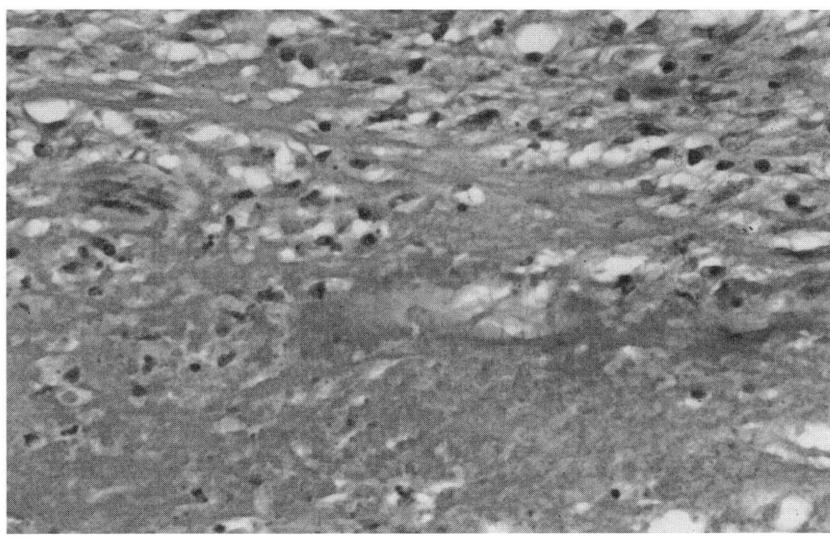

Figure 11 Toxocariasis. (**A**) Enucleated eye with a preretinal inflammatory mass, total retinal detachment, and subretinal exudate. (**B**) Peripheral granuloma with central necrosis and the presence of a distorted wall consistent with a larva (hematoxylin and eosin, $\times$ 240).

except that retinal detachment is absent and the lesion is more circumscribed (Fig. 12) (1). Such lesions can raise a suspicion of retinoblastoma, and indeed, this was the presumptive diagnosis in 20 of the 46 eyes sectioned by Wilder (164) in her study, which established nematode infestation as the cause.

3. *Chronic endophthalmitis*. According to early descriptions of ocular toxocariasis chronic endothalmitis was by far the most common form of presentation, accounting for about two-thirds of reported cases (2). Typically, a focus of granulomatous inflammation forms within the retina, with a central zone of necrosis in which a *Toxocara* larva may be found (Fig. 13); eosinophils are a prominent component of the cellular infiltrate and may exert a cytotoxic effect on the larva (131). The retina is usually detached as a result of serous exudation, the latter sometimes containing cholesterol crystals. This invites comparison with Coats disease, and a study of several such globes by Ashton (2) revealed a small granulomatous nodule surrounding a nematode larva in one instance, even though other parts of the same eye showed no sign of inflammation.

Less common ocular disease in toxocariasis includes optic neuritis with retinal detachment and vitritis, anterior chamber involvement and the presence of presumed *T. canis* larva within a clear cornea (144). The role of *Toxocara* in diffuse chorioretinitis remains speculative.

Pathology: Artificially induced ocular toxocariasis in laboratory animals suggests that the inflammation promoted by *T. canis* is caused by products of viable larvae (161) and that, once initiated, it can proceed in the absence of the parasite. The larva, having initiated a tissue response, moves away, making identification of parasites in the subsequent

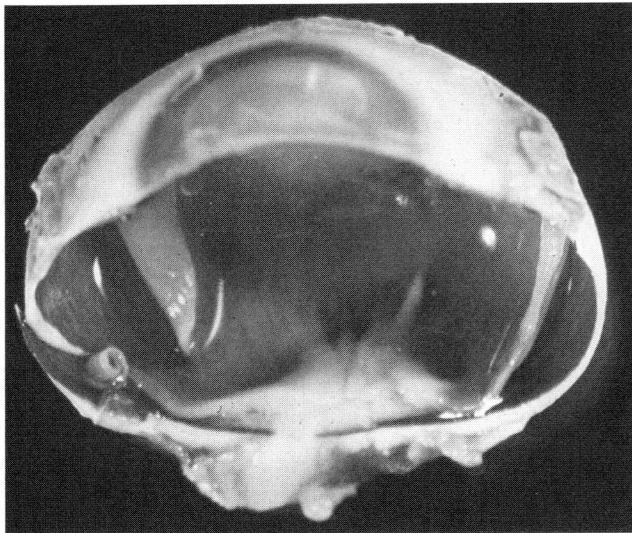

Figure 12 Toxocariasis. Posterior retinal granuloma.

granulomatous phase a relatively unlikely event (61). Indeed, the migratory behavior of the larva in conjunction with sloughing of its sheath may be a means of evading serious damage from the host's immune reaction (61,161). A remarkable case in whom eight distinct posterior segment lesions were examined histologically was reported by Lyness et al. (92): a larva was found in only one of them, and from the character of the inflammatory response it seemed possible that the entire sequence was attributable to a single larva that had initiated a local reaction and repeatedly moved to other locations before succumbing.

The classical lesion was described by Wilder as "eosinophilic abscesses sometimes surrounded by epithelioid and giant cells" (164). Multiple sections in similar cases have revealed tubular hyaline structures representing residual capsular sheaths (Fig. 11B) and, rarely, a well-preserved larva. In eyes with active inflammation the vitreous is infiltrated by numerous eosinophils. The average width of a second-stage larva of *T. canis* is approximately 18 to 21 μm. Enucleation and cytologic specimens in longstanding cases showed a mononuclear infiltrate containing lymphocytes and plasma cells.

Immunodiagnosis: As might be anticipated, *Toxocara* larvae stimulate IgG, IgM, and IgE production (34,158). In the past, most immunologic-based serological tests lacked sensitivity and cross-reacted with other antihelminthic antibodies. An ELISA has become the test of choice for the diagnosis of toxocariasis (122). Sensitivity and specificity have reached values >90% when the cutoff of titers is lowered from 1:32 to 1:8 (32,146). In cases with negative or low anti-*Toxocara* ELISA values in the serum, vitreous and aqueous specimens may demonstrate higher values (136). This is suggestive of local antibody production within the eye. The ratio between vitreous and serum values or the presence of higher titers from the vitreous may help in the diagnosis when eosinophils are not demonstrated in vitreous cytology.

Gnathostomiasis

Human infestation by the spiruroid nematode, *Gnathostoma spinigerum*, is well recognized in Southeast Asia, parts of China, and particularly Japan

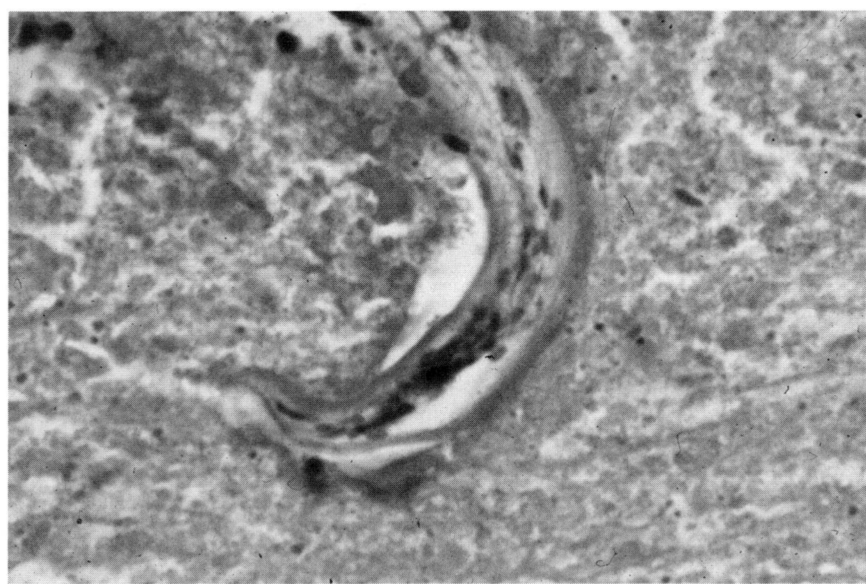

Figure 13 Toxocariasis. Section of a *Toxocara canis* larva within an area of necrosis in a preretinal granuloma (hematoxylin and eosin, × 200).

and Thailand, where it can be endemic. It is one of the helminths associated with VLM, starting with nausea and epigastric discomfort some 24 to 48 hours after eating infected food and proceeding to cause a migratory cutaneous swelling. The latter, that is usually painless, together with conspicuous eosinophilia, is generally diagnostic. Liver dysfunction and a potentially fatal myeloencephalitis may also develop.

The life cycle involves a sequence of intermediate hosts and the definitive host, in which sexual reproduction and the formation of ova occur in any one of a number of carnivores, including dogs, cats, and larger feline species. Indeed, it seems that the first description of the parasite, in 1836, was in the stomach wall of a tiger (117). The human is an accidental host. Ova in the feces of infected animals hatch in water at about 27°C to form larvae that are ingested by freshwater microcrustaceans of the genus *Cyclops*. Here they develop into second-stage larvae before the first intermediate host is devoured by a second host, usually a fish or a frog but even chickens and ducks, where they penetrate the gastric wall, parasitize the muscle tissues, molt to create third-stage larvae, and encyst. Maturation to adult worms takes place only in the stomach of the definitive host and so depends, in turn, on the fish or frog being eaten. The already complex life cycle can be further compounded if the second intermediate host is consumed by a third host, such as rats, snakes, or poultry. Paratenic hosts of this sort can themselves become infected, and although they do not promote larval maturation, they can be a source of human disease should infected poultry be eaten in an adequately cooked state. Raw fish is probably the most frequent source of human infection.

In humans, the third-stage, permanently migrating larvae can survive for several years, but maturation to the adult worm is very rare (28). Cutaneous swelling may recur intermittently over many years. Cerebral involvement is often fatal.

Ocular lesions: The paucity of published reports of ocular gnathostomiasis (67,142,169), which is incidental to the vagaries of the wandering larvae and may not be manifest until long after the initial infection (157), is likely to be an understatement of its incidence. Eyelid swelling appears to be the most common sequence, but orbital cellulitis, uveitis, intraocular hemorrhage, and central retinal artery occlusion are also reported (85). Viable larvae measuring about 5 mm in length may be seen in the anterior chamber and are presumed to have entered the eye via the optic nerve or by direct penetration of the sclera. In two cases described by Kittiponghansa et al. (85), the larvae produced multiple holes in the iris, a fibrinous exudative response, and an acute rise in intraocular pressure (IOP) that resolved after surgical removal of the offending worm. When the track of the larvae is such as to traverse the vitreous, however, fibrous bands may form and ultimately give rise to retinal detachment (157).

Filariasis

Filarial nematodes are thread-like worms especially adapted for survival in the tissues of hosts during all stages of development. The females are ovoviviparous and produce first-stage larvae known as microfilariae, which can remain without further maturation in the blood or skin for about one week. Filarial parasites may be classified according to the habitat of the adult worms in the vertebral host. The cutaneous group includes *Loa loa*, *Onchocerca volvulus*, and *Mansonella streptocerca*. The lymphatic group includes *Wuchereria bancrofti*, *Brugia malayi*, and *B. timori*. The body cavity group includes *M. perstans* and *M. ozzardi*.

Much of the disease attributable to filarial infection appears to have an immunological pathogenesis, allergic reactions being excited by dying worms and microfilariae (83). Raised serum levels of IgG and IgE are common, and eosinophilia is usual. In addition, there is evidence that the immune response may have a cumulative protective effect, since microfilarial numbers usually diminish with increasing age in patients living in endemic areas where repeated infection is common (112). Studies in laboratory animals suggest that any immunity is likely to be aimed at the microfilariae rather than the adult worm (31). The limited information available points to the importance of cell-mediated mechanisms in this context (6), antibodies appearing to have little protective function.

Bancroftian Filariasis

W. bancrofti is prevalent in many tropical areas of the world, with males measuring up to 4 cm and females up to 10 cm in length. Adult worms reside in the lymphatics of the limbs and groin, where they are prone to cause elephantiasis and, in males, hydroceles. The female is viviparous, and emerging larvae, which are sheathed, enter the circulating blood with a nocturnal periodicity. When ingested by a suitable species of mosquito feeding on the skin, the larvae undergo further stages of development, becoming capable of infecting other individuals when they are disgorged in the saliva of the feeding insect. Infective larvae in human tissue migrate to the draining lymph nodes and, after a further two molts, develop into mature worms.

Ocular Lesions: Involvement of the eyes may be direct. Direct invasion of the inner eye by first-stage larvae (microfilariae) is a result of hematogenous dissemination and is accompanied by a granulomatous iridocyclitis should the anterior chamber be infected, or a subretinal inflammatory lesion (135). Allergic reactions in the tissues appear to be linked with death of the parasite (108), and it is conceivable that the paucity of ocular involvement by *Wuchereria* is an index of the infrequency with which microfilariae leave the circulation, becoming stranded in the extravascular structures of the eye. The adult worm, responsible for most of the manifestations of bancroftian filariasis, may on very rare occasions invade the eye.

Conjunctival edema may accompany recurrent allergic episodes, provoked by death of adult worms in the tissues, in which the principal elements are lymphangiitis, lymphadenitis, and fever. Microfilariae cannot be demonstrated, and the conjunctiva is probably responding to circulating antigen–antibody complexes.

Malayan Filariasis

B. malayi is a filarial nematode similar to *Wuchereria* in many respects but restricted to Southeast Asia and Southern India. Isolated accounts of outer eye involvement have appeared, including one case in whom intertwined male and female worms were identified in the bulbar conjunctiva (75). Anterior uveitis related to the presence of an adult worm in the anterior chamber has also been described (134), the parasite being presumed to have entered the eye by way of the iris vessels.

Loiasis

Loiasis is prevalent in tropical West and Central Africa and is caused by the filarial roundworm *L. loa*. The adult worms reside in the subcutaneous connective tissue, where the viviparous female produces sheathed microfilariae measuring 200 to 300 μm in length and 6 to 8 μm in width. Many microfilariae enter the bloodstream, being most readily detected during the daylight hours, and transmission is by the bite of blood-sucking mangrove flies of the genus *Chrysops*. In the fly the larvae undergo two molts to become third-stage larvae and ready to be reintroduced into human tissue. Bites usually occur around the ankles, and larvae slowly mature over 6 to 12 months into adult worms that migrate through the subcutaneous tissues and survive for up to 20 years.

Allergic responses are provoked by the liberation of microfilariae from the female worms and are probably IgE-mediated, in the form of transient painless edematous swellings in the subcutaneous tissue (Calabar swellings); sometimes the lesions are associated with intense itching and fever. A pronounced eosinophilia of 20,000 to 50,000 mm^3 is usual.

Ocular lesions: Not uncommonly, adult worms migrate across the conjunctiva, earning them the name of African eye worm, and this is likely to be attended by intense pain and itching, which persists until the worm moves into the deeper and less richly innervated tissues of the orbit. *L. loa,* which has been likened to a piece of fishing line and may measure up to 7 cm in length and about 0.5 mm in diameter, can often be removed surgically from the conjunctiva. Worms dying in the conjunctival habitat are associated with an inflammatory nodule characterized histologically by a granuloma in which macrophages, lymphocytes, plasma cells, eosinophils, epithelioid cells, including giant cell forms are grouped around a nidus of coagulative eosinophilic necrosis; a dead gravid female nematode may also be demonstrable (123). The significance of the inflammation being related to female worms is that, as with subcutaneous swellings elsewhere, the source of the antigenic stimulation is considered the ova and first-stage larvae (54).

Rarely, microfilariae invade the globe, Toussaint and Danis (155) having described the clinical and histological findings in one such case; extensive retinal hemorrhage and serous exudation, with the formation of capillary microaneurysms, were associated with microfilarial embolism of the retinal vessels, and many venous channels were surrounded by a mantle of lymphocytes. Müller (103) comments on the similarity of the choroidoretinal lesions seen in another case to those of onchocerciasis and suggests that this mode of presentation may be more common than is generally recognized. Migration into the vitreous and the anterior chamber by adult *L. loa* has also been described (114,148).

Onchocerciasis

Onchocerciasis, or river blindness, is prevalent in much of West and Central Africa and Central America and affects about 18 million people worldwide (110,163). Numerically, it is by far the most important helminth infection in the ophthalmic context, with some 500,000 people possibly having eye lesions as a result of onchocercal infection. The control of the vector and administration of drugs with wider impact beyond specific filarial parasites have been one of major achievements of last decades (100).

Humans are the natural host of the adult worm (*O. volvulus*), which resides in the subcutaneous tissues and is eventually destined to be incarcerated within a nodule of dense fibrous tissue known as an onchocercoma. The fertilized viviparous female releases large numbers of microfilariae, which migrate through the superficial dermis (Fig. 14). Further development is dependent on the larvae being ingested by blackflies (*Simulium* sp.) feeding on the skin. After molting twice, third-stage larvae can infect other individuals the next time the fly bites. Flies of the *Simulium* genus breed on the banks of streams, where there is well-oxygenated running water, and have characteristic feeding habits. Members of the *S. damnosum* complex, the usual vector in Africa, tend to bite the feet and legs, whereas *S. ochraeum,* occurring in Central America,

(A) 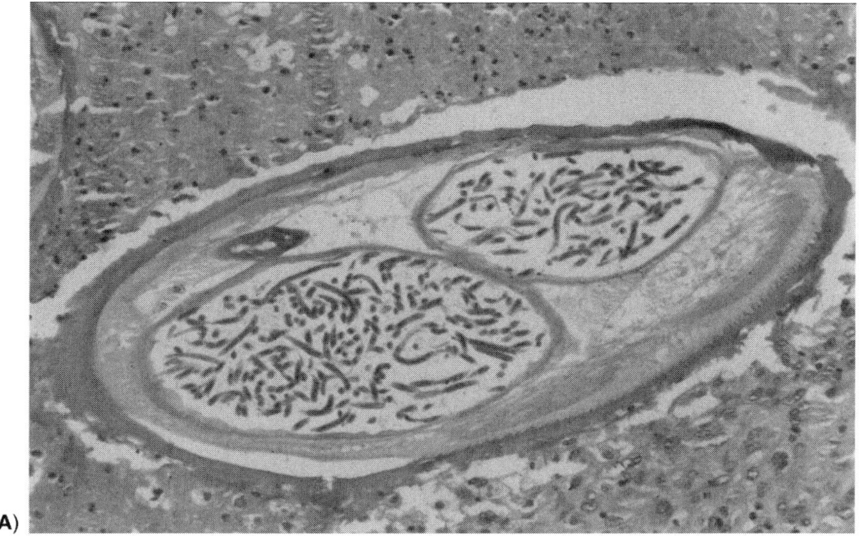

(B) 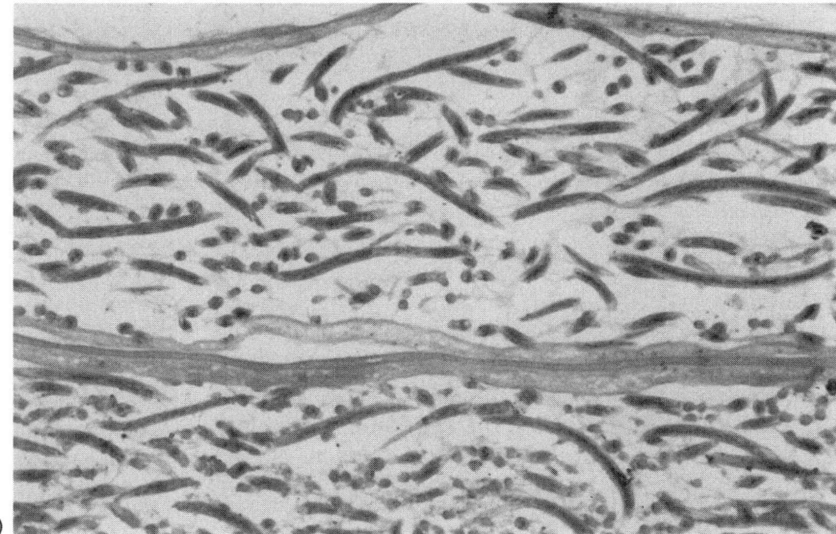

Figure 14 Onchocerciasis. (**A**) Nodule with adult female *Oncocerca* worms (hematoxylin and eosin, × 60). (**B**) Longitudinal section of the midbody of a gravid female with numerous microfilariae (hematoxylin and eosin, × 120).

bites much higher. This is related to the risk of incurring ocular complications, since microfilariae migrating from nodules on the upper part of the body have a greater chance of reaching the eye than those emanating from lower nodules.

Microfilariae within the skin are often associated with an itchy rash with multiple papules, proceeding, through intradermal edema, to atrophy and loss of skin elasticity. Lymphadenopathy is also present, and it is probable that some of the skin changes are a manifestation of hypersensitivity to microfilarial antigens. *O. cervicalis*, *O. gutturosa*, *O. dewittei*, and *O. lupei*, which normally infect horses, cattle, and wild boar, respectively, may be responsible for aberrant, zoonotic, subconjunctival infections in man (147).

Immunology. Raised levels of all the major antibody classes have been reported in patients with onchocerciasis, but their significance is uncertain. The difficulty is occasioned in part by the dubious specificity of the antibodies, given an appreciable degree of antigen sharing between the various filarial worms and the frequency with which patients are infected with more than one parasite at any one time. Probably the most reliable evidence is the IgE responses (162), but even then its pathogenetic relevance is not clear since there is little correlation between circulating antibody levels and disease activity (94). On the other hand, allegedly parasite-specific IgM levels have been claimed to bear an inverse relationship to the microfilarial density in the skin. Antibody generation appears to be a response to dying microfilariae (22) and to be the basis of the anaphylactic reactions that can attend filaricide treatment with diethylcarbamazine or ivermectin (33,68).

The filariae harbor abundant intracellular *Wolbachia* bacteria. *Endobacteria* contribute to the pathogenesis of onchocerciasis, and molecules have been identified that promote inflammatory or counter-inflammatory immune mechanisms, divert the host's immune response or procure evasion of the parasite (16). Cell-mediated responses have been found to be depressed in patients with heavily infected skin (111); conversely, it has been suggested that patients in Yemen developing an unusual form of onchocerciasis known as "sowdah," with few microfilariae in the tissues and pronounced lymphocytic and plasma cell infiltration, have a high level of T cell activity (140). Significantly, perhaps, these patients rarely develop eye lesions.

Ocular lesions: Involvement of the eyeball is due to microfilarial invasion of either anterior or posterior segments. Anterior segment lesions are related to the presence of microfilariae that reach the cornea and anterior chamber from the periorbital skin and conjunctiva (Fig. 15). The microfilariae are 200 to 400 μm in length and 5 to 10 μm in width and have no sheaths. Live microfilariae within the cornea are without effect, but eventually a punctate keratitis may develop in which the minute opacities are almost certainly a response to dying larvae. Eye lesions usually are related to duration and severity of infection and area caused by an abnormal host immune response to microfilariae. Light microscopy of experimentally-induced lesions (56) shows lymphocytes and eosinophils aggregated around necrotic remnants of individual microfilariae (Fig. 15). Such lesions, which possibly represent an immune reaction to specific microfilarial antigens (54), may resolve completely. Sclerosing keratitis, which may supervene, appears to be the outcome of more intense and recurrent infection, a contention supported by experimental studies (38), and is characterized by the formation of a fibrovascular pannus with a variable amount of leukocytic infiltration. Duke (42) drew attention to the greater incidence of corneal lesions in patients from the savanna regions of West Africa compared with rain forest areas. Experimental studies in the rabbit, involving the injection of equal numbers of microfilariae from volunteers living in each of these regions into the corneoscleral limbus, indicate that such a topographical difference is a function of the parasite and is probably related to strain variations (44,56). Patterns of onchocercal eye disease are associated with parasite strain differences at the DNA level (110). The significance of a finding that autoantibodies to corneal extracts develop in guinea pigs injected with *O. lienalis* (39) has yet to be determined, although both humoral and cell-mediated reactions are involved (37).

The more severe degrees of corneal and conjunctival involvement may be accompanied by a nongranulomatous iridocyclitis in which lymphocytes predominate and is probably an indirect response to antigen diffusing from infected corneal tissue. *G. iritis* has been described, however, and appears to be a response to direct invasion of the anterior uvea (132). Anterior and posterior synechiae with secondary cataract formation may develop in more severely affected cases.

Posterior segment lesions appear to be a function of heavy *O. volvulus* infection and may progress with alarming rapidity (139). They are the major cause of onchocercal visual impairment in rain forest areas (110). The precise mode of entry to the posterior segment is

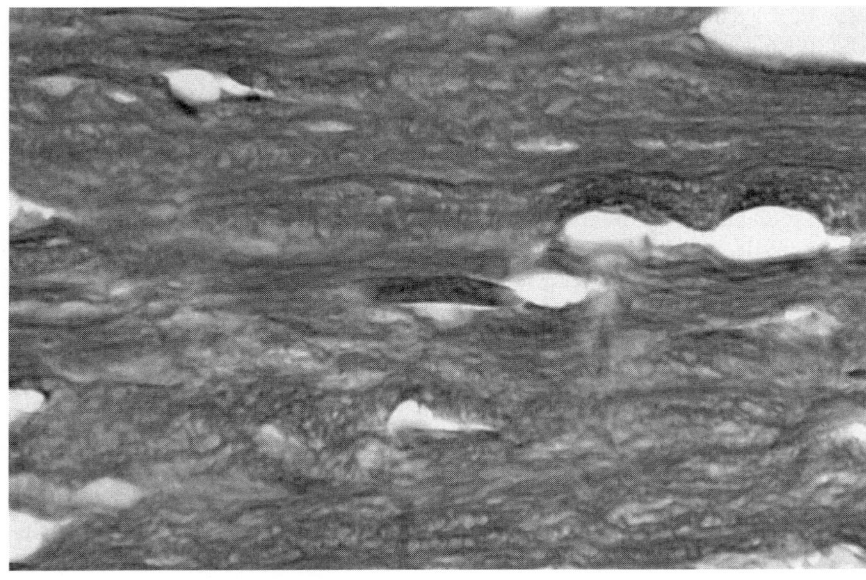

Figure 15 Onchocerciasis. Section of the cornea with a microfilaria within the collagenous corneal lamellae (hematoxylin and eosin, × 240).

arguable: microfilariae may enter from the orbit along the sheaths of ciliary blood vessels and nerves (42,43,109) or via the bloodstream. Microfilarial invasion of the choroid is associated with a diffuse lymphocytic, plasma cell, and eosinophil reaction attended by both focal hyperplasia and a degeneration of the RPE (57) to create a "pigmentary retinopathy." In some patients pigmentary degeneration is pronounced and is associated with marked retinal atrophy, so that the underlying choroidal vasculature is laid bare to produce a virtually pathognomonic fundus appearance (12,129).

The mechanism of the retinal changes is obscure, and a description of circulating autoantibodies to arrestin (retinal S antigen) and interphotoreceptor retinoid binding protein (27,88) is as likely to be an epiphenomenon as it is to be causal. A finding of rather more interest is that there is an apparent sharing of antigens between the microfilariae of *O. volvulus* and the RPE (15,17). The possible contribution of nonimmune processes also needs consideration, especially as clinically recognizable pigmentary changes preceded demonstrable antibody or cell-mediated responses in monkeys inoculated intravitreally with live microfilariae (138). What these other mechanisms might be, however, is obscure. Even more patients with posterior segment involvement develop optic atrophy, and whereas retinal changes are involved in some cases, direct invasion of the optic nerve is likely to be responsible in others (12). Microfilariae have been demonstrated in both the nerve (132) and its sheath (118).

Nodules surrounding adult worms have been described in the orbit, usually the anterior part, as a rare event. In one such case a gravid female was surrounded by a leukocytic reaction that included eosinophils, lymphocytes, plasma cells, and macrophages, with multinucleated giant cell forms inside a dense fibrous capsule (Fig. 14); microfilariae could be seen within the collagenous tissue (55).

Dirofilariasis

Although several members of the genus *Dirofilaria* have been recognized in humans, the most usual being *Dirofilaria immitis*, *D. repens*, *D. ursi*, and *D. tenuis* (*D. conjunctivae*), infection is rare and accidental, and man is an unsuitable host for completion of the worm life cycle. *Dirofilaria* are widely distributed throughout the world. *D. immitis* is indigenous in the canine population of North America, where in some parts up to 50% of dogs are infected with the parasite. Transmission is normally from dog to dog through mosquitoes feeding on the skin. Adult female worms measure 25 to 30 cm in length and 0.2 to 0.4 cm in width, males being shorter, only 4 to 5 cm.

(**A**)
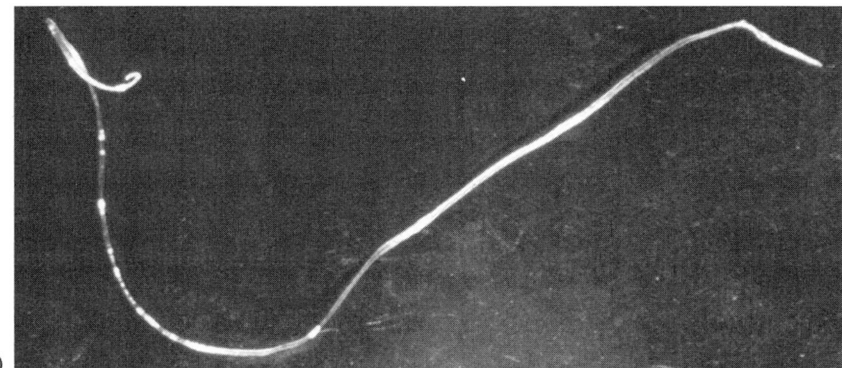

(**B**)
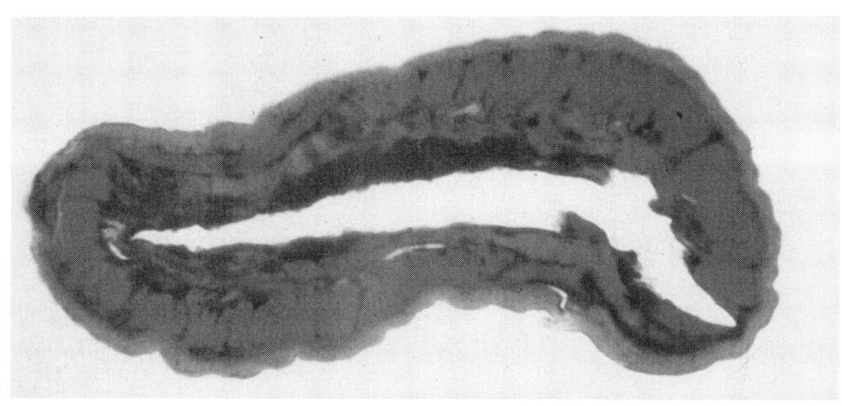

Figure 16 Dirofilariasis. (**A**) *Dirofilaria* excised from the eyelid. (**B**) Cross-section of the worm with lateral cords and muscle (Masson trichrome stain, × 120).

Ocular lesions: Ocular involvement in humans is extremely rare and is probably the result of being bitten near the eye by infected mosquitoes (Fig. 16) (52). In such circumstances the infective larvae may mature into adult worms, which as long as they remain viable cause little disturbance, but in the dying phase promote inflammatory nodules in the subconjunctival stroma (133) or a necrotizing granuloma in the orbit or eyelid (Fig. 17) (20,152). Ciliary body and iris involvement has been described in one patient, and intravitreous disease by *D. repens* (66). Eosinophils are prominent in both blood and tissues.

Parastrongyliasis

The *Angiostrongylus* genus includes nematodes recently reclassified within the genus *Parastrongylus* in which humans act as accidental hosts. Human infection occurs by the ingestion of infective larvae in slugs, snails or on vegetation. They may cause eosinophilic meningitis (*Angiostrongylus cantonensis*), subcutaneous nodules and inflammatory bowel disease (*A. costaricensis*). Ocular involvement has been reported from Sri Lanka (36).

Dracunculiasis

Also known as the Guinea worm, *Dracunculus medinensis* is a tissue dwelling spiruroid nematode found in many parts of West and East Africa, South America, and South Asia. Humans are the natural host, the mature female worm migrating to the skin to provoke the formation of a blister that is liable to burst on contact with water. First-stage larvae released from the ruptured blister may then be ingested by crustaceans of the genus *Cyclops* to undergo further development. The cycle is completed by drinking contaminated water. Subsequently the postgravid adult worm dies and is either destroyed or calcified. Related species of *Dracunculus* infest a number of other mammals, especially mink, raccoons, and otters in North America (102).

Ocular lesions: Rarely, the mature worms migrate to the eyelids, conjunctiva and orbit, where they stimulate an initial granulomatous inflammatory reaction (23) that is frequently followed by abscess formation (Fig. 18). It is possible that part of the inflammation is due to secondary bacterial infection incurred by disruption of the covering epithelium as the female *Dracunculus* makes her way to the surface. Ultimately, a giant cell reaction to residues of the calcified dead worm may be seen (23,104). In some infected individuals, periorbital edema can occur as part of a generalized cutaneous hypersensitivity reaction to the parasite just before it emerges.

Thelaziasis

Parasites of the genus *Thelazia*, commonly named eyeworms, are nematodes which infect the eyes and associated tissues of mammals, including humans (115). Transmission of eyeworms occurs via nonbiting diptera (*Musca* sp.) that feed on the ocular secretions, tears and conjunctiva of animals. Among several species *Thelazia callipaeda* is responsible for human and canid ocular infection in the Far East, and *Thelazia californiensis* parasitizes several ruminants, including deer, as well as dogs in North America (62).

Human infection is accidental and very rare (84). In such cases adult worms (males measure 4–13 mm and females 7–19 mm) may develop in the conjunctival sac from implanted larvae and promote intense inflammation with epiphora, conjunctivitis, keratitis, corneal opacity, and ulcers (46). *T. callipaeda* is the

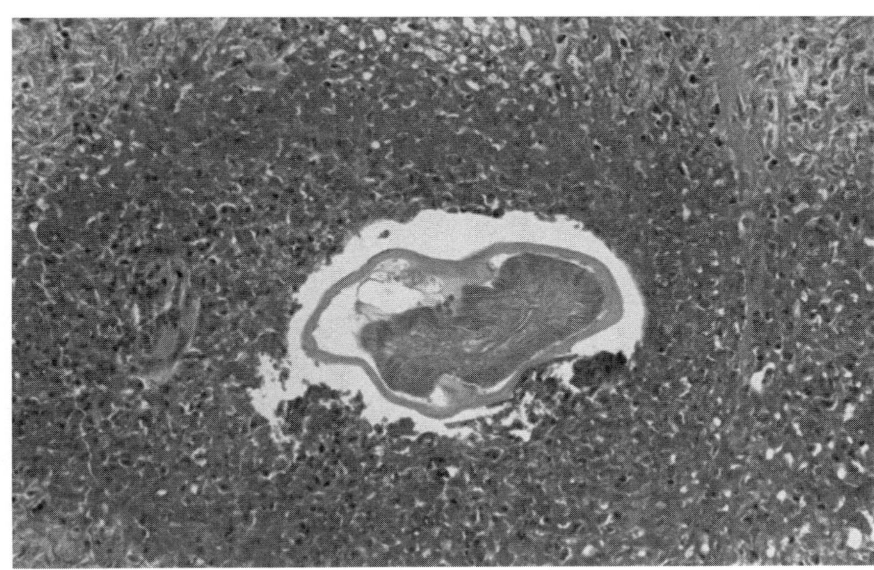

Figure 17 Dirofilariasis. Abscess of the eyelid with fragment of a worm surrounded by eosinophilic necrosis (hematoxylin and eosin, ×120).

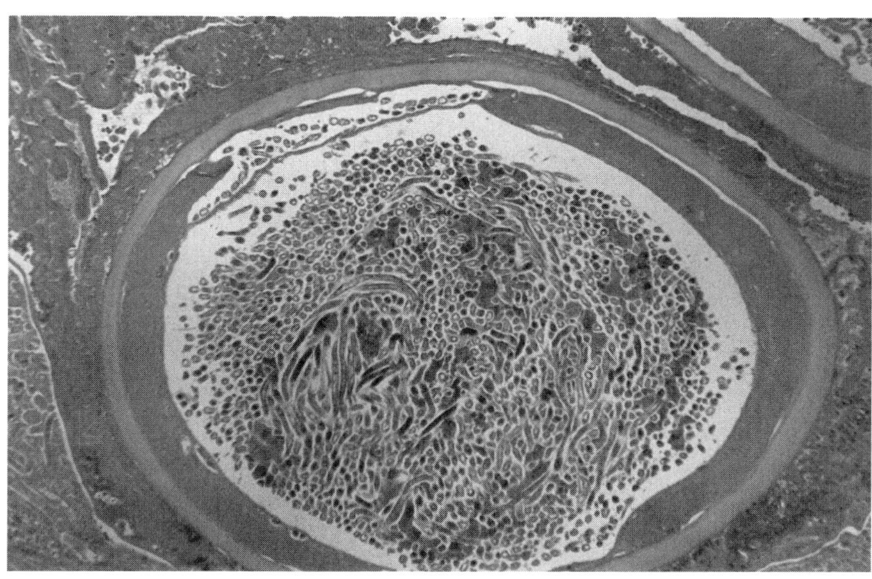

Figure 18 Dracunculiasis. Transverse section of a gravid female from a soft tissue lesion (hematoxylin and eosin, × 60).

species most likely to cause scarring since it burrows into the tissue, whereas *T. californiensis* confines its movements to the surface and provokes only minor irritation (145).

Trichinosis

Trichinosis (trichinellosis) is caused by nematodes of the genus *Trichinella*. The application of molecular and biochemical methods in conjunction with experimental studies on biology have resulted in the identification of seven *Trichinella* species, which have distinct epidemiological and geographical distributions (86,124). In addition to the classical agent *T. spiralis* (found throughout the world in many carnivorous and omnivorous animals), four other species of *Trichinella* are now recognized as causing infection in humans, including *T. pseudospiralis* (mammals and birds throughout the world), *T. nativa* (arctic bears), *T. nelsoni* (African predators and scavengers), and *T. britovi* (carnivores of Europe and western Asia) (21). *T. spiralis* is a parasitic nematode of carnivorous animals of widespread distribution. Living in the gut mucosa, larvae from the ovoviviparous female penetrate into the submucosa and are carried in the circulatory system to various organs, including the myocardium, brain, lungs, retina, lymph nodes, pancreas, and cerebrospinal fluid (CSF). However, only the larvae that invade the skeletal muscle survive. The life cycle is completed when infected meat is eaten by other carnivores and in humans it usually results from consuming undercooked meat (most frequently pork) or game. The species of *Trichinella* involved, as well as the number of parasites ingested, together with sex, age, ethnic group, and immune status of the host are important factors in clinical disease in humans. Cell-mediated responses to the adult worm within the intestines are associated with goblet cell proliferation, which, by coating the worm with mucus, promotes its expulsion (10). The larva may damage the muscle cells directly, or indirectly stimulating the infiltration of inflammatory cells, primarily eosinophils. Cellular responses during this stage are probably responsible for the marked eosinophilia characteristic of patients with trichinosis (81). IgG, IgM, and IgE antibodies directed against larval antigens are also formed, and although there is evidence of antibody-dependent cytotoxicity, the larvae are able to survive through a capacity for encystment. The classical clinical triad includes myalgias, periorbital edema, and eosinophilia. The diagnosis is made on the basis of these clinical manifestations, hypereosinophilia, total IgE, and muscle enzyme level increase. Indirect hemagglutination, bentonite flocculation, indirect immunofluorescence, latex agglutination, and ELISA are the more commonly used tests, the last being the most sensitive (105). The definitive diagnosis requires surgical biopsy of the involved muscle. A muscle biopsy is useful for genetic typing (by random amplified polymorphic DNA analysis of the parasite) (8).

Ocular lesions: Ocular signs (edema of the eyelids, chemosis, conjunctivitis, conjunctival hemorrhages, disturbed vision, and ocular pain) at the parenteral stage may help in the clinical diagnosis. Periorbital edema is peculiar to trichinellosis, ranging from 17% to 100% of patients in over 2000 trichinellosis cases reviewed. This edema probably results from of an allergic response (149,151). Most infected individuals, however, have few symptoms, but of those presenting with clinical signs, about one-third include an ocular disturbance. As a rule this results from a larval infestation of the extraocular muscles and presents as a painful limitation of eye movements associated with proptosis and chemosis. The affected muscles are swollen, and as the myositis progresses, they lose their cross-striations before forming a basophilic halo of necrotic tissue around the responsible larvae. These changes develop within the first two to three weeks after larval invasion, but subsequently, as chronic inflammatory cells accumulate, individual larvae, with the exception of *T. pseudospiralis* and *T. papuae*, become encysted within two weeks depending on the *Trichinella* species involved. By about the fifth week the myositis subsides, and within a few months the cysts often become calcified, although the enclosed larvae may survive for several years. Rare retinal hemorrhages and papilledema have also been described (48) and may be the result of several factors such as vasculitis, granulomatous inflammatory reaction, and neural damage by eosinophil degranulation products (eosinophil derived-neurotoxin and major basic protein).

REFERENCES

1. Ashton N. Larval granulomatosis of the retina due to *Toxocara*. Br J Ophthalmol 1960; 44:129–48.
2. Ashton N. *Toxocara canis* and the eye. In: Rycroft PV, ed. Proceedings of Second Corneo-Plastic Conference, London 1967. Pergamon Press, Oxford 1969:579–91.
3. Ashton N, Brown N, Easty D. Trematode cataract in freshwater fish. J Small Anim Pract 1969; 10:471–78.
4. Ashton N, Cook C. Allergic granulomatous nodules of the eyelid and conjunctiva. Am J Ophthalmol 1979; 87:1–28.
5. Badir G. Schistosomiasis of the conjunctiva. Bull Ophthalmol Soc Egypt 1949; 39:52–60.
6. Bagai RC, Subrahmanyam D. Nature of acquired resistance to filarial infection in albino rats. Nature 1970; 228:682–3.
7. Bajaj MS, Pushker N. Optic nerve cysticercosis. Clin Experiment Ophthalmol 2002; 30:140–3.
8. Bandi C, La Rosa G, Bardin MG, et al. Random amplified polymorphic DNA fingerprints of the eighth taxa of trichinella and their comparison with allozyme analysis. Parasitology 1995; 110:401–7.
9. Bass JL, Mehta KA, Glickman LT, Blocker R, Eppers BM. Asymptomatic toxocariasis in children: a prospective study and treatment trial. Clin Pediatr (Phila) 1987; 26:441–6.
10. Bell RG, McGregor DD, Adams LS. Studies on the inhibition of rapid expulsion of *Trichinella spiralis* in rats. Int Arch Allergy Appl Immunol 1982; 69:73–80.
11. Binford CH, Connor DH. Pathology of Tropical and Extraordinary Diseases. Vol II. Washington, DC: Armed Forces Institute of Pathology 1976:340–550.
12. Bird AC, Anderson J, Fuglsang H. Morphology of posterior segment lesions of the eye in patients with onchocerciasis. Br J Ophthalmol 1976; 60:2–20.
13. Boase AJ. Coenurus cyst of the eye. Br J Ophthalmol 1956; 40:183–5.
14. Bradley JE, Jackson JA. Immunity, immunoregulation and the ecology of trichuriasis and ascariasis. Parasite Immunol 2004; 26:429–41.
15. Bradley JE, Nirmalan N, Klager SL, Faulkner H, Kennedy MW. River blindness: a role for parasite retinoid-binding proteins in the generation of pathology? Trends Parasitol 2001; 17:471–5.
16. Brattig NW. Pathogenesis and host responses in human onchocerciasis: impact of *Onchocerca filariae* and *Wolbachia endobacteria*. Microbes Infect 2004; 6:113–28.
17. Braun G, McKechnie DM, Connor V, et al. Immunological cross reactivity between a cloned antigen *of Onchocerca volvulus* and a component of the retinal pigment epithelium. J Exp Med 1991; 174:169–111.
18. Bresson-Hadni S, Vuitton DA, Bartholomot B, et al. A twenty-year history of *Alveolar echinococcosis*: analysis of a series of 117 patients from eastern France. Eur J Gastroenterol Hepatol 2000; 12:327–36.
19. Brown DH. Ocular *Toxocara canis* II: clinical review. J Pediatr Ophthalmol 1970; 17:182–91.
20. Brumback GF, Morrison HM, Weatherby NF. Orbital infection with *Dirofilaria*. South Med J 1968; 61:188–92.
21. Bruschi F, Murrell KD. New aspects of human trichinellosis: the impact of new Trichinella species. Postgrad Med J 2002; 78:15–22.
22. Bryceson ADM, Warrell DA, Pope HM. Dangerous reactions to treatment of onchocerciasis with diethylcarbamazine. Br Med J 1977; 1:742–4.
23. Burnier M Jr, Hidayat AA, Neafie R. Dracunculiasisis of the orbit and eyelid: light and electron microscopic observations of two cases. Ophthalmology 1991; 98: 919–24.
24. Burren CH. The distribution of *Toxocara* sp. larvae in the central nervous system of the mouse. Trans R Soc Trop Med Hyg 1971; 65:450–3.
25. Capron A, Dessaint J-P, Capron M, Joseph M, Torpier G. Effector mechanisms of immunity to schistosomes and their regulation. Immunol Rev 1982; 61:41–66.
26. Cardenas F, Plancarte A, Quiroz H, Rabiela MT, Gomez-Leal A. *Taenia crassiceps*: Experimental model of intraocular cysticercosis. Exp Parasitol 1989; 69:324–9.
27. Chan C-C, Nussenblatt RB, Kim MK, Palestine AG, Awadzi K, Ottesen EA. Immunopathology of onchocerciasis 2. Antiretinal auto antibodies in serum and ocular fluids. Ophthalmology 1987; 94:439–43.
28. Chitanondh H, Rosen L. Fatal eosinophilic encephalomyelitis caused by the nematode *Gnathostoma spinigerum*. Am J Trop Med Hyg 1967; 16:638–45.
29. Chowdhury AB, Kean BH, Browne HG. Inoculation of helminth eggs into animal eyes. Am J Pathol 1960; 36:125–33.
30. Cunha de Souza E, Lustosa da Cunha S, Gass JDM. Diffuse unilateral subacute neuroretinitis in South America. Arch Ophthalmol 1992; 110:1261–3.
31. Denham DA, Ponnudurai T, Nelson GS, Rogers R, Guy F. Studies with *Brugia pahangi* II: The effect or repeated infection on parasite levels in cats. Int J Parasitol 1972; 2:401–7.
32. de Savigny DH, Voller A, Woodruff AW. Toxocariasis: serological diagnosis by enzyme immunoassay. J Clin Pathol 1979; 37:284–8.
33. De Sole G, Remme J, Awadzi K, et al. Adverse reactions after large-scale treatment of onchocerciasis with ivermectin: combined results from eight community trials. Bull World Health Organ 1989; 67:707–19.
34. Despommier D. Toxocariasis: clinical aspects, epidemiology, medical ecology, and molecular aspects. Clin Microbiol Rev 2003; 16:265–72.
35. Dickinson AJ, Rosenthal AR, Nicholson KG. Inflammation of the retinal pigment epithelium: a unique presentation of ocular schistosomiasis. Br J Ophthalmol 1990; 74:440–2.

36. Dissanaike AS, Ihalamulla RL, Naotunne TS, Senarathna T, Withana DS. Third report of ocular parastrongyliasis (angiostrongyliasis) from Sri Lanka. Parassitologia 2001; 43:95–7.
37. Donnelly JJ, Rockey JH, Bianco AE, Soulsby EJL. Ocular immunopathologic findings of experimental onchocerciasis. Arch Ophthalmol 1984; 102:628–34.
38. Donnelly JJ, Taylor HR, Young E, Khatami M, Lok JB, Rockey JH. Experimental ocular onchocerciasis in cynomolgus monkeys. Invest Ophthalmol Vis Sci 1986; 27:492–9.
39. Donnelly JJ, Xi M-S, Haldar JP, Hill DE, Lok JB, Khatami M, Rockey JH. Autoantibody induced by experimental onchocerca infection: effect of different routes of administration of microfilariae and of treatment with diethycarbamazine citrate and ivermectin. Invest Ophthalmol Vis Sci 1988; 29:827–31.
40. Drouet PL, Thomas C, Cordier J, Algan B. Origine parasitaire de certaines hémorragies récidivantes du vitré. Bull Mem Soc Fr Ophtalmol 1949; 62:250–3.
41. Dubey JP. *Toxocara cati* and other intestinal parasites of cats. Vet Rec 1966; 79:506–8.
42. Duke BOL. Onchocerciasis. Br Med Bull 1971; 25:66–71.
43. Duke BOL. Route of entry of *Onchocerca volvulus* microfilariae into the eye. Trans R Soc Trop Med Hyg 1976; 70:90–1.
44. Duke BOL, Anderson J. A comparison of the lesions produced in the cornea of the rabbit eye by microfilariae of the forest and Sudan-savanna strains of *Onchocerca volvulus* from Cameroon I: the clinical picture. Z Tropenmed Parasitol 1972; 25:354–68.
45. Duke BOL, Garner A. Reactions to subconjunctival inoculation of *Onchocerca volvulus* microfilariae in preimmunized rabbits. Z Tropenmed Parasitol 1975; 26:435–48.
46. Duke-Elder S. Diseases of the Outer Eye: System of Ophthalmology, Vol 8, Kimpton, London 1965:416–7.
47. Editorial. Immunopathology of schistosomiasis. Lancet 1987; 2:194–5.
48. Edwards JD. The ocular manifestations of trichinosis. Trans Ophthalmol Soc UK 1954; 74:495–1.
49. Ellis GS, Pakalnis VA, Worley G, et al. *Toxocara canis* infestation: clinical and epidemiological associations with seropositivity in kindergarten children. Ophthalmology 1986; 93:1032–7.
50. Epstein E, Proctor NSF, Heinz HJ. Intraocular *Coenurus* infestation. S Afr Med J 1959; 33:602–4.
51. Finkelman FD, Pearce EJ, Urban JF Jr, Sher A. Regulation and biological function of helminth-induced cytokine responses. In: Ash C, Gallagher RB, eds. Immunoparasitology Today. Elsevier Trends Journals, Cambridge, pp. A62–A65.
52. Font RL, Neafie RC, Perry HD. Subcutaneous dirofilariasis of the eyelid and ocular adnexa: report of six cases. Arch Ophthalmol 1980; 98:1079–82.
53. Fox AS, Kazacos AR, Gould NS, Heydemann PT, Thomas C, Boyer KM. Fatal eosinophilic meningoencephalitis and visceral larva migrans caused by the raccoon ascarid *Baylisascaris procyonis*. N Engl J Med 1985; 312: 1619–23.
54. Gallin MY, Murray D, Lass JH, Grossniklaus HE, Greene BM. Experimental interstitial keratitis Induced by *Onchocerca volvulus* antigens. Arch Ophthalmol 1988; 106:1447–52.
55. Garner A. Pathology of pseudotumours of the orbit: a review. J Clin Pathol 1973; 26:639–48.
56. Garner A, Duke BOL, Anderson J. A comparison of the lesions produced in the cornea of the rabbit eye by microfilariae of the forest and Sudan-savanna strains of *Onchocerca volvulus* from Cameroon II. The pathology. Z Tropenmed Parasitol 1973; 24:385–96.
57. Garner A. Pathology of ocular onchocerciasis. Trans R Soc Trop Med Hyg 1976; 70:374–7.
58. Gass DM, Braunstein RA. Further observations concerning the diffuse unilaterlal subacute neuroretinitis syndrome. Arch Ophthalmol 1983; 101:1689–97.
59. Gass JDM, Scelfo R. Diffuse unilateral subacute neuroretinitis. J R Soc Med 1978; 71:95–111.
60. Gavin PJ, Kazacos KR, Shulman ST. Baylisascariasis. Clin Microbiol Rev 2005; 18:703–18.
61. Ghafoor SYA, Smith HV, Lee WR, Quinn R, Girdwood RWA. Experimental ocular toxocariasis. Br J Ophthalmol 1984; 68:89–96.
62. Giangaspero A, Traversa D, Otranto D. Ecology of Thelazia spp. in cattle and their vectors in Italy. Parassitologia. 2004; 46:257–9.
63. Gibbons LM, Jacobs DE, Sani RA. *Toxocara malaysiensis* n. sp. (Nematoda: Ascaridoidea) from domestic cat (*Felis catus* Linnaeus 1758). J Parasitol 2001; 87:660–5.
64. Glickman LT, Schantz PM. Epidemiology and pathogenesis of zoonotic toxocariasis. Epidemiol Rev 1981; 3: 230–50.
65. Goldberg MA, Kazacos KR, Boyce WM, et al. Diffuse unilateral subacute neuroretinitis: morphologic, serologic, and epidemiologic support for *Baylisascaris* as a causative agent. Ophthalmology 1993; 100:1965–1701.
66. Gorezis S, Psilla M, Asproudis I, Peschos D, Papadopoulou C, Stefaniotou M. Intravitreal dirofilariasis: a rare ocular infection. Orbit. 2006; 25:57–9.
67. Gyi K. Intra-ocular gnathostomiasis. Br J Ophthalmol 1960; 44:42–5.
68. Hawking F. Diethylcarbamazine: a review of the literature with special reference to its pharmacodynamics, toxicity, and use in the therapy of onchocerciasis and other filiarial infections. Bull WHO 1978; 142:4–82.
69. Ibechukwu BI, Onwukeme KE. Intraocular coenurosis: a case report. Br J Ophthalmol 1991; 75:430–1.
70. Irvine WC, Irvine AR. Nematode endophthalmitis: *Toxocara canis*. Am J Ophthalmol 1959; 47:185–91.
71. Jakobiec FA, Gess L, Zimmerman LE. *Granulomatous dacryoadenitis* caused by *Schistosoma haematobium*. Arch Ophtalmol 1977; 95:278–80.
72. Jakubzick C, Kunkel SL, Joshi BH, Puri RK, Hogaboam CM. Interleukin-13 fusion cytotoxin arrests *Schistosoma mansoni* egg-induced pulmonary granuloma formation in mice. Am J Pathol 2002; 161:1283–97.
73. Jeffrey MP. Ocular disease caused by nematodes. Am J Ophthalmol 1955; 40:41–53.
74. John T, Barsky HJ, Donnelly JJ, Rockey JH. Retinal pigment epitheliopathy and neuroretinal degeneration in ascarid-infected eyes. Invest Ophthalmol Vis Sci 1987; 28:1583–98.
75. Joon-Wah M, Singh D, Sukoharyono J, Suranandami S. *Brugia malayi* infection of the human eye: a case report. Southeast Asian J Trop Med Public Health 1974; 5: 226–9.
76. Kagan IG, Agasin M. *Echinococcus* antigens. Bull WHO 1968; 39:13–24.
77. Kaliaperumal S, Rao VA, Parija SC. Cysticercosis of the eye in South India-a case series. Indian J Med Microbiol 2005; 23:227–30.
78. Kaplan MH, Whitfield JR, Boros DL, Grusby MJ. The cells are required for the *Schistosoma mansoni* egg-induced granulomatous response. J Immunol 1998; 160:1850–6.
79. Kazacos KR. Visceral and ocular larva migrans. Semin Vet Med Surg (Small Anim) 1991; 6:227–35.
80. Kazacos KR, Vestre WA, Kazacos EA. Raccoon ascarid larvae *(Baylisascaris procyonis)* as a cause of ocular

larva migrans. Invest Ophthalmol Vis Sci 1984; 25: 1177–83.

81. Kazura JW. Trichinosis. In: Warren KS, Mahmoud AAE, eds. Tropical and Geographical Medicine. McGraw-Hill, New York 1984:427–30.
82. Kephardt GM, Andrade ZA, Gleich GJ. Localization of eosinophil major basic protein onto eggs of *Schistosoma mansoni* in human pathologic tissue. Am J Pathol 1988; 133:389–96.
83. King CL, Nutman TB. Regulation of the immune response in lymphatic filariasis and onchocerciasis. In: Ash C, Gallagher RB eds. Immunoparasitology Today. Elsevier Trends Journals, Cambridge 1991:A54–A58.
84. Kirschner BI, Dunn JP, Ostler HB. Conjunctivitis caused by Thelazia californiensis. Am J Ophthalmol 1990; 110:573–4.
85. Kittiponghansa S, Prabriputaloong A, Pariyanonda S, Ritch R. Intracameral gnathostomiasis: a cause of anterior uveitis and secondary glaucoma. Br J Ophthalmol 1987; 71:618–22.
86. Kociecka W. Trichinellosis: human disease, diagnosis and treatment. VetParasitol 2000; 93:365–83.
87. Kuchle M, Knorr HLJ, Medenblik-Frysch S, et al. Diffuse unilateral subacute neuroretinitis syndrome in a German most likely caused by the raccoon roundworm, *Baylisascaris procyonis*. Graefes Arch Clin Exp Ophthalmol 1993; 231:48–51.
88. van der Lejit A, Doekes G, Hwan BS, Vetter CM, Rietveld E, Stilma IS, Kijlstra A. Humoral autoimmune response against S-antigen and IRBP in ocular onchocerciasis. Invest Ophthalmol Vis Sci 1990; 31:1374–80.
89. Leon LA, Almeida R, Mueller JF. A case of ocular sparganosis in Ecuador. J Parasitol 1972; 58:184–5.
90. Lightowlers MW, Gottstein B. Echinococcosis/hydatidosis: antigens, immunological and molecular diagnosis. In: Thompson RCA, Lymbery AJ, eds. *Echinococcus* and hydatid disease. CAB International, Wallingford, UK 1995; 355–410.
91. Litricin O. *Echinococcus cyst* of the eyeball. Arch Ophthalmol 1953; 50:506–9.
92. Lyness RW, Earley OE, Logan WC, Archer DB. Ocular larva migrans. Br J Ophthalmol 1987; 71:396–401.
93. Macchioni G. A new species: *Toxocara lyncis*, in the caracal (*Lynx caracal*). Parasitology 1999; 41:529–32.
94. Mackenzie CD, Burgess PA, Sisley BM. Onchocerciasis. Immunodiag Parasitic Dis 1986; 1:255–89.
95. Mackenzie CD, Jungery M, Taylor PM, Ogilvie BM. Activation of complement, the induction of antibodies to nematode surfaces and the effect of these factors and leucocytes on worm survival in vitro. Eur J Immunol 1980; 70:594–601.
96. Maguire AM, Green WR, Michels RG, Erozan YS. Recovery of intraocular *Toxocara canis* by pars plana vitrectomy. Ophthalmology 1990; 97:675–80.
97. Manschot WA. *Coenurus* infestation of eye and orbit. Arch Ophthalmol 1976; 94:961–4.
98. Mitchell G. E Co-evolution of parasites and adaptive immune responses. In *Immunoparasitology Today*, Ash C, Gallagher RB, eds. Elsevier Trends Journals, Cambridge 1991:A2–A5.
99. Mizgajska H. Eggs of *Toxocara* spp. in the environment and their public health implications. J Helminthol 2001; 75:147–51.
100. Molyneux DH, Nantulya V. Public-private partnerships in blindness prevention: reaching beyond the eye. Eye 2005; 19:1050–6.
101. Morales AC, Croxatto JO, Crovetto L, Ebner R. Hydatid cysts of the orbit. Ophthalmology 1988; 95:1027–32.
102. Müller R. *Dracunculus* and dracunculiasis. Adv Parasitol 1971; 9:73–151.
103. Müller R. Worms and Human Disease. 2nd Ed. Wallingford, Oxon: CABI Publishing, 2002.
104. Müller R. The pathology of experimental *Dracunculus* infection and its relevance to chemotherapy. In: Soulsby EJL, ed. Pathophysiology of Parasitic Infection. Academic Press, New York 1976:133–48.
105. Murrell KD, Bruschi F. Clinical trichinellosis. Prog Clin Parasitol 1994; 4:117–50.
106. Nathwani D, Laing RB, Currie PF. 1992. Covert toxocariasis as a cause of recurrent abdominal pain in childhood. Br J Clin Pract 1992; 46:271.
107. Naumann GOH, Knoee HLJ. DUSN occurs in Europe. Ophthalmology 1994; 101:971–2.
108. Nelson GS. The pathology of filarial infections. Helminthol Abstr 1966; 35:311–36.
109. Neumann E, Gunders AE. Pathogenesis of the posterior segment lesion of ocular onchocerciasis. Am J Ophthalmol 1973; 75:82–9.
110. Newland HS, White AT, Greene BM, Murphy RP, Taylor HR. Ocular manifestations of onchocerciasis in a rain forest area of West Africa. Br J Ophthalmol 1991; 75: 163–9.
111. Ngu JL, Blackett K. Immunological studies in onchocerciasis in Cameroon. Trop Geogr Med 1976; 28:111–20.
112. Ogilvie BM, Worms MJ. Immunity to nematode parasites of man with special reference to *Ascaris* hookworms and filariae. In: Cohen S, Sadun E, eds. Immunology of Parasitic Infections. Blackwell, Oxford 1976:381–407.
113. Oldham JN. Observations on the incidence of *Toxocara* and toxocariasis in dogs and cats from the London area. J Helminthol 1965; 39:251–6.
114. Osuntokun O, Olurin O. Filarial worm (*Loa loa*) in the anterior chamber: report of two cases. Br J Ophthalmol 1975; 59:166–7.
115. Otranto D, Traversa D. Thelazia eyeworm: an original endo- and ecto-parasitic nematode. Trends Parasitol 2005; 21:1–4.
116. Ottesen EA. Filariasis now. Am J Trop Med Hyg 1989; 41 (Suppl.):9–17.
117. Owen R. Anatomical descriptions of two species *of Entozoa* from the stomach of a tiger *(Felis tigris* Linn.), one of which forms a new genus of *Nematoidea, Gnathostoma*. Proc Zool Soc Lond 1836; 47:123–6.
118. Paul EV, Zimmerman LE. Some observations on the ocular pathology of onchocerciasis. Hum Pathol 1970; 1: 581–94.
119. Perkins ES. Pattern of uveitis in children. Br J Ophthalmol 1966; 50:169–85.
120. Piessens WF, Ratiwayonto S, Tuti S, et al. Antigen-specific suppressor cells and suppressor factors in human filariasis with *Brugia malayi*. N Engl J Med 1980; 302: 833–7.
121. Pittella JEH, Orefice F. Schistosomotic choroiditis II: report of first case. Br J Ophthalmol 1985; 69:300–2.
122. Pollard ZF, Jarret WH, Hagler WS, et al. ELISA for diagnosis of ocular toxocariasis. Ophthalmology 1979; 86:743–9.
123. Poltera AA. The histopathology of ocular loaiasis in Uganda. Trans R Soc Trop Med Hyg 1973; 67:819–29.
124. Pozio E, La Rosa G, Rossi P, et al. Biological characterizations of trichinella isolates from various host species and geographical regions. J Parasitol 1992; 78:647–53.
125. Pushker N, Bajaj MS, Betharia SM. Orbital and adnexal cysticercosis. Clin Experiment Ophthalmol 2002; 30: 322–33.

126. Rathinam S, Fritsche TR, Srinivasan M, et al. An outbreak of trematode-induced granulomas of the conjunctiva. Ophthalmology 2001; 108:1223–9.
127. Read RW, Zhang J, Albini T, et al. Splendore-Hoeppli phenomenon in the conjunctiva: immunohistochemical analysis. Am J Ophthalmol 2005; 140:262–6.
128. Ree GH, Voller A, Rowland HAK. Toxocariasis in the British Isles 1982–3. Br Med J 1984; 288:628–9.
129. Ridley H. Ocular onchocerciasis including an investigation in the Gold Coast. Br J Ophthalmol (Suppl.) 1945; 10:1–58.
130. Rockey JH, Donnelly JJ, Stromberg BE, Soulsby EJL. Immunopathology of *Toxocara canis* and *Ascaris* serum infections of the eye: the role of the eosinophil. Invest Ophthalmol Vis Sci 1979; 18:1172–84.
131. Rockey JH, John T, Donnelly JJ, et al. In vitro interaction of eosinophils from ascarid-infected eyes with *Ascaris suum* and *Toxocara canis* larvae. Invest Ophthalmol Vis Sci 1983; 24:1346–57.
132. Rodger FC. Blindness in West Africa. HK. London: Lewis, 1959.
133. Romano A, Sachs R, Lengy J. Human ocular dirofilariasis in Israel. Isr J Med Sci 1976; 12:208–14.
134. Rose L. Filarial worm in anterior chamber of eye in man. Arch Ophthalmol 1966; 75:13–15.
135. Ruiz-Barranco F, de Vicente Esquinas M. Quiste parasitario intraocular emigrante. Arch Soc Esp Oftal 1976; 36:185–92.
136. Sabrosa NA, de Souza EC. Nematode infections of the eye: toxocariasis and diffuse unilateral subacute neuroretinitis. Curr Opin Ophthalmol 2001; 12:450–4.
137. Schantz PM, Glickman LT. Roundworms in dogs and cats: veterinary and public health considerations. Compend Contin Educ Pract Vet 1981; 3:773–84.
138. Semba RD, Donnelly JJ, Young E, et al. Experimental onchocerciasis in cynomolgus monkeys. IV. Chorioretinitis elicited by *Onchocerca volvulus* microfilariae. Invest Ophthalmol Vis Sci 1991; 32:1499–507.
139. Semba RD, Murphy RP, Newland HS, et al. Longitudinal study of lesions of the posterior segment in onchocerciasis. Ophthalmology 1990; 97:1334–41.
140. Semnani RT, Nutman TB. Toward an understanding of the interaction between filarial parasites and host antigen-presenting cells. Immunol Rev 2004; 201:127–38.
141. Sen DK, Mullen R, Gupta PV, Chilana JS. Cestode larva (sparganum) in the anterior chamber of the eye. Trop Geogr Med 1989; 41:270–3.
142. Sen K, Ghose N. Ocular gnathostomiasis. Br J Ophthalmol 1945; 29:618–26.
143. Sher A, Moser G. Schistosomiasis: immunologic properties of developing schistosomula. Am J Pathol 1981; 102:121–6.
144. Shields JA. Ocular toxocariasis: a review. Surv Ophthalmol 1984; 28:361–81.
145. Singh TS, Singh KN. Thelaziasis: report of two cases. Br J Ophthalmol 1973; 77:528–9.
146. Smith HV. Antibody reactivity in human toxocariasis. In: Lewis JW, Maizels RM, eds. *Toxocara* and toxocariasis: clinical, epidemiological, and molecular perspectives. Institute of Biology and the British Society for Parasitology, London, UK 1993:91-109.
147. Sreter T, Szell Z, Egyed Z, Varga I. Subconjunctival zoonotic onchocerciasis in man: aberrant infection with *Onchocerca lupi*? Ann Trop Med Parasitol 2002; 96:497–502.
148. Stemmle J, Markwalder KA, Zinkernagel AS, Wirth MG, Grimm F, Hirsch-Hoffmann S, Thiel MA. *Loa loa* infection of the eye - a case series. Klin Monatsbl Augenheilkd 2005; 222,226–30.
149. Tabbara KF, Shoukrey N. Trichinosis. In: Gold DH, Weingeist TA eds. The Eye in Systemic Disease, JB Lippincott, Philadelphia 1990:191–2.
150. Tansurat P. Sparganosis. In: Marcial-Rojas RA ed. Pathology of Protozoal and Helminthic Diseases with Clinical Correlation. Williams and Wilkins, Baltimore 1971:585–91.
151. Tassi C, Pozio E, Felecia D, et al. Evaluation of some immunological parameters in trichinellosis patients with periorbital edema. Clin Chem Enzymol Comms 1991; 4:1–7.
152. Thomas D, Older JJ, Kandawalla NM, Torczynski E. The *Dirofilaria* parasite in the orbit. Am J Ophthalmol 1976; 82:931–3.
153. Thompson DE, Bundy DAP, Cooper ES, et al. Epidemiological characteristics of *Toxocara canis* zoonotic infection of children in a Caribbean community. Bull World Health Organ 1986; 64:283–90.
154. Tost F, Hellman A, Ockert G. *Toxocara canis* infection: environmental, parasitologic and epidemiologic studies. Ophthalmology 1998; 95:486–9.
155. Toussaint D, Danis P. Retinopathy in generalized *Loa loa* filariasis. Arch Ophthalmol 1965; 74:470–6.
156. Tsang VCW, Wilson M. *Taenia solium* cysticercosis: an under-recognized but serious public health problem. Parasitol Today 1995; 11:124–6.
157. Tudor RC, Blair E. *Gnathostoma spinigerum:* an unusual cause of ocular nematodiasis in the Western hemisphere. Am J Ophthalmol 1971; 72:185–90.
158. Voller A, Bartlett A, Bidwell DE. Enzyme immunoassay for parasitic diseases. J R Soc Trop Med Hyg 1976; 70:98–105.
159. Vosgien I. Le circus cellulosae chez l'homme et chez les animaux. Bull Soc Centr Vet 1912; 12:270–7.
160. Warren KS. Regulation of the prevalence and intensity of schistosomiasis in man: immunology or ecology. J Infect Dis 1973; 127:595–609.
161. Watzke RC, Oaks JA, Folk JC. *Toxocara canis* infection of the eye: Correlation of clinical observations with developing pathology in the primate model. Arch Ophthalmol 1984; 102:282–91.
162. Weiss N, Speiser F, Hussain R. IgE antibodies in human onchocerciasis: application of a newly developed radioallergosorbent test (RAST). Acta Trop (Basel) 1981; 38:353–62.
163. World Health Organization. WHO Expert Committee on Onchocerciasis: Third Report. World Health Organization, Geneva, 1987. Technical Report Series No.: 752.
164. Wilder HC. Nematode endophthalmitis. Trans Am Acad Ophthalmol Otolaryngol 1950; 55:99–109.
165. Wilkinson CP, Welch RB. Intraocular *Toxocara*. Am J Ophthalmol 1971; 71:921–30.
166. Williams PH, Templeton AC. Infection of the eye by tapeworm *Coenurus*. Br J Ophthalmol 1971; 55:766–9.
167. Williams DF, Williams GA, Caya JG, et al. Intraocular *Echinococcus multilocularis*. Arch Ophthalmol 1987; 105:1106–9.
168. Wilson M, Bryan RT, Fried JA, et al. Clinical evaluation of cysticercosis enzyme-linked immunoelectrotransfer blot in patients with neurocysticercosis. J Infect Dis 1991; 164:1007–9.
169. Witenberg G, Jacoby J, Stechelmacher S. A case of ocular gnathostomiasis. Ophthalmologica 1950; 119:114–22.
170. Woodruff AW. Toxocariasis. Br Med J 1970; 3:663–9.
171. Yokota T, Coffman RL, Hagiwara H, et al. Isolation and characterization of lymphokine cDNA clones encoding mouse and human IgA-enhancing factor activities: Relationship to interleukin 5. Proc Natl Acad Sci USA 1987; 84:7388–92.

14

Ocular Diseases Due to Arthropods

Mary K. Klassen-Fischer and Ronald C. Neafie
Armed Forces Institute of Pathology, Washington, D.C., U.S.A.

INTRODUCTION

Arthropods (phylum Arthropoda) are invertebrates with jointed appendages and exoskeletons, and include insects, arachnids, and a variety of organisms in other classes. They frequently serve as vectors of infectious diseases, but they may also cause disease by biting, stinging, producing toxins, or directly invading tissue. Ocular diseases directly due to arthropods are uncommon.

OPHTHALMOMYIASIS

Myiasis is infection by larval dipterans, or fly maggots. Some fly species are obligatory parasites in the larval stage and cause invasive myiasis. These parasitic species have elaborate means of invading tissue and tend to have specific hosts. Other species are saprophytic flies, which normally thrive on dead tissue, and can cause opportunistic infections of wounds. Saprophytic flies can also cause imperceptible myiasis by depositing eggs into an orifice, such as the nose or an eye, of an incapacitated or sleeping person who is unable to drive off flies (2).

Some flies that cause invasive myiasis include *Dermatobia hominis* (human botfly), *Hypoderma bovis* (cattle gadfly), *H. tarandi* (reindeer warble fly), *H. lineatum*, *Oestrus ovis* (Fig. 1), *Gasterophilus intestinalis*, and *Cuterebra* (4,5,7,8,15,16,23,27,28). Flies reported to cause myiasis include blow flies (Calliphoridae) of the genera *Calliphora*, *Phaenicia*, *Lucilia*, *Phormia*, *Cochliomyia*, *Chrysomyia*, and *Sarcophaga* (2,29). The most accurate way to identify fly larvae is to rear them to the adult stage, although this is usually not practical. Fly larvae themselves are best studied intact where the overall morphologic features can be observed, especially the posterior spiracles (Fig. 2). They can also be identified when processed in the laboratory although determining species is usually impossible. In these instances, geographic considerations are of great importance. In hematoxylin–eosin-stained sections, fly larvae can be identified by the presence of a thick cuticle with spines, striated muscle, and tracheae (Fig. 3). Fly larvae can also be

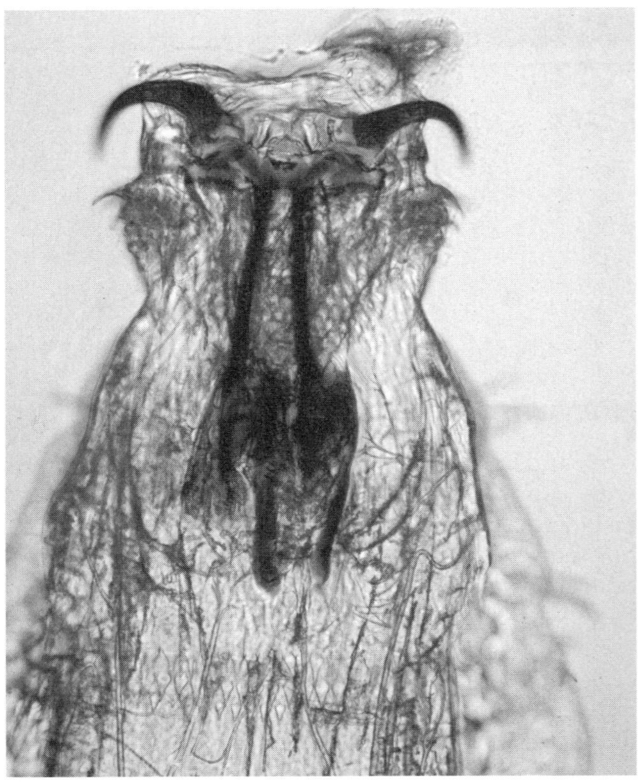

Figure 1 *Oestrus ovis*, first-stage larva removed from margin of eyelid. Note prominent pair of oral hooks at the anterior end (×290).

distinguished from other arthropods by the absence of legs and antennae.

Ocular myiasis can be caused by either parasitic or saprophytic flies. Within the eyelid it is called ophthalmomyiasis externa, and within the globe itself, ophthalmomyiasis interna.

Ophthalmomyiasis Externa

The sheep nasal botfly, *O. ovis*, which normally completes its life cycle in the nasal passages of sheep and goats, is a frequent cause of ophthalmomyiasis externa in humans (Fig. 1) (4,23,28). It is found in North America, Europe, and Asia. The adult female fly deposits a first-stage larva with each strike to the eyes, nares, or mouth of sheep or goats. Larvae bore into the mucosa and migrate to the frontal sinuses or nasopharynx. Those deposited in or near the eye migrate to the conjunctiva, eyelid, or lacrimal duct.

Because humans are an unnatural host, larvae of *O. ovis* do not mature beyond the first stage. Patients present with a sudden onset of redness, tearing, and a foreign-body sensation in the affected eye (4). The symptoms are those of catarrhal conjunctivitis (23). The condition is self-limiting and rarely causes residual damage, but may be complicated by secondary bacterial infection (23). Pain and tissue destruction may develop if the larvae are numerous, requiring enucleation of the eye. Invasion of the corneal stroma may cause transient iridocyclitis, though significant direct damage to the cornea is unusual. Rarely, larvae enter the nose and nasal sinuses through the lacrimal duct, cause extensive necrosis or penetrate the orbit (23,27).

In one report of nine cases of ophthalmomyiasis externa due to *D. hominis*, seven patients had palpebral myiasis (including one with three larvae)

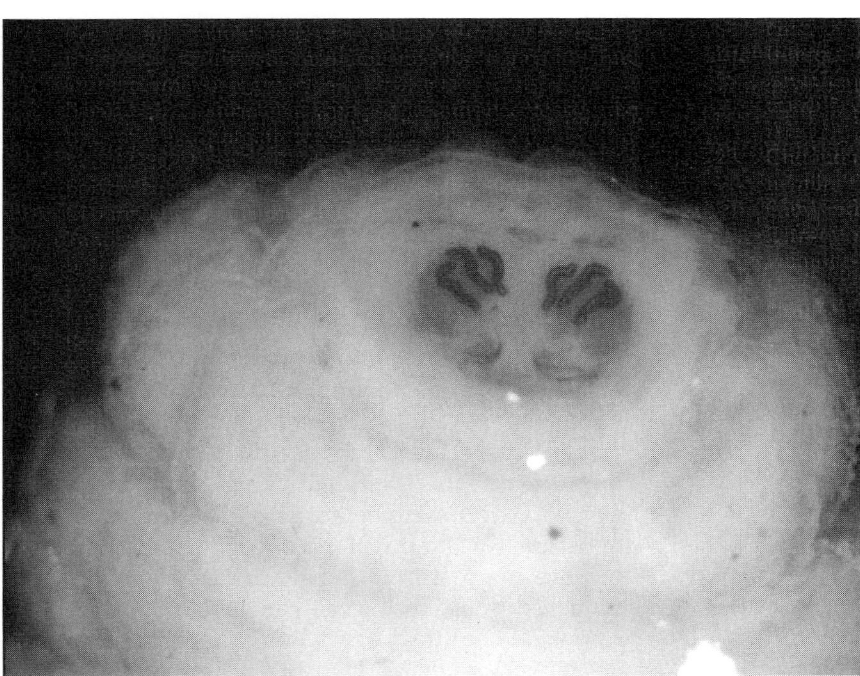

Figure 2 Posterior spiracles of mature third-stage *Cordylobia anthropophaga* larva. Note the moderately sinuous pattern of the respiratory slits (×90).

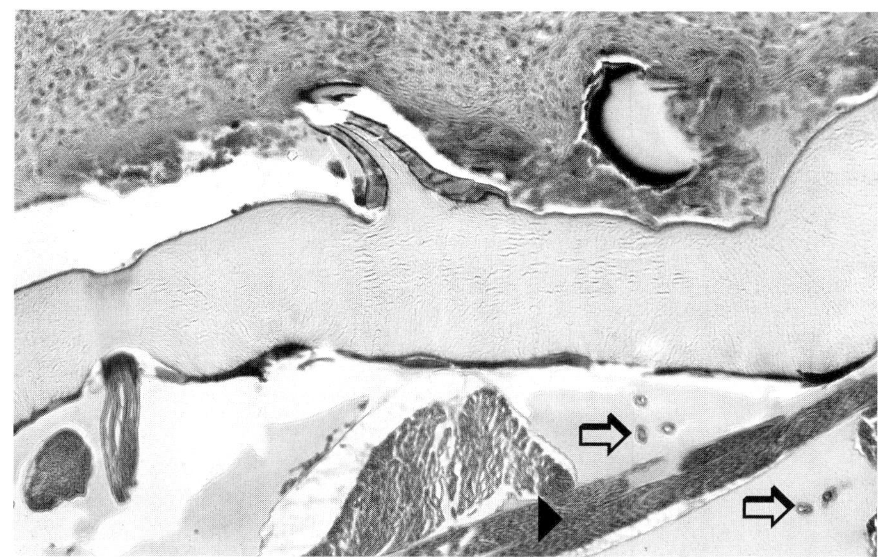

Figure 3 Stained section through body wall of mature third-stage *Dermatobia hominis* larva. Note thick cuticle with spines, striated muscle (*arrowhead*), and tracheae (*arrows*) (Movat, ×115).

and two had conjunctival myiasis (7). All had palpebral edema. The larval posterior spiracles, through which the organism breathes, were seen on the palpebral skin or free margin or on the conjunctiva. In three cases, movements were seen.

Patients with diminished consciousness in some hospital settings need protection from flies. One debilitated patient had nine larvae of the facultative fly, *Sarcophaga crassipalpis*, on the eyelid, cornea, and bulbar conjunctiva (29). Clinical signs included inflammation of the eyelid and conjunctival congestion. The larvae were removed and reared to the third instar stage (the period of growth after the second molt after hatching) or the adult stage for accurate identification of the species.

Ophthalmomyiasis Interna

Ophthalmomyiasis interna results from penetration of the globe by larvae of certain flies that burrow through the sclera. It occurs more frequently during childhood when the sclera is relatively soft, causing severe intraocular inflammation (8). Larvae entering the anterior chamber provoke acute iridocyclitis that ends in severe cases with extensive scarring and phthisis bulbi. In one case, a second-stage larva of *H. lineatum* caused severe uveitis, phthisis bulbi and complete loss of vision (8). Larvae penetrating the posterior sclera inhabit the subretinal space, where they may produce characteristic linear tracks in the retinal pigment epithelium, and subretinal and vitreous hemorrhage (5,8,12). The resulting acute exudative choroiditis may result in traction detachment of the overlying retina (8). Histologic sections show a perivascular inflammatory infiltrate with prominent eosinophils.

Hypoderma sp. is a common cause of ophthalmomyiasis interna in humans. *H. bovis* (northern cattle grub) infects humans, cattle, and deer in North America, Europe, and Asia (15). Adult female flies lay one or more eggs at each strike on an animal. First-stage larvae emerge, crawl down the hairs, and penetrate the skin through hair follicles or minor breaks in the skin. The larvae migrate to the animal's back, mature within warbles to the third instar stage, and drop to the ground and pupate in a life cycle that takes one year.

H. bovis larvae rarely develop fully in humans. They usually die before reaching the third instar stage, provoking an intense inflammatory response and a tender swelling. Edema may involve much of the head and face. Invasion of the orbit by first-stage *Hypoderma* sp. larvae may irreversibly damage the eye as described above (8).

The reindeer warble fly (*H. tarandi*) is a common cause of internal posterior ophthalmomyiasis in northern Scandinavia (16). Larvae invade the vitreous or, in some cases, the anterior chamber and produce opacity due to leukocytic exudation (18). This species also causes ophthalmomyiasis externa presenting as an eyelid tumor (16).

G. intestinalis, the common horse bot fly, is an accidental parasite of humans. There is a report of a *G. intestinalis* larva in the posterior chamber of the eye (15), and the larva dying there doing no permanent damage.

DEMODEX INFECTION

Demodex folliculorum and *D. brevis* mites belong to the family Arachnida. They are common in histologic sections of skin, especially of the face. *D. folliculorum*

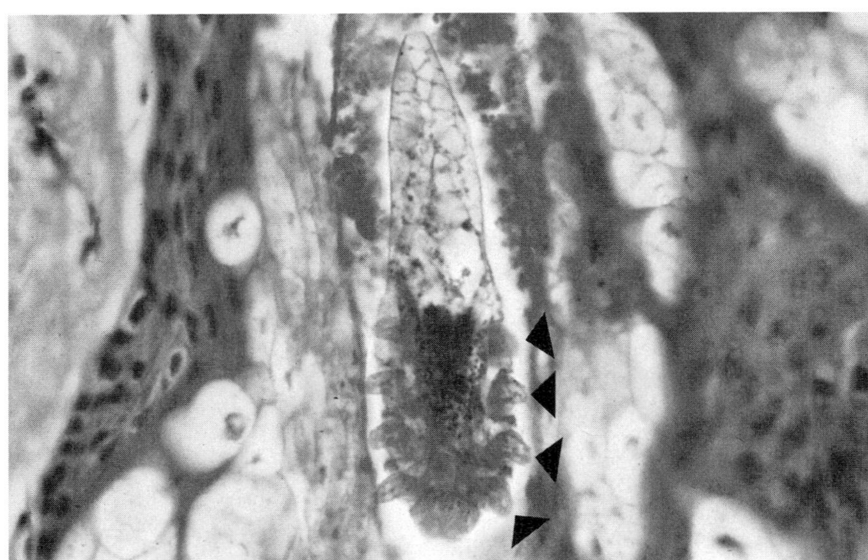

Figure 4 *Demodex folliculorum* in hair follicle of skin from cheek. Note four pairs of legs (*arrowheads*) (hematoxylin and eosin, ×485).

mites in all stages inhabit hair and eyelash follicles; *D. brevis* is present in the eyelash sebaceous glands, small hair sebaceous glands, and in the lobules of the meibomian glands but is very rare in eyelash specimens (9,11). In one large histologic study, *Demodex* mites were not seen in meibomian glands (24). The mites feed on epithelial cells and sebaceous secretions and can cause an accumulation of keratin and lipid-containing debris around the base of the hair shaft or eyelash (9). When many mites are present, the formation of the superficial lipid layer of the tear film is affected. Large populations of *D. brevis* may destroy the glandular cells, produce granulomas in the eyelid, and plug the ducts of the meibomian or sebaceous glands.

There is no consensus to what degree *Demodex* mites cause or contribute to disease (1). They may obstruct the hair follicles, but whether or not they directly cause folliculitis is controversial. There is some evidence that patients with blepharitis have an increased prevalence of *Demodex* mites relative to the general population, but in one study, no difference in the prevalence of *D. folliculorum* was found in eyelash samples from patients with chronic seborrheic blepharitis compared to controls (17). In another study, the number of mites per eyelash was significantly higher in patients with retained cylindrical dandruff (4.1) versus in those without (0.2) (11). Although secondary bacterial infection may cause inflammation, mechanical injury incurred by movement of

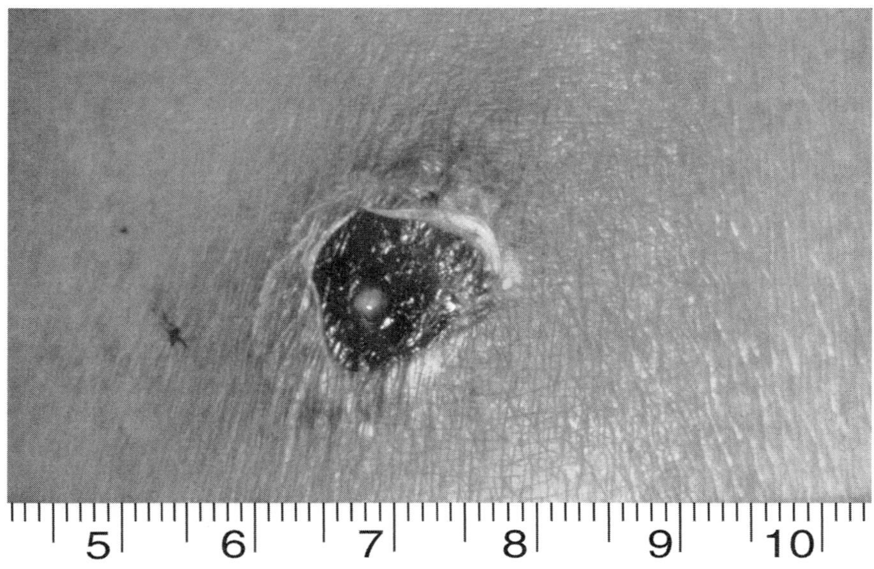

Figure 5 Brown recluse spider bite. There is a plaque with purulent exudate, black eschar, and surrounding erythema.

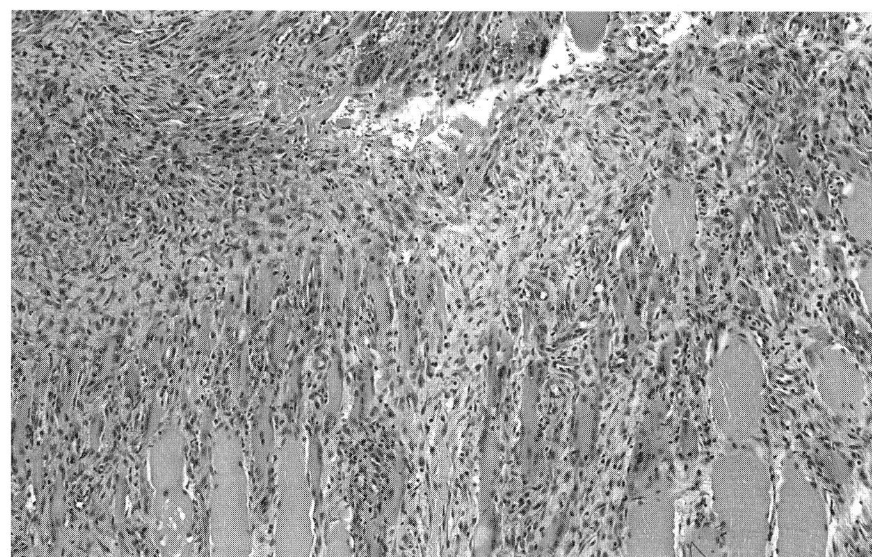

Figure 6 Brown recluse spider bite of thigh depicting chronic inflammation of muscle (hematoxylin and eosin, ×90).

the gravid female in the act of egg-laying can also be involved (10). Histopathologic changes include hyperkeratosis, chronic perifolliculitis, follicular distension, hyperplasia, and melanocyte aggregation (9,24). Eyelid hygiene with shampoo reduces the number of mites but does not eradicate them (11).

D. folliculorum is an elongated mite about 300 μm long and 50 μm wide. *D. brevis* is somewhat smaller. The cuticle is transversely striated. There are four pairs of short stumpy legs on the anterior one-third of the body that frequently can be observed in histologic sections (Fig. 4).

ARTHROPOD ASSAULT

Arthropods assault the skin by biting or stinging depending on the species. Biting arthropods release secretions into the skin to facilitate blood-sucking. Inflammatory responses occur as a hypersensitivity response to these secretions. Stinging arthropods release various venoms into the skin that also promote inflammation. Retained portions of arthropod mouth parts or stingers can cause a foreign-body inflammatory response.

Spider bites such as those caused by the black widow and brown recluse are rarely fatal, but can cause significant lesions (Fig. 5). They cause necrosis and inflammation of the skin, subcutaneous tissue, and underlying muscle (Fig. 6).

The histopathologic changes caused by arthropod bites are nonspecific. Typically, there is a wedge-shaped perivascular dermal inflammatory infiltrate consisting of eosinophils, lymphocytes, and histiocytes, sometimes with spongiosis, edema, and an extravasation of erythrocytes. Such skin lesions may persist for several years and may be difficult to distinguish from other dermatological conditions, including tumors or lymphoma. In general, the diagnosis of exposure to an arthropod venom or toxin is based on the clinical history. In some cases, capturing the arthropod for identification is useful.

Louse Infection

The pubic louse (*Phthirus pubis*), and less commonly the head louse (*P. capitis*), may infest eyebrows and eyelashes. Mature lice deposit eggs (nits) on eyelids or periorbital skin. Larval stages last about 10 days. Lice use the terminal claws on their legs to cling to hairs and eyelashes near the epidermal surface (Fig. 7).

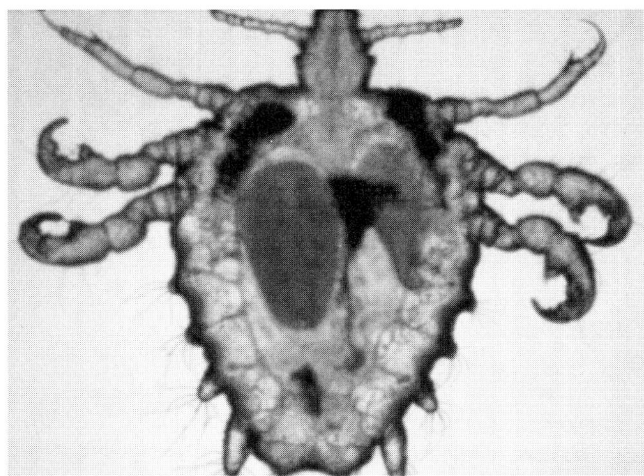

Figure 7 The pubic louse *Phthirus pubis* is 1.5 to 2.0 mm long and 1.5 mm wide. Note the second and third pairs of legs that are provided with powerful claws adapted for clinging to hairs (× 30).

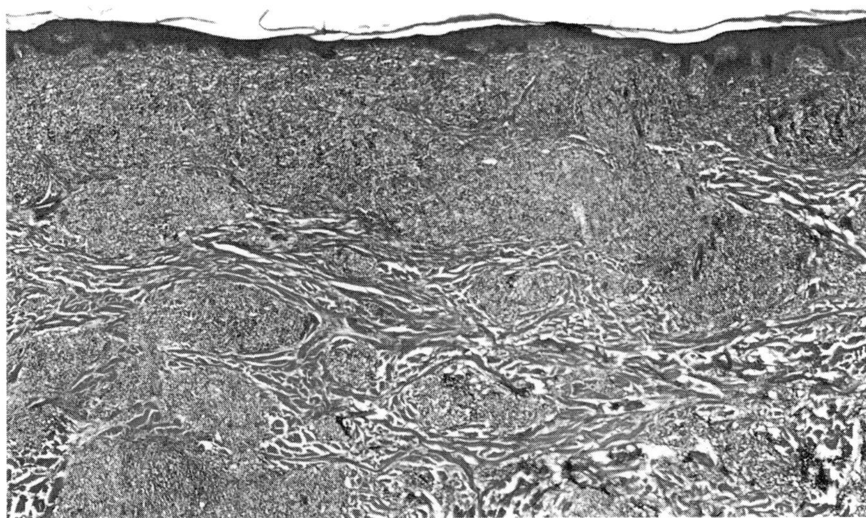

Figure 8 Tick bite reaction causing severe local inflammation of skin that may mimic lymphoma (hematoxylin and eosin, ×15).

A louse bite results in itching, scratching and sometimes secondary infection may develop. Persistent blepharoconjunctivitis may be an inflammatory response to the parasite's excreta. In some cases, the chief complaint may simply be foreign bodies on the eyelashes (14). Palpebral *P. pubis* infection may be associated with genital infection, other sexually transmitted diseases, or sexual abuse in children. Treatment sometimes involves removal of the parasites and cutting the lashes at the base (14).

Tick Bite

Ticks are arthropods with eight legs in the adult stage. Tick bites to the eyelid are unusual in humans. The salivary secretions of ticks and other blood-sucking arthropods cause local inflammation (Fig. 8). In one case, a *Hyalomma* sp. tick became embedded in the meibomian gland orifice and presented as a mass at the eyelid margin (26).

Hymenopteran Sting

The inflammatory response to the stings of ants, bees, and wasps is similar in the eyelid to that in other parts of the body. Unusual reactions to hymenopteran stings, such as ocular myasthenia gravis and optic neuritis, have been rarely reported (3,25). The pathogenesis of myasthenia gravis shortly after a wasp sting is unknown, but it may have been an immediate hypersensitivity reaction or a direct effect of the toxic venom on acetylcholine synthesis, release, or degradation. Also, it may have resulted from a latent or subclinical myasthenia gravis at the time of the sting (3).

Black Fly Bite

Black flies are well known as vectors of onchocerciasis (see Chapter 13). Their bites also cause a noninfectious disease called simuliidosis or simuliosis. Only the females take a blood meal and worldwide are perhaps the most troublesome insect pest of humans and animals (Fig. 9). The saliva contains factors that may induce a delayed type hypersensitivity reaction. When black flies bite around the eyes, the

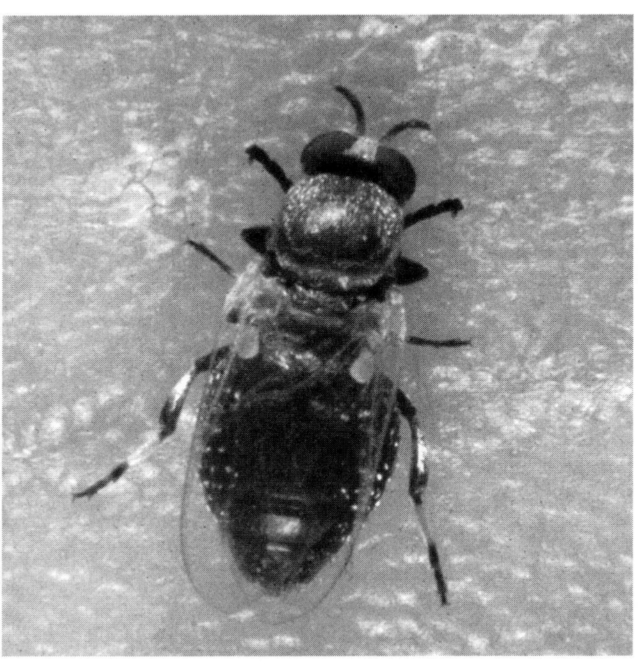

Figure 9 Female *Simulium damnosum* feeding on a human volunteer (×30).

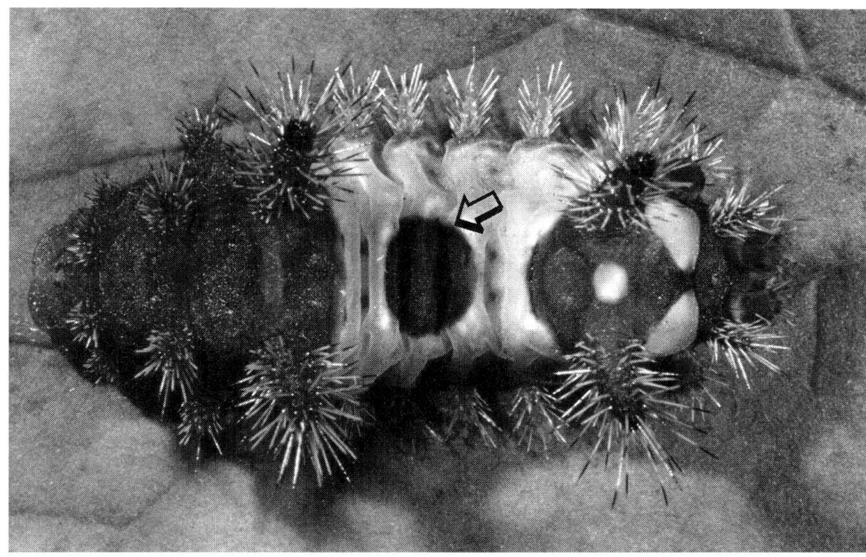

Figure 10 The saddleback caterpillar (*Sibine* sp.) can be identified by its characteristic dorsal patch resembling a saddlecloth. A dark spot (*arrow*) resembles a saddle (×7.5).

surrounding tissue may become so swollen that vision is obscured.

Millipede Exposure

Millipedes are slow-moving, predominantly saprophagous arthropods found in dark, damp places around the world. Most species are innocuous, but some species, mostly found in the tropics, can cause skin or eye irritation. A few species are capable of producing secretions containing hydrogen cyanide, benzoquinones, and a variety of other organic molecules that can cause superficial chemical burns on human skin and damage to the eyes. Exposure of the eye to the secretions of *Polyconoceras* (*Salpidobolus*), a species of millipede in Papua New Guinea, causes severe pain, periorbital erythema and edema, conjunctivitis or keratitis (13). Most exposures occur in children during the rainy season. Patients recover fully with standard topical ophthalmic therapy, despite anecdotal unpublished reports of blindness.

Blister Beetle Exposure

Blister beetles are insects, such as *Paederus* sp. in Africa, that extrude toxin when they are handled. Severe periorbital dermatitis or keratoconjunctivitis (Nairobi eye, Christmas eye, or *Paederus* ophthalmia) may occur when a beetle accidentally flies into the eye and extrudes the vesicating toxin or when the toxic chemical is transferred to the eye by the fingers (22).

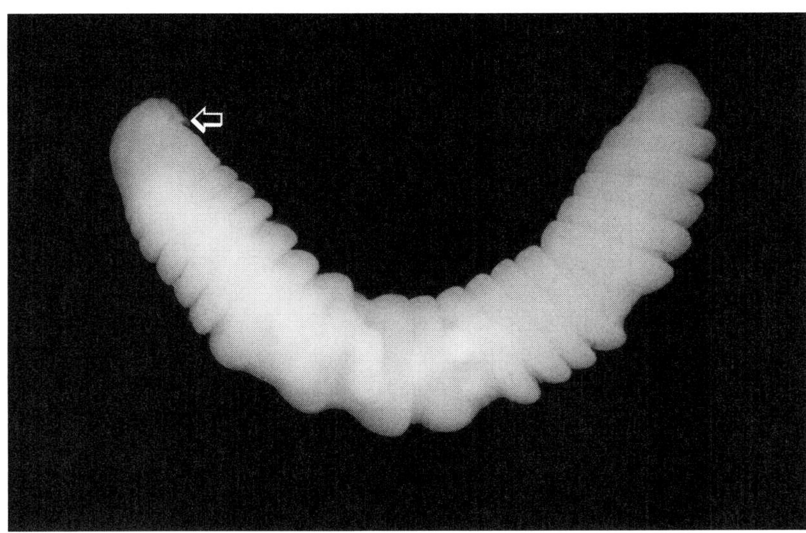

Figure 11 *Armillifer armillatus* larva removed from conjunctiva. Note pseudosegmentation and small hook (*arrow*) at the anterior end (×12).

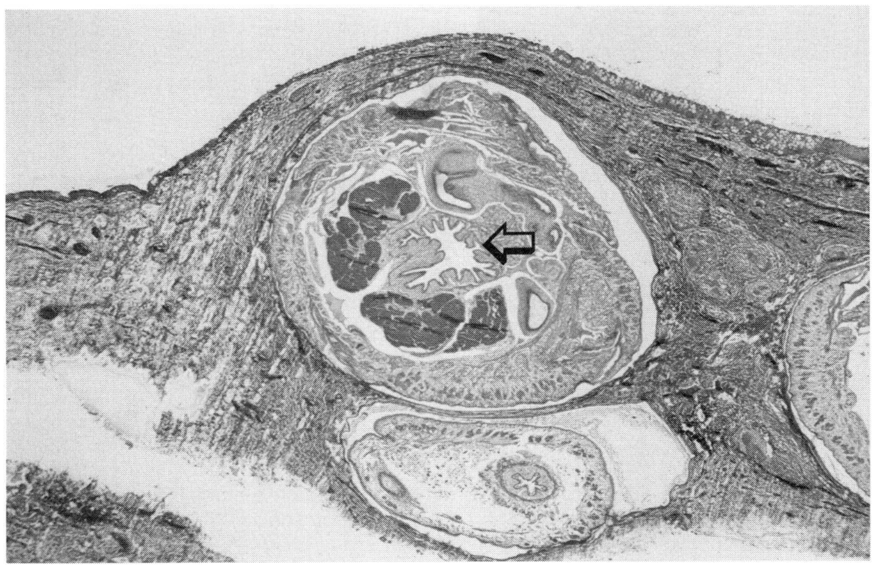

Figure 12 *Armillifer armillatus* larva in conjunctival nodule. Note digestive tube (*arrow*) in the center with adjacent acidophilic glands on the left (hematoxylin and eosin, ×24).

Caterpillar Exposure

The larvae ("caterpillars") of some moths (order Lepidoptera) have hairs that can cause cutaneous reactions. The saddleback caterpillar (*Sibine* sp.) is one of these that can cause pain and necrosis. They are found throughout much of the United States and can be identified by their characteristic green dorsal patch resembling a saddlecloth and a brown spot resembling a saddle (Fig. 10). The mucous membranes of the eye, upper respiratory tract, and the oropharynx may also be affected. Contact of caterpillar hairs with the conjunctiva, cornea, or iris results in marked congestion, pain, itching, photophobia, and even vascularization of the cornea. Painful pseudotubercles may form around the hairs.

Whether the reaction is mechanical due to the nettling hairs or spines entering the skin or due to a toxin or both is unknown (6). Contact of skin with nettling hairs of caterpillars, such as the brown moth *Euproctis chrysorrhoea*, causes a marked erythematous wheal-like urticarial reaction that gradually becomes more infiltrated and develops into erythematous papules or vesicles. The extension of the reaction beyond the area of contact and the occurrence of constitutional symptoms suggest a toxin. Immunological studies suggest an allergic reaction (21). Biochemical analysis of an extract of the nettling hairs revealed a potent esterolytic enzyme (6). The nettling hairs induce the formation of spherocytes when mixed in vitro with human erythrocytes.

PENTASTOMIASIS

Pentastomes, or tongue worms, are cosmopolitan parasitic arthropods that may accidentally infect humans. Only larval pentastomes cause disease in humans. Ocular pentastomiasis is extremely rare. The larval stage of *Linguatula serrata*, which accounts for most of the rare infections in the United States, has been found in the conjunctiva, eyelids, and the anterior chamber, where it is prone to provoke acute iridocyclitis with ocular pain, conjunctivitis, and visual difficulties (19,20). In Africans, *Armillifer armillatus* causes most infections in humans, and larvae have invaded the subconjunctiva and the anterior chamber (20). The eye is

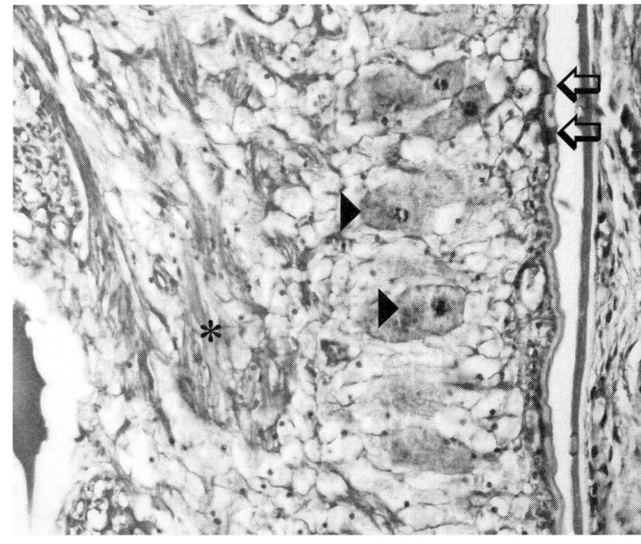

Figure 13 *Armillifer armillatus* larva in conjunctival nodule. Note sclerotized openings (*arrows*) in cuticle, subcuticular glands (*arrowheads*), and striated muscle (*asterisk*) (Movat ×330).

probably infected by direct contact with water containing pentastomid eggs. Larval pentastomes are elongate, pseudosegmented parasites that have hooks at the anterior end (Fig. 11). The cuticle may have spines as in *L. serrata* or be smooth as in *A. armillatus*. Larval pentastomes in tissue sections can be identified by the presence of a digestive tube, prominent acidophilic glands, striated muscle, and a cuticle with sclerotized openings (Figs. 12 and 13).

ACKNOWLEDGMENT

The authors acknowledge Jose F. Rodriguez for his technical assistance with the images.

REFERENCES

1. Baima B, Sticherling M. Demodicidosis revisited. Acta Derm Venereol 2002; 82:3–6.
2. Beckendorf R, Klotz SA, Hinkle N, Bartholomew W. Nasal myiasis in an intensive care unit linked to hospital-wide mouse infestation. Arch Intern Med 2002; 162:638–40.
3. Brumlik J. Myasthenia gravis associated with wasp sting. J Am Med Assoc 1976; 235:2120–21.
4. Cameron JA, Shoukrey NM, Al-Garni AA. Conjunctival ophthalmomyiasis caused by the sheep nasal botfly (*Oestrus ovis*). Am J Ophthalmol 1991; 112:331–4.
5. Custis PH, Pakalnis VA, Klintworth GK, et al. Posterior internal ophthalmomyiasis: identification of a surgically removed *Cuterebra* larva by scanning electron microscopy. Ophthalmology 1983; 90:1583–90.
6. de Jong MC, Bleumink E, Nater JP. Investigative studies of the dermatitis caused by the larva of the brown-tail moth (*Euproctis chrysorrhoea* Linn.). I. Clinical and experimental findings. Arch Dermatol Res 1975; 253:287–300.
7. Denion E, Dalens PH, Couppie P, et al. External ophthalmomyiasis caused by *Dermatobia hominis*: a retrospective study of nine cases and a review of the literature. Acta Ophthalmol Scand 2004; 82:576–84.
8. Edwards KM, Meredith TA, Hagler WS, Healy GR. Ophthalmomyiasis interna causing visual loss. Am J Ophthalmol 1984; 97:605–10.
9. English FP, Nutting WB. Demodicosis of ophthalmic concern. Am J Ophthalmol 1981; 91:362–72.
10. English FP, Nutting WB, Cohn D. Demodectic oviposition in the eyelid. Aust NZ J Ophthalmol 1985; 13:11–3.
11. Gao YY, DiPascuale MA, Li W, et al. High prevalence of *Demodex* in eyelashes with cylindrical dandruff. Invest Ophthalmol Vis Sci 2005; 46:3089–94.
12. Gass JD, Lewis RA. Subretinal tracks in ophthalmomyiasis. Trans Sect Ophthalmol Am Acad Ophthalmol Otolaryngol 1976; 81:483–90.
13. Hudson BJ, Parsons GA. Giant millipede 'burns' and the eye. Trans R Soc Trop Med Hyg 1997; 91:183–5.
14. Ikeda N, Nomoto H, Hayasaka S, Nagaki Y. *Phthirus pubis* infestation of the eyelashes and scalp hairs in a girl. Pediatr Dermatol 2003; 20:356–7.
15. James MT. The flies that cause myiasis in man. Washington, DC: United States Government Printing Office, 1947.
16. Kearney MS, Nilssen AC, Lyslo A, et al. Ophthalmomyiasis caused by reindeer warble fly larva. J Clin Pathol 1991; 44: 276–84.
17. Kemal M, Sumer Z, Toker MI, et al. The prevalence of *Demodex folliculorum* in blepharitis patients and the normal population. Ophthal Epidemiol 2005; 12:287–90.
18. Kirillichev AI. The presence of gadfly larva in the globe (Russian). Oftalmol Zh 1975; 30:619–20.
19. Lazo RF, Hidalgo E, Lazo JE, et al. Ocular linguatuliasis in Ecuador: case report and morphometric study of the larva of *Linguatula serrata*. Am J Trop Med Hyg 1999; 60:405–9.
20. Meyers WM, Neafie RC, Connor DH. Pentastomiasis. In: Binford CH, Connor DH, eds. Pathology of Tropical and Extraordinary Diseases: An Atlas. Vol. 2. Washington, DC: Armed Forces Institute of Pathology, 1976:546–50.
21. Perlman F, Press E, Googins JA, et al. Tussockosis: reactions to Douglas fir tussock moth. Ann Allergy 1976; 36:302–7.
22. Poole TR. Blister beetle periorbital dermatitis and keratoconjunctivitis in Tanzania. Eye 1998; 12:883–5.
23. Reingold WJ, Robin JB, Leipa D, et al. *Oestrus ovis* ophthalmomyiasis externa. Am J Ophthalmol 1984; 97:7–10.
24. Roth AM. *Demodex folliculorum* in hair follicles of eyelid skin. Ann Ophthalmol 1979; 11:37–40.
25. Russell FE. Envenomation and diverse disease states (Letter). J Am Med Assoc 1977; 238:581.
26. Samaha A, Green WR, Traboulsi EI, Ma'luf R. Tick infestation of the eyelid. Am J Ophthalmol 1998; 125:263–4.
27. Sigauke E, Beebe WE, Gander RM, et al. Case report: ophthalmomyiasis externa in Dallas County, Texas. Am J Trop Med Hyg 2003; 68:46–7.
28. Stevens JD, McCartney AC, Howes R. *Oestrus ovis* ophthalmomyiasis acquired in the UK: case report and scanning electron microscopic study. Br J Ophthalmol 1991; 75:702–3.
29. Uni S, Shinonaga S, Nishio Y, et al. Ophthalmomyiasis caused by *Sarcophaga crassipalpis* (Diptera: Sarcophagidae) in a hospital patient. J Med Entomol 1999; 36:906–8.

15

Ocular Trauma

J. Douglas Cameron
Department of Ophthalmology, Mayo Clinic, Rochester, Minnesota, U.S.A.

INTRODUCTION

Trauma is any forcible disruption of tissues by a source of external energy. The energy is conserved during the traumatic episode but may be transferred to another object and may be converted to a different type of energy. The most common external energy type causing trauma is kinetic energy; however, thermal energy, electrical energy, chemical energy, and ionizing radiation may also cause tissue damage (38).

No two traumatic episodes are exactly alike. A surgical procedure is a carefully planned event taking into account the risk–benefit ratio to the patient, robust general health, a sterile site, optimally crafted instruments, minimal tissue disruption, minimal duration of procedure, careful reconstitution of tissues to optimize the repair process, a reasonable expectation of the pace of return of normal function, and an awareness of the most common complications and remedies for those complications.

Accidental injury, in contrast, is of no benefit to the patient and is associated with considerable risk of loss of ocular function. Accidents happen to persons irrespective of the presence or absence of systemic disease at the time of injury. The "instruments" of injury are often crude (rocks), hot (high-velocity missiles), infected (vegetable matter and fingernails), or metabolically reactive (pure copper metal fragment). The "instruments" often travel through infected media of the skin surface or conjunctival sac and carry microbes into vulnerable tissues. Tissues may be mechanically disrupted in a small area (foreign-body entrance site) that may be easily repaired or may be chemically disrupted at a molecular level over a huge surface area (alkali injury) such that repair by intrinsic systems and therapeutic strategies are generally ineffective and may even potentiate tissue damage.

CLASSIFICATION OF INJURIES

The abundance of unpredictable variables has led to difficulties in classifying which types of injuries might be managed by currently available treatments.

Also the lack of standardization of definitions of trauma-related injury has hampered prospective evaluation of novel treatment strategies.

Recently The Ocular Trauma Classification Group (29) devised a system to categorize mechanical ocular injuries based on features at the initial eye examination that have proven to be of prognostic significance. The classification is based on the single most important feature of an ocular injury, i.e., whether or not the architectural integrity of the cornea and sclera has been interrupted.

An injury is defined as clinical evidence of tissue interruption. A "closed globe injury" is one in which the eye wall is intact. An "open globe injury" is one in which the eye wall is not intact. A contusion is a closed globe injury caused a blunt object. The injury may be at the site of impact (*coup*) or opposite the site of injury (*contra coup*). A rupture is a full-thickness wound caused by a blunt object. A laceration is a full-thickness wound caused by a sharp object. A penetrating injury is a single full-thickness wound of the eye wall, usually caused by a sharp object. There is no "exit" wound. A perforating injury consists of two full-thickness wounds (entrance and exit) usually caused by a single missile. The terms "perforating" and "penetrating" are not used in reference to tissues other than the eye wall. Other clinical factors are also assessed including the grade of injury (visual acuity), the presence or absence of a relative afferent pupillary defect, and the zone of injury (tissue type involved and location relative to the corneoscleral limbus). This classification system is limited to mechanical injuries but similar systems have been proposed for chemical (28,46) and thermal injury (39) to guide management.

This chapter discusses the cellular and tissue damage and subsequent reaction that occur in various types of injury. The manner and degree of cell death is determined by the type and extent of the injury. The response of the tissue to cell death and architectural disruption is determined primarily by the cellular environment of the injured tissue.

MECHANICAL INJURY

Overview

Mechanical ocular injury results from the transfer of kinetic energy from an external object to the tissues of the eye. Kinetic energy is the energy that a body possesses as a result of its motion and is determined in part by the mass of the object. The energy attained is proportional to the square of the velocity attained, so that a slowly moving object develops only a small amount of kinetic energy and therefore may inflict insignificant damage. A high-velocity object develops a large amount of kinetic energy and therefore may perforate the eye wall and fracture bone.

Dense tissues absorb more energy than less dense tissues and are therefore more efficient media for the transfer of energy, i.e., they retard the transfer of force. Kinetic energy is able to compress, distort, and disrupt tissues. Disruption occurs when the energy delivered exceeds the native tensile strength of the tissue and is prone to occur at sites where tissue planes are anchored. Shearing forces are more likely to develop at interfaces between tissues of differing density.

Anatomic Considerations

The globe is composed of many different tissue types arranged in planes and anchored at specific points. The entire anterior segment is anchored directly or indirectly to the scleral spur a dense, circumferential band of collagen that is part of the internal sclera immediately posterior to the trabecular meshwork (Fig. 1). The structure is clinically visible only by gonioscopy and only in individuals with an "open angle" configuration. Histologically, the configuration is relatively well demarcated (the scleral roll) in childhood but over time it blends with the surrounding tissue (the scleral spur). The longitudinal muscle of the ciliary body inserts directly into the scleral spur. The iris does not insert into the scleral spur but is indirectly anchored through its attachment with the anterior face of the ciliary body. The posterior boundary of the trabecular meshwork inserts into the scleral spur. The structures of the posterior segment are also anchored indirectly by the scleral

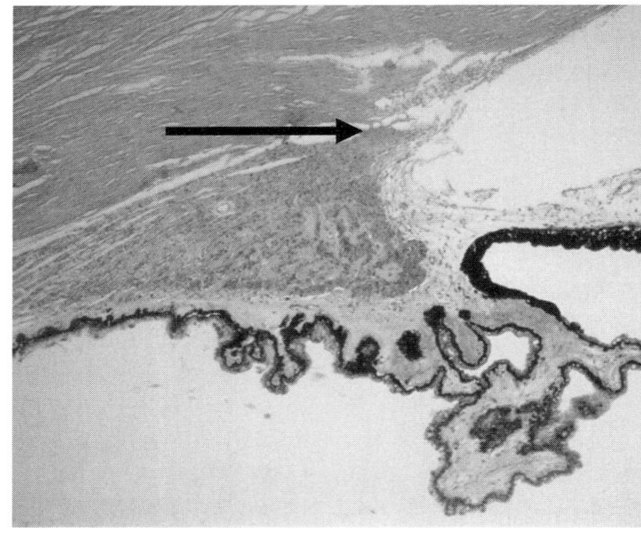

Figure 1 The scleral spur (*arrow*) is a collagenous structure of the internal sclera posterior to the trabecular meshwork. The longitudinal muscle of the ciliary body directly inserts into the scleral spur anchoring the anterior choroid. The internal muscles of the ciliary body do not insert into the scleral spur and are vulnerable to displacement (hematoxylin and eosin, ×100).

spur. The anterior part of the choroid is limited by the scleral spur and the equatorial choroid is anchored at the ostia of the vortex veins. The posterior choroid is anchored at the optic disc. The anterior choroid supports the origin of the zonules at the anterior border of the vitreous face. The vitreous base adheres firmly to the pars plana epithelium and internal peripheral retina where it straddles the ora serrata over a distance of 4 mm. The neurosensory retina is also anchored at the ora serrata (Fig. 2).

Other anchored structures include the insertion of the zonules into the equatorial area of the lens and the anterior vitreous face to the posterior capsule of the crystalline lens. Additional areas of increased adhesion include the vitreoretinal attachments at the optic disc, at the margin of the fovea and overlying retinal blood vessels.

The eye is composed of several planes of extracellular matrix (ECM), such as Descemet membrane, the lens capsule, and Bruch membrane. The components of the basement membrane are relatively elastic but will rupture at a lower energy level than the surrounding fibrous ECM. The optic nerve axons have essentially no tensile strength since they are composed to a large extent of lipid. With elongation of the optic nerve during anterior displacement of the globe the optic nerve axons will rupture before the arachnoid mater or dura mater, both of which possess considerable innate tensile strength.

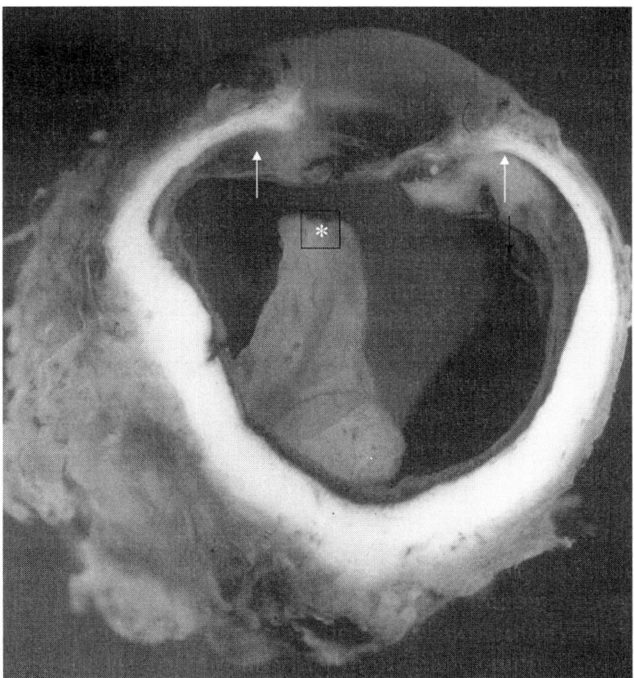

Figure 2 Compression of the globe has caused the retina (*) to become totally disinserted from the ora serrata (*arrows*). An example of total retinal dialysis.

Disruption of the globe is also more likely at areas where the eye wall is relatively thin. Conjunctiva and Tenon capsule insert into the external scleral sulcus at the corneoscleral limbus. The trabecular meshwork and the canal of Schlemm are located in the internal scleral sulcus. Between the sulci the thickness of the sclera is reduced from approximately 1000 μm to approximately 650 μm. Similarly the sclera at the insertion of the four rectus muscles and the superior oblique muscles thinned to accommodate the muscle tendon. The insertion of the inferior oblique muscle is directly from muscular fibers into the sclera and there is no thinning in this area. Any site of previous surgery such as a radial keratotomy and penetrating keratoplasty is also a location of potential disruption of the eye wall.

The globe is anchored in the orbit by the medial and lateral canthal ligaments. Extreme anterior excursion of the globe is limited both by the extraocular rectus muscle insertions in the sclera and by the insertion of the dura of the optic nerve into the posterior sclera in the region of the circle of Zinn-Haller. Excursion of the globe posteriorly, vertically or laterally, is limited by the apex and walls of the orbit.

Closed Globe Injury

Blunt ocular trauma distributes energy over a larger area than penetrating trauma. Multiple sites of injury tend to be produced from rapid deceleration and acceleration, shearing, crushing or compression, and multiple mechanisms usually operate simultaneously.

Injuries at low kinetic energy involving contact of a blunt object with the anterior surface of the globe, particularly if the force is tangential, are likely to cause abrasions of either the corneal or conjunctival surface. The resulting death of surface cells will stimulate replacement from limbal stem cells. With the loss of the major barrier to microbes (particularly *Pseudomonas aeruginosa*) there is a substantial risk of infection until the surface barriers are reestablished. There is also a risk of a faulty production of basement membrane by regenerating epithelial cells as in persons with diabetes mellitus leading to faulty cell adhesion and possible recurrent erosion (indirect trauma-related loss of surface epithelium). Defective basement membrane can be identified clinically as intraepithelial linear opacities. Injuries of greater kinetic energy may disrupt Bowman membrane (a structure with no regenerative potential) and the anterior corneal stroma, resulting in a focal corneal scar or an epithelial facet (17).

Cornea

More severe blunt injury to the cornea, e.g., bungee cord injuries, may generate waves of sufficient energy to disrupt corneal endothelial cells. This may produce only localized damage in the form of traumatic corneal rings or cause generalized damage with diffuse stromal edema and corneal opacification (3). Repair depends on the presence of a sufficient corneal endothelial cell reserve to cover Descemet membrane by enlargement and spreading of remaining viable endothelial cells. Marked deformation of the eye, as during obstetrical delivery, may cause horizontal expansion of the cornea and rupture of Descemet membrane. The ruptures may be single or multiple and are often oriented vertically. Free strands of Descemet membrane may project into the anterior chamber. The injury initially causes corneal edema that may resolve as the adjacent, uninjured corneal endothelium spreads. Ultimately this type of injury may cause astigmatism, with amblyopia (22).

In injuries with higher kinetic energy there is a risk of perforating the eye wall. An air pellet (BB missile) has been found to penetrate a normal porcine cornea at a muzzle velocity of approximately 75 m/sec (31). Muzzle velocity is the speed at which a projectile leaves the muzzle of a gun and is a relative measure of kinetic energy. Muzzle velocities for an average pistol are about 330 m/sec, but some military weapons have a muzzle velocity of about 1800 m/sec, i.e., greater than the speed of sound (340 m/sec). A velocity of more than 46 m/sec is necessary to penetrate skin and objects moving faster than 60 m/sec will fracture bone. Once the cornea is perforated the intraocular pressure (IOP) tends to be reduced toward atmospheric pressure (Fig. 3).

If energy is applied to the globe, such that the eye wall is not penetrated, the wall is deformed, often with the cornea and lens–iris diaphragm retrodisplaced to the plane of the ocular equator (36). The globe is a hollow sphere filled with noncompressible fluid and the pressure relationships within the eye are subject to the laws of any hydraulic system. Increased external pressure will result in markedly increased IOP. During scleral depression to examine the peripheral retina the IOP of the human eye increases from an average of 18 to 60–350 mmHg, exceeding both the diastolic and systolic blood pressures. During a routine enucleation the IOP has been measured at 150 to >500 mmHg (12). External pressure will increase the pressure in the anterior chamber, presumably >500 mmHg, compressing the iris against the anterior surface of the lens and creating a relative pupillary block of posteriorly-directed fluid. Increased IOP becomes transferred to the weak, vulnerable areas of the anterior chamber, i.e., the trabecular meshwork, the face of the ciliary body, and the iris root.

The most clinically apparent injury in this setting is hyphema. The source of bleeding is often not clinically visible but it is most likely the result of shearing forces disrupting branches of the major arterial circle of the ciliary body. Adding extravasated blood to the limited volume of the normal anterior chamber (0.3 mm^3) (11) will increase intracameral pressure and aid in hemostasis. Ultimate damage to the tissues of the anterior chamber depends on the volume of hemorrhage, the state of health of the corneal and trabecular endothelial cells, and the length of time normal aqueous humor dynamics are interrupted.

Small volumes of extravasated blood are rapidly cleared through the trabecular meshwork and perhaps through the vascular system of the iris stroma. Larger volumes of hemorrhage may physically occlude the trabecular meshwork, interrupting the flow of aqueous humor and increasing IOP. The aqueous humor supplies nutrients to the lining of the posterior chamber, the lens epithelium, the corneal endothelium and the trabecular endothelium. Degeneration of supportive surface cells may lead to cataract, corneal endothelial and trabecular meshwork decompensation, and permanent scarring. A clinical clue to the relative state of health of anterior chamber surface cells is indicated by the degree of oxygenation of the extravasated blood. Deoxygenation (blackball or eight-ball hemorrhage) indicates severe nutritional stress.

An increasing duration of hyphema accentuates the risk of several types of tissue damage. The natural history of extravasated blood is to become organized by fibrous metaplasia of blood-borne monocyte macrophages. The organization leads to a permanent fibrous mass that may contain cholesterol from degenerating erythrocytes that is evident in tissue sections by characteristic clefts. Degenerating blood also establishes

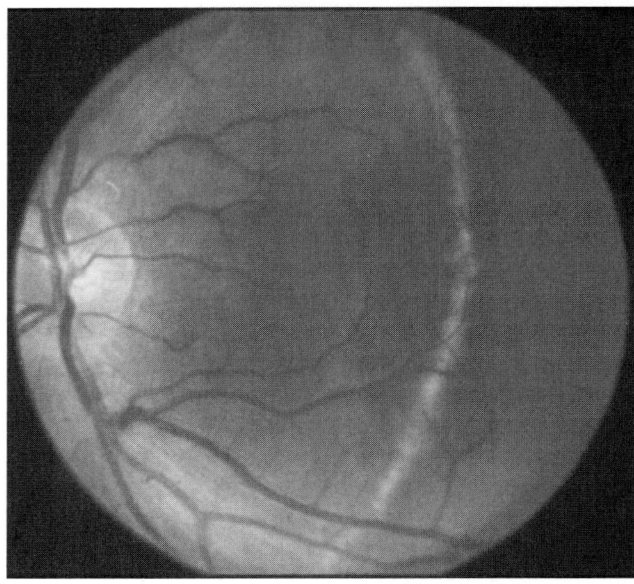

Figure 3 Rupture of Bruch membrane is concentric to the optic disc and visible because of reflection of light from the sclera.

the risk of hemosiderosis bulbi and ferrous ions released from degenerating hemoglobin are toxic to all epithelial and endothelial cells. Iron accumulating in the lens epithelium will create a rust-like opacity under the anterior lens capsule. Endothelial cells of the cornea and trabecular meshwork that have survived the initial traumatic insult may degenerate because of intracellular ferritin interfering with essential metabolic functions. Degenerating erythrocytes release denatured hemoglobin that is soluble in aqueous humor and is able to diffuse across an intact Descemet membrane and accumulate within the corneal stroma. The molecules are distributed in a gradient that is most concentrated in the posterior and central cornea. At a certain concentration denatured hemoglobin will precipitate in the corneal stroma creating a reddish-orange opacity (corneal blood staining). Denatured stromal hemoglobin can be cleared peripherally through the limbal vascular arcades. However, there is no efficient mechanism of clearing the central cornea due to lack of veins and lymphatic channels.

A plane of relative weakness exists between the longitudinal muscle of the ciliary body, stabilized anteriorly at its attachment to the scleral spur, and the oblique and circular muscle bundles that are not stabilized by direct attachment to the scleral spur. The tremendous force generated by high anterior chamber IOP will cause fluid to dissect along the plane between the longitudinal muscle of the ciliary body and the remainder of the ciliary musculature, causing posterior displacement of the poorly supported internal muscle fibers of the ciliary body. With clear media this area of displacement can be recognized by focal deepening of the anterior chamber and by gonioscopic views of internal sclera posterior to the scleral spur. This rent in the anterior ciliary body does not substantially influence IOP in either direction. However, if there is sufficient pressure to rupture the relatively robust structure of the ciliary musculature, presumably there is enough energy to damage the delicate trabecular beams that are only microns away from the face of the ciliary body. The damage is presumed because it is not clinically visible by any diagnostic method. The presence of a clinically detectable recession of the anterior chamber angle is functionally important therefore because of the near certainty of trabecular damage that will raise IOP.

Another vulnerable structure is the insertion of the longitudinal muscle of the ciliary body into the scleral spur. Rupture at this point (cyclodialysis) will allow aqueous humor to enter the suprachoroidal space which, unlike the juxtacanalicular apparatus of the trabecular meshwork, has no significant barriers to diffusion of this fluid. The IOP may be reduced to the point that it adversely affects vision.

Iris

The root of the iris is an extremely delicate structure where it inserts into the face of the ciliary body. It is composed of a small number of collagenous strands, arterioles and venules of the anterior ciliary circulation, and the iris pigment epithelium. The iris pigment epithelium has essentially no tensile strength, and the consistency of the iris is that of wet tissue paper. Tears through the sphincter pupillae are common. The iris can be disinserted from the ciliary body and displaced centrally (iridodialysis). Damage to the iris blood vessels can compromise the blood-aqueous barrier leading to fibrin accumulation in the anterior chamber. The adhesive properties of the fibrin-rich aqueous humor may lead to anterior and posterior synechiae. Extensive interruption of the blood supply of the iris in this setting may lead to total iris atrophy.

Severe compression of the posterior iris to the anterior surface of the lens may transfer melanin pigment from the iris pigment epithelium to the lens capsule (Vossius ring). The pigment may be dispersed into the convection current of the aqueous humor and manifest as anterior chamber pigment dispersion.

Lens and Zonules

Posterior displacement of the crystalline lens focuses energy at the insertion of the zonules into the lens capsule. Rupture of zonular support leads to displacement of the lens into either the anterior or posterior chamber in a position where aqueous humor flow may be interrupted by obstruction of the pupil. The lens capsule may be ruptured allowing instantaneous hydration of the lens cortex resulting in opacification.

Retina and Choroid

One of the most common posterior segment *contracoup* injuries in closed globe trauma is opacification of the deep layers of the retina (commotio retinae, Berlin edema). A pressure wave generated anteriorly traverses the globe and shears the photoreceptor outer segments. The internal portion of the retina is intact without any edema, as indicated by normal retinal blood vessels overlying the deeper opacity. Any damage to the underlying retinal pigment epithelium (RPE) may result in atrophic changes. The photoreceptor outer segments generally repair spontaneously (40).

Any shock waves passing in the vicinity of the globe may be of such magnitude to cause rapid distortion of the globe and extensive disruption of neurosensory retina, RPE, and choroid (retinitis sclopeteria). Bullets passing near but not through the globe are the usual cause. The retina may remain attached if the cortical vitreous remains intact. Hemorrhage and physical disruption result in extensive chorioretinal scarring and loss of vision (traumatic retinopathy) (25).

Direct deformation of the posterior segment places stress on Bruch membrane which has limited extensibility and limited tensile strength relative to the sclera and tends to rupture in a pattern concentric with the optic disc. The rupture is clinically apparent because of exposure of the underlying sclera (Fig. 4). The overlying neurosensory retina that is not clinically visible also ruptures, but is manifest by immediate and permanent loss of visual field peripheral to the defect. The clinical outcome is highly dependent on the position of the rupture relative to the fovea centralis, and ruptures through the papulomacular bundle will result in the most severe loss of vision. The rupture stimulates fibrovascular repair with blood vessels originating in the chorioid. The rent in Bruch membrane therefore establishes a lifelong risk of additional visual loss due to hemorrhage from subretinal neovascularization (1,16).

In experimental models of blunt-force injury compression of the globe may reduce the anterior–posterior length of the eye by 59% (7). To compensate for the presence of noncompressible intraocular contents there is marked lateral expansion of the equatorial sclera. This is followed by a compensatory overshoot of 112% as the globe rebounds toward its normal spherical shape, followed by diminishing oscillations of compression and rebound expansion. The strongest anchoring points of the retina are at the ora serrata, the vitreous base, and the scleral canal. The retina is thickest at the scleral canal particularly in the region of the papulomacular bundle and the superior and inferior poles of the optic disc. Similarly the neurosensory retina at the ora serrata is protected by the strong attachment of the vitreous base that extends 2 mm anterior and 2 mm posterior to the ora serrata. The area of the retina that is most vulnerable is the relatively thin peripheral retina just posterior to the vitreous base. Possibly because the temporal eye is less protected than the nasal side by the orbital rim, retinal breaks tend to be at the site of injury with temporal injuries (*coup* injury) and opposite the site of injury nasally (*contracoup injuries*). Severe distortion may rupture of the pars plana anterior to the vitreous base and cause total avulsion of the vitreous base. Giant retinal tears may not become clinically detectable until a reduction in vitreous volume following injury (traumatic syneresis) allows displacement of the retina from its normal position (5).

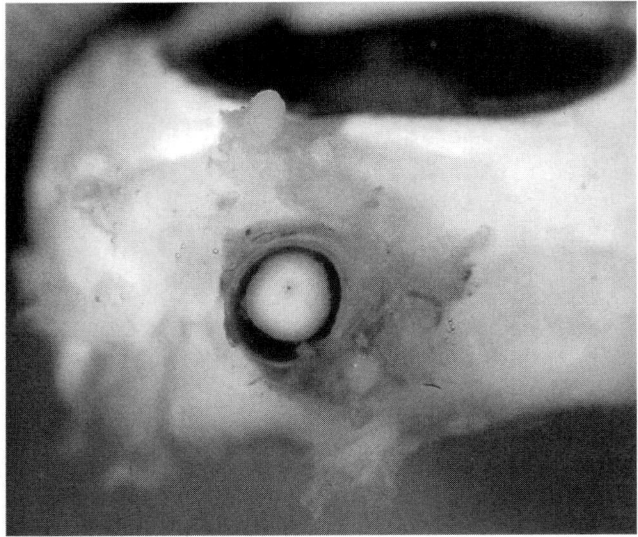

Figure 4 Subdural and subarachnoid hemorrhage of the optic nerve is evident in this autopsy case of a child who died shortly after being injured. The optic nerve is normal.

A full-thickness macular hole is a round break involving all layers of the retina. Concussion during blunt trauma may only partially separate the vitreous from the fovea, and traction on the retina by the vitreous may result in a retinal hole (20).

There are several entities in which the eye is affected by damage inflicted on nonocular tissue. Purtcher retinopathy consists of inner retinal ischemia in the distribution of the radial peripapillary circulation, which has a near-linear distribution along the superior and inferior temporal vascular arcades. Because of a limited number of collateral channels in the internal retina where the nerve fiber layer is thickest the system is vulnerable to ischemia and the development of infarcts in the inner retina. This type of retinal infarction has been identified with closed chest trauma, acute pancreatitis, amniotic embolism, connective tissue disease, and retrobulbar anesthesia, among others. The mechanism of occlusion is controversial and may involve leukocyte aggregations and complement activation.

Terson syndrome is an intracranial subarachnoid hemorrhage leading to hemorrhage in the retina and vitreous. The most common cause is rupture of an intracranial aneurysm. Extravasated blood travels through the subarachnoid space of the brain into the contiguous space surrounding the optic nerve. Increased subarachnoid pressure exceeds the intraluminal pressure of the central retinal vein but not the central retinal artery causing sequestration of blood within the intraocular venous compartment. Intraocular hemorrhage results from distention and rupture of retinal capillaries and is most often seen in the posterior retina. It may break through the internal limiting membrane (ILM) into the vitreous.

The Shaken-Impact Syndrome

The shaken-impact syndrome (acceleration–deceleration syndrome, child abuse) is described in infants generally under the age of three years. The primary presenting features are subdural hemorrhage, metaphyseal and rib fractures, and retinal hemorrhages.

Generally the historical information offered does not correlate with the degree of injury. The mechanism of injury is controversial but it is thought to be due to rotational kinetic forces generated by acceleration and deceleration of an infant's head. The head of an infant is larger in proportion to the body than that of an older child or adult and is poorly supported by the underdeveloped upper body musculature. This is particularly obvious when the child is intentionally shaken or the child's head strikes a hard surface. During extreme excursions of the head, the eyes are displaced anteriorly in the orbit reflecting the inertia imparted by the high water content of the vitreous. Shearing forces are generated that rupture blood vessels in the subarachnoid space and in the subdural space of the optic nerve resulting in hemorrhage (Fig. 5). Compression of the venous system leads to intraocular hemorrhage. The dura mater of the optic nerve inserts into the sclera in the region of small caliber circumferential blood vessels in the sclera that supply blood to the optic nerve head (circle of Zinn–Haller). A rupture of the dura mater and the shearing of blood vessels within it lead to intrascleral hemorrhage, a finding only seen at autopsy. Intrascleral hemorrhage in the region of Zinn–Haller has only been reported in the setting of shaken-impact syndrome (9). Hemorrhage in the retina may be found at any level of the retina and in the vitreous, and unlike Terson syndrome, may extend to the ora serrata. Attempts have been made to date the hemorrhages to prove that the injuries are the result of multiple episodes, although there is no method of precisely dating a hemorrhage based on histologic findings (14). Traction detachment of the macula and retinoschisis has also been observed. It is unusual to find any sign of trauma, including cataract, in the anterior segment. Extensive shearing forces generated in the brain may lead to cerebral atrophy and death if the infant lives for several months (15).

Open Globe Injuries

The eye wall may be interrupted when distortional forces or IOP exceed its tensile strength or a foreign object passes through the tissue. The globe is a hollow sphere containing noncompressible fluid and the normal IOP is in the range 10 to 21 mmHg. The rupture point of the living eye has not been determined, but pressures of >500 mmHg have been measured that did not disrupt the collagenous framework of the eye wall, although various internal structures may have been adversely affected. There are sites of vulnerability of the eye wall where rupture is more likely as described above.

Eye wall rupture begins, or is more clinically obvious, at the corneoscleral limbus, particularly temporally. The laceration often extends posteriorly through one of the rectus muscle insertions, again most often temporally, and may reach the insertion of the inferior oblique muscle. The clinical signs of a ruptured globe include severe periocular hemorrhage, profound loss of vision, an IOP of <5 mmHg, an unusually deep or shallow anterior chamber, irregular pupil, afferent pupillary defect and opaque media.

Extravasated blood is usually present in the wound associated with herniated uveal tissue and these may be difficult to separate (Fig. 6). The uveal tract readily herniates through the eye wall because it is attached to the sclera at only three sites: the scleral spur, the ampullae of the vortex veins and at the optic canal. With large ruptures, especially when associated

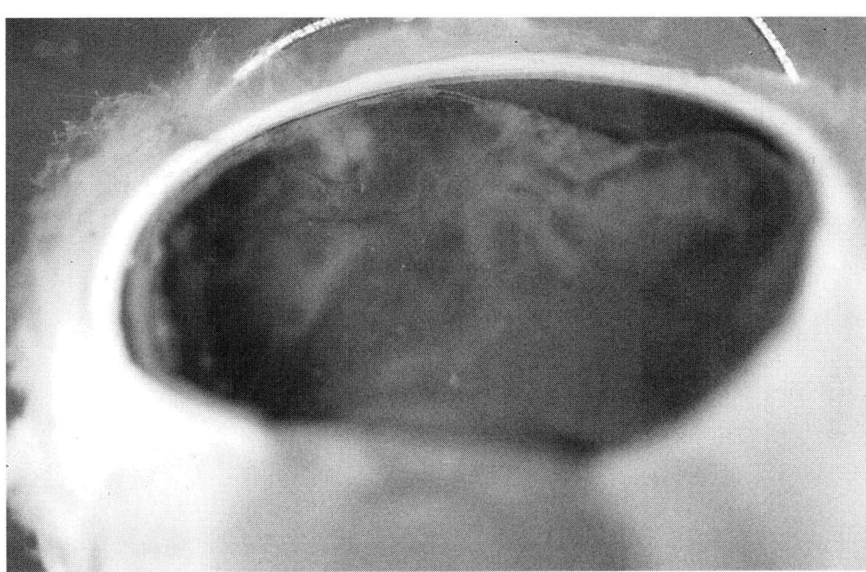

Figure 5 Diffuse intraretinal hemorrhage as well as elevation of the posterior retina is present in this case of child abuse homicide.

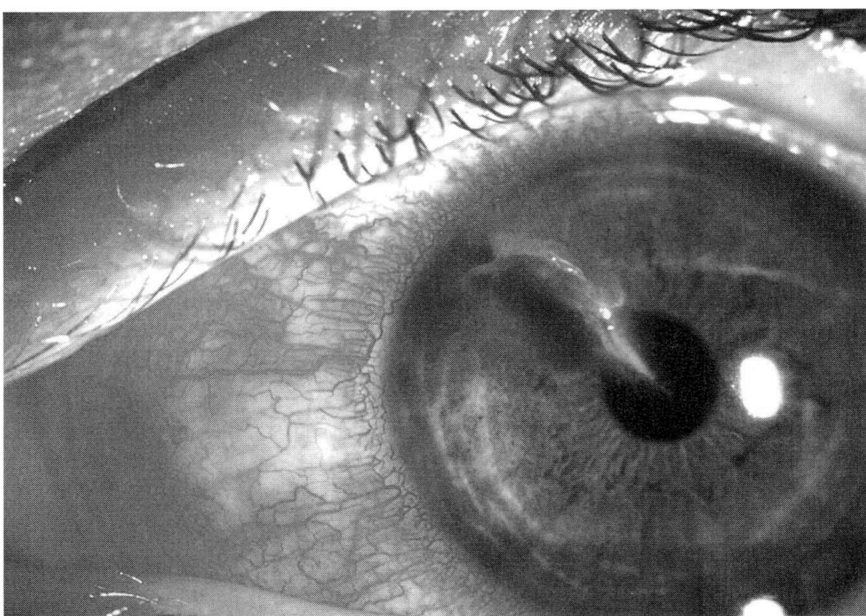

Figure 6 Lacerated cornea. The pupil is distorted because the iris is drawn into the wound. In this case the vision and intraocular pressure may be normal, but there is a major risk of infection being wicked into the eye by the exposed iris tissue.

with high IOP and suprachoroidal hemorrhage, the entire contents of the globe may be expelled.

Cornea

Rupture of the cornea often produces a stellate irregular wound as a result of multiple force vectors acting on a curved surface, and tissues may be lost during the traumatic episode. Surgical repair is often difficult and often causes extensive corneal opacification and irregular astigmatism.

Lens

The entire crystalline lens of a younger person may be expelled through a 3-mm corneoscleral limbal rupture.

Uvea

Iris is often forced into the wound causing a temporary seal but this is unstable and cannot effectively resist microbial invasion. Posterior wounds are often associated with choroidal hemorrhage, choroidal effusion, retinal dialysis and retinal detachment, all of which may not be clinically visible because of opaque media.

Penetrating Injury

A penetrating injury caused by a foreign object passing through the eye wall distributes energy over a smaller area than that found with either a closed globe injury or a ruptured globe. Tissue damage is directly related to the amount of kinetic energy the missile loses at the site of impact and the velocity of the missile is more a determining factor than its mass or composition. The transferred energy of the missile

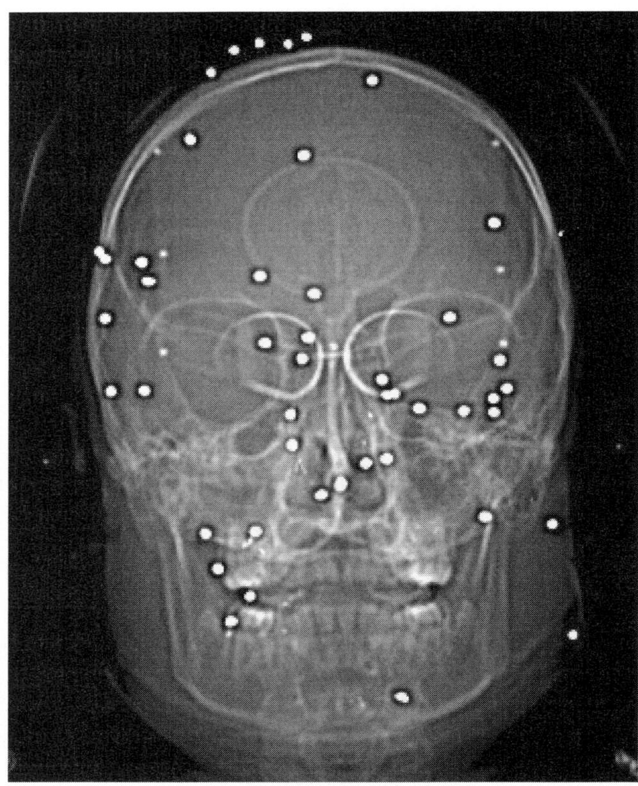

Figure 7 This 11-year-old boy was shot in the face during a hunting accident. The pellets had enough muzzle velocity to penetrate the skin and perforate one of his eyes.

crushes and lacerates tissue as the shock waves sequentially compress and expand the tissue along the route of the wave.

The entrance wound is usually anterior, creating corneal wounds that may be difficult to detect clinically. Clinical signs include loss of aqueous humor and a shallow anterior chamber, rents in the iris, irregular pupil, cataract, and anterior herniation of vitreous. The wound may create a fistula allowing surface epithelium to gain entrance to the eye. This epithelial ingrowth can be limited by a healthy endothelium (contact inhibition of movement) but often the endothelium is also damaged. Surface epithelium growing over the trabecular meshwork will cover the trabecular beams and obstruct aqueous humor outflow. Surface epithelium grows abundantly over the anterior surface of the iris and may extend posteriorly if there is access through the vitreous face. The epithelial ingrowth may be accompanied by fibrous tissues leading to fibrosis of the trabecular meshwork. Once this occurs the condition is irreversible.

Sclera

The missile may enter through the sclera with its path extending into the vitreous cavity. Often materials in the scleral wound become incarcerated interfering with repair but allowing growth of episcleral fibrovascular tissues into the eye along a vitreous scaffold. The injury is often accompanied by hemorrhage and the blood-retinal barrier is damaged. Both features allow inclusion of circulating cells that have the potential of transforming into fibroblasts. As in other sites, granulation tissue forms and matures into a fibrovascular scar. Because of the action of myofibroblasts the repaired tissue contracts and produces traction on the surrounding vitreous. This tension is transmitted to the retina creating a tractional retinal detachment. The tension lines are usually oriented along the route of the missile, although the fibrous tissue may form along the anterior border of the vitreous to create a cyclitic membrane that displaces the ciliary body centrally and causes hypotony.

INTRAOCULAR FOREIGN BODIES

Overview

No matter what its composition, the presence of an intraocular foreign body adds markedly to the complexity and possible unfavorable outcome of an episode of ocular trauma (Fig. 7). Even totally inert material, such as glass in the anterior chamber, can lead to corneal decompensation. A foreign body composed of pure copper can totally destroy an eye over a short period of time.

Foreign bodies, such as skin, cilia, or vegetable material, may be carried into the eye when penetrated by twigs, thorns, and other sharp objects, and when fragments of glass, metal, or rock enter the eye as projectiles. A small inert foreign body may remain for a long period of time inside the eye without provoking a clinically detectable reaction.

Certain ocular tissues react to a foreign body more violently than others. For example, a foreign body in the highly vascular uveal tissue is more likely to provoke an inflammatory response than one lodged in the avascular lens or vitreous. To a large extent the shape and sharpness of the extraneous object determine its irritating and damaging effects, especially if it remains mobile within the eye. As in other tissues, foreign bodies within the eye tend to migrate toward the surface. Aside from gravity, the movements of intraocular foreign bodies may be related to the contraction of the extra- and intraocular muscles, the currents of the intraocular fluid, and the movements of the eyelids (44). Some materials, especially vegetable or animal matter, can set up a marked granulomatous response, whereas more inert objects, such as the precious metals gold, silver, and platinum, may merely become surrounded by a fibrous capsule. Relatively inert substances, such as stone, rock, clay, carbon, glass, and some plastics, do not necessarily interact with the tissues but may damage the eye during entry and by migration once within the eye. The presence of glass in the anterior chamber angle can cause recurrent iridocyclitis, probably by mechanical irritation and edema of the cornea if it traumatizes the corneal endothelium; on the retina it may provoke a mild inflammatory response, leading to its encapsulation by glial proliferation. Certain metals may be sterile at the time of entry, especially if hot, but may still prove toxic to ocular tissues. The most important elements in this category are copper and iron and their alloys. However, lead, zinc, nickel, aluminum, and mercury can all incite inflammatory reactions, especially if lodged in the posterior segment (8).

Copper

Copper and its alloys produce a purulent reaction, the severity of which depends on the degree to which the copper is bound. The copper-containing foreign body therefore usually leads to hypopyon, a vitreous abscess, retinal detachment, and finally phthisis bulbi. Alternatively, if the reaction is less pronounced, the retina may slowly degenerate. When a foreign body is composed of a copper alloy, there is slow diffusion of copper throughout the ocular tissues and a greenish-blue ring may appear in the peripheral cornea at the level of Descemet membrane and the deep stroma (8). In addition, a sunflower-shaped lens opacity, discoloration of the iris, zonules, and vitreous framework, and tiny metallic flecks on the retina (chalcosis) are likely to develop. The sunflower cataract, which is characterized by a colorful display of powdery opacities forming a central disc with radiating petal-like spokes, results from deposition of copper in the deeper layers of the anterior lens capsule. It is controversial as to whether copper is present in the lens epithelium (8).

Rosenthal et al. (34,35) have shown that pure copper or a 60% alloy of this metal may fail to provoke an inflammatory response in rabbits if the metallic object is located anteriorly in the vitreous and away from the retina. In this position, cuprous ions would be present in low concentration at the retinal surface. However, pure copper adjacent to the retina initiates a purulent response followed by encapsulation in glial tissues. In the same position, a 60% copper alloy produces a less intense acute reaction followed by a chronic inflammatory response, again with encapsulation of the foreign body. Copper enters the retina either within macrophages or by diffusion, which can lead to retinal disorganization, loss of cells in the inner nuclear and ganglion cell layers, and gliosis. This reaction is localized to the region of the foreign body. A particle that remains shiny confers a good prognosis since it indicates that a chemical reaction is not taking place. Encapsulation serves to protect the eye from the deleterious effects of copper in some cases. Increased levels of copper in the aqueous humor often reflect the intraocular diffusion of copper. Eventual migration of copper-containing particles and extrusion through the sclera have been described (35).

Iron

An iron-containing foreign body may cause severe damage to ocular structures and an electroretinogram (ERG) may be useful in detecting the onset of retinopathy. The mildest effect of iron is a reversible increase in the amplitude of the "a" wave (which arises from the inner segments of the photoreceptors) and/or the "b" wave (originating in the vicinity of the bipolar cells of the retina and thought to arise from the Müller cells) when the eye appears normal (26). With more toxic doses the amplitude of the ERG diminishes and some of this decrease may also be reversible. The photoreceptors are primarily injured, but the Müller cells appear intact microscopically. Even after the foreign body is removed, the ERG can continue to deteriorate, possibly because enough iron remains in the tissue to continue its toxic action.

The pathogenesis of the retinal degeneration is not certain but Burger and Klintworth (2) demonstrated selective necrosis of the outer retina in the absence of vascular narrowing. Placing iron wires into the vitreous of rabbits, they found early changes in the visual receptor cells, with pyknosis followed by karyorrhexis and a macrophage response. Breakup of the normal lamellar arrangement of the photoreceptor discs also occurred. The processes of the RPE that are normally applied to the outer segments became disorganized. Müller cells, which appeared resistant to the effects of iron, filled the void with their processes.

It is noteworthy that retinal injury occurs early but iron staining is late and the stainable iron is not found in areas where there is most damage to the retina. The inner layers, especially the ILM and the nerve fiber layer, often show moderate staining but appear normal by light and transmission electron microscopy (TEM), as does the RPE. It has been suggested that the innocuous form of stored iron stains most prominently but iron attached to and inactivating vital enzymes may not stain. In other words, the appearance of iron pigments in a tissue may imply a greater capacity for detoxifying iron and withstanding its effects, rather than a special sensitivity (49). Free ions and/or an iron–glycosaminoglycan complexes diffuse to various parts of the eye, where the iron is bound to cell enzymes. The relatively resistant uvea stores the iron, whereas the retina, less able to detoxify it, is poisoned at an early stage. Mascuiulli et al. (26) found less toxicity with ferric than with ferrous ions but determined that oxidation or reduction of ions can occur following injection of the material into the eye. Burger and Klintworth (2) speculate that the reason for the susceptibility of photoreceptors to iron compounds reflects the high glycolytic activity of the retina, which makes it more susceptible to agents that interfere with the responsible enzyme systems.

Encapsulation of an iron-containing foreign body may protect the ocular tissues somewhat. As the ocular structures become discolored, the foreign body may diminish in size and even disappear completely. Iron diffuses throughout the eye, to be taken up by epithelial cells of the ciliary body and lens, smooth muscle, keratocytes, and others. The cornea, iris, vitreous, and retina eventually become brownish in color. The lens becomes yellow at first just beneath the capsule, where the iron is concentrated by the anterior epithelium, and later becomes brown throughout. Eventually a mature cataract develops and histochemical methods for the demonstration of iron point to a diffuse involvement.

Retinal detachment or chorioretinal adhesion may also occur. The ciliary epithelium stains heavily for iron but must continue to secrete aqueous humor because glaucoma occurs so regularly. Glaucoma is a frequent late event after injury to the trabecular meshwork and an infiltration of iron-laden macrophages into the anterior chamber angle. Siderosis bulbi secondary to massive hemophthalmos can produce similar discoloration of the ocular tissues and the intravitreal injection of hemoglobin can produce damage to the outer retina.

Organic Matter

Vegetable matter, such as cotton fibers and wood, often provokes a granulomatous response followed by fibrous or glial tissue proliferation. The inflammation, in the absence of an infectious process, may be immediate or delayed. Occasionally, skin or bone may enter the eye as a complication of an explosion injury, but these are relatively inert. Rarely, cilia are carried into the anterior segment of the eye. They may be free in the anterior chamber or partially or completely in contact with or incarcerated in iris, cornea, or lens. They usually excite no response, although an early or late inflammatory reaction may occur, which can be severe enough to lead to destruction of the globe. Why a quiet eye develops severe inflammation years after implantation of a cilium is not well understood. A granuloma can also form and occasionally cysts may be associated with the cilia, possibly originating from the follicle at its base. Cysts may also form in the absence of cilia, presumably from the implantation of nonkeratinizing or keratinizing epithelium (derived from conjunctiva or skin). Such cysts may occur following any penetrating injury of the globe.

Hairs or spines of insects and plants may enter the conjunctiva and cornea and may cause a severe reaction (47). They may fall into the conjunctival sac, be blown in or rubbed in, as caterpillar hairs are sharply pointed (see Chapter 14), and may contain barbs that point away from the base. They are also brittle and may break easily. The barbed hairs enter the tissue at the proximal end and migrate base first. Their passive movement may be related to blinking, ocular movements, pulse, and perhaps to the movement of the ciliary musculature and continued rubbing. The hairs of plants and seeds may produce a similar picture. In addition to mechanical damage there is apparent toxicity of the hair itself, which is thought to be due to the protoplasm of the cell rather than from venom secreted by the cell. A purulent keratoconjunctivitis and iridocyclitis can occur as the caterpillar hairs burrow inward. After one or two months, nodules occur in the conjunctiva and perhaps on the iris. They may be found in association with vitritis, choroiditis, and retinal perivasculitis. Although the inflammation eventually subsides, an endophthalmitis may lead to loss of the eye. Weinberg et al. (48) reported in some young patients the presence of filamentous foreign material in a subconjunctival location surrounded by granulomatous inflammation. It was derived from blankets, sweaters, or stuffed animals.

Other

At one time some golf balls contained a liquid center surrounded by a bound rubber string under extremely high pressure. Cutting such a golf ball or unwinding the rubber band beneath the outer shell result in the ejection of the central material, usually containing a mixture of zinc and barium sulfates, with an explosive force (19). The contents can penetrate the conjunctiva or skin. A white caseous conjunctival lesion can result, which when examined microscopically is found to contain black birefringent particles, usually within macrophages, and a mild inflammatory response.

THERMAL INJURY

Ocular tissue may be damaged by both heat and freezing, and, indeed, the scarring that may occur has been utilized therapeutically to obtain an adhesion between the choroid and the retina. The untoward effects of penetrating diathermy include necrosis of all layers of the globe, with extensive episcleral, scleral, and choroidal inflammatory reactions, as well as shrinkage, thinning, and weakening of the sclera. Cryothermy as in cryotherapy appears to be much less destructive. Although the cellular elements in the sclera may diminish, there is no shrinkage and the sclera retains its strength. The sensory retina undergoes coagulative necrosis, and the RPE becomes vacuolated with dispersion of its granules. Pigment clumping occurs, and the atrophic retinal and choroidal layers become joined together in scar tissue (6,28).

CHEMICAL INJURIES

Overview

Chemical injuries to ocular tissues are particularly destructive because the damage is directed mainly toward the most fundamental structural and functional element of all cells, the plasma membrane. Biochemical activities of all cells occur in an aqueous medium and intracellular biological reactions must be separated from the biochemical reactions in the extracellular environment. This segregation of biochemical activities is accomplished by interposition of a lipoproteinous membrane across which aqueous solutes cannot pass. The cellular internal environment is able to effect and is affected by the external environment through specialized regions of the plasma membrane that generally function as receptor sites for various protein signals (cytokines).

Strong acids and alkalis destroy the plasma membrane of cells and expose cytoplasmic contents. An alkaline agent, such as ammonia, dissociates in an aqueous environment into anionic hydroxyl group (OH^-) and cations (NH^{4+}). The cation generally determines the characteristics of penetration of the compound into tissue. The more dissociated the compound and the smaller the molecule, the more rapid and deep the penetration. Saponification is the process by which the hydroxyl anions are able to disrupt a

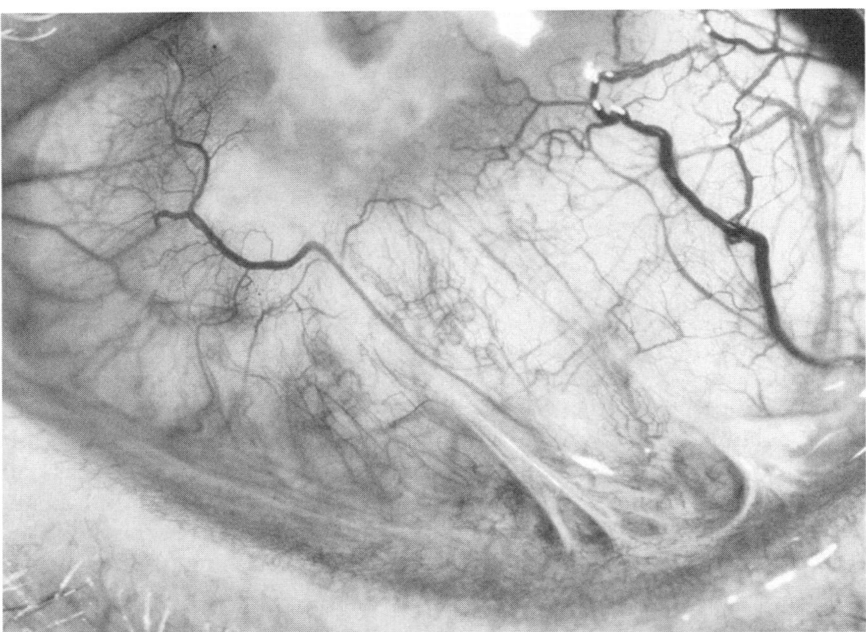

Figure 8 End-stage effects of alkali burn. The conjunctiva is totally nonfunctional; it has lost its ability to form tears due to the direct effect of the alkali and the inflammation that followed. The cornea is nonfunctional due to the direct effect of the alkali and the fibrosis and vascularization that followed.

plasma membrane and combine with its lipids to form small spherules (micelles) that make the lipid soluble and mobile in a fluid environment. The cell membrane loses its ability to isolate the internal biochemistry of the cell. The cell membrane becomes porous, the cell swells, and ceases to function as internal degeneration proceeds. Surface debris is generally carried away from the site of injury by mechanical forces (e.g., the wiping motion of the eyelid margin). Debris sequestered within tissues or tissue cavities is generally removed via phagocytosis by polymorphonuclear leukocytes (PMNs) and monocytes. Ironically in the setting of alkali-damaged tissues, particularly the cornea, participation of PMNs is stimulated and adds to the degree of tissue destruction.

Alkali Injuries

Alkali injuries are generally more serious than acid injuries but both agents have a high potential for immediate and delayed tissue destruction (Fig. 8). Ammonia hydroxide (NH_4OH) is the most dangerous of commonly encountered compounds. It is a small molecule that can penetrate to the level of the anterior chamber in seconds. Household ammonia is a 7% aqueous solution. Anhydrous ammonia (a 100% concentration) is commonly used as an agricultural fertilizer. It has a boiling point of $-33^{\circ}C$ and must be maintained a high pressure to remain in a liquid state. The highly volatile mixture is injected under high pressure into the soil to add nitrogen. Accidental contact with the face and the upper respiratory tract make anhydrous ammonia one of the most dangerous chemicals used in agriculture.

The most commonly encountered alkali compound leading to injury is lime [$Ca(OH)_2$], a component of many building materials. Even though the degree of penetration is low, lime particles may be sequestered in the upper fornix of the conjunctiva and, if not promptly removed, function as an ongoing source of alkali.

Immediate damage by alkaline agents affects such vital structures as the corneal and conjunctival epithelium, the peripheral nerve axons and endings, keratocytes, corneal endothelial cells, and most importantly, the vascular endothelial cells. Total loss of vascular endothelium leads to intravascular coagulation and ischemia distal to the point of obstruction. Partial damage leads to changes in the vascular endothelial luminal surface leading to intravascular thrombosis. Even mild damage changes the competence of the blood vessels and compromises the blood-aqueous and blood-retinal barriers of the eye. Total physical loss of the conjunctiva and its blood vessels may be present within minutes of the initial injury.

Loss of corneal epithelium is crucial for determining short- and long-term effects. Absence of the corneal epithelium subjects the corneal stroma to the potential of both drying and swelling. The risk of microbial infection is significant. Damage to epithelial basement membrane may delay epithelial healing and damage to limbal stem cells, and conjunctival epithelium reduces or eliminates a potential source of cells for reepithelialization.

Alkali destroys keratocytes but it also damages the ECM of Bowman layer and the corneal stroma. Collagen fibers that are perfectly uniform in their native state are denatured and become shorter and thicker, thereby reducing the ability to transmit light. Proteoglycans that uniformly separate the collagen fibers by altering water content are also chemically altered to allow increased and nonhomogeneous hydration and therefore spacing.

Alkali reaching the anterior chamber easily overwhelms the buffering capacity of the aqueous humor. Normal convection currents in the anterior chamber distribute alkali to the corneal epithelium (increased corneal hydration), trabecular epithelium (destruction of trabecular beams), juxtacanalicular connective tissue (failure of filtration), iris stroma (breakdown of blood-aqueous barrier, synechia formation), sphincter pupillae and dilator pupillae (nonreactive pupil), lens epithelium and cortex (cataract), ciliary epithelium (decreased oxygen and nutrients including ascorbic acid), vitreous (biochemical depot acting as a sustained release source), and retina (neurosensory dysfunction). Recovery of function is difficult if not impossible.

The key to recovery is the extent of initial damage. Several clinical classification schemes have been proposed to guide therapeutic management (28).

The most important process relates to the corneal epithelium and reflects its intimate relationship with the keratocytes of the corneal stroma and responding inflammatory cells, particularly the PMNs. Because of its vulnerable position of the corneal surface, cellular turnover is rapid, calling upon replacement cells produced by the stem cells of the corneoscleal limbus (palisades of Vogt). The epithelial cells of the cornea are distinctly different from those of the conjunctival epithelium. The conjunctival epithelium is directly supported by blood vessels and its surface is lubricated by the production of mucus. Stem cells for the conjunctival epithelium are thought to exist in the fornices.

The corneal epithelium is a stratified squamous epithelium and is a major refracting surface of the globe (45 out of a total of 60 diopters), participates in nutrition of the underlying stroma, and protects the stroma from noxious agents in the environment, particularly microbial organisms. The apical portions of the cells are specialized to allow adhesion of tear film elements such as mucous, and prevent adhesion of microbial organisms. The base of the cell adheres to a basement membrane that it produces, and attachment is maintained through proteins of the anchoring complex. Small numbers of epithelial cells can be replaced by sliding of adjacent undamaged cells. The anchoring complexes must be sequentially altered to allow the position of the cell to change. The cell moves over existing, possibly damaged, basement membrane supplemented by a temporary surface composed of fibronectin. Larger epithelial defects must be replaced by cells derived from the stem-cell population. When there is extensive damage conjunctival epithelium can cover the corneal surface but its phenotype remains that of conjunctival epithelium and it induces fibrovascular pannus on the anterior corneal surface.

A fundamental function of the repair process is to remove damaged ECM. Matrix metalloproteinases (MMPs) form a group of proteases that are able to precisely cleave specific categories of ECM molecules. Large, damaged molecules are reduced in size allowing diffusion to lymphatic channels or phagocytosis. Collagenase (MMP-1) is not normally present in the corneal stroma because the turnover of ECM proceeds at an extremely slow rate. ECM protein damaged by alkali is a signal to migrating epithelial cells to send a stimulus (cytokine) to keratocytes to secrete collagenase and other proteolytic enzymes. Once the epithelial surface is re-established keratocytes cease producing collagenase and begin to repair the ECM. The presence of debris is also a signal that attracts PMNs to the site, usually from corneoscleral limbal blood vessels, although transit through tears and aqueous humor also occurs. The PMNs internalize debris and degrade it with intracellular proteases. If the amount of debris is overwhelming, the PMNs will indiscriminately release all contained enzymes, including collagenase, at the site of injury (exocytosis).

Delayed epithelialization of an alkali-damaged corneal surface creates serious consequences for the integrity of the corneal stroma. Delay may be due to direct damage to basement membrane by the alkali, proteolytic destruction of fibronectin by PMNs, PMNs directly affecting the advancing epithelial cells, or substantial damage to the stem cell population. If the epithelial defect persists the cytokine signals to fibroblasts to produce collagenase remain and extensive loss of ECM to the point where ulceration or perforation is possible. Persistent and ongoing damage also recruits additional PMNs into the area of injury accelerating the cycle of damage–recruitment–-damage, which will continue until epithelial continuity is restored.

Adding to the complications of stromal lysis, reformation of ECM is also faulty. Ascorbate is normally secreted by the ciliary epithelium but with alkali damage this epithelium, intraocular ascorbate levels drop precipitously, limiting collagen formation. Ascorbate is a water-soluble vitamin that is essential to the formation of collagen type I and deficiency is characterized by the production of abnormal collagen of diminished tensile strength and increased susceptibility to degradation.

Acid Injuries

The most commonly encountered acid injuring the eye is sulfuric acid used in storage batteries and as a cleaning agent. The reaction with water is exothermic and can add thermal injury to chemical damage. Hydrofluoric acid is used in the manufacture of glass and, because of its small molecular size and ability to penetrate deeply into tissues, may be as destructive as alkaline agents.

The major effect of acidic agents is to cause surface rather than deep penetrating and sustained injury as is found with alkali agents. Acidic agents tend to cause denaturation of surface proteins. The denatured proteins tend become a barrier to diffusion and protect the underlying tissue from damage. Acid injuries are similar to surface thermal burns.

ELECTRICAL INJURIES

Electrical injury from high-tension wires and from lightning may induce lens opacities beneath the anterior and posterior capsules by damaging the epithelium and posterior subcapsular fibers, respectively. Cataracts resulting from lightning are usually bilateral, whereas those associated with electrical injuries are primarily anterior and usually unilateral, although not always on the side of the injury. The opacities occur after a variable latent period (rapid after lightning but usually 1–18 months following electrical injury). The configuration of the opacity depends to some extent on the age of the victim, with younger lenses being more susceptible to damage. Initially, vacuoles and punctate or linear opacities create a spongy appearance; the cataract subsequently either matures over a period of months or remains stationary. Conjunctival hyperemia, subconjunctival hemorrhage, opacities of the corneal stroma, iridocyclitis of varying severity, retinal (especially macular) and optic disc edema, whitish punctate or pigmentary retinal changes, chorioretinal atrophy, and retinal hemorrhage or retinal detachment have all been reported.

ULTRASOUND INJURIES

Sonic energy is a form of mechanical energy transmitted through a material medium, unlike electromagnetic radiation which can traverse a vacuum. Sound waves travel in straight lines, exhibit interference, diffraction, and dispersion, and are refracted or reflected at the interfaces between media of different density. The biological action of ultrasonic waves is not fully understood. The frequency of the waves and the intensity and duration of the stimulus produce certain thermal, mechanical, and chemical effects. The vibrations raise tissue temperature, especially at tissue interfaces, where energy absorption and reflection take place selectively. Disruptive forces occur at high-energy levels and can lead to necrosis. Necrosis and ulceration of the corneal epithelium and stromal leukomata can result from a thermal burn. Selective heating of the peripheral cornea with focused ultrasound was used to altering the corneal curvature however, with repair changes in corneal curvature reverted to pretreatment dimensions. Lens changes may also occur with ultrasound; low-frequency, high-intensity waves can produce turbidity in the deep cortex that may be transient.

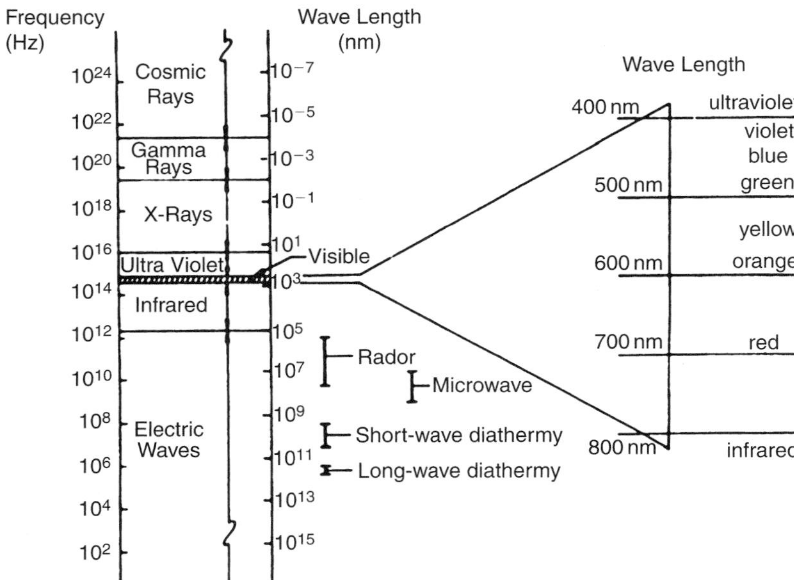

Figure 9 The electromagnetic spectrum. *Source*: Reproduced from Klintworth GK, Landers MB III. *The Eye*. Baltimore: Williams and Wilkins, 1976.

The turbidity appears not to be due to an elevated temperature. A second type of cataract that is thought to be thermal can also develop after radiation of high frequency and intensity. This is localized at first but eventually enlarges to include the entire lens with a loss of lens fiber architecture. Exposure of the retina and choroid to low-frequency ultrasonic transscleral waves can produce chorioretinal adhesions (21).

RADIATION INJURY

Radiation is a form of energy composed of electromagnetic waves (photons), usually of ultrashort wavelength, or accelerated subatomic particles that originate from internal changes in atoms and molecules and travel through space (Fig. 9). Radiation injury is any abnormality of form or function caused by electromagnetic waves or accelerated subatomic particles. Radiation is measured as the quantity of energy per mass of tissue. The international unit is the Grey (Gy) which is 1 J/kg where 1 Gy is equal to 100 rad in earlier terminology. One Gy produces 10^5 ionizing events per cell that may result in 1000 to 2000 breaks of single-stranded DNA or 40 breaks of double-stranded DNA (4).

As radiation travels through materials there are random collisions of photons or subatomic particles with atoms and molecules of the material. When radiation traverses a cell there may be hundreds of collision sites along its path. Collisions with atomic nuclei may (such as α particles) which in turn can damage molecules at additional sites (direct ionization). Photons interact with electrons (particularly those associated with water) resulting in a transfer of energy to produce chemical intermediates (hydroxyl radicals) that can disrupt biological molecules (indirect ionization).

Only collisions that alter the structure of vital molecules in cells or the DNA of the nucleus have the potential for significantly altering cell function. With high doses of radiation, hundreds of sites of damage may occur. Cell death is more likely to follow a double-stranded break in DNA than single-stranded breaks. Any damage to DNA is significant because of the limited capacity for repair. With low-dose radiation, DNA repair enzymes can mend most breaks within 24 hours, although the higher the dose, the slower the rate of repair. Damage caused by large particles is more difficult to repair than that caused by photons. Sublethal damage to DNA may be expressed in the form of mutations or even alterations in the structure and number of chromosomes. Most vital molecules in a cell are redundant, and replacement by the cell biosynthetic apparatus is possible.

Radiation affects reproductive integrity by producing necrosis, apoptosis, accelerated senescence, and terminal differentiation. Cells undergoing mitosis are more susceptible to damage than differentiated cells, although lymphocytes and oocytes can be damaged during the interphase stage of the cell cycle. Cells that are damaged are often progenitor cells, and a radiated cell may enter one more cycles of reproduction before all the progeny are rendered sterile. The effect of cell death in a cell system with progenitor cells may not be apparent until there is tissue failure due to a lack of cells to replace senescent cells.

Radiation effects are randomly distributed throughout tissues: some radiated cells will be adversely affected while others will be undamaged. Tissues that are particularly sensitive are the stem cells of the epidermis (hyperemia and exfoliation), bone marrow (anemia and immune deficiency), and intestinal epithelium (dysentery-like diarrhea). The adverse effects of acute radiation are manifestations of a failure of the most vulnerable body systems. Other parts of the body such as the liver and vascular endothelium are more resistant, although many of the late signs of radiation injury relate to vaso-occlusive disease from failure of vascular endothelial cells to regenerate. The brain is particularly sensitive to vascular injury. Early on there may be cerebral edema due to disruption of the blood–brain barrier, followed by damage to oligodendroglia that may cause focal demyelination. Later still there may be frank coagulative necrosis followed by gliosis or fibrosis (30). The signs of damage to other tissues may also appear years or decades after radiation injury in the form of localized necrosis or reactive fibrosis. Tissues already exposed to radiation may be more resistant to subsequent episodes of exposure.

Of all the tissues of the eye, the lens is the most sensitive to radiation and the sclera is the least sensitive. The sclera is able to tolerate 1000 Gy as may occur in brachytherapy for choroidal melanoma. The lens, however, is only able to tolerate <5.5 Gy, prompting attempts to shield the lens or exclude the lens from the field of radiation when treating retinoblastoma (37). The neurosensory retina is able to tolerate 50 Gy. However, the vascular endothelium of the retina is damaged by doses in excess of 3 cGy. The conjunctiva and eyelid are relatively resistant, although keratoconjunctivitis sicca and loss of eyelashes may occur following radiation (27).

Radiation cataracts result from radiation energy damaging the dividing cells at the lens equator. Damaged cells migrate to the posterior pole of the lens, but because of structural abnormalities of the constituent crystallins do not transmit light and form a layer of opaque cells inside the posterior capsule, i.e., a posterior subcapsular cataract. Risk factors include young age and high dose.

Retinal abnormalities were found shortly after radiation injury from the atomic bomb blasts of Hiroshima and Nagasaki (10). These lesions, including intraretinal ischemia and hemorrhage, were thought to be due to a generalized pancytopenia. Most effects of radiation on the retina are delayed and are similar to the vaso-occlusive events of diabetic retinopathy (18). The initial damage includes direct and indirect ionization events in vascular endothelial cells with focal loss of capillary endothelial cells and pericytes. Retinal ischemia is compensated somewhat by endothelial proliferation, although subretinal neovascularization and intravitreal vascular proliferation are uncommon. Infarcts due to occlusions of the choriocapillaris appear clinically as retinal exudates that may be mistaken for recurrent retinoblastoma. The clinical signs of retinopathy become apparent six months to many years after radiation and tend to be slowly but relentlessly progressive (23).

The optic nerve contains functioning oligodendroglia that can be damaged by radiation causing demyelination. The vascular system of the optic nerve is also vulnerable to radiation damage which may present as a painless but progressive loss of vision (33).

Ultraviolet (UV) radiation is the 400 to 100 nm portion of the electromagnetic spectrum. High-wavelength energy such as UV radiation does not penetrate deeply into tissues. The wavelengths between 280 and 100 nm (UVB) are particularly important because the energy is absorbed at tissue surfaces sufficient to cause "sunburn" and to induce cutaneous neoplasia (45).

The cornea absorbs UV radiation in the range 360 to 210 nm. High-dose UV radiation may damage corneal epithelial renewal mechanisms manifested by delayed (8–12 hours) corneal necrosis, superficial exfoliation and exposure of sensory nerve endings (solar keratopathy, welder keratopathy, snow blindness) (41). Chronic anterior segment exposure to UV light causes degeneration of the supportive collagen (elastoid degeneration) of the conjunctiva, as seen in the pinguecula and pterygium (see Chapter 30).

That energy in the visible light spectrum (480–720 nm) can injure the retina, particularly the photoreceptors and the RPE, has been shown in monkeys and other animals. Friedman and Kuwabara (13) observed that threshold lesions (an indirect ophthalmoscope was used) were associated with rises in temperature of only 2.5 to 3°C and that heating the animal to 42.5°C in the dark failed to result in retinal damage. This suggested to them that the effect of light might be potentiated by heat and that the susceptibility of these tissues to the damaging effects of intense light is probably determined by the rate of metabolism, which in turn is related to the temperature. Tso et al. (42) extended these studies to five months following injury in rats. Initially they found retinal edema and degeneration of photoreceptor outer segments, but later they saw evidence of repair and regeneration of photoreceptor cells and RPE. An oval area of variable pigmentation corresponding to an accumulation of pigment-laden macrophages was observed in the macular region at a later time. Finally, an elevated pigmented scar containing proliferated RPE with some regeneration of rod and cone outer segments developed in the macular area. Similar irradiation under conditions of hypothermia produced less damage. Tso et al. (43) found similar damage and repair in the monkey eye, in which outer segment material and melanosomes were identified within macrophages.

Solar retinopathy is characterized by macular edema and depigmentation and is produced by multiple wavelengths emanating from the sun. It is generally noted during psychotic episodes or coincident with injudicious observation of a solar eclipse. Damage to the naked eye may be due to potentially reversible thermal damage, even though the retina is relatively well protected by the "heat–sink" of the choriocapillaris. Concentrating light energy by viewing through a telescope may induce a photocoagulation-like disruption of the choriocapillaris (24,32).

ACKNOWLEDGMENT

Donald Morris wrote comparable parts of this chapter for the first and second editions.

REFERENCES

1. Aguilar J, Green WR. Choroidal rupture: a histopathologic study of 47 cases. Retina 1984; 4:269–75.
2. Burger P, Klintworth GK. Experimental retinal degeneration in the rabbit produced by intraocular iron. Lab Invest 1974; 30:9–19.
3. Cibis G. Traumatic corneal endothelial rings. Arch Ophthalmol 1978; 96:485–8.
4. Connell P, Martel M, et al. Principles of radiation oncology. In: DeVita V, Hellman S, Rosenberg S, eds. Cancer: Principles and Practice of Oncology. Philadelphia, PA: Williams & Wilkins, 2005.
5. Cox M, Freeman H. Retinal detachment due to ocular penetration. I. Clinical characteristics and surgical results. Arch Ophthalmol 1978; 96:1354–61.
6. Curtin V, Fujino T, et al. Comparative histopathology of cryosurgery and photocoagulation. Arch Ophthalmol 1966; 75:674–82.
7. Delori F, Pomerantzell O, et al. Deformation of the globe under high-speed impact: its relation to contusion injuries. Invest Ophthalmol Vis Sci 1969; 8:290–301.
8. Duke-Elder S, MacFaul P. Injuries, Part I. London: Klimpton, 1972.
9. Elner S, Elner V, et al. Ocular and associated findings in suspected child abuse. Arch Ophthalmol 1991; 108:321–2.
10. Fick J. Ocular lesions following the atomic bombing of Hiroshima and Nagasaki. Am J Ophthalmol 1948; 31: 137–54.
11. Fontana S, Brubaker R. Volume and depth of the anterior chamber in the normal aging human eye. Arch Ophthalmol 1980; 98:1083–88.
12. Fraunfelder F, Boozman F. No-touch technique for intraocular malignant melanomas. Arch Ophthalmol 1977; 95:1616–20.

13. Friedman E, Kuwabara T. The retinal pigment epithelium. IV. The damaging effects of radiant energy. Arch Ophthalmol 1968; 80:265–79.
14. Gilliland MG, Folberg R, Hayreh SS. Age of retinal hemorrhages by iron detection: an animal model. Am J Forensic Med Pathol 2005; 26:1–4.
15. Green W. Retina. In: Spencer W, ed. Ophthalmic Pathology: A Text and Atlas. Philadelphia, PA: WB Saunders and Company, 1996:869–72.
16. Gross J, King L, et al. Subfoveal neovascular membrane removal in patients with traumatic choroidal rupture. Ophthalmology 1996; 103:579–85.
17. Hamil M. Mechanical injury. In: Krachmer J, Mannus M, Holland E, eds. Cornea. Chap. 100, Vol. I. Philadelphia, PA: Elsevier Mosby, 2005:1245–51.
18. Hayreh S. Post-irradiation retinopathy: a fluorescence fundus angiographic study. Br J Ophthalmol 1970; 54: 705–14.
19. Johnson F, Zimmerman L. Barium sulfate and zinc sulfate deposits resulting from golf ball injury to the conjunctiva and the eyelid. Am J Clin Pathol 1965; 44:533–8.
20. Johnson R, Gass J. Idiopathic macular holes: observations, stages of formation, and implications for surgical intervention. Ophthalmology 1988; 95:917–24.
21. Karlin D. Chorioretinal lesions in rabbits produced by low frequency ultrasound. Am J Ophthalmol 1969; 68:84–91.
22. Lloyd R. Birth injuries of the cornea and allied conditions. Am J Ophthalmol 1938; 21:359–65.
23. Maguire A, Schachat A. Radiation retinopathy. In: Schachat A, ed. Retina. Chap. 83. Philadelphia, PA: Elsevier Mosby, 2006:1483–9.
24. Mainster M, Turner P. Retinal injuries from light: mechanisms, hazards and prevention. In: Schachat A, ed. Retina. Chap. 109. Philadelphia, PA: Elsevier Mosby, 2006:1857–70.
25. Martin D, Awh C, et al. Treatment and pathogenesis of traumatic chorioretinal rupture (scloptaria). Am J Ophthalmol 1994; 117:190–200.
26. Mascuiulli L, Anderson D, et al. Experimental ocular siderosis in the squirrel monkey. Am J Ophthalmol 1972; 74:638–61.
27. Murphree A, Samuel M, et al. Retinoblastoma. In: Hinton D, Schachat A, eds. Retina. Chap. 22, Vol. 1. Philadelphia, PA: Elsevier Mosby, 2006:557–607.
28. Pfister R, Pfister D. Alkali injuries of the eye. In: Krachmer J, Mannus M Holland E, eds. Cornea. Chap. 103, Vol. I. Philadelphia, PA: Elsevier Mosby, 2005:1285–93.
29. Pieramici D, Sternberg PJ, et al. A system for classifying mechanical injuries of the eye (globe). The Ocular Trauma Classification Group. Am J Ophthalmol 1997; 123:820–31.
30. Posner J. Nonmetastatic effects of cancer: the nervous system. Goldman L, Bennett J, eds. Cecil Textbook of Medicine. Chap. 195. Philadelphia, PA: WB Saunders & Company, 2000.
31. Powley KD, Dahlstrom DB, et al. Velocity necessary for a BB to penetrate the eye: an experimental study using pig eyes. Am J Forensic Med Pathol 2004; 25:273–5.
32. Pruet R. Traumatic maculopathies. Freeman H, ed. Ocular Trauma. Chap. 32. New York: Appleton-Century-Crofts, 1979:316–8.
33. Rao N, Spenscer W. Optic nerve. In: W. Spencer, ed. Ophthalmic Pathology: A Text and Atlas. Philadelphia, PA: WB Saunders & Company, 1996:560–2.
34. Rosenthal R, Appleton B. Histochemical localization of intraocular copper foreign bodies. Am J Ophthalmol 1975; 78:613–25.
35. Rosenthal R, Appleton B, et al. Intraocular copper foreign bodies. Am J Forensic Med Pathol 1974; 78:671–8.
36. Schepens C. Pathogenesis of traumatic rhegmatogeneous retinal detachment. Freeman H, ed. Ocular Trauma. New York: Appleton-Century-Crofts, 1979:273–84.
37. Schipper J, Tan K, et al. Treatment of retinoblastoma by precision megavoltage radiation therapy. Radiother Oncol 1985; 3:117–32.
38. Serway RA, Jewett JW, eds. Physics for Scientists and Engineers. Belmont, CA: Thompson-Brooks/Cole, 2004.
39. Settle J. Burns. In: Mason J, Purdue, eds. The Pathology of Trauma. Chap. 14. London: Arnold, 2000:212–29.
40. Slipperley J, Qugley H, et al. Traumatic retinopathy in primates: the explanation of commotio retinae. Arch Ophthalmol 1978; 96:2267–73.
41. Spencer W, ed. Cornea. Ophthalmic Pathology: A Text and Atlas. Philadelphia, PA: WB Saunders & Company, 1996: 233–4.
42. Tso M, Fine B, et al. Photic maculopathy produced by the indirect ophthalmoscope. I. Clinical and histologic study. Am J Ophthalmol 1972; 73:686–9.
43. Tso M, Wallow I, et al. Different susceptibility of rod and cone cells to argon laser. Arch Ophthalmol 1973; 89: 228–34.
44. Tulloh C. Migration of intraocular foreign bodies. Br J Ophthalmol 1956; 40:173–7.
45. Upton A. Radiation injury. In: Goldman L, Bennett J, eds. Cecil Textbook of Medicine. Philadelphia, PA: WB Saunders & Company, 2000:62–7.
46. Wagoner MD. Chemical injuries of the eye: current concepts in pathophysiology and therapy. Surv Ophthalmol 1997; 41: 275–313.
47. Watson P, Sevel D. Ophthalmia nodosa. Br J Ophthalmol 1966; 50:209–17.
48. Weinberg J, Eagle RC, et al. Conjunctival synthetic fiber granuloma: a lesion that resembles conjunctivitis nodosa. Ophthalmology 1984; 91:867–72.
49. Wise J. Treatment of experimental siderosis bulbi, bitreous hemorrhage, and corneal blood staining with deferoxamine. Arch Ophthalmol 1966; 75:698–707.

16

Wound Healing

J. Douglas Cameron
Department of Ophthalmology, Mayo Clinic, Rochester, Minnesota, U.S.A.

INTRODUCTION

The majority of ocular tissues, particularly those that transmit and process visible light, cannot be restored if injured or destroyed. Tissues such as the retina, vitreous and corneal stroma are formed only during embryologic development and are not replaced after birth. With the sole exception of the corneal epithelium, injured ocular tissue can only be repaired with less functional tissue that can neither transmit light efficiently nor process light signals.

Ocular trauma may occur either as the result of unplanned accidental injury (see Chapter 15) or as a planned event, i.e., ocular surgery. Accidental injury is highly variable in cause, extent, and outcome, whereas surgical procedures are planned to maximize benefit and minimize compromise of ocular function. The fundamental repair processes are the same in each situation. However, the natural history of repair of surgical procedures is much more predictable than the natural history of accidental injury. Management of both situations depends on intimate knowledge of the mechanisms of tissue damage and the stages and pace of the repair process. Deviations from the expected natural history can be recognized early and corrected. A clinical example is penetrating keratoplasty wound dehiscence requiring additional wound suturing.

While the repair process is similar for all ocular tissues, specific features in each tissue are clinically significant. For example, the crystalline lens repair process is limited to epithelial cell fibrous metaplasia (transformation of lens epithelial cells to collagen-producing, contractile myofibroblasts). The repair process of the retina is limited to gliosis of the neurosensory retina and fibrous metaplasia of the retinal pigment epithelium (RPE). These processes restore architectural but not functional integrity.

CUTANEOUS WOUNDS

Repair of Cutaneous Wounds

The model for all tissue repairs is the skin, as in a simple linear incision to the level of the subcutaneous fat (16). When an incision is not sutured the open wound fills with blood that will coagulate and form a protective surface for tissue exposed by the injury. Coagulated blood protects the deep tissue from dehydration and the introduction of microbes and toxic substances in the environment, as well as provisional scaffold for repair. Early in the repair process platelets from extravasated blood interact with thrombin and collagen to release mediators such as adenosine diphosphate (ADP), fibrinogen, fibronectin, transpondin and von Willebrand factor. Initially, stimulation of the repair process is dependent upon protein signals resulting from cell death.

Inflammatory cells enter the wound from damaged blood vessels probably stimulated by hypoxia. Initially, polymorphonuclear leukocytes (PMNs) populate the wound to inactivate and clear bacteria and to begin tissue debridement primarily through the action of proteolytic enzymes. PMNs also produce platelet-like growth factors such as connective tissue-derived growth factor, which is related to platelet-derived growth factor (PDGF). At approximately 24 to 48 hours the PMNs are replaced by monocytes, which transform into macrophages to continue the clearing of debris. Macrophages also elaborate numerous cyokines that modulate the healing process locally.

Undamaged surface epithelial cells at the margins of the wound migrate into the wound to establish more permanent protection from the environment. Before epithelial cell movement occurs there is a delay of several hours when the cell changes shape, forms lamellipodia from its plasma membrane in the direction of the wound, increases the number of gap junctions, and changes its complement of cell surface integrin receptors to utilize a transitional substrate of fibronectin. The surface epithelium migrates into the wound as undifferentiated squamous cells, which produce proteolytic enzymes (including collagenase types I and IV) that allow migration between the blood clot and necrotic dermis and the deeper viable dermis. Once the total surface is covered the squamous cells proliferate and mature into differentiated, polarized, keratin-producing cells. Formation of a new basement membrane containing laminin is one of the events that terminates the migration/proliferation process of the epithelium. The overlying clot, its function completed, will be shed along with the first turnover of keratin.

Epithelial cells protect the underlying tissue but contribute little to the mechanical strength of the wound and the tensile strength of the repair tissue is determined by the activity of fibroblasts. Fibroblasts are found normally in all supportive tissues of the body and additional fibroblasts may be recruited from monocytes in the peripheral blood. Fibroblasts are capable of producing many types of extracellular matrix including collagen, glycosaminoglycans (GAGs), cartilage and even bone, depending on the tissue environment. Early in the course of repair, the first matrix produced is rich in collagen type III and hyaluronic acid. The delicate nature of collagen type III and the high water content of hyaluronic acid facilitate movement of cells through a low viscosity matrix. Both macromolecules are found during embryonic development, when movement of cells is vital, and not in normal adult tissues, where tensile strength and stability are desirable.

The wounded area remains active over a considerable time, constantly degrading and reforming tissue in a process known as remodeling. The initial response is modified to accommodate local tissue requirements, i.e., an approximation of the pre-wounded state. The cellular component is modified by apoptosis and the matrix is modified by several proteolytic enzyme systems, the principal one being the matrix metalloproteinase system. A provisional matrix of fibronectin is organized early in the repair process and fibroblasts migrate along this pathway. Fibronectin is replaced by collagen type III, which is in turn replaced by collagen type I. Fibroblasts will then contract and their orientation will reflect the pattern established in the matrix. Wound contraction is generally more important in the repair of deep wounds rather than shallow wounds (16). The remodeling process will continue as long as the tissue is viable but any interference with this process, as in scurvy, may cause substantial damage to tissues.

Undamaged, surrounding blood vessels support the repair process via angiogenesis (see Chapter 68). Endothelial cells at the terminal end of damaged blood vessels form a solid bulb of undifferentiated endothelial cells that migrate into the wound guided by chemotactic factors. When two endothelial bulbs fuse to form a vascular arcade, a common lumen is established and blood will flow. The direction of flow will determine acquisition of venular and arteriolar characteristics. The endothelium is more porous than in normal capillary networks, allowing transudation of plasma and diapedesis of inflammatory cells. The adventitial support of the newly formed blood vessels is not as strong as in native vessels and they are more friable and likely to bleed.

Granulation tissue (named because of its granular macroscopic appearance) is composed of delicate collagenous strands and other matrix components, newly formed blood vessels and edema, as well as acute and chronic inflammatory cells. Variations of this basic repair process are found in every tissue except the central nervous system (CNS), where astrocytes are the counterparts of fibroblasts. These glial cells repair by producing robust intracellular structural elements and are not capable of secreting extracellular architectural proteins; a CNS "scar" is composed of reactive astrocytes.

Constant communication between the squamous epithelium and the dermal fibroblasts is accomplished by cytokines, primarily transforming growth factor β1 (TGFβ1). Cytokines are produced by both squamous cells and fibroblasts and influence the behavior of each other. Once epithelial migration stops through contact inhibition, fibroblasts become "activated." That is, the fibroblasts change from a resting state with a few cytoplasmic organelles to an active state in which the number and complexity of organelles is increased. Fibroblasts produce and secrete matrix precursors, which self-assemble outside the cell into mature structural components. The tissue environment will determine such characteristics as fibril orientation and strength and ultimately the organization and surface contour of the tissue. The fundamental goals of wound suturing are to minimize the amount of clot formation, limit the extent of epithelial migration, and reestablish tissue strength and contours.

It is important to note that collateral injury to skin adnexal structures, such as hair follicles, is not repaired. These highly differentiated structures will simply involute and their remnants may be incorporated into the repaired matrix. Loss of adnexal structures and alteration of pigment production by epithelial melanocytes will make the site of a cutaneous injury obvious permanently.

Fetal wound repair is characterized by an absence of scar formation. Among the differences from adult repair are the unique nature of embryonic fibroblasts and the extracellular matrix they produce. Also there is minimal participation of the inflammatory component seen in adult healing, particularly the cytokine TGFβ (1).

Abnormalities of Cutaneous Wound Repair

Abnormalities of skin repair are not common but can be dramatic. A keloid is a bulky scar that distorts tissue far beyond the original site of injury and alterations of a histamine control pathway in cutaneous repair are thought to be the major defect. The scar contains a reduced number of myofibroblasts and the collagen is much thicker than that produced by normal wound repair and rarely remodels to a functional size or contour. A hypertrophic scar results from a disorderly proliferation of fibroblasts and blood vessels. An alteration of the quantity of GAGs is commonly observed. This type of wound alteration, however, tends to remain at the site of injury and will remodel toward a functionally acceptable volume and contour.

CORNEAL WOUNDS

Repair of Corneal Wounds

Wound repair of the cornea is unique because of a lack of direct blood vessel participation in the process. Similar control mechanisms and extracellular matrix molecules participate in corneal wound healing as in the skin, although repair materials are delivered via several conduits, including tears, aqueous humor and corneoscleral limbal blood vessels.

Repair of the anterior portion of a corneal wound is similar to that observed in skin. If only the epithelium is damaged and Bowman layer is preserved, epithelial migration quickly covers the wounded area and reestablishes functional properties. In this case the normal anatomy is restored and there is no clinical sign of a functional defect (i.e., the wound is "healed"). If the wound penetrates through Bowman layer the wounded area remains clinically visible (an epithelial facet). Epithelium fills the defect in Bowman layer and any anterior stromal defect to reestablish the anterior corneal contour. Bowman layer is composed of densely packed collagen type I and, because it is acellular, it is not capable of reacting. In epithelial facet formation the wound is not extensive enough to stimulate the full repair response and the epithelial plug remains as a clinically visible nebular scar. An epithelial facet is commonly caused by injury with a small metallic foreign body (e.g., automobile muffler rust).

With penetration of a wound to the level of the deep stroma, the repair process of the cornea begins to differ from cutaneous repair. Because the corneal stroma is relatively dehydrated exposure to aqueous humor will cause immediate swelling. In the case of a small penetrating or perforating wound of the cornea, particularly if the orientation of the wound is oblique to the surface, e.g., a clear cornea cataract incision, the swelling may be sufficient to close the wound and maintain a watertight seal that will sustain normal intraocular pressure.

Corneal fibroblasts (keratocytes) within 100 μm of the wound will be destroyed, probably through mechanical disruption of their delicate dendritic processes. The wound edge remains intact despite the death of the keratocytes because of the density and organization of the corneal stroma and corneal epithelial cells will migrate over the edge. Once the entire surface is covered by migrated cells contact inhibition of movement occurs and the epithelium begins to differentiate and fill in the defect. The external surface of the cellular mass will duplicate the radius of curvature of the surrounding tissue to restore the anterior refracting surface of the cornea.

As found in the skin, corneal epithelium will stimulate keratocytes to repair the extracellular matrix of the wound. Multiple growth factors regulate the process including epidermal growth factor, TGFs, acidic fibroblast growth factor, basic fibroblast growth factor, keratocyte growth factor, hepatocyte growth factor, PDGF, insulin-like growth factor 1, insulin like growth factor 2, and connective tissue growth factor (40). The collagen and proteoglycans produced in the repair process are similar, but not identical, to the native extracellular matrix. The repair tissue cannot transmit light as efficiently as the original extracellular matrix and will remain as a visible scar.

Repair of the corneal endothelial surface in a perforating corneal wound is different from cutaneous repair but similar to that of single cell layers elsewhere (crystalline lens, RPE, pleural mesothelium). With interruption of the monolayer, cells in the center of the wound are destroyed and viable cells at the periphery migrate or spread to cover the defect. Corneal endothelial cells generally do not proliferate at a site of injury, except to a limited extent in young people. Some of the cells assume characteristics of fibroblasts rather than endothelial cells (fibrous metaplasia) and are capable of producing extracellular matrix similar to that of the posterior cornea. The matrix contributes to the tensile strength of the damaged posterior cornea. With maturation of the repair site, cells that resemble native endothelial cells produce a basement membrane and establish a diffusion gradient between the corneal stroma and endothelium (7).

There is a region in the posterior one-third of the corneal stroma where neither the anterior corneal repair process nor the fibrous metaplasia of the corneal endothelium is operative. In this region there are insufficient keratocytes to repair the matrix and fibrous metaplasia of the endothelium does not extend into it. After injury, the posterior corneal stroma never regains significant tensile strength.

Repair of a full-thickness corneal wound that is not complicated by microbial infection or incarceration of other tissue components is identified histologically by defects in Bowman layer, qualitative differences in extracellular matrix along the course of the stromal wound and an interruption of Descemet membrane. Because of the natural elasticity of Descemet membrane the cut edges may curl anteriorly toward the stroma. A new thin basement membrane may cover the posterior stroma in wounds that have been present for some time.

Abnormalities of Corneal Wound Repair

The completeness of the repair process is dependent upon the orientation of the wound relative to the visual axis. The full repair process is present in penetrating keratoplasty wounds. With partial thickness wounds, such as that used in radial keratotomy, the process is incomplete and the scar tends to be weak. With lamellar wounds, such as those produced with laser-assisted in situ keratomileusis (LASIK), the wound heals in the region of Bowman layer but the interlamellar portion does not heal (10,36) creating a potential space. This may result in complications such as delayed flap separation, intralamellar fluid accumulation with or microbial infection (8,18).

Abnormalities of Corneal Repair in Keratoplasty Procedures

Occasionally fibrous metaplasia of the endothelium is not confined to the graft–host interface but extends to the visual axis causing decreased vision. This forms a retrocorneal membrane (posterior collagenous layer).

The repair of a horizontal wound in the setting of refractive surgical procedures such as LASIK differs from the perpendicular wound of a penetrating keratoplasty. To change the optical characteristics of the cornea, a horizontally oriented, hinged corneal flap approximately 100 μm thick is created in the central anterior cornea. The flap is raised and excimer laser energy is applied in the visual axis to remove a calculated amount of stromal tissue. The anterior curvature of the cornea is thus altered to reduce its optical power in the case of myopic refractive error. The peripheral edges of the lamellar wound (at the level of Bowman layer) heal in the same manner as the most superficial portion of a penetrating wound, with mobilization of epithelium and a fibrous response from the corneal stroma. The lamellar wound only extends to the mid stroma and therefore the corneal endothelium does not participate in the repair process. There is no mechanism to heal the extensive interface between the posterior surface of the lamellar flap and the excimer-treated posterior corneal stroma. Experimental models of corneal wound healing indicate that only 50% of the normal tensile strength of an intralamellar wound return when the repair process is complete (25,26). From autopsy studies of human eyes that have been treated with LASIK, the tensile strength at the intralamellar interface is <2% of the original tensile strength for periods of up to two years following the procedure (37).

The degree of return of architectural strength following refractive surgery depends on the procedure. A high risk of corneal rupture during accidental trauma in patients who have undergone radial keratotomy has been reported (4,24,34). The risk of corneal rupture in such procedures as anterior lamellar keratectomy and LASIK appears to be minimal (33). However, the lack of healing of the central lamellar wound in LASIK, together with the creation of a potential space in the corneal stroma, has led to the development of many new complications. There is a risk of traumatic dislocation of a lamellar flap due to the application of tangential forces on its surface (27,28). The potential space is also a platform for an inflammatory reaction (diffuse lamellar keratopathy), microbial infection (17), and intralamellar collection of fluid associated with increased intraocular pressure. Similar potential problems exist for other surgical procedures such as deep lamellar endothelial keratoplasty (3,5) and femtosecond laser keratectomy (38).

CORNEOSCLERAL LIMBAL WOUNDS

Repair of Corneoscleral Limbal Wounds

Wound repair at the corneoscleral limbus is a combination of events found in subepithelial repair of the skin and repair of posterior, peripheral corneal tissue. Prior to the introduction of clear corneal cataract incisions, corneal surgical wounds entered the sclera peripheral to the limbus, extended across the surgical limbus to the peripheral cornea and into the anterior chamber through peripheral Descemet membrane. In this situation, the posterior corneal wound is repaired in the manner of a posterior perforating wound with fibrous metaplasia of the endothelium and the episcleral wound is repaired by granulation tissue. The scleral and peripheral corneal wounds are slowly and incompletely repaired. This type of wound response is still used in glaucoma filtration surgery.

Abnormalities of Corneoscleral Limbal Wound Repair

One of the major complications of corneal wounds in general, and limbal wounds in particular, is the migration of surface epithelial cells through a fistula of the corneoscleral coat to anterior chamber surfaces (epithelial ingrowth). Large traumatic wounds are more likely to be associated with epithelial ingrowth but some risk exists even for surgical wounds through peripheral corneal tissue ("clear cornea cataract incision") (42). Inhibition of migration of surface epithelial cells is normally accomplished by contact with healthy cells such as the corneal endothelium (6). If the endothelium is damaged or lost, epithelial cells can proliferate over the posterior surface of the cornea creating a translucent zone with a well-demarcated border where surface epithelium and corneal endothelium abut. Trabecular beams are similarly at risk. Surface epithelial cells will modulate the matrix over which they migrate to resemble the surface with which they are originally associated. In the area of the trabecular meshwork the result is scarring to the point that aqueous humor filtration is interrupted. Even physical removal of the surface epithelial cells will not restore the function of the meshwork. There is no barrier to proliferation over the anterior or posterior surface of the iris or any other acellular surface within the eye (39,44). Intracameral mucus has been observed when conjunctival epithelial cells are included among the invading squamous cells (22).

The invading epithelial cells may maintain a sheet-like configuration on anterior chamber surfaces or may form a cyst containing desquamated epithelial debris. The cyst may dissociate from the surface and float freely in the anterior chamber. Surgical removal of a cyst may be beneficial by reducing the amount of squamous epithelium in the anterior chamber; however, surgical rupture of the cyst may disseminate squamous cells onto uninvolved tissues.

Similarly, highly reactive fibrous tissue from the episclera may migrate through an open wound (fibrous ingrowth) and cause fibrosis and distortion of the anterior chamber and filtration angle. Surgical removal of anterior chamber fibrous tissue is extremely difficult.

Delicate blood vessels may persist in a corneoscleral limbal wound and project from the internal cornea into the anterior chamber as delicate vascular arcades. These, like all neovascular channels, have a tendency to hemorrhage. Multiple episodes of microhyphema (the sputtering hyphema of Swann) are reported by patients as intermittent red or pink vision and there may be an associated episodic increase in intraocular pressure.

Brown–McLean syndrome is the result of a decompensated peripheral cornea caused by intraoperative or postoperative iris contact. The condition usually begins inferiorly with edema of the peripheral 2 to 3 mm of the cornea but the edema may spread circumferentially (35).

CRYSTALLINE LENS WOUNDS

Repair of Crystalline Lens Wounds

Limited wounds of the lens may be repaired via fibrous metaplasia of the lens epithelium, but to no clinical advantage because the repair process produces opaque tissue. With any injury of the epithelium the surrounding cells proliferate and form fibroblast-like cells that are able to produce a collagenous extracellular matrix. The fibroblasts mature into myofibroblasts that contract and distort the original lens capsule, further limiting meaningful transmission of light. With scar maturation the internal epithelial cells return to a cuboidal configuration and produce lens capsule basement membrane.

Abnormalities of Crystalline Lens Wound Repair

Fragments of the lens that are dissociated from the main body of the lens may undergo a similar process to form a small group of reactive lens epithelial cells surrounded by basement membrane (Elschnig pearls). The cells in the reactive tissue are markedly enlarged, and nucleated similar to those seen in posterior subcapsular cataracts (bladder cells/Wedl cells). A Soemmerring ring is the result of the same process causing opacification of the equatorial lens remnants after injury. Usually the axial area is clear because lens tissue is missing.

Attempts at wound repair by residual lens epithelial cells, particularly those in the equatorial region, are responsible for opacification of the posterior capsule following extracapsular cataract extraction or phacoemulsification and posterior chamber intraocular lens insertion.

RETINAL WOUNDS

Repair of the Retinal Wounds

The retina is capable of repair but architectural characteristics may be reestablished without function. Only two cell types are sufficiently pliable to participate in a repair reaction, the glial cells (primarily Müller cells) of the neurosensory retina and the RPE. With thermal (argon laser) or mechanical injury to the retina the highly differentiated components of the neurosensory retina will be destroyed or will involute. The change in retinal architecture will stimulate glial cell proliferation, and if the internal limiting membrane (ILM) is intact, the repair process will be limited to the neurosensory retina. Similarly damage to the RPE will cause surviving cells to proliferate and migrate into the wounded area with fibrous metaplasia. During this process intracellular melanin granules may be lost and will not be reproduced in the reactive cells. If Bruch membrane is intact the metaplastic epithelial cells will migrate into the subretinal space. When the retina and its ILM are intact, and Bruch membrane is sound, and there is not excessive intraretinal hemorrhage, the glial cells and metaplastic RPE migrate toward each other to form desmosomal attachments and create an intraretinal adhesion. Such an adhesion is the surgical goal for photocoagulation of retinal tears threatening detachment. This process is also operative in panretinal photocoagulation for proliferative diabetic retinopathy.

Abnormalities of Retinal Wound Repair

If the ILM is interrupted by the application of photocoagulation, glial cells may proliferate on to the retinal surface or along a scaffold of detached vitreous. Contraction of the cellular elements of the repair tissue will then alter the contour of the internal retinal surface and adversely affect transmission of light (epiretinal membrane formation). Similarly, if Bruch membrane is interrupted by photocoagulation or other factors, repair may be complicated by fibrovascular ingrowth from the choroid into the subretinal space in a manner that is histologically identical with the subretinal neovascularization associated with histoplasmosis or choroidal rupture.

EPISCLERAL TISSUE WOUNDS

Episcleral Tissue Wound Repair

Strabismus procedures and retinal detachment repair are strongly influenced by fibrovascular tissue. Unlike the sclera and the choroid that are generally passive because of the lack of reactive fibroblasts, the episcleral tissue responds promptly and exuberantly. This reaction allows rapid stabilization for rectus muscle reattachment and scleral buckles.

Abnormalities of Episcleral Wound Repair

The episcleral reactivity creates operative difficulties, however, if a second operation is necessary at the same site because of fibrous adhesions between the sclera and surrounding soft tissue. Tissue planes may be substantially altered or inaccessible. Fibrous reactive tissue may also gain entry to the eye through retinal reattachment drainage sites or vitrectomy ports. Once inside the eye the fibrous tissue will proliferate and contract often causing irreparable tractional retinal detachment.

Scleral buckles are generally stable within weeks of placement, although chronic inflammation may persist near the buckles for years. Remodeling of the tissue, as elsewhere, is continuous and extrusion of the buckling element anteriorly through the conjunctiva or internally across the sclera into the subretinal or vitreous space may occur. The smaller the diameter of the surgical device, the greater the risk of migration.

CREATION OF SURGICAL WOUNDS

Surgical wounds are the result of precise delivery of kinetic energy to tissue that is of less functional significance than the tissue affected by disease. For example, there is minimal or no loss of vision when an incision is placed at the periphery of the cornea to remove a cataract. The incision is outside the 4 mm central functional zone of the cornea in an area that, although transparent, mainly functions as a "carrier" for the central optical zone.

Incision

A steel blade is an efficient instrument to deliver energy to tissue. The edge is beveled to give the greatest concentration of energy per unit area. If the energy applied is greater than the tissue tensile strength, the tissue will separate in a predictable and precise manner. A diamond blade is better than a steel blade because of its denser and more stable crystal structure and it has a finer, more durable edge. A trephine is a cylinder with a sharpened edge that can remove a precise, reproducible cross-sectional area of tissue, as in penetrating keratoplasty. The instrument is more complicated than a simple linear knife edge because the location of the bevel on the inside or outside of the trephine blade will determine its course through tissue. Similarly, adding two blades together with a hinge to form a scissor will also change the wound profile. More compression occurs near the hinge of the scissor than near the tips of the blades (14).

A stream of water under high pressure can also be used to deliver energy and separate tissue. Water jets have been used in industry to cut metal and to process meat. The energy has been applied experimentally to produce a corneal tissue flap for refractive surgery, with wound surface characteristics that are similar to those created by a steel microtome. Also, various types of laser, particularly the femtosecond laser, have been used to make intrastromal incisions for both refractive surgery and for surgical treatment of diseased endothelial cells.

Thermal Application

Extreme changes of temperature will alter the structure and function of living tissue. Heat damages tissues by disrupting cell membranes and by denaturing and shrinking extracellular matrix components, particularly collagen. Extreme heat will oxidize (carbonize) tissue to ash. Cautery is used to shrink blood vessels and induce intravascular coagulation to control intraoperative bleeding.

Diathermy is essentially completion of an electric circuit by incorporation of tissue. The tissue acts as a resistor and generates heat in the electric field. The amount of heat in the tissue will be affected by conduction, convection, and heat capacity (15). Diathermy has been used to create intraretinal adhesions by transscleral application, but it is only applicable over a small surface area and the tight adhesions of small diameter may actually promote retinal tears. Also transscleral diathermy may cause lysis of scleral collagen and focal weakening of the scleral coat (11). For these reasons diathermy is rarely used today in ocular surgery.

Cold does not produce as much tissue damage as heat. Cold produces intracellular ice crystals that disrupt cell membranes and organelles, but the extracellular matrix is minimally altered by the degree and duration of cold used for surgical purposes (13). Cryoprobes were once used to remove cataracts (intracapsular cataract extraction). An ice ball was created on the anterior surface of the lens creating sufficient adhesion to mechanically remove the lens. If the application site also involved the margin of the pupil, the ice ball could be melted and the instrument moved to another location without clinical damage to the iris tissue. Cryotherapy is now the primary method of creating intraretinal adhesions of the peripheral retina in reattachment procedures. Because the frozen cells are destroyed, cryotherapy is also used to destroy aqueous humor-producing cells of the pars plicata in intractable glaucoma and atypical melanocytes and frank melanoma cells in extensive primary acquired melanosis with atypia. Neither the structure of the ciliary body nor the conjunctival substantia propria is significantly altered.

Light Amplification by Stimulated Emission of Radiation

Light amplification by stimulated emission of radiation (laser) is a system of converting one form of energy (light or electrical) with variable characteristics to a projectable form of energy of uniform wavelength and polarity. In all laser systems energy is applied to a specific medium in a chamber with reflective surfaces and high energy photons are concentrated as they are reflected by the surfaces during multiple passes through the medium. Each pass increases the concentration of photons oriented in the same manner to produce a narrow coherent (near monochromatic) beam as the energy is released from the optical chamber (32). Different laser wavelengths affect tissue differently.

Visible spectrum (400–760 nm) lasers (e.g., argon laser, 488 nm) photocoagulate tissue. The energy of the laser beam is absorbed by tissue and the tissue temperature is increased, potentially to the point of protein denaturation or carbonization. Melanin and hemoglobin are the most likely proteins to absorb energy in this spectrum. Far infrared laser (CO_2 laser, 10,600 nm) energy is absorbed by water, producing intracellular steam by photovaporization. Cells are disrupted by heat and the mechanical effects of an expanding gas. Infrared lasers in the 760–10,000 nm spectrum [e.g., neodymium-doped yttrium aluminium garnet (Nd:YAG), 1064 nm] alter tissue by photodisruption. The energy of the laser beam is not absorbed by tissue but reaches a threshold to produce an explosion causing tissue to vaporize and form plasma, a random gas of electrons and protons stripped from atoms by high energy fields. A gas–liquid phase change occurs, giving rise to cavitation or gas bubble formation, similar to a bolt of lightning. The plasma collapses to produce an acoustic shock wave that can disrupt an opacified posterior capsule (32). Far ultraviolet laser (e.g., excimer laser, 193 nm) is absorbed by tissue and intermolecular bonds are disrupted (photoablation). The action is very precise and there is minimal collateral damage from heat production. The broken bonds cannot recombine and the tissue decomposes. During absorption excess energy is produced and molecular fragments are ejected from the application site forming a plume. The fragments are composed of free radicals, simple carbons, and simple hydrocarbons.

Many types of lasers are used in ophthalmology. The most commonly used laser is the argon laser. The generator medium is a gas that produces wavelengths of 488 nm (green) and 514.5 nm (red) and tissue is altered by photocoagulation. For the Nd:YAG laser the generator medium is a solid producing a beam at 1064 nm. Photodisruption of tissue occurs both by a thermal effect (1500°C) and a shock wave. Excimer (excited diamer) laser has a generator medium of two rare gas halides, argon and fluorine. The molecules spontaneously dissociate to produce a beam of 193 nm wavelength and the tissue is altered by photoablation. The holmium laser (holmium: yttrium–aluminum–garnet) was once used for laser correction of hyperopia. The beam had a wavelength of 2060 to 2120 nm causing photocoagulation. The femtosecond laser produces infrared wavelengths (1053 nm) in short bursts (femtosecond = 10^{-15} seconds). The beam can penetrate deeply into the cornea and create a tissue plane by photocoagulation. Collateral heat damage is minimized by the short duration of the pulse.

Implantable Devices

Intraocular lenses were conceived when Ridley observed that intraocular foreign bodies made of polymethymethacrylate (PMMA) from World War II British fighter plane canopies showed nearly complete biocompatibility, i.e., there was no tissue reaction. It was further established by Ridley that an intraocular lens made of PMMA was biostable and was not degraded by soft tissue lytic enzymes.

The design and placement of intraocular lenses has changed markedly over the past 60 years. Initially, nearly spherical lenses were placed in the lens capsule after cataracts were removed by the extracapsular technique. When intracapsular cataract extraction became popular intraocular lenses were either sutured to the iris or placed in the anterior chamber. Currently, because of the return to extracapsular cataract surgery, the intraocular lens is characteristically placed in the posterior chamber and within the lens capsule. Initially, 180° limbal incisions were necessary to implant the lens. Now different materials are used for intraocular lens construction that are pliable and can be folded in a manner that allows introduction through a 3.5-mm incision in peripheral clear cornea.

Complications of intraocular lenses may involve all regions of the eye but certain lens designs may exhibit characteristic problems. Physical contact of the synthetic lens with the corneal endothelium during insertion or subsequent dislocation of the lens anteriorly may compromise endothelial function to the point of corneal decompensation (pseudophakic bulbous keratopathy). Similarly contact with the delicate trabecular meshwork by supporting devices for anterior chamber lenses may cause secondary trabecular scarring. A combination of uveitis, glaucoma, and hyphema, all due to mechanical contact with the trabecular meshwork, became known as the uveitis-glaucoma-hyphema (UGH) syndrome. Iris-supported intraocular lenses were attached to delicate iris tissue either with sutures or metal clips. The contact points of the support devices were capable of causing pressure necrosis of the iris, leading to dislocation of the lens. The lenses were unstable and tended to cause movement of the iris with any movement of the eye. The pressure wave thus generated was thought to instigate cystoid macular edema, a cause of potentially severe visual loss. Variations in lens manufacture have also caused reactions due to retained materials on the surface of the lens and retention of sharp contours. Intraocular lens dislocation was a significant problem with the early heavy lenses and remains a problem when zonular support is weak, e.g., in the exfoliation syndrome (2).

Glaucoma filtering devices are used in cases where a traditional fistula is not likely to succeed, such as neovascular glaucoma. Traditional medical therapy is ineffective because of the neovascular membrane over the meshwork and standard fistulae are quickly occluded by a process similar to granulation tissue formation. An inert tube, usually made of silicon, may be inserted into the anterior chamber and the aqueous humor is allowed to exit into the soft tissues of the orbit. The earliest glaucoma filtration devices were short and terminated in anterior episcleral tissue where they stimulated a repair reaction that often occluded the outflow. Current devices have a longer tube that terminates in a large synthetic reservoir located near the equator of the eye on the episcleral surface. In this location the episcleral tissue reaction is beneficial because it anchors the reservoir in the desired location. The free end of the drainage tube empties into the reservoir where it is protected from the fibrous reaction (29,30). As with any other synthetic device in soft tissue, migration is a possible but unusual complication. Along with extrusion there is also a risk of developing endophthalmitis (19).

The refractive power of the cornea can be altered by changing the shape or the refractive index of the cornea. In an experimental model, Choyce inserted high refractive index polysulfone lenses into the cornea of cats but the surgical strategy turned out to be impractical because the device was impermeable to the flow of nutrients across the cornea and resulted in necrotizing ulceration of the anterior and posterior stroma. This type of device has not been used in humans (23).

Circular arcs or linear blocks of PMMA have been inserted into the cornea in a specific pattern to change the shape of the cornea. The anticipated advantages of this type of system were that it would not interfere with the flow of nutrients and that the material could be easily removed. This device has been used in humans, although there have been reports of intrastromal keratocyte activation and extracellular matrix production (41).

A keratoprosthesis is a synthetic device used to replace severely scarred and vascularized corneas where there is a substantial risk of corneal graft rejection, as is found in pemphigoid and Stevens–Johnson syndrome (12). The device consists of a central optic made of PMMA or other polymers. The main problem with this device has been adequate incorporation of the synthetic optic into the diseased host tissue to prevent extrusion (21).

Artificial retinal implants are now being developed. Several strategies have been investigated: a light-driven microphotodiode implanted in the subretinal space (9), an epiretinal microcontact device connected by a cable to a receiver outside the eye (20), and an epiretinal implant with wireless connections to an external receiver (43). The devices are intended to help persons with outer retinal degenerative diseases, such as retinitis pigmentosa and age-related macular degeneration, and they are not able to replicate inner retinal or optic nerve function. As of this time, light stimulation but not form recognition has been achieved. The long-term stability of retinal cell interaction with any of these devices has not yet been established (31).

REFERENCES

1. Adzick NS, Lorenz HP. Cells, matrix, growth factors, and the surgeon. The biology of scarless fetal wound repair. Ann Surg 1994; 220:10–8.
2. Apple D, Mamalis N, Loftfield K, et al. Complications of intraocular lenses. A historical and histopathological review. Surv Ophthalmol 1984; 29:1–54.
3. Azar D, Jain S, Sambursky R. A new surgical technique of microtome-assisted deep lamellar keratoplasty with a hinged flap. Arch Ophthalmol 2000; 118:1112–5.
4. Binder P, Waring GO 3rd, Arrwosmith PN, Wang C. Histopathology of traumatic corneal rupture after radial keratotomy. Arch Ophthalmol 1988; 106:1584–90.
5. Busin M, Arffa RC, Sebastiani A. Endokeratoplasty as an alternative to penetrating keratoplasty for the surgical treatment of diseased endothelium. Ophthalmology 2000; 107:2077–82.
6. Cameron J, Flaxman B, Yanoff M. In vitro studies of corneal epithelial endothelial interactions. Invest Ophthalmol Vis Sci 1974; 13:575–9.
7. Cameron JD. Chapter 8: Corneal reaction to injury. In: Cornea JH, Krachmer MJ, Mannus E, Holland J, eds. Philadelphia: Elsevier Mosby, 2005:115–31.
8. Chang M, Jain S, Azar D. Infections following laser in situ keratomeliusis: an integration of the published literature. Surv Ophthalmol 2004; 49:269–80.
9. Chow AY, Pardue MT, Pearlman JI, et al. Subretinal implantation of a semiconductor-based photodiodes: durability of novel implant designs. J Rehabil Res Dev 2002; 39:313–21.
10. Dawson D, O'Brien T, Edelhauser H. Long-term corneal keratocyte defects after PRK and LASIK: in vivo evidence of stress-induced premature cellular senescence. Am J Ophthalmol 2006; 141:918–20.
11. DeGuillebon H, Ishii Y. Scleral changes during diathermy application. Influence of the electrode type. Arch Ophthalmol 1970; 83:752–9.
12. Dohlman C, Terada H. Keratoprosthesis in pemphigoid and Stevens–Johnson syndrome. Adv Exp Med Biol 1998; 438:1021–5.
13. Eisner G. Tissue tactics. Application of cold. In: Eye Surgery: An Introduction to Operative Technique. Berlin: Springer-Verlag, 1990:114–5.
14. Eisner G. Tissue tactics. The division of tissues. In: Eye Surgery: An Introduction to Operative Technique. Berlin: Springer-Verlag, 1990:64–79.
15. Eisner G. Tissue tactics. Application of heat. In: Eye Surgery: An Introduction to Operative Technique. Berlin: Springer-Verlag, 1990:109–13.
16. Falanga V. Mechanisms of cutaneous wound repair. In: Freedberg IM, et al., eds. Fitzpatrick's Dermatology in General Medicine. New York: McGraw-Hill, 200:3236–46.
17. Freitas D, Alvarenga D. An outbreak of *Mycobacterium chelonae* infection after LASIK. Ophthalmology 2003; 110: 276–85.
18. Galal A, Rtola A, Belda J, et al. Interface corneal edema secondary to steroid-induced elevation of intraocular pressure simulating diffuse lamellar keratitis. J Refract Surg 2006; 22:441–7.
19. Gedde SJ, Scott IU, Tabandeh H, et al. Late endophthalmitis associated with glaucoma drainage implants. Ophthalmology 2001; 108:1323–7.
20. Humayun M, Weiland JD, Fujii GY et al. Visual perception in a blind subject with a chronic microelectronic retinal prosthesis. Vision Res 2003; 43:2573–81.
21. Ilhan-Sarac O, Akpek EK. Current concepts and techniques in keratoprosthesis. Curr Opin Ophthalmol 2005; 16: 246–50.
22. Layden W, Torcznski E, Font R. Mucogenic glaucoma and goblet cell cyst of the anterior chamber. Arch Ophthalmol 1978; 96:2259–63.
23. Lindstrom RL, Lane SS, Cameron JD, et al. Intracorneal lenses. Trans New Orleans Acad Ophthalmol 1988; 36: 279–96.
24. Luttrull JK, Jester JV, Smith RE. The effect of radial keratotomy on ocular integrity in an animal model. Arch Ophthalmol 1982; 100:319–20.
25. Maurice DM, Monroe F. Cohesive strength of corneal lamellae. Exp Eye Res 1990; 50:59–63.
26. Maurice OM. The biology of wound healing in the corneal stroma. Castroviejo Lecture. Cornea 1987; 6:162–8.
27. Melki S, Talamo J. Late traumatic dislocation of laser in situ keratomileusis corneal flaps. Ophthalmology 2000; 107:1236–9.
28. Melki S, Azar D. LASIK complications: etiology management and prevention. Surv Ophthalmol 2001; 46:95–116.
29. Minckler DS. Advances with aqueous shunts—1990 to 2001. J Glaucoma 2001; 10:S85–7.
30. Minckler DS, Vedula SS, Li TJ, et al. Aqueous shunts for glaucoma. Cochrane Database Syst Rev 2006; 2: CD004918.
31. Palanker D, Huie P, Baqnkov A, et al. Migration of retinal cells through a perforated membrane: implications for a high-resolution prosthesis. Invest Ophthalmol Vis Sci 2004; 45:3266–70.

32. Patel C, Wood OR II. Fundamentals of lasers. In: Karlin DB, ed. Lasers in Ophthalmic Surgery. Cambridge, MA: Blackwell Science, 1995:1–30.
33. Peacock LW, Slade SG, Martiz J, et al. Ocular integrity after refractive procedures. Ophthalmology 1997; 104:1079–83.
34. Pearlstein E, Agapitos PJ, Cantrill HL, et al. Ruptured globe after radial keratotomy. Am J Ophthalmol 1988; 106:755–6.
35. Reed JW, Cain LR, Weaver RG, Oberfeld SM. Clinical and pathologic findings of aphakic peripheral corneal edema: Brown–McLean syndrome. Cornea 1992; 11:577–83.
36. Schmack I, Dawson DG, McCarey BE, et al. Cohesive tensile strength of human LASIK wounds with histologic, ultrastructural, and clinical correlations. J Refract Surg 2005; 21:433–45.
37. Schmack I, Dawson DG, McCarey BE, et al. Functional attributes of human LASIK corneas—strength and haze measurements. In: Combined Meeting of the AAOP/EOPS/IOPS, New Orleans, October 23, 2004.
38. Soong H, Mian S. Femtosecond laser-assisted posterior lamellar keratoplasty. Ophthalmology 2005; 112:44–9.
39. Stark W. Management of epithelial ingrowth and cysts. Dev Ophthalmol 1981; 5:64–73.
40. Tuli S, Goldstein M, Schultz GS. Chapter 9: Corneal reaction to injury. In: Cornea JH, Krachmer MJ, Mannus E, Holland J, eds. Philadelphia: Elsevier Mosby, 2005:133–50.
41. Twa MD, Ruckhofer J, Dash RL, et al. Histologic evaluation of corneal stroma in rebbits after intrastromal corneal ring implantation. Cornea 2003; 22:146–52.
42. Vargas LG, Vroman DT, Solomon KD, et al. Epithelial downgrowth after clear corneal pacoemulsification: a report of two cases. Ophthalmology 2002; 109:2331–5.
43. Walter P, Kisvarday ZF, Gortz M, et al. Cortical activation via an implanted wireless retinal prosthesis. Invest Ophthalmol Vis Sci 2005; 46:1780–5.
44. Zavala E, Binder P. The pathologic findings of epithelial ingrowth. Arch Ophthalmol 1980; 98:2007–14.

17

Overview of Aging

Mitchell T. Heflin
Center for Aging and Human Development, Duke University, Durham, North Carolina, U.S.A.

Helen Lum
Durham Veterans Administration Medical Center, Durham, North Carolina, U.S.A.

INTRODUCTION

Over the course of the twentieth century, the number of Americans over the age of 65 years increased from 3 million to over 35 million. Concurrently, the population of those over age 85 years has grown from 100,000 to over 4 million and, by the end of the last century, represented the fastest growing segment of society. By 2030, some estimate that the percentage of the overall population over age 65 will reach 70 million, just over 20% of the total population and that 10 million of these people will be over age 85 years (Fig. 1). As the "Baby Boomer" generation reaches the ranks of the oldest-old in 2050, their numbers may swell to over 20 million (Fig. 2). A recent report from the National Institute on Aging entitled *65+ in the United States: 2005*, also points out that this phenomenon is not isolated to the United States. Across the globe, the percentage of the population over 65 years will increase by 25% to 50% over the next 25 years (19).

CAUSE OF ENLARGING AGED POPULATION

What accounts for this explosion in the older adult population? While some attribute it to a declining birth rate, most believe that it reflects the health-care successes of the twentieth century. Fries (13), in his landmark paper, pointed out that the extension of the human lifespan reflects "the elimination of premature death, particularly neonatal mortality." Additionally, improvements in other aspects of public health, including nutrition, less crowded living arrangements, safe drinking water, immunizations, and antibiotics, have led to lower rates of mortality throughout childhood and early adulthood. As a result, people survive to adulthood and late life more often. The survival curves depicted in Figure 3 clearly demonstrate the change in shape of the overall graph from nearly linear in 1900 to rectangular in the late twentieth century, with most mortality being

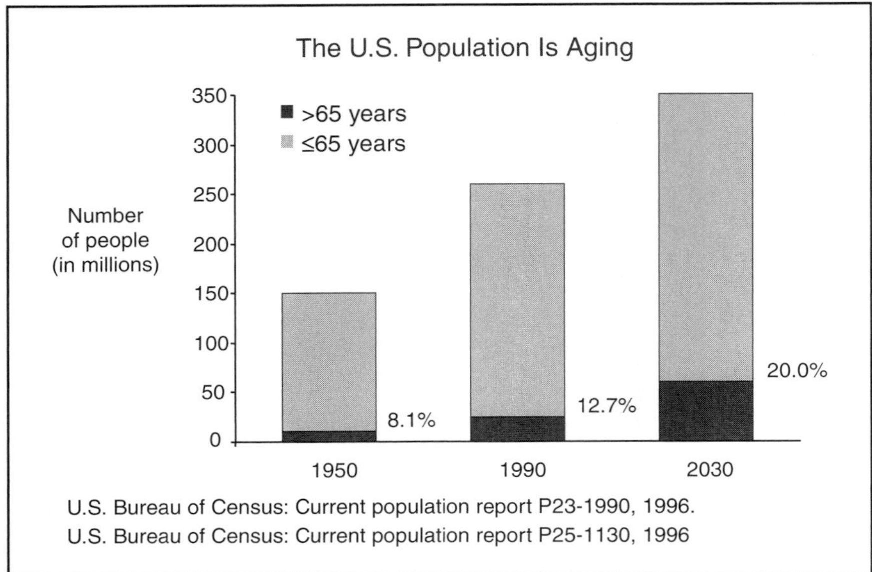

Figure 1 Estimates of the U.S. population size in 1950, 1990, and 2030.

compressed into late life. While the life expectancy at birth over the same period has risen dramatically from 47 years to nearly 77 years, the maximum lifespan of Americans has remained remarkably stable. In fact, many believe that the median life expectancy of certain societies will plateau around age 85 sometime in the early twenty-first century as premature deaths are minimized (13).

What, then, is it about human biology and aging that limits our ability to extend life? As advances in medicine deliver more and more individuals to old age, we are encountering the limits of the organism at the cellular, tissue and organ level to cope with stress and recover completely. Williamson (45) defines this process of biologic aging as "Adult life changes in structure and function, leading to decreased reserve capacity, and increased vulnerability to age related diseases and the overall forces of mortality, ultimately leading to death." In the end, changes at the most basic levels lead to an impaired ability to deal with the crises of living. Across cell types and organ systems, certain consistent age-related alterations in function have been observed. First, variability at the organ and individual levels decreases as evidenced by less

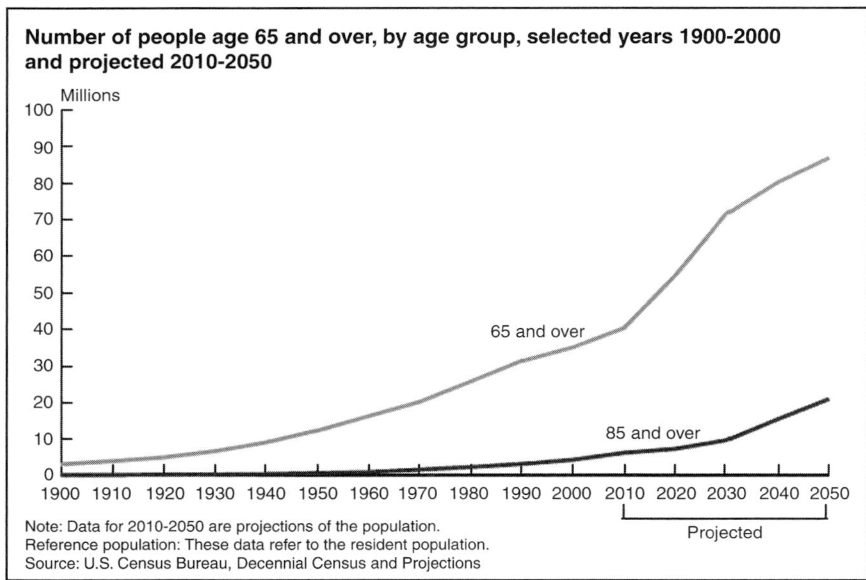

Figure 2 Projection of individuals aged over 65 and 85 years from 1900 to 2050. *Source*: From U.S. Census Bureau.

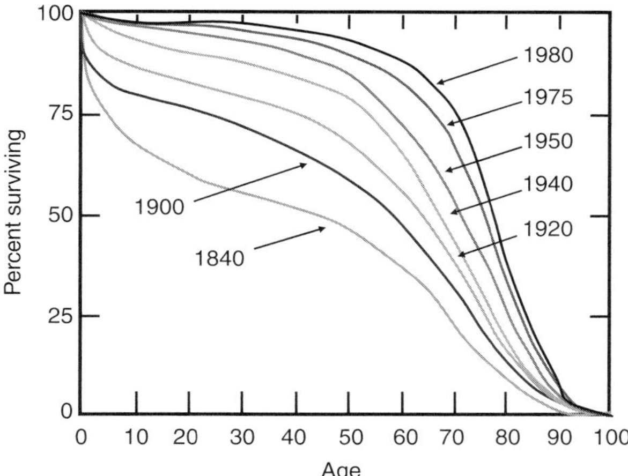

Figure 3 Survival curves for the United States. Population: 1840–1980. *Source*: From U.S. Bureau of Health Statistics.

fluctuation in heart rate or hormone secretion. Second, these declines are most evident under stress. Ultimately, systems are slower to react and recover. The result is an impaired ability to deal with any demands beyond a narrow range outside the normal. Fries points out that organ reserve decreases almost linearly beginning at 30 years of age, such that by the eighth and ninth decades, the ability of an organ system to "restore homeostasis" is significantly impaired. In fact, this progressive narrowing in reserve has been most accurately termed "homeostenosis" and is often depicted as a steady tapering in the reserve available in multiple organ systems as time progresses (Fig. 4) (12). In this situation, an

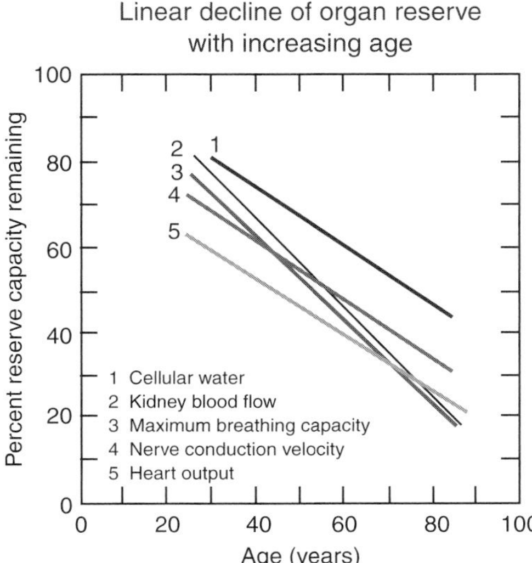

Figure 4 Linear decline of organ reserve with increasing age. *Source*: From Ref. 3.

individual may function within the normal range without difficulty, but stress such as acute illness may exceed their capacity to restore function and recover health. The result, at best, may be a decline in health and ability, and at worst, death.

THEORIES OF AGING

At the biologic level, science provides a number of plausible explanations for observed changes with aging. Theories of senescence can be grouped into two major categories. *Error or damage theories* propose that an organism ages over time due to persistent threat from damaging agents and an ever declining ability to respond to or repair this damage. *Program theories* postulate that age, particularly maximal age, is determined by genetic and developmental factors that influence the biologic life course. It is likely that aging is a result of a complex combination of both types of events (6).

The free radical theory of aging proposes that oxidative metabolism generates an abundance of oxygen free radicals, which are highly reactive and indiscriminately damage the entire spectrum of molecules, including proteins, DNA, and lipids. This injury, in turn, leads to cell dysfunction and, ultimately, to tissue and organ disrepair. Part of this theory originally postulated that smaller species with higher metabolic rates live shorter lives due to more rapid accumulation of byproducts. While this portion of the theory has been debunked, many still contend that limiting the production of oxidants can contribute to improved health, if not extended life. Another theory asserts that the accumulation of glucose-related molecules on proteins contributes to their dysfunction and degradation. These "glycosylated" molecules become more abundant over time and lead to impairment at the tissue and organ level. Theory proponents point to the many chronic problems including diabetic retinopathy that routinely arises in patients with longstanding diabetes mellitus (see Chapter 67) as proof of the significance of this phenomenon. No direct evidence exists, however, to support either the theory itself or a potential means of intervention (31).

A separate line of reasoning posits that human lifespan and aging result from genetic-based timing mechanisms. The oldest of these theories suggests that evolutionary pressures are biased for traits that promote health and reproduction in early adulthood, occasionally at the expense of health and function in late life. Further, little selective pressure exists against negative traits that emerge in late life, leaving humans prone to the ill effects of aging. On this front, geneticists have identified among species of fruit flies and certain nematodes, specific genes that, when activated, result in a significant prolongation in the organism's lifespan. Work is also underway to discover similar genetic sequences among mammalian models (29).

While much attention has focused on the discovery of the "senescence gene," study of the enzyme telomerase has also generated excitement and speculation. All cells are programmed to die at some point (apoptosis) (see Chapter 2) to be replaced by younger cells. These divisions and replacements are limited by the number of generations intrinsic to a specific cell line, the so-called Hayflick phenomenon. Biologists theorize that, from an evolutionary perspective, humans are designed to survive to approximately age 40 years and therefore are equipped with an appropriate number of cell divisions. As detailed above, advances in medicine and public health have extended the median life expectancy and, as a result, more people are encountering problems related to exhausting their allotted number of cell divisions (replicative aging). DNA in the telomeres at the end of chromosomes tracks the inevitable loss of chromosomal material with replication. As telomeres shorten, cell aging and demise eventually occur. Telomerase, composed of proteins and RNA, prevents telomere shortening and may extend the number of replications allotted to a cell and thereby extend the lifespan of the organ. This advantage must be weighed against the price of "immortality," namely the increased risk of malignancy (47).

Perhaps the most intriguing development in the last quarter century involves the purposeful reduction of food intake, termed caloric restriction. Caloric restriction is the only intervention that has been shown to reproducibly extend the maximal life span. In rats, maximum lifespan increases an average of 20 months with a 40% reduction in calories. Rhesus monkeys enrolled in a trial of caloric restriction appear to have a lower disease burden and mortality than controls after 15 years. The mechanism is not well understood, but may be metabolically mediated. In observational studies in humans, those with lower average body temperature, lower insulin levels and higher dehydroepiandrosterone sulfate levels (all changes found in calorically restricted monkeys) appeared to survive longer. Efforts are underway now to find chemical agents that mimic these metabolic effects (36).

AGING CHANGES IN DIFFERENT ORGANS

To understand the changes in the individual's ability to cope with physiologic stress with age, one must also examine the changes at the level of the organ system. In this chapter, we review age-related changes in the major organ systems at the cellular and physiologic levels and comment specifically on the incidence of relevant diseases and ailments in that system. As will be evident, while normal aging is not itself a diagnosis, it is, indeed, fertile ground for disease, and, in particular, chronic disease.

Immunology and Hematology Systems

Many experts implicate immunosenescence in the increased incidences of malignancy, infection, and autoimmune diseases with aging. While not clear, direct evidence exists to connect specific changes in the immune system with these conditions, a basic understanding of these changes is important.

Decline in T-cell immunity reflects the most pronounced alterations. Change is most evident in the decline in delayed-type hypersensitivity reactions, important in responses to specific antigens and immunizations. Specifically, T-cell proliferation is impaired as evidenced by a decreased ability to recruit peripheral blood mononuclear cells. This may result in a decreased response to immunizations, such as influenza or tetanus, and an attenuated reaction to purified protein derivative of tuberculin (9). Some hypothesize that this decrease is related to the normal thymic involution with age or a preferential accumulation of memory T cells out of proportion to naïve T cells. Changes in levels of certain interleukins may be important as well. Decreases in interleukin 2 (IL2) or changes in the IL2 receptor may attenuate T-cell proliferation with aging. On the other hand, increases in interleukin 6 (IL6), an important mediator of inflammation, may contribute to age-related increases in rates of certain diseases (32).

Age-related changes in B-cell activity are also pronounced. These changes include: (*i*) lower antibody production in response to infection or immunization, (*ii*) altered levels of immunoglobulins with increases in specific classes, (*iii*) decreased affinity of antibodies, and (*iv*) increased levels of autoantibodies. A lowered production of antibodies may have important implications for the effectiveness of certain vaccinations, particularly those for which the initial dose is delivered in late life (e.g., pneumococcal vaccine). Older adults also have a higher prevalence of monoclonal gammopathies, many of which have no clear clinical significance (32).

At least some of the changes in cell-mediated and humoral immunity may be related to changes in signal activation as well as alterations in rates of apoptosis (programmed cell death), allowing either the accumulation of dysfunctional cells or the disproportionate early death of undifferentiated cells.

Changes in immune function with aging are difficult to study given the high rates of concurrent illness, both acute and chronic, in this population. In addition, the effects of medications, environmental factors and psychosocial stressors are also unpredictable and poorly understood. Perhaps it is most important to understand that physiologic stress may have a substantial adverse impact on immunity among older adults and, as a result, further amplify the phenomenon of homeostenosis.

In the absence of comorbid illness, there appears to be little effect of aging on the hematologic system. A very modest increase in the prevalence of anemia with advancing age likely reflects an impaired response to stimulation of progenitor cells in the presence of hematopoietic stress. This may, indeed, be primarily related to changes in a variety of growth factors described above, including increased levels of IL6 with underproduction of other factors, leading to dysregulation of hematopoiesis (2).

Neurologic System

The impact of aging on the brain and neuromuscular systems may be the most clinically evident and most highly feared. The typical caricature of the older adult depicts many stereotypical changes, including decline in hearing and vision, poor memory, and impaired balance. While many older adults are spared these ailments, this picture of aging does reflect many of the predictable decrements in neurologic function with aging.

With respect to special senses, older adults experience declining vision, hearing, taste, and smell. Common vision problems include reduced visual acuity, particularly hyperopia and impaired accommodation and directional gaze. Aging changes in the eye include posterior vitreous detachment (PVD), vitreous liquefaction (syneresis), and asteroid hyalosis (see Chapter 29). PVD can lead to retinal breaks and retinal detachment (see Chapter 28). Age-related atrophy of the lacrimal gland can lead to a dry eye especially in women (see Chapter 30). Premature aging is feature of Pelizaeus-Merzbacher disease and Cockayne syndrome (see Chapter 70) With respect to auditory function, progressive high-frequency hearing loss affects over 25% of older adults, most often due to loss of hair cells, termed presbycusis. Other more serious age-related ocular abnormalities are cataract (see Chapter 22 and 23) and age-related maculopathy (see Chapter 18). Moreover primary open angle glaucoma becomes more prevalent as individuals become older (see Chapter 20 and 21).

Changes in the neuromuscular system have some of the most important implications for the older adult. Muscle mass, strength, and fine motor coordination all decline with age. These changes are likely multifactorial related to disuse, neuronal loss (particularly within the anterior horn cells and posterior columns) with decreased deep tendon reflexes and impaired vibratory sense, and myopathic changes. As a result, gait and balance are often impaired. This phenomenon is reflected in a stooped posture with shortened step length and height, and an impaired ability to compensate when walking. Falls and injuries related to falls increase steadily with aging, such that over 30% of community dwelling adults over age 65 suffer a fall each year and 10% of these result in significant injury. One of the most ominous of these injuries, hip fracture, occurs in only 1% of falls, but results in significant disability, cost, and a higher risk of mortality, particularly in the visually impaired.

Cognitive changes with aging are perhaps the most commonly parodied. Many people still refer to "senility" as a normal part of aging. While dementia and related disorders are very common (affecting up to 40–50% of adults aged 85 and over), it is important to distinguish normal aging from disease in this case, given the implications for prognosis and planning. As a gross measure of impact, brain weight declines with age—with an average loss of up to 250 g between ages 30 and 60. Pathologically, there is an increased occurrence of amyloid plaques and neurofibrillary tangles, although these entities still occur much more often among those with dementia. Declining brain function is also reflected in impaired glucose metabolism. Age, indeed, does have specific clinical affects on cognition. Most obviously, processing speeds are slowed, particularly with respect to new learning and problem-solving skills. In addition, beyond age 60, people begin to exhibit reduced verbal function and memory, although in the normal adult these are very subtle and minimally progressive. A key point of differentiation between the changes of normal aging and dementia is that these changes should not, in the absence of other confounding conditions, such as delirium or depression, affect normal and customary function. Indeed, studies have even revealed improvements with age in certain areas, including judgment, organization, and efficiency in reasoning (1).

Endocrine System

The aging endocrine system presents an intriguing model for the overall changes in homeostatic regulation described earlier. In a normal, unstressed state in the disease-free individual, little change is evident, particularly in the levels and activity of most hormones. However, with illness or other challenges, abnormalities become obvious and important. Another key concept is that clinical presentations of endocrinologic disorders may be atypical, blunted, or even undetectable when compared with those of younger persons. Several examples of these principles are detailed below.

Hypothalamic–pituitary–adrenal axis function appears to be well preserved with normal aging. Prolonged elevation of glucocorticoid secretion with stress may have adverse effects, ultimately, on immune function and glucose metabolism. While primary Cushing syndrome is relatively rare in older adults, chronic administration of exogenous glucocorticoids is common. The ravages that steroids cause to the entire body are particularly severe and debilitating in older adults, including osteoporosis, glucose intolerance, neuropsychiatric symptoms, cataracts, glaucoma, and myopathy. Likewise, the most common cause of adrenal insufficiency in older adults is the suppression of normal adrenal function due to chronic glucocorticoid administration. The presentation of this syndrome can be nonspecific, including generalized weakness, weight loss, dizziness, falls, or overall failure to thrive.

With respect to the sympathetic nervous system and adrenal medulla, levels of norepinephrine and epinephrine rise with age, primarily due to increased secretion. However, the resultant physiologic response is muted due to decreased receptor and postreceptor activation despite increased circulating hormone levels. The clinical implication may be a blunted response to stimuli such as hypoglycemia, hypoxia, or systemic infection. The renin–angiotensin–aldosterone system also changes significantly with age. Decreased levels of renin contribute to lower levels of aldosterone, which in turn leads to an increased propensity for salt-wasting among older adults. This phenomenon has important implications. Along with impaired thirst and antidiuretic hormone response, older adults may become volume-depleted more rapidly and have a greater propensity to develop hyperkalemia.

Decline in growth hormone (GH) is also observed with aging, such that among adults in their 70s and 80s about 50% have little or no detectable GH secretion. This may contribute to changes in body composition, including decreased muscle mass and strength, further contributing to the risk for falls and fractures. Lower levels of testosterone among older men, in addition to lowering libido and sexual function, may contribute to changes in cognition and loss of bone and muscle mass.

With respect to thyroid function, circulating triiodothyronine (T3) and thyroxin (T4) levels remain near-normal with aging, but with illness, the levels of both are lower and specifically the conversion of T4 to T3 is impaired and results in a marked decline in the latter—a condition often referred to as sick euthyroid. Thyroid disorders are common among older adults, but often difficult to diagnose. The presentation can be nonspecific with weight loss, apathy, and weakness as possible clinical manifestations of both hypo- and hyperthyroidism.

Alterations in glucose metabolism with aging are primarily manifested with stress. In normal older adults, glucose tolerance testing reveals a higher elevation in serum glucose levels among older adults compared to younger ones. Obesity, decreased activity, comorbid illness and medication may all contribute to the impaired response to endogenous insulin observed with aging. Of course, the most important consequence is the much higher incidence of diabetes mellitus—found in up to 20% of adults over age 65. The implications of this diagnosis for overall health, including vision, renal function, cardiovascular disease, cognition, and disability, are well documented.

Finally, aging results in a number of important changes in calcium homeostasis leading to reduced bone mass and an increase in fracture risk among older adults. Decreased intake and impaired absorption of calcium and a high prevalence of hypovitaminosis D lead to lower levels of serum calcium in older adults. Most often, the body compensates by increasing secretion of parathyroid hormone (PTH). This homeostatic mechanism, however, results in an increase in bone demineralization and a resultant reduction in bone mass. This clinical circumstance is exaggerated with abnormal elevations in PTH due to primary, secondary, or tertiary hyperparathyroidism (Fig. 5) (16).

Cardiovascular System

Cardiovascular disease dramatically increases with age and is a major cause of morbidity and mortality in the elderly (22). Eighty-three percent of all

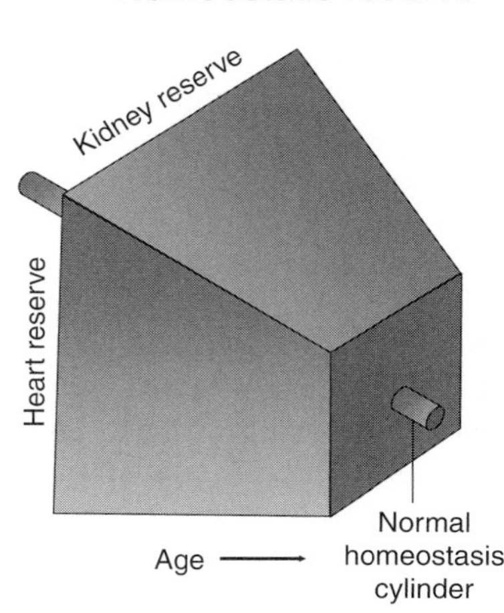

Figure 5 Homeostatic reserve. *Source*: From Ref. 12.

cardiovascular deaths in the United States occur in patients over 65 years old (21). Among the leading causes of cardiovascular disease are uncontrolled hypertension, coronary artery disease, and stroke. These diseases often result from structural changes in arteries and the heart's anatomy, leading to impairment of the body's compensatory mechanisms.

Over time, large arteries stiffen and thicken. The luminal diameter also increases. This phenomenon is a result of accumulated fragmentation in elastin fibers, increased crosslinking of collagen in the subendothelium, combined with progressive calcification. Arterial wall stiffness and thickness leads to an increase in arterial systolic pressure and impedance to left ventricular ejection. This increased afterload is likely the stimulus for left ventricular hypertrophy. Both systolic blood pressure and mean blood pressure increase with age, along with a widening of the pulse pressure.

Similar to large arteries, the walls of the small arteries thicken and the luminal diameters increase, causing increased impedance. These gradual changes are reflected in a slow decline in the diastolic pressure—most often noted between the ages of 60 and 80 years old. Additionally, in small arteries, it is believed that there is an age-related decrease in the basal level of nitric oxide as well as a muted response to this intrinsically potent vasodilator (41). An increase in impedance along with a decrease in vascular conductance leads to greater peripheral vascular resistance. At the capillary level, age-related increased peripheral vascular resistance has been associated with decreased perfusion during times of stress like ischemia or heat (26). At the venous level, the age-related declining response to nitric oxide is thought to be responsible for the inability of older adults to respond to hypovolemic circulatory stress (33).

Like the vasculature, the heart also experiences structural changes with age. Myocytes hypertrophy but decline in number. There is also an age-related enlargement of the atria; particularly, the left atrium. In addition, the heart becomes more fibrotic as collagen filaments, fibronectin and integrins increase. Sympathetic as well as parasympathetic neurons decrease with age. Valves, such as the aortic and mitral valves, become more calcified and stiff. At rest, these structural changes are hardly noticeable. There is no change in the resting left ventricular ejection fraction, heart rate, or cardiac output. However, under conditions in which the heart must perform at a faster rate, there is significant compromise. Fewer myocytes along with increased wall stiffness make the heart less contractile. Loss of innervation leads to decreased neuromuscular control. Consequently, the heart is unable to "squeeze" as hard and as fast as is needed during times of stress or even routine exercise.

Renal System

During the 1990s, the United States experienced a near doubling of the number of patients with end-stage kidney disease. The number of incident cases increased from 53,000 in 1991 to 93,000 in 2000 (14). According to Luke and Beck (27), the average age of patients starting dialysis is 62 years old. According to the National Center for Chronic Disease Prevention and Health Promotion, kidney disease is the ninth leading cause of death in the United States (34). Aging of the renal system is characterized by structural changes in the renal vasculature, tubules and glomeruli. These changes manifest as an age-related decline in renal blood flow and impaired tubular function.

Over time, the renal arteries undergo wall thickening much like the cardiovascular and pulmonary arteries. The smaller renal arteries become more tortuous and irregular with age. These changes lead to increased vascular resistance. Simultaneously, there is a steady decline in the total number of nephrons starting at age 40. By the fifth decade, sclerotic glomeruli are evident. Light microscopy shows focal sclerosis and partial thickening of the glomerular basement membrane (44). Age-related glomerulosclerosis is thought to be triggered by the decompensation of podocytes, cells that form the filtration barrier in the glomerulus (43). With the loss of glomeruli, the attached renal tubules degenerate and become replaced by connective tissue. There is a net "generalized tubular interstitial fibrosis."

Along with increased renal vascular resistance in both the afferent and efferent arterioles, there is a 10% per decade decrease in renal blood flow (44). This leads to a decline in renal efficiency for handling fluids and electrolytes. Age-related changes in the glomerular filtration rate seem to be variable despite the gradual decline in renal blood flow. In a longitudinal study done between 1958 and 1981, it was noted that 30% of the population showed no glomerular filtration rate decline with age. Five to ten percent of the population had a higher than expected decline in glomerular filtration rate. The remaining majority demonstrated the expected loss of 10% of their glomerular filtration rate per year after the fourth decade (25). The variability in glomerular filtration rate suggests that drug dosing, fluid replacement, or electrolyte correction need careful consideration in the elderly. In particular, health-care providers must be cognizant of the route of clearance of medications and familiarize themselves with those drugs eliminated principally or exclusively by the kidneys (Table 1). Many of these drugs are taken by elderly patients who also happen to have age-related eye diseases.

Table 1 Drugs Whose Renal Elimination is Impaired with Advancing Age

ACE inhibitors	Flouroquinolones
Acetazolamide	Furosemide
Amantadine	Lithium
Aminoglycosides	Metformin
Chlorpropamide	Procainamide/NAPA
Cimetidine	Ranitidine
Digoxin	Vancomycin

Abbreviations: ACE, angiostensin converting enzyme; NAPA, *N*-acetyl-procainamide.

Respiratory System

Pulmonary function progressively declines throughout life and can be associated with respiratory symptoms, disease, and increased mortality (4,9,15). The source of this decline is a combination of structural changes in the vasculature and musculature of the pulmonary system. This leads to a decrease in physiologic reserves in that pulmonary function is compromised if an acute insult such as pneumonia or pulmonary embolism occurs.

Changes in the pulmonary vasculature are reminiscent of those seen in the cardiovascular system. For instance, autopsy reports show that the intimal thickening in pulmonary arteries is similar to that seen in the systemic vasculature (41). This is accompanied by impaired regulation of blood flow. As in the cardiovascular system, this impairment is caused by decreased receptor-mediated responsiveness (41). In addition to vasculature changes, there is an age-related decline in the function of respiratory musculature. For example, diaphragm strength is 25% less in the healthy older person as compared to a young adult (42). Chest wall compliance also decreases with age (8).

The age-related structural changes in the pulmonary vasculature and musculature result in significant functional changes. Pulmonary artery wall thickening leads to a progressive increase in pulmonary artery pressure. According to Davidson and Fee (7), there is a 60% increase in mean pulmonary artery pressure from age 40 to 70. This can lead to pulmonary blood flow resistance, cardiac decompensation, and even hypoxemia if pulmonary ventilation and perfusion become severely mismatched. The decreased receptor-mediated responsiveness of aged pulmonary vasculature can result in diminished reactions to important environmental cues like hypoxia and hypercarbia.

Although there is documented decline in respiratory musculature, the total lung capacity, or volume of air within the respiratory system, is minimally changed with age. This is a reflection of the body's adaptive system. The total lung capacity is a balance between the force of the inspiratory muscles and the elastic recoil of the lung along with the stiff chest wall. With age, inspiratory muscles weaken. However, the elastic recoil also decreases, making the lungs easier to expand. The chest wall becomes stiffer over time and provides resistance. In addition to weakened respiratory muscles, there is a decrease in diffusing capacity by approximately 5% per decade after age 40 (8). These changes contribute to reduced physiologic reserves and may further impair exercise tolerance.

Gastrointestinal System

A 2004 survey of gastroenterology resource utilization in the United States reported more than 10 million office visits per year by patients over 65 years of age (38). This finding initially appears enigmatic since the function of the gastrointestinal tract is commonly believed to remain relatively intact with aging. A plausible explanation is the accretion of small effects from multiple chronic diseases and years of environmental as well as lifestyle exposures.

There are many age-related changes that occur within the mouth. Teeth discolor and become more likely to fracture as dental pulp recedes from the crown and the root canal narrows. Muscles of the tongue, like other skeletal muscles, decline in mass. Fat and fibrous tissue replace up to 25% of the secretory parenchyma of the salivary glands (5). Compensatory mechanisms minimize the impact of these changes such that swallowing and phonation are not clinically diminished in the healthy elderly patient. However, if patients have a superimposing neurologic or muscular illness like Parkinson disease, stroke, diabetic neuropathy, myasthenia gravis, amyotrophic lateral sclerosis or polymyositis, the age-associated oropharyngeal changes predispose to dysphagia, aspiration and malnutrition (18,40).

In 1964, Soergel et al. coined the term presbyesophagus to describe esophageal dysfunction associated with age (40). Among the findings were decreased amplitude of peristaltic contractions, incomplete sphincter relaxation, delayed esophageal emptying, frequent tertiary contractions, and esophageal dilatation. However, the incidence of presbyesophagus in patients with neither diabetes mellitus nor neurologic disease appears to be small (5). The current consensus suggests that esophageal dysmotility is more often a result of underlying chronic diseases like diabetes mellitus or side effects of medications than just normal aging.

Over the past 20 years, the incidence of peptic ulcers has decreased in all age groups except in the elderly (40). This is likely associated with a decline in gastric motility and luminal changes. In the stomach, decline in motility and emptying is caused by age-related autonomic nervous system dysfunction (5). In addition, the elderly often take anticholinergic medications, which further contribute to delayed emptying. This prolongs the "gastric contact time" of noxious agents, like nonsteroidal antiinflammatory

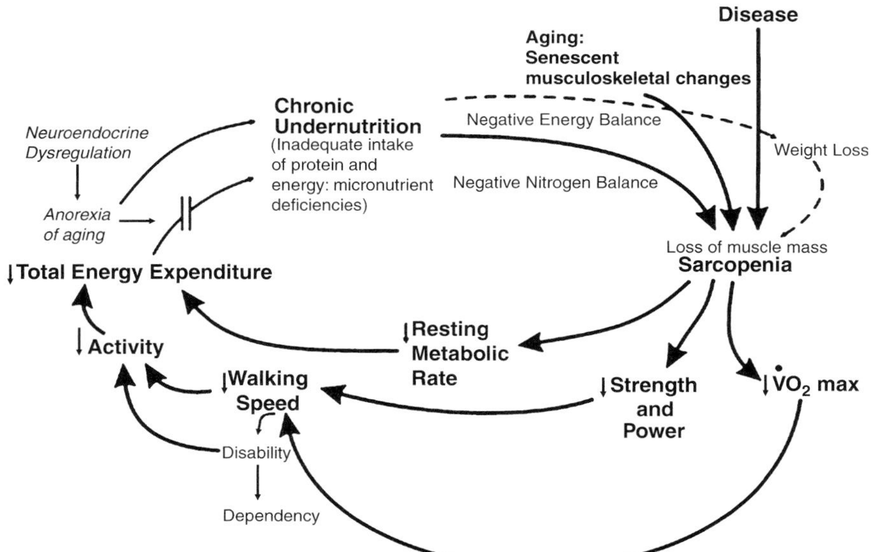

Figure 6 Cycle of frailty. Hypothesized as consistent with demonstrated pairwise associations and clinical signs and symptoms of fragility. *Source*: From Ref. 11.

drugs. Age-related gastric luminal changes include decreased prostaglandin and bicarbonate secretion, slowed mucosal cell proliferation, and impaired gastric blood flow. These changes collectively decrease the gastric mucosal defense against injury.

The liver, gallbladder, and pancreas experience an age-related decline in organ size, blood flow, and cell proliferation. Between age 70 and 90, the liver decreases from 2.5% of body weight to 1.6% as the overall number of hepatocytes decrease (28). Cytochrome p450 activity decreases with age, contributing to a slower metabolism of certain drugs. Thus caution must be used while prescribing hepatically cleared medications in the elderly.

Like the stomach, the small intestine and colon experience age-related decline in motility and luminal changes. In normal healthy elderly, these deficits do not change the overall daily function of the gut. However, when superimposed on chronic illnesses or polypharmacy, the elderly become more susceptible to disorders such as diverticulosis, altered bowel habits and colon cancer.

The Frailty Syndrome

What, ultimately, are the clinical implications of the changes described above? Fries' description of "homeostenosis" provides a link between the biological changes of aging and the increased vulnerability of humans to illness and functional decline in late life—a state commonly referred to as "frailty." Fried et al.'s recent definition of frailty moves beyond restraints of chronologic age, comorbidity, and disability to identify a unique clinical entity with independent predictive capacity (11). The "cycle of frailty" ties together the individual system-specific changes and identifies key events or clinical presentations that create a specific phenotype (Fig. 6). The authors define five key elements to this hypothetical cycle, including: (*i*) weight loss, (*ii*) weakness, (*iii*) poor endurance, (*iv*) slowness, and (*v*) inactivity.

Frailty is defined as the presence of three or more of these conditions. Using the Cardiovascular Health Study database, they examined the frequency and predictive capacity of these elements on health, ability, and mortality. Among over 5000 community dwelling adults over age 65, the prevalence of frailty by this definition was 6.9% and the four-year incidence was 7.2%. By this definition, frailty independently predicts falls, declines in mobility, loss of ability to perform activities of daily living, hospitalization, and death. This definition seems to provide a defined link between disease and disability in late life and, perhaps, a target for intervention to prevent the onset of functional decline, i.e., a means of further compressing comorbidity and disability in late life.

REFERENCES

1. Adams RD, Victor M, Ropper AH. Neurology of Aging in Principles of Neurology. 6th ed. New York: McGraw-Hill, 1997.
2. Ajmani RS, Riftkind JM. Hemorheological changes during human aging. Gerontology 1998; 44:111–20.
3. Baker GT, Martin GR. Molecular and Biologic Factors in Aging: The Origins, Causes, and Prevention of Senescence in Geriatric Medicine, 3rd ed. New York: Springer-Verlag, 1996.
4. Bang KM, Gergen PJ, Kramer R, Cohen B. The effect of pulmonary impairment on all-cause mortality in a national cohort. Chest 1993; 103:536–40.
5. Blechman MB, Gelb AM. Aging and gastrointestinal physiology. Gastroenterology 1999; 15:429–38.

6. Cristafolo VJ, Tresini M, Francis MK, Volker C. Biological theories of senescence. In: Bengston VL, Schaie W, eds. Handbook of Theories of Aging. Chap. 6. New York: Springer, 1999:98–112.
7. Davidson WR, Fee EC. Influence of aging on pulmonary hemodynamics in a population free of coronary artery disease. Am J Cardiol 1990; 65:1454–8.
8. Enright P. In: Hazzard WR, Blass JP, Halter JB, Ouslander JG, Tinetti ME, eds. Aging of the Respiratory System in Principles of Geriatric Medicine and Gerontology. Chap. 41, 5th ed. New York: McGraw-Hill, 2003:511–33.
9. Enright PL, Kronmal RA, Higgins MW, et al. Prevalence and correlates of respiratory symptoms and disease in the elderly. Chest 1994; 106:827–34.
10. Fietta A, Merlini C, Dos Santos C, et al. Influence of aging on some specific and nonspecific mechanisms of the host defense system in 146 healthy subjects. Gerontology 1994; 40:237–45.
11. Fried LP, Tangen CM, Walston J. Frailty in older adults: evidence for a phenotype. J Gerontol A Biol Sci Med Sci 2001; 56:146–56.
12. Fries JF, Crapo LM. Vitality and Aging: Implications of the Rectangular Curve. San Francisco, CA: WH Freeman, 1981.
13. Fries JF. Aging, natural death, and the compression of morbidity. N Engl J Med 1980; 303:130–5.
14. Gilbertson DT. Projecting the number of patients with end-stage renal disease in the United States to the year 2015. J Am Soc Nephrol 2005; 16:3736–41.
15. Griffith KA, Sherrill DL, Siegel EM, et al. Predictors of loss of lung function in the elderly. Am J Respir Crit Care Med 2001; 163:61–8.
16. Gruenewald DA, Matsumoto AM. Aging of the Endocrine System in Principles of Geriatric Medicine and Gerontology. 4th ed. New York: McGraw-Hill, 1999.
17. Hall KE. In: Hazzard WR, Blass JP, Halter JB, Ouslander JG, Tinetti ME, eds. Effect of Aging on Gastrointestinal Function in Principles of Geriatric Medicine and Gerontology. Chap. 41. New York: McGraw-Hill, 2003:593–600.
18. Hall KE, Proctor DD, Fisher L, et al. American gastroenterological association future trends committee report: effects of aging of the population on gastroenterology practice, education, and research. Gastroenterology 2005; 129:1305–38.
19. He W, Sengupta M, Velkoff VA, DeBarros KA. 65+ in the United States: 2005. Washington, DC: United States Department of Health and Human Services, 2005.
20. Hornick TR, Kowal J. Clinical epidemiology of endocrine disorders in the elderly. Endocrinol Metab Clin North Am 1997; 26:145–63.
21. Hoyert DL, Heven MP, Murphy SL, et al. Deaths: Final Data for 2003. National Statistics Report. April 19, 2006.
22. Kannel WB. Incidence and epidemiology of heart failure. Heart Fail Rev 2000; 5:167–73.
23. Lee TM, Su SF, Chou TF, et al. Loss of preconditioning by attenuated activation of myocardial ATP-sensitive potassium channels in elderly patients undergoing coronary angioplasty. Circulation 2002; 105:334–40.
24. Leipzig RM. In: Cassel CK, Leipzig R, Cohen HJ, et al., eds. Evidence-based Medicine and Geriatrics in Geriatric Medicine: An Evidence-based Approach. Chap. 1, 4th ed. New York: Springer, 2003:3–14.
25. Lindeman RD, Tobin J, Shock NW. Longitudinal studies on the rate of decline in renal function with age. J Am Geriatr Soc 1985; 33:278–85.
26. Longobardi G, Abete P, Ferrara N, et al. Warm-up phenomenon in adult and elderly patients with coronary artery disease: further evidence of the loss of "ischemic preconditioning" in the aging heart. J Gerontol 2000; 55A:M124–9.
27. Luke RG, Beck LH. Gerontologizing nephrology. J Am Soc Nephrol 1999; 10:1824–7.
28. Mezey E. In: Hazzard WR, Blass JP, Halter JB, Ouslander JG, Tinetti ME, eds. Hepatic, Biliary and Pancreatic Disease in Principles of Geriatric Medicine and Gerontology. Chap. 41, 5th ed. New York: McGraw-Hill, 2003:601–12.
29. Miller RA. Genetic approaches to the study of aging. J Am Geriatr Soc 2005; 53:S284–6.
30. Miller RA. The aging immune system: primer and prospectus. Science 1996; 273:70–4.
31. Miller RA. In: Hazzard WR, Blass JP, Halter JB, Ouslander JG, Tinetti ME, eds. The Biology of Aging and Longevity in Principles of Geriatric Medicine and Gerontology. Chap. 1, 4th ed. New York: McGraw-Hill, 1999:3–16.
32. Murasko DM, Bernstein ED. In: Hazzard WR, Blass JP, Halter JB, Ouslander JG, Tinetti ME, eds. Immunology of Aging in Principles of Geriatric Medicine and Gerontology. Chap. 3, 4th ed. New York: McGraw-Hill, 1999:35–52.
33. Olsen H, Vernersson E, Lanne T. Cardiovascular response to acute hypovolemia in relation to age: implications for orthostasis and hemorrhage. Am J Physiol Heart Circ Physiol 2000; 278:H222–32.
34. Pirtle CJ, Schoolwerth AC, Giles WH, et al. State-Specific Trends in Chronic Kidney Failure—United States, 1990–2001. CDC MMWR 2004; 53:918–20.
35. Rivard A, Fabre JE, Silver M, et al. Age-dependent impairment of angiogenesis. Circulation 1999; 99:111–20.
36. Roth GS. Caloric restriction and caloric restriction mimetics: current status and promise for the future. J Am Geriatr Soc 2005; 53:S280–3.
37. Russell, Robert M. Changes in gastrointestinal function attributed to aging. Am J Clin Nutr 1992; 55:1203S–7S.
38. Russo MW, Wei JT, Thiny MT, et al. Digestive and liver diseases statistics. Gastroenterology 2004; 126:1448–53.
39. Shaker R, Staff D. Esophageal disorders in the elderly. Gastroenterol Clin North Am 2001; 30:335–61.
40. Shamburek RD, Farrar JT. Disorders of the digestive system in the elderly. N Engl J Med 1990; 322:438–43.
41. Taffet GE, Lakatta EG. In: Hazzard WR, Blass JP, Halter JB, Ouslander JG, Tinetti ME, eds. Aging of the Cardiovascular System in Principles of Geriatric Medicine and Gerontology. Chap. 33, 5th ed. New York: McGraw-Hill, 2003:403–21.
42. Tolep K, Higgins N, Muza S, et al. Comparison of diaphragm strength between healthy adult elderly and young men. Am J Respir Crit Care Med 1995; 152:677–82.
43. Wiggins JE, Goyal M, Sanden SK, et al. Podocyte hypertrophy, "adaptation," and "decompensation" associated with glomerular enlargement and glomerulosclerosis in the aging rat: prevention by calorie restriction. J Am Soc Nephrol 2005; 16:2953–66.
44. Wiggins J. In: Hazzard WR, Blass JP, Halter JB, Ouslander JG, Tinetti ME, eds. Changes in Renal Function in Principles of Geriatric Medicine and Gerontology. Chap. 44, 5th ed. New York: McGraw-Hill, 2003:543–9.
45. Williamson J. Geriatric medicine: whose specialty? Ann Intern Med 1979; 91:774–7.
46. Wilson JAP. Cassel CK, Leipzig R, Cohen HJ, et al., eds. Gastroenterolgic Disorders in Geriatric Medicine: An Evidence-Based Approach. Chap 56, 4th ed. New York: Springer, 2003:835–51.
47. Wright WE, Shay J. Telomere biology in aging and cancer. J Am Geriatr Soc 2005; 53:S292–4.

18

Age-Related Macular Degeneration

Lyndell L. Lim and Robyn H. Guymer
Centre for Eye Research Australia, University of Melbourne, East Melbourne, Victoria, Australia

INTRODUCTION

Age related macular degeneration (AMD) is a progressive late onset disease affecting the central macula, which is responsible for fine central vision needed for driving, reading, and recognizing people's faces. It is the leading cause of irreversible blindness in western countries. Combined data from three predominantly Caucasian communities (U.S.A., the Netherlands, and Australia) indicates the prevalence for late AMD is 0.2% in the 55 to 64 age-group, rising sharply to 13% in the >85 years age group (158,210). The prevalence increases rapidly with age such that for the >90 age group, more than two thirds of individuals have early AMD changes, and one quarter have significant visual loss from late AMD (22). It is estimated that the number of people with AMD will double by year 2020 (217). Current treatment options for AMD are limited, mostly to the late neovascular stage of the disease, with no treatment currently available for the late atrophic form of disease.

DEFINITION

AMD is a progressive, degenerative disorder affecting the macula that predominantly occurs in persons >50 years of age. It is diagnosed and classified by its clinical appearance. Early AMD, or "age related maculopathy" is characterized by the presence of drusen, which are yellow subretinal deposits often associated with pigmentary abnormalities of the retina and retinal pigment epithelium (RPE) at the macula. People with drusen are usually asymptomatic, although on questioning, patients may volunteer some difficulty with dark adaptation and reading for prolonged periods of time. The main concern with early AMD, however, is the increased risk of progression to advanced, vision threatening, late AMD.

Advanced or late AMD refers to the sight-threatening complications of this disease. There are two main manifestations of late AMD—geographic atrophy (GA) and choroidal neovascularization (CNV).

CNV in exudative, or "wet," AMD is responsible for the majority of severe visual loss, and is an abnormal vascular complex (the CNV) growing from the choroid between the retina and its underlying supportive tissues. The result is usually a rapid impairment of retinal function with visual distortion and vision loss. By contrast, GA in non-exudative, or "dry," AMD is the result of the underlying supporting tissues of the retina (the RPE) becoming thinned and atrophic, causing slow loss of overlying photoreceptors and thus of retinal function.

PREVALENCE

Early signs of AMD are present in 15% of the population over 50 years but the prevalence is very much age dependent, affecting 30% of people in their 70s, increasing to 60% for those in their 90s. The prevalence of late AMD, whether CNV or GA, with its associated severe vision loss, also increases dramatically with age, affecting <1% of those younger than 65 years, but affecting 25% in the over 90 age group. In more than half of cases there is bilateral visual loss. Overall, the prevalence of CNV and GA AMD has been found to be 1.2% and 0.6%, respectively in a population-based American study (126), with similar rates (1.2% and 0.45%, respectively) found in a similar Australian study (158). These results are comparable with other large epidemiological studies around the world (29,171,210,226).

HISTOPATHOLOGY

Aging Changes of the Retina

The RPE

Normal RPE: The RPE is metabolically highly active with specialized functions to sustain the photoreceptor cells and, in particular, outer segment renewal. Unlike other phagocytes, the RPE cells remain in situ for a lifetime, and loss of RPE cells with age results in an increasing metabolic demand on each remaining cell (4). These cells discharge cytoplasmic material into the inner portion of Bruch membrane to achieve cytoplasmic renewal, a mechanism common to all metabolically active but non-dividing cells (53,113,114,184,191).

Throughout life the RPE cells phagocytose and degrade the shed tips of rod outer segments. Engulfed rod outer segments are contained in a phagocytic vacuole (phagosome), and a primary lysosome fuses with the vacuole to deliver degradative enzymes, forming a secondary lysosome, or phagolysosome. The undigested end products within the phagolysosome, called residual bodies, are autofluorescent granules (23,24,43,49). These residual bodies are thought to have a finite half-life (227), with some of the products resulting from degradation of the contents of these intracytoplasmic vesicles being recycled, and the remainder extruded through the basal surface of the RPE into Bruch membrane to diffuse into the choroidal circulation.

Aging changes: RPE changes with age are characterized by the accumulation of residual bodies that contain lipofuscin. These are similar to the "age pigment" found in other organs, including the brain (215). The lipofuscin in the RPE exhibits autofluorescence, and can be measured using a confocal scanning laser ophthalmoscope (47,227,228). Early measurements confirm that levels increase with age. The RPE residual body content also increases with age, and the relationship is best approximated by a nonlinear mathematical model that when graphed describes a parabola (a quadratic model) although the relationship between the two is not precise (166).

It is not known if the accumulation of lipofuscin-containing residual bodies leads to RPE functional compromise, but it is a possibility. After the seventh decade the RPE basement membrane thickens, and the number and complexity of basal convolutions of the RPE lessen. These changes have been interpreted as indicating RPE cellular stress, and their presence correlates closely with the risk of CNV, one of the forms of advanced AMD (80,195,220).

Bruch Membrane

Normal Bruch membrane: Bruch membrane is crucial because of its strategic location. It is interposed between the RPE and metabolically active photoreceptors and their major source of nutrition, the choriocapillaris. In addition to acting as a support element and an attachment site for the RPE, Bruch membrane provides a semipermeable filtration barrier through which major metabolic exchange takes place. Nutrients pass from the choriocapillaris to the photoreceptors and the RPE, while cellular breakdown products travel in the opposite direction (21).

Bruch membrane can be divided ultrastructurally into five layers: (*i*) the basement membrane of the RPE, which forms the innermost layer, (*ii*) an inner collagenous zone (ICZ), (*iii*) an elastic zone, (*iv*) an outer zone of collagen (OCZ), and (*v*) an outermost basement membrane elaborated by the endothelial cells of the choriocapillaris (105). The interfiber matrix of Bruch membrane is composed largely of heparan sulfate and chondroitin/dermatan sulfate (101).

Diffusion through Bruch membrane depends on the local concentration of salts, glucose, and the pH. Any alteration in the structure or composition of Bruch membrane may influence its diffusion properties and ultimately the function of the RPE and outer retina.

Age Changes

Bruch membrane has long been known to change in thickness, ultrastructure, and histochemistry with age (105,195). These changes occur in both the posterior pole and the periphery but are generally greater at the posterior pole (106,164,183). Alteration in the extracellular matrix (ECM) and the biophysical properties of Bruch membrane lead to altered nutrition and consequent abnormal functioning of the RPE and photoreceptors. It has been suggested that these changes in Bruch membrane have a major influence on the development and subsequent outcome of disease (16).

Changes in collagen, elastin, and glycosaminoglycan (GAG) components:
As Bruch membrane ages, an almost linear decline occurs in the solubility of collagen from nearly 100% in the first decade of life to 40–50% in the ninth decade in both the macula and the peripheral retina (122). This decrease in solubility is thought to result from an increase in the cross-linking of collagen fibers that would have an effect on permeability and may change the nature of the ECM. With age there is also an increase in amino acids such as tyrosine, methionine, and phenylalanine in the macular region of Bruch membrane that indicates deposition of non-collagenous proteinaceous material and may reflect debris accumulation (122).

A deposition of fibrous long space collagen (LSC) occurs in Bruch membrane, and its significance to disease has been the subject of great debate (155). Most attention has been devoted to LSC located between the plasma membrane and the basement membrane of the RPE, where it makes up part of the basal laminar deposits (BLDs), and is implicated in the pathogenesis of AMD. LSC in Bruch membrane is presumed to be a product of the RPE cells and has generally been regarded as a sign of cellular distress (194,219). However, the finding of LSC in the OCZ in the majority of young eyes (90,219) suggests that LSC is a normal feature that may be the result of constant collagen turnover. This form of collagen exhibits a 100 nm period and is especially frequent in a wide variety of tumors, especially schwannomas, and in non-neoplastic scars, in the trabecular meshwork, as well in the cornea in several diseases. Vascular endothelial cells produce enzymes that degrade collagen, and it has been proposed that a constant formation and degradation of collagen occurs normally. The apparent shift of LSC production from the choriocapillaris and outer choroid in the young to the RPE and inner choroid in older adults may be relevant to the pathogenesis of AMD (90).

The elastic tissue elements in Bruch membrane, which form a continuous meshwork of intersecting elastic fibers, also change with age. The fiber number increases, and the immature elastic elements (oxytalan) mature (5). Calcification also occurs, rendering Bruch membrane brittle (144).

Overall, the debris in Bruch membrane that accumulates with age may reflect RPE metabolic activity in general rather than being directly derived from outer segment material, as neither rhodopsin epitopes nor phagosomal enzyme activity have been shown in the Bruch membrane deposits (54). On the other hand, docosahexaenoic acid has been detected in this debris and is found in quantity only in the outer segments (184). This implies that material derived from the rod outer segments partly contributes toward the debris.

Change in lipid composition of Bruch membrane:
Lipids progressively accumulate in Bruch membrane with age and analyses of Bruch membrane have revealed little or no lipid in human eyes younger than 50 years, but the amount of lipid in this structure increases exponentially in persons more than 50 years old (106,206). These lipids consist of phospholipids, triglycerides, fatty acids, and free cholesterol (106). Higher quantities of lipid have been consistently extracted from Bruch membrane beneath the macula compared to the peripheral part of the retina, and the magnitude of the difference increased with age (106).

If these extracellular deposits of lipid are derived from blood, a large proportion of them would be expected to be composed of cholesterol and cholesterol esters, with more than 90% of phospholipid being phosphatidylcholine. However, different studies found very little cholesterol ester in Bruch membrane with no more than 50% of the phospholipid present being phosphatidylcholine. This is in keeping with the theory that the abnormal material is cellular in origin, rather than being derived from plasma, thereby differing from other extracellular lipid deposits, such as those in atherosclerosis and arcus senilis (14,106,206).

More recent studies of normal aged Bruch membrane have also revealed the presence of lipoprotein-like-particles containing apoB, apoA-I, and cholesterol (140), where the isolated esterified cholesterol was found to not only be different from plasma cholesterol but also to lack the two most abundant fatty acid residues of outer segment phospholipids (cholesteryl docohexanoate or cholesteryl stearate). Therefore, the lipid accumulation in Bruch membrane seems more likely to be of ocular and cellular origin but perhaps further processed by an intermediate cellular mechanism. This interpretation is supported by other studies analyzing the lipid content in eyes with AMD with similar findings (40,41).

Choriocapillaris

Normal Choriocapillaris: Choroidal blood flow is very high, achieving high oxygen tension in the outer retina, which is necessary to maintain the photoreceptor dark current in the dark-adapted state (212). The capillary bed is sinusoidal, and the endothelial cells are fenestrated. Material from the RPE is believed to diffuse through Bruch membrane and be cleared by the choriocapillaris. The mechanism whereby debris is cleared remains unknown, although many believe that this occurs by passive diffusion. Nutrients required by the RPE and photoreceptors travel in the opposite direction.

Age changes: With age, the cross-sectional area of the choriocapillaris is reduced and the normal sinusoidal capillaries are replaced by a tubular system (183). In 10 decades the density of the choriocapillaris decreases by 45%, and its diameter decreases by 34%, whereas the thickness of Bruch membrane increases by 135% (183). These changes could account for the perfusion defect seen on fluorescein angiography (FA) in some cases of AMD (173,180,181). It is not possible to determine if Bruch membrane thickening precedes choriocapillaris changes in AMD, and a causal relationship between the two structures has not yet been proven.

An initial abnormality in the choriocapillaris could lead to a reduction in clearance of waste material from Bruch membrane into the choroidal circulation. Alternatively, the diffuse deposits in Bruch membrane may induce secondary changes in the capillaries by acting as a barrier to diffusion between the RPE and choroid. There is good evidence that diffusible agents from the RPE regulate the morphologic attributes of the choriocapillaris, so the interposition of a diffusion barrier between the two structures may alter the accessibility of these molecules to the capillaries, resulting in reversion of the vessels to the more common tubular arrangement of capillary beds (98,136,180). This concept has been illustrated by the expression at high levels of tissue inhibitor of metalloproteinase-3 (TIMP-3) in Bruch membrane (38,229) and the demonstration that TIMP-3 influences endothelial function (7).

Early AMD

Drusen are the clinical hallmark of early AMD and are seen ophthalmoscopically as pale deposits at the level of Bruch membrane. However, the formation of BLD has been described as the earliest change seen in AMD and is generally clinically undetectable. It could be argued that some of these changes (such as early, non-confluent BLDs) are simply part of the normal physiologic aging process in the retina—but exactly when these deposits become a pathological process as part of early AMD is unclear.

The BLDs

Unlike drusen, which are located external to the basement membrane of the RPE, BLDs are situated between the RPE and its basement membrane. BLDs are typically seen in the seventh decade and two forms have been described—early and late.

The early form of BLD has a patchy distribution and histologically appears as a pale staining eosinophilic material with faint banding. When viewed by transmission electron microscopy (TEM), three phenotypes have been described—fibrillar, amorphous and polymerized (192). Despite similarities with RPE basement membrane, BLD is biochemically distinct, as shown by its lack of staining with ^{3}H-proline, a typical tracer for basement membrane collagen (103). Therefore, BLD is regarded as the result of a faulty degradative process in stressed RPE cells rather than from enhanced synthesis (103,192).

The late form of BLD is characterized by a continuous, diffuse thickening internal to the RPE basement membrane. It is characteristic of early AMD (195). By light microscopy, it resembles a thick hyalinized Bruch membrane (Fig. 1), but by TEM, this form of BLD is composed of amorphous material with a flocculent appearance (192) and forms a layer on the internal surface of the early form of BLD. The presence of late BLD is thought to indicate altered metabolism of severely stressed RPE and is mainly found over regressing drusen.

Drusen

Drusen were originally described as being composed of polymorphous material of vesicular, granular, and filamentous appearance. They are the result of focal deposits of a material similar to BLD in discrete mounds between the basement membrane of the RPE and the inner collagenous layer of Bruch membrane.

Historically they have been divided into hard and soft drusen, according to the nature of their margins. Hard drusen are defined as measuring 63 μm in diameter, being discrete, and having distinct margins. Histologically they are composed of dense hyaline material continuous with the inner collagenous layer of Bruch membrane (79). Ultrastructurally, they consist of finely granular or amorphous material with a variable number of pale and bristle-coated vesicles, tube-like structures and abnormal collagen (105). Their presence alone in small numbers has been thought not to signify increased risk of visual loss and is not included as a criterion for the diagnosis of early AMD (18,80). However, persons with large areas of small hard drusen (> 0.9 optic disc areas) have a two to three times increased risk of developing large soft drusen and pigmentary changes that lead to an increased risk of developing advanced AMD (132).

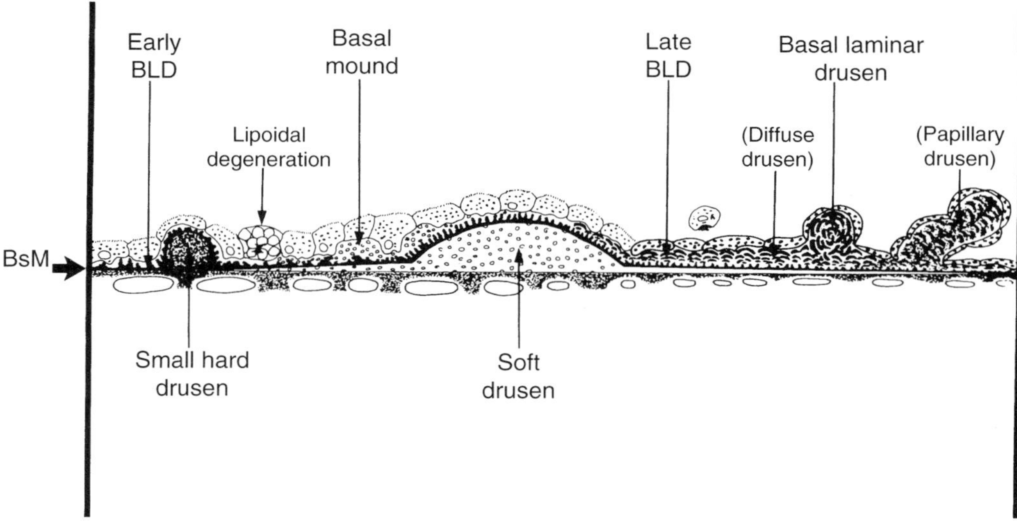

Figure 1 Schematic ultrastructural appearance of the various deposits accumulating under the RPE during the evolution of AMD. The relationship to the RPE basement membrane is shown. BLD is internal to the BsM; typical drusen are external. Membranous coils are found both internal to the BsM as mounds at the base of the RPE and external to the BsM as soft drusen. Hard drusen consist predominantly of amorphous material. *Abbreviations*: AMD, age related macular degeneration; BLD, basal laminar deposit; BsM, basement membrane; RPE, retinal pigment epithelium.

Soft drusen have indistinct edges, tend to be large, and may be confluent. They are thought to form from clusters of small, hard drusen (soft clusters) or in late life from a focal accentuation of the membranous debris within Bruch membrane (soft membranous drusen) (193,195,196). Histologically, these drusen are composed of pale staining amorphous material.

Irregular pigmentation at the level of the RPE is also commonly seen in subjects with drusen and is classified as part of early AMD. Areas of focal hyperpigmentation histologically correspond with clumps of pigmented cells in the outer layers of the retina and in the subretinal space, while small areas of hypopigmentation/atrophy represent atrophy of the RPE overlying areas of Bruch membrane thickening (28).

Although drusen and their presence in AMD have been well described histologically, the exact composition of drusen and the mechanism of their deposition are still unclear, although recent proteomic work has contributed greatly to our understanding of their composition and possible mechanisms of their formation and this is discussed in greater detail below.

To date, there are two main theories of drusen formation that can be loosely described as "transformation/degeneration" of RPE versus "excess production/deposition."

Transformation/degeneration theory: This theory was first proposed by Donders (48), who postulated that drusen were directly derived from the nuclear remnants of dead RPE cells. The lack of structures resembling outer segments, phagosomes, or lipofuscin granules, however, is thought to make this unlikely (30). Even so, this basic premise forms part of a recent hypothesis that inflammation plays an integral role in drusen formation.

This inflammatory hypothesis of drusen biogenesis is based upon newer methods of drusen analysis that have revealed the exact composition of drusen more clearly. Histochemical and immunocytochemical studies have shown that drusen are composed of a variety of lipids, polysaccharides, GAGs and many proteins, including apoE and acute phase proteins such as C-reactive protein (CRP), fibrinogen, and vitronectin (9,10,92,163,170).

In one inflammatory model, it is proposed that the debris that accumulates in compromised RPE cells is the critical seeding event for drusen formation, the cellular debris constituting a chronic inflammatory stimulus that becomes the target of encapsulation by a variety of inflammatory mediators (10). This theory is supported by the presence of acute phase proteins and complement components such as C3 and C5 in drusen, as well as the finding that neural retina, RPE and choroidal cells are all capable of producing complement fragments that are required to initiate the complement cascade (8,163,170), resulting in the initiation of an inflammatory response.

Further evidence supporting the role of inflammation in the pathogenesis of AMD are recent linkage studies and genome wide scans that have identified several genetic variations [single nucleotide polymorphisms (SNPs)] within the complement factor H (*CFH*) gene that appear to greatly increase the risk of developing AMD (50,93,94,133). As *CFH* is a key regulator of the complement cascade that results in inflammation and the destruction of infected and dysplastic cells, defects in *CFH* as a result of these SNPs may result in excess stimulation of the complement cascade, thereby increasing cellular damage and subsequent drusen formation. This, in combination with the discovery of *CFH* in drusen, choroid and RPE using immunohistochemical methods in samples from patients with AMD, further strengthens an inflammatory hypothesis (93,133).

In addition to these findings, studies using immunocytochemistry, confocal imaging and other similar techniques have identified amyloid-beta (Aβ) in drusen, where the Aβ is co-localized with complement factors (11,45,117). Aβ is a major component of plaques in Alzheimer disease, another disease of aging where oxidative stress and inflammation are thought to play a part. As the formation of plaques in Alzheimer disease has been thought to be triggered by Aβ, the finding of this same protein in drusen both increases support for the inflammatory hypothesis and opens up further possibilities regarding their formation, such as a possible shared causation with Alzheimer disease.

Excess production/deposition theory: The second theory of drusen formation is based upon the idea that drusen material is shed as parcels of cytoplasm "pinched off" from the basal surface of the RPE. This "budding" is thought to be a means of either removing damaged cellular components or byproducts of phagocytic processing. This debris then accumulates with degradation and fragmentation of the budded portion (30,53,113,123,184,191). The unsaturated fatty acids from the photoreceptor outer segments are liable to free radical damage, particularly in the high oxygen tension of RPE and outer segments (235). It is postulated that the substrate for degradation may be altered by peroxidation, resulting in cross-linked compounds making them less susceptible to complete degradation by lysosomal enzymes and hence build up as drusen. The ability of highly active free radical scavenging systems in the outer retina to counteract this may alter with age (178).

Direct proteomic analysis of drusen has also revealed the presence of crosslinked common drusen proteins such as TIMP-3 and vitronectin, suggesting an oxidative basis to drusen development, where these proteins become crosslinked and bound to Bruch membrane, possibly as a result of reduced mechanisms in the retina to deal with oxidative stress as a result of aging (38). This finding may link both theories, with debris and bound down proteins from incomplete degradation being one of the stimuli for inflammation and drusen formation.

What is known is that the presence of drusen contributes to the overall risk of the development of advanced, sight-threatening AMD. However, at what stage the universal deposition of material with age becomes abnormal and predisposes to disease is not clear. The risk of visual loss in subjects with drusen has been estimated by several studies, the most recent being the large prospective age-related eye disease study (AREDS) study involving over 3000 subjects followed for five years. In this study, the area of retina affected by drusen had the highest correlation with progression to advanced AMD. Other risk factors included large drusen and the presence of pigmentary changes at the macula (42).

Large, prospective, population based studies have confirmed the progression of large drusen to advanced AMD. The Beaver Dam Eye study found that 14% of eyes with soft drusen developed advanced AMD over 10 years (130), the Blue Mountains Eye Study found that eyes with soft drusen were six times more likely to develop advanced AMD than those without soft drusen (230), and the Vision Impairment Project found a 9.5 times increased risk of progression in eyes with soft drusen or pigmentary abnormalities over five years (161).

Advanced AMD

There are two main subtypes of advanced AMD—"dry," or GA, and "wet," which includes CNV, pigment epithelial detachments and their complications, namely disciform scars.

Geographic Atrophy

GA is the end stage of atrophic, or "dry," AMD. Clinically, it has been defined as a well-demarcated, typically oval area of atrophy characterized by hypopigmentation due to the absence of the RPE that measures at least 175 μm in diameter. The absence of the RPE in these areas results in the increased visibility of the underlying choroidal vessels (Fig. 2).

Histologically, affected areas have an absence of RPE cells and photoreceptors, and in long standing cases, atrophy of the underlying choriocapillaris, characterized by a loss of the capillaries and attenuation or flattening of the larger vessels, is also seen. Areas bordering GA have a reduced number of photoreceptors with fragmented outer segments and stunted inner segments, whilst the RPE contains hyperpigmented cells alternating with attenuated cells.

The cause of GA is still to be fully elucidated. Earlier theories have proposed that the aging changes seen in the choriocapillaris and Bruch membrane (as discussed earlier) may affect water movement and reduce diffusion through Bruch membrane, resulting in a global reduction of metabolic exchange between the RPE and the choriocapillaris (55). Impairment of metabolic exchange between choroid and RPE could therefore compromise photoreceptor function and

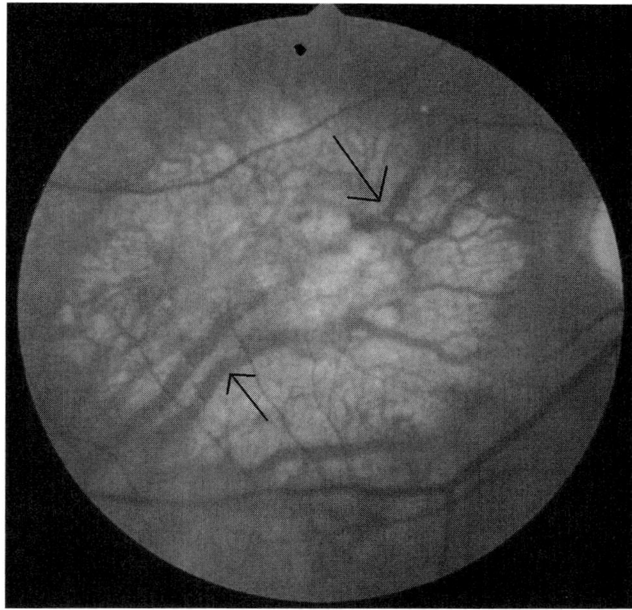

Figure 2 Geographic atrophy affecting the right eye. Note the increased visibility of the underlying choroidal vessels (*black arrows*) due to the absence of the retinal pigment epithelium.

eventually lead to cell death. This would lead initially to loss of retinal sensitivity seen in early AMD and subsequently to the loss of photoreceptors seen in GA (17,33). This concept is supported by the observation that patients with prolonged choroidal perfusion on their angiogram, which is thought to indicate diffuse thickening of Bruch membrane, are at three times greater risk of losing vision due to GA than in those without this clinical sign (180).

More recently, studies involving the measurement of RPE autofluorescence using the confocal laser scanning ophthalmoscope have revealed high levels of autofluorescence at the edges of GA, such areas then becoming atrophic within 1 year (108). Irregular autofluorescence in the unaffected eye of those with unilateral GA was also found to predict the later development of GA in the unaffected eye (108,109). As this autofluorescence is due to the accumulation of lipofuscin in the RPE, several theories have been proposed as to how this accumulation leads to RPE cell death and the resulting clinical appearance of GA.

One theory suggests that lipofuscin itself is toxic to RPE cells and leads directly to their death (19,109). This is based on the finding that lipofuscin is a photosensitizer and therefore may have direct cellular toxicity through its ability to act as a free radical generator (25). A2-E, a component of lipofuscin, has also been shown to be potentially toxic to RPE cells by causing the leakage of toxic intracellular lysosomes (200). The precipitating event in the development of GA in this model is RPE cell death, leading to photoreceptor death and later choriocapillaris atrophy. This sequence of events is further supported by studies that have shown the development of choroidal degeneration in areas where the RPE has been selectively destroyed (136).

Another theory postulates that the accumulation of lipofuscin potentiates RPE cell damage (79) and later death of both the RPE cell and its overlying photoreceptors (19,109). This is based on studies that found that A2-E can act as a lysosomal hydrolase inhibitor and therefore interfere with RPE lysosomal degradation (23,51,107). The inhibition of lysosomal enzymes has recently been shown in rats to increase the accumulation of lipofuscin in the RPE, which in turn decreases the ability of the RPE cells to recycle materials, leading to the shortening and loss of photoreceptor outer segments (167). These changes correlate well with the histological appearance of the retina on the edges of established GA in humans and in aging retina (as discussed previously).

Clinically, GA has been seen to develop de novo, in areas of fading drusen and in resolved RPE detachments (RPED). The most common pattern is the development of GA in areas of regressing drusen. In this pattern, focal, discrete areas of GA form in areas previously occupied by drusen and later enlarge and coalesce to often involve the fovea, resulting initially in paracentral scotomas and later, a central scotoma with marked visual acuity loss. RPED, which are covered in more detail below, can also eventually resolve or collapse, frequently resulting in a residual area of RPE atrophy.

Pigment Epithelial Detachments

Clinically, several different types of RPED have been described, including drusenoid, serous, hemorrhagic, and fibrovascular, the fibrovascular subtype being a form of occult CNV (see below) (16,31,97). The presence of large confluent hypofluorescent, hydrophobic soft drusen is a well recognized predisposing factor for the formation of RPED (36,80).

Drusenoid RPED is the result of the coalescence of large areas of soft drusen, resulting in the detachment of the overlying RPE and is not associated with new blood vessels. They are generally associated with a better prognosis than other types, as they tend to progress slowly without causing many visual symptoms. Over time, this type of RPED has been found to either remain stable as a persistent drusenoid RPED, but may progress to GA or CNV, resulting in severe visual loss (16,31,97,186).

Serous RPED are due to the accumulation of fluid beneath the RPE as a result of altered fluid dynamics across the RPE and Bruch membrane. This may be due to CNV, or altered permeability of Bruch membrane. Clinically, they appear as a well demarcated, dome shaped elevation of the RPE that transilluminates as a result of the fluid collection (Fig. 3). FA of these lesions reveals a characteristic, rapid hyperfluorescence within the RPED as it fills with fluorescein, followed by late pooling of the dye within the well-defined borders of the RPED (Fig. 4A, B). The natural history of this type of RPED tends to be worse than for drusenoid RPEDs, with far less remaining stable and a far greater percentage progressing to GA, CNV or a disciform scar (26). Hemorrhagic RPED are the result of hemorrhage from associated CNV, resulting in the collection of blood beneath the RPE. It should be noted, however, that a recently described entity, idiopathic polypoidal choroidal vasculopathy (IPCV), also causes hemorrhagic RPED, although it remains to be determined if IPCV is part of the AMD spectrum.

RPED as the result of CNV in "wet" AMD have been well described (68). In these cases, CNV develops in the sub-RPE space and may eventually result in excess fluid exudation, and occasionally hemorrhage, detaching the overlying RPE and neural retina. Clinically and angiographically, notched, or ring-like RPEDs are seen, depending on the site of exudation from the CNV (68).

In some cases, the RPE overlying the serous fluid may also become tense and rips, resulting in a denuded area as the free edge of the torn RPE rolls up upon itself. This is usually associated with a sudden, marked loss of vision. These rips are thought to result from tangential forces across the taut, elevated RPE, with the rip occurring at the junction between attached and detached RPE (80). Therefore, the most highly elevated type of RPEDs are the most likely to tear (36). RPE rips can also occur after photocoagulation (66), photodynamic therapy (22,56) or from contraction of an adjacent or associated CNV (67,80).

All RPEDs were initially postulated to result from an alteration in the physical attachment of the RPE from the progressive accumulation of debris on the inner surface of Bruch membrane. Fluid was then considered to accumulate beneath the RPE after passing through Bruch membrane from the

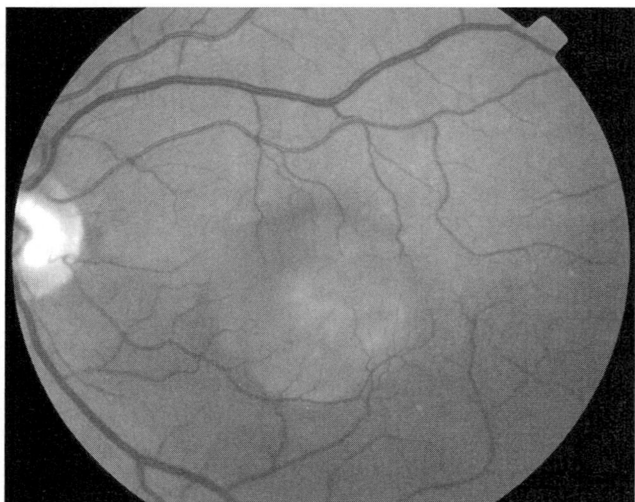

Figure 3 Serous detachment of the retinal pigment epithelium affecting the left eye.

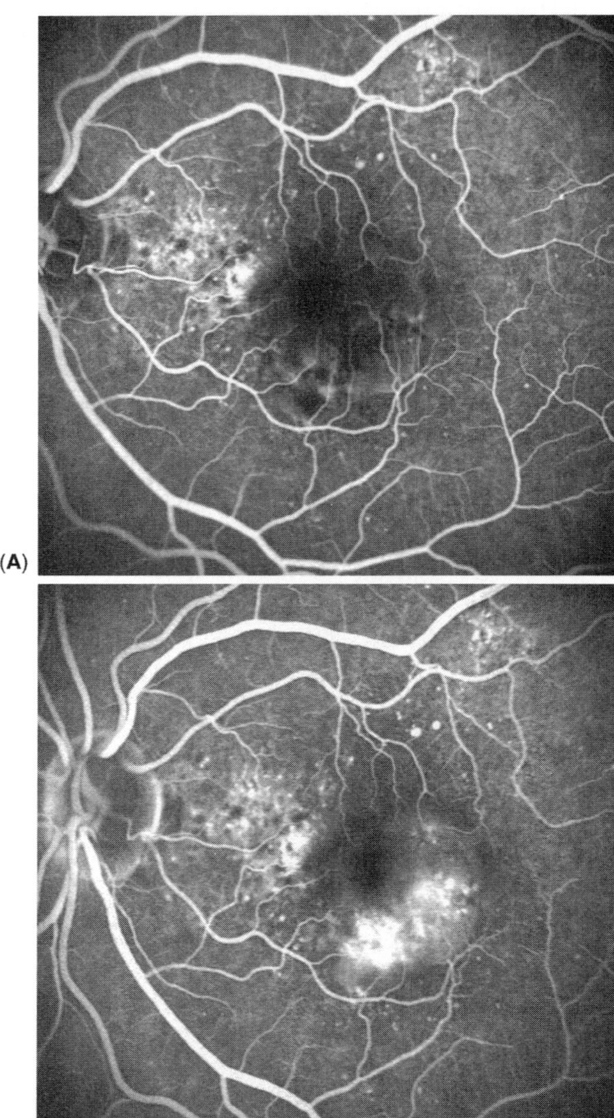

Figure 4 (**A**) Early phase of a FFA of the same serous RPED illustrated in Figure 3. (**B**) Late phase of the FFA demonstrating pooling of fluorescein within the RPED. *Abbreviations*: FFA, fundus fluorescein angiogram; RPED, retinal pigment epithelium detachment.

choriocapillaris (65). However, this explanation requires either high hydrostatic pressure in the choroid compared to the subretinal space or, alternatively, flow induced by an osmotic pressure gradient from the choroid into the subpigment epithelial space. The little evidence that exists does not support either of these proposals (57). Another proposal was that exudation from CNV growing through Bruch membrane provided an alternative source of sub-RPE fluid (67). However, CNV is not universal in RPEDs (13), implying that it is not always the initiating event in the pathogenesis of the lesion.

An alternative concept is that the sub-RPE fluid is derived from the vitreous rather than from the choroid (16). It is widely accepted that fluid is pumped from the vitreous through the retina into Bruch membrane due to active movement of ions by the RPE. Therefore, if Bruch membrane became hydrophobic due to lipid accumulation or other degenerative or aging changes discussed previously, then resistance to water flow could cause fluid to collect between the RPE and Bruch membrane.

It is evident that decreased hydraulic conductivity of Bruch membrane would be an essential prerequisite for fluid to accumulate in the sub-pigment epithelial space and such decreased conductivity has been demonstrated. A linear decrease in hydrophobic conductivity of Bruch membrane was demonstrated in samples obtained from human donors of increasing age (102). This is further supported by the observation that subjects with unilateral RPE rips are at an increased risk of a rip in the other eye (35), thereby implying that the same changes to Bruch membrane occur on both eyes.

Choroidal Neovascularization

The CNV is the process leading to "wet" AMD. It is the result of abnormal choroidal vessels growing through Bruch membrane and proliferating beneath either the RPE or the neurosensory retina. These abnormal vessels then either leak and/or bleed. The result is a rapid impairment of retinal function resulting in visual distortion and vision loss.

Histologically, CNV starts as an ingrowth of capillaries through Bruch membrane and are typically associated with basal laminar or linear deposits (78). With time, these capillaries mature into arteries and veins, followed by fibrosis (79,80). Gass initially subdivided CNV into two groups, based on where these vessels were found within the retina (69). CNV type I referred to vessels located in the sub-RPE space (between the RPE and Bruch membrane), whilst CNV type II were vessels located in the subsensory retinal space (between the neural retina and the underlying RPE). CNV type I was thought to be due to diseased RPE, where its attachment to the underlying Bruch membrane is loosened, thereby allowing vessels to infiltrate the sub-RPE space. This type of CNV was typically thought to occur in diseases such as AMD. CNV type II was attributed to conditions causing a breach in the RPE that allowed the ingrowth of vessels from the choroid into the sub-retinal space. Examples of this type of CNV included CNV secondary to laser burns, choroiditis scars (as in the ocular histoplasmosis syndrome (see Chapter 11), and past central serous retinopathy, where there has been a clear break in the RPE.

Clinically, the CNV is often seen as a grey-green membrane beneath the sensory retina. Serous detachment of the retina or subretinal hemorrhage is often associated, due to fluid leakage or hemorrhage from the CNV itself (Fig. 5). In severe bleeding, large areas of subretinal hemorrhage may occur (Fig. 6) (80) with associated sudden and catastrophic central visual loss. The blood may also extend into the vitreal cavity, resulting in a vitreal hemorrhage.

Based on the pattern of leakage from the abnormal vascular complex as seen on fundus FA, CNV is classified into "classic" and "occult" varieties, which are important when considering treatment options. "Classic" CNV are lesions with a well defined, often lacy hyperfluorescence in the early phases of the angiogram and late fluorescein leakage in the mid to late phases. In contrast, "occult" CNV is defined as either a fibrovascular RPE detachment or a lesion that demonstrates late-phase leakage from an undertermined source. Of these two types of CNV,

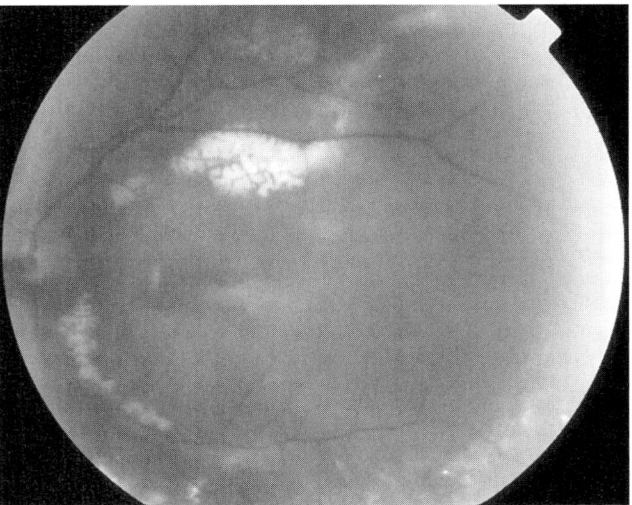

Figure 5 Fundus photograph of the left eye demonstrating a large serous retinal detachment secondary to choroidal neovascularization. Note the areas of hard exudate towards the periphery of the detachment.

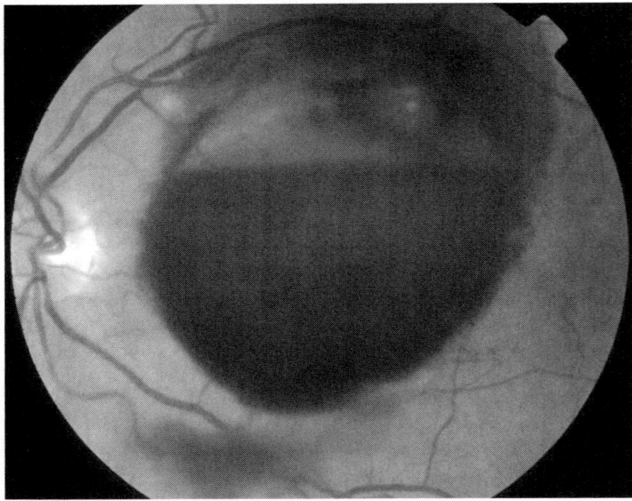

Figure 6 Large area of subhyaloid and associated subretinal hemorrhage resulting in severe central loss of vision.

predominantly classic lesions are usually thought to result in more rapid visual loss, whereas the progression of visual loss in mainly occult lesions tend to be more insidious. In both types of CNV, visual loss results from leakage from the newly formed blood vessels or hemorrhage or both.

With the advent of submacular surgery, when CNV is surgically excised from beneath the retina, correlation between the clinical and histological appearance of CNV in AMD has become possible. Several studies have now confirmed that well-defined, "classic" CNV on fundus fluorescein angiogram (FFA) correlates best with CNV type II, with the fibrovascular complex situated in the subretinal space; whilst ill-defined "occult" CNV on FFA corresponded best with CNV type I, where most fibrovascular tissue was located in the sub-RPE space (84,139). These studies also found that conditions resulting in a breach in the RPE were almost always associated with classic CNV type II, whilst CNV due to AMD could either be classic type II, occult type I, or a combination of both (27,83–85).

Histologic analyses of CNV with cell markers have disclosed that the cellular components of these membranes include RPE, inflammatory cells, vascular endothelium, glial cells, myofibroblasts and fibrocytes (82,145). Extracellular components have included several types of collagen (collagen types I, III, IV, and V), fibronectin, laminin, GAGs and lipid (82).

The formation of a disciform scar is always associated with poor central vision and is considered to be the end stage of CNV. Clinically, a disciform scar appears predominantly as pale, subretinal tissue (Fig. 7) and may be associated with serous and/or hemorrhagic detachment of the retina and RPE (79).

Histologically, disciform scars predominantly develop from CNV, where it is thought that leakage and hemorrhage from the abnormal vascular complex leads to fibrous tissue proliferation and a fibrovascular scar with endothelium lined vascular channels (79,145). The scar itself often has two components—one within layers of Bruch membrane and the other between the neural retina and RPE (79,80,195).

At present, the determinants of Bruch membrane changes that predispose to neovascularization are not clear. Inward growth of choroidal new vessels through Bruch membrane is the common endpoint in several retinal diseases leading to disciform scarring and visual loss. It is likely that blood vessel growth is suppressed by the metabolic environment of Bruch membrane, which is likely to be influenced by diffusible agents produced by the RPE (124,175). New vessel formation is thought to occur as a consequence of an imbalance in the stimulating and inhibiting influences of growth factors, and any disruption to their diffusion through Bruch membrane to the choroid could alter this balance (71,72).

Cells invading Bruch membrane may also alter it and release angiogenic factors. Macrophages increase in number (124) and are thought by some to be the factor common to all diseases with neovascularization (15). Macrophages promote the growth of endothelial cells, pericytes and fibroblasts, and macrophage derived prostaglandins, especially prostaglandin E, may be a strong stimulus to neovascularization (182). Activated macrophages secrete enzymes such as collagenases and elastases, and may erode Bruch membrane by a combination of mechanical disruption, phagocytosis, and extracellular release of

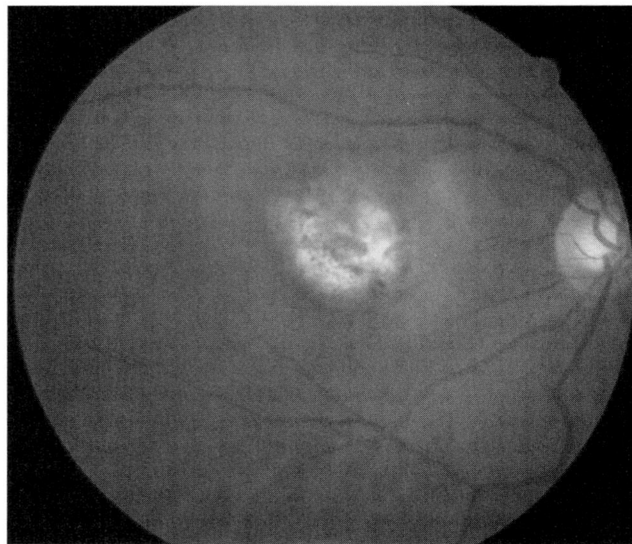

Figure 7 Disciform scar—end stage AMD. *Abbreviation*: AMD, age related macular degeneration.

enzymes. This erosion first involves the OCZ then the ICZ of Bruch membrane, with the elastic layer being more resistant. This cellular response with increasing age is not seen until Bruch membrane has membranous debris present beneath the RPE basement membrane and seems to occur preferentially beneath hard drusen. This may be related to the fact that the RPE is often anchored over hard drusen whilst it becomes separated from Bruch membrane by membranous soft deposits, so that any diffusible factors from the RPE will have maximal effect where it remains attached (124). Other cells such as monocytes, lymphocytes, fibroblasts and mast cells may also play a role in Bruch membrane damage and the promotion of new vessels to invade (100,174).

Endothelial cell processes have also been found to invade Bruch membrane normally (90) and perhaps angiogenesis is just an exaggeration of this normal phenomenon. Endothelial budding through the capillary basement membrane is the initial step in neovascularization in other human tissues. This budding is thought to be initiated by endothelial membrane-associated metalloproteinases that digest collagen types IV and V found in basement membranes (121). Endothelial cells also produce two proteases, plasminogen activator and latent collagenases that facilitate connective tissue invasion (100). The disruption of the basement membrane locally is believed to facilitate an outgrowth of capillary sprouts (121).

The mechanisms that initiate and modulate the normal rate of basement membrane dissolution and endothelial cell protrusion, and the conversion of this phenomenon to neovascularization are unknown. The choriocapillaris responds to its environment which has been amply demonstrated in vitro and in vivo (7,71,137). The process thereafter is likely to be determined by the relative concentrations of various growth factors, and the nature of the collagen and inter-fiber matrix of Bruch membrane. Some have suggested that the basement membrane may bind these factors, thereby modulating their immediate effect (72). Ample evidence suggests the existence in Bruch membrane of many factors with the potential to modify cell behavior (53,144,195,219).

Angiogenic growth factors that may have a role in the formation of CNV secondary to AMD thus far include vascular endothelial growth factor (VEGF), basic fibroblast growth factor (FGF2), nitric oxide, angiopoietins, and pigment epithelium-derived growth factor (PDGF). Of these, the role of VEGF appears to be the most prominent (see Chapter 68).

VEGF is a pro-angiogenic growth factor that is essential for normal embryonic tissue growth and is expressed by RPE cells in a paracrine fashion in the normal maintenance of the underlying choriocapillaris. However, abnormally increased levels of VEGF have been found to be responsible for the development of pathologic ocular neovascularization in conditions such as proliferative diabetic retinopathy. Elevated intra-ocular levels of VEGF have also been implicated in the development of CNV secondary to AMD (111,134,146). VEGF expression is increased by tissue hypoxia and oxidative stress, and these factors have also been implicated in the pathogenesis of AMD. However, the exact mechanism of VEGF over-expression in AMD remains to be fully elucidated.

Nevertheless, treatments aimed at reducing intra-ocular levels of VEGF in the form of various anti-VEGF monoclonal antibodies have recently been tested in multi-center, controlled clinical trials with some efficacy in the treatment of CNV in AMD (77). This success suggests that VEGF and other angiogenic growth factors play a significant role in the propagation and possibly the initiation of CNV.

These considerations imply that CNV as part of age-related macular disease may occur as a distortion of a normal mechanism, rather than as a process unique to the aging eye.

ETIOLOGY AND PATHOGENESIS

The cause and pathogenesis of AMD is still unknown. Several theories have been proposed and the most widely considered are discussed below. The general consensus is that AMD has a multi-factorial causation, where both genetic and environmental factors play a part.

Genetics

AMD is generally regarded as a complex genetic disorder wherein environmental risk factors impact on a genetic background. The genetic basis of AMD has really only been established over the last 15–20 years. There is now abundant evidence from family, sibling and twin studies to support a genetic basis for AMD.

Other conditions with established Mendelian inheritance and phenotypic features in common with AMD have also been investigated and the causative genes found, with the hope that the genes responsible for these diseases would also be good candidate genes for AMD. These include Sorsby fundus dystrophy (MIM #136900; *TIMP3* gene) (232), Stargardt disease (MIM #248200; *ABCA4* gene) (6) and Best disease (MIM #153700; *VMD2*/Bestrophin gene) (see Chapter 35) (179). Unfortunately, none of the causative genes found in each of these diseases has been conclusively linked to the pathogenesis of AMD.

Other diseases where the phenotype is most similar to AMD are Doyne honeycomb retinal dystrophy (MIM #126600), which is characterized by drusen at the macula as well as around the optic nerve head, and Malattia levantinese (MIM #126600), where drusen form a classic radial pattern at the macula. Investigation into these conditions have revealed that the same genetic mutation results in both phenotypic forms, with Doyne honeycomb retinal dystrophy and Malattia levantinese sharing the same gene mutation on chromosome 2 (81,99). The *FBLN3* (*EFEMP1*) gene that encodes for fibulin 3 (also known as the epidermal growth factor containing fibrillin-like ECM protein-1) has been found to accumulate within and beneath RPE cells in the areas of drusen seen in Malattia levantinese and Doyne honeycomb retinal dystrophy (154). This accumulation is due to misfolding of the mutant protein, resulting in its impaired secretion from the RPE. However, mutations of the *FBLN3* gene do not appear to have a role in typical AMD.

Further research has implicated other genes in the fibulin family, especially those that code for fibulin 5 (*FBLN5*) and fibulin 6 (*FBLN6*) in AMD. The fibulins are a family of proteins involved in the organization and stability of various extracellular proteins, including elastin, which is a major component of Bruch membrane (see Chapter 36). A study on one large family with an AMD phenotype revealed a mutation in *FBLN6* (199).

More recent research has disclosed missense mutations in the *FBLN5* gene, which is involved in the binding and organization of elastin fibers (118). Such mutations have been found in association with cutis laxa (MIM #219100), a connective tissue disease characterized by loose skin and variable systemic involvement (143,157). An analysis for sequence variations in five members of the fibulin gene family in a large group of AMD subjects revealed that a missense mutation in *FBLN5* was associated with a particular phenotype of AMD characterized by basal laminar drusen and varying degrees of RPED (213). This suggests that this molecular abnormality may result in alterations in the ECM of Bruch membrane, thereby impairing the attachment of RPE to it and also predisposing to the formation of drusen. However, only seven out of 402 cases of AMD were identified as having this mutation. Although another study has identified other missense mutations in this same gene in patients with AMD, these were only identified in three out of 514 cases (147). Therefore the possible association of mutations in the *FBLN5* gene in AMD still requires further investigation.

The first gene to be relatively consistently linked to AMD was the apolipoprotein E (*APOE*) gene, which has also been associated with Alzheimer disease and cardiovascular disease. Studies have shown that the presence of the E4 alleles of the *APOE* gene decreases the risk of AMD, suggesting a protective effect, whilst the presence of the E2 alleles may increase the risk of AMD. These allelic associations are opposite to those found in cardiovascular disease and Alzheimer disease, where the E4 alleles appears to be the "at risk" allele whilst the E2 alleles is protective. The significance of this finding is unexplained.

Although apoE is associated with the RPE, and Bruch membrane and apoE immunoreactivity occurs in most types of drusen (9), exactly how the *APOE* gene is involved in the pathogenesis of AMD is still unclear, with further research needed to establish how the alleles interact in the lipid pathway to influence AMD development. However, recent findings in a murine model where aged mice with an *APOE* phenotype were fed a high fat, cholesterol rich diet were found to develop lesions mimicking human AMD further supports a role of the *APOE* gene in AMD pathogenesis (150), and the existence of this animal model will allow further research into its role.

More recently, several groups have identified a number of genetic variations, known as SNPs (see Chapter 31) within the *CFH* gene on chromosome 1 (1q32) that appears to greatly increase an individual's risk of developing AMD (50,93,94,133). Previous genome wide studies identified chromosome 1 (1q32) as being likely to carry a candidate gene for AMD (1,116,233) and subsequently several research teams have confirmed this link between *CFH* and AMD. A further large, prospective, population-based study has also confirmed these findings, where the presence of the allele *CFH* Y402H increased the risk of all types of AMD, particularly in those >75 years of age and homozygotes (46).

Furthermore, other genes associated with the complement pathway have since been found that may also be associated with AMD, namely the complement factor B and complement component two genes (74). A hypothetical gene, *LOC387715*, has also been proposed to play a role, particularly in smokers (198).

Overall, the *CFH* gene has the strongest association with AMD thus far and adds weight to the hypothesis that uncontrolled inflammation plays a role in the pathogenesis of AMD.

Environmental Risk Factors

The greatest risks for developing AMD are increasing age and a family history of AMD (207,210). The most consistently found modifiable risk factor, however, is smoking, where there is a two to five times increased risk of incident AMD, or progression from early AMD to CNV in current smokers (156,207,210). Other studies have implicated hypertension, carotid/cardiovascular disease, and high cholesterol levels (2,148,156,210,225).

Several large population based studies have demonstrated that smoking is associated with AMD

(156,207). In one study, a dose-response relationship was demonstrated between neovascular AMD and smoking (226), whilst another found that people who smoked more were more likely to show progression of their AMD (131). This risk decreases once a smoker ceases smoking (129,226). To date, smoking represents the most important, and only universally agreed upon modifiable risk factor for AMD.

Evidence linking AMD to systemic hypertension are conflicting. Some studies have found that the prevalence of early AMD progressively increased in relationship to the duration of systemic hypertension (211) or elevated systolic or diastolic blood pressure (75,224). The AREDS, indicated a positive association between diastolic BP, history of hypertension and use of anti-hypertensive medication, with wet AMD but not dry AMD (112). The Macular Photocoagulation Study Group found in a prospective study that patients with unilateral CNV were more likely to experience progression of CNV in the fellow eye if they were hypertensive (149). However, a number of more recent studies have failed to confirm any significant link between AMD and hypertension (44,104,127,208).

Several studies (Blue Mountains Eye Study, Beaver Dam Eye Study, and the French "Pathologies Oculaires Liees a l'Age" study) have found a positive relationship between early AMD and a high body mass index (BMI) (44,104,125,197,208).

A number of studies have also linked increased cholesterol or total dietary fat intake to both early and late AMD when analyzed as the risk associated with the highest versus lowest quartiles of intake (112,152,202,203). Conversely, increased intake of long chain omega-3 poly unsaturated fatty acids and fish have been associated with reduced risk of early AMD (202,209).

Although AMD shares risk factors with atherosclerosis, the actual association between AMD and atherosclerosis is inconsistent. Some studies have demonstrated positive links between AMD and atherosclerosis (32,223,225). An example is the Rotterdam Eye Study that demonstrated a positive association between AMD and carotid artery atherosclerotic plaques (225), a finding that is supported by other studies linking AMD to cardiovascular disease and cerebrovascular disease (32,223). However, other studies have found no such association (44,125,149,209,218).

Theories of Causation

Vascular Theory

Friedman (59) was one of the first to propose a hemodynamic model for AMD. In this model, AMD is a vascular disorder characterized by the impairment of choroidal perfusion of the RPE, resulting in the failure of the choriocapillaris to clear lipoproteins produced by the RPE (59,60,62,63). The result is considered to be an accumulation of lipoproteins as basal deposits and drusen in Bruch membrane.

This model also suggests that there is a progressive accumulation of lipid in ocular tissues such as sclera and Bruch membrane, occurring as a general aging change that results in decreased compliance of ocular tissues and an unduly rigid Bruch membrane that is more prone to breakage and fracture. This is based on the theory that the major layers of the eye wall are analogous to those of the arterial wall, as both share the same connective tissues (elastin and collagen) (62), with Bruch membrane being equivalent to the wall of a capillary. This notion was supported by Curcio et al. (39), who described Bruch membrane as a specialized arterial intima based on its aging changes and lipid deposition, as both the arterial intima and Bruch membrane are located between two diffusion barriers (the endothelial cell and elastic lamina for the arterial intima, and the choriocapillaris endothelium and RPE for Bruch membrane). This was based upon their finding that Bruch membrane accumulates esterified and non-esterified fatty acids in a linear manner with increasing age, much like the arterial intima. Therefore, the aging changes seen in Bruch membrane and the lipid accumulation in ocular tissues are thought to be analogous to the accumulation of lipid and stiffening of large systemic arteries seen in atherosclerosis.

An added consequence of the stiffening of ocular tissues and blood vessels is thought to be impaired choroidal perfusion from decreased ocular blood flow and elevated hydrostatic pressure across the choriocapillaris. The result is further lipid deposition. This, in combination with breaks in Bruch membrane and VEGF, is thought to cause CNV (63).

The strengths of this model is that it neatly explains the association between cardiovascular disease (CVD) and AMD, as both have been found to share similar risk factors (hypertension, smoking, obesity, and high dietary fat intake), with some studies showing an increased prevalence of AMD in those with CVD (2,148,156,210,225). Decreased choroidal blood flow and increased lipid content of Bruch membrane with increasing age has also been well documented (34,37,61,86,87,159,160).

However, increased hydrostatic pressure in the choriocapillaris and increased scleral rigidity has not yet been conclusively demonstrated, nor does this model explain the racial differences in the incidence of AMD. The link between AMD and CVD and their risk factors is also yet to be conclusively proven.

Oxidation Theory

Cumulative oxidative damage has been implicated in many age related diseases with oxidative stress accepted by many as a reasonable basis for the aging process. It is not surprising, therefore that these same processes have been implicated in the pathogenesis of AMD.

Oxidative damage to tissues results from the production of reactive oxygen intermediates that include free radicals, hydrogen peroxide, superoxide anion and singlet oxygen. Reactive oxygen intermediates are produced during oxidative metabolism and photochemical reactions. Their production is particularly increased by irradiation exposure, aging and inflammation. These reactive oxygen intermediates, when generated, are able to cause cytoplasmic and nuclear damage. This damage includes processes such as protein cross-linking and fragmentation, DNA oxidation and alterations, and degradation of cellular membranes, which are particularly susceptible to oxidation due to their high polyunsaturated fatty acid (PUFA) content (photoreceptor outer segments have a PUFA content of approximately 50%). An accumulation of reactive oxygen intermediates are thought to trigger cell death via apoptosis (236,237).

Several factors combined expose the retina to a high production of reactive oxygen intermediates, placing it at particularly high risk of cumulative oxidative damage. Firstly, it has the highest metabolic demand and oxygen consumption of any tissue. Due to the nature of its function, the retina has a high irradiation/light exposure and contains many photosensitizers, or chromophores such as rhodopsin, melanin and lipofuscin. Also, the process of phagocytosis and recycling of shed photoreceptors discs is an oxidative process in itself.

Several antioxidant processes protect the retina from its high exposure to reactive oxygen intermediates. Common antioxidants found in most cells are the water soluble vitamin C and glutathione, whilst the main lipid soluble antioxidants are vitamin E and carotenoids. In the retina, the most prominent of these are the macular pigments, lutein and zeaxanthin. These pigments quench singlet oxygen but also have their greatest absorption peak in the short wavelength (blue light) spectrum of visible light. This is thought to protect the RPE from oxidative damage as blue light has been implicated in the increased oxidative toxicity of lipofuscin (see below). The progressive accumulation of cellular damage therefore occurs when these native antioxidants become overwhelmed by the rate of production of free radicals.

Several animal experiments have shown that photo-oxidative damage may play a role in the pathogenesis of AMD. One of the first was by Wiegand et al., when albino rats were exposed to constant illumination (234). This resulted in the selective destruction of retinal photoreceptors due to damage and loss of their PUFA content. Other studies have since shown similar findings from constant illumination (76,165) leading to the suggestion that long-term exposure to sunlight may lead to the development of AMD via the accumulation of photo-oxidative damage to photoreceptors, choriocapillaris and the RPE.

Further clinical evidence that may support this mechanism is the finding that those with a past history of cataract surgery may have a higher risk of progressing to end stage AMD in comparison to those who had not had surgery (58,231). Mechanisms that have been proposed to account for this include a possible increased exposure and susceptibility of the eye to phototoxic damage and post-operative inflammation resulting in the induction of angiogenesis (128,216,221). These findings, however, are far from conclusive with other studies having conflicting results (12). In addition, as most of these studies were population based observational studies, their results do not exclude the possibility that end-stage AMD and cataracts may share other common, unaccounted for risk factors.

Aside from the direct toxicity via the reactive oxygen intermediates, particularly superoxide anions, lipofuscin is a photosensitizer and it has been implicated in direct cellular toxicity. Production of these anions has been found to be greatest when lipofuscin is exposed to short wavelength (blue) light. From these findings, it appears that the accumulation of lipofuscin by the RPE with increasing age is detrimental to the tissue itself, as it leads to further oxidative damage, compromise and possibly, an increased risk of progressing to AMD (188,189). Studies with cultured RPE cells have supported this theory, where blue light exposure in combination with lipofuscin resulted in the loss of cells and signs of RPE cellular stress (membrane blebbing and increased vacuolation) in those cells that remained (236). It is interesting to note that these morphologic changes mirror those seen with aging.

RPE cellular stress as a result of cumulative oxidation damage due to high internal production of reactive oxygen intermediates has also been proposed as a possible mechanism that may lead to AMD through the gradual loss of RPE cells. As already mentioned, central to the function of RPE cells is the phagocytosis and recycling of photoreceptor outer segments, a process that creates high oxidative stress. It is thought that this may in turn lead to eventual damage of mitochondrial membranes, thereby triggering RPE cell death via apoptosis (236).

All of these oxidative theories point towards a possible common pathway for the development of AMD where native antioxidant properties are exhausted or overwhelmed by the volume of free radicals produced, leading to a progressive accumulation of oxidative damage within retinal cells and eventual cell death. Clinical research has therefore been focussed on the possible beneficial effect of increasing retinal stores of antioxidants.

Epidemiological data regarding the possible protective effect of a diet rich in antioxidants have been conflicting (52,151,153,218,222). More recently, a large randomized controlled trial of high dose dietary supplements of antioxidant vitamins C, E, and beta-carotene in combination with zinc and copper (the AREDS study) has reported a small benefit in preventing the vision threatening complications of AMD in a subgroup of people with AMD (2). The doses used in this study were 500 mg vitamin C, 400 IU vitamin E, 15 mg beta-carotene, 80 mg zinc, and 2 mg copper daily. Benefit in the numbers progressing to CNV was seen in only one subgroup of subjects, those considered to be at greatest risk of progressing. The findings from this study and the benefits of mass subscribing of these supplements are however subject to debate (70, 142,205).

No benefits were seen for subjects in any of the earlier stages of the disease, and there was an increase, albeit not significant, in the rate of development of GA in the treated group. This formulation should also not be given to smokers, as two large Scandinavian studies have found that beta-carotene increases their risk of developing lung cancer (4,168,169). After this became known smokers in the AREDS study were no longer retained in a test group receiving beta-carotene. There may also be some reason to be concerned about the long term, high dietary supplementation of zinc (110,190,214). Consequently, the long term benefits of these antioxidant dietary supplements are far from definitive.

Research has also been directed toward dietary supplements of the macular pigments lutein and zeaxanthin, which are the main components of the pigment found at the macula and have antioxidant and blue light-filtering properties. Recent population studies have shown that patients with higher plasma levels of lutein and zeaxanthin had half the risk of both early and late AMD in comparison to those with low plasma levels (52,64). Subjects with a high dietary intake of spinach and collard greens (dark-green leafy vegetables) that are rich in carotenoids also had a significantly lower risk of wet AMD (201) It is noteworthy that this effect has not been shown with carrots, which are low in lutein and zeaxanthin., despite being an important source of carotenoids with vitamin A activity. In addition, people with a greater macular pigment density have been found to retain more visual sensitivity at an older age (96). Whilst dietary supplementation of lutein and zeaxanthin has been shown to increase macular pigment density (95), results of prospective treatment trials are required before any definite conclusions can be made and such trials are currently being planned.

Inflammation

Inflammation has been recently implicated in a number of degenerative diseases associated with aging, including atherosclerosis and Alzheimer disease (3,73,92,172,177,187). The role of inflammation in AMD pathogenesis is a rapidly evolving area, particularly with the *CFH* gene discovery in 2005, and has been reviewed extensively (92,177).

A number of recent epidemiological studies have found an association between AMD and increased levels of blood inflammatory markers. For example, AMD has been linked to high leukocyte count (20,127), high plasma fibrinogen level (208), oxidized LDL, and elevated CRP (204).

With regard to CRP, elevated levels of this inflammatory marker have been found to be an independent risk factor for the development of CVD (138,141) and recently it has been associated with increased risk of advanced AMD (204). This further implicates the possible role of inflammation in the pathogenesis in both of these diseases, particularly given the direct pro-inflammatory actions of CRP on vascular endothelial cells (141).

The role of inflammation as a possible basis for the development of AMD has already been discussed with regard to drusen formation, where two inflammatory cell types—macrophage and dendritic cells—may play a role in AMD pathogenesis. Immunohistochemical analyses suggest the presence of both of these cells in the core of drusen (92,162). In atherosclerosis, oxidized LDL is thought to be the stimulus which causes activation of dendritic cells and macrophages, leading to inflammation and eventually pathologic changes (73,187). Hageman et al. proposed that a similar initial event may occur in drusen biogenesis leading to chronic inflammation (92).

A number of drusen-associated constituents are also active participants in the humoral and cellular immune response (92). Autoantibodies have been detected in the sera of AMD patients, some of which are directed specifically against drusen, RPE and retina components (88,92,176). Inflammatory cells may be involved in the breakdown of Bruch membrane, RPE atrophy, and CNV (177). Accumulation of inflammatory cells has also been demonstrated in choroidal vessels associated with drusen and disciform scars (78,177).

Macrophages may also have a role in the genesis of CNV (89,177), and it is their high sensitivity to oxygen tension (135) that has made some authors suggest that tissue hypoxia secondary to vascular compromise could be the initiating event causing macrophage accumulation and stimulation of angiogenesis (177). The role of macrophages in the erosion of the Bruch membrane via the secretion of proteolytic enzymes has already been discussed. This, in combination with their ability to secrete angiogenic growth factors and interact with VEGF and intercellular adhesion molecules further strengthens the theory that such inflammatory cells may have a key role in the genesis of CNV.

Several papers have reported a possible protective effect of statins in AMD, as this class of drug has anti-inflammatory effects in addition to their lipid lowering properties (91).

The recent finding implicating the *CFH* gene in AMD (50,93,94,133) greatly strengthens the inflammatory theory of AMD, as SNPs within this gene could result in decreased regulation of the complement cascade and uncontrolled inflammation. Further, supporting genetic findings in favor of this inflammatory theory is the recent link between variants encoding Toll-like receptor 4 (a key mediator in pro-inflammatory pathways that provides a link between innate and adaptive immunity) and an increased susceptibility to developing AMD (238). In addition, a recent large, prospective population-based study has found that not only did the presence of the *CFH* gene increase the risk of all forms of AMD, this risk increased exponentially in those who had the SNP and were also smokers (46). As smoking is known to activate the complement pathway, the progression of AMD in those with impaired *CFH* may therefore be accelerated. These findings add further weight to the theory that AMD may have an inflammatory pathogenesis.

However, what triggers the inflammatory pathway is still not known. The fact that the *CFH* gene is involved in the alternative complement pathway has led some to speculate that organisms may act as a trigger, and indeed some work has implicated Chlamydia in AMD (115,119,120,185). It is possible that a number of organisms could be the trigger that activates the alternate complement pathway which is then unable to terminate effectively in those with defective *CFH*, leading to chronic inflammation and disease. We await further research into the triggers of this inflammatory process.

REFERENCES

1. Abecasis GR, Yashar BM, Zhao Y, et al. Age-related macular degeneration: a high-resolution genome scan for susceptibility loci in a population enriched for late-stage disease. Am J Hum Genet 2004; 74:482–94.
2. Age-Related Eye Disease Study Research Group. A randomized, placebo-controlled, clinical trial of high-dose supplementation with vitamins C and E, beta carotene, and zinc for age-related macular degeneration and vision loss: AREDS report no. 8. Arch Ophthalmol 2001; 119:1417–36.
3. Akiyama H, Barger S, Barnum S, et al. Inflammation and Alzheimer's disease. Neurobiol Aging 2000; 21: 383–421.
4. Albanes D, Heinonen OP, Taylor PR, et al. Alpha-tocopherol and beta-carotene supplements and lung cancer incidence in the alpha-tocopherol, beta-carotene cancer prevention study: effects of base-line characteristics and study compliance. J Natl Cancer Inst 1996; 88: 1560–70.
5. Alexander RA, Garner A. Elastic and precursor fibres in the normal human eye. Exp Eye Res 1983; 36:305–15.
6. Allikmets R, Singh N, Sun H, et al. A photoreceptor cell-specific ATP-binding transporter gene (ABCR) is mutated in recessive stargardt macular dystrophy. Nat Genet 1997; 15:236–46.
7. Anand-Apte B, Pepper MS, Voest E, et al. Inhibition of angiogenesis by tissue inhibitor of metalloproteinase-3. Invest Ophthalmol Vis Sci 1997; 38:817–23.
8. Anderson DH, Hageman GS, Mullins RF, et al. Vitronectin gene expression in the adult human retina. Invest Ophthalmol Vis Sci 1999; 40:3305–15.
9. Anderson DH, Ozaki S, Nealon M, et al. Local cellular sources of apolipoprotein E in the human retina and retinal pigmented epithelium: implications for the process of drusen formation. Am J Ophthalmol 2001; 131: 767–81.
10. Anderson DH, Mullins RF, Hageman GS, Johnson LV. A role for local inflammation in the formation of drusen in the aging eye. Am J Ophthalmol 2002; 134:411–31.
11. Anderson DH, Talaga KC, Rivest AJ, et al. Characterization of beta amyloid assemblies in drusen: the deposits associated with aging and age-related macular degeneration. Exp Eye Res 2004; 78:243–56.
12. Armbrecht AM, Findlay C, Aspinall PA, et al. Cataract surgery in patients with age-related macular degeneration: one-year outcomes. J Cataract Refract Surg 2003; 29: 686–93.
13. Barondes MJ, Pagliarini S, Chisholm IH, et al. Controlled trial of laser photocoagulation of pigment epithelial detachments in the elderly: 4 year review. Br J Ophthalmol 1992; 76:5–7.
14. Bazan HE, Bazan NG, Feeney-Burns L, Berman ER. Lipids in human lipofuscin-enriched subcellular fractions of two age populations. Comparison with rod outer segments and neural retina. Invest Ophthalmol Vis Sci 1990; 31:1433–43.
15. BenEzra D. Neovasculogenic ability of prostaglandins, growth factors, and synthetic chemoattractants. Am J Ophthalmol 1978; 86:455–61.
16. Bird AC, Marshall J. Retinal pigment epithelial detachments in the elderly. Trans Ophthalmol Soc UK 1986; 105: 674–82.
17. Bird AC. Doyne Lecture. Pathogenesis of retinal pigment epithelial detachment in the elderly; the relevance of Bruch's membrane change. Eye 1991; 5(Pt. 1):1–12.
18. Bird AC, Bressler NM, Bressler SB, et al. An international classification and grading system for age-related maculopathy and age-related macular degeneration. The International ARM Epidemiological Study Group. Surv Ophthalmol 1995; 39:367–74.
19. Bird AC. The Bowman lecture: towards an understanding of age-related macular disease. Eye 2003; 17:457–66.
20. Blumenkranz MS, Russell SR, Robey MG, et al. Risk factors in age-related maculopathy complicated by choroidal neovascularization. Ophthalmology 1986; 93:552–8.

21. Bok D. Retinal photoreceptor-pigment epithelium interactions: Friedenwald lecture. Invest Ophthalmol Vis Sci 1985; 26:1659–94.
22. Boscia F, Furino C, Sborgia L, et al. Photodynamic therapy for retinal angiomatous proliferations and pigment epithelium detachment. Am J Ophthalmol 2004; 138:1077–9.
23. Boulton M, McKechnie NM, Breda J, et al. The formation of autofluorescent granules in cultured human RPE. Invest Ophthalmol Vis Sci 1989; 30:82–9.
24. Boulton M, Docchio F, Dayhaw-Barker P, et al. Age-related changes in the morphology, absorption and fluorescence of melanosomes and lipofuscin granules of the retinal pigment epithelium. Vision Res 1990; 30: 1291–303.
25. Boulton M, Dontsov A, Jarvis-Evans J, et al. Lipofuscin is a photoinducible free radical generator. J Photochem Photobiol B 1993; 19:201–4.
26. Braunstein RA, Gass JD. Serous detachments of the retinal pigment epithelium in patients with senile macular disease. Am J Ophthalmol 1979; 88:652–60.
27. Bressler NM, Bressler SB, Gragoudas ES. Clinical characteristics of choroidal neovascular membranes. Arch Ophthalmol 1987; 105:209–13.
28. Bressler NM, Silva JC, Bressler SB, et al. Clinicopathologic correlation of drusen and retinal pigment epithelial abnormalities in age-related macular degeneration. Retina 1994; 14:130–42.
29. Buch H, Nielsen NV, Vinding T, et al. 14-year incidence, progression, and visual morbidity of age-related maculopathy: the Copenhagen city eye study. Ophthalmology 2005; 112:787–98.
30. Burns RP, Feeney-Burns L. Clinico-morphologic correlations of drusen of Bruch's membrane. Trans Am Ophthalmol Soc 1980; 78:206–25.
31. Casswell AG, Kohen D, Bird AC. Retinal pigment epithelial detachments in the elderly: classification and outcome. Br J Ophthalmol 1985; 69:397–403.
32. Chaine G, Hullo A, Sahel J, et al. Case-control study of the risk factors for age related macular degeneration. France-DMLA Study Group. Br J Ophthalmol 1998; 82: 996–1002.
33. Chen JC, Fitzke FW, Pauleikhoff D, Bird AC. Functional loss in age-related Bruch's membrane change with choroidal perfusion defect. Invest Ophthalmol Vis Sci 1992; 33:334–40.
34. Chen SJ, Cheng CY, Lee AF, et al. Pulsatile ocular blood flow in asymmetric exudative age related macular degeneration. Br J Ophthalmol 2001; 85:1411–5.
35. Chuang EL, Bird AC. Bilaterality of tears of the retinal pigment epithelium. Br J Ophthalmol 1988; 72:918–20.
36. Chuang EL, Bird AC. The pathogenesis of tears of the retinal pigment epithelium. Am J Ophthalmol 1988; 105:285–90.
37. Ciulla TA, Harris A, Kagemann L, et al. Choroidal perfusion perturbations in non-neovascular age related macular degeneration. Br J Ophthalmol 2002; 86:209–13.
38. Crabb JW, Miyagi M, Gu X, et al. Drusen proteome analysis: an approach to the etiology of age-related macular degeneration. Proc Natl Acad Sci USA 2002; 99:14682–7.
39. Curcio CA, Millican CL, Bailey T, Kruth HS. Accumulation of cholesterol with age in human Bruch's membrane. Invest Ophthalmol Vis Sci 2001; 42:265–74.
40. Curcio CA, Presley JB, Malek G, et al. Esterified and unesterified cholesterol in drusen and basal deposits of eyes with age-related maculopathy. Exp Eye Res 2005; 81:731–41.
41. Curcio CA, Presley JB, Millican CL, Medeiros NE. Basal deposits and drusen in eyes with age-related maculopathy: evidence for solid lipid particles. Exp Eye Res 2005; 80:761–75.
42. Davis MD, Gangnon RE, Lee LY, et al. The Age-Related Eye Disease Study severity scale for age-related macular degeneration: AREDS Report No. 17. Arch Ophthalmol 2005; 123:1484–98.
43. Deguchi J, Yamamoto A, Yoshimori T, et al. Acidification of phagosomes and degradation of rod outer segments in rat retinal pigment epithelium. Invest Ophthalmol Vis Sci 1994; 35:568–79.
44. Delcourt C, Michel F, Colvez A, et al. Associations of cardiovascular disease and its risk factors with age-related macular degeneration: the POLA study. Ophthalmic Epidemiol 2001; 8:237–49.
45. Dentchev T, Milam AH, Lee VM, et al. Amyloid-beta is found in drusen from some age-related macular degeneration retinas, but not in drusen from normal retinas. Mol Vis 2003; 9:184–90.
46. Despriet DD, Klaver CC, Witteman JC, et al. Complement factor H polymorphism, complement activators, and risk of age-related macular degeneration. J Am Med Assoc 2006; 296:301–9.
47. Docchio F, Boulton M, Cubeddu R, et al. Age-related changes in the fluorescence of melanin and lipofuscin granules of the retinal pigment epithelium: a time-resolved fluorescence spectroscopy study. Photochem Photobiol 1991; 54:247–53.
48. Donders F. Beitrage zur pathologischen Anatomie des Auges. Albrecht von Graefes Archiv. fur Ophthalmologie 1855; 2:106–18.
49. Dorey CK, Wu G, Ebenstein D, et al. Cell loss in the aging retina. Relationship to lipofuscin accumulation and macular degeneration. Invest Ophthalmol Vis Sci 1989; 30:1691–9.
50. Edwards AO, Ritter R III, Abel KJ, et al. Complement factor H polymorphism and age-related macular degeneration. Science 2005; 308:421–4.
51. Eldred GE, Lasky MR. Retinal age pigments generated by self-assembling lysosomotropic detergents. Nature 1993; 361:724–6.
52. Eye Disease Case-Control Study Group. Antioxidant status and neovascular age-related macular degeneration. Arch Ophthalmol 1993; 111:104–9.
53. Feeney-Burns L, Ellersieck MR. Age-related changes in the ultrastructure of Bruch's membrane. Am J Ophthalmol 1985; 100:686–97.
54. Feeney-Burns L, Gao CL, Tidwell M. Lysosomal enzyme cytochemistry of human RPE, Bruch's membrane and drusen. Invest Ophthalmol Vis Sci 1987; 28:1138–47.
55. Fisher RF. The influence of age on some ocular basement membranes. Eye 1987; 1(Pt. 2):184–9.
56. Fossarello M, Peiretti E, Zucca I, Serra A. Unfavorable effect of photodynamic therapy for late subretinal neovascularization with chorioretinal anastomoses associated with idiopathic multiple serous detachments of the retinal pigment epithelium. Eur J Ophthalmol 2004; 14:568–71.
57. Foulds WS. Doyne Memorial Lecture, 1976: clinical significance of trans-scleral fluid transfer. Trans Ophthalmol Soc UK 1976; 96:290–308.
58. Freeman EE, Munoz B, West SK, et al. Is there an association between cataract surgery and age-related macular degeneration?: data from three population-based studies. Am J Ophthalmol 2003; 135: 849–56.

59. Friedman E, Smith TR, Kuwabara T. Senile choroidal vascular patterns and drusen. Arch Ophthalmol 1963; 69:220–30.
60. Friedman E, Ivry M, Ebert E, et al. Increased scleral rigidity and age-related macular degeneration. Ophthalmology 1989; 96:104–8.
61. Friedman E, Krupsky S, Lane AM, et al. Ocular blood flow velocity in age-related macular degeneration. Ophthalmology 1995; 102:640–6.
62. Friedman E. The role of the atherosclerotic process in the pathogenesis of age-related macular degeneration. Am J Ophthalmol 2000; 130:658–63.
63. Friedman E. Update of the vascular model of AMD. Br J Ophthalmol 2004; 88:161–3.
64. Gale CR, Hall NF, Phillips DI, Martyn CN. Lutein and zeaxanthin status and risk of age-related macular degeneration. Invest Ophthalmol Vis Sci 2003; 44: 2461–5.
65. Gass JD. Pathogenesis of disciform detachment of the neuroepithelium. Am J Ophthalmol 1967; 63(Suppl. L): 1–139.
66. Gass JD. Retinal pigment epithelial rip during krypton red laser photocoagulation. Am J Ophthalmol 1984; 98: 700–6.
67. Gass JD. Pathogenesis of tears of the retinal pigment epithelium. Br J Ophthalmol 1984; 68:513–9.
68. Gass JD. Serous retinal pigment epithelial detachment with a notch: a sign of occult choroidal neovascularization. Retina 1984; 4:205–20.
69. Gass JDM, ed. Stereoscopic Atlas of Macular Diseases: Diagnosis and Treatment. 4th ed. St. Louis, MO: Mosby, 1997.
70. Gaynes BI. AREDS misses on safety. Arch Ophthalmol 2003; 121:416–7.
71. Glaser BM, Campochiaro PA, Davis JL Jr, Sato M. Retinal pigment epithelial cells release an inhibitor of neovascularization. Arch Ophthalmol 1985; 103:1870–5.
72. Glaser BM. Extracellular modulating factors and the control of intraocular neovascularization: an overview. Arch Ophthalmol 1988; 106:603–7.
73. Glass CK, Witztum JL. Atherosclerosis: the road ahead. Cell 2001; 104:503–16.
74. Gold B, Merriam JE, Zernant J, et al. Variation in factor B (BF) and complement component 2 (C2) genes is associated with age-related macular degeneration. Nat Genet 2006; 38:458–62.
75. Goldberg J, Flowerdew G, Smith E, et al. Factors associated with age-related macular degeneration: an analysis of data from the first National Health and Nutrition Examination Survey. Am J Epidemiol 1988; 128:700–10.
76. Gottsch JD, Bynoe LA, Harlan JB, Rencs EV, Green WR. Light-induced deposits in Bruch's membrane of protoporphyric mice. Arch Ophthalmol 1993; 111:126–9.
77. Gragoudas ES, Adamis AP, Cunningham ET Jr, et al. Pegaptanib for neovascular age-related macular degeneration. N Engl J Med 2004; 351:2805–16.
78. Green WR, Key SN III. Senile macular degeneration: a histopathologic study. Trans Am Ophthalmol Soc 1977; 75:180–254.
79. Green WR, McDonnell PJ, Yeo JH. Pathologic features of senile macular degeneration. Ophthalmology 1985; 92: 615–27.
80. Green WR, Enger C. Age-related macular degeneration histopathologic studies: the 1992 Lorenz E. Zimmerman Lecture. Ophthalmology 1993; 100:1519–35.
81. Gregory CY, Evans K, Wijesuriya SD, et al. The gene responsible for autosomal dominant Doyne's honeycomb retinal dystrophy (DHRD) maps to chromosome 2p16. Hum Mol Genet 1996; 5:1055–9.
82. Grossniklaus HE, Martinez JA, Brown VB, et al. Immunohistochemical and histochemical properties of surgically excised subretinal neovascular membranes in age-related macular degeneration. Am J Ophthalmol 1992; 114:464–72.
83. Grossniklaus HE, Hutchinson AK, Capone A Jr, et al. Clinicopathologic features of surgically excised choroidal neovascular membranes. Ophthalmology 1994; 101: 1099–111.
84. Grossniklaus HE, Gass JD. Clinicopathologic correlations of surgically excised type 1 and type 2 submacular choroidal neovascular membranes. Am J Ophthalmol 1998; 126:59–69.
85. Grossniklaus HE, Green WR. Histopathologic and ultrastructural findings of surgically excised choroidal neovascularization. Submacular Surgery Trials Research Group. Arch Ophthalmol 1998; 116:745–9.
86. Grunwald JE, Hariprasad SM, DuPont J. Effect of aging on foveolar choroidal circulation. Arch Ophthalmol 1998; 116:150–4.
87. Grunwald JE, Hariprasad SM, DuPont J, et al. Foveolar choroidal blood flow in age-related macular degeneration. Invest Ophthalmol Vis Sci 1998; 39: 385–90.
88. Gurne DH, Tso MO, Edward DP, Ripps H. Antiretinal antibodies in serum of patients with age-related macular degeneration. Ophthalmology 1991; 98:602–7.
89. Guymer R, Luthert P, Bird A. Changes in Bruch's membrane and related structures with age. Prog Retin Eye Res 1999; 18:59–90.
90. Guymer RH, Bird AC, Hageman GS. Cytoarchitecture of choroidal capillary endothelial cells. Invest Ophthalmol Vis Sci 2004; 45:1660–6.
91. Guymer RH, Chiu AW, Lim L, Baird PN. HMG CoA reductase inhibitors (statins): do they have a role in age-related macular degeneration? Surv Ophthalmol 2005; 50: 194–206.
92. Hageman GS, Luthert PJ, Victor Chong NH, et al. An integrated hypothesis that considers drusen as biomarkers of immune-mediated processes at the RPE-Bruch's membrane interface in aging and age-related macular degeneration. Prog Retin Eye Res 2001; 20: 705–32.
93. Hageman GS, Anderson DH, Johnson LV, et al. A common haplotype in the complement regulatory gene factor H (HF1/CFH) predisposes individuals to age-related macular degeneration. Proc Natl Acad Sci USA 2005; 102:7227–32.
94. Haines JL, Hauser MA, Schmidt S, et al. Complement factor H variant increases the risk of age-related macular degeneration. Science 2005; 308:419–21.
95. Hammond BR, Jr., Johnson EJ, Russell RM, et al. Dietary modification of human macular pigment density. Invest Ophthalmol Vis Sci 1997; 38:1795–801.
96. Hammond BR Jr, Wooten BR, Snodderly DM. Preservation of visual sensitivity of older subjects: association with macular pigment density. Invest Ophthalmol Vis Sci 1998; 39:397–406.
97. Hartnett ME, Weiter JJ, Garsd A, Jalkh AE. Classification of retinal pigment epithelial detachments associated with drusen. Graefes Arch Clin Exp Ophthalmol 1992; 230: 11–9.
98. Henkind P, Gartner S. The relationship between retinal pigment epithelium and the choriocapillaris. Trans Ophthalmol Soc UK 1983; 103:444–7.

99. Heon E, Piguet B, Munier F, et al. Linkage of autosomal dominant radial drusen (malattia leventinese) to chromosome 2p16-21. Arch Ophthalmol 1996; 114:193–8.
100. Heriot WJ, Henkind P, Bellhorn RW, Burns MS. Choroidal neovascularization can digest Bruch's membrane: a prior break is not essential. Ophthalmology 1984; 91: 1603–8.
101. Hewitt AT, Nakazawa K, Newsome DA. Analysis of newly synthesized Bruch's membrane proteoglycans. Invest Ophthalmol Vis Sci 1989; 30:478–86.
102. Hillenkamp J, Hussain AA, Jackson TL, et al. The influence of path length and matrix components on ageing characteristics of transport between the choroid and the outer retina. Invest Ophthalmol Vis Sci 2004; 45:1493–8.
103. Hirata A, Feeney-Burns L. Autoradiographic studies of aged primate macular retinal pigment epithelium. Invest Ophthalmol Vis Sci 1992; 33:2079–90.
104. Hirvela H, Luukinen H, Laara E, Sc L, Laatikainen L. Risk factors of age-related maculopathy in a population 70 years of age or older. Ophthalmology 1996; 103: 871–7.
105. Hogan MJ. Role of the retinal pigment epithelium in macular disease. Trans Am Acad Ophthalmol Otolaryngol 1972; 76:64–80.
106. Holz FG, Piguet B, Minassian DC, et al. Decreasing stromal iris pigmentation as a risk factor for age-related macular degeneration. Am J Ophthalmol 1994; 117:19–23.
107. Holz FG, Schutt F, Kopitz J, et al. Inhibition of lysosomal degradative functions in RPE cells by a retinoid component of lipofuscin. Invest Ophthalmol Vis Sci 1999; 40: 737–43.
108. Holz FG, Bellman C, Staudt S, et al. Fundus autofluorescence and development of geographic atrophy in age-related macular degeneration. Invest Ophthalmol Vis Sci 2001; 42:1051–6.
109. Holz FG, Pauleikhoff D, Klein R, Bird AC. Pathogenesis of lesions in late age-related macular disease. Am J Ophthalmol 2004; 137:504–10.
110. Huang X, Cuajungco MP, Atwood CS, et al. Alzheimer's disease, beta-amyloid protein and zinc. J Nutr 2000; 130: 1488S–1492S.
111. Husain D. RA, Cuthbertson RA. Vascular endothelial growth factor (VEGF) expression is correlated with choroidal neovascularisation in a monkey model. IOVS 1997; 38(Suppl.):501.
112. Hyman L, Schachat AP, He Q, Leske MC. Hypertension, cardiovascular disease, and age-related macular degeneration. Age-Related Macular Degeneration Risk Factors Study Group. Arch Ophthalmol 2000; 118:351–8.
113. Ishibashi T, Patterson R, Ohnishi Y, et al. Formation of drusen in the human eye. Am J Ophthalmol 1986; 101: 342–53.
114. Ishibashi T, Sorgente N, Patterson R, Ryan SJ. Pathogenesis of drusen in the primate. Invest Ophthalmol Vis Sci 1986; 27:184–93.
115. Ishida O, Oku H, Ikeda T, et al. Is Chlamydia pneumoniae infection a risk factor for age related macular degeneration? Br J Ophthalmol 2003; 87:523–4.
116. Iyengar SK, Song D, Klein BE, et al. Dissection of genomewide-scan data in extended families reveals a major locus and oligogenic susceptibility for age-related macular degeneration. Am J Hum Genet 2004; 74:20–39.
117. Johnson LV, Leitner WP, Rivest AJ, et al. The Alzheimer's A beta-peptide is deposited at sites of complement activation in pathologic deposits associated with aging and age-related macular degeneration. Proc Natl Acad Sci USA 2002; 99:11830–5.
118. Johnson LV, Anderson DH. Age-related macular degeneration and the extracellular matrix. N Engl J Med 2004; 351:320–2.
119. Kalayoglu MV, Galvan C, Mahdi OS, et al. Serological association between Chlamydia pneumoniae infection and age-related macular degeneration. Arch Ophthalmol 2003; 121:478–82.
120. Kalayoglu MV, Bula D, Arroyo J, et al. Identification of Chlamydia pneumoniae within human choroidal neovascular membranes secondary to age-related macular degeneration. Graefes Arch Clin Exp Ophthalmol 2005; 243:1080–90.
121. Kalebic T, Garbisa S, Glaser B, Liotta LA. Basement membrane collagen: degradation by migrating endothelial cells. Science 1983; 221:281–3.
122. Karwatowski WS, Jeffries TE, Duance VC, et al. Preparation of Bruch's membrane and analysis of the age-related changes in the structural collagens. Br J Ophthalmol 1995; 79:944–52.
123. Killingsworth MC. Age-related components of Bruch's membrane in the human eye. Graefes Arch Clin Exp Ophthalmol 1987; 225:406–12.
124. Killingsworth MC, Sarks JP, Sarks SH. Macrophages related to Bruch's membrane in age-related macular degeneration. Eye 1990; 4(Pt. 4):613–21.
125. Klein BE, Klein R, Lee KE, Jensen SC. Measures of obesity and age-related eye diseases. Ophthalmic Epidemiol 2001; 8:251–62.
126. Klein R, Klein BE, Linton KL. Prevalence of age-related maculopathy: The Beaver Dam Eye Study. Ophthalmology 1992; 99:933–43.
127. Klein R, Klein BE, Franke T. The relationship of cardiovascular disease and its risk factors to age-related maculopathy: The Beaver Dam Eye Study. Ophthalmology 1993; 100:406–14.
128. Klein R, Klein BE, Jensen SC, Cruickshanks KJ. The relationship of ocular factors to the incidence and progression of age-related maculopathy. Arch Ophthalmol 1998; 116:506–13.
129. Klein R, Klein BE, Moss SE. Relation of smoking to the incidence of age-related maculopathy. The Beaver Dam Eye Study. Am J Epidemiol 1998; 147:103–10.
130. Klein R, Klein BE, Tomany SC, et al. Ten-year incidence and progression of age–related maculopathy: The Beaver Dam eye study. Ophthalmology 2002; 109:1767–79.
131. Klein R, Klein BE, Tomany SC, Moss SE. Ten-year incidence of age-related maculopathy and smoking and drinking: the Beaver Dam Eye Study. Am J Epidemiol 2002; 156:589–98.
132. Klein R, Peto T, Bird A, Vannewkirk MR. The epidemiology of age-related macular degeneration. Am J Ophthalmol 2004; 137:486–95.
133. Klein RJ, Zeiss C, Chew EY, et al. Complement factor H polymorphism in age-related macular degeneration. Science 2005; 308:385–9.
134. Kliffen M, Sharma HS, Mooy CM, Kerkvliet S, de Jong PT. Increased expression of angiogenic growth factors in age-related maculopathy. Br J Ophthalmol 1997; 81:154–62.
135. Knighton DR, Hunt TK, Scheuenstuhl H, Halliday BJ, Werb Z, Banda MJ. Oxygen tension regulates the expression of angiogenesis factor by macrophages. Science 1983; 221:1283–5.
136. Korte GE, Reppucci V, Henkind P. RPE destruction causes choriocapillary atrophy. Invest Ophthalmol Vis Sci 1984; 25:1135–45.

137. Korte GE, Chase J. Additional evidence for remodelling of normal choriocapillaris. Exp Eye Res 1989; 49:299–303.
138. Kuvin JT, Karas RH. The effects of LDL reduction and HDL augmentation on physiologic and inflammatory markers. Curr Opin Cardiol 2003; 18:295–300.
139. Lafaut BA, Bartz-Schmidt KU, Vanden Broecke C, et al. Clinicopathological correlation in exudative age related macular degeneration: histological differentiation between classic and occult choroidal neovascularisation. Br J Ophthalmol 2000; 84:239–43.
140. Li CM, Chung BH, Presley JB, et al. Lipoprotein-like particles and cholesteryl esters in human Bruch's membrane: initial characterization. Invest Ophthalmol Vis Sci 2005; 46:2576–86.
141. Li JJ, Chen XJ. Simvastatin inhibits interleukin-6 release in human monocytes stimulated by C-reactive protein and lipopolysaccharide. Coron Artery Dis 2003; 14:329–34.
142. Lim L, Guymer RH. AMD: to supplement or not? Clin Exp Ophthalmol 2004; 32:341–3.
143. Loeys B, Van Maldergem L, Mortier G, et al. Homozygosity for a missense mutation in fibulin-5 (FBLN5) results in a severe form of cutis laxa. Hum Mol Genet 2002; 11:2113–8.
144. Loffler KU, Lee WR. Basal linear deposit in the human macula. Graefes Arch Clin Exp Ophthalmol 1986; 224: 493–501.
145. Lopez PF, Grossniklaus HE, Lambert HM, et al. Pathologic features of surgically excised subretinal neovascular membranes in age-related macular degeneration. Am J Ophthalmol 1991; 112:647–56.
146. Lopez PF, Sippy BD, Lambert HM, et al. Transdifferentiated retinal pigment epithelial cells are immunoreactive for vascular endothelial growth factor in surgically excised age-related macular degeneration-related choroidal neovascular membranes. Invest Ophthalmol Vis Sci 1996; 37:855–68.
147. Lotery AJ, Baas D, Ridley C, et al. Reduced secretion of fibulin 5 in age-related macular degeneration and cutis laxa. Hum Mutat 2006; 27:568–74.
148. Macular Photocoagulation Study Group. Laser photocoagulation for juxtafoveal choroidal neovascularization: five-year results from randomized clinical trials. Arch Ophthalmol 1994; 112:500–9.
149. Macular Photocoagulation Study Group: Risk factors for choroidal neovascularization in the second eye of patients with juxtafoveal or subfoveal choroidal neovascularization secondary to age-related macular degeneration. Arch Ophthalmol 1997; 115:741–7.
150. Malek G, Johnson LV, Mace BE, et al. Apolipoprotein E allele-dependent pathogenesis: a model for age-related retinal degeneration. Proc Natl Acad Sci USA 2005; 102: 11900–5.
151. Mares-Perlman JA, Brady WE, Klein R, et al. Serum antioxidants and age-related macular degeneration in a population-based case–control study. Arch Ophthalmol 1995; 113:1518–23.
152. Mares-Perlman JA, Brady WE, Klein R, et al. Dietary fat and age-related maculopathy [see comment]. Arch Ophthalmol 1995; 113:743–8.
153. Mares-Perlman JA, Klein R, Klein BE, et al. Association of zinc and antioxidant nutrients with age-related maculopathy. Arch Ophthalmol 1996; 114:991–7.
154. Marmorstein LY, Munier FL, Arsenijevic Y, et al. Aberrant accumulation of EFEMP1 underlies drusen formation in Malattia leventinese and age-related macular degeneration. Proc Natl Acad Sci USA 2002; 99:13067–72.
155. Marshall GE, Konstas AG, Lee WR. Collagens in ocular tissues. Br J Ophthalmol 1993; 77:515–24.
156. McCarty CA, Mukesh BN, Fu CL, et al. Risk factors for age-related maculopathy: the visual impairment project. Arch Ophthalmol 2001; 119:1455–62.
157. Midwood KS, Schwarzbauer JE. Elastic fibers: building bridges between cells and their matrix. Curr Biol 2002; 12: R279–81.
158. Mitchell P, Smith W, Attebo K, Wang JJ. Prevalence of age-related maculopathy in Australia. The Blue Mountains Eye Study. Ophthalmology 1995; 102:1450–60.
159. Mori F. The role of choroidal haemodynamic abnormalities in the pathogenesis of age related macular degeneration. Br J Ophthalmol 2001; 85:1399–400.
160. Mori F, Konno S, Hikichi T, et al. Pulsatile ocular blood flow study: decreases in exudative age related macular degeneration. Br J Ophthalmol 2001; 85:531–3.
161. Mukesh BN, Dimitrov PN, Leikin S, et al. Five-year incidence of age-related maculopathy: the visual impairment project. Ophthalmology 2004; 111:1176–82.
162. Mullins R, Aptsiauri, N, Hageman, G. Dendritic cells and proteins associated with immune-mediated processes are associated with drusen and may play a central role in drusen biogenesis. IOVS 2000; 41:S24.
163. Mullins RF, Russell SR, Anderson DH, Hageman GS. Drusen associated with aging and age-related macular degeneration contain proteins common to extracellular deposits associated with atherosclerosis, elastosis, amyloidosis, and dense deposit disease. FASEB J 2000; 14: 835–46.
164. Newsome DA, Huh W, Green WR. Bruch's membrane age-related changes vary by region. Curr Eye Res 1987; 6: 1211–21.
165. Noell WK, Walker VS, Kang BS, Berman S. Retinal damage by light in rats. Invest Ophthalmol 1966; 5: 450–73.
166. Okubo A, Rosa RH Jr, Bunce CV, et al. The relationships of age changes in retinal pigment epithelium and Bruch's membrane. Invest Ophthalmol Vis Sci 1999; 40: 443–9.
167. Okubo A, Sameshima M, Unoki K, et al. Ultrastructural changes associated with accumulation of inclusion bodies in rat retinal pigment epithelium. Invest Ophthalmol Vis Sci 2000; 41:4305–12.
168. Omenn GS, Goodman GE, Thornquist MD, et al. Risk factors for lung cancer and for intervention effects in CARET, the beta-carotene and retinol efficacy trial. J Natl Cancer Inst 1996; 88:1550–9.
169. Omenn GS, Goodman GE, Thornquist MD, et al. Effects of a combination of beta carotene and vitamin A on lung cancer and cardiovascular disease. N Engl J Med 1996; 334:1150–5.
170. Ozaki S, Johnson LV, Mullins RF, et al. The human retina and retinal pigment epithelium are abundant sources of vitronectin mRNA. Biochem Biophys Res Commun 1999; 258:524–9.
171. Pagliarini S, Moramarco A, Wormald RP, et al. Age-related macular disease in rural southern Italy. Arch Ophthalmol 1997; 115:616–22.
172. Parums DV, Brown DL, Mitchinson MJ. Serum antibodies to oxidized low-density lipoprotein and ceroid in chronic periaortitis. Arch Pathol Lab Med 1990; 114:383–7.
173. Pauleikhoff D, Chen JC, Chisholm IH, Bird AC. Choroidal perfusion abnormality with age-related Bruch's membrane change. Am J Ophthalmol 1990; 109:211–7.
174. Penfold P, Killingsworth M, Sarks S. An ultrastructural study of the role of leucocytes and fibroblasts in the

breakdown of Bruch's membrane. Aust J Ophthalmol 1984; 12:23–31.

175. Penfold PL, Killingsworth MC, Sarks SH. Senile macular degeneration: the involvement of giant cells in atrophy of the retinal pigment epithelium. Invest Ophthalmol Vis Sci 1986; 27:364–71.
176. Penfold PL, Provis JM, Furby JH, Gatenby PA, Billson FA. Autoantibodies to retinal astrocytes associated with age-related macular degeneration. Graefes Arch Clin Exp Ophthalmol 1990; 228:270–4.
177. Penfold PL, Madigan MC, Gillies MC, Provis JM. Immunological and aetiological aspects of macular degeneration. Prog Retin Eye Res 2001; 20:385–414.
178. Penn JS, Anderson RE. Effect of light history on rod outer-segment membrane composition in the rat. Exp Eye Res 1987; 44:767–78.
179. Petrukhin K, Koisti MJ, Bakall B, et al. Identification of the gene responsible for best macular dystrophy. Nat Genet 1998; 19:241–7.
180. Piguet B, Palmvang IB, Chisholm IH, et al. Evolution of age-related macular degeneration with choroidal perfusion abnormality. Am J Ophthalmol 1992; 113:657–63.
181. Polkinghorne PJ, Capon MR, Berninger T, et al. Sorsby's fundus dystrophy: a clinical study. Ophthalmology 1989; 96:1763–8.
182. Polverini PJ, Cotran PS, Gimbrone MA Jr, Unanue ER. Activated macrophages induce vascular proliferation. Nature 1977; 269:804–6.
183. Ramrattan RS, van der Schaft TL, Mooy CM, et al. Morphometric analysis of Bruch's membrane, the choriocapillaris, and the choroid in aging. Invest Ophthalmol Vis Sci 1994; 35:2857–64.
184. Reme CE. Autography in visual cells and pigment epithelium. Invest Ophthalmol Vis Sci 1977; 16:807–914.
185. Robman L, Mahdi O, McCarty C, et al. Exposure to chlamydia pneumoniae infection and progression of age-related macular degeneration. Am J Epidemiol 2005; 161: 1013–9.
186. Roquet W, Roudot-Thoraval F, Coscas G, Soubrane G. Clinical features of drusenoid pigment epithelial detachment in age related macular degeneration. Br J Ophthalmol 2004; 88:638–42.
187. Ross R. Atherosclerosis is an inflammatory disease. Am Heart J 1999; 138:S419–20.
188. Rozanowska M, Jarvis-Evans J, Korytowski W, et al. Blue light-induced reactivity of retinal age pigment: in vitro generation of oxygen-reactive species. J Biol Chem 1995; 270:18825–30.
189. Rozanowska M, Korytowski W, Rozanowski B, et al. Photoreactivity of aged human RPE melanosomes: a comparison with lipofuscin. Invest Ophthalmol Vis Sci 2002; 43:2088–96.
190. Rulon LL, Robertson JD, Lovell MA, et al. Serum zinc levels and Alzheimer's disease. Biol Trace Elem Res 2000; 75:79–85.
191. Rungger-Brandle E, Englert U, Leuenberger PM. Exocytic clearing of degraded membrane material from pigment epithelial cells in frog retina. Invest Ophthalmol Vis Sci 1987; 28:2026–37.
192. Ryan SJ, ed. Retina. St. Louis, MO: Mosby, 1989.
193. Sarks JP, Sarks SH, Killingsworth MC. Evolution of soft drusen in age-related macular degeneration. Eye 1994; 8: 269–83.
194. Sarks SH. New vessel formation beneath the retinal pigment epithelium in senile eyes. Br J Ophthalmol 1973; 57:951–65.
195. Sarks SH. Ageing and degeneration in the macular region: a clinico-pathological study. Br J Ophthalmol 1976; 60:324–41.
196. Sarks SH. Council Lecture: drusen and their relationship to senile macular degeneration. Aust J Ophthalmol 1980; 8:117–30.
197. Schaumberg DA, Christen WG, Hankinson SE, Glynn RJ. Body mass index and the incidence of visually significant age-related maculopathy in men. Arch Ophthalmol 2001; 119:1259–65.
198. Schmidt S, Hauser MA, Scott WK, et al. Cigarette smoking strongly modifies the association of LOC387715 and age-related macular degeneration. Am J Hum Genet 2006; 78:852–64.
199. Schultz DW, Klein ML, Humpert AJ, et al. Analysis of the ARMD1 locus: evidence that a mutation in HEMICENTIN-1 is associated with age-related macular degeneration in a large family. Hum Mol Genet 2003; 12: 3315–23.
200. Schutt F, Bergmann M, Holz FG, Kopitz J. Isolation of intact lysosomes from human RPE cells and effects of A2-E on the integrity of the lysosomal and other cellular membranes. Graefes Arch Clin Exp Ophthalmol 2002; 240:983–8.
201. Seddon JM, Ajani UA, Sperduto RD, et al. Dietary carotenoids, vitamins A, C, and E, and advanced age-related macular degeneration. Eye Disease Case-Control Study Group. J Am Med Assoc 1994; 272: 1413–20.
202. Seddon JM, Rosner B, Sperduto RD, et al. Dietary fat and risk for advanced age-related macular degeneration. Arch Ophthalmol 2001; 119:1191–9.
203. Seddon JM, Cote J, Rosner B. Progression of age-related macular degeneration: association with dietary fat, transunsaturated fat, nuts, and fish intake. Arch Ophthalmol 2003; 121:1728–37 [erratum appears in Arch Ophthalmol 2004; 122:426].
204. Seddon JM, Gensler G, Milton RC, et al. Association between C-reactive protein and age-related macular degeneration. J Am Med Assoc 2004; 291:704–10.
205. Seigel D. AREDS investigators distort findings. Arch Ophthalmol 2002; 120:100–1.
206. Sheraidah G, Steinmetz R, Maguire J, et al. Correlation between lipids extracted from Bruch's membrane and age. Ophthalmology 1993; 100:47–51.
207. Smith W, Mitchell P, Leeder SR. Smoking and age-related maculopathy. The Blue Mountains Eye Study. Arch Ophthalmol 1996; 114:1518–23.
208. Smith W, Mitchell P, Leeder SR, Wang JJ. Plasma fibrinogen levels, other cardiovascular risk factors, and age-related maculopathy: The Blue Mountains Eye Study. Arch Ophthalmol 1998; 116: 583–7.
209. Smith W, Mitchell P, Leeder SR. Dietary fat and fish intake and age-related maculopathy. Arch Ophthalmol 2000; 118:401–404.
210. Smith W, Assink J, Klein R, et al. Risk factors for age-related macular degeneration: pooled findings from three continents. Ophthalmology 2001; 108:697–704.
211. Sperduto RD, Hiller R. Systemic hypertension and age-related maculopathy in the Framingham study. Arch Ophthalmol 1986; 104:216–9.
212. Steinberg RH. Monitoring communications between photoreceptors and pigment epithelial cells: effects of "mild" systemic hypoxia: Friedenwald lecture. Invest Ophthalmol Vis Sci 1987; 28:1888–904.

213. Stone EM, Braun TA, Russell SR, et al. Missense variations in the fibulin 5 gene and age-related macular degeneration. N Engl J Med 2004; 351:346–53.
214. Suh SW, Jensen KB, Jensen MS, et al. Histochemically-reactive zinc in amyloid plaques, angiopathy, and degenerating neurons of Alzheimer's diseased brains. Brain Res 2000; 852:274–8.
215. Taubold RD. Studies on chemical nature of lipofusion (age pigment) isolated from normal human brain. Lipids 1975; 10:383–90.
216. Taylor HR, Munoz B, West S, et al. Visible light and risk of age-related macular degeneration. Trans Am Ophthalmol Soc 1990; 88:163–73; discussion 173–8.
217. Taylor HR. Fred Hollows lecture: eye care for the community. Clin Exp Ophthalmol 2002; 30:151–4.
218. The Eye Disease Case-Control Study Group. Risk factors for neovascular age-related macular degeneration. Arch Ophthalmol 1992; 110:1701–8.
219. van der Schaft TL, de Bruijn WC, Mooy CM, et al. Is basal laminar deposit unique for age-related macular degeneration? Arch Ophthalmol 1991; 109:420–5.
220. van der Schaft TL, de Bruijn WC, Mooy CM, de Jong PT. Basal laminar deposit in the aging peripheral human retina. Graefes Arch Clin Exp Ophthalmol 1993; 231:470–5.
221. van der Schaft TL, Mooy CM, de Bruijn WC, et al. Increased prevalence of disciform macular degeneration after cataract extraction with implantation of an intraocular lens. Br J Ophthalmol 1994; 78:441–5.
222. Van den Langenberg GM, Mares-Perlman JA, Klein R, et al Associations between antioxidant and zinc intake and the 5-year incidence of early age-related maculopathy: The Beaver Dam Eye Study. Am J Epidemiol 1998; 148:204–14.
223. Van Newkirk MR, Nanjan MB, Wang JJ, et al. The prevalence of age-related maculopathy: the visual impairment project. Ophthalmology 2000; 107:1593–600.
224. Vidaurri JS, Pe'er J, Halfon ST, et al. Association between drusen and some of the risk factors for coronary artery disease. Ophthalmologica 1984; 188:243–7.
225. Vingerling JR, Dielemans I, Bots ML, et al. Age-related macular degeneration is associated with atherosclerosis: The Rotterdam Study. Am J Epidemiol 1995; 142:404–9.
226. Vingerling JR, Hofman A, Grobbee DE, de Jong PT. Age-related macular degeneration and smoking: The Rotterdam Study. Arch Ophthalmol 1996; 114:1193–6.
227. von Ruckmann A, Fitzke FW, Bird AC. Distribution of fundus autofluorescence with a scanning laser ophthalmoscope. Br J Ophthalmol 1995; 79:407–12.
228. von Ruckmann A, Fitzke FW, Bird AC. Fundus autofluorescence in age-related macular disease imaged with a laser scanning ophthalmoscope. Invest Ophthalmol Vis Sci 1997; 38:478–86.
229. Vranka JA, Johnson E, Zhu X, et al. Discrete expression and distribution pattern of TIMP-3 in the human retina and choroid. Curr Eye Res 1997; 16:102–10.
230. Wang JJ, Foran S, Smith W, Mitchell P. Risk of age-related macular degeneration in eyes with macular drusen or hyperpigmentation: the Blue Mountains Eye Study cohort. Arch Ophthalmol 2003; 121:658–63.
231. Wang JJ, Klein R, Smith W, et al. Cataract surgery and the 5-year incidence of late-stage age-related maculopathy: pooled findings from the Beaver Dam and Blue Mountains eye studies. Ophthalmology 2003; 110: 1960–7.
232. Weber BH, Vogt G, Pruett RC, et al. Mutations in the tissue inhibitor of metalloproteinases-3 (TIMP3) in patients with Sorsby's fundus dystrophy. Nat Genet 1994; 8:352–6.
233. Weeks DE, Conley YP, Tsai HJ, et al. Age-related maculopathy: a genomewide scan with continued evidence of susceptibility loci within the 1q31, 10q26, and 17q25 regions. Am J Hum Genet 2004; 75: 174–89.
234. Wiegand RD, Giusto NM, Rapp LM, Anderson RE. Evidence for rod outer segment lipid peroxidation following constant illumination of the rat retina. Invest Ophthalmol Vis Sci 1983; 24:1433–5.
235. Wing GL, Blanchard GC, Weiter JJ. The topography and age relationship of lipofuscin concentration in the retinal pigment epithelium. Invest Ophthalmol Vis Sci 1978; 17:601–7.
236. Winkler BS, Boulton ME, Gottsch JD, Sternberg P. Oxidative damage and age-related macular degeneration. Molecular Vision 1999; 5:32.
237. Wu J, Seregard S, Spangberg B, et al. Blue light induced apoptosis in rat retina. Eye 1999; 13:577–83.
238. Zareparsi S, Buraczynska M, Branham KE, et al. Toll-like receptor 4 variant D299G is associated with susceptibility to age-related macular degeneration. Hum Mol Genet 2005; 14:1449–55.

19

The Aging Lens

Elaine R. Berman[†]
Hadassah-Hebrew University Medical School, Jerusalem, Israel

[†]Deceased.

INTRODUCTION

Aging is intimately associated with lens opacification (cataract), and the latter is often perceived as an accelerated form of aging. A broad spectrum of biochemical and structural changes occur in the lens during normal development, maturation, and aging. Among the most prominent in the aging lens are increases in weight, thickness, coloration, nontryptophan fluorescence, and light absorbance (18,19). Absorbance of light at <400 nm is more than double at 76 years of age than at 42 years of age (Fig. 1). Other important age-related changes include increased glycation of crystallins and cleavage of fiber cell membrane protein MP26. There are also significant decreases in enzyme activities. A large body of information has accumulated during the past two decades on these changes, and for clarity of presentation, this discussion is limited to age-related changes found in clear noncataractous lenses.

Lens fiber cells are not shed, nor do they degenerate; rather, they are continually displaced inwardly toward the center as they mature. Hence, the proteins in old (nuclear) lens fiber cells are as old as the organism itself. Because of the loss of intracellular organelles, there is only minimal protein synthesis in the nuclear region; metabolic activity in the lens appears to be confined mainly to the superficial cortical and epithelial layers. Morphologic changes in the lens with aging are covered in Chapter 23.

Aging of the lens is a normal, and complex, physiological process. Age-related changes in the lens are studied using three types of experimental approach: (*i*) comparisons of nuclear (old) and cortical (new) regions of single lenses; (*ii*) analysis of concentric microdissected layers of individual lenses; and (*iii*) comparisons of specific components in individual lenses of various ages. The last two approaches (described here) have been integrated into a single technique by several laboratories (28,29,33,43).

FIBER CELL PLASMA MEMBRANES AND CYTOSKELETON

Main Intrinsic Protein

Main intrinsic protein (MP26), also known as aquaporin 0 is the most abundant component of lens fiber

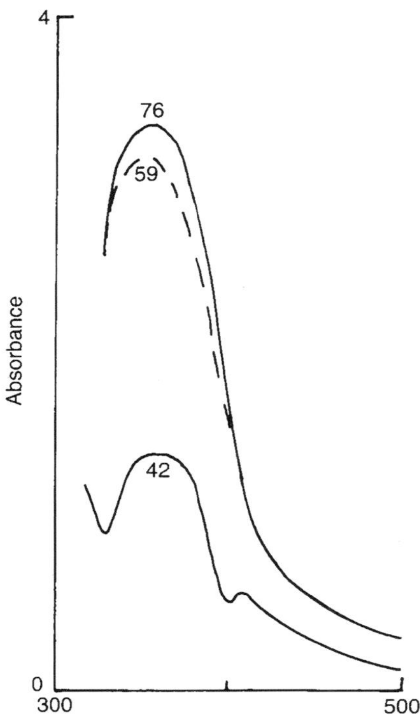

Figure 1 Absorbance of light from 300 to 500 nm by human lens. The numbers on the curves represent average ages in years. *Source*: From Ref. 18.

cell plasma membranes. Although an age-related conversion of MP26 to MP22 in human and bovine fiber cell plasma membranes has been recognized for many years (3,10,21), the site(s) of cleavage could not be established with certainty in early studies. More recently, antisera made against the C- and N-terminal peptides of bovine MP26 have been used as probes to identify subtle covalent changes in the molecule not recognizable by conventional polyclonal antisera (59). These studies demonstrated an age-dependent production of 15 and 20 kDa polypeptides at the N-terminus of the molecule, while cleavage of MP26 to form MP22 was shown to occur at the C-terminus. Thus, both ends of the MP26 molecule are degraded in vivo in an age-dependent manner, possibly by proteolytic cleavage.

Other Membrane Proteins

There is also evidence for proteolytic breakdown of other proteins of higher molecular weight in older plasma membrane fibers. Radioimmunoassays for 57, 70, 82, and 100 kDa proteins in cortical and nuclear regions of sheep lens suggest that each of these proteins follows a specific and characteristic pattern of degradation (24). A recently described 115 kDa extrinsic membrane protein, possibly a component of the beaded filament, also appears to be degraded in bovine lens in an age-related manner (15). Immunoreactive fragments not arising as artifacts during the isolation procedure are more abundant in the old (nuclear) region than in the cortex.

Cytoskeletal Components

Cytoskeletal components of the lens undergo numerous morphological and biochemical changes with aging, although many of the details are not yet clear (1,18). In general, it appears that degradation of cytoskeletal proteins commences with the formation of mature secondary fibers. On the whole, spectrin, vimentin, and actin are gradually lost from the deep cortical and nuclear fiber cells, although these proteins persist in the superficial cortical cells. The intermediate filament of the lens, vimentin, has been detected morphologically in an 80-year-old human lens, but only in the epithelial cells (32). Biochemical analysis of different fiber cell layers of human lens have revealed a marked decrease in vimentin in the deep layers of the cortex and the complete absence of it and other cytoskeletal components from adult human nucleus; cytoskeletal components are detectable in newborn lens, however.

CRYSTALLINS AND ENZYME ACTIVITIES

Overview

Age-related changes in the lens crystallins occur as a result of both differential synthesis during development and postsynthetic modifications throughout life (18,20). Although the post-synthetic changes occur predominantly in the nuclear region and changes resulting from differentiation are expressed mainly in outer cortical crystallins, there is nevertheless a considerable overlap. The documented age-related changes occurring in the crystallins include loss of sulfhydryl and formation of disulfide bridges, cross-linking, accumulation of high-molecular-weight aggregates, increase in insoluble protein associated with browning and nontryptophan fluorescence, photo-oxidation of tryptophan, production of photosensitizers, generation of free radicals, proteolysis of polypeptide chains, and nonenzymatic glycation.

The distribution of water-soluble, urea-soluble, and urea-insoluble proteins has been examined in concentric microdissected layers of human noncataractous lenses ranging from 1.8 to 65 years of age (27). Using the dry weight of lens tissue as a reference, the amounts of these proteins were similar in cortical and nuclear regions until the age of 30 years. However, after 40 years of age the insoluble protein increased continuously from cortex to nucleus; the increase in nuclear protein insolubilization in lenses of fifth to sixth decade individuals involves mainly the urea-insoluble fraction, whereas in younger lenses this increase is due mainly to urea-soluble proteins. The disappearance of 20 to 22 kDa soluble proteins from the deep cortex and nucleus was noted in all lenses, except those of a 1.8-year-old infant (27). This striking loss of soluble 20 to 22 kDa polypeptide has also been observed by other investigators (8,33). Thus nuclear protein insolubilization and loss of soluble 20 to 22 kDa crystallins is considered a major age-related change in the lens.

McFall-Ngai et al. (33) examined the soluble crystallins in clear postmortem human lenses ranging in age from newborn to 70 years old. Protein analysis of serial sections taken through the optical axis of the lens showed a complex pattern of both gradual and abrupt changes in crystallin concentrations in cortical and nuclear regions with aging. Similar to the observations of Li et al. (27), these investigators found a striking age-related loss of 19 to 21 kDa γ-crystallins in both cortical and nuclear regions. These γ-crystallins have anomalous electrophoretic behavior on sodium dodecyl sulfate (SDS) gels if not subjected to prior heat denaturation. This may have resulted from age-related modifications in their charge characteristics (66). Three populations of γ-crystallins are readily resolved and identified in young lenses, but with increasing age, two of the species are no longer separable. There is an age-related increase in heterogeneity of the γ-crystallins; moreover, they become more acidic with age.

Similar changes can be induced in unmodified γ-crystallin (obtained from the expression of a gene construct integrated into mouse L cells) after exposure to ascorbic acid in the presence of iron and oxygen (47). The alterations of γ-crystallin in this system indicate an ascorbic acid-induced oxidation and imply that a similar mechanism may explain the changes occurring in vivo in aging γ-crystallins. Other studies using antisera to synthetic peptides corresponding to the N- and C-terminal regions of human γ_{I-II}crystallin gene (49) demonstrate extensive covalent modifications during aging in normal human lenses (58). Whether these apparent covalent modifications of the N- and C-terminal regions of γ-crystallins are mediated by endogenous lens proteinases or oxidative changes, or both, remains to be established.

The γ-crystallins contain six or seven cysteine sulfhydryl residues per monomer, and a marked loss in protein thiol occurs in the nucleus of older rodent lenses (25). The γ-crystallins undergo increasing insolubilization with age, thought to result from oxidation of thiol groups and the formation of disulfides bonds. Support for this concept has come from Raman spectroscopy, an important tool not only for monitoring the conversion of sulfhydryl (–SH) groups to disulfide (–SS–) bonds but also for measuring the degree of hydration or dehydration in the lens nucleus. There is now direct evidence for an age-related conversion of –SH to –SS– in the nucleus of rodent lenses (42,65). Not only exposed but also buried protein sulfhydryl groups are converted to disulfide bonds; this transformation correlates with the hard, relatively dehydrated nucleus found in the aging rodent lens. Biochemical studies show that the –SS– bonds formed in aging rat lenses are intramolecular, not intermolecular (22). There are no substantial changes in the molecular weight distribution of the proteins, and it has been suggested that the γ-crystallin molecules assume a more compact spatial arrangement in the nucleus as a result of intramolecular disulfide bond formation. This is in contrast to human and guinea pig lenses, in which the age-related loss of –SH is not accompanied by the formation of –SS– bonds (64). The loss of sulfhydryl in this case may be the result of increased oxidation of glutathione (GSH) formation of protein sulfhydryl, and reduction of the mixed disulfide by GSH reductase and nicotinamide adenine dinucleotide phosphate (NADPH) to yield the original protein sulfhydryl and oxidized GSH. The latter is then thought to be extruded from the lens.

Confocal Raman microspectroscopy was used recently to study the secondary and tertiary conformations of crystallins in human lenses from donor eyes ranging in age from 20 to 75 years (52). This highly discriminative and sensitive method revealed an increased content of aromatic amino acid side chains and a more pronounced β-sheet conformation in the nuclear regions than in the cortex. The former reflects a change in crystallin composition and the latter, a true age-related post-translational change in the secondary conformation of crystallins. Comparisons of cortical and nuclear spectra support biochemical studies showing extensive photooxidation of tryptophan to *N*-formylkynurenine and other photosensitizers in nuclear crystallins.

Although β-crystallins are the most abundant soluble polypeptides in the lens, relatively little is known regarding their age-related synthesis. The basic principal polypeptide (βB_p or βB_2) is the major β-crystallin in bovine and human lens (18). It bears extensive amino acid sequence similarity with γ_{II}crystallin; moreover, bovine βB_2 displays unusual heat stability (34). Human βB_2-crystallin is also heat stable; this polypeptide is synthesized in new cortical fiber cells throughout life, but its concentration in old nuclear fiber cells decreases significantly with age. Post-translational changes result in a decrease in the molecular mass of βB_2 from 26 to 22 to 23 kDa, a consequence of in vivo proteolysis of the N-terminal region of the molecule (60). The cleavage occurs mainly in young lenses (0–10 years), with very little detectable in older lenses (>40 years).

Other changes in human β-crystallins include an age-related decrease in a 29 kDa polypeptide and an increase in the 27 kDa polypeptide, but only until about age 5 years; afterward there is a slow decrease until age 86 years (2). At all ages, the 29 kDa β-crystallin is detectable in the superficial fiber cells. The 27 kDa polypeptide shows a changing distribution pattern during aging, however, persisting in the superficial cortex but showing marked losses in the deep cortical and nuclear regions in older lenses.

The foregoing discussion has centered on age-related changes in human and rodent crystallins, but significant conformational changes detectable by ultraviolet (UV) fluorescence and circular dichroism have also been reported in bovine lens crystallins (30). With increasing age, bovine α-crystallin, but not β- or γ-crystallin, undergoes changes in tertiary structure involving tryptophan, tyrosine, and cysteine residues. There are also striking decreases in tryptophan fluorescence and increases in non-tryptophan fluorescence. Other studies on bovine lens crystallins have revealed a gradual decrease in the proportion of soluble α-crystallin in the lens nucleus (9). In addition, and similar to the human lens, both the charge and size heterogeneity of monomeric bovine lens γ-crystallins increase with age. Analysis of concentric layers of lenses from prenatal to 15-year-old cattle show that whereas γ-crystallins account for about 22% of the proteins synthesized prenatally, this value drops to about 4% at birth; the major monomeric species at that time is βs-crystallin (43).

High-Molecular-Weight Aggregates

A high-molecular-weight class of crystallin, composed mainly of α-crystallin polypeptides, was first identified in bovine lens by Spector et al. (55). It accumulates in an age-dependent manner in most animal lenses (43), as well as in the human lens (23). The age-related increase in the concentration of high-molecular-weight aggregates is primarily in the nuclear region of normal lenses (53,54). The bonds holding the aggregates are weak, noncovalent linkages that can be disrupted by detergents and other agents. These aggregates are thought to be intermediates in the formation of water-insoluble (urea-soluble) protein, but this has not been proven.

Despite extensive investigation, neither the precise chemical nature of high-molecular-weight aggregates nor the mechanism of their formation is known with certainty. High-molecular-weight fractions isolated from the nucleus of calf and adult bovine lenses display age-related differences in tertiary structure as manifested by their UV fluorescence and circular dichroism properties (35). The aggregates in bovine lens are poly disperse populations of different conformations; because of the apolar (hydrophobic) nature of the predominant α-crystallin polypeptides, their association in high-molecular-weight aggregates is mainly through noncovalent interactions.

The high-molecular-weight aggregates of human lens appear to have a more complex composition; the presence of 43 kDa polypeptide in disulfide-linked aggregates has been described by Spector (53,54). Several degraded proteins are also found in high-molecular-weight aggregates from human lens; one of them, a 9.6 kDa polypeptide, is a cleavage product of the α-crystallin A chain. It increases during aging from 7% of the water-soluble proteins to 36% of the water-insoluble proteins. In further studies, the proteins of human lenses of various ages have been separated into three fractions: water soluble, urea soluble, and urea insoluble (56). The amounts of degraded polypeptides smaller than 18 kDa increase with age; moreover, the polypeptides isolated from either water-soluble or urea-soluble fractions self-aggregate during storage, resulting in the formation of polymers ranging in size from 18 to 1500 kDa. These findings, as well as others showing that the degraded polypeptides are immunoreactive toward both α- and γ-crystallins, suggest that an age-related polymerization of degraded polypeptides into high-molecular-weight aggregates leads to their insolubilization. The origin of the degraded polypeptides has not been established, but they may be derived through the activation of endogenous proteinases. Among the endogenous substances that may control proteinase activity in human lens is a trypsin inhibitor activity associated mainly with the α-crystallins in young lenses (51,57). With increasing age, it associates with the aggregates. Beyond the age of 60 years, the inhibitor activity is found mainly in the water-insoluble fraction.

LENS METABOLISM

Overview

It has long been recognized that lens metabolism decreases with age; this includes not only the proliferative capacity of the epithelial cells but also the specific activities of most lens enzymes (Table 1). The extent of the demonstrable age-related decrease depends in part on how the enzyme activity is expressed (as wet weight of tissue, as milligrams of protein, or as total activity per lens). Moreover, with any of these parameters used as reference for

Table 1 Lens Enzymes Showing Decreased Activity in Aging

Enzyme(s)	Species	References
Glycolytic or oxidative	Rat	41–43
Methionine adenosyltransferase	Rat	44
Superoxide dismutase	Human	45,46
Endopeptidases	Human	47
Exopeptidases	Human	47
Glutathione peroxidase	Human	48
	Monkey[a]	49
Glutathione reductase	Monkey	49
	Rabbit	50
	Human	45

[a] Glutathione peroxidase activity in monkey lens increases until adulthood and then declines.

calculation, the enzyme activity varies considerably according to whether young (cortical) or old (nuclear) regions are chosen for analysis.

Glycolytic and Oxidative Enzymes

The catalytic activities of glycolytic and oxidative enzymes in the rat lens are higher in the equatorial (young) region than in the nuclear (old) region (18). Many enzymes also display altered electrophoretic mobility with aging; moreover, certain enzymes lose their catalytic activity even though they are immunologically detectable. The specific activities of most glycolytic enzymes in whole rat lens decline with age when calculated on the basis of wet weight of tissue and plotted on a semilogarithmic scale (11). However, the specific activities of the same group of enzymes calculated per milligram of protein remains fairly constant with age, except of aldolase. Aldolase displays a marked decline in specific activity in the aging rat lens, possibly the result of a post-translational modification, such as denaturation, that leads to its inactivation (13). The same may be true for glyceraldehyde 3-phosphate dehydrogenase, a key enzyme in both glycolysis and the pentose phosphate pathway. Another enzyme, glucose 6-phosphate dehydrogenase (G6PD), also undergoes changes with age. By using an antibody prepared against denatured G6PD that does not recognize "native" G6PD, antigenically cross-reactive but catalytically inactive G6PD molecules have been shown to accumulate in the rat lens nucleus (14). Superoxide dismutase (SOD) is present at low but detectable levels in the lens, and the SOD activity declines markedly with age in both the nuclear and equatorial regions (48).

The activities of enzymes of GSH synthesis, GSH synthetase, and γ-glutamylcysteine synthetase decline sharply with age in human, bovine, rabbit, and dog lenses (50). For other enzymes in GSH metabolism, however, such as GSH reductase, there are species variations in age-related changes in activity (37,45). In the human lens, GSH reductase activity is lost slowly and gradually throughout life (44). GSH reductase activity in cultured epithelial cells from 8-year-old rabbits is 50% lower than in cells cultured from 4-day-old rabbits (46). However, the levels of GSH peroxidase, hexokinase, and G6PD are comparable in young and old lens epithelial cells from rabbits.

Glycation Reactions

The nonenzymatic glycation (or glycosylation) of a protein occurs by condensation of the aldehyde moiety of a sugar with a protein amino group to form a covalent adduct (5,19). Sugar molecules can condense readily with the α-amino group of an amino acid when available and, although somewhat less reactive, with e-amino groups as well. The initial product formed is a labile Schiff base, which undergoes Amadori rearrangement to a ketoamine, the first step in the nonenzymatic browning of food (the Maillard reaction) (5). This important reaction is now believed to be involved in aging and in cataract formation in the lens. Under physiological conditions, in the final stages of the Maillard reaction, extensive condensation leads to alterations in protein conformation and formation of high-molecular-weight cross-linked aggregates. These proteins are far less water soluble than the parent proteins. The extent to which this reaction proceeds, either in vivo or in vitro, depends on the concentration of glucose present, the number of potentially reactive amino groups on the protein, and other less well defined factors (5,18).

The ε-amino groups of lysine in bovine lens crystallins, particularly the high-molecular-weight aggregates of α-crystallin, are glycated nonenzymatically in vivo in an age-related manner (12). Moreover, incubation of human and bovine lens proteins with reducing sugars in the absence of oxygen leads to the formation of fluorescent yellow pigments and non-disulfide protein-cross-links (36). The pigment formed is strikingly similar to that found in diabetic lenses and in cataractous human lenses. Both these observations imply the existence of a Maillard reaction in the lens.

Human lens crystallins, soluble and insoluble, contain an average of 0.028 nmol glycated lysine per nmol crystallin monomer (16). Similar levels of glycation are found in the soluble and the insoluble crystallins. Glycation of human lens crystallins increases with age in a linear manner: 1.3% of lysine residues are glycated in the infant lens and 2.7% in the 50-year-old lens, and by theoretical extrapolation of the data, approximately 4.2% of human lens crystallins would be glycated in older age groups. These are surprisingly low values; despite their longevity, lens proteins undergo far less glycation than proteins that turn over rapidly, such as hemoglobin or serum albumin. The relatively slow rate of glycation of lens crystallin may be the consequence of several factors: (*i*) the concentration of glucose in the lens is relatively low (1 mM in normal humans); (*ii*) the predominantly β-pleated structures of the crystallins provide only a limited number of exposed lysine residues for glycation; and (*iii*) lens crystallins have a smaller percentage of lysine residues than highly glycated proteins, such as hemoglobin or albumin, and some of their α-amino groups may be blocked.

In addition to glucose, ascorbic acid (Fig. 2) is also capable of forming adducts with bovine lens crystallins (6). The reaction with ascorbate is faster than that occurring with glucose, although the fluorescence spectra are similar. In both cases the brown coloration that forms appears to represent a nonenzymatic Maillard-type reaction. Ascorbic acid is present at higher concentrations than glucose in normal lens. Hence, it may play an important role in the glycation of lens crystallins, and recent findings support this view. The browning and aggregation of bovine β- and γ-crystallins, but not α-crystallin, can be produced in vitro in the presence of either ascorbic acid or dehydroascorbic acid (39). Under similar experimental conditions, glucose, even at concentrations as high as 100 mM over a six week period, is ineffective in generating cross-linked proteins. The physiological importance of ascorbate glycation is that it occurs under low oxygen tension with as little as 2 mM ascorbic acid, the average concentration in normal lens. The glycating species is the oxidized form of ascorbic acid, since the formation of covalent adducts, as well as cross-linked proteins, is inhibited by GSH and other reducing agents (40). These interesting findings suggest that in vitro, and possibly in vivo, GSH may inhibit glycation by maintaining ascorbic acid in the reduced state, a form that is not active in glycation. In aging and in cataractous lenses, in which the concentrations of oxidized ascorbic acid are presumably normal but the levels of GSH may be low or depleted, increased glycation is expected. Other studies show that incubation of calf lens extracts with 20 mM ascorbic acid induces the formation of high-molecular-weight aggregates (41); the cross-linking by ascorbate appears to be between the βH- and α-crystallins. The principal ascorbate-modified amino acid is lysine; in addition, a small amount of glycated arginine was detected. The mechanism of glycation by ascorbate is still unknown, but studies using a model system have shown that ascorbic acid auto-oxidation by GSH is enhanced in the presence of metal ions, suggesting involvement of oxygen free radicals (62,63). Whether glycation in vivo proceeds through the formation of an ascorbyl free radical generated by GSH in the presence of endogenous metal ions remains to be established.

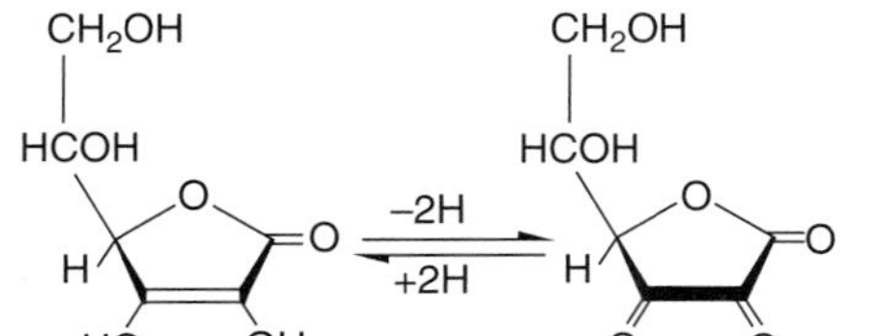

L-ascorbic acid (reduced) (ASA) ⇌ **L-dehydroascorbic acid (oxidized) (DHA)**

Figure 2 Structures of L-ascorbic acid and L-dehydroascorbic acid. The reduced form (ASA) with an enediol structure at carbon atoms 2 and 3 is unstable and in solution at physiological pH is readily oxidized to dehydroascorbic acid (DHA), possibly through an ascorbyl radical intermediate. The equilibrium concentrations of each species depends on the levels of oxygen present; in the lens, where oxygen levels are low, the reduced species (ASA) is probably the major species. *Source*: From Berman ER. Biochemistry of the Eye. New York: Plenum Press, 1991.

Photochemical Changes

The increase in refractive index in aging human lens is accompanied by increased yellow coloration and nontryptophan fluorescence. One of the factors inducing these changes is thought to be the amount of UV radiation absorbed by the lens throughout the lifetime of the individual (18,26). Two mechanisms have been proposed to account for these changes: one is a direct process in which radiation is absorbed by endogenous chromophores, such as tryptophan and other aromatic amino acids, and the other is an indirect process, that is, absorption by extraneous photosensitizing compounds, such as drugs. The level of fluorogens (UV-absorbing chromophores) is relatively low in normal lenses below 10 years of age, but these substances steadily increase, especially in the nucleus, as the lens ages.

Tryptophan residues in the lens are thought to be the major photochemically active species in UV-induced changes in the aging lens; pigment formation and protein aggregation involve singlet oxygen and other reactive free radicals. Brown nuclear cataracts are an accelerated form of the normal aging process in which photochemically induced fluorescent pigments accumulate mainly in the nuclear region (19,26). The age-related yellowing of the human lens is in fact beneficial to vision, since it allows the lens to act as a filter in protecting the aging retina from cumulative photochemical damage. However, the increasing amount of UV radiation absorbed by the lens during the lifetime of the individual may be a risk factor in the development of cortical cataracts (see Chapter 24).

Whether tryptophan plays a direct or indirect role in chromophore production during aging has not been established with certainty. Kynurenine derivatives, products of tryptophan oxidation, can function as photosensitizers and have been detected in both clear and cataractous aging lenses. Nevertheless, this does not always correlate with increased nuclear pigmentation during aging (7); no corresponding increase in tryptophan or oxidation products derived from it could be detected in extracts from either cortical or nuclear regions of pigmented human lenses when calculated as a function of age (7). Instead, a particular fluorophore (excitation and emission maxima of 345 and 425 nm, respectively) increases significantly in clear old lenses and in those with nuclear cataracts. This fluorophor is not an oxidation product of free tryptophan; it appears to be associated with the γ-crystallins and may represent an oxidized fragment of this crystallin.

A yellow pigment that fluoresces at 440 nm with excitation at 370 nm is thought to arise from either UV-oxidized tryptophan residues (67) or a Maillard reaction following glycation of lens crystallins. This nontryptophan fluorescence has been examined further using a new fluorometric technique developed by Liang et al. (31). The method utilizes front-surface illumination of samples oriented 60° relative to the incident beam; this minimizes reflected light and therefore can be used with solid or turbid samples. Studies on insoluble crystallins from old and young bovine lenses show a red shift of tryptophan fluorescence, indicating a less hydrophobic environment with aging. Moreover, tryptophan residues are more exposed in older samples as a result of unfolding of crystallins (30). Another age-related difference is the appearance of a 370/440 nm non-tryptophan fluorescence peak in insoluble powdered samples from old bovine lenses. This peak, which is also present in human lenses, shows a shift to longer wavelengths in 60- to 75-year-old lenses.

Two metabolically generated fluorophores have been detected in the human lens using a newly developed Raman imaging system. One is a 441.6 nm excited green fluorophor (64) and the other a 488.0 nm excited fluorophor (4). The latter is detectable in human lenses after 10 years of age.

REFERENCES

1. Alcala J, Maisel H. Biochemistry of lens plasma membranes and cytoskeleton. In: Maisel H, ed. The Ocular Lens: Structure, Function, and Pathology. New York: Marcel Dekker, 1985:169–222.
2. Alcala J, Katar M, Rudner G, Maisel H. Human beta crystallins: Regional and age related changes. Curr Eye Res 1988; 7:353–9.
3. Alcala J, Valentine J, Maisel H. Human lens fiber cell plasma membranes. I. Isolation, polypeptide composition and changes associated with ageing. Exp Eye Res 1980; 30: 659–77.
4. Barron BC, Yu N-T, Kuck JFR Jr. Distribution of a 488.0-nm-excitedfluorophor in the equatorial plane of the human lens by a laser Raman microprobe: a new concept in fluorescence studies. Exp Eye Res 1988; 47:901–4.
5. Baynes JW, Watkins NJ, Fisher CI. The Amadori product on protein: Structure and reactions. In: JW Baynes, V Monnier, eds. The Maillard Reaction in Ageing, Diabetes and Nutrition. New York: Alan Liss, 1989:43–67.
6. Bensch KG, Fleming JE, Lohmann W. The role of ascorbic acid in senile cataract. Proc Natl Acad Sci U.S.A. 1985; 82: 7193–6.
7. Bessems GJH, Hoenders HJ. Distribution of aromatic and fluorescent compounds within single human lenses. Exp Eye Res 1987; 44:817–24.
8. Bessems GJH, Hoenders HJ, Wollensak J. Variation in proportion and molecular weight of native crystallins from single human lenses upon aging and formation of nuclear cataract. Exp Eye Res 1983; 37:621–31.
9. Bessems GJH, de Man BM, Bours J, Hoenders HJ. Age-related variations in the distribution of crystallins within the bovine lens. Exp Eye Res 1986; 43:1019–30.
10. Bouman AA, de Leeuw ALM, Broekhuyse RM. Lens membranes. XII. Age-related changes in polypeptide composition of bovine lens fiber membranes. Exp Eye Res 1980; 31:495–503.
11. Bours J, Fink H, Hockwin O. The quantification of eight enzymes from the ageing rat lens, with respect to sex differences and special reference to aldolase. Curr Eye Res 1988; 7:449–55.
12. Chiou S-H, Chylack LT Jr, Tung WH, Bunn HE. Nonenzymatic glycosylation of bovine lens crystallins: effect of aging. J Biol Chem 1981; 256:5176–80.
13. Dovrat A, Gershon D. Studies on the fate of aldolase molecules in the aging rat lens. Biochim Biophys Acta 1983; 757:164–7.
14. Dovrat A, Scharf J, Eisenbach L, Gershon D. G6PD molecules devoid of catalytic activity are present in the nucleus of the rat lens. Exp Eye Res 1986; 42:489–96.
15. FitzGerald PG. Age-related changes in a fiber cell-specific extrinsic membrane protein. Curr Eye Res 1988; 7:1255–62.
16. Garlick RL, Mazer JS, Chylack LT Jr, et al. Nonenzymatic glycation of human lens crystallin: Effect of aging and diabetes mellitus. Clin Invest 1984; 74:1742–9.
17. Geller AM, Kotb MYS, Jernigan HM Jr, Kredich NM. Methione adenosyltransferase and S-adenosylmethionine in the developing rat lens. Exp Eye Res 1988; 47: 197–204.
18. Harding J. Cataract, Biochemistry, Epidemiology and Pharmacology. London: Chapman and Hall, 1991.
19. Harding JJ, Crabbe MJC. The lens: Development, proteins, metabolism and cataract. In: Davson H, ed. The Eye. 3rd ed. Orlando, FL: Academic Press, 1984; lb: 207–492.
20. Harding JJ, Dilley KJ. Structural proteins of the mammalian lens: a review with emphasis on changes in development, aging and cataract. Exp Eye Res 1976; 22:1–73.

21. Horwitz J, Robertson NP, Wong MM, et al. Some properties of lens plasma membrane polypeptides isolated from normal human lenses. Exp Eye Res 1979; 28:359–65.
22. Hum TE, Augusteyn RC. The nature of disulphide bonds in rat lens proteins. Curr Eye Res 1987; 6:1103–8.
23. Jedziniak JA, Nicoli DE, Baram H, Benedek GB. Quantitative verification of the existence of high molecular weight protein aggregates in the intact normal human lens by light-scattering spectroscopy. Invest Ophthalmol Vis Sci 1978; 17:51–7.
24. Kistler J, Kirkland B, Gilbert K, Bullivant S. Aging of lens fibers: mapping membrane proteins with monoclonal antibodies. Invest Ophthalmol Vis Sci 1986; 27:772–80.
25. Kuck JFR, Yu N-T, Askren CC. Total sulfhydryl by Raman spectroscopy in the intact lens of several species: Variations in the nucleus and along the optical axis during aging. Exp Eye Res 1982; 34:23–37.
26. Lerman S. Ocular phototoxicity. N Engl J Med 1988; 319: 1475–7.
27. Li L-K, Roy D, Spector A. Changes in lens protein in concentric fractions from individual normal human lenses. Curr Eye Res 1986; 5:127–35.
28. Li L-K, So L. Age dependent lipid and protein changes inindividual bovine lenses. Curr Eye Res 1987; 6:599–605.
29. Li L-K, So L, Spector A. Membrane cholesterol and phospholipidin consecutive concentric sections of human lenses. J Lipid Res 1985; 26:600–9.
30. Liang JN, Bose SK, Chakrabarti B. Age-related changes in protein conformation in bovine lens crystallins. Exp Eye Res 1985; 40:461–9.
31. Liang JN, Pelletier MR, Chylack LT Jr. Front surface fluorometric study of lens insoluble proteins. Curr Eye Res 1988; 7:61–7.
32. Maisel H, Ellis M. Cytoskeletal proteins of the aging human lens. Curr Eye Res 1984; 3:369–81.
33. McFall-Ngai MJ, Ding L-L, Takemoto LJ, Horwitz J. Spatial and temporal mapping of the age-related changes in human lens crystallins. Exp Eye Res 1985; 41:745–58.
34. McFall-Ngai M, Horwitz J, Ding L-L, Lacey L. Age-dependent changes in the heat-stable crystallin, βBp, of the human lens. Curr Eye Res 1986; 5:387–94.
35. Messmer M, Chakrabarti B. High-molecular-weight protein aggregates of calf and cow lens: Spectroscopic evaluation. Exp Eye Res 1988; 47:173–83.
36. Monnier VM, Cerami A. Nonenzymatic browning in vivo: possible process for aging of long-lived proteins. Science 1981; 211:491–3.
37. Monnier VM, Cerami A. Detection of nonenzymatic browning products in the human lens. Biochim Biophys Acta 1983; 760:97–103.
38. Ohrloff C, Hockwin O, Olson R, Dickman S. Glutathione peroxidase, glutathione reductase and superxide dismutase in the aging lens. Curr Eye Res 1984; 3:109–15.
39. Ortwerth BJ, Feather MS, Olesen PR. The precipitation and cross-linking of lens crystallins by ascorbic acid. Exp Eye Res 1988; 47:155–68.
40. Ortwerth BJ, Olesen PR. Glutathione inhibits the glycation and crosslinking of lens proteins by ascorbic acid. Exp Eye Res 1988; 47:737–50.
41. Ortwerth BJ, Olesen PR. Ascorbic acid-induced cross-linking of lens proteins: evidence supporting a Maillard reaction. Biochim Biophys Acta 1988; 956:10–22.
42. Ozaki Y, Mizuno A, Itoh K, lriyama K. Inter- and intramolecular disulfide bond formation and related structural changes in the lens proteins: a Raman spectroscopic study in vivo of lens aging. J Biol Chem 1987; 262: 15545–51.
43. Pierscionek B, Augusteyn RC. Protein distribution patterns in concentric layers from single bovine lenses: changes with development and ageing. Curr Eye Res 1988; 7:11–23.
44. Rathbun WB, Bovis MG. Activity of glutathione peroxidase and glutathione reductase in the human lens related to age. Curr Eye Res 1986; 5:381–5.
45. Rathbun WB, Bovis MG, Holleschau AM. Glutathione peroxidase, glutathione reductase and glutathione-S-transferase activities in the rhesus monkey lens as a function of age. Curr Eye Res 1986; 5:195–9.
46. Reddan JR, Giblin FJ, Dziedzic DC, et al. Influence of the activity of glutathione reductase on the response of cultured lens epithelial cells from young and old rabbits to hydrogen peroxide. Exp Eye Res 1988; 46: 209–21.
47. Russell P, Garland D, Zigler JS Jr, et al. Aging effects of vitamin C on a human lens protein produced in vitro. FASEB J 1987; 1:32–5.
48. Scharf J, Dovrat A, Gershon D. Defective superoxide dismutase molecules accumulate with age in human lenses. Graefes Arch Clin Exp Ophthalmol 1987; 225: 133–6.
49. Schoenmakers JGG, Den Dunnen JT, Moormann RJM, et al. The crystallin gene families. In: Nugent, J Whelan, eds. Human Cataract Formation, Ciba Foundation Symposium 106,1. London: Pitman, 1984:208–18.
50. Sethna SS, Holleschau AM, Rathbun WB. Activity of glutathione synthesis enzymes in human lens related to age. Curr Eye Res 1982/1983; 2:735–42.
51. Sharma KK, Olesen PR, Ortwerth BT. The binding and inhibition of trypsin by ct-crystallin. Biochim Biophys Acta 1987; 915:284–91.
52. Siebinga I, Vrensen GFJM, Otto K, et al. Ageing and changes in protein conformation in the human lens: a Raman microspectroscopic study. Exp Eye Res 1992; 54: 759–67.
53. Spector A. The search for a solution to senile cataracts. Invest Ophthalmol Vis Sci 1984; 25:130–46.
54. Spector A. Aspects of the biochemistry of cataract. In: Maisel H, ed. The Ocular Lens. Structure, Function, and Pathology. New York: Marcel Dekker, 1985:405–38.
55. Spector A, Freund T, Li L-K, Augusteyn RC. Age-dependent changes in the structure of alpha crystallin. Invest Ophthalmol 1971; 10:671–86.
56. Srivastava OP. Age-related increase in concentration and aggregation of degraded polypeptides in human lenses. Exp Eye Res 1988; 47:525–43.
57. Srivastava OP, Ortwerth BJ. The effects of aging and cataract formation on the trypsin inhibitor activity of human lens. Exp Eye Res 1989; 48:25–36.
58. Takemoto L, Kodama T, Takemoto D. Covalent changes at the N- and C-terminal regions of gamma crystallin during aging of the normal human lens. Exp Eye Res 1987; 45:201–14.
59. Takemoto L, Takehana M. Major intrinsic polypeptide (MIP26K) from human lens membrane: Characterization of low-molecular-weight forms in the aging human lens. Exp Eye Res 1986; 43:661–7.
60. Takemoto L, Takemoto D, Brown G, et al. Cleavage from the N-terminal region of βBp crystallin during aging of the human lens. Exp Eye Res 1987; 45:385–92.
61. Taylor A, Davies KJA. Protein oxidation and loss of protease activity may lead to cataract formation in the aged lens. Free Radic Biol Med 1987; 3:371–7.
62. Winkler BS. In vitro oxidation of ascorbic acid and its prevention by GSH. Biochim Biophys Acta 1987; 925: 258–64.

63. Wolff SF, Wang G-M, Spector A. Pro-oxidant activation of ocular reductants. 1. Copper and riboflavin stimulate ascorbate oxidation causing lens epithelial cytotoxicity in vitro. Exp Eye Res 1987; 45:777–89.
64. Yu N-T, Cai MZ, Ho DJ-Y, Kuck JFR Jr. Automated laser-scanning-microbeam fluorescence/Raman image analysis of human lens with multichannel detection: evidence for metabolic production of a green fluorophor. Proc Natl Acad Sci USA 1988; 85:103–6.
65. Yu N-T, DeNagel DC, Pruett PL, Kuck JFR Jr. Disulfide bond formation in the eye lens. Proc Natl Acad Sci USA 1985; 82:7965–8.
66. Zigler JS Jr, Russell P, Takemoto LI, et al. Partial characterization of three distinct populations of human-y-crystallins. Invest Ophthalmol Vis Sci 1985; 26:525–31.
67. Zigman S. Photobiology of the lens. In: Maisel H, ed. The Ocular Lens: Structure, Function, and Pathology. New York: Marcel Dekker, 1985:301–47.

20

Anterior Segment Changes in Glaucoma

Ian Grierson
Unit of Ophthalmology, School of Clinical Sciences, University of Liverpool, Liverpool, U.K.

INTRODUCTION

"Glaucoma" is a generic term used to describe a variety of pathophysiological processes in which the intraocular pressure (IOP) usually reaches a level sufficient to cause damage to the eye. The crucial defects occur in the retina and optic nerve (see Chapter 21). There are exceptions, however, and glaucoma can occur in individuals whose IOP falls in or close to the normal range (normotensive glaucoma). Alternatively, a population is recognized with IOP above the normal range but without signs of glaucomatous damage and a low glaucoma conversion rate (ocular hypertensives). Pathologically elevated IOP is typically the consequence of blockage or alteration of the outflow system.

NORMAL OUTFLOW PATHWAY

The circulating intraocular fluid, the aqueous humor, is produced at the ciliary processes by a combination of energy-dependent secretion and pressure-dependent ultrafiltration. On the other hand, drainage from the eye is entirely a result of pressure-dependent bulk flow. The characteristic of a bulk flow system is that flow depends on a pressure gradient overcoming the intrinsic resistance of the tissue to allow outflow to occur at the same rate as inflow. The analogy of a faucet dripping into a sink with a partially blocked drain is of some value. The sink will fill with water until a pressure head develops that is sufficient to drive water out at the same rate that it drips into the sink. In the normal human population, the inflow of aqueous humor is between 2 and 4 μl/min, the average IOP is approximately 16 mmHg, and the episcleral venous pressure is of the order of 9 mmHg. Therefore, a pressure head of 7 mmHg is needed to overcome the intrinsic resistance of the outflow system to allow the egress of aqueous humor at the rate of 2 to 4 μl/min and thus maintain ocular equilibrium.

There are two major routes of aqueous humor drainage: the conventional outflow pathway and the uveoscleral pathway. The conventional outflow pathway is located at the corneoscleral limbal region of the eye (Fig. 1) and is by far the more important in humans. It is thought to account for around 90% of total drainage (16,17,50), although this might be an overestimate. It consists of the trabecular meshwork (TM), Schlemm canal, and a series of collector vessels leading the aqueous humor to the intrascleral plexus and ultimately to the episcleral venous system. The remaining 10% of drainage is mainly by the uveoscleral route, whereby aqueous humor passes across the face of the ciliary muscle, into the suprachoroid, and through the scleral coat to end in the vortex system. A compromised conventional outflow system is the principal cause of pathologically elevated IOP.

Conventional Outflow Pathway

The TM consists of two anatomical regions: the uveal meshwork and the corneoscleral meshwork (Fig. 2). Uveal trabeculae are cordlike structures that form the layers immediately adjacent to the chamber angle. These trabeculae consist of collagenous cores surrounded by endothelium, and they merge posteriorly with the ciliary muscle. Openings through the uveal layers can measure in excess of 70 μm in diameter (Fig. 3A) and are so large that the resistance offered to aqueous humor passage must be negligible. The corneoscleral trabeculae are made up of the same elements as those present in the uveal trabeculae, but they form layers of flattened sheets (Fig. 3B), have fewer and smaller openings for aqueous humor passage, and link posteriorly with the scleral spur rather than the ciliary muscle (Fig. 2). The inner wall of Schlemm canal (preferably called the drainage wall) consists of an endothelial monolayer that is linked to the corneoscleral trabeculae by a loose connective tissue zone called the juxtacanalicular connective tissue (JCT), the cribriform zone, or the endothelial meshwork (Fig. 4). The JCT, a term first introduced by Fine (41), is used here. The JCT is more cellular and far less dense than the outer (structural) wall of Schlemm canal. Up to the JCT, aqueous humor has been passing through endothelium-lined channels filled with nothing but aqueous humor. By way of comparison, the pathways through the JCT are narrow (4–7 μm diameter) and extremely tortuous and are filled with extracellular matrix (ECM) materials (Fig. 4). The coarse extracellular framework materials are for the most part organized into "plaques" (147,150) consisting of columns of elastic like tissue. The fine framework materials are glycosaminoglycans (GAGs) and glycoproteins, which usually need either immunochemical or histochemical staining for visualization. From a functional point of view, the distribution of GAGs may be of crucial importance because they are hydrophilic and retard the progress of aqueous humor. Therefore, the GAGs located within the narrow, tortuous spaces of the JCT are likely to make a major contribution to the resistance to aqueous humor outflow (27,37,71) and determine preferential flow pathways (74).

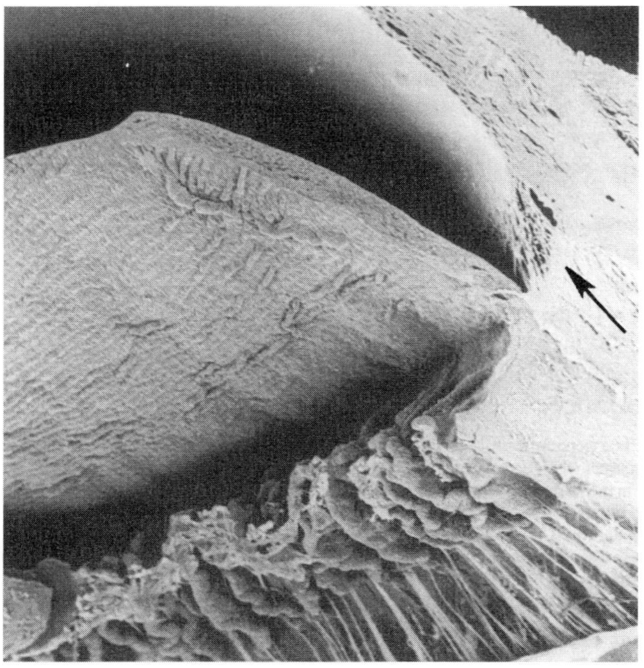

Figure 1 Chamber angle by scanning electron microscopy. The trabecular meshwork is marked by an arrow (×24).

Once the JCT has been negotiated, aqueous humor passes through the endothelial monolayer into Schlemm canal. The endothelium on the inner or drainage aspect of the canal has similarities to the endothelium of a lymphatic vessel. The monolayer, unlike the endothelium on the outer or structural aspect of the canal, lacks a true basement membrane. Instead it relies on cell–cell associations, with processes extending from the JCT cells for adhesion (67). Undoubtedly this is a modification to facilitate drainage.

The precise route by which aqueous humor passes through the endothelial monolayer into Schlemm canal is still controversial. Considerable study has been made of transendothelial pathways, often referred to as giant vacuoles, which can be up to and beyond 15 μm in diameter (Fig. 5) (36,60,62,80,83,176). At one time they were thought to be intracellular vesicles that were transported across the endothelium, but serial reconstruction has shown them to be complex invaginations (64,171). They are pressure dependent (60,83,171) and temperature

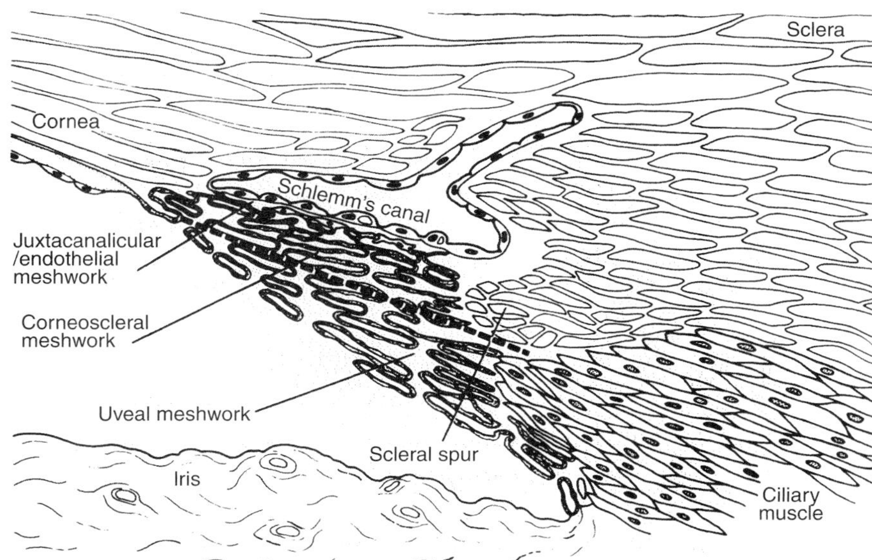

Figure 2 Anatomy of the outflow apparatus.

independent (180) and form as well in postmortem eyes (83) as in vivo (60,61). The invagination can be compared to an open parachute: the force that opens the parachute and gives it shape is air pressure, whereas the force that gives the invagination its shape is hydrostatic pressure (Fig. 5). The guide ropes of the invagination are cellular process connections with the underlying JCT cells, and if these are lost for whatever reason invaginations do not form.

Tripathi (176) was able to show that some, although not all, of the invaginations had openings on the luminal aspect. The luminal opening or pore, in conjunction with the invagination, is thought to serve as a transcellular route by which aqueous humor gains entry to Schlemm canal. Scanning electron microscopy (SEM) has disclosed approximately 4,000 pores in the whole of Schlemm canal, with sizes ranging between 0.2 and 3.0 μm (63,69). Taking into consideration the size and frequency of the invaginations and pores, it appears unlikely that the transcellular channels offer more than a token resistance to aqueous humor outflow (15,38,121,171). They are far too frequent and far too large. The question has arisen of why only some of the invaginations have pores and the rest are merely cul-de-sacs (Fig. 4)? The answer is not known, but it has been assumed that they represent different stages in a developmental cycle (64,176).

The cell–cell junctioning in the canal monolayer is extremely weak and is no barrier to tracer particles. More detailed investigations using freeze fracture (134) and tracer injection at physiological pressures (35) have highlighted the paracellular outflow route and suggest that it is far more influential than previously thought. Quantitative studies are required to determine precisely the relative contributions to drainage made by the transcellular and paracellular pathways (4,35). What is clear, however, is that the endothelial monolayer is extremely leaky and likely to contribute little to the resistance to outflow in the normal eye (4).

Some 25 to 35 collector channels drain the aqueous humor, from the lumen of Schlemm canal to the subconjunctival vessels and the episcleral venous system. Most collector channels reach the episclera via the intrascleral plexus, but some channels bypass the intrascleral plexus, and these are called aqueous veins. The collector channels have rather large diameters (20–90 μm) in terms of the dimensions of the outflow system as a whole, and classical literature indicates a contribution of only 25% of the total resistance (52). Monkey research calculates the resistance that lies beyond the TM and Schlemm canal to be merely 10% (111). Thus, it would seem that the only region in the conventional outflow system to offer major resistance to drainage in the normal eye is the JCT.

In terms of function, both the uveoscleral and conventional outflow routes are pressure-sensitive and have the facility to allow the passage of an increased volume of fluid in response to an elevation in the IOP. The conventional outflow system is particularly pressure sensitive, however, as a result of dramatic configurational changes in response to pressure change. Above normal IOP the TM is distended, making flow easier; beneath normal it becomes compacted, making flow more difficult. The closer to Schlemm canal, the more dramatic the TM changes become (60,83).

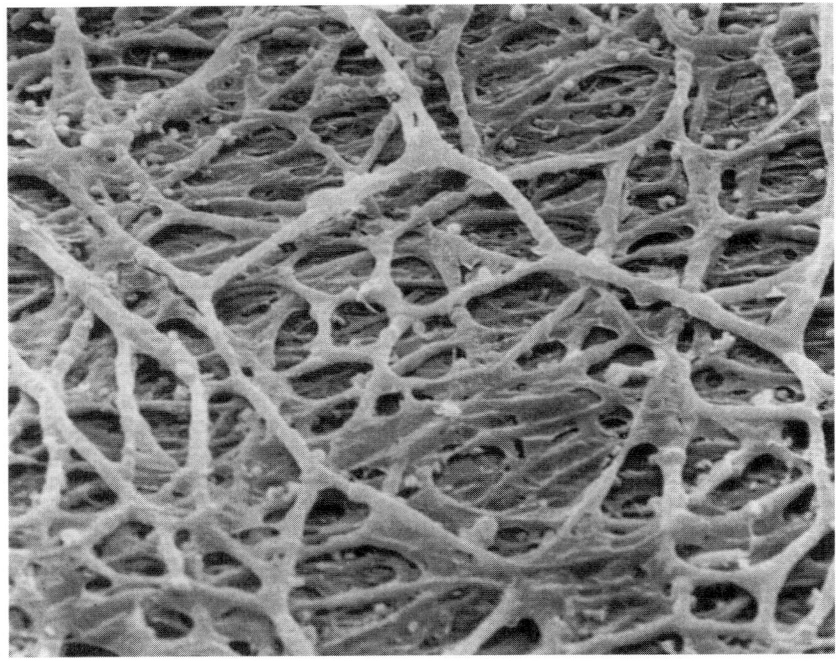

(A)

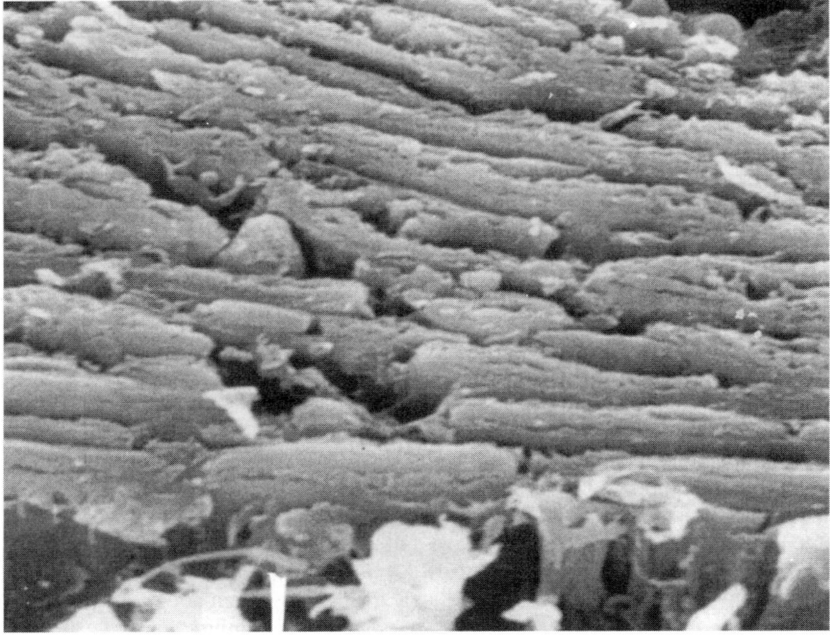

(B)

Figure 3 (**A**) Uveal trabeculae in flat preparation and (**B**) corneoscleral trabeculae in cross section as seen by scanning electron microscopy: (**A**), ×250; (**B**) ×300.

The conventional outflow system can be considered a "dampening device." In other words, in addition to acting as a drain, it serves to dampen any major fluctuations in IOP by allowing rapid egress of fluid in response to minor pressure elevation (63,68,69). Diurnal variation is only a few millimeters of Hg in the normal eye. Patients with mean IOP beyond 22 mmHg are suspected of having primary open-angle glaucoma (POAG), and those with diurnal pressure variations beyond 5 mmHg are even more likely to be glaucomatous. Thus there is blockage in the outflow system of patients with POAG, and affected patients are also less capable of making the passive morphological change from a low to a high flow configuration when the outflow system is faced with an increased drainage demand (36,63,68,69).

The Meshwork Cell

For many years the behavioral, functional, and metabolic activities of the cells in the TM were either

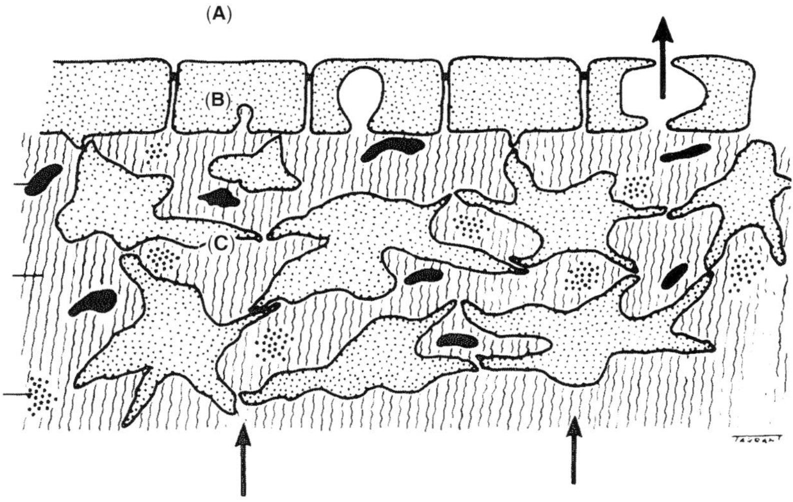

Figure 4 Main structural features in the drainage wall of Schlemm canal: (A) Schlemm canal; (B) endothelium lining the canal; (C) Juxtacanalicular Connective Tissue.

dismissed or ignored. It was assumed that whatever activity TM cells had was virtually lost after embryological development. It was for the most part the work of Rohen and his group that highlighted the fact that TM cells were not the functionally inert cells they were once presumed to be (55,77,147). Physiological, immunological, cell biological, genomic and proteomic studies among others have helped to define the functional characteristics of the cells that line the small and delicate trabecular pathways (Table 1).

TM cells, by covering the trabeculae, maintain the trabeculae as separate and distinct units, but as a consequence they must bear much of the stress and strain to which the delicate tissue is subjected throughout life. The dramatic change in shape of the TM and the TM cells (which develop elongated processes) in response to elevated IOP testifies to the elasticity of these cells and the wear and tear to which they are subjected (61,186). Contraction of the adjacent ciliary muscle also stretches the TM and produces marked shape changes and similar extension of meshwork cells (65). Simple stretching of the TM cells has been shown by genomic analysis to up and down regulate a battery of genes (183). TM cells, like corneal endothelium, have a nonthrombogenic surface, and platelets do not bind to them. This may be of importance when there is bleeding into the anterior chamber (132).

That TM cells are phagocytic was first shown by Rohen and Van der Zypen in 1968 (149), and in human tissue by Grierson and Lee in 1973 (59,66). They demonstrated that monkey TM cells were able to phagocytose a wide range of particulate materials when they were introduced into the outflow system (149) and these findings were supported by numerous other groups (55). Phagocytosis resulted in the eventual migration of some of the TM cells from their normal position on the trabeculae. Subsequently, phagocytosis of materials ranging from erythrocytes and melanin to carbon and iron have been shown in

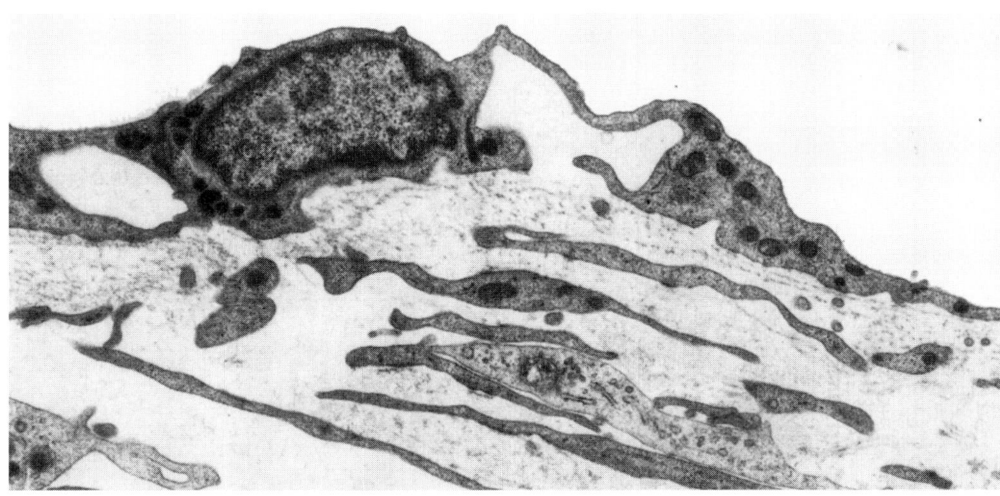

Figure 5 Transmission electron micrograph showing an invagination (gaint vacuole) in the endothelium lining the canal (×15,200).

Table 1 Suggested Activities of Meshwork Cells

Cover the trabeculae (maintain trabecular integrity)
Nonthrombogenic surface properties (like corneal endothelium)
Load bearing (stress and strain)
Phagocytosis
Migratory
Possible antigen processing (express class II antigens)
Synthesis of extracellular materials
Degradation of extracellular materials (GAGs in particular)
Synthesis of growth factors
Free radical defense
Contractility

human, monkey, and nonprimate species both in vitro and in vivo. Indeed, it has been suggested that TM cells are the reticuloendothelial cells of the eye (147). TM cells have Fc receptors, and Lynch and coworkers (110) showed that human TM cells express class I (HLA-ABC) and class II (HLA-DR) histocompatibility antigens. Cultured TM cells exhibit stimulated migratory behavior in response to components of aqueous humor (21,55) and to aqueous humor itself (77). TM cells therefore have several characteristics in common with macrophages, but their phagocytosis is by no means as effective or efficient. Nonetheless, the TM has been considered a biological filter because TM phagocytes can remove debris from the circulating aqueous humor (147).

TM cells can synthesize a variety of ECMs, including collagens, glycoproteins, and GAGs (27,58,179,195). Of particular interest are the key biologically active proteins such as fibronectin, laminin, fibrillin, SPARC, thrombospondins, myocilin to name a few. It is likely that there is a low level of remodeling in the trabeculae, such that extracellular elements are degraded and others synthesized. The TM structure can therefore be considered to be maintained in a state of dynamic catabolic–synthetic equilibrium. Nowhere is the equilibrium more important than in the JCT beneath Schlemm canal. Juxtacanalicular connective tissue cells have the functionally important role of maintaining the composition, distribution, and quantity of the ECMs in the narrow spaces through which aqueous humor must pass. The canal monolayer on the TM side does not have a basement membrane, and the invagination and transcellular channel system in particular for the passage of aqueous humor has relatively large openings. It is likely that there is continuous erosion of ECM from the JCT through the transcellular channels of the canalicular endothelium. The cells of the JCT may have the role of replacing and modifying the ECM to compensate for the gradual erosion of materials through the canal endothelium.

Detoxification may be another key role for the TM cell. Hydrogen peroxide is a known constituent of aqueous humor and can have a severe damaging effect on cells by the means of free radical attack. Interestingly, TM cells have a battery of protective enzymes that includes catalase, glutathione peroxidase, glutathione reductase, and glucose-6-phosphate dehydrogenase. Perfusion studies with hydrogen peroxide show that the TM can remove it effectively and has a pronounced ability to defend itself against the effects of free radical assault (126). Perhaps this is a necessary defense mechanism for TM cells, but its relevance to the outflow system in health and disease remains unclear (53).

TM cells have a well-developed cytoskeleton (153,175) in which contractile components are prominent such as myosin, actin, and α-smooth muscle actin. As a result TM cells are capable of producing a contraction when exposed to ATP (70), endothelin-1, and exhibit all the characteristics of smooth muscle cells both in vitro and in ex vivo preparations (186). Cytochalasin B, H-7, and latrunculin (which have a variety of effects on actin) and a range of cytoskeletal active agents dramatically increases the facility of aqueous humor outflow (175), suggesting that contractile TM cells influence the caliber of the pathways for aqueous humor passage and perhaps antagonize the actions of the ciliary muscle (186).

Age Changes in the Outflow System

The impetus for research into the aging outflow system has come from the need to have a baseline for evaluation of glaucoma specimens. Changes in the past that were thought to be glaucomatous have subsequently also been shown to be prominent in the aging outflow system. It is more than likely that in POAG, at least, many of the alterations are merely an exaggeration of the normal aging process.

Alvarado and colleagues (6,7) were the first to establish quantitatively that TM cells diminish throughout life (Fig. 6). Grierson and Howes (56) calculated that at 20 years of age humans have around 750,000 TM cells, which is reduced to about 400,000 at 80 years of age, with a loss rate of 6,000 cells per year. TM cells are lost from every region, and there is even cell loss from Schlemm canal, albeit less than 500 endothelial cells per year. The reason cells are lost from the outflow system remains open to speculation. It seems likely that strong contact inhibition of cellular division exists in the normal TM and guarantees that replacement is restricted. Factors responsible for cell loss are likely to be both genetic and environmental. The many possible environmental factors that may contribute to cell loss include apoptotic death promoted by mechanical wear and tear or toxins in the aqueous humor (1). Also TM cell migration due to chemoattractants in the aqueous humor has been highlighted (55,77).

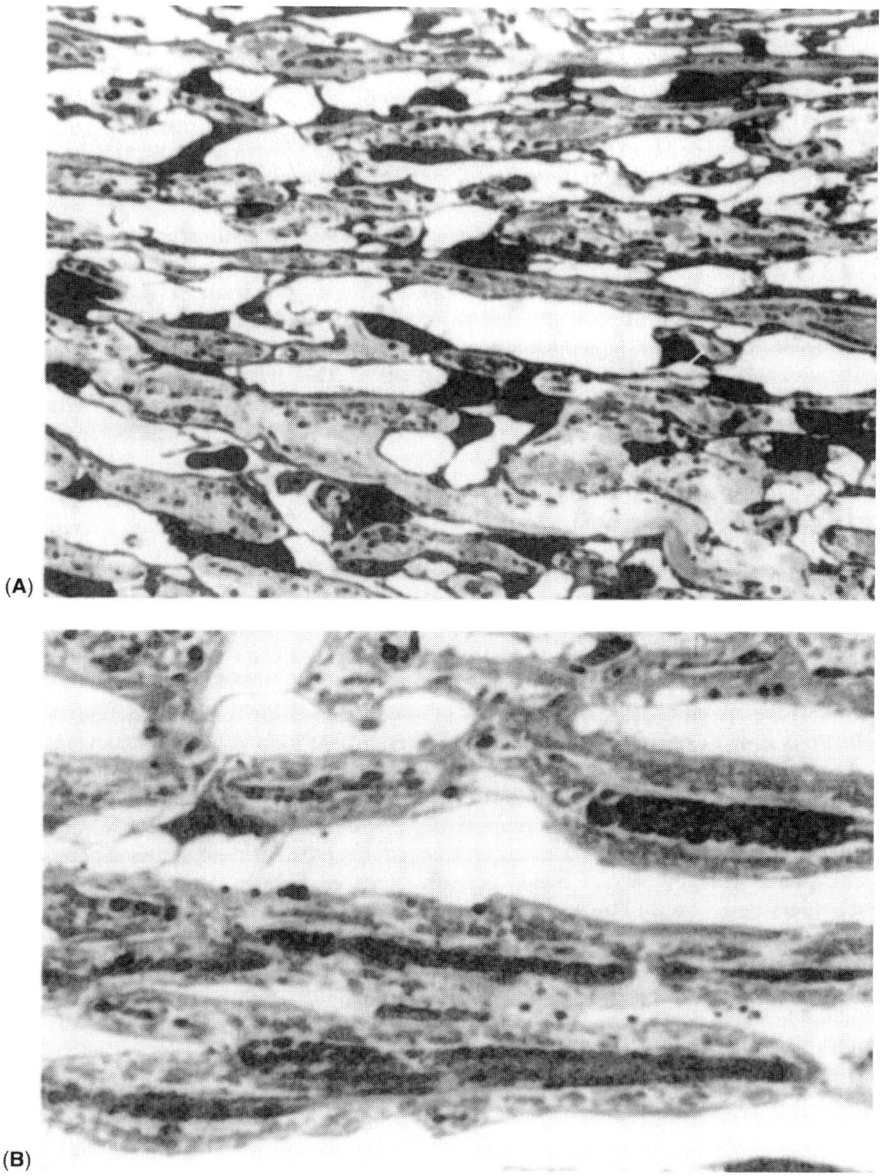

Figure 6 Corneoscleral trabeculae from (**A**) a 33-year-old subject and (**B**) a 76-year-old subject (light micrographs, ×1,300).

In the many morphological investigations of age changes in the outflow system, emphasis has been placed on the accumulation of ECM in the uveal and corneoscleral trabeculae, causing them to thicken with age. The extracellular core of uveal trabeculae consists mainly of collagen fibrils and elasticlike material and is covered by TM cells resting on a basement membrane. With increasing age, the elastic component of the core becomes more obvious and the basement membrane of the uveal trabeculae becomes irregular and multilayered. These changes are thought to be related to the loss of cell cover as the cell population becomes depleted in older people. Even where the cell cover is present it is often only loosely associated with the ECM core.

Corneoscleral trabeculae alter similarly with aging. The cell cover becomes more and more incomplete, and where cells are present they are often poorly attached. They accumulate melanin in the cytoplasm by phagocytosis of pigment that is slowly released into the aqueous humor from the iris epithelium throughout life (31,54,119). The basement membrane thickens, and elasticlike material is more prominent. McMenamin and colleagues (117,119) reported a linear increase in trabecular thickness with age. Thickening is very variable in different regions of the same eye, however.

The original trabecular collagen core remains much the same size, but a new layer forms between the original core and the basement membrane, which

Tripathi (176) called the cortical zone (Fig. 6). The developing cortical region in the aging outflow system is rich in elasticlike material and other ECM (Fig. 6). The increasing prominence of the elasticlike material with aging is not because of an increase in the electron-dense center of the material but a three-fold increase in the surrounding electron-lucent sheath (108). Biochemical extraction studies show that a proportion of the protein-bound methionine in the trabeculae is converted into methionine sulfoxide during aging, and the process is thought to relate to the alteration of ECM and the thickening of the sheathing substance (79).

Fusion of adjacent trabeculae is rare in young eyes but increases substantially in both the corneoscleral and uveal meshwork in persons over the age of 50 years. The absence of a cellular cover because of cell loss is thought to be the predisposing factor (55). For that matter, spreading of surviving cells and activation due to pigment phagocytosis and/or loss of trabecular adhesion may result in reactive repair processes that contribute to trabecular thickening (55).

Considerable research effort has centered on aging changes in the JCT, which is not surprising given its important contribution to the resistance to aqueous humor outflow. The number of JCT cells drops by about 40% throughout life (56), and some research groups believe that the amount of ECM in this region increases. Current findings suggest that there may not be an overall increase in ECM but an alteration of the type and disposition of material present (71). Electron-dense plaques of elasticlike material increase with advancing age (117,119), and as in the trabeculae, this is probably due to an increase in the sheath rather than the elastic core (108).

McMenamin and colleagues (117,119) have shown that ground substances consisting of granular material and immature collagen are common in those under 40 years of age but are much decreased in the elderly. GAGs in the JCT are thought to increase with aging, but study has been hampered by their labile nature and difficulties associated with quantitative analysis (71). The glycoproteins fibronectin and laminin are present here; fibronectin is fairly ubiquitous in the meshwork, but laminin is exclusive to the JCT (112). Myocilin is located both in the cells and as part of the ECM in the JCT. A similar cellular and ECM distribution is seen in the trabecular regions of the meshwork. As yet no age-related alterations in distribution and quantity have been observed (28).

The age-related decrease in cell number in the endothelial monolayer of Schlemm canal seems to be accompanied by an increase in the amount of subendothelial ECM. Counts have been made of the number of invaginations in the endothelium at various ages and the invaginations clearly diminish with increasing age (18,57,119). Perhaps the increase in subendothelial deposits is related to a dearth of transcellular flow channels. Some believe that Schlemm canal is more septated in the elderly (119). Undoubtedly some individuals after the sixth decade have several smaller channels instead of a single canal, but this alteration is not apparent universally. Grierson and colleagues (57) were unable to show a statistically significant increase in the numbers of bifurcations and septae with age.

Several of the age changes described, such as loss of cellularity in the meshwork, trabecular thickening, trabecular fusions, altered JCT matrix, and depleted invaginations in the canal endothelium, could be expected to impair the drainage function of the outflow system. Indeed, resistance increases with age (50) but not dramatically. Because there is ample spare capacity within the system. IOP rises marginally because the increase in resistance is compensated for by a reduction in the rate of aqueous humor production. Clearly, aging changes at the ciliary processes to some extent compromise the mechanisms for aqueous humor formation.

CLASSIFICATION OF GLAUCOMA

Glaucoma is generally classified into five major groups. Two primary forms are recognized: one in which the pathological processes occur within the outflow apparatus, *primary open-angle glaucoma* (chronic simple glaucoma), and another in which there is occlusion of the angle by iridotrabecular contact, *primary closed-angle glaucoma.* In a wide variety of pathological situations, the outflow apparatus is obstructed as a result of other disease processes that do not lead to angle closure, and these comprise the group included in *secondary open-angle glaucoma.* Conversely, when a disease leads to iridotrabecular contact and occlusion of the angle, the process is referred to as *secondary angle-closure glaucoma.* In the fifth major group, *congenital glaucoma,* aqueous humor outflow is obstructed at birth or in infancy by a malformation in the outflow system and chamber angle (goniodysgenesis). This group can be subdivided into those cases in which the abnormality occurs only in the angular tissues, *primary congenital glaucoma,* and *secondary congenital glaucoma,* in which the angle malformation is associated with other ocular and/or systemic abnormalities.

Primary Open-Angle Glaucoma

As yet the pathogenesis of POAG is poorly understood and the earliest events are particularly controversial. Too often in the past simple aging changes have been mistaken for glaucomatous features. Age-related and glaucoma-related alterations are intimately linked, and it is unwise to study the latter without intimate knowledge of the former. Controversies have arisen because of the quality of material available for investigation but that has improved immeasurably in recent years. Postmortem donor eyes from POAG patients and specimens from glaucoma surgery are studied but both have to be interpreted with care. Histopathological and experimental investigations have highlighted a range of sometimes related and sometimes contradictory observations and findings (Table 2). The possible glaucoma features listed in Table 2 is by no means complete but serves to illustrate a complex and somewhat subtle development of biologic and histopathologic events that culminates in compromised drainage of aqueous humor.

The alterations can be simplified to being either occlusion of aqueous humor flow pathways, alteration in ECM materials, or loss of cell function and death. Most are likely components of the pathological process, but which if any is the initial precipitating lesion is not known. An appreciation of the sequence of many pathological events has been obscured because of the tendency of investigators to "pool" specimens and seek common factors that might relate to the disease process. By doing so, the stage of glaucomatous development and the regimen of antiglaucoma therapy adopted before surgery is ignored in individual specimens. In a study conducted by our own group (54,55,71), we collected trabeculectomy specimens that came with full patient details, and of these a proportion were derived from an institution at which surgery was frequently the first form of antiglaucoma treatment. These patients either had no or minimal antiglaucoma medication. Other trabeculectomy specimens in our study followed failure of a single or series of medications to control IOP. Our collection of trabeculectomy specimens therefore came from patients with POAG at a relatively early stage of development, as well as those with advanced glaucoma.

Some collector channels were occluded and Schlemm canal was replaced in some specimens (Fig. 7), but these were from the group in whom IOP could not be controlled after these patients received maximal medical therapy and probably represented the end stage of the pathological process. Langham (97) suggested that collector vessels may lose tone and narrow sufficiently to elevate IOP pathologically. However, it seems improbable that

Table 2 Documented Features of the Outflow System in Primary Open-Angle Glaucoma

Excessive depletion of meshwork cells causing decompensation (6,55,71,72)
Progressive narrowing of the lumina of collector channels (97,98)
Alteration and closure of Schlemm canal (3,44,124,125)
Loss of invagination and flow channels from the canal endothelium (178)
Breakdown in meshwork cell to canal endothelial cross talk leading to reduced drainage (5)
Accumulation of ECMs, including GAGs, glycoproteins, and small proteins in the JCT (71,102,107,114,136,144,148,151)
Thickening and fusion of trabeculae (8,10,55)
Increase in thrombospondin-1 (46)
Colchin deposition in the meshwork (14)
Abnormal oculomedin expression (48)
Hyperpigmentation of meshwork cells (31,54)
Change in the actin content and distribution in meshwork cells (177)
Alterations in meshwork myocilin (82,89)
Failure of phagocytosis [discussed and not supported either by Grierson and Hogg (54,55) or Epstein and Rhoden (35);see also (113).
Changes in meshwork cell stress proteins and proteasome inhibition (20)
Abnormalities in NO or NO-containing meshwork cells (123)
Meshwork cell senescence in the outflow pathway (102)

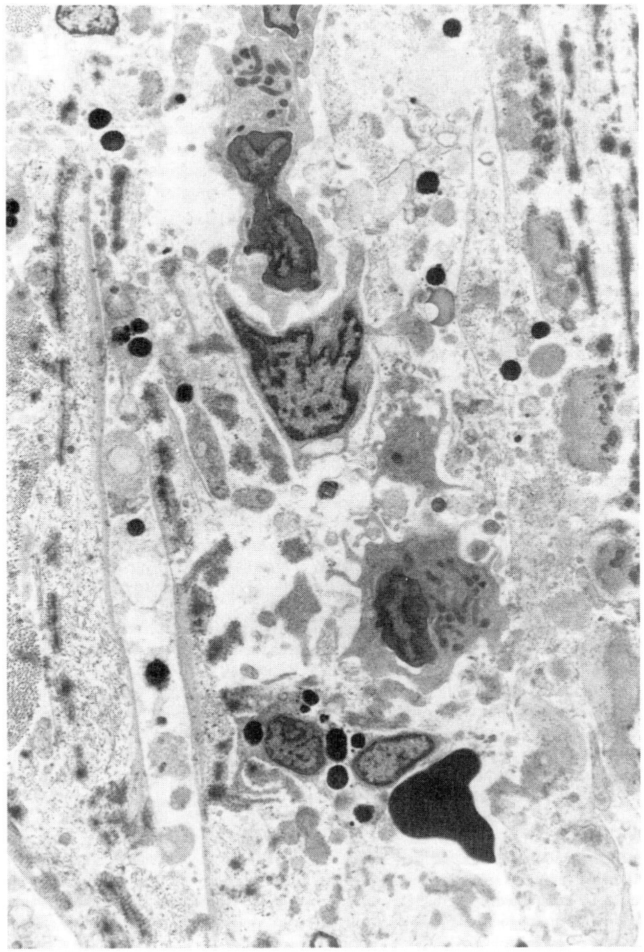

Figure 7 Transmission electron micrograph of the Schlemm canal region in advanced primary open-angle glaucoma in which there is canal replacement by fibrocellular material (×11,200).

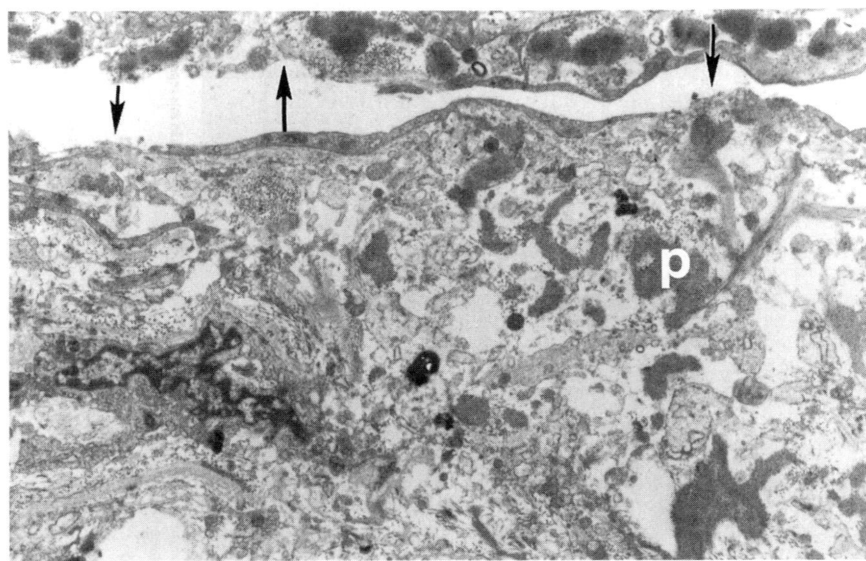

Figure 8 Transmission electron micrograph showing part of Schlemm canal in primary open-angle glaucoma. The canal is narrow, and the endothelial monolayer is discontinuous (*arrows*). Plaque material is indicated (p) (×7,600).

narrowing could raise IOP substantially in early disease. A narrowing of 50% elevates IOP a mere 1 to 2 mmHg (124). Fine et al. (41,42) observed replacement of Schlemm canal by fibrocellular tissue (Fig. 7) and attributed this to local hyperplasia of endothelial cells, but simple breakdown of the canal endothelium with subsequent loss of organization may be more likely. Deficits and areas of thinning of the canal endothelium are evident even in trabeculectomy specimens obtained from persons without prior antiglaucoma medication (Fig. 8), whereas extensive fibrocellular replacement of Schlemm canal is rarely seen, and then only in those with chronic poorly controlled glaucoma (54). Although it is conceivable that the small deficits (Fig. 8) are precursors of zones of extensive fibrocellular replacement (Fig. 7), the deficits may result from surgical trauma, because they have not been observed in enucleated glaucomatous eyes. Closure of Schlemm canal remains a possible mechanism of increased outflow resistance and canalicular narrowing has been quantitatively demonstrated in POAG (3), but we think it is unlikely to be an early event although key information is still lacking.

Tripathi (178) did not find ultrastructural changes in the TM of glaucoma subjects whose IOP was well controlled by topical medication at the time of their deaths. In contrast to age-matched controls, he noticed a virtual absence of invaginations in the endothelium of Schlemm canal. Others have also found endothelial invaginations to be extremely rare in trabeculectomy specimens. A failure in the transcellular channel aqueous humor drainage system would have a dramatic effect on IOP and is worth considering as a possible early lesion in POAG. However, despite there being some resilience to pressure change in the invagination/pore system (36), the pressure head that normally maintains the integrity of the invaginations is not so evident in postmortem eyes, which soften rapidly after death, or in trabeculectomy specimens, in which the pressure head is lost before fixation.

Many authors (8,10,46,71,107,109,114,141–143, 145,148,150,151) and others postulate an accumulation of ECM in the JCT of eyes with POAG and have proposed that the fundamental defect in POAG begins at the JCT because this is the site of maximum resistance to normal aqueous humor outflow. The ECM may accumulate (Fig. 9) because of either excessive synthesis by JCT cells or failure of the JCT catabolic or phagocytic mechanism by which debris and excess ECM are degraded.

At least one of the ECM components, the sheath covering of the plaques of elastic-like material, that increases with age shows a marked increase in POAG (71,108,145,148,167), and this seems not to be secondary to medication and to be an early change (71,148). On the other hand, Eithier et al. (37) demonstrated with flow models that changes to coarse ECM materials are unlikely to influence outflow dynamics substantially. Indeed, the collagen content of the JCT may decrease in POAG. Undoubtedly the key materials in this tissue are the fine matrix components, the GAGs and glycoproteins (114,151). The former require special techniques for electron microscopic demonstration and an effective quantitative morphometric study of GAGs in POAG has yet to be conducted conclusively (71). However an excessive accumulation of ECMs in the JCT that compromises aqueous humor drainage would explain how a subtle

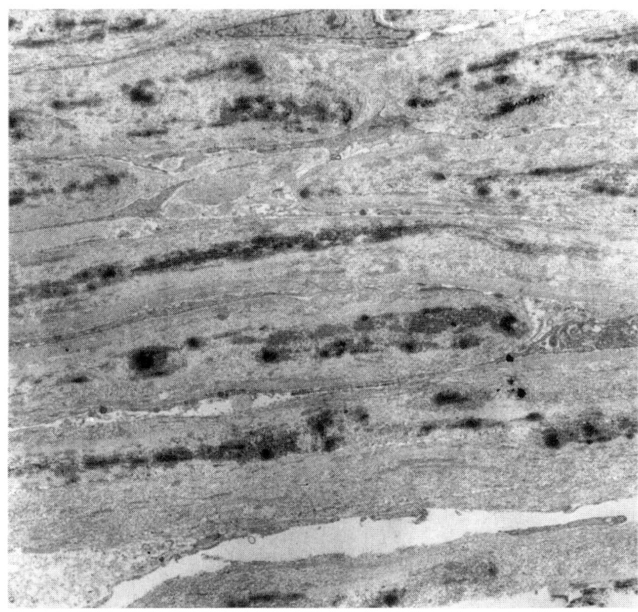

Figure 9 Transmission electron micrograph of corneoscleral trabeculae in primary open-angle glaucoma. In this region the trabeculae are fused together in the absence of a cell cover (×4,500)

alteration could have a marked effect on IOP, but it still remains to be established whether this occurs and, if it does, whether it is a primary or a secondary event.

Some investigators have been unimpressed with JCT alterations and believe that the cardinal abnormalities must occur elsewhere (5–7,42,44,71). In the TM the trabeculae have been thought to thicken excessively in POAG (166), but this also happens in aging. Trabecular thickening, beyond that expected from the normal age-related process, is a sporadic patchy finding that, if it occurs at all, is a manifestation of advanced POAG. Fine et al. (42) highlighted another aspect of trabecular disorganization, namely, trabecular fusion resulting in the loss of drainage pathways. They noted that this change was more pronounced in the posterior TM close to the scleral spur. The result of marked trabecular fusion in this region is an extended and enlarged scleral spur. Fusions of this type are more dramatic than those seen in aging (Figs. 6 and 9) and are found in areas where there is a marked depletion in TM cells.

Alvarado et al. (6) first demonstrated that patients with POAG have considerably fewer cells in the TM than age-matched normal controls. The cell loss was regional in the sense that the cellularity was markedly decreased in the TM but was virtually unaffected in the JCT. The cell loss was of such consistency that cellularity was proposed as a possible predictor of whether a specimen was glaucomatous. Our studies (54,55,71), confirmed much of the Alvarado (6) data showing that TM cells are lost in POAG beyond the level expected from normal aging (Figs. 9 and 10); a finding also supported by others (72).

Our series of trabeculectomies came both from patients that had previous failed maximum medical therapy and an important group where trabeculectomy was essentially the first form of antiglaucoma treatment (Fig. 10). In the group in whom trabeculectomy followed maximum medical therapy, the TM cell count was almost half that of an age-matched control group of normals. The difference was less marked in the patients who had little or no previous antiglaucoma medication but was still highly significant [see also (54,55,71)]. Clearly TM cell loss is part of the histopathology of POAG development in the outflow tissues and not simply a side effect of protracted medication. It is also suspected that a lower cell population is an early manifestation of POAG (6,71).

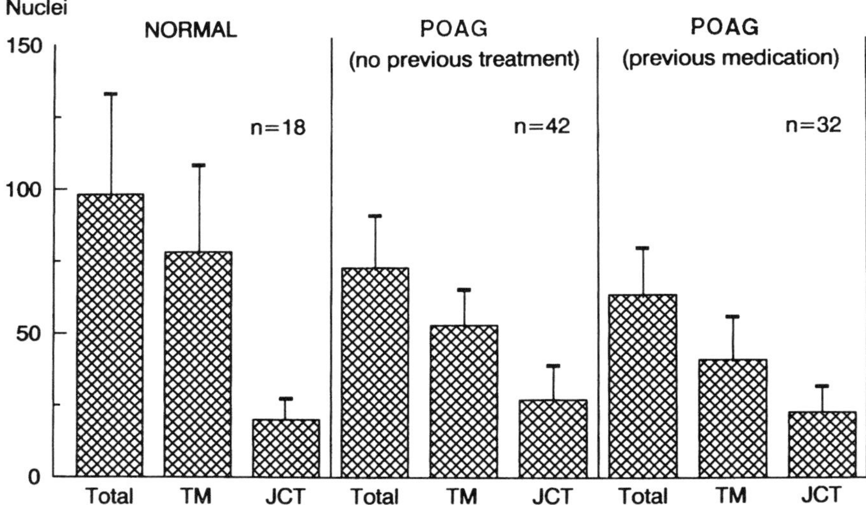

Figure 10 Histogram showing age-matched normals, primary open-angle glaucoma (POAG) at an early stage of the disease with no previous treatment before surgery, and a final group with maximal medical therapy before surgery. The columns (plus standard deviations) are of nuclei from the meshwork. The total numbers are significantly lower in the POAG groups than the normal. This is a result of cell loss from the trabecular meshwork (TM), not the juxtacanalicular connective tissue (JCT) (student's *t*-test).

Apoptotic cell death and migration of TM cells away form the outflow tissues in conjunction with poor replacement potential seem the likely mechanisms for cell loss (55). The causative processes leading to excessive cell loss may include wear and tear (55), altered growth factor balances (107,189), oxidative stress (47,53,126), and natural cellular senescence (102).

That the POAG TM is often more pigmented than normal has been observed by several authors but was demonstrated quantitatively by Grierson (31,54). Whether this is due to an excessive loss of melanin from the iris of POAG patients, free melanin being retained longer within the trabecular meshes, remains to be determined. Although heightened TM cell phagocytosis in POAG, once the more likely suspect, is now out of favor (113). Proliferation of flattened sheets of cells from the region of Schwalbe line onto the anterior surface of the TM was noted by Fine et al. (42) in eyes with POAG and are presumably stimulated to form by the absence of a cellular cover on the trabecular cords.

In conclusion, it seems that early changes in POAG are likely to be in the ECM of the JCT, such that IOP is elevated and there is a decrease in TM cellularity over and above the normal age-related loss. The JCT alterations are likely to account for any canal narrowing that takes place and ultimately for canal replacement. TM cell loss is probably responsible for the other TM changes, that is, trabecular fusion, trabecular thickening, and the spreading of peripheral corneal endothelium onto the uveal meshwork. It remains to be determined whether cell loss or JCT matrix alterations are the primary event and how the two interrelate. The importance and role of myocilin (89,169), thrombospondin-1 (46), colchin (14), oculomedin (48), and other biologically significant materials (the genes of many of which are associated with disease-causing mutations) in the outflow tissues in health and glaucoma have still to be determined but represent fascinating future research directions.

Primary Closed-Angle Glaucoma

In primary closed-angle glaucoma, contact between the peripheral iris and the inner surface of the TM prevents the outflow of aqueous humor in the region of attachment (Fig. 11A) (103–105). Histological reports (87,99,167) are sparse but such as are available describe contact over the total inner surface of the aqueous humor outflow system in end-stage closed-angle glaucoma.

Iris bombé, or anterior bowing of the iris, occurs in acute primary-angle closure glaucoma when the pressure in the posterior chamber is higher than in the anterior chamber. This results from restricted aqueous humor flow through the pupil (pupil block) and is associated with a shallow anterior chamber and hypermetropia.

A similar iris bombé mechanism may take place in pupil block secondary to inflammatory adhesions between the iris and lens (seclusio pupillae), by the formation of a pupillary membrane (occlusio pupillae), by pupillary obstruction of formed vitreous in aphakia, by a dislocated crystalline lens, or by a prosthetic intraocular lens.

In individuals with a deep anterior chamber, the lines of force during pupillary movements are limited to a radial direction in the flat plane of the iris diaphragm. In an individual with a shallow anterior chamber, the forces of dilatation and constriction can be resolved into both radial and posterior components. In semidilatation of the pupil, the posterior vector is maximal and blockage results from pressure of the pupil against the lens. This position commonly triggers iris bombé, which closes the iridocorneal drainage angle and provokes an acute rise in IOP. The time scale of the rate of increase can vary but in its most rapid form can reach 60 to 70 mmHg within minutes. If the iris bombé is not released pharmacologically within hours, permanent iridocorneal adhesions may result (peripheral anterior synechiae), although it is possible for attacks lasting some days to resolve without long-term sequelae.

Intermittent subclinical attacks of iris bombé can lead to the gradual development of synechiae, and this results in a type of chronic angle-closure glaucoma referred to as "creeping" angle-closure glaucoma (104,105). It is generally accepted that iridotrabecular contact is most commonly found in the upper part of the anterior chamber angle, from which point the attachment progresses in an inferior direction (13,194). The outflow system where there is angle closure is associated with compression of the trabeculae and reduction of Schlemm canal to a narrow slit. However, there is also evidence to suggest that permanent angle damage can happen without clinically identifiable synechiae. In these regions intertrabecular spaces are open but an influx of inflammatory cells is often seen. The TM cells can be replete with melanin granules of iris epithelial origin (99).

A more unusual type of angle closure occurs in individuals in whom the anterior chamber is of normal depth in the central part but narrow at the periphery: the plateau iris (131,184). When the pupil dilates the iris crowds the angle, leading to its obstruction. This condition is often only diagnosed retrospectively when a peripheral iridectomy performed for supposed pupil block glaucoma fails to prevent another acute attack. The ciliary processes may provide structural support to prevent the bunched up iris from "falling away from the TM after iridectomy" (131).

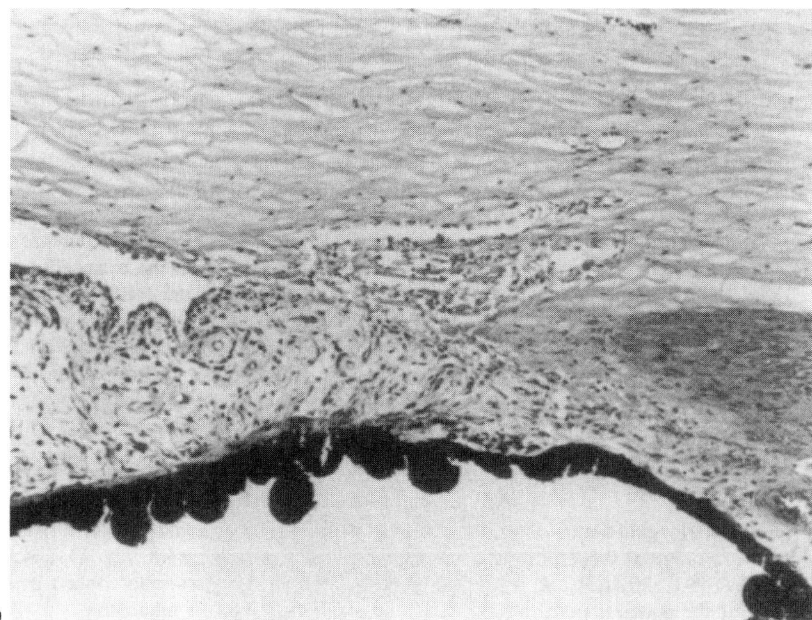

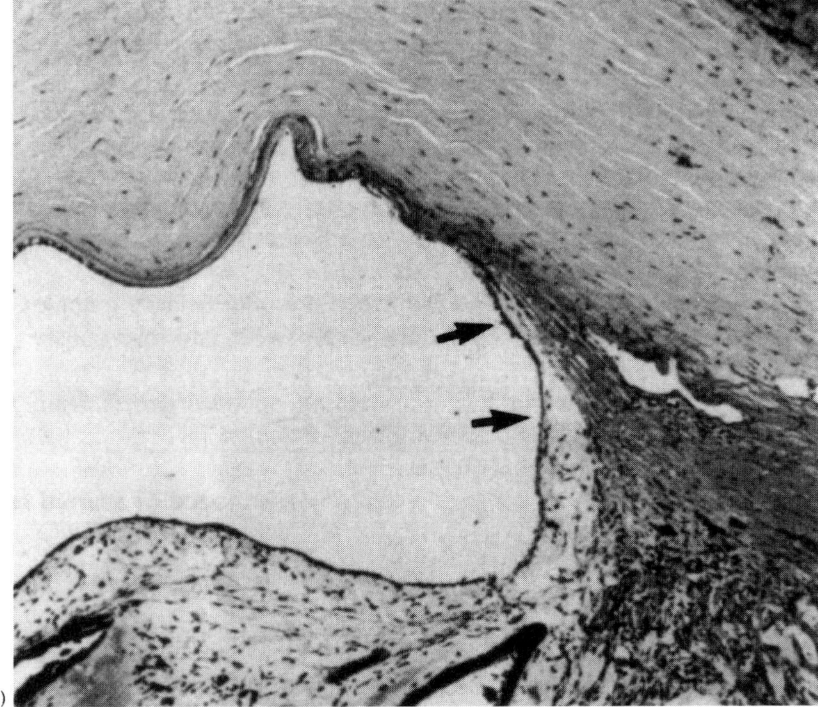

Figure 11 (**A**) Light micrograph showing the anterior chamber angle in early iridotrabecular contact. (hematoxylin and eosin, × 96). (**B**) Light micrograph showing persistence of iris tissue (*arrows*) on the inner surface of the trabecular meshwork in a case of closed-angle glaucoma after a Scheie operation (hematoxylin and eosin, × 85).

The pathological effects of iridotrabecular contact have not been extensively investigated. In our limited experience, we have demonstrated iris debris on the inner surface of the TM after an anterior chamber angle was surgically released. Alternatively, a fold of iris may remain adherent to the TM while giving the appearance of an open angle (Fig. 11B). Such observations may help to explain unsatisfactory surgical results.

Secondary Open-Angle Glaucoma

An increase in outflow resistance can develop when cells, cellular debris, or ECM enters an open anterior chamber angle and obstructs outflow pathways that were previously normal. The process is never entirely mechanical, and secondary changes occur in the native TM cells, in the trabecular framework, and in the extracellular tissues of the outer layers. The reactive changes in these structures to the obstructing material vary according to the dimensions, the chemical nature, and the quantity of material to which the tissue is exposed. It is important to reiterate that, although the outflow system has a potential for self-cleaning, it has a limited capacity and can be overloaded. The secondary open-angle glaucoma group can be subdivided according to the nature of the infiltrating material (Table 3).

Hemolytic and Ghost Cell (Erythroclastic) Glaucoma

Small quantities of blood are cleared rapidly from the anterior chamber, and their effects on aqueous humor dynamics are minimal. In part this is because of the operation of effective mechanisms for the lysis of platelets and fibrin (129,154) in the aqueous humor. In addition, intact erythrocytes and leukocytes are sufficiently malleable to negotiate the tortuous pathways through the TM. The lining endothelium of Schlemm canal does not present a barrier because blood cells can pass through invaginations and transcellular channels with apparent ease (80). This sequence of events changes when the volume of blood is excessive and the fibrinolytic mechanism is depleted. An even more complex situation occurs when the blood has been subjected to stagnation and lysis, for example in the entry of blood into the anterior chamber from a long-standing vitreous hemorrhage (25,26,40). Fenton and Zimmerman (40), who introduced the term "hemolytic glaucoma," considered that the increased outflow resistance was due to obstruction by large macrophages filled with erythrocyte debris; these cells appear to lose their malleability until the ingested products of erythrocytes are degraded (66) (Fig. 12). However emphasis also has been placed on lysed erythrocytes (ghost cells or erythroclasts) as agents of blockage. Unlike erythocytes, ghost cells are spherical and rigid, so that they are unable to pass through the outflow system, and their accumulation in the inner layers of the TM causes obstruction (ghost cell glaucoma) (25,96). Indeed, the injection of autologous ghost red blood cells into the anterior chamber of primate eyes produces chronic glaucoma (133).

The situation is complicated by the fact that the native TM cells have an impressive capacity to phagocytose intact and fragmented red cells (55,66). There is also evidence to indicate that engorged TM cells may separate from the trabecular beams, so that the latter swell and become disorganized, further aggravating the already increased impedance. Finally, in the late stages of exposure to breakdown products of blood or metallic iron, the outflow system becomes heavily impregnated with stainable iron that may or may not be tissue toxic. From the pathogenetic point of view, we think it is a mistake to make too much of a distinction between hemolytic and ghost cell glaucoma. Lee (99) stated "In my own files it has not been possible to find a completely monocellular ghost cell infiltrate in the TM and there has always been an admixture of macrophages in cases of such severity that enucleation has been required." This also has been our experience.

Table 3 Various Types of Secondary Open-Angle Glaucoma

Type of glaucoma	Infiltrating material
Hemolytic glaucoma	Macrophages with debris from erythrocytes
Ghost cell glaucoma	Rigid membranous spheres produced by red cell lysis (erythroclasts) and macrophages
Inflammatory open-angle glaucoma	Inflammatory cells
Glaucoma due to direct invasion by viable tumor cells	Tumor cells
Phacolytic glaucoma	Macrophages containing lens material, lens fragments, and high-molecular-weight proteins
Capsular glaucoma	Pseudoexfoliative material and melanin granules
Pigmentary glaucoma, pigment dispersion syndrome	Melanin granules, clump cells, and macrophages
Melanomalytic glaucoma	Macrophages containing necrotic debris from melanomas, cellular debris, and melanin granules
Corticosteroid glaucoma	Filamentous material
Posttraumatic glaucoma	Red blood cells entering a damaged or scarred outflow system

Glaucoma Secondary to Inflammation

Glaucoma is commonly associated with chronic uveitis, occurring in some 25% of cases (130,170). This is particularly true of children with systemic uveitis syndromes, especially those with pauciarticular juvenile chronic arthritis (85), in which it is a devastating complication. Nongranulomatous trabeculitis, as might occur in association with a viral infection (99), Fuchs heterochromic iridocyclitis (84,99) and scleritis or episcleritis (187), is associated with a lymphoplasmacytoid infiltration of the outflow tissues.

The secondary open-angle glaucoma that develops in some of the above patients may be attributed to simple mechanical obstruction by an inflammatory infiltrate dominated by lymphocytes and plasma cells, but this is probably an oversimplification. Conceivably, the release of hydrolytic enzymes, growth factors, cytokines, free radicals, and other materials from inflammatory cells and damaged tissues are also involved through effects on the endothelial cells of the outflow system. Irrespective of the mechanism,

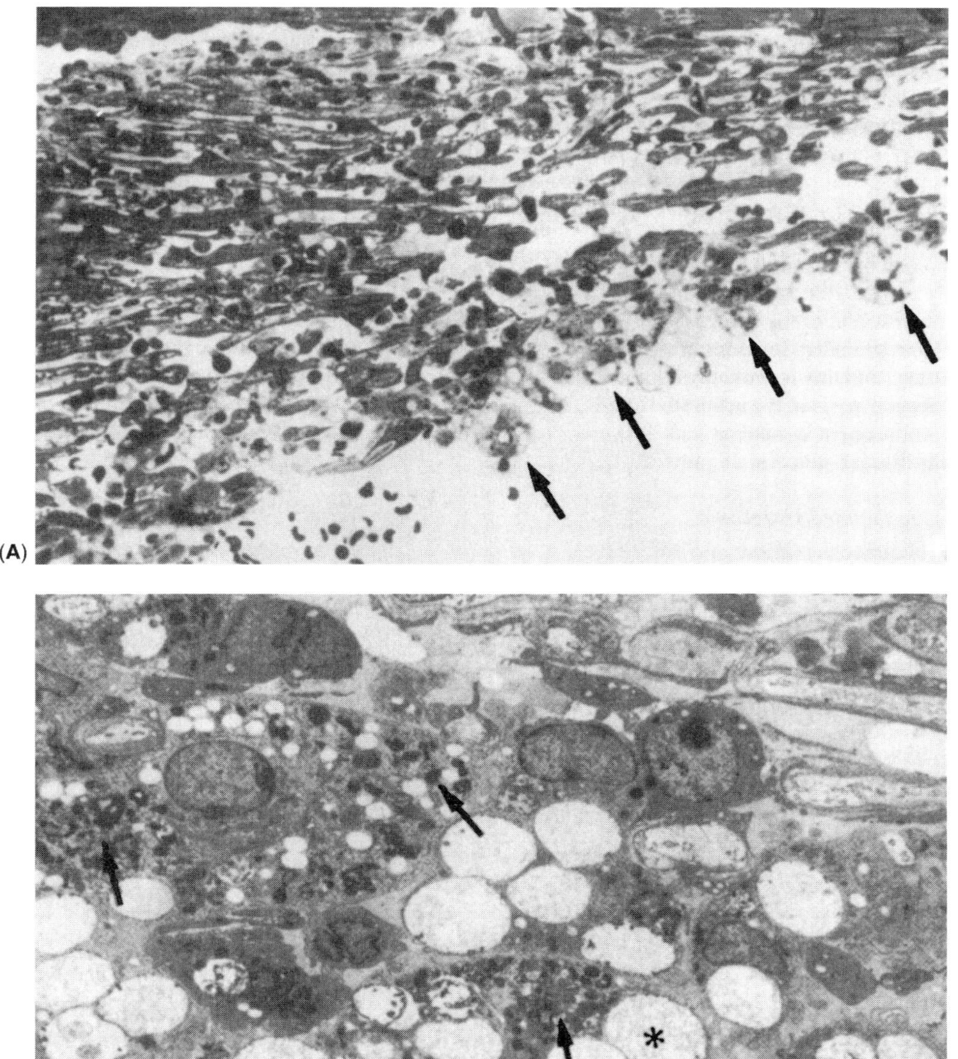

Figure 12 (**A**) Outflow system after exposure to blood for 14 days. Giant macrophages containing red cell debris line the inner surface of the trabecular meshwork (*arrows*) (Toluidine blue, ×140). (**B**) Electron micrograph shows lysed red cells (*asterisks*) and hemoglobin debris (*arrows*) within the macrophages (×1,400).

these effects are eventually manifest as degeneration in the trabeculae, tissue remodelling and reactive fibrosis. Extensive use of corticosteroids is associated with the management of some of the inflammatory glaucoma patients (170) and the ocular hypertensive effect of these needs to be taken into consideration.

Secondary open angle glaucoma due to sarcoidosis (73) involves a TM infiltration dominated by lymphocytes but the key pathological event is fibrosis of the outflow system particularly around Schlemm canal. Even infiltration of neoplastic lymphocytes in leukemic glaucoma probably produces a biological reactive response from the outflow tissues contributing to pressure rise (158).

Glaucoma Secondary to Neoplasms

Cells from intraocular neoplasms, such as retinoblastoma and malignant melanoma, shed into the intraocular cavities, may be carried into the outflow system (99,192,194). If a sufficient number of these cells are trapped within the TM a secondary open-angle glaucoma supervenes. In an eye containing a diffuse (or ring) melanoma of the iris or ciliary body adjacent to the outflow system, the tumor cells may directly invade the TM or proliferate along its inner surface (32). Of a retrospective histopathologic sequential series of 169 patients with microscopically proven iris melanoma, 30% presented with tumor-induced secondary elevated IOP (160).

The process of tumor cell infiltration, through the circulating aqueous humor or by direct invasion, does not appear to be particularly destructive to the trabecular tissues: the tumor cells are often seen in close relation to apparently normal TM cells.

A somewhat different process occurs in melanomalytic glaucoma (99,118,181), in which tumor cells are not primarily responsible for trabecular blockade although usually some are to be found in the TM. Lysis and breakdown of necrotic anterior uveal melanomas lead to obstruction of the TM by large melanin-laden macrophages, cellular debris, and free melanin granules. In addition, tumor necrosis releases enzymes and metabolic products complicating the situation. Melanin phagocytosis by native TM is observed but this is surprisingly modest in some cases (99). This form of glaucoma is rare as is a variant called melanocytomalytic glaucoma (43) where macrophages and tumor debris from a necrotic iris melanocytoma produces obstruction.

Cataract-Associated Glaucoma

Obstructed aqueous humor outflow may follow the release of protein and other materials from a cataractous lens, particularly when it is hypermature, into the anterior chamber (34,45). Such phacolytic glaucoma can be attributed to occlusion of the intratrabecular spaces by a massive infiltration of exogenous macrophages, which are engorged with lens material and extracellular fragments of lens fibers, and possibly, by the accumulation of heavy-molecular-weight lens protein (33,34). Light microscopy does not reveal obvious deleterious effects on the trabecular tissues. Many of the macrophages are too large to enter the outflow pathways. In addition, macrophages accumulate in the iris stroma, along the inner surface of the posterior retina, and even on the optic disc. The more complex situation of lens-induced uveitis is dealt with elsewhere (see Chapter 4).

α-Chymotrypsin once used to facilitate intracapsular cataract extraction by the chemical dissolution of zonular fibers was occasionally complicated by a transient but severe postoperative glaucoma (90) produced by zonular material packing the intertrabecular spaces (8).

Phacomorphic Glaucoma

Phacomorphic glaucoma is induced by changes in the lens shape or position. Some hypermature cataracts may imbibe water and swell, with consequent anterior displacement of the iris and shallowing of the anterior chamber. This may cause lens-pupil block and a secondary angle-closure glaucoma. In extreme cases, the anterior chamber may be completely obliterated by a swollen lens, and this may lead to synechial closure of the drainage angle. When the lens is subluxed or frankly dislocated, lens-pupil block may occur, or alternatively, the entire lens may end up in the anterior chamber. In addition to the secondary glaucoma, there is direct trauma to the corneal endothelium. In this situation phacomorphic glaucoma is prevented if timely removal of the lens is performed.

Capsular Glaucoma

In many patients with the pseudoexfoliation syndrome (PXE) (see Chapter 25) a "capsular glaucoma" develops that is similar in its clinical manifestations to POAG. Clinicopathological evidence indicates that the quantity of exfoliated material (Fig. 13) in the outflow system is related to the severity of the glaucoma (138,157). Attention has also been drawn to the prominence of melanin pigment in the TM cells of the outflow system, and this has been attributed to the breakdown of iris pigment epithelium that occurs in PXE. However, any relationship between pigment presence in the outflow pathways and disease severity has not been identified (157).

The concept that this form of glaucoma is due primarily to an overload of the outflow system by PXE material and melanin pigment granules has been challenged (194). Thus, it has been proposed that patients with PXE suffer from a coincidental POAG. The observed morphology, according to this hypothesis, is explained as an enhancement of a preexisting obstruction of the outflow system due to POAG by the accumulation of PXE material. What is clear however is that only some of the PXE material is washed into the TM from outside the outflow system; much of it is synthesized by TM cells themselves and accumulates in the walls of Schlemm canal (157).

PXE is a general disorder of the ECM both within and outside the eye. The PXE material appears to be made up of microfibrils (Fig. 13) of noncollagenous basement substance combined with elastic fibrillar components (138) such as fibrillin-1 and arises from the iris, ciliary body, zonules, and lens epithelia and from the endothelium of iris vessels among others. It has also been found in extraocular tissues of the orbit, in the conjunctiva (165), and elsewhere.

Pigmentary Glaucoma

In a small percentage of young, mainly Caucasian, myopic males and, more rarely, females, there is excessive release of iris epithelial melanin granules into the aqueous humor to produce pigment dispersion syndrome. Such liberated pigment can obstruct the aqueous humor outflow and give rise to one of the most common forms of secondary open-angle glaucoma usually referred to as pigmentary glaucoma. The risk of developing pigmentary glaucoma from

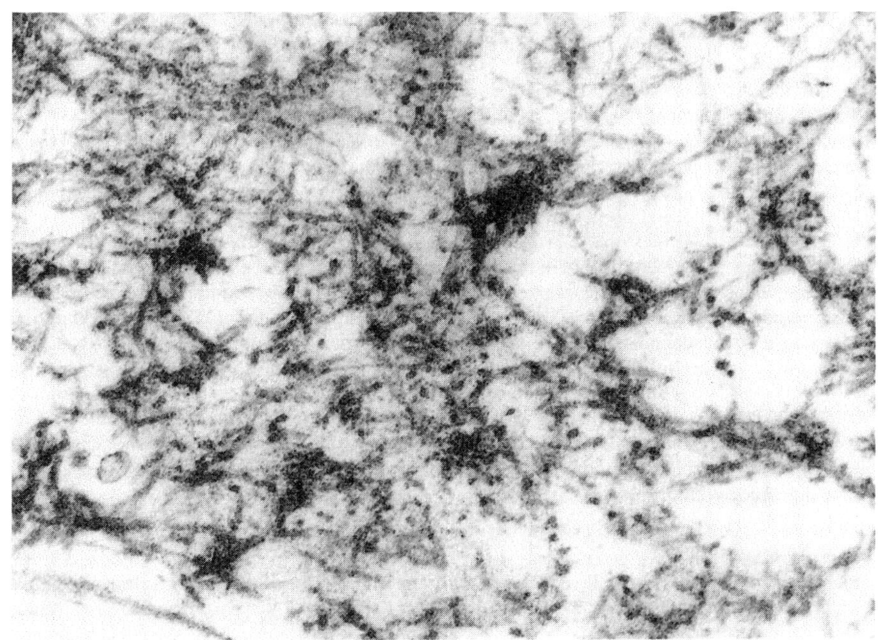

Figure 13 Pseudoexfoliation material present in an intertrabecular space by transmission electron microscopy (×31,900).

pigment dispersion is about 10% in 5 years (161). Melanin release was once thought to be caused by iris epithelial atrophy but friction between the zonular fibers and peripheral iris that causes abrasion of the iris pigment epithelium is now far more widely accepted (22,23,39). That radial transillumination defects are found in the midperipheral iris in close approximation to anterior packets of zonular fibers lends support to the mechanical nature of the lesion. In addition the depth of the anterior chamber in patients with the pigment dispersion syndrome has been found, particularly in the midperiphery, to be excessive.

In pigmentary glaucoma the outflow system becomes heavily pigmented (39) and in such cases, up to 95% of the cells of the TM contain melanin (54). Numerous melanin-laden cells, similar to the heavily pigmented rounded cells normally found just anterior to the sphincter muscle of the iris (clump cells of Koganei), accumulate in the outer layers of the TM (137). In addition, melanin granules accumulate in a vertical line behind and within the corneal endothelium (Krukenberg spindle) (12).

Infusion of melanin granules into the outflow system under experimental conditions indicates that the glaucomatous process is not one of simple pigment blockage mechanism (33). Since the TM has a marked capacity for melanophagocytosis, activated cells in this tissue may detach from the trabeculae and accumulate in the outer TM and possibly contribute to the blockage in a more effective manner than melanin granules alone (23). Although the evidence for melanin and melanomacrophage accumulation in the JCT is not strong; indeed, some morphometric studies show the opposite (122). Most pigment is found in the trabecular part of the TM (Fig. 14). Clinically, there does not appear to be a direct correlation between the amount of pigment visible in the angle and the extent of IOP elevation. Consequently, some eyes with heavy deposition have normal or only slightly elevated IOP.

The theories of the pathogenesis of pigmentary glaucoma have been reviewed by numerous people (39,99,122,143). Some authorities consider the glaucoma to be a destructive effect of the melanin infiltrate or to be due to mechanical obstruction of the extracellular spaces in the TM by melanin-containing macrophages (native or otherwise), but this view is not universally accepted. Others propose that individuals suffering from pigmentary glaucoma have a preexisting congenital abnormality in the outflow pathway, the assumption being that this abnormality alone is not manifest as a congenital glaucoma but is precipitated by pigment deposition in a developmental defect (101). Another suggestion is that POAG is the underlying disease in pigmentary glaucoma.

Corticosteroid Glaucoma

Corticosteroid glaucoma is a well-recognized entity in which signs of raised IOP (clinically similar to those of POAG) develop in individuals who have been treated with topical or systemic corticosteroids (88). Following the isolation of the TM inducible

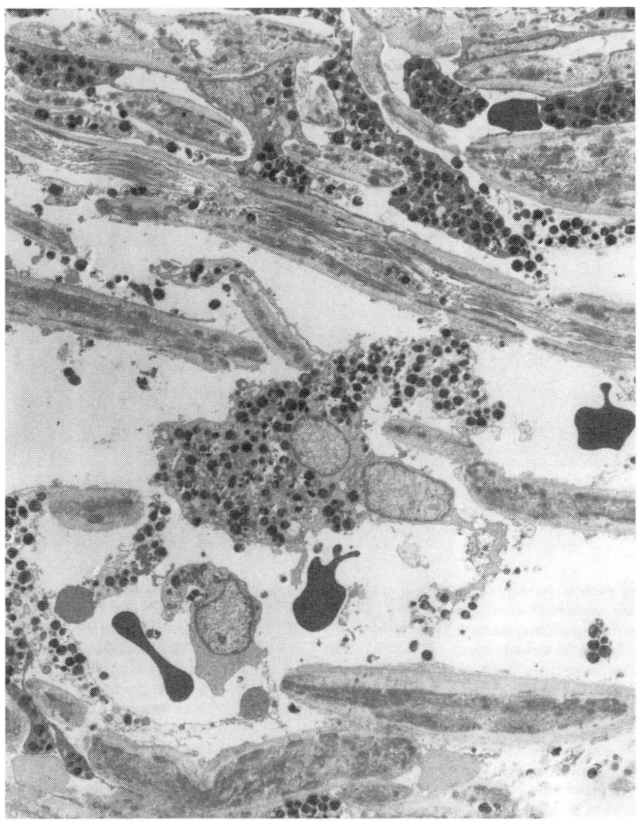

Figure 14 Pigmentary glaucoma. The corneoscleral meshwork as seen by transmission electron microscopy. Mobile pigmented cells abound (×2,500).

glucocorticoid response gene (169) or more usefully called the myocilin gene (*TIGR/MYOC*) there has been a surge of interest in steroid effects on the outflow tissues. Corticosteriod treatment seems to produce elevated IOP in around 30% or so of the normal population and more than 90% of POAGs. Thus administration of corticosteroid has the potential to produce a drug-induced secondary glaucoma and in POAG patients, to make their condition worse.

The molecular basis for this type of glaucoma is now better understood but there are still many unknowns. Certainly TM cells have functional receptors for glucocorticoids (185). Indeed an alternative splicing variant of the human glucocorticoid receptor GRbeta, that has been implicated in a number of steroid-resistant diseases, seems to be decreased in those sensitive to steroid-induced IOP elevation (196). On steroid exposure, the cells of the TM show an apparent increase in the content of mitochondria and rough endoplasmic reticulum (RER) (146). Clearly a significant induction of myocilin mRNA is associated with steroid exposure (30) and the protein is evident both with in TM cells and in the ECM of the outflow tissues. In addition it has been a long held belief steroid treatment can produce a broad-based change in the synthesis of ECM components, perhaps including a shift from GAG to collagen production (75,164). In addition to change in synthetic activity, other suggested behavioral alterations in steroid treated TM cells include the development of geodesic arrangements of actin within the cytoplasm (29), defective TM cell contractility, perhaps diminished lytic/phagocytic activity and increased apoptosis.

All or some of the above would have negative implications for the facility of outflow and so contribute to elevated IOP. Despite the lack of a clear understanding of the pathobiology of steroid-induced glaucoma many scientists feel that study of this condition will further our understanding of POAG. It does not seem to be anyway close to being a perfect drug-related model of POAG however. The fine structure of the outflow apparatus in corticosteroid glaucoma has differences from that seen in POAG. Most obvious is the presence of a fingerprint arrangement of basement membrane-like material that is a characteristic ECM feature of corticosteroid glaucoma (93,145,146). In addition there is a buildup of a dense feltwork of fibrillar material in the spaces of the juxtacanalicular meshwork (93,146) not seen either in the normal or the POAG meshwork (Fig. 15). The fingerprint and feltwork materials may well be related but they are undoubtedly entirely different from the plaque deposits that build up in the JCT of POAG patients (93,150).

Silicone oil glaucoma

Silicone oil is employed as a retinal tamponade in the management of complicated cases of retinal detachment. Secondary glaucoma is a complication of some eyes following intraocular silicone oil administration (99,106). Emulsification of the silicone oil is an adverse event and histological studies have shown obstruction of the TM by minute silicone bubbles, silicone-laden macrophages, and pigmented cells (99,127). A multitude of factors, such as inflammation, pupil block, and peripheral anterior synechiae, may lead to secondary glaucoma in these complicated eyes that have undergone previous surgery, but in some cases preexisting lesions may account for the glaucoma rather than the silicone oil itself.

Traumatic Secondary Open-Angle Glaucoma

Physical trauma to the globe by concussion or perforating injuries can lead to a secondary open-angle glaucoma. In the acute situation, the elevation in IOP may be due to the release of a number of

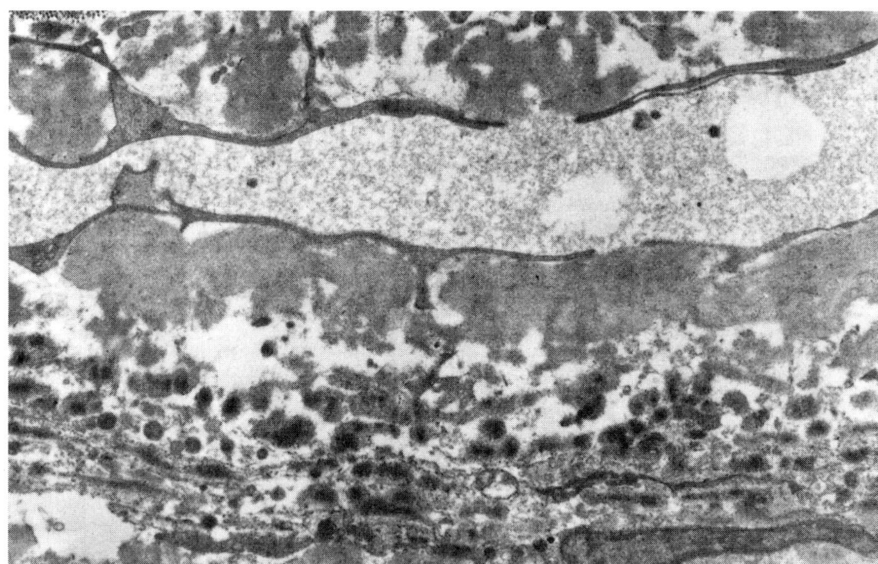

Figure 15 Corticosteroid glaucoma. A dense felt work of material collects on both sides of Schlemm canal (transmission electron microscopy, ×6,500).

inflammatory mediators, in addition to mechanical blockage by inflammatory cells in the outflow system. Concussion injuries may cause glaucoma for a variety of reasons. The TM may become disorganized, with fusion of the trabecular beams (76). In addition, the ciliary body may be torn or separated from the sclera (cyclodialysis). If blood vessels are torn, the wound and ensuing hemorrhage resolve with fibroblastic proliferation and scar formation. This may contract and distort the anterior segment structures and lead to secondary closed-angle glaucoma.

A simple tear in the ciliary body may cause the outflow system to collapse and degenerate (possibly because the trabeculae are no longer supported by the ciliary muscle). The endothelium of the cornea may proliferate and become transformed into spindle cells that extend into the uveal trabeculae, and occasionally endothelial cells migrate across the anterior chamber angle on the iris and lay down ectopic Descemet membrane (139). If this "endothelial downgrowth" is sufficiently extensive or if the outflow system is severely disorganized, glaucoma ensues. When the peripheral cornea or corneoscleral limbus is damaged by a perforating wound, the TM becomes invaded by fibroblasts. Occlusion of the intertrabecular spaces by fibroblasts and the consequent deposition of collagen are followed by an irreversible obstruction to outflow.

Very rarely, corneal or conjunctival epithelium may be introduced into the anterior chamber, either by implantation or by proliferation through a residual defect in the cornea. Indeed, this "epithelial downgrowth" may even follow intraocular surgery. This displaced epithelium can grow across the surface of the intraocular tissues (Fig. 16). The formation of an impermeable cellular layer on the inner surface of the TM obstructs the outflow should a large proportion of the angle be involved.

Secondary Closed-Angle Glaucoma

An investigation of 646 consecutive surgical eye specimens showed secondary glaucoma to be the main non-neoplastic (91). This is a frequent

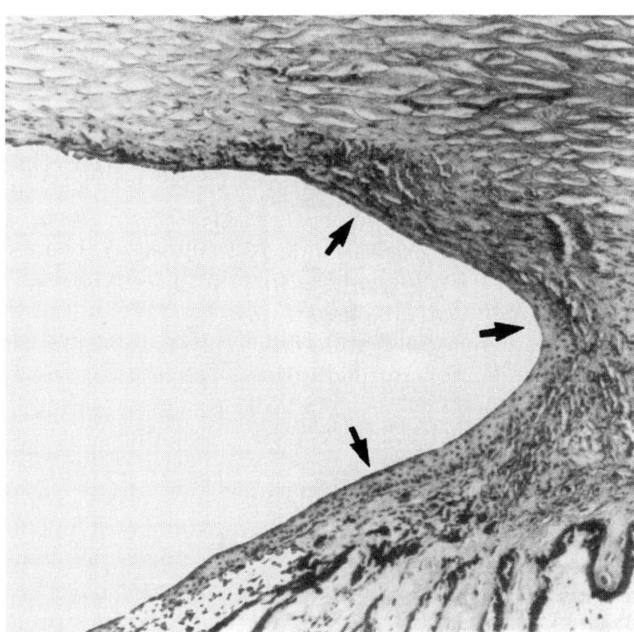

Figure 16 Light micrograph of an epithelial downgrowth (*arrows*) lining the chamber angle (hematoxylin and eosin, ×90).

termination of inflammatory, ischemic, and neoplastic disease, and the glaucoma responds poorly, if at all, to treatment. The blindness and intractable pain that characterize the most severe form of this type of glaucoma are often referred to as "absolute glaucoma." The pathogenic processes that lead to the secondary closed-angle glaucoma often cannot be determined by a morphological evaluation of the enucleated globe. Nevertheless, the mechanisms of secondary angle-closure glaucoma can be considered in terms of four processes.

Hypotonic Collapse of the Anterior Camber

Peripheral anterior synechiae and central posterior synechiae can form during ocular hypotony that follows, for example, traumatic or infectious perforations of the corneoscleral coats of the globe. Loss of IOP allows the anterior segment structures to come into contact at the critical iridocorneal and iridolenticular sites, and adhesion is enhanced by the associated exudation of plasma. Incarceration of the iris supplements the tendency to iridocorneal contact. If the IOP is not restored by rapid surgical closure of the penetrating ocular wound, fibrous adhesions form and lead to glaucoma.

Disturbance of the Lens-Iris Diaphragm

The lens may be dislocated in an ocular concussion or in more severe injuries to the eye (139), and in these situations mechanical pupillary block or angle deformation obstructs aqueous humor outflow secondarily. Such uncomplicated situations are rare, and in most traumatic cases, the effects of hemorrhage or angle recession are additional. Apart from trauma, lens displacement and pupil block are terminal features of advanced retinal detachment resulting from a variety of causes. Intraocular tumors may also present with a secondary closed-angle glaucoma (192). The most severe form a pupillary block glaucoma is appropriately termed malignant glaucoma. This can occur spontaneously with or without the use of miotics (159), but it presents most commonly after a surgical procedure for the treatment of glaucoma. This is particularly likely to occur in small eyes with a short axial length and a prominent ciliary body, demonstrable on ultrasonography. The lens is displaced anteriorly in malignant glaucoma, a "direct lens-block angle closure mechanism" (100). The sequence of events leading to the development of malignant glaucoma remains debatable. The lens displacement has been attributed to constriction of the ciliary body around the lens by overaction of the sphincter component of the ciliary muscle (ciliolenticular block) and to an accumulation of aqueous humor within the vitreous.

Disturbance of the Vitreous-Iris Diaphragm in Aphakia

Aphakic glaucoma was an important clinical entity that embraced several pathogenic mechanisms, when intracapsular cataract surgery was in common use. Glaucoma is far less common with current extracapsular procedures with intraocular lens implantation whether it is phacoemulsification (PHACO) or extracapsular cataract extraction (ECCE). Secondary glaucoma incidence with either PHACO or ECCE is quoted at around 0.5% by some authorities but becomes higher when secondary pseudophakic glaucoma develops late onset (after 1 year) (92). Secondary pseudophakic glaucoma (182) is more likely particularly if there has been a rupture of the posterior lens capsule with vitreous loss. Inadequate wound closure and fistula formation bring about the events seen in hypotonic collapse of the anterior chamber.

An alternative process for the formation of iridocorneal contact occurs if iris tissue is incarcerated in the corneal wound or if fibrous tissue grows into the angle from an inadequately opposed wound. Also, the surgical procedure may be followed by uveitis and secondary inflammatory adhesions. In ECCE and PHACO these adhesions are likely to be between the iris and the anterior capsular remnants or, more rarely, the intraocular lens, with subsequent pupil block. Finally, iridovitreal adhesions can cause pupil block and forward protrusion of the iris and vitreous, and the latter may also occlude the intended drainage pathway provided by an iridectomy. Obliteration of aqueous humor flow through the pupil leads rapidly to an accumulation of aqueous humor behind the iris, which enhances the bombé mechanism.

Iridocorneal Adhesion by Membrane Contraction

The formation of a fibrovascular adhesion between the iris and the cornea (Fig. 17) or between the iris and lens gives rise to an extremely serious clinical situation (neovascular glaucoma), which responds poorly to treatment and may necessitate enucleation. The cause and pathogenesis of neovascularization of the iris (rubeosis iridis) have been the subject of extensive investigation. The fibrovascular membrane passes onto the surface of the iris, sometimes across the pupil and across the TM, occluding the anterior chamber angle. The iris pigment epithelium is drawn around the pupil and distorts the sphincter pupillae (ectropion uveae).

Additional, rare causes of secondary angle-closure glaucoma include the iridocorneal endothelial (ICE) syndrome and senile iridoschisis. Three entities—iris nevus syndrome, Chandler syndrome, and essential iris atrophy—comprise the ICE syndrome (193). In the iris nevus syndrome (Cogan–Reese

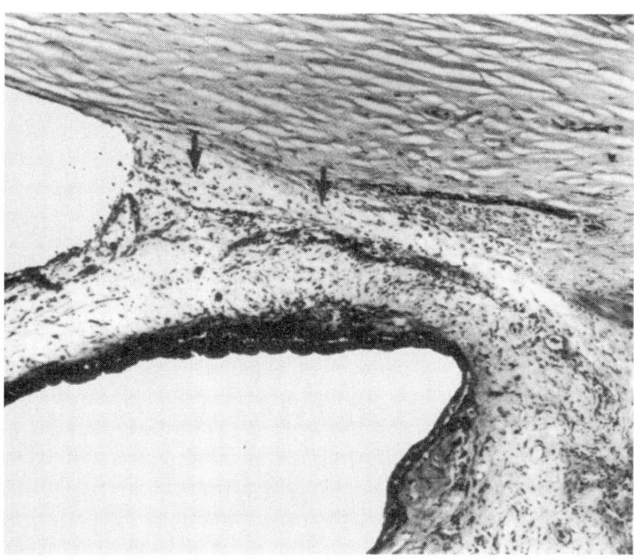

Figure 17 Light micrograph showing occlusion of the angle by fibrovascular tissue (*arrows*) in neovascular glaucoma (hematoxylin and eosin, ×81).

syndrome), a diffuse iris "nevus" is associated with peripheral anterior synechiae and heterochromia iridis (155). In Chandler syndrome an endothelial dystrophy of the cornea is associated with mild to moderate atrophy of the iris stroma without hole formation and peripheral anterior synechiae (144). Essential or progressive iris atrophy is characterized by atrophy of the iris stroma with pupillary distortion and peripheral anterior synechiae (156). In each subgroup of the ICE syndrome, morphological studies have disclosed in some cases the presence of a membrane across the inner surface of the TM, in addition to peripheral anterior synechiae. This downgrowth is thought to be the most important feature of the syndrome (24,95). Patients with Chandler syndrome tend to have more severe corneal edema than the rest of the group of patients with ICE syndrome, and secondary glaucoma is worse in those with essential iris atrophy or the iris nevus syndrome (188).

Senile iridoschisis is another cause of secondary angle-closure glaucoma (194). Senile iridoschisis is a bilateral disease in which splitting of the iris stroma leads to peripheral anterior synechiae. Elderly males and females are affected equally in this disease. The means whereby the iris disorder leads to angle closure glaucoma is obscure.

Congenital Glaucoma

By designation, congenital glaucoma refers to glaucoma caused by an obstruction of the aqueous humor drainage attributable to a developmental anomaly, even though ocular hypertension may not be present at birth but only emerge sometime in infancy or early childhood. The forms of glaucoma that occur in infancy and childhood fall into three broad groups (9,94,120,140,190).

Primary Congenital Glaucoma

This includes those cases in which a malformation of the anterior chamber angle tissues is the sole manifestation of the disease. This group may be further subdivided into infantile (up to 3 years) and juvenile forms (3–20 years).

Infantile Glaucoma Associated with Other Anomalies

In this group the chamber angle malformation is associated with other malformations within the eye or with generalized disorders, as in the phakomatoses (see Chapter 55). Not only may there be a malformation of the angular tissues, but in addition, obstruction to aqueous humor outflow results from the formation of secondary synechiae.

Glaucoma in Infancy and Childhood: Secondary Types

Many pathological conditions that cause glaucoma in adults, such as trauma, inflammation, and neoplasms, may occur early in life, when the pathogenetic processes are essentially the same.

The nature of the developmental disturbances of the tissues of the anterior chamber angle in congenital glaucoma is incompletely understood. This lack of understanding is partly due to the difficulty encountered in the acquisition of suitable material for investigation. When available, globes or trabeculectomy specimens have been obtained at an advanced stage, and interpretation has been rendered difficult by previous surgical intervention.

Any understanding of the pathogenesis of congenital glaucoma requires some knowledge of the normal development of the outflow system. It is believed that the TM cells are derived from the neural crest (140) although it is not clear whether this is also the case for Schlemm canal which may well be mesodermal. It has been proposed that the growth factor TGFβ has a crucial role to play in the development of the TM (81). The growth factor enhances *Foxc1* and induces *Pitx2* and these transcription factors are essential to proper developmental progression of neural crest cells.

To explain the formation of the anterior chamber angle, two theories based on light microscopic observations have been advanced. The first assumes that the tissue between the trabecular anlage and the developing iris atrophies (94). That enzymatic action contributes to the formation of the chamber angle and the intertrabecular spaces is supported by the finding of abundant macrophages in the angular region of the developing cat eye (137) and the presence of necrotic cells, frequently associated with macrophages, in the developing rat chamber angle (135). Detailed human studies, however, cast doubt on this mechanism. Neither Wulle (191) or McMenamin and colleagues (115,116) were able to find convincing evidence of cell necrosis or atrophy. In addition a study of mouse development was unable to detect evidence of cell death or atrophy during trabecular channel and beam formation (163). An alternative proposal is that a cleft is formed in the angle region by a differential growth rate in the angular tissues (see also Chapter 51) (2,94). The use of transmission electron microscopy (TEM) on carefully prepared material revealed that separation of the tissues takes place by a subtle realignment of the cells, which lose their intercellular attachments and are gradually separated by the confluence of extracellular spaces (162). Death of cells and phagocytic activity are thought not to be features of this second alternative process.

Closure of Schlemm canal has been noted only rarely and may be a feature of early-onset congenital glaucoma or a secondary development in the pathogenesis of late-onset congenital glaucoma; presumably related to budding failure in the former and compromised drainage in the latter. Some level of faulty canal development, such as backward displacement or narrowing, may be present without impairing aqueous humor drainage. The absence of invaginations (giant vacuoles) from the canal endothelium has been noted in congenital glaucoma (6,162), but this may be due to loss of pressure head at fixation.

Corneoscleral trabeculae are thickened and poorly formed, often in conjunction with a maldeveloped scleral spur. An important feature of congenital glaucoma is a grossly thickened JCT (9,172). Tawara and Inomata (172) considered that as trabecular formation advances from the anterior chamber angle toward Schlemm canal, the cleavage process becomes interrupted so that the undifferentiated JCT is abnormally large. Given the importance of the JCT in provoking resistance to drainage, an enlarged JCT would lead to elevated IOP.

An interesting feature of the study by Smelser and Ozanics (162) was the tentative confirmation of the classic view that the canal of Schlemm forms by budding of endothelial cells from the intrascleral venous plexus, a derivation that may explain the specific functional properties of the monolayer.

The histological study of the iridocorneal angle in congenital (infantile) glaucoma in material obtained postmortem has not yielded uniform results. The following features have been described (Fig. 18): (*i*) rudimentary development of a scleral spur, (*ii*) persistence of pectinate ligaments, (*iii*) closure of Schlemm canal, (*iv*) abnormal narrowing and backward displacement of Schlemm canal, (*v*) absence of invaginations from the endothelium of Schlemm canal, (*vi*) enlarged JCT with accumulated ECM, (*vii*) retarded differentiation of the corneoscleral mesh work, (*viii*) thickening of trabeculae, (*ix*) abnormal and extensive insertion of the longitudinal ciliary muscle fibers into the uveal meshwork, and (*x*) the presence of a membrane across the inner surface of the meshwork.

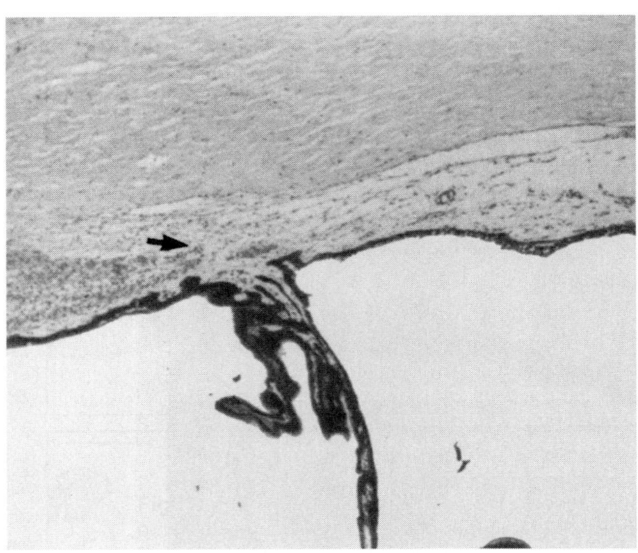

Figure 18 Light micrograph of the chamber angle in Rieger anomaly, showing iridocorneal strands, hypoplasia of the trabecular meshwork, and scleral spur. The ciliary muscle extends more anteriorly than normal (*arrow*) (hematoxylin and eosin, ×60). *Source*. Courtesy of the late Dr. T. Kuwabara.

Maumenee (120), in support of earlier investigations, stressed the apparent failure of the iris root to separate from the trabeculae and the displacement of the scleral spur associated with an anterior attachment of the ciliary muscle into the uveal and corneoscleral trabeculae. In all but one case in Maumenee's series, the canal of Schlemm was open, and in none of the cases was there evidence of a persistent membrane across the inner surface of the meshwork. It is at this point that there is a discrepancy between histopathology and the observations made by gonioscopy in congenital glaucoma. Gonioscopy often reveals an apparent semitransparent membrane in the anterior chamber angle, imaginatively likened to a "morning mist," and this has been suggested to represent either a residual endothelial membrane (Barkan membrane) (11) or condensed pectinate ligaments (188). A scanning electron microscopic study has shown only condensation of uveal trabecular beams in a case in which a Barkan membrane was observed on gonioscopy (8,11). Openings in the anterior chamber angle region are evident in an 18-week human fetus (and earlier), corresponding to the start of aqueous humor formation (129). Perhaps aqueous humor flow through the openings contributes to angle formation and trabecularization by limiting matrix formation and thus enhancing the cleavage process.

Failure of cleavage and goniodysgenesis are generally favored as the major pathogenetic processes in congenital glaucoma. Dysgenesis can extensively involve the anterior segment (94), and the term "anterior chamber cleavage syndrome" was coined for the spectrum of abnormalities. Various eponymously labeled anomalies (such as the Peters, Axenfeld, von Hippel, and Rieger anomalies) include malformations of the posterior cornea, iris hypoplasia and irido- and lenticulocorneal contact, in addition to goniodysgenesis (see Chapter 52). Accumulated evidence also implicates chamber angle malformations in the glaucoma associated with neurofibromatosis, aniridia, and encephalo-oculofacial angiomatosis, as well as the Marfan and Lowe syndromes. It is worth noting that in the neural crest-derived dysgenesis syndromes like the Axenfeld-Rieger group may in part be due to a loss of TGFβ signalling in key neural crest tissues (81).

Mutations in the *CYP1B1* gene are most often associated with infantile congenital glaucoma (78) whereas myocilin gene *(TIGR/MYOC)* mutations, among others, can have a role in juvenile glaucoma (onset between 3 and 20 years) (see Chapter 34). Interestingly given that the *MYOC* gene is also the trabecular glucocorticoid response gene, ultrastructural studies of the outflow system in juvenile glaucoma show features in common with steroid glaucoma and POAG. The ECM of the TM has fingerprint-like basement membrane aggregates characteristic of the steroid treated outflow system and also there is an accumulation of plaque material as seen in aging and POAG (49). There seems to be some structural abnormality in that the TM is smaller than in normal eyes (173).

EFFECTS OF RAISED INTRAOCULAR PRESSURE ON THE TISSUES OF THE ANTERIOR SEGMENT

Several factors influence the effects of a raised IOP on the anterior segment tissues, the most important of which are the duration, as well as the rate and magnitude, of the increase in IOP. The gradual increase in IOP occurring in POAG more easily permits reflex vasomotor adjustments than the rapid and extreme ocular hypertension associated with acute primary closed-angle glaucoma. In the latter situation, the biochemical abnormalities that accompany reflex ischemia and acidosis, or reflex vasodilatation and plasma leakage, may cause serious and often irreparable damage to cells exposed to this unfavorable environment (19). The resistance of the tissues to these insults also depends on the viability of the cellular constituents and their innate capacity for repair.

The corneal endothelium is a principal target for these harmful mechanisms. Corneal edema is a common clinical manifestation of the raised IOP, although there is a marked variation in individual response to a given pressure level. Hence, it is presumed that the functional integrity of the corneal endothelium is better preserved in some individuals than in others. Nevertheless, decompensation of the corneal epithelium occurs ultimately, and by light microscopy this is seen as flattening and attenuation of the monolayer, with presumably apoptotic loss of individual cells. Since in the human eye the corneal endothelium has little regenerative capacity, the remaining cells stretch to maintain a single layer. The ultrastructural architecture of the corneal endothelial cells may be slightly attenuated, or there may be extremely advanced degeneration, with swelling of organelles, cytoplasrnic vacuolation, and dilatation of the intercellular clefts. Aqueous humor passes easily through the dilated intercellular spaces, and the damaged endothelial cells are unable to transport fluid back into the anterior chamber. The flow of aqueous humor into the corneal stroma increases as a result of this loss of endothelial function, and marked changes are found in the tissue when it is subject to ultrastructural investigation (51). The collagen fibers become deformed, and lakes of extracellular fluid appear between the lamellae and adjacent to the contracted keratocytes. The functional effect of stromal fiber separation is to disturb the refractive index of the tissue. It is also possible that changes in the hydration of the stromal proteoglycans contribute to corneal opacification.

The early alterations in the corneal epithelium are valuable in diagnostic histopathology and include swelling and loss of staining intensity of the basal layer of the epithelial cells. This is followed by widening of the extracellular spaces (spongiosis), presumably due to intercellular edema, and basal separation. TEM has shown that the desmosomes connecting adjacent epithelial cells are usually intact and the detached epithelium continues to secrete a basal lamina (86). Such edematous separation of the epithelium constitutes bullous keratopathy and is followed by an ingrowth of a pannus of fibroblasts, which deposit collagen between the epithelium and Bowman layer. Infection is a common accompaniment, which encourages leukocytic infiltration and neovascular proliferation from the periphery. This process may destroy Bowman zone as it grows into the corneal tissue (degenerative pannus).

The effects of glaucoma on the lens are selective and make an interesting comparison with the total involvement that follows a disturbance in hydration of the corneal tissues. The entity of subcapsular flecking (*Glaukomflecken*), which is the only well-established lenticular manifestation of glaucoma, is peculiar in that focal necrosis of the lens epithelium and adjacent cortex occurs within the pupillary area in acute glaucoma. The patchy nature of this cellular destruction suggests that only a proportion of the cells are unable to survive the hostile environment associated with severe acute glaucoma. The sparing of all but the central part of the anterior lens remains unexplained. In a study of the ultrastructural changes in glaucomatous subcapsular flecks, Brini and Flament (19) were impressed by dilatation of the RER and an excess of glycogen granules in the surviving epithelial cells, and this was attributed to an alteration in epithelial metabolism during the episode of ocular hypertension. These authors also demonstrated a recovery process manifest as further growth of young lens fibers onto the outer surface, which can have the effect of burying the necrotic lens cells.

The iris and ciliary body are markedly susceptible to high IOP levels. In routine histological material, diffuse atrophy of the stroma and the smooth muscle in the anterior uveal tissue is common. Ischemic necrosis and atrophy of the sphincter pupillae are diagnostic features of acute glaucoma. In addition, the ciliary processes become stunted and the normal vessels are replaced by hyalinized connective tissue; the fortuitous effect of this degenerative change is presumed to be a reduction in the volume of aqueous humor inflow.

The relative significance of primary neural mechanisms or vasoconstrictor ischemic atrophy in the causation of the uveal atrophy has not been fully elucidated. Fluorescein angiography (FA) has demonstrated a loss of the capillary network of the iris after an episode of acute angle closure (152). In the normal eye, blood flow ceases in the iris vessels when the IOP is greater than the diastolic pressure in the ophthalmic artery (152). Mydriasis, on the other hand, is abolished only when IOP is greater than the systolic pressure in the ophthalmic artery. This observation suggests that a neural or an unknown mechanism may exert an effect on the function of the iris musculature. In addition eyes with end stage glaucoma exhibit fewer and smaller capillaries in the choroid and decreased choroidal vein and artery density compared with controls (168).

The response of the corneoscleral envelope to raised IOP depends on the physical and anatomical properties of the tissue and on regional susceptibilities. In the eye of the infant or child with congenital glaucoma, the cornea and sclera stretch almost uniformly to an extreme degree, enlarging the eye (buphthalmos). In the adult eye, focal segments of scleral stretching tend to occur at sites of neural or vascular penetration, where the tissue is inherently weaker. The sclera is lined by uveal tissue, and the staphylomata are most commonly found at the corneoscleral limbus (intercalary), the ciliary body (ciliary), the equator (equatorial), and the site of entry of the posterior ciliary arteries and nerves.

It is appropriate at the end of this discussion to return to the outflow system in considering the effects of raised IOP on the anterior segment tissues. A paradoxical situation occurs in both open- and closed-angle glaucoma because, in each basic pathological process, the flow of aqueous humor across the TM is reduced. Since the metabolic support of the native cells of the TM is dependent on the adequate aqueous perfusion, it is highly probable that aqueous stasis plays an important secondary role in the advanced degeneration observed in the TM at the end stage of glaucoma (10,54,99,174).

REFERENCES

1. Agarwal R, Talati M, Lambert W, et al. Fas-activated apoptosis and apoptosis mediators in human trabecular meshwork cells. Exp Eye Res 1999; 68:583–90.
2. Allen L, Burian HM, Braley AE. A new concept of the development of the anterior chamber angle. Arch Ophthalmol 1955; 53:783–98.
3. Allingham RR, de Kater AW, Ethier CR. Schlemm's canal and primary open angle glaucoma: correlation between Schlemm's canal dimensions and outflow facility. Exp Eye Res 1996; 62:101–9.
4. Allingham RR, de Kater AW, Ethier CR, et al. The relationship between pore density and outflow facility in human eyes. Invest Ophthalmol Vis Sci 1992; 33:1661–9.
5. Alvarado JA, Alvarado RG, Yeh RF, et al. A new insight into the cellular regulation of aqueous outflow: how trabecular meshwork endothelial cells drive a mechanism that regulates the permeability of Schlemm's canal endothelial cells. Br J Ophthalmol 2005; 89:1500–5.
6. Alvarado J, Murphy C, Juster R. Trabecular meshwork cellularity in primary open angle glaucoma and non-glaucomatous normals. Ophthalmology 1984; 91:564–79.
7. Alvarado J, Murphy C, Polansky J, Juster R. Age related changes in trabecular meshwork cellularity. Invest Ophthalmol Vis Sci 1981; 21:114–21.
8. Anderson DR. Pathology of the glaucomas. Br J Ophthalmol 1972; 56:146–157.
9. Anderson DR. The development of the trabecular meshwork and its abnormality in primary infantile glaucoma. Trans Am Ophthalmol Soc 1981; 79:458–85.
10. Ashton N. Discussion on the trabecular structure in relation to the problem of glaucoma. Proc R Soc Med 1958; 52:69–72.
11. Barkan O. Pathogenesis of congenital glaucoma. Gonioscopic and anatomic observations of the angle of

the anterior chamber in the normal eye and in congenital glaucoma. Am J Ophthalmol 1955; 40:1–11.
12. Becker B, Podos SM. Kruckenberg's spindles and primary open angle glaucoma. Arch Ophthalmol 1966; 76:635–639.
13. Bhargava SK, Leighton DA, Phillips CI. Early closed angle glaucoma. Arch Ophthalmol 1973; 89:361–72.
14. Bhattacharya SK, Peachey NS, Crabb JW. Cochlin and glaucoma: a mini-review. Vis Neurosci 2005; 22:605–13.
15. Bill A. The drainage of aqueous humor. Invest Ophthalmol 1975; 14:1–39.
16. Bill A, Phillips CI. Uveoscleral drainage in human eyes. Exp Eye Res 1971; 72:275–81.
17. Bito LZ. The physiology and pathophysiology of the intraocular fluids. Exp Eye Res 1977; 25 Suppl:273–89.
18. Boldea RC, Roy S, Mermoud A. Ageing of Schlemm's canal in nonglaucomatous subjects. Int Ophthalmol 2001; 24:67–77.
19. Brini A, Flament J. Cataracta glaucomatosa acuta. Exp Eye Res 1973; 76:19–28.
20. Caballero M, Liton PB, Epstein DL, Gonzalez P. Proteasome inhibition by chronic oxidative stress in human trabecular meshwork cells. Biochem Biophys Res Commun 2003; 308:346–52.
21. Calthorpe CM, Grierson I. Fibronectin induces migration of bovine trabecular meshwork cells in vitro. Exp Eye Res 1990; 51:39–48.
22. Campbell DG. Pigmentary dispersion and glaucoma: A new theory. Arch Ophthalmol 1979; 97:1667–72.
23. Campbell DG, Schertzer RM. Pathophysiology of pigment dispersion syndrome and pigmentary glaucoma. Curr Opin Ophthalmol 1995; 6:96–101.
24. Campbell DG, Shields MB, Smith TR. The corneal endothelium and the spectrum of essential iris atrophy. Am J Ophthalmol 1978; 86:317–24.
25. Campbell DG, Simmons RJ, Grant MW. Ghost cells and glaucoma. Am J Ophthalmol 1976; 57:441–50.
26. Campbell DG, Simmons RJ, Tolentino FI, McMeel JW. Glaucoma occurring after closed vitrectomy. Am J Ophthalmol 1977; 83:63–9.
27. Chapman SA, Bonshek RE, Stoddart RW, et al. Glycans of the trabecular meshwork in primary open angle glaucoma. Br J Ophthalmol 1996; 80:435–44.
28. Cheng, LE, Ueda, J., Wentz-Hunter, K., Yue, BY. Age independent expression of myocilin in the human trabecular meshwork. Int J Mol Med 2002; 10:33–40.
29. Clark AF, Brochie D, Read AT, et al. Dexamethasone alters F-actin architecture and promotes cross-linked network formation in human trabecular meshwork cells. Cell Motil Cytoskeleton 2005; 60:83–95.
30. Clark AF, Steely HT, Dickerson JE, Jr, et al. Glucocorticoid induction of the glaucoma gene MYOC in human and monkey trabecular meshwork cells and tissues. Invest Ophthalmol Vis Sci 2001; 42:1769–80.
31. Cracknell KP, Grierson I, Hogg P, et al. Melanin in the trabecular meshwork is associated with age, POAG but not Latanoprost treatment. A masked morphometric study. Exp Eye Res, 2006; 82:986–93.
32. Demirci H, Shields CL, Eagle RC Jr, Honavar S. Ring melanoma of the anterior chamber angle: a report of fourteen cases. Am J Ophthalmol 2001; 132:336–42.
33. Epstein DL, Freddo TF, Anderson PJ, et al. Experimental obstruction to aqueous outflow by pigment particles in living monkeys. Invest Ophthalmol Vis Sci 1986; 27: 387–95.
34. Epstein DL, Jedziniak JA, Grant WM. Identification of heavy-molecular-weight soluble protein in aqueous humor in human phacolytic glaucoma. Invest Ophthalmol Vis Sci 1978; 77:398–402.
35. Epstein DL, Rohen JW. Morphology of the trabecular meshwork and inner wall endothelium after cationized ferritin perfusion in the monkey eye. Invest Ophthalmol Vis Sci 1991; 32:160–71.
36. Ethier CR, Coloma FM, de Kater AW, Allingham RR. Retroperfusion studies of the aqueous outflow system. Part 2: Studies in human eyes. Invest Ophthalmol Vis Sci 1995; 36:2466–75.
37. Eithier CR, Kamm RD, Palaszewski BA, et al. Calculations of flow resistance in the juxtacanalicular meshwork. Invest Ophthalmol Vis Sci 1986; 27:1741–50.
38. Epstein DL, Rohen JW. Morphology of the trabecular meshwork and inner-wall endothelium after cationized ferritin perfusion in the monkey eye. Invest Ophthalmol Vis Sci 1991; 32:160–71.
39. Farrar SM, Shields MB. Current concepts in pigmentary glaucoma. Surv Ophthalmol 1993; 37:233–52.
40. Fenton RH, Zimmerman LE. Hemolytic glaucoma: an unusual cause of acute open angle secondary glaucoma. Arch Ophthalmol 70:236–39.
41. Fine BS. Observations on the drainage angle in man and rhesus monkeys: A concept of the pathogenesis of chronic simple glaucoma. Invest Ophthalmol Vis Sci 1964; 5:609–46.
42. Fine BS, Yanoff M, Stone RA. A ciinicopathological study of four cases of primary open-angle glaucoma compared to normal eyes. Am J Ophthalmol 1981; 91:88–105.
43. Fineman MS, Eagle RC Jr, Shields JA, et al. Melanocytomalytic glaucoma in eyes with necrotic iris melanocytoma. Ophthalmology 1998; 105:492–6.
44. Fink AI, Felix MD, Fletcher RC. Schlemm's canal and adjacent structures in glaucomatous patients. Am J Ophthalmol 1972; 74:893–906.
45. Flocks M, Littwin CS, Zimmerman LE. Phacolytic glaucoma. Arch Ophthalmol 1955; 54:37–45.
46. Flugel-Koch C, Ohlmann A, Fuchshofer R, et al. Thrombospondin-1 in the trabecular meshwork: localization in normal and glaucomatous eyes, and induction by *TGF*-beta 1 and dexamethasone in vitro. Exp Eye Res 2004; 79:649-63.
47. Freedman S, Anderson PJ, Epstein DL. Superoxide dismutase and catalase in the calf trabecular meshwork. Invest Ophthalmol Vis Sci 1985; 26:1330–5.
48. Fujiwara N, Matsuo T, Ohtsuki H. Protein expression, genomic structure, and polymorphisms of oculomedin. Ophthalmic Genet 2003; 24:141–51.
49. Furuyoshi N, Furuyoshi M, Futa R, et al. Ultrastructural changes in the trabecular meshwork of juvenile glaucoma. Ophthalmologica 1997; 211:140–6.
50. Gabelt BT, Kaufman, PL. Changes in aqueous humor dynamics with age and glaucoma. Prog Retin Eye Res 2005; 24:612–37.
51. Goldman JN, Benedek GB, Dohlman CH, Cravitt B. Structural alterations affecting transparency in swollen human corneas. Invest Ophthalmol 1968; 7:510–9.
52. Grant M. Experimental aqueous perfusion in enucleated human eyes. Arch Ophthalmol 1963; 69:783–801.
53. Green K. Free radicals and aging of anterior segment tissues of the eye: a hypothesis. Ophthalmic Res 1995; 27:143–9.
54. Grierson I. What is open angle glaucoma? Eye 1987; 1:15–28.
55. Grierson I, Hogg P. The proliferative and migratory activities of trabecular meshwork cells. Prog Ret Eye Res 1996; 15:33–67.
56. Grierson I, Howes RC. Age-related depletion of the cell population in the human trabecular meshwork. Eye 1987; 1:204–10.

57. Grierson I, Howes RC, Wang Q. Age-related changes in the canal of Schlemm. Exp Eye Res 1984; 39:505–12.
58. Grierson I, Kissun R, Ayad S, et al. The morphological features of bovine meshwork cells in vitro and their synthetic activities. Graefes Arch Clin Exp Ophthalmol 1985; 223:225–36.
59. Grierson I, Lee WR. Erythrocyte phagocytosis in the human trabecular meshwork. Br J Ophthalmol 1973; 57: 400–15.
60. Grierson I, Lee WR. Changes in the monkey outflow apparatus at graded levels of intraocular pressures: A qualitative analysis by light microscopy and scanning electron microscopy. Exp Eye Res 1974; 19:21–33.
61. Grierson I, Lee WR. Pressure-induced changes in the ultrastructure of the endothelium lining Schlemm's canal. Am J Ophthalmol 1975; 80:863–84.
62. Grierson I, Lee WR. Pressure effects on the distribution of extracellular materials in the rhesus monkey outflow apparatus. Graefes Arch Clin Exp Ophthalmol 1977; 203: 155–68.
63. Grierson I, Lee WR. Pressure effects on flow channels in the lining endothelium of Schlemm's canal. Acta Ophthalmol (Copenh.) 1978; 56:935–52.
64. Grierson I, Lee WR, Abraham S. Pathways for the drainage of the aqueous humour into Schlemm's canal. Trans Ophthalmol Soc U.K. 1977; 97:719–26.
65. Grierson I, Lee WR, Abraham S. Effects of pilocarpine on the morphology of the outflow apparatus. Br J Ophthalmol 1978; 75:302–13.
66. Grierson I, Lee WR, Abraham SA. Further observation on the process of haemophagocytosis in the human outflow system. Graefes Arch Clin Exp Ophthalmol 1978; 208: 49–64.
67. Grierson I, Lee WR, Abraham S, Howes RC. Associations between cells in the walls of Schlemm's canal. Graefes Arch Clin Exp Ophthalmol 1978; 208:33–47.
68. Grierson I, Lee WR, McMenamin PG. The morphological basis of drug action on the outflow system of the eye. Res Clin Forums 1981; 3:7–25.
69. Grierson I, Lee WR, Moseley H, Abraham S. The trabecular wall of Schlemm's canal: a study of the effects of pilocarpine by scanning electron microscopy. Br J Ophthalmol 1979; 63:9–16.
70. Grierson I, Millar L, Jiang De Y, et al. Investigations of cytoskeletal elements in cultured bovine meshwork cells. Invest Ophthalmol Vis Sci 1986; 27:1318–30.
71. Grierson I, Swalem A, Davies H, et al. Pathological dilemmas in the outflow system in primary open-angle glaucoma. Acta Ophthalmol Scand 1997 220(Suppl):7–12: discussion 13–4.
72. Hamard P, Valtot F, Sourdille P, et al. Confocal microscopic examination of trabecular meshwork removed during ab externo trabeculectomy. Br J Ophthalmol 2002; 86:1046–52.
73. Hamanaka T, Takei A, Takemura T, Oritsu M. Pathological study of cases with secondary open-angle glaucoma due to sarcoidosis. Am J Ophthalmol 2002; 134:17–26.
74. Hann CR, Bahler CK, Johnson DH. Cationic ferritin and segmental flow through the trabecular meshwork. Invest Ophthalmol Vis Sci 2005; 45:1–7.
75. Hernandez MR, Weinstein BJ, Wenk EJ, et al. The effect of dexamethasone on the incorporation of precursors of extracellular matrix components in the outway pathway region of the rabbit eye. Invest Ophthalmol Vis Sci 1983; 24:704–9.
76. Herschler J. Trabecular damage due to blunt anterior segment injury and its relationship to traumatic glaucoma. Trans Am Acad Ophthalmol Ololaryngol 1977; 85:239–48.
77. Hogg P, Calthorpe M, Batterbury M, Grierson I. Aqueous humor stimulates the migration of human trabecular meshwork cells in vitro. Invest Ophthalmol Vis Sci 2000; 41:1091–8.
78. Hollander DA, Sarfarazi M, Stoilov I, et al. Genotype and phenotype correlations in congenital glaucoma: CYP1B1 mutations, goniodysgenesis and clinical characteristics. Am J Ophthalmol 2006; 142:993–1004.
79. Horstmann HJ, Rohen JW, Sames K. Age-related changes in the composition of proteins in the trabecular meshwork of the human eye. Mech Ageing Dev 1983; 21: 121–36.
80. Inomata H, Bill A, Smelser GK. Aqueous humor pathways through the trabecular meshwork and into Schlemm's canal in the cynomolgus monkey (Macaca irus): An electron microscopic study. Am J Ophthalmol 1972; 75:760–89.
81. Ittner LM, Wurdak H, Schwerdtfeger K, et al. Compound developmental eye disorders following inactivation of TGFbeta signalling in neural-crest stem cells. J Biol 2005; 4:11.1–11.6.
82. Joe MK, Sohn S, Hur W, et al. Accumulation of mutant myocilins in ER leads to ER stress and potential cytotoxicity in human trabecular meshwork cells. Biochem Biophys Res Commun 2003; 19:592–600.
83. Johnstone MA, Grant WM. Pressure-dependent changes in structures of the aqueous outflow system of human and monkey eyes. Am J Ophthalmol 1973; 75:365–83.
84. Jones NP. Glaucoma in Fuchs' heterochromic uveitis: aetiology, management and outcome. Eye 1991; 5:662–7.
85. Kanski JJ, Shun-Shin GA. Systemic uveitis syndrome in childhood: an analysis of 340 cases. Ophthalmology 1984; 91:1247–52.
86. Kenyon KR. Synthesis of basement membrane by the corneal epithelium in bullous keratopathy. Invest Ophthalmol 1969; 8:156–68.
87. Kerman BM, Christensen RE, Foos RY. Angle closure glaucoma: a clinicopathologic correlation. Am J Ophthalmol 1973; 76:887–95.
88. Kersey JP, Broadway DC. Corticosteroid-induced glaucoma: a review of the literature. Eye 2006; 20:407–16.
89. Kim BS, Savinova OV, Reedy MV, et al. Targeted disruption of the myocilin gene (Myoc) suggests that human glaucoma-causing mutations are gain of function. Mol Cell Biol 2001; 21:7707–13.
90. Kirsch RE. Glaucoma following cataract extraction associated with the use of alpha-chymotrypsin. Arch Ophthalmol 1964; 72:612–620.
91. Kitzmann AS, Weaver AL, Lohse CM, et al. Clinicopathologic correlations in 646 consecutive surgical eye specimens, 1990–2000. Am J Clin Patbol 2003; 119: 594–601.
92. Kooner KS, Cooksey JC, Perry P, Zimmerman TJ. Intraocular pressure following ECCE, phacoemulsification, and PC-IOL implantation. Ophthalmic Surg 1988; 19:643–6.
93. Kubota T, Okabe H, Hisatomi T, Yamakiri K, Sakamoto T, Tawara A. Ultrastructure of the trabecular meshwork in secondary glaucoma eyes after intravitreal triacinolone acetonide. J Glaucoma 2006; 15:117–9.
94. Kupfer CA. A note on the development of the chamber angle. Invest Ophthalmol 1969; 8:69–74.
95. Kupfer CA, Chan CC, Burnier M Jr, Kaiser-Kupfer MI. Histopathology of the ICE syndrome. Trans Am Ophthalmol Soc 1992; 90:149–56.

96. Lambrou FH, Aiken DG, Woods WD, Campbell DG. The production and mechanism of ghost cell glaucoma in the cat and primate. Invest Ophthalmol Vis Sci 1985; 26: 893–7.
97. Langham ME. Pharmacology of aqueous humour outflow. Exp Eye Res 1977; (Suppl.):311–322.
98. Larina, JN. State of the intrascleral passages of aqueous humor outflow in glaucoma. Vestn Oftalmol 1967; 80: 18–23.
99. Lee WR. Doyne Lecture. The pathology of the outflow system in primary and secondary glaucoma. Eye 1995; 9: 1–23.
100. Levene R. A new concept of malignant glaucoma. Arch Ophthalmol 1972; 87:497–506.
101. Lichter PR, Shaffer RN. Iris processes and glaucoma. Am J Ophthalmol 1970; 70:905–11.
102. Liton PB, Challa P, Stinnett S, et al. Cellular senescence in the glaucomatous outflow pathway. Exp Gerontol 2005; 40:745–8.
103. Lowe RF. Primary creeping angle-closure glaucoma. Br J Ophthalmol 1964; 48:544–50.
104. Lowe RF. The natural history and principles of treatment of primary angle closure glaucoma. Am J Ophthalmol 1966; 67:642–51.
105. Lowe RF. Etiology of the anatomical basis for primary angle closure glaucoma. Br J Ophthalmol 1970; 54:161–9.
106. Lucke K, Strobe B, Foerster M, Laqua H. Secondary glaucoma after silicone oil surgery. Klin Monatsbl Augenheilkd 1990; 196:205–9.
107. Lütjen-Drecoll E. Morphological changes in glaucomatous eyes and the role of TGFbeta2 for the pathogenesis of the disease. Exp Eye Res 2005; 81:1–4.
108. Lütjen-Drecoll E, Dietl T, Futa R, Rohen JW. Age changes of the trabecular meshwork: A preliminary morphometric study. In The Structure of the Eye, Vol. IV, JG. Holly field, Ed. Elsevier Biomedical Press, New York, 1982; 341–8,.
109. Lütjen-Drecoll E, Futa R, Rohen JW. Ultrahistochemical studies on tangential sections of the trabecular meshwork in normal and glaucomatous eyes. Invest Ophthalmol Vis Sci 1981; 27:563–73.
110. Lynch MG, Peeler JS, Brown RH, Niederkorn JY. Expression of HLA class I and II antigens on cells of the human trabecular meshwork. Ophthalmology 1987; 94: 851–7.
111. Maepeu O, Bill A. Pressures in the episcleral veins, Schlemm's canal and trabecular meshwork in monkeys: Effects of changes in intraocular pressures. Exp Eye Res 1989; 49:645–63.
112. Marshall GE. Konstas, AG, Lee, WR. Immunogold localization of type IV collagen and laminin in the aging human outflow system. Exp Eye Res 1990; 51:691–9.
113. Matsumoto Y, Johnson DH. Trabecular meshwork phagocytosis in glaucomatous eyes. Ophthalmologica 1997; 211:147–52.
114. McCarty MF. Primary open-angle glaucoma may be a hyaluronic acid deficiency disease: potential for glucosamine in prevention and therapy. Med Hypotheses 1998; 51:483–4.
115. McMenamin PG. A morphological study of the inner surface of the anterior chamber angle in pre- and postnatal human eyes. Curr Eye Res 1989; 8:727–39.
116. McMenamin PG. Human foetal iridocorneal angle: a light and scanning electron microscopic study. Br J Ophthalmol 1989; 73:871–9.
117. McMenamin PG, Lee WR. Age related changes in the extracellular materials in the inner wall of Schlemm's canal. Graefes Arch din Exp Ophthalmol 1980; 212:159–72.
118. McMenamin PG, Lee WR. Ultrastructural pathology of melanomalytic glaucoma. Br J Ophthalmol 1986; 70: 895–906.
119. McMenamin PG, Lee WR, Aitken DAN. Age-related changes in the human outflow apparatus. Ophthalmology 1986; 93:194–209.
120. Maumenee AE. Further observations on the pathogenesis of congenital glaucoma. Am J Ophthalmol 1963; 55:1163–76.
121. Moseley H, Grierson I, Lee WR. Mathematical modelling of aqueous humour outflow from the eye through the pores in the lining endothelium of Schlemm's canal. Clin Phys Physiol Meas 1983; 1:47–63.
122. Murphy CG, Johnson M, Alvarado JA. Juxtacanalicular tissue in pigmentary and primary open angle glaucoma. The hydrodynamic role of pigment and other constituents. Arch Ophthalmol 1992; 110:1779–85.
123. Nathanson JA, McKee M. Alterations of ocular nitric oxide synthase in human glaucoma. Invest Ophthalmol Vis Sci 1995; 36:1774–84.
124. Nesterov AP. Role of blockade of Schlemm's canal in pathogenesis of primary open-angle glaucoma. Am J Ophthalmol 1970; 70:691–96.
125. Nesterov AR, Batmanov YE. Schlemm's canal and scleral spur in normal and glaucomatous eyes. Am J Ophthalmol 1974; 78:634–8.
126. Nguyen KR, Chung ML, Anderson PJ, et al. Hydrogen peroxide removed by the calf aqueous outflow pathway. Invest Ophthalmol Vis Sci 1988; 29:976–81.
127. Ni C, Wang W-J, Albert DM, Schepens CL. Intravitreous silicone oil injection: histopathologic findings in an eye after 12 years. Arch Ophthalmol 1983; 101:1399–401.
128. Pandolfi M, Astedt B. Outflow resistance in the foetal eye. Acta Ophthalmol (Copenh) 1971; 49:344–50.
129. Pandolfi M, Kwaan HC. Fibrinolysis in the anterior segment of the eye. Arch Ophthalmol 1967; 77:99–104.
130. Panek WC, Holland GN, Lee DA, Christensen RE. Glaucoma in patients with uveitis. Br J Ophthalmol 1990; 74:223–7.
131. Pavlin CJ, Ritch R, Foster FS. Ultrasound biomicroscopy in plateau iris syndrome. Am J Ophthalmol 1992; 113:390–5.
132. Polansky JR, Wood IS, Maglio MT, Alvarado JA. Trabecular meshwork cell culture in glaucoma research. Ophthalmology 1984; 97:580–95.
133. Quigley HA, Addicks EM. Chronic experimental glaucoma in primates. I. Production of elevated intraocular pressure by the anterior chamber injection of autologous ghost red cells. Invest Ophthalmol Vis Sci 19:126–138.
134. Raviola G, Raviola E. Paracellular route of aqueous outflow in the trabecular meshwork and canal of Schlemm. Invest Ophthalmol Vis Sci 1981; 27:52–72.
135. Remé C, Urner V, Acberhard B. The development of the chamber angle in the rat eye. I. Morphological characteristics of developmental stages. Graefes Arch Clin Exp Ophihalmol 1983; 220:139–53.
136. Richardson TM, Hutchinson BT, Grant WM. The outflow tract in pigmentary glaucoma. Arch Ophthalmol 1977; 95: 1015–25.
137. Richardson TM, Marks MS, Ausprunk DM, Miller M. A morphological and morphometric analysis of the aqueous outflow system of the developing cat eye. Exp Eye Res 1985; 41:31–51.
138. Ritch R, Schlotzer-Schrehardt U, Konstas AG. Why is glaucoma associated with exfoliation syndrome? Prog Retin Eye Res 2003; 22:253–75.
139. Rodman HI. Chronic open angle glaucoma associated with dislocation of the lens: a new pathologic concept. Arch Ophthalmol 1963; 69:445–54.

140. Rodrigues M, Font RL. Neural crest origin of human trabecular meshwork and its implications for the pathogenesis of glaucoma. Am J Ophthalmol 1989; 108:469–70.
141. Rodrigues MM, Katz SI, Foidart J, Spaeth GL. Collagen, factor VIII antigen, and immunoglobulins in the human aqueous drainage channels. Ophthalmology 1980; 57: 337–45.
142. Rodrigues MM, Spaeth GL, Sivalingam E, Weinreb S. Histology of 150 trabeculectomy specimens in glaucoma. Trans Ophthalmol Soc UK 1976; 96:245–55.
143. Rodrigues MM, Spaeth GL, Weinreb S, Sivalingam E. Spectrum of trabecular pigmentation in open-angle glaucoma: a clinico-pathologic study. Trans Am Acad Ophthalmol Ololaryngol 1976; 96:258–76.
144. Rodrigues MM, Streeten BW, Spaeth GL. Chandler's syndrome as a variant of essential iris atrophy. Arch Ophthalmol 1978; 96:643–52.
145. Rohen JW, Futa R, Lütjen-Drecoll E. The fine structure of the cribriform meshwork in normal and glaucomatous eyes as seen in tangential sections. Invest Ophthalmol Vis Sci 1981; 21:574–85.
146. Rohen JW, Linner E, Witmer R. Electron microscopic studies on the trabecular meshwork in two cases of corticosteroid glaucoma. Exp Eye Res 1973; 77:19–31.
147. Rohen JW, Lütjen-Drecoll E. Biology of the trabecular meshwork. In Basic Aspects of Glaucoma Research, E. Lütjen-Drecoll, ed. Schattauer-Verlag, Stuttgart 1982; 141–66.
148. Rohen JW, Lütjen-Drecoll E, Flugel C, Meyer M, Grierson I. Exp Eye Res 1993; 56:683–92.
149. Rohen JW, Van der Zypen, E. The phagocytic activity of the trabecular meshwork endothelium. Graefes Arch Clin Exp Ophthalmol 1968; 175:143–60.
150. Rohen JW, Witmer R. Electron microscopic studies on the trabecular meshwork in glaucoma simplex. Graefes Arch Clin Exp Ophthalmol 1972; 183:251–66.
151. Russell P, Koretz J, Epstein DL. Is primary open angle glaucoma caused by small proteins? Med Hypotheses 1993; 41:455–8.
152. Rutkowski PC, Thompson HS. Mydriasis and increased intraocular pressure. I. Pupillographic studies. II. Iris fluorescein studies. Arch Ophthalmol 1972; 87:21–9.
153. Ryder MI, Weinreb RN, Alvarado J, Polansky J. The cytoskeleton of the cultured human trabecular cell. Invest Ophthalmol Vis Sci 1988; 29:251–60.
154. Saiduffazar H. Fibrinolytic activity in the aqueous humor. Exp Eye Res 1970; 10:293–6.
155. Scheie H, Yanoff M. Iris nevus (Cogan-Reese) syndrome: a case of unilateral glaucoma. Arch Ophthalmol 1975; 95: 963–970.
156. Scheie HG, Yanoff M, Kellog WT. Essential iris atrophy. Arch Ophthalmol 1975; 94:1315–20.
157. Schlotzer-Schrehardt U, Naumann GO. Trabecular meshwork in pseudoexfoliation syndrome with and without open-angle glaucoma. A morphometric, ultrastructural study. Invest OphthalmolVis Sci 1995; 36:1750–64.
158. Schuman JS, WangN, Eisenberg DL. Leukemic glaucoma the effects on outflow facility of chronic lymphocytic leukaemia lymphocytes. Exp Eye Res 1995; 61:609–17.
159. Schwartz AL, Anderson DR. Malignant glaucoma in an eye with no antecedent operation or mitotics. Arch Ophthalmol 1975; 93:379–81.
160. Shields CL, Materin MA, Shields JA, et al. Factors associated with elevated intraocular pressure in eyes with iris melanoma. Br J Ophthalmol 2001; 85:666–9.
161. Siddiqui Y, Ten Hulzen RD, Cameron JD, et al. What is the risk of developing pigmentary glaucoma from pigment dispersion syndrome? Am J Ophthalmol 2003; 136:794–9.
162. Smelser GV, Ozanics VMS. The development of the trabecular meshwork in the primate eye. Am J Ophthalmol 1971; 77:366–385.
163. Smith RS, Zabaleta A, Savinova OV, John SW. The mouse anterior chamber angle and trabecular meshwork develop without cell death. BMC Dev Biol 2001; 1:3.
164. Southren AL, Gordon GG, Munnangi PR, et al. Altered cortisol metabolism in cells cultured from trabecular meshwork specimens obtained from patients with primary open-angle glaucoma. Invest Ophthalmol Vis Sci 1983; 24: 1413–7.
165. Speakman JJ, Ghosh M. The conjunctiva in senile lens exfoliation. Arch Ophthalmol 1976; 94:1757–9.
166. Speakman JS, Leeson TS. Site of the obstruction to aqueous outflow in chronic simple glaucoma. Br J Ophthalmol 1962; 46:321–35.
167. Spencer WH. Ophthalmic Pathology. An Alias and Textbook. Philadelphia: W.B. Saunders, 1985.
168. Spraul CW, Lang GE, Lang GK, Grossniklaus HE. Morphometric changes in the choriocapillaris and the choroidal vasculature in eyes with advanced glaucomatous changes. Vision Res 2002; 42:923–32.
169. Stone EM, Fingret JH, Alward WL, et al. Identification of a gene that causes primary open angle glaucoma. Science 1997; 31:668–70.
170. Sung VC, Barton K. Management of inflammatory glaucomas. Curr Opin Ophthalmol 2004; 15:136–40.
171. Svedbergh B. Effects of artificial intraocular pressure elevation on the corneal endothelium in the vervet monkey (*Cercopithecus ethiops*). Acta Ophthalmol (Copenh) 1975; 53:839–55.
172. Tawara A, Inomata H. Developmental immaturity of the trabecular meshwork in congenital glaucoma. Am J Ophthalmol 1981; 92:508–25.
173. Tawara A, Inomata H. Developmental immaturity of the trabecular meshwork in juvenile glaucoma. Am J Ophthalmol 1984; 98:82–97.
174. Teng CC, Katzin HM, Chi HH. Primary degeneration in the chamber angle as an etiological factor in wide-angle glaucoma. Am J Ophthalmol 1957; 45:193–203.
175. Tian B, Geiger B., Epstein DL, Kaufman PL. Cytoskeletal involvement in the regulation of aqueous humor outflow. Invest Ophthalmol Vis Sci 2000; 41:619–23.
176. Tripathi RC. Mechanism of the aqueous outflow across the trabecular wall of Schlemm's canal. Exp Eye Res 1971; 11:116–21.
177. Tripathi RC. Comparative physiology and anatomy of the aqueous outflow pathway. In Davson H, Graham LT eds. The Eye: Comparative Physiology, Vol. 5. New York: Academic Press, 1974: 163–356.
178. Tripathi RC. Pathologic anatomy of the outflow pathway of aqueous humour in chronic simple glaucoma. Exp Eye Res 1977; (Suppl):403–7.
179. Ueda J, Wentz-Hunter K, Yue BY. Distribution of myocilin and extracellular matrix components in the juxtacanalicular tissue of human eyes. Invest Ophthalmol Vis Sci 2002; 43:1068–78.
180. Van Buskirk EM, Grant WM. Influence of temperature and the question of involvement of cellular metabolism in aqueous outflow. Am J Ophthalmol 1974; 77:565–72.
181. Van Buskirk EM, Leure-duPree AE. Pathophysiology and electron microscopy of melanomalytic glaucoma. Am J Ophthalmol 1978; 85:160–6.
182. van Oye R, Gelisken O. Pseudophakic glaucoma. Int Ophthalmol 1985; 8:183–6.
183. Vittal V, Rose A, Gregory KE, Kelley MJ, Acott TS. Changes in gene expression by trabecular meshwork cells

in response to mechanical stretching. Invest Ophthalmol Vis Sci 2005; 46:2857–68.

184. Wand M, Grant WM, Simmons RJ, Hutchinson BT. Plateau iris syndrome. Trans Am Acad Ophthalmol Otolaryngol 1977; 83:122–30.
185. Weinreb RN, Bloom E, Baxter JD, Alvarado J, Lan N, O'Donnell J, Polansky JR. Detection of glucocorticoid receptors in cultured human trabecular cells. Invest Ophthalmol Vis Sci 1981; 27:403–7.
186. Wiederholt M, Thieme H, Stumpff F. The regulation of trabecular meshwork and ciliary muscle contractility. Prog Retin Eye Res 2000; 19:271–95.
187. Wilhelmus KR, Grierson I, Watson PG. Histopathologic and clinical associations of scleritis and glaucoma. Am J Ophthalmol 1981; 91:697–705.
188. Wilson MC, Shields MB. A comparison of the clinical variants of the iridocorneal endothelial syndrome. Arch Ophthalmol 1989; 107:1465–8.
189. Wordinger RJ, Clark AF, Agarwal R, et al. Cultured human trabecular meshwork cells express functional growth factor receptors. Invest Ophthalmol Vis Sci 1998; 39:1575–89.
190. Worst JGF. Congenital glaucoma: remarks on the aspect of chamber angle. Ontogenetic and pathogenetic background and mode of action on goniotomy. Invest Ophthalmol 1968; 7:127–34.
191. Wulle KG. The development of the productive and draining system of the aqueous humour in the human eye. Adv Ophthalmol 1972; 26:296–355.
192. Yanoff M. Glaucoma mechanisms in ocular malignant melanoma. Am J Ophthalmol 1970; 70:898–904.
193. Yanoff M. Iridocorneal endothelial syndrome: unification of a disease spectrum. Surv Ophthalmol 1979; 24:1–2.
194. Yanoff M, Fine BS. Ocular Pathology, 5th ed. New York: Elsevier Mosby, 2002.
195. Yun AJ, Murphy CG, Polansky JR, Newsome DA, Alvarado JA. Proteins secreted by human trabecular cells. Invest Ophthalmol Vis Sci 1989; 50:2012–22.
196. Zhang X, Clark AF, Yorio, T. Regulation of glucocorticoid responsiveness in glaucomatous trabecular meshwork cells by glucocorticoid receptor-beta. Invest Ophthalmol Vis Sci 2005; 46:4607–16.

21

Posterior Segment Changes in Glaucoma

Stuart J. McKinnon
Departments of Ophthalmology and Neurobiology, Duke University, Durham, North Carolina, U.S.A.

INTRODUCTION

In humans, the optic nerve primarily transmits visual information from the retina to the lateral geniculate nucleus. Afferent fibers of the optic nerve also synapse in accessory central nervous system (CNS) centers such as the Edinger-Westphal nucleus, which controls pupillary reflexes. The optic nerve originates from axons of the retinal ganglion cells (RGCs) in the innermost cell layer of the retina. These un-myelinated axons then course posteriorly in bundles of the nerve fiber layer and meet at the rim of the optic nerve head. The bundles then bend approximately 90° and pass through the lamina cribrosa, a circular, fenestrated connective tissue extension of the sclera, into the orbit where the fibers become myelinated. For 20 mm to 30 mm behind the eye, the nerve has a sinuous course to allow movement of the globe. The intra-orbital optic nerve is covered by an outer dura mater and an inner arachnoid sheath, both of which are attached to the sclera around the lamina cribrosa. The 10 mm long intra-cranial portion begins at the optic foramen, through which the optic nerve fibers then pass posteriorly and medially to the optic chiasm where they partially decussate. The mixed fibers continue in the optic tracts, to terminate primarily in the lateral geniculate nuclei.

Axons of neighboring RGCs are formed into nerve fiber bundles by processes of Müller cells and astrocytes (74). Axons from the peripheral retina lie more deeply in the nerve fiber layer and more central axons run perpendicularly through the nerve fiber layer to lie anteriorly and closer to the vitreo-retinal interface (Fig. 1). Axons from RGCs located in the superior and inferior temporal retina occupy superior and inferior lateral positions within the optic nerve, whereas axons from the nasal hemiretina assume more medial positions (52,75). Axons from more peripheral RGCs tend to lie at the circumference of the optic nerve, and axons from more posterior RGCs run more centrally within the nerve (92). Nerve fibers that originate within 0.5 mm of the fovea are called papillomacular fibers. Nasal papillomacular fibers pass directly to the optic disc, whereas the temporal

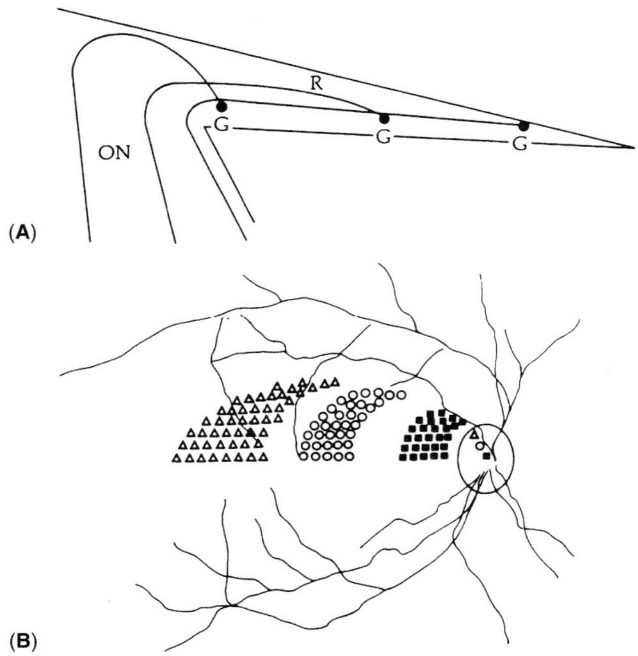

Figure 1 Vertical and topographic diagram of organization of axons within the retinal nerve fiber layer of rhesus monkeys. (**A**) Axons from retinal ganglion cells (*cells labeled* G) travel toward the optic nerve (ON) where they make an approximate 90° bend to enter the nerve head. Axons from peripheral retinal ganglion cells (*to right*) are located in deeper positions within the nerve fiber layer. Axons from more central retinal ganglion cells travel upward to be located in more superficial layers. (**B**) Within the optic nerve head (*large oval*), axons from the peripheral retina (*triangles*) are located in circumferential positions. Axons from central retina (*circles*) are located in intermediate positions, and axons from peripapillary retina (*squares*) are located centrally. *Source*: From Ref. 52.

papillomacular fibers pass above and below the macula and enter the optic nerve head temporally. Fibers originating from the superotemporal retina but outside the macula are termed superior arcuate fibers and enter the optic disc between 12 and 1 o'clock positions. Fibers originating from the inferotemporal retina outside the macula are termed inferior arcuate fibers and enter the disc between the 5 and 6 o'clock positions (63). The arcuate and papillomacular fibers are topographically segregated into superior and inferior arcades by the horizontal meridian, an imaginary line through the macula and the optic disc. In the peripheral retina, the nerve fiber layer thickness is extremely thin, whereas close to the optic disc the fiber bundles become more compact and the nerve fiber layer increases in thickness to 200 to 300 μm, being thickest in the superotemporal and inferotemporal areas due to a greater number of fibers from the arcuate bundles (75). The highly ordered topography of nerve fibers in the retina is crucial to understanding the location and progression of visual field defects seen in glaucoma.

The primary constituents of the optic nerve head are the axons of the RGC, representing about 70% of the volume. Connective tissue, neuroglia, and blood vessels make up the remaining 30% (50). These connective tissue components undergo several changes in glaucoma. In humans, the lamina cribrosa consists of 8 to 12 interconnected planar lamellae composed mainly of collagen types I and III, and elastin. The lamellae are composed of inter-connecting beams (Fig. 2), whose fibers are oriented longitudinally within an extracellular matrix (ECM) containing glycosaminoglycan (GAGs) (56). Elastin fibers also form a ring around the scleral canal (71). The amount of collagen in the lamina cribrosa increases with age. The average thickness of the lamina is about 250 μm and it contains numerous pores through which the optic nerve fiber bundles pass (Fig. 2). The anterior lamina contains fewer pores (average of 392) than the posterior lamina (average of 540). The pores of the lamina between the collagen beams are narrowest in the superior and inferior quadrants, where axonal loss typically occurs initially in glaucoma. The proportion

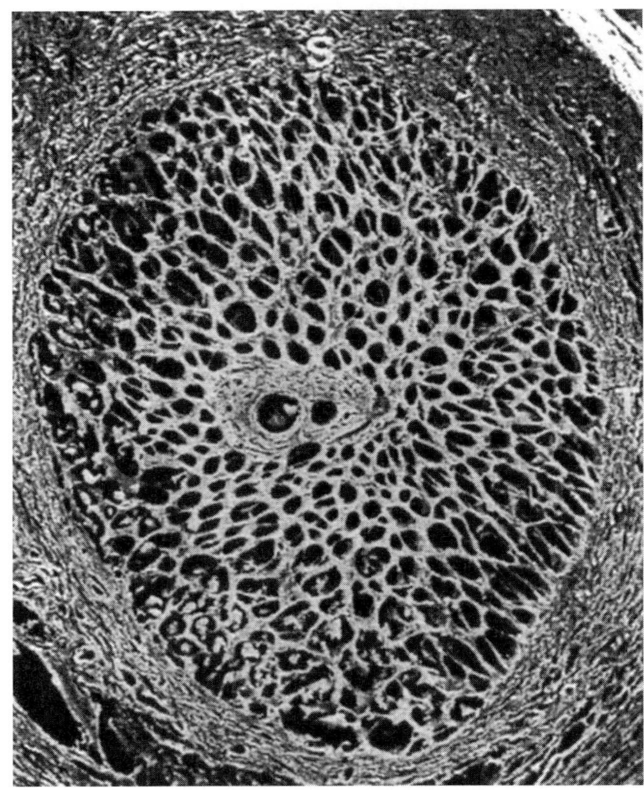

Figure 2 Scanning electron micrograph of a cross section of the human lamina cribrosa after trypsin digest, dissection, and embedding in plastic, demonstrating inter-connecting collagen. These pores in the lamina offer a conduit for nerve fibers and provide structural support. Blood vessels feeding the nerve fibers are located within the collagen beams. *Source*: From Ref. 22.

of the cribiform area occupied by pores at the level of the choroid is independent of age. The proportion of the cribiform area occupied by pores at the scleral level, however, shows a highly significant decline after adulthood is reached, suggesting a net loss of about 5% per decade (equivalent to about 6000 axons per year) and about 20% of optic nerve fiber mass by the age of 74 years. Age-related loss of axons is accompanied by progressive alterations in the collagen of the lamina cribrosa. In older patients with glaucoma these age-related changes may contribute to more rapid progression of vision loss (64).

OPTIC NERVE DAMAGE IN GLAUCOMA

The clinical manifestations of glaucoma are detected by visual function testing and by examination of the optic nerve head. Visual field tests are employed to detect peripheral vision loss, a functional consequence of loss of RGC axons. Loss of sensitivity nasally ("nasal step") is commonly detected first, followed by arcuate hemifield loss. In the final stages, macular field loss and loss of central vision occur. Progressive changes in the optic nerve include posterior displacement of the nerve head surface and excavation of prelaminar tissues beneath the anterior scleral ring. Other optic neuropathies caused by ischemia, inflammation, or compression usually result in atrophy and pallor of the optic nerve head, but lack the typical clinical excavation of rim tissue found in glaucoma.

The optic nerve damage is a sequel to the loss of RGCs and their axons in the retina. The underlying mechanism for this remains controversial and there are two traditional theories to explain the damage to RGCs. The mechanical hypothesis relates the ganglion cell damage to changes in the connective tissue structure of the optic nerve head. Misalignment of the connective tissue beams in the lamina leads to kinking of the bundles of ganglion cell axons and mechanical obstruction of rapid-phase axonal transport (69). The alternative vascular hypothesis states that ischemia, in combination with elevated intraocular pressure (IOP), causes ganglion cell death. Metabolic tracers have been shown to accumulate in the lamina cribrosa in inverse proportion to the perfusion pressure in cat eyes (76) and interruption of blood flow in the short posterior arteries causes blockage of axonal transport in primates (77). However, more inclusive theories treat the optic nerve head as a bio-mechanical structure, suggesting that IOP-related connective tissue stress and strain contribute to the pathophysiology of the optic nerve head (10).

Axonal Transport Blockade

RGCs possess extremely long axons, and cell homeostasis depends on the continuous bi-directional movement of materials within these axons, a process termed axonal transport. These materials, consisting of mitochondria, microtubules, vesicles and other elements, allow metabolic support and communication between neurons. Orthograde or anterograde axonal transport away from the cell body serves to maintain cell membranes and synaptic function. Orthograde transport consists of a slow phase, in which soluble protein and mitochondria move at 1 mm to 5 mm per day, and a rapid phase, in which microsomal material moves at 400 mm/day (68). Retrograde transport towards the cell body serves communication and recycling functions. It occurs at about half the rate of rapid orthograde transport (50–260 mm/day) and returns up to 50% of cytoplasmic material from the distal axon to the cell body (51).

Orthograde axonal transport within RGCs has been investigated after an intra-vitreal injection of tritiated leucine into monkey eyes subjected to acute elevations of IOP. After diffusion and incorporation into ganglion cells, axonal movement of the radiolabeled leucine was quantified by autoradiography or scintillation counting. The greatest accumulation of radioactivity was seen within the lamina cribrosa, with signal also being seen within the optic nerve tract and dorsal lateral geniculate nucleus (dLGN). Retrograde transport within optic nerve axons was studied after injection of horseradish peroxidase (HRP) into the dLGN and optic tract. HRP accumulation was seen in and around the lamina in eyes subjected to increased IOP (Fig. 3). In eyes exposed to an acute IOP elevation, complete blockade of orthograde or retrograde transport was not demonstrated. Upon histologic examination, enlarged and distended axons filled with HRP reaction product were noted. Serial reconstructions of the optic nerve heads from hypertensive eyes showed orthograde and retrograde label accumulation most often in the inferior temporal quadrant, and least often in the superior nasal quadrant (61). Further studies have shown that a progressive accumulation of label occurs at the scleral lamina cribrosa from 3 to 8 hours after IOP elevation in monkeys. Examination by transmission electron microscopy (TEM) revealed axons distended by smooth surfaced vesicles and mitochondria after two hours of acute pressure elevation (68).

Optic Nerve Head Perfusion

The vascular supply of the optic nerve head has three sources. Distal retinal nerve fiber layer bundles are supplied from retinal arterioles, the pre-laminar nerves is supplied from peripapillary choroid, and the laminar nerve is supplied from branches of the short posterior ciliary arteries (Fig. 4). Capillaries in the optic nerve head are morphologically identical to blood vessels of similar size in the retina and brain (2).

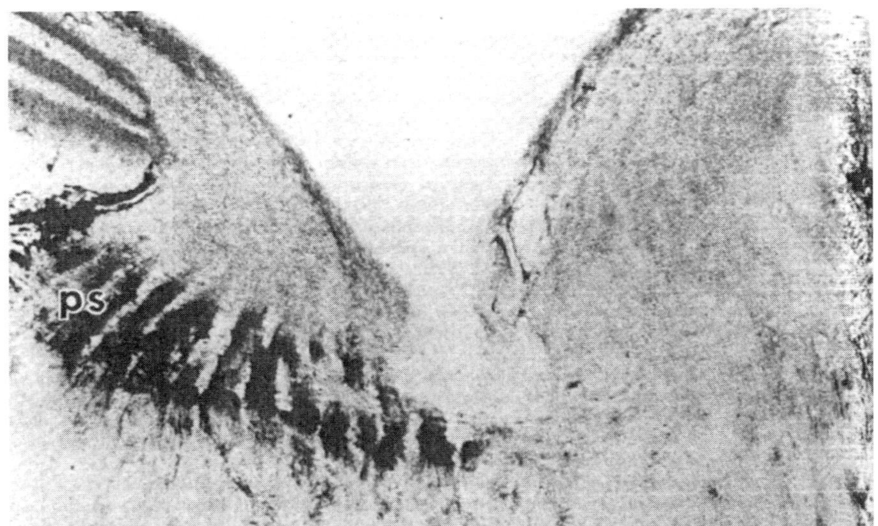

Figure 3 Axonal transport blockade. Photomicrograph of optic nerve head of rhesus monkey eye subjected to increased intraocular pressure for 23 hours by anterior chamber cannulation. Horseradish peroxidase was injected into the lateral geniculate nucleus and tritiated leucine was injected into the vitreous approximately 24 hours before enucleation. Accumulation of both labels (*dark materials*) was noted in the pars scleralis (ps) temporally. *Source*: From Ref. 53.

In the anterior lamina cribrosa, capillaries are located within glial and collagenous zones (51) and extensively anastomose (43). Glial cell processes lining pores of the lamina cribrosa lack tight junctions, allowing low-molecular-weight molecules such as fluorescein to pass from the choroid into the nerve fiber bundles (7). Injections of lanthanum or HRP into the vitreous at normal IOP show some molecular passage into the optic nerve head tissues (67). This apparent lack of a true blood–brain barrier in the lamina cribrosa may permit injury to the optic nerve from blood-borne agents (30).

Frank occlusion of the capillaries running within each laminar beam may occur due to tensile compressive or shear strains. It has been hypothesized that IOP-related strain within the peripapillary sclera exerts compressive effects on volume flow within the branches of the posterior ciliary arteries that penetrate to the choroid, pre-laminar, laminar or post-laminar regions. IOP-related strain within each individual laminar beam may have acute compressive effects on laminar capillary volume flow.

Although ischemia occurs in optic nerve heads of some patients with glaucoma (53), there is little experimental evidence to show that elevated IOP causes primary loss of nerve head capillaries with subsequent loss of axons. Ischemia has been proposed as the cause of optic nerve head cupping in glaucoma, and fluorescein angiography is one of several techniques used to study optic nerve blood flow in normal subjects and glaucoma patients. The retinal circulation and intra-retinal transit times in patients with glaucoma are slower than normal, and filling of nerve head blood vessels is delayed. Localized relative and absolute filling defects correlate with visual field loss (22).

The optic nerve head vasculature has an autoregulatory capability and can alter flow in response to changes in IOP, systemic blood pressure, or metabolic need. In a study using microspheres in monkeys, moderate IOP elevations had mild effects on retinal

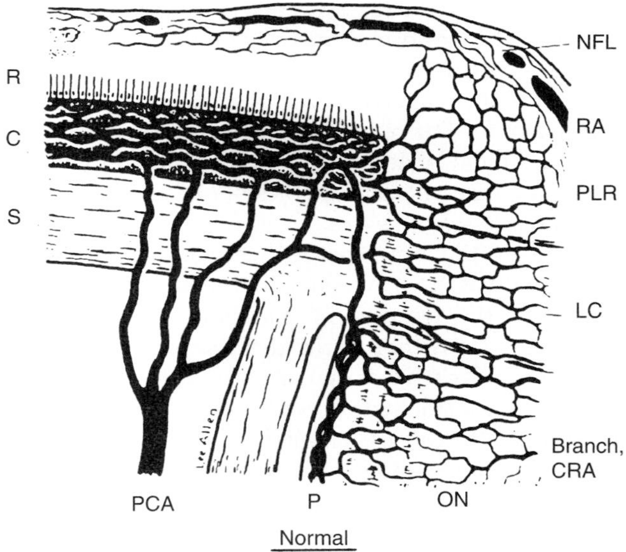

Figure 4 Blood supply of the optic nerve and the adjacent retina. Retinal nerve fibers are supplied by retinal arterioles, prelaminar nerve fibers are supplied by peripapillary choroidal blood vessels, and the laminar nerve fibers are supplied by centripetal branches of the short posterior ciliary arteries. *Abbreviations*: C, choroid branch; CRA, centripetal branch of central retinal artery; LC, lamina cribrosa; NFL, nerve fiber layer; ON, optic nerve; P, pia; PCA, posterior ciliary artery; PLR, pre-laminar region; R, retina; RA, retinal arteriole; S, sclera. *Source*: From Ref. 22.

and pre-laminar blood flow but no effect on retrolaminar flow. As IOP increased, retinal and pre-laminar flow was directly related to the perfusion pressure, and retrolaminar flow increased. At IOPs high enough to stop retinal and pre-laminar blood flow, the anterior lamina was underperfused and the posterior lamina was overperfused. Optic nerve blood flow has been found not to be more pressure-sensitive than retinal blood flow (26). However, ECM changes and thickening of astrocyte and endothelial cell basement membranes from chronic activation in glaucoma have been postulated to reduce nutrient diffusion to axons even when capillary perfusion may be normal (10).

Peripapillary Atrophy

Peripapillary chorioretinal atrophy has been described as a loss of retinal pigment epithelium (RPE) adjacent to the optic disc and obliteration of smaller peripapillary choroidal blood vessels. Peripapillary changes have been noted more often in glaucoma patients (3) and a significant correlation exists between the location of peripapillary atrophy and the visual field defect (31). Peripapillary atrophy is described in two areas, a peripheral zone "alpha" with irregular RPE pigmentation, and a more central zone "beta" with marked atrophy of the RPE, and visible choroidal vessels and sclera (Fig. 5). Jonas et al. measured peripapillary regions in 582 eyes of 321 patients with primary open-angle glaucoma (POAG) and 390 eyes of 231 normal patients (36). In POAG eyes, both zones were significantly larger and more frequent than normal. The size and frequency of peripapillary atrophy correlated with the stage of the glaucoma. In early glaucoma, changes in the nasal peripapillary sector were most marked. Significant findings were enlargement of zone alpha, occurrence of zone alpha anywhere in the nasal sector, and most importantly, occurrence of zone beta anywhere. In further studies, peripapillary atrophy increased with decreasing neuroretinal rim area, and was associated with shallow glaucomatous cupping and diffuse nerve fiber loss (37).

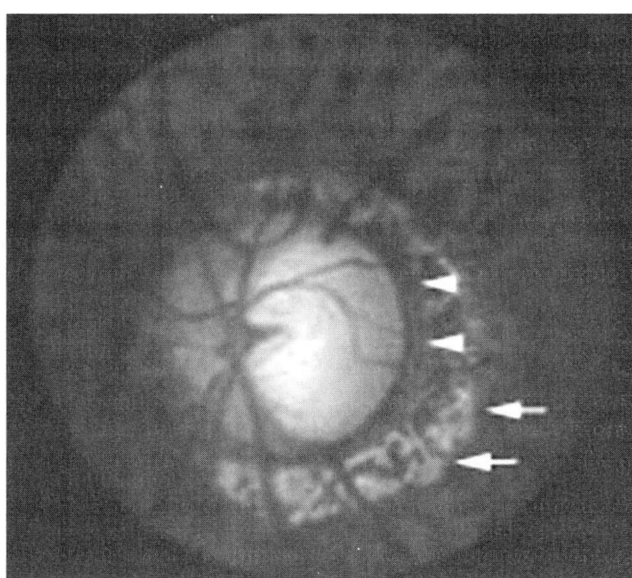

Figure 5 An optic nerve head with glaucomatous damage demonstrates peripapillary atrophy in the more central "zone beta" (*arrowheads*) and more peripheral "zone alpha" (*arrows*). The presence of zone beta peripapillary atrophy in any sector correlates with glaucomatous cupping and nerve fiber loss.

Optic Disc Hemorrhages

Optic disc or peripapillary hemorrhages occur at the neuroretinal rim, and due to their location in the nerve fiber layer, are flame-shaped (Fig. 6). Various mechanisms have been proposed to explain the occurrence of optic disc hemorrhages, including ischemia, vascular abnormalities, and mechanical trauma at the level of the lamina cribrosa. The most likely explanation involves continuing axonal atrophy, with posterior deformation of the lamina cribrosa and rupture of stretched capillaries. Hemorrhages occur in the optic nerve head in 0% to 0.7% of healthy eyes. Their occurrence in glaucomatous eyes was first noted in

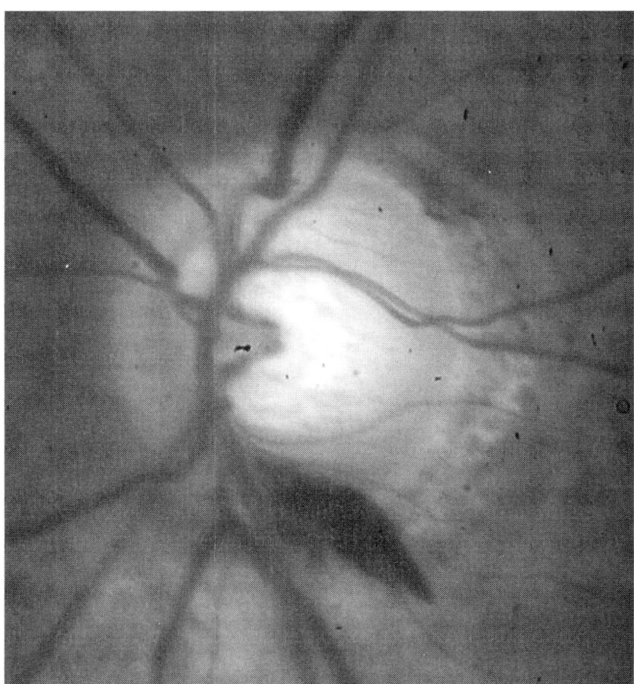

Figure 6 An optic disc hemorrhage is seen in the inferotemporal quadrant. The hemorrhage is located in the peripapillary nerve fiber layer and correlates with progression of visual field loss and optic nerve damage in corresponding areas.

1889 by Bjerrum, and the association between optic disc hemorrhages and glaucoma was firmly established by Drance et al. (17). In various forms of glaucoma the incidence of optic disc hemorrhages varies from 2% to 42%, and they are more common in eyes with low-tension glaucoma (83). Optic disc hemorrhages are thought to signal active injury and in chronic open-angle glaucoma and ocular hypertension visual field loss progresses more often in eyes with optic disc hemorrhages than in those without (18). In one study, 36% of eyes with optic disc hemorrhages were associated with a concentric enlargement of the optic cup and 31% had notching of the neural rim at the location of the optic disc hemorrhage (1). A study of glaucomatous eyes showed that 63% of visual fields and 79% of optic discs progress after optic disc hemorrhage, and a majority of the changes corresponded clinically to the area of hemorrhage on the optic disc (83).

Extracellular Matrix Changes

Tissue damage involves repair and remodeling processes that are regulated by interactions between cells and their ECM support. Astrocytes reside in the optic nerve head and actively participate in the remodeling of the ECM in glaucoma. Enhanced expression of collagen type IV is seen in pre-laminar astrocytes and de novo expression of elastin is seen in laminar astrocytes (89). Collagen type IV was considerably increased in quantity throughout the lamina in eyes with all degrees of glaucoma damage. Collagen type IV has been immunolocalized to the septal margins of laminar beams and to thickened astrocyte basement membranes. Large quantities of collagen type I, collagen type III, and collagen type IV have been found between the disorganized laminar beams (57). Collagen type IV and other basement membrane macromolecules appear to extend into nerve bundles, filling spaces left by degenerating axons (32). In young adults, thin elastic fibers run longitudinally in the core of the beams. With normal aging, elastic fibers assume a tubular shape surrounded by collagen. In mild glaucoma, tubular elastic fibers have not been recognized. In advanced glaucoma, masses of non-fibrillary elastin are characterized by loss of collagen fibers, thickened basement membranes, and bundles of microfibrils (33). Elastic fibers also show loss and fragmentation at the bottom of the cup and disorganization in the peripheral walls of the optic cup (57). Matrix metalloproteinases (MMPs) are proteolytic enzymes that effect tissue remodeling in the optic nerve head. MMP substrates include molecules involved in intercellular adhesion, cell-matrix interaction, and cell signalling. Inhibition of MMP activity in the optic nerve head could be used as a therapy in the treatment of glaucoma, as retinas from MMP-9 knockout mice preserve of RGCs after optic nerve ligation (13).

Biomechanical Changes in the Optic Nerve Head

The load bearing tissues of the optic nerve head consist of the connective tissues of the peripapillary sclera, the lamina cribrosa, and the scleral canal. The ECM of the sclera and lamina resist compressive and shear stresses. Stiffness and strength are influenced by collagen fiber diameter and cross-linking, as well as interactions with other ECM components. Tissue elasticity results from collagen and elastin (10). A considerable amount of lamina cribrosa deformation occurs at normal or subnormal IOPs. Eyes fixed at 5 mmHg demonstrate continuous vertical columns of axonal bundles passing through the lamina (93). The lamina and scleral canal wall act like an expansible trampoline at low IOP levels, with the scleral canal expanding and the lamina cribrosa becoming more stretched as IOP is elevated to 10 mmHg (8).

Normal monkey optic nerve heads exhibit a posterior deformation of approximately 30 μm after acute elevations of IOP of 10–45 mmHg. In monkey eyes subjected to chronic IOP elevations, optic nerve head surface compliance, or ease of deformability, increased significantly 1 to 2 weeks after onset. This early hypercompliance is thought to be a separate manifestation of connective tissue damage. After 3 to 6 weeks of chronic elevated IOP, the viscoelastic properties of monkey peripapillary sclera are also altered (9). Computer modeling has been used to examine the forces induced in the sclera and lamina cribrosa by elevated IOP. The architecture of the lamina cribrosa has been modeled computationally using finite element analysis, in which three-dimensional geometries are modeled that approximate tissue characteristics of the laminar components. Large stress and strain concentrations and gradients, up to 33 times greater than background, were seen affecting individual laminar beams (6). In human eyes judged to have an early stage of glaucoma, a compressive rearrangement of the successive laminar sheets has been seen in eyes with increased IOP but with normal visual acuity and visual fields (Fig. 7).

Disruption of collagen precedes changes in elastin and remodeling of the ECM. Other changes in laminar structure occur at later stages, including posterior displacement of the posterior limit of the superior and inferior lamina (70).

Apoptosis in Glaucoma

Several studies directly implicate apoptosis in ganglion cell death due to glaucoma. Rat eyes subjected to 4 months of IOP elevation display DNA fragmentation and a reduction in mitochondrial membrane

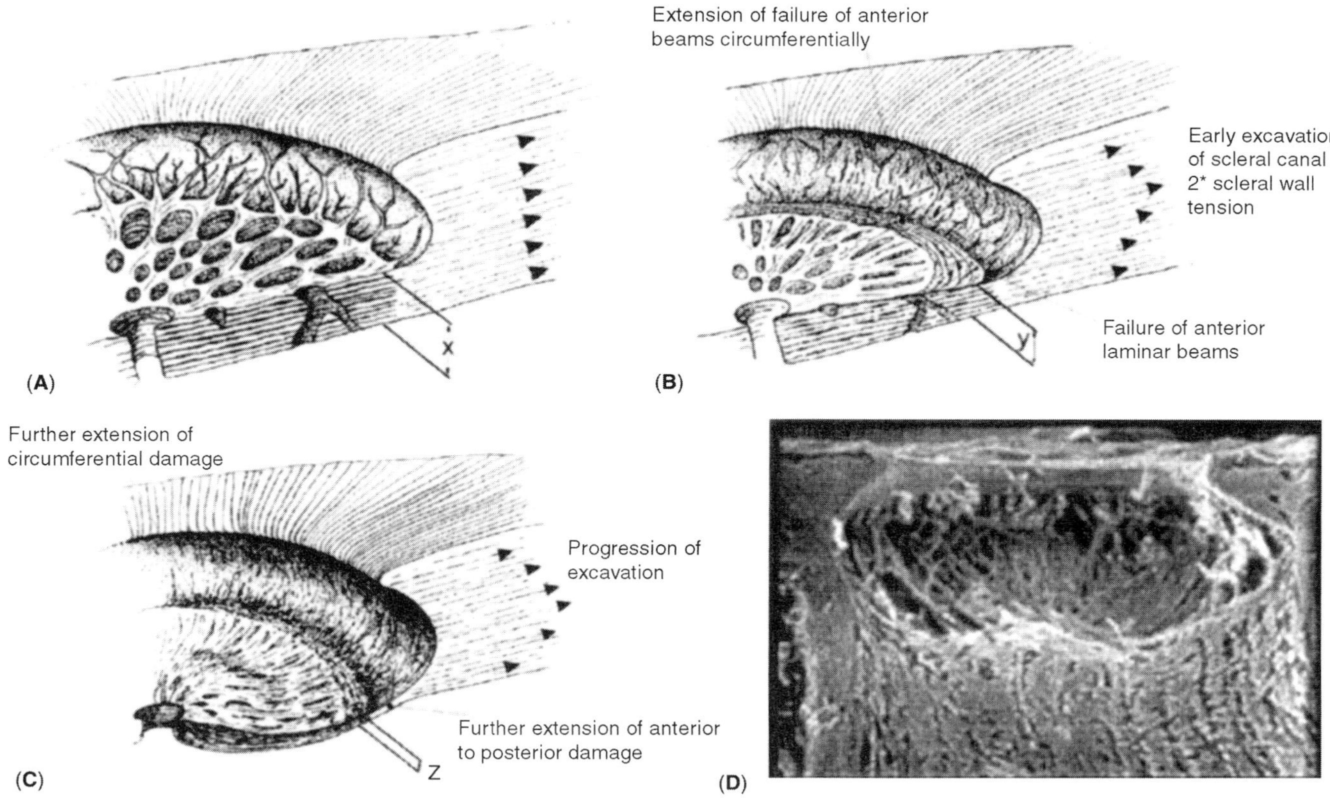

Figure 7 Progression of posterior deformation and excavation of optic nerve head tissues. (**A**) Sagittal representation of the scleral canal and lamina cribrosa with normal laminar thickness (X) and directions of scleral wall tension (*arrow heads*). (**B**) Early failure of anterior laminar plates results in thinning (Y), excavation, and circumferential extension. (**C**) Further progression causes more thinning of the lamina (Z). The remaining lamina is posteriorly deformed and the scleral wall is forced under the anterior scleral rim. (**D**) Pronounced laminar thinning and excavation are seen in an end-stage optic nerve head. *Source*: From Ref. 10.

potential of RGCs consistent with apoptosis (see Chapter 2) (54). RGCs in rabbits and monkeys subjected to conditions of experimental glaucoma and optic nerve transection die by apoptosis (25,72). Apoptotic RGCs are present in significantly greater numbers of human retinas with glaucoma, when compared to age-matched control retinas (39).

Caspase-8, which is involved in the "extrinsic" pathway of apoptosis, is activated in rat glaucoma models (47). Due to its apical position in the apoptotic cascade, caspase-8 is thus an attractive target to prevent RGC death in glaucoma. In experimental rat glaucoma under high IOP conditions, caspases-8 and -9 are transcriptionally up-regulated, and caspase-9, which participates in the "intrinsic" pathway of apoptosis is activated in RGCs (34).

TRIGGERS OF RETINAL GANGLION CELL APOPTOSIS

Specific triggers of apoptosis have been implicated in glaucoma, including blockage of axonal transport of neurotrophic factors, excitotoxicity, exposure to cytokines, immunologic modulation, and derangement of vasoactive regulators such as endothelin and nitric oxide.

Neurotrophin Deprivation

Survival of neurons is dependent on the trophic support of their innervating targets, a concept embodied in the "neurotrophin hypothesis". Only those neurons that are successful in establishing correct synaptic connections with their targets obtain trophic factor support, allowing their survival. Vertebrate neuronal cell death induced by trophic factor deprivation requires the participation of caspases (24). This demonstration was the first functional evidence that trophic factor deprivation activates apoptosis in vertebrate neurons.

The most extensively studied of these factors belong to the nerve growth factor family, that includes nerve growth factor, brain-derived neurotrophic factor (BDNF), neurotrophin 3, neurotrophin 4, and neurotrophin 5. This family of growth factors are ligands that bind to tyrosine kinase receptor A (TRKA), tyrosine kinase receptor B (TRKB) and tyrosine kinase receptor C (TRKC), that are retrogradely transported to the cell body of the neuron. The neurotrophin receptor TRKB is a membrane bound receptor that when bound by BDNF, activates tyrosine kinases, stimulating cell survival pathways by triggering phosphatidylinositol 3-kinase and extra-cellular signal regulated kinase cascades (82). Embryonic development of mouse RGCs is strongly influenced by neurotrophic factor expression, as is apoptosis of adult RGCs (16). BDNF is a survival factor for RGCs in vitro (49), and it is expressed in the retinorecipient layers of the superior colliculus in rats (44). BDNF has been shown to be retrogradely transported to the retina, suggesting that target-derived BDNF is a major source of the neurotrophin for RGCs (73).

To investigate the possibility that RGC death is initiated by a blockade of retrograde axonal transport of neurotrophins arriving from central target cells, studies of ultra-structural alterations and the immunohistochemical localization of BDNF, TRKA, TRKB, and TRKC in optic nerve heads of rats with acute IOP elevation equaling retinal artery perfusion pressure have been performed. BDNF and the TRKB receptor are localized in monkey eyes with unilateral, chronic experimental glaucoma and with optic nerve axotomy. TRKB labeling in elevated IOP eyes is significantly greater than in their paired control eyes. Of six monkeys with experimental glaucoma, the glaucomatous optic nerve heads demonstrated alterations in TRKB labeling consisting of increased axonal labeling in the nerve head compared to the superficial retina and the myelinated nerve, focal labelled fibers in the nerve head, prominent glial labeling not detected in normal eyes. BDNF labeling showed similar focal an accumulations in the same areas as TRKB. The differences between control and glaucoma eyes were significant (66). Interruption of BDNF retrograde transport and an accumulation of TRKB at the optic nerve head in acute and chronic glaucoma models suggest a role for neurotrophin deprivation in the pathogenesis of RGC death in glaucoma (Fig. 8) (66).

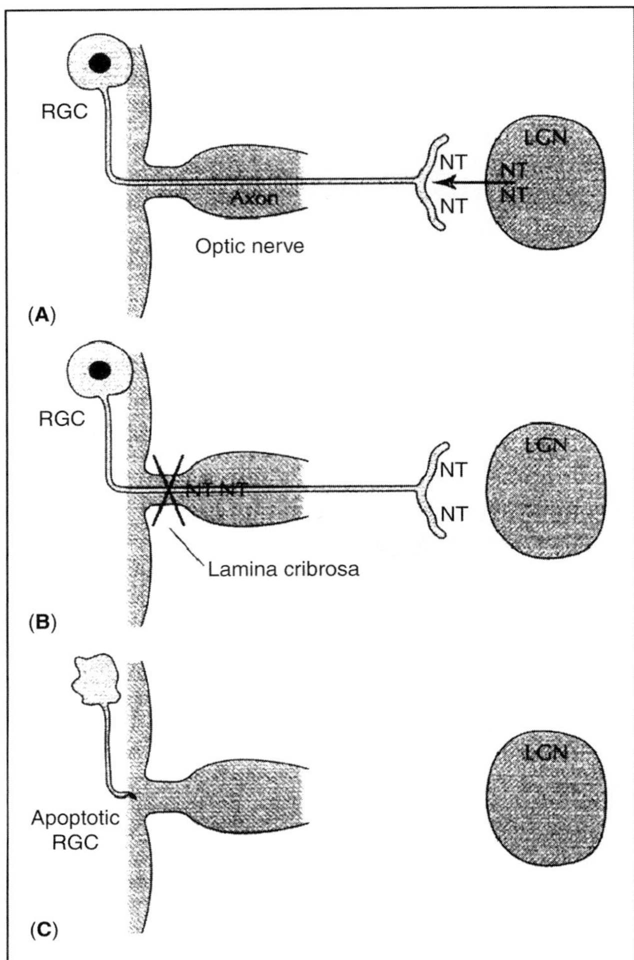

Figure 8 Retrograde transport block of neurotrophins in glaucoma. (**A**) In humans, the lateral geniculate nucleus (LGN) produces neurotrophins (NT) that flow to the cell body of the retinal ganglion cell (RGC) by retrograde transport. (**B**) Retrograde transport blockade at the lamina cribrosa deprives the RGC of required growth factors. (**C**) RGC death occurs by apoptosis. *Source*: From Ref. 46.

Excitotoxicity

Pathologic increases in intracellular calcium ion concentration have also been implicated in RGC loss. Adrenergic receptor agonists and antagonists are used in the treatment of glaucoma and decrease IOP by decreasing aqueous production and increasing aqueous outflow. Betaxolol, a β_1-blocker, inhibits glutamate-receptor stimulated increases of intra-cellular calcium in RGCs. Brimonidine, an α_2-agonist, has been shown to be neuroprotective in animal models of retinal and optic nerve injury by inhibiting calcium influx and up-regulating neurotrophins such as BDNF (4). Intervention with Ca^{2+}-channel blockers decreases retinal neuronal apoptosis in animal and cell culture models (41).

Glutamate. Glutamate is an excitatory amino acid neurotransmitter that exerts its neurotoxic effect through the *N*-methyl-D-aspartate (NMDA) receptor (19). In one study samples of vitreous obtained from humans with glaucoma and from monkeys with experimental glaucoma had elevated glutamate levels compared to controls (20), but this observation has recently been questioned (12). Memantine is a selective NMDA receptor blocker that inhibits excessive levels of glutamatergic activity with less effect on normal glutamatergic signalling. Overaction of NMDA-type glutamate receptors contributes to excitotoxic RGC injury in a number of animal models. Memantine prevents RGC death from NMDA-induced neurotoxicity in vitro in a dose-dependent manner, and protects RGCs in laser photocoagulation models of rat (28) and monkey (29) glaucoma.

Nitric Oxide

Nitric oxide is an important signalling molecule that acts in many tissues to regulate a diverse range of physiological processes including vasodilation, neuronal function, inflammation, and immune function. Nitric oxide has also been demonstrated to be involved in the regulation of apoptosis. Nitric oxide generated by inducible nitric oxide synthase (iNOS) from macrophages and/or perivascular cells can generate toxic free radicals such as peroxynitrite. Selective inhibition of iNOS preserves normal iNOS production by scavenging excessive peroxynitrite, or by inhibiting the metabolic pathways triggered by peroxynitrite. iNOS has been localized in optic nerve heads from human glaucomatous eyes and from rat eyes with chronic IOP elevation (60). In an experimental rat model of glaucoma, oral treatment with iNOS inhibitors provided significant neuroprotection of RGCs (61,62). However, another study in a rat glaucoma model showed no increase in iNOS protein or mRNA expression in glaucomatous eyes when compared to controls, and no neuroprotective effect of pharmacologic iNOS inhibition (65).

Endothelin

Endothelin 1 (EDN1) is a potent vasoconstricting peptide that has been noted in plasma and aqueous humor of glaucoma patients (38,85). EDN1 affects the vasculature through two major receptors, EDNRA and EDNRB. The EDNRB receptor, primarily located on glial cells in the CNS, can participate in neuronal disease (79). EDN1 may reduce blood flow in the optic nerve due to vasoconstriction, or may mediate neuronal damage through the EDNRB receptor on the glial cells. A retrobulbar infusion of EDN1 in primates causes a significant focal loss of RGC axons, but the location has been variable within the optic nerve of individual animals. There is also significant variability between animals in response to EDN1 induced ischemia (14).

Tumor Necrosis Factor-α

Tumor necrosis factor-α (TNFα) is a protein cytokine recognized as a multi-functional pro-inflammatory mediator, and binds to members of the superfamily of TNF receptors. A so-called death domain in the cytoplasmic portion of each TNF receptor recruits adaptor proteins that bind to and activate caspase-8, forming an active signalling complex that is known to activate caspase-3 and to induce cell death (21). The finding of caspase-8 activation in glaucoma implicates the extrinsic apoptosis pathway in RGC death due to exposure to elevated IOP involving TNF receptor superfamily members (47). In vitro studies using primary co-cultures of RGCs and glial cells have shown that elevated IOP or ischemia, two prominent stress factors identified in the eyes of patients with glaucoma, can initiate the apoptotic cell death cascade in RGCs, through TNFα secreted by activated glial cells. Immunohistochemical studies in human eyes obtained post-mortem have revealed increased immunostaining for TNFα and TNFα receptor-1 in glaucomatous optic nerve heads compared to age matched control eyes, being most prominent in post-laminar glial cells and pial septa (88,94). Death of RGCs in culture is attenuated approximately 66% by inhibiting bioactivity of TNFα (87). These observations provide direct evidence that TNFα has an essential role in glaucomatous neurodegeneration. Also, optineurin, a protein of unknown function that has been implicated in the TNFα signalling pathway, is speculated to play a neuroprotective role in the retina (78). Mutations in the *OPTN* gene that encode for optineurin are associated with adult-onset open-angle glaucoma (see Chapter 34).

Calcineurin

Calcineurin is a widely-expressed Ca^{2+}/calmodulin-dependent protein phosphatase that when cleaved, leads to apoptotic neuronal death in the CNS. In a rat glaucoma model calcineurin is cleaved to a constitutively active form that is detected in RGCs exposed to elevated IOP but not in control RGCs, including RGCs after optic nerve crush. Oral treatment of rats with increased IOP with the calcineurin inhibitor FK506 tends to reduce RGC loss and promote optic nerve preservation (35).

Amyloid

Glaucoma and Alzheimer disease (AD) (see Chapter 70) are chronic neurodegenerative conditions that share certain morphologic similarities. Eyes from AD patients are reported to show loss of large magnocellular RGCs, the cell type that dies earliest in glaucoma (80). Neurofilament triplet proteins that are components of neurofibrillary tangles in AD also localize to large RGCs in an experimental model of glaucoma in the monkey (90). Synaptic dysfunction in AD is associated with deficient glutamate transport function (42) and caspase activity (45) leading to increased susceptibility to excitotoxic injuries.

Amyloid precursor protein (APP), which plays a role in synaptic homeostasis (58), is expressed normally in several areas of the CNS including RGCs, and is packaged in small transport vesicles for rapid anterograde transport in the optic nerve to the plasma membranes in axons, dendrites, and synapses, where it plays an important homeostatic role (55,58). Synaptic dysfunction in AD is associated with deficient glutamate transport function and susceptibility to excitotoxic injury (42), findings also noted in glaucoma (59). Cleavage of APP by β- and γ-secretases causes the formation of amyloid-β, a component of the amyloid plaques of AD. Amyloid-β is neurotoxic and also stimulates a TNFα-dependent expression of inducible nitric oxide synthase and neuronal apoptosis (15).

RGC death in glaucoma involves abnormal processing of APP and upregulation of amyloid-β (47). A study of nursing home patients in Germany found a statistically significant increase in the prevalence of glaucoma in patients diagnosed with AD (12/49 or 24.7%) compared with a matched control group without AD (12/186 or 6.5%) (5). This suggests that RGC death in glaucoma may involve chronic amyloid-β neurotoxicity, in a manner that mimics AD at the molecular level. With the loss of the protective effect of APP and the upregulation of toxic APP fragments that include amyloid-β, RGCs ultimately die from chronic caspase activation, loss of synaptic homeostasis, amyloid-β cytotoxicity and other excitotoxic events (48).

Autoimmunity

Autoimmune mechanisms may also contribute to glaucomatous optic neuropathy. Elevated serum levels of autoantibodies to antigens of the optic nerve and retina and abnormal T-cell subsets have been reported in glaucoma (27). Heat shock protein and crystalline expression is up-regulated in the retina and optic nerve head in glaucoma (91). Active immunization with myelin or myelin-derived peptides has been shown to reduce RGC loss in rat models of optic nerve crush and ocular hypertension (23,40,81). Antibody profiles against optic nerve antigens in patients with glaucoma have been analyzed, and significantly increased titers to α-fodrin have been detected in the sera of normal tension glaucoma patients. Fodrin is a major neuronal cytoskeleton protein, and links actin filaments to the plasma membrane. Fodrin is a target of caspase-3 and is cleaved early in apoptosis, leading to structural rearrangements such as membrane blebbing (27). Fodrin cleavage has been reported in neurodegenerative diseases such as AD, and α-fodrin is cleaved by caspase-3 in a rat model of chronic IOP elevation (84).

Heat-Shock Proteins

Heat-shock proteins (HSPs) (see Chapter 36) are induced when a cell experiences various types of environmental stress such as heat, cold, and oxygen deprivation. They also act as molecular "chaperones," shuttling proteins from one compartment to another inside the cell, and also transport old proteins for degradation. Patients with glaucoma have been noted to have increased antibody titers to HSPs (hsp27), which may pre-dispose toward retinal or optic nerve damage due to antibody attenuation of endogenously released retinal HSPs (86). Overproduction of certain HSPs (hsp70) is neuroprotective in several models of RGC and nervous system injury (11).

REFERENCES

1. Airaksinen PJ, Mustonen E, Alanko HI. Optic disc hemorrhages. Analysis of stereophotographs and clinical data of 112 patients. Arch Ophthalmol 1981; 99:1795–801.
2. Anderson DR, Braverman S. Reevaluation of the optic disk vasculature. Am J Ophthalmol 1976; 82:165–74.
3. Anderson DR. Correlation of the peripapillary damage with the disc anatomy and field abnormalities in glaucoma. Doc Ophthalmol 1983; 35:1–10.
4. Baptiste DC, Hartwick AT, Jollimore CA, et al. Comparison of the neuroprotective effects of adrenoceptor drugs in retinal cell culture and intact retina. Invest Ophthalmol Vis Sci 2002; 43:2666–76.
5. Bayer AU, Ferrari F. Severe progression of glaucomatous optic neuropathy in patients with Alzheimer's disease. Eye 2002; 16:209–12.
6. Bellezza AJ, Hart RT, Burgoyne CF. The optic nerve head as a biomechanical structure: initial finite element modeling. Invest Ophthalmol Vis Sci 2000; 41:2991–3000.
7. Ben-Sira I, Riva CE. Fluorescein diffusion in the human optic disc. Invest Ophthalmol 1975; 14:205–11.
8. Burgoyne CF, Quigley HA, Thompson HW, et al. Measurement of optic disc compliance by digitized image analysis in the normal monkey eye. Ophthalmology 1995; 102:1790–9.
9. Burgoyne CF, Quigley HA, Thompson HW, et al. Early changes in optic disc compliance and surface position in experimental glaucoma. Ophthalmology 1995; 102: 1800–9.
10. Burgoyne CF, Downs JC, Bellezza AJ, et al. The optic nerve head as a biomechanical structure: a new paradigm for understanding the role of IOP-related stress and strain in the pathophysiology of glaucomatous optic nerve head damage. Progress in Retinal and Eye Research 2005; 24: 39–73.
11. Caprioli J, Ishii Y, Kwong JM. Retinal ganglion cell protection with geranylgeranylacetone, a heat shock protein inducer, in a rat glaucoma model. Trans Am Ophthalmol Soc 2003; 101:39–50.
12. Carter-Dawson L, Crawford ML, Harwerth RS, et al. Vitreal glutamate concentration in monkeys with experimental glaucoma. Invest Ophthalmol Vis Sci 2002; 43: 2633–7.
13. Chintala SK, Zhang X, Austin JS, et al. Deficiency in matrix metalloproteinase gelatinase B (MMP-9) protects against retinal ganglion cell death after optic nerve ligation. J Biol Chem 2002; 277:47461–8.
14. Cioffi GA, Wang L, Fortune B, et al. Chronic ischemia induces regional axonal damage in experimental primate optic neuropathy. Arch Ophthalmol 2004; 122:1517–25.
15. Combs CK, Karlo JC, Kao SC, et al. beta-Amyloid stimulation of microglia and monocytes results in TNFalpha-dependent expression of inducible nitric oxide synthase and neuronal apoptosis. J Neurosci 2001; 21: 1179–88.

16. Cui Q, Harvey AR. NT-4/5 reduces naturally occurring retinal ganglion cell death in neonatal rats. Neuroreport 1994; 5:1882–4.
17. Drance SM, Begg IS. Sector haemorrhage–a probable acute ischaemic disc change in chronic simple glaucoma. Can J Ophthalmol 1970; 5:137–41.
18. Drance SM, Fairclough M, Butler DM, et al. The importance of disc hemorrhage in the prognosis of chronic open angle glaucoma. Arch Ophthalmol 1977; 95:226–8.
19. Dreyer EB, Pan ZH, Storm S, et al. Greater sensitivity of larger retinal ganglion cells to NMDA-mediated cell death. Neuroreport 1994; 5:629–31.
20. Dreyer EB, Zurakowski D, Schumer RA, et al. Elevated glutamate levels in the vitreous body of humans and monkeys with glaucoma. Arch Ophthalmol 1996; 114: 299–305.
21. Enari M, Hug H, Nagata S. Involvement of an ICE-like protease in Fas-mediated apoptosis. Nature 1995; 375:78–81.
22. Fechtner RD, Weinreb RN. Mechanisms of optic nerve damage in primary open angle glaucoma. Surv Ophthalmol 1994; 39:23–42.
23. Fisher J, Levkovitch-Verbin H, Schori H, et al. Vaccination for neuroprotection in the mouse optic nerve: implications for optic neuropathies. J Neurosci 2001; 21:136–42.
24. Gagliardini V, Fernandez PA, Lee RK, et al. Prevention of vertebrate neuronal death by the crmA gene. Science 1994; 263:826–8.
25. Garcia-Valenzuela E, Shareef S, Walsh J, et al. Programmed cell death of retinal ganglion cells during experimental glaucoma. Exp Eye Res 1995; 61:33–44.
26. Geijer C, Bill A. Effects of raised intraocular pressure on retinal, prelaminar, laminar, and retrolaminar optic nerve blood flow in monkeys. Invest Ophthalmol Vis Sci 1979; 18:1030–42.
27. Grus FH, Joachim SC, Bruns K, et al. Serum autoantibodies to alpha-fodrin are present in glaucoma patients from Germany and the United States. Invest Ophthalmol Vis Sci 2006; 47:968–76.
28. Gu Z, Yamamoto T, Kawase C, et al. Neuroprotective effect of N-methyl-D-aspartate receptor antagonists in an experimental glaucoma model in the rat. Nippon Ganka Gakkai Zasshi 2000; 104:11–16.
29. Hare W, WoldeMussie E, Lai R, et al. Efficacy and safety of memantine, an NMDA-type open-channel blocker, for reduction of retinal injury associated with experimental glaucoma in rat and monkey. Surv Ophthalmol 2001; 45 (Suppl. 3):S284–9.
30. Hayreh SS. Pathogenesis of cupping of the optic disc. Br J Ophthalmol 1974; 58:863–76.
31. Heijl A, Samander C. Peripapillary atrophy and glaucomatous visual field defects. Doc Ophthalmol 1985; 42: 403–7.
32. Hernandez MR, Andrzejewska WM, Neufeld AH. Changes in the extracellular matrix of the human optic nerve head in primary open-angle glaucoma. Am J Ophthalmol 1990; 109:180–8.
33. Hernandez MR. Ultrastructural immunocytochemical analysis of elastin in the human lamina cribrosa. Changes in elastic fibers in primary open-angle glaucoma. Invest Ophthalmol Vis Sci 1992; 33:2891–903.
34. Huang W, Dobberfuhl A, Filippopoulos T, et al. Transcriptional up-regulation and activation of initiating caspases in experimental glaucoma. Am J Pathol 2005; 167: 673–81.
35. Huang W, Fileta JB, Dobberfuhl A, et al. Calcineurin cleavage is triggered by elevated intraocular pressure, and calcineurin inhibition blocks retinal ganglion cell death in experimental glaucoma. Proc Natl Acad Sci USA 2005; 102: 12242–7.
36. Jonas JB, Nguyen XN, Gusek GC, et al. Parapapillary chorioretinal atrophy in normal and glaucoma eyes. I. Morphometric data. Invest Ophthalmol Vis Sci 1989; 30: 908–18.
37. Jonas JB, Fernandez MC, Naumann GO. Glaucomatous parapapillary atrophy. Occurrence and correlations. Arch Ophthalmol 1992; 110:214–22.
38. Kaiser HJ, Flammer J, Wenk M, et al. Endothelin-1 plasma levels in normal-tension glaucoma: abnormal response to postural changes. Graefes Arch Clin Exp Ophthalmol 1995; 233:484–8.
39. Kerrigan LA, Zack DJ, Quigley HA, et al. TUNEL-positive ganglion cells in human primary open-angle glaucoma. Arch Ophthalmol 1997; 115:1031–5.
40. Kipnis J, Yoles E, Porat Z, et al. T cell immunity to copolymer 1 confers neuroprotection on the damaged optic nerve: possible therapy for optic neuropathies. Proc Natl Acad Sci USA 2000; 97:7446–51.
41. Krieglstein J, Lippert K, Poch G. Apparent independent action of nimodipine and glutamate antagonists to protect cultured neurons against glutamate-induced damage. Neuropharmacology 1996; 35:1737–42.
42. Li S, Mallory M, Alford M, et al. Glutamate transporter alterations in Alzheimer disease are possibly associated with abnormal APP expression. J Neuropathol Exp Neurol 1997; 56:901–11.
43. Lieberman MF, Maumenee AE, Green WR. Histologic studies of the vasculature of the anterior optic nerve. Am J Ophthalmol 1976; 82:405–23.
44. Ma YT, Hsieh T, Forbes ME, et al. BDNF injected into the superior colliculus reduces developmental retinal ganglion cell death. J Neurosci 1998; 18:2097–2107.
45. Masliah E, Mallory M, Alford M, et al. Caspase dependent DNA fragmentation might be associated with excitotoxicity in Alzheimer disease. J Neuropathol Exp Neurol 1998; 57:1041–52.
46. McKinnon SJ. Glaucoma, apoptosis, and neuroprotection. Curr Opin Ophthalmol 1997; 8:28–37.
47. McKinnon SJ, Lehman DM, Kerrigan-Baumrind LA, et al. Caspase activation and amyloid precursor protein cleavage in rat ocular hypertension. Invest Ophthalmol Vis Sci 2002; 43:1077–87.
48. McKinnon SJ. Glaucoma: ocular Alzheimer's disease? Front Biosci 2003; 8:s1140–56.
49. Meyer-Franke A, Kaplan MR, Pfrieger FW, et al. Characterization of the signaling interactions that promote the survival and growth of developing retinal ganglion cells in culture. Neuron 1995; 15:805–19.
50. Minckler DS, McLean IW, Tso MO. Distribution of axonal and glial elements in the rhesus optic nerve head studied by electron microscopy. Am J Ophthalmol 1976; 82:179–87.
51. Minckler DS, Bunt AH, Johanson GW. Orthograde and retrograde axoplasmic transport during acute ocular hypertension in the monkey. Invest Ophthalmol Vis Sci 1977; 16:426–41.
52. Minckler DS. The organization of nerve fiber bundles in the primate optic nerve head. Arch Ophthalmol 1980; 98: 1630–6.
53. Minckler DS, Spaeth GL. Optic nerve damage in glaucoma. Surv Ophthalmol 1981; 26:128–48.
54. Mittag TW, Danias J, Pohorenec G, et al. Retinal damage after 3 to 4 months of elevated intraocular pressure in a rat glaucoma model. Invest Ophthalmol Vis Sci 2000; 41:3451–9.
55. Morin PJ, Abraham CR, Amaratunga A, et al. Amyloid precursor protein is synthesized by retinal ganglion cells,

rapidly transported to the optic nerve plasma membrane and nerve terminals, and metabolized. J Neurochem 1993; 61:464–73.
56. Morrison JC, Jerdan JA, Dorman ME, et al. Structural proteins of the neonatal and adult lamina cribrosa. Arch Ophthalmol 1989; 107:1220–4.
57. Morrison JC, Dorman-Pease ME, Dunkelberger GR, et al. Optic nerve head extracellular matrix in primary optic atrophy and experimental glaucoma. Arch Ophthalmol 1990; 108:1020–4.
58. Moya KL, Benowitz LI, Schneider GE, et al. The amyloid precursor protein is developmentally regulated and correlated with synaptogenesis. Dev Biol 1994; 161: 597–603.
59. Naskar R, Vorwerk CK, Dreyer EB. Concurrent downregulation of a glutamate transporter and receptor in glaucoma. Invest Ophthalmol Vis Sci 2000; 41:1940–4.
60. Neufeld AH, Hernandez MR, Gonzalez M. Nitric oxide synthase in the human glaucomatous optic nerve head. Arch Ophthalmol 1997; 115:497–503.
61. Neufeld AH, Sawada A, Becker B. Inhibition of nitric-oxide synthase 2 by aminoguanidine provides neuroprotection of retinal ganglion cells in a rat model of chronic glaucoma. Proc Natl Acad Sci USA 1999; 96:9944–8.
62. Neufeld AH, Das S, Vora S, et al. A prodrug of a selective inhibitor of inducible nitric oxide synthase is neuroprotective in the rat model of glaucoma. J Glaucoma 2002; 11: 221–5.
63. Ogden TE. Nerve fiber layer of the primate retina: morphometric analysis. Invest Ophthalmol Vis Sci 1984; 25:19–29.
64. Ogden TE, Duggan J, Danley K, et al. Morphometry of nerve fiber bundle pores in the optic nerve head of the human. Exp Eye Res 1988; 46:559–68.
65. Pang IH, Johnson EC, Jia L, et al. Evaluation of inducible nitric oxide synthase in glaucomatous optic neuropathy and pressure-induced optic nerve damage. Invest Ophthalmol Vis Sci 2005; 46:1313–21.
66. Pease ME, McKinnon SJ, Quigley HA, et al. Obstructed axonal transport of BDNF and its receptor TrkB in experimental glaucoma. Invest Ophthalmol Vis Sci 2000; 41:764–74.
67. Peyman GA, Apple D. Peroxidase diffusion processes in the optic nerve. Arch Ophthalmol 1972; 88:650–4.
68. Quigley H, Anderson DR. The dynamics and location of axonal transport blockade by acute intraocular pressure elevation in primate optic nerve. Invest Ophthalmol 1976; 15:606–16.
69. Quigley HA, Guy J, Anderson DR. Blockage of rapid axonal transport. Effect of intraocular pressure elevation in primate optic nerve. Arch Ophthalmol 1979; 97: 525–31.
70. Quigley HA, Hohman RM, Addicks EM, et al. Morphologic changes in the lamina cribrosa correlated with neural loss in open-angle glaucoma. Am J Ophthalmol 1983; 95:673–91.
71. Quigley HA, Brown A, Dorman-Pease ME. Alterations in elastin of the optic nerve head in human and experimental glaucoma. Br J Ophthalmol 1991; 75:552–7.
72. Quigley HA, Nickells RW, Kerrigan LA, et al. Retinal ganglion cell death in experimental glaucoma and after axotomy occurs by apoptosis. Invest Ophthalmol Vis Sci 1995; 36:774–86.
73. Quigley HA, McKinnon SJ, Zack DJ, et al. Retrograde axonal transport of BDNF in retinal ganglion cells is blocked by acute IOP elevation in rats. Invest Ophthalmol Vis Sci 2000; 41:3460–6.
74. Radius RL, Anderson DR. The histology of retinal nerve fiber layer bundles and bundle defects. Arch Ophthalmol 1979; 97:948–50.
75. Radius RL, Anderson DR. The course of axons through the retina and optic nerve head. Arch Ophthalmol 1979; 97: 1154–8.
76. Radius RL, Bade B. Pressure-induced optic nerve axonal transport interruption in cat eyes. Arch Ophthalmol 1980; 99:2163–5.
77. Radius RL. Distribution of pressure-induced fast axonal transport abnormalities in primate optic nerve. An autoradiographic study. Arch Ophthalmol 1981; 99:1253–7.
78. Rezaie T, Child A, Hitchings R, et al. Adult-onset primary open-angle glaucoma caused by mutations in optineurin. Science 2002; 295:1077–9.
79. Rogers SD, Demaster E, Catton M, et al. Expression of endothelin-B receptors by glia in vivo is increased after CNS injury in rats, rabbits, and humans. Exp Neurol 1997; 145:180–95.
80. Sadun AA, Bassi CJ. Optic nerve damage in Alzheimer's disease. Ophthalmology 1990; 97:9–17.
81. Schori H, Kipnis J, Yoles E, et al. Vaccination for protection of retinal ganglion cells against death from glutamate cytotoxicity and ocular hypertension: implications for glaucoma. Proc Natl Acad Sci USA 2001; 98:3398–403.
82. Segal RA, Greenberg ME. Intracellular signaling pathways activated by neurotrophic factors. Annu Rev Neurosci 1996; 19:463–89.
83. Siegner SW, Netland PA. Optic disc hemorrhages and progression of glaucoma. Ophthalmology 1996; 103: 1014–24.
84. Tahzib NG, Ransom NL, Reitsamer HA, et al. Alpha-fodrin is cleaved by caspase-3 in a chronic ocular hypertensive (COH) rat model of glaucoma. Brain Res Bull 2004; 62:491–5.
85. Tezel G, Kass MA, Kolker AE, et al. Plasma and aqueous humor endothelin levels in primary open-angle glaucoma. J Glaucoma 1997; 6:83–9.
86. Tezel G, Seigel GM, Wax MB. Autoantibodies to small heat shock proteins in glaucoma. Invest Ophthalmol Vis Sci 1998; 39:2277–87.
87. Tezel G, Wax MB. Increased production of tumor necrosis factor-alpha by glial cells exposed to simulated ischemia or elevated hydrostatic pressure induces apoptosis in cocultured retinal ganglion cells. J Neurosci 2000; 20:8693–700.
88. Tezel G, Li LY, Patil RV, et al. TNF-alpha and TNF-alpha receptor-1 in the retina of normal and glaucomatous eyes. Invest Ophthalmol Vis Sci 2001; 42:1787–94.
89. Varela HJ, Hernandez MR. Astrocyte responses in human optic nerve head with primary open-angle glaucoma. J Glaucoma 1997; 6:303–13.
90. Vickers JC, Hof PR, Schumer RA, et al. Magnocellular and parvocellular visual pathways are both affected in a macaque monkey model of glaucoma. Aust N Z J Ophthalmol 1997; 25:239–43.
91. Wax MB. Is there a role for the immune system in glaucomatous optic neuropathy? Curr Opin Ophthalmol 2000; 11:145–50.
92. Wolff E, Penman GG. The position occupied by the peripheral retinal fibers in the nerve fiber layer and the nerve head. Acta 16th Concilium Ophthalmol (1950) 1951: 625–35.
93. Yan DB, Coloma FM, Metheetrairut A, et al. Deformation of the lamina cribrosa by elevated intraocular pressure. Br J Ophthalmol 1994; 78:643–8.
94. Yan X, Tezel G, Wax MB, et al. Matrix metalloproteinases and tumor necrosis factor alpha in glaucomatous optic nerve head. Arch Ophthalmol 2000; 118:666–73.

22

Structure and Biochemistry of the Lens

John J. Harding
Nuffield Laboratory of Ophthalmology, University of Oxford, Oxford, U.K.

INTRODUCTION

The crystalline lens, with its unusually high protein content and unique arrangement of structural fibers, provides, together with the cornea, the refractive index necessary to focus images on the retina. To achieve this, the lens must be perfectly transparent. Loss of transparency, or cataract, is the most common cause of blindness and visual impairment worldwide. Cataract formation is a multifactorial process, resulting from a wide variety of physical, biochemical, metabolic, and structural changes occurring in both the nuclear and cortical regions of the lens. Cataracts are intimately associated with normal aging processes in the lens, and with advancing age most individuals develop some degree of lens opacification.

A full appreciation of the multitude of changes that can lead to lens opacification is of necessity based on an understanding of the normal lens. Hence the present chapter provides a general survey of the normal lens, physical properties, biochemistry, and metabolism, with emphasis on the mammalian lens and human lens in particular. Chapter 24 summarizes current research on experimentally induced cataractogenesis, biochemical studies on inherited cataract in animal models and in human cataract, and epidemiological studies. Many of these and other associated topics have been reviewed in a number of comprehensive publications (9,19,58,59,61,85). This chapter is based on the chapter by Elaine Berman in the previous edition (15). It also borrows heavily from my chapter in Biochemistry of the Eye (59).

ANATOMY AND STRUCTURE OF NORMAL LENS

The lens is built up of two cell types: a single layer of epithelial cells on the anterior surface underlying the capsule and fiber cells that occupy the rest of the lens and comprise the major cellular component of the tissue (Fig. 1). Beginning in the embryo and continuing throughout life, the epithelial cells undergo mitosis near the equator and differentiate into elongated fiber cells. This process is characterized by a massive accumulation of soluble crystallins and de novo

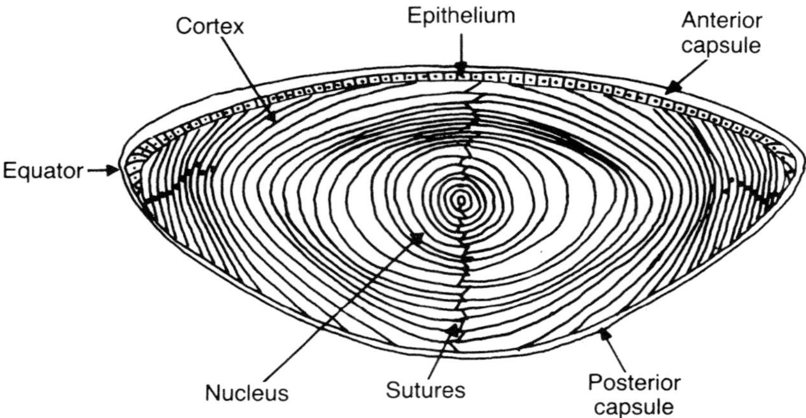

Figure 1 Section through the lens. *Source*: Drawing by John Cronin.

synthesis of MP26 (Aquaporin 0, discussed in the section on Lens Fiber Cell Plasma Membrane), lipids, and other components required for formation of the rapidly elongating fiber cell plasma membrane. Electrical and metabolic communications between the fiber cells are established by junctional complexes that have some of the characteristics of gap junctions found in other tissues. With their differentiation into mature fiber cells, there is a concomitant loss of nuclei and other intracellular organelles. Mitochondria and nuclei are lost simultaneously (10). DNA, RNA and oxidative phosphorylation are also lost. Organelle loss is similar in part to apoptosis, but the two are distinctly different.

New fiber cells are laid down as concentric layers on previously formed embryonic fibers. Thus, the nucleus contains the oldest cells and the cortex the newest cells. There are no distinct morphological markers or barriers between these regions; rather, general physiological and biochemical gradients distinguish the transition from cortical to nuclear zones. The fiber cells meet in a region called the lens suture. There is little or no turnover of protein in the lens nucleus; most if not all of the detectable protein synthesis occurs in the epithelium and in developing fiber cells in the peripheral cortex. Given the essential absence of new protein synthesis in the bulk of the lens, that is, in the fiber cells, posttranslational changes play a major role in modifying the protein composition of the mature lens.

The lens grows throughout life leaving the oldest cells further and further from the source of nutrients (19,59). Differentiation of epithelial to fiber cells is induced by fibroblast growth factor (FGF) aided by insulin-like growth factor (IGF) (127,96).

PHYSICAL BASIS OF TRANSPARENCY AND STATE OF WATER

The lens is transparent because it neither absorbs nor scatters significant amounts of light in the visible region of the spectrum. The cytoplasm contains about 35% solids, consisting almost entirely of soluble proteins, the crystallins. Small-angle X-ray scattering and light-scattering studies of lens extracts over a wide range of concentrations show convincingly that lens transparency is the result of the short-range spatial order of the lens proteins (42). When concentrated as in the lens, α-crystallin the main potential light scatterer shows an even distribution which reduces light scattering and favors transparency (19).

The human lens is almost colorless at birth and becomes increasingly yellow with age. Approximately half of the total water of the lens is *water of hydration*, defined as bound water associated with the nonfreezable water content of the lens (87). With age, the total water content in the nucleus and intermediate layers of human lens gradually decreases, although cortical layers remain essentially unchanged. The nonfreezable water content decreases with age throughout the lens.

ACCOMMODATION

The young lens has an adjustable focus but this is lost by middle age. It depends on the ciliary muscle pulling on the zonules to flatten the lens and then the elasticity of the lens for recovery of the more rounded shape (9,59).

BIOCHEMISTRY OF NORMAL LENS

Low-Molecular-Weight Solutes

Various low-molecular-weight solutes of human and animal lens were listed in the previous edition and earlier reviews (15,58). Clearly the lens has most of the small molecules found in all other tissues. Glutathione (GSH), a tripeptide with a thiol group (Fig. 2), is a key component of the lens redox system. Most GSH in the lens, as in other cells, is in the reduced form, and it is

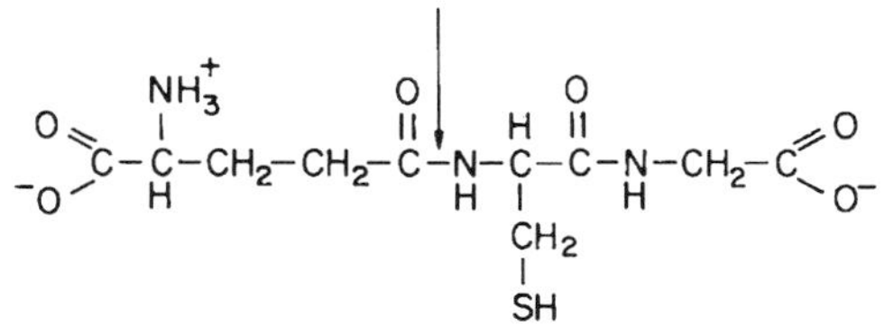

Figure 2 Structure of glutathione (GSH), a tripeptide of γ-glutamate, cysteine, and glycine. The peptide bond in GSH indicated by the arrow is atypical for most peptides because it is between the nitrogen atom of cysteine and the carboxyl group of the δ-carbon of glutamate rather than with the usual α-carbon carboxyl group. *Source*: From Ref. 14.

thought to play an important role in protecting the tissue from oxidative damage. It could also protect the lens against electrophilic attack. GSH protects Na^+-K^+-ATPase thus helping to maintain cation levels in lens (59). Ascorbic acid is present at high levels in the lens and may function as an antioxidant. However, ascorbic acid displays prooxidant properties under some conditions (166). Ascorbate also induces cross-linking, cleavage, and insolubilization of crystallins (51,111–113); there is compelling evidence that it plays an important role in the Maillard-type browning reaction found in aging lenses and in cataracts (12,61).

Many metabolites of glucose are present in lens, as are the related pathways. Three inorganic ions, K^+, Na^+, and Ca^{2+}, show important metabolic fluxes in normal lens, and Ca^{2+} especially has been implicated in cataract formation and other lens abnormalities (63).

The Crystallins

The principal components of lens fiber cells are the crystallins. Three crystallins (α, β, and γ) have been recognized for nearly a century, but more recently other crystallins have been identified (Table 1) (19,59). All mammalian lenses examined to date have α, β, and γ crystallins; many of them have been sequenced, and cDNA and genomic clones are being used to examine the relationships within and between the various families.

It is now known that β- and γ-crystallins are related so that the lens crystallins consist of two superfamilies, α and βγ crystallins (19). α-Crystallin is synthesized in epithelial cells whereas βγ-crystallins appear only after differentiation to fiber cells starts (19). The molecular architecture of some βγ-crystallins has been studied by X-ray crystallographic techniques and their structural motifs have been established. This information is not available for α-crystallin. Several detailed reviews are available on lens crystallins, their composition and structure, and, most importantly, the primary gene products and posttranslational modifications (19,59,61,94,140).

Some properties of the major families of crystallins are summarized in Table 1. This review will concentrate on mammalian crystallins (α, β, γ) with γ-crystallin being monomeric and the others aggregated.

α-Crystallins

In the native state, the α-crystallins are the largest of the lens crystallins, with molecular masses ranging from about 600 to 900 kDa and constituent subunit masses of 20 kDa. The subunits are of two types αA and αB with each also present in phosphorylated and truncated forms (19,59). The αA and αB polypeptides isolated from over 40 species show about 60% sequence homology and probably arose by a single duplication of an ancestral α-crystallin gene that gave

Table 1 Some Properties of the Crystallins

Molecular form	Mol. wt (KDa)	Subunit wt. (kDa)	Secondary structure	Thiol content	N-terminal amino add	Occurrence
α Aggregate	700	20	Some β	Low	Masked	All vertebrates
β Aggregate	40-200	23-35	Mostly β	High	Masked	All vertebrates
γ Monomer	20	20	Mostly β	High	Gly or Ala	Vertebrates (not birds or reptiles)
δ Tetramer	200	49	Mostly α	Low	Probably masked	All birds and reptiles
ε Tetramer	150	38	α and β			Some birds and reptiles
ρ Monomer	39	39	Mostly β			Frogs
τ Monomer or dimer	48 or 100	48	Mostly α			Lampreys, some fishes, birds, and reptiles
ξ, Tetramer	150	38	α and β			Guinea pig, camel, elephant, shrew
λ Monomer	36	36	α and β			Rabbit, hare
SUI Dimer	60	30	α and β		Gly	Squid, octopus
Ω Tetramer	230	59			Masked	Octopus
π Tetramer	120	37				Diurnal gecko

Abbreviations: Gly, glycine; Ala, alanine.
Source: Adapted from Ref. 58 for additions see text.

rise to separate αA and αB genes. Unexpectedly, sequence data on small heat-shock proteins of *Drosophila* (73) and on p40 antigen of *Schistosoma mansoni* (107) have revealed highly conserved regions similar to the C-terminal sequences of α-crystallins.

The phosphorylated polypeptides αA and αB arise by direct phosphorylation of the primary gene products, αA and αB (142). Serine residue in position 122 (Ser-122) is the principal phosphorylation site in the α-crystallin A chain, but there are additional sites as well (30,156). The B chain appears to be phosphorylated at two sites: Ser-59 and Ser-43 or Ser-45. Despite extensive amino acid sequence similarity between the A and B chains, the phosphorylation sites are different, being located near the C and N terminals, respectively. The biological significance of phosphorylation of α-crystallins is not known but may be related to their different functional roles in the lens (31).

Absence of an X-ray structure for α-crystallin led to many proposed models for its structure (59) but the best evidence so far, from cryo-electron microscopy, is that the aggregated protein exists as a roughly spherical molecule with a cavity in the center (57). Recent X-ray and neutron scattering studies support the view that there is access to the cavity (126). Careful electrospray mass spectrometry was applied to determine the exact mass of aggregates of αB-crystallin and hence the number of subunits (4). The results confirmed the polydispersity of α-crystallin and showed that the most common aggregates had 28 and 29 subunits. There was no evidence for substructures such as hexamers, tetramers or dimers as had been postulated previously.

Since the last edition was written the major advance in α-crystallin research has been the discovery that it has the properties of a molecular chaperone, that is a protein that protects other vulnerable proteins (9,19,43,68,69). Indeed α-crystallin is now established as the leading member of the family of small heat shock proteins with which it shares sequence homology. This is consistent with its structure having a cavity and with its distribution in tissues beyond the lens. The first evidence for its chaperone properties came from the demonstration that it could prevent the heat-induced aggregation of other proteins including crystallins (69). Subsequently it was shown that it could prevent reduction-induced aggregation of insulin (47) and chemically-induced inactivation of a variety of enzymes (68). Other proteins did not share the chaperone activity. Examples of the chaperone effects of α-crystallin are listed in Table 2 (59).

The issue of stoichiometry was more readily addressed by enzyme activity experiments. For some enzymes a single α-crystallin aggregate could protect one or two molecules of enzyme, which supports the view that the target proteins are protected in the cavity, but in respect of GSH reductase and fumarase it appears that one aggregate can protect up to seven molecules of enzyme in which case there must be some binding to the outside (68). The uncertainty over whether binding is on the outside or inside is compounded by our ignorance of the specific part of the polypeptide chains involved in binding. The chaperone properties of many mutant α-crystallins has been investigated but with little insight (43). A more promising approach induced binding of the target to the chaperone site and led to production of a mini-chaperone peptide (137).

Table 2 Protective Effect of α-Crystallin

	Temp (°C)	Species (a)
Heat-induced aggregation of:		
β_L-Crystallin	*55*	Bovine
β_H-Crystallin	60	Bovine
γ-Crystallin	66	Bovine
ξ-Crystallin	55	Bovine
Alcohol dehydrogenase	48	Bovine
α-Glucosidase	48	Bovine
Glutathione S-transferase	48	Bovine
Enolase	48	Bovine
Citrate synthase	42	Bovine (αB)
Guanidine-dialysis precipitation	25	Bovine
Rhodanese	47	Bovine
Glycation-induced inactivation of:		
Glucose-6-phosphate dehydrogenase	37	Bovine
Glutathione reductase	37	Human
Malate dehydrogenase	37	Bovine
Steroid-induced inactivation of catalase	37	Bovine
Aggregation of reduced insulin	25 (25-40)	Bovine
Aggregation of UV-irradiated γ-crystallin	15-56	Bovine

Source: From Ref. 43. See Ref. 43 for more information.

Ideas on the mechanism of the chaperone function of α-crystallin were thrown into disarray by two papers showing that neither dissociation nor the native aggregate was required for function (5,70).

The chaperone activity of α-crystallin increases with temperature (43). Decreased chaperone activity with aging and cataractogenesis are discussed in Chapters 19 and 36.

β- and γ-Crystallins

The β- and γ-crystallins comprise about two-thirds of adult vertebrate lens crystallins; their nomenclature is operational, being derived from conventional gel-filtration profiles (61). The α-crystallins are found in the first peak eluted from gel filtration columns, whereas the heterogeneous βH (heavy) and βL (light) fractions are eluted in the second and third peaks, respectively; the last peak contains the monomeric γ-crystallins. Further biochemical, physicochemical, and immunological criteria are used to resolve and characterize the major aggregates and to elucidate their subunit structures.

A large number of β- and γ-crystallins are available in highly purified form, and recently many of their cDNAs and genes have been cloned. The gene and the protein structures deduced from X-ray crystallography show conclusively that an ancestral βγ gene was duplicated to produce both the family of β-crystallin subunits and a closely related family of γ-crystallin monomers (19). More specifically, cDNA and amino acid sequence studies have established a remarkably close structural relationship between two members of these families, βB_2 and γB (formerly called γII). The highly conserved regions in these two crystallins are clearly seen when aligned according to their four motifs (19,61). Moreover, bovine γB, bovine βB_2, and the major murine β-crystallin β_{23} all have two symmetrical domains, each folded into two similar "Greek key" motifs (19). The two-domain structure of γB-crystalin is shown in Figure 3.

The β- and the γ-crystallin gene families contain eight and six primary gene products respectively, and together they comprise the βγ-crystallin superfamily (19). The highly homologous γ-crystallin genes are closely linked gene clusters: the five or six human γ-crystallin genes are located on the long arm of chromosome 2 (2q33-36) (42,138). The rat γ-crystallin genes are located on chromosomes 9 (19). The γ-crystallin genes have one major exon coding for each of the two domains in the molecule. In contrast, owing to the extensive heterogeneity of the β-crystallins, their genes are predicted to be dispersed throughout the genome (67). There appear to be two linked βB_2 genes, one of which has been mapped to chromosome 22 (22q11.2–q12.2) (67). The β-crystallin genes have one exon for each motif. Recently γN-crystallin was discovered with one exon for the N-terminal domain and two for the C-terminal domain (166). It was proposed as a "missing link" between the β-crystallins and the γ-crystallins.

The β-crystallins are extremely complex, consisting of a heterogeneous group of polymers ranging in size from about 50 to 200 kDa . Each of the six or seven polypeptides in this group is composed of varying numbers of 23 to 35 kDa subunits. In addition, a low-molecular-weight 21 kDa monomer γs was for many years classified with the β-crystallins. However, cDNA sequencing shows that although it has some characteristics of both members of the βγ superfamilies, it is more closely related to the γ than to the β-crystallins (18,19). The tail of βS-crystallin is flexible and its N-terminus is acetylated (32).

The confused nomenclature of the βγ-crystallins was apparent in the last edition (15) and discussed

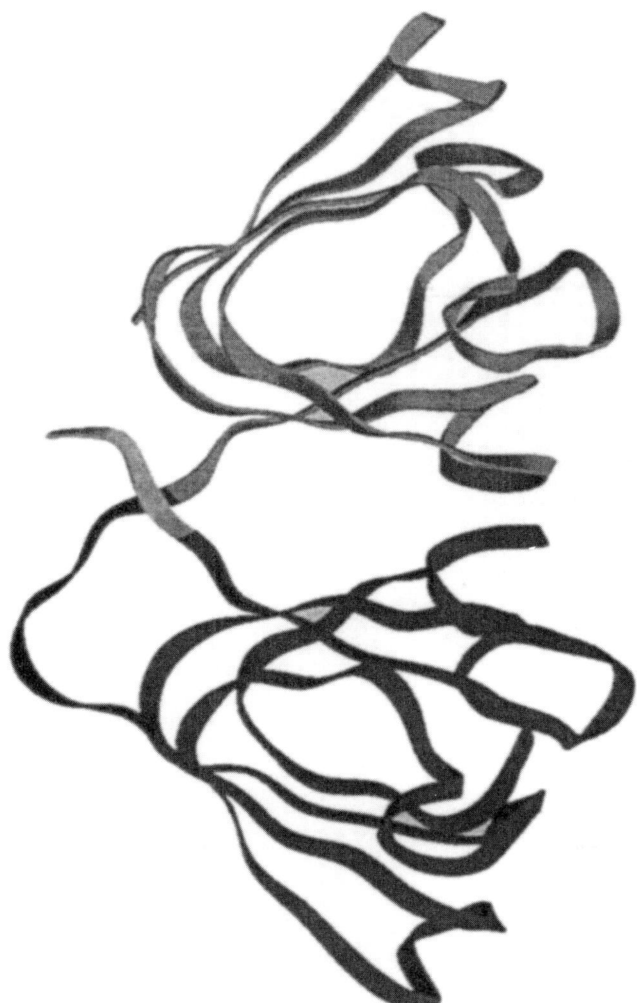

Figure 3 Structure of γB-crystallin. *Source*: Courtesy of Drs. B. Norledge and C. Slingsby.

subsequently (59) but remains still partly because the best characterized γ-crystallins were the bovine crystallins, whereas the nomenclature was based on amino acid sequences of the rat proteins based on cDNA. The rat sequences were later found to have errors (89) so the nomenclature is more dubious than ever. Some of the original bovine sequences also had to be revised and that led to revised relationships to the rat sequences (59). Eight β-crystallins have been characterized as primary gene products and classified into βA (acidic) and βB (basic) crystallins. The basic β-crystallins have both N- and C-terminal peptides extending from their four-motif core structures, together with a few small insertion sequences, whereas the acidic β-crystallins lack prominent C-terminal extensions but have many insertions (19).

Structure predictions for other βγ-crystallins have been published but the X-ray structure was determined only for βB2-crystallin (11). It had been expected that this β-crystallin would have a structure like γII-crystallin but with tails added so it was a surprise to find that although the βB2-polypeptides had two domains like γ-crystallin, its domains were separated (Fig. 4). Each domain of one polypeptide interacts with the opposite domain of a second polypeptide to form a dimer corresponding to the molecular mass of βL-crystallin. The connecting peptide of βB2-crystallin is longer than that of γ-crystallin allowing the separation of the domains. βL-crystallin contains polypeptides other than βB2, which is assumed to be present partly as heterodimers with other β-crystallin polypeptides.

The γ-crystallins comprise a group of six homologous 21 kDa monomeric proteins. Although prominent in the lenses of most vertebrates, they are absent in birds and possibly in some reptiles. The phosphorylated γ-crystallins are greatly enriched in the lens nucleus. The first lens crystallin to be sequenced was γ_{II}-crystallin (36); subsequently, complete primary sequences as well as the three-dimensional structures of other γ-crystallins have been determined (19,133). The secondary structures of the γ-crystallins are very similar, all being highly symmetrical and having β-pleated sheet structures. Their three-dimensional structures consist of four antiparallel β-helical motifs arranged as two symmetrical globular domains

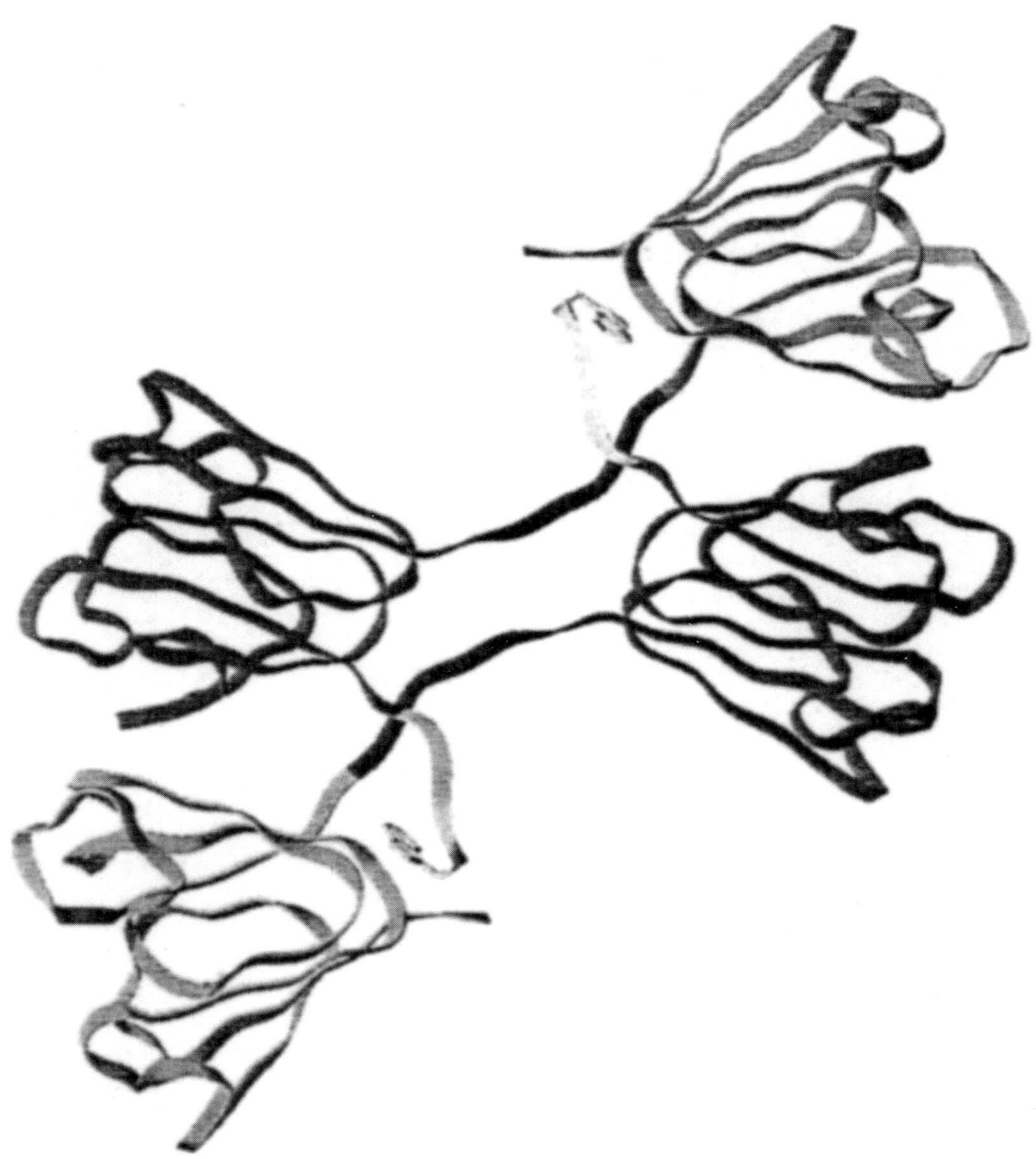

Figure 4 The structure of the βB2-crystallin dimer. *Source*: From Ref. 59. Figure provided by Brian Norledge and Christine Slingsby.

(Fig. 3). There are no free loops or tails. At high resolution 73 water molecules can be seen in the first shell around the molecule with a further 49 molecules in a second shell (105). Each domain consists of two nearly identical Greek key motifs. There are differences in core packing, however, and in the number of exposed hydrophobic residues and ion pairs in mammalian γ-crystallins (146). In addition, despite their structural resemblance and high degree of amino acid sequence similarity, inherent differences in their tertiary structures exist; for example, bovine γ-crystallins II, III, and IV display striking differences in denaturation behavior and susceptibility to proteolysis. Studies on the evolution of the βγ crystallins at both the gene and protein levels suggest a division of γ-crystallins into two major groups: γ-crystallins I–III, on the one hand, and IV–VI on the other (19). The latter are most abundant in young lenses.

The γ-crystallins of all species have a remarkably high thiol content, and this class of crystallins, perhaps more than others, is thought to play an important role in lens transparency. Amino acid analyses and X-ray crystallography reveal that γ_{II} the major γ-crystallin in bovine lens and the most extensively studied, contains seven cysteine residues, six of them located in the N-terminal domain (146,165). Measurements of the reactivities of the sulfhydryl groups of γ_{II}-, γ_{III}-, and γ_{IV}-crystallins toward a thiol-specific fluorescent probe have demonstrated two classes of reactive cysteines with marked differences in spatial arrangements and microenvironments (101). A search for GSH attached to human lens proteins showed it on cysteine (Cys) of γS-crystallin, notably attached to Cys-82 and in a region covering Cys-22, Cys-24 and Cys-26 (35). Cys-24 of human γS-crystallin was identified as the most accessible of all cysteines in γ-crystallins by modeling (143).

The α-, β- and γ-crystallins are the major proteins of mammalian lens and are clearly sufficient as structural proteins for a transparent refracting tissue (59). All undergo a variety of post-translational modifications even in clear lenses and at an early age (19,44). These changes become more relevant in cataractogenesis (see Chapter 24) (58). There are other crystallins present in limited numbers of species that are of less interest in a review concentrating on the mammalian lens but have an intrinsic fascination in that many of them are variants of enzymes.

δ-Crystallins

The δ-crystallins are the major soluble proteins of avian and reptile lenses, replacing γ-crystallins in these species, although they are completely different proteins (19). They account for about 70% of the crystallins in the developing chicken lens. The δ-crystallin mRNA disappears a few months after hatching, however, and the protein is no longer synthesized in mature chicken lens (19). The native molecule is a 200 kDa tetramer consisting of major 48 kDa and minor 50 kDa subunits (Table 1). Rather unexpectedly, mRNA produced from chicken δ_1-crystallin cDNA synthesizes both subunits, yet two closely related δ-crystallin genes (δ_1 and δ_2) are present in the chicken (19).

The X-ray structure of turkey δ-crystallin at 0.25 nm resolution shows that it is almost entirely α-helical with negligible β-sheet unlike the major mammalian crystallins (139). A major assembly of 20 helices forms the center of the tetramers which have a potential to form tubules as in arginosuccinate lyase.

Crystallins as Functional Enzymes

The unexpected evolutionary relationships between the α-crystallins and nonlenticular proteins, such as small heat-shock proteins and *Schistosoma* p40 antigen, were noted earlier. Even more remarkable are several other observations on lens crystallins as functional enzymes (Table 3). δ_2-Crystallin of chicken has considerable sequence similarity to yeast and human argininosuccinate lyase (a urea cycle enzyme) (116,164); and indeed δ2-crystallin has arginosuccinate lyase activity. Chick lens has a specific activity for arginosuccinate lyase 80 times that of liver (116). The duck lens δ-crystallin is even more active.

ε-Crystallin, a major component of duck lens, expresses a high level of lactic dehydrogenase (LDH) activity that appears to be identical to one of the isoenzymatic forms of LDH (duck heart LDH-B4) (163).

Table 3 The Strange Relations of Lens Crystallins

Crystallin	Relations	Active
α	Heat shock proteins	–
	Antigens of *Schistosoma* and *Mycobacterium*	–
βγ	Bacterial protein S	–
δ	Arginosuccinate lyase	Duck (chicken)
ε	Lactate dehydrogenase	Duck and other
ρ	Aldo-keto reductases, prostaglandin-F synthase	–
τ	α-Enolase	Reptiles, birds, fish, lamprey
λ	Hydroxyacyl CoA dehydrogenase	–
π	Glyceraldehyde 3-phosphate dehydrogenase	Diurnal geckos
ξ	Alcohol/polyol dehydrogenase NADPH; quinone oxidoreductase	
Squid lens polypeptides	Glutathione S-transferase	No

Source: Adapted from Ref. 58; for additions see text.

Other examples include turtle τ-crystallin and squid S_{III}-crystallin (Table 3), which have sequence similarities and enzymatic properties of enolase and GSH S-transferase, respectively (164). In addition, π-crystallin of *Rana pipiens* manifests approximately 40% to 50% amino acid sequence similarities to rat lens nicotinamide adenine dinucleotide phosphate (NADPH)-dependent aldehyde reductase and to human liver aldose reductase (25). Similarities have also been found between the 225 C-terminal amino acid sequences of the European common frog ε-crystallin and bovine lung prostaglandin F synthase; the finding of 77% identical and/or conserved substitutions without deletions or additions suggests that the proteins may be identical (160).

The long-held view that lens crystallins are "lens specific" may have to be revised. A provocative hypothesis implies that certain crystallins were recruited from nonlenticular tissues as lens proteins during evolution because of their thermodynamic stability (164). Carried further, it has been predicted that nonlenticular functions may someday be found for all lens crystallins (116,164).

Genes for Lens Proteins

The evolution of the eye has puzzled scientists since the days of Darwin. The evolution of the lens seems at first to be an easier problem but remains the subject of much debate (39). The development of the whole eye depends on master genes probably the homeobox genes *Pax-6*, *Six-3*, *Msx-1*, and *Msx-2* (66,149). Mutations of *Pax-6* are associated with small eyes or absence of eyes in mice.

Several hereditary cataracts have been related to mutated crystallins but it is likely that the problem is the accumulation of aberrant protein rather than the lack of an essential component (see Chapter 33). Some evolutionary changes such as gene duplication, exon duplication, intron loss, divergent evolution, insertion of extra DNA sequences and sliding of splice, translation and initiation sites have been demonstrated within crystallin genes (19).

The *CRYAA* and *CRYAB* genes arose by duplication from a common ancestor before the divergence that led to cartilaginous fish and higher vertebrates and it can be argued that this ancestor was a heat-shock protein as αB-crystallin is now (39). The αB-crystallin gene has a heat shock element in its 5′ flanking region just like the small heat shock protein genes and therefore can be induced by heat.

Hypertonic stress induces αB-crystallin in kidney cortex endothelial cells and retinal pigment epithelium (RPE) but in lens cells the results were less clear (59). The *CRYAA* and *CRYAB* are on different chromosomes, chromosomes 21 and 11, respectively, in humans (59). In rodents and some other mammals such as hedgehog and bat a longer version of αA-crystallin, called αA^{Ins}-crystallin is found. This polypeptide is simply the αA-chain with an insert of 22 amino acids and is produced as a minor component by alternative splicing (39).

αA-crystallin is found almost only in lens. The cis regulatory elements responsible for the lens-specific expression have been localized to the 5′-flanking region by studies in cell culture and in transgenic mice (29). At least two separate regions are involved. The proximal domain of the promoter (sequence –88 to +46) contains elements for lens specificity and for the initiation of expression at an appropriate stage during development. The distal domain is essential in chick lens epithelia but not in rabbit lens cells. The apparent heat-shock responsive element is at positions –60 to –89 in the human *CRYAA* crystallin gene, and at –344 to –363 in the equivalent murine gene, but these elements are not functional.

αB-crystallin has been found in many tissues including heart, skin, brain, retina, muscle, kidney and lung (29,39). Increased expression is found in several pathological conditions of the central nervous system, including Alexander disease, scrapie, Parkinson disease, Alzheimer disease, and Creuzfeld–Jakob disease (see Chapter 70). Regulatory elements have been identified in the 5′-flanking sequence of the human and murine αB-crystallin gene that control expression in the lens but other sequences may control expression in other tissues. The heat-responsive element is also found in the 5′-flanking sequence.

The human *CRYBB1*, *CRYBB2*, *CRYBB3*, *CRYBA4* genes are clustered on chromosome 22 (39). The *CRYBA1* gene is on chromosome 17. Six of the rat γ-crystallin genes (A–F) are in a cluster on chromosome 9 (19). The human *CRYBA2* and *CRYGA*, *CRYGB*, *CRYGC*, and *CRYGD* genes are on chromosome 2 (42,71) while the mouse genes are on chromosome 1 and the bovine genes are on chromosome 8 (59).

Genes for β-crystallins have one exon for each of the four Greek key motifs in the protein but genes for γ-crystallin have a single exon for each domain of two motifs (19). This difference suggests that the β- and γ-crystallin gene families diverged at the time of a single domain ancester, although no monomeric single domain crystallins are known to exist naturally (19).

The βA1 and βA3-chains are identical except for an additional 17 amino acids at the N-terminus of the βA3-chain (59). Both polypeptides are translated from a single mRNA with two start codons. The alternate splicing site has been identified in species from frog and chicken to mice and men (39). The β-crystallin gene family must date back more than 350 million years. The pattern of expression of the βγ-crystallin genes changes during development.

A deletion of 12 nucleotides from the βB2-crystallin gene appears to be the cause of Philly cataract in mouse. The absence of four amino acids leads to a protein that is unable to fold, which in turn leads to all the biochemical changes found in Philly cataract (see Chapter 24).

In rodents all the tail-less γ-crystallin genes are expressed but in human lens only two major γ-crystallins are produced in significant amounts. The promoters for the other four genes are absent or weak and the fourth unexpressed gene produces an unstable mRNA (39).

There are two delta-crystallin genes producing δ1- and δ2-crystallins (see above). The two have homologous sequences with δ2-crystallin corresponding to arginosuccinate lyase. δ1-crystallin is highly expressed in lens with the major determinant of the lens specificity being an enhancer located in the third intron (62).

ε-Crystallin is produced from the same gene as the lactate dehydrogenase isoenzyme B4 and similarly τ-crystallin and α-enolase are produced by the same gene (19,59). In these cases the enzymes have been recruited as crystallins without gene duplication and sequence divergence.

The major intrinsic membrane protein in the lens, MIP or MP26, is homologous to other membrane proteins. The *MIP* gene for human MP26 has been assigned to the long arm of chromosome 12 (12cen-q14) (141). The MIP sequence contains a twofold repeat (29). Regulatory elements in the 5′-flanking sequence of the gene are responsible for the lens-specific expression of MIP.

Lens Fiber Cell Plasma Membrane

The lens cell membranes show up clearly in electron micrographs but because they are thin and in an almost regular arrangement they do not decrease transparency (59). Adjacent cells are locked together by multiple interdigitations. The membranes serve to separate the contents of a cell from its neighbors but they include pumps, channels and junctions that provide links for specific materials to pass through. There are some specialized proteins in lens membranes but in addition all the major proteins of the erythrocyte membrane are present (3).

The major feature of lens membranes is the gap junctions. These are channels between cells thought to provide electrical continuity and the passage of metabolites. The lens membranes are enormously rich in gap and other junctions, covering more than 60% of the surface of fiber cells. The gap junction is a highly specialized organelle which unlike other channels spans the plasma membrane of two adjacent cells (24). The two cells each contribute half the channel called a connexon which has a 2 to 3 nm diameter pore. Each connexon consists of six connexin protein molecules. Connexins range in size from 16 to 70 kDa in subunit mass. Connexin 50 is the protein identified in outer cortical fiber cell membranes as MP70. Further into the lens the gap junctions consist of MP38, a cleavage product of MP70. The other junctions (12 nm thick) consist of MIP (or MP26) the major intrinsic protein of lens fiber membranes. MP26 has been highly conserved throughout evolution (61).

The passage of glucose is made possible by specific glucose transporters found in membrane preparations from both cortex and nucleus (98). Other metabolites may have their own specific transport systems. Alternatively passage from epithelium to fiber cells at least may be by endocytosis (23). There are other channels apart from gap junctions to provide electrical conductance (59).

MIP (also called MP26 and aquaporin-0) has sequence homology with CHIP 28 from erythrocyte and both proteins form water channels. About 50% of total protein of the fiber cell membrane is MIP, but it is absent from the epithelial cells. Thus it is an excellent marker for differentiation (59). Its amino acid sequence has been determined and it has a molecular mass of 28.2 kDa (55). It has transmembrane α-helical segments surrounding the water pore (54). It is found only in lens. It has bound lipid and is cleaved in vitro to a shortened version, MP22 (2). It can be phosphorylated on serine by cAMP-dependent protein kinases (50,59,83). This phosphorylation may be mediated by G proteins acting through a Ca^{2+}-calmodulin adenylate cyclase system or possibly by an endogenous protein kinase C (88). The Ca^{2+}- and phospholipid-dependent enzyme appears to phosphorylate serine residues in the C-terminal region of MP26. Both phosphorylating systems are known to alter junctional permeability in other tissues, and they may be acting in concert in the lens to regulate the phosphorylation of MP26, which in turn could control the permeability of lens gap junctions. γE-crystallin binds to MIP/aquaporin-0 in the plasma membrane but any role in controlling permeability has yet to be investigated (46).

When incorporated into reconstituted membranes MIP exhibits channel-like properties (86,90, 175). Molecules up to 1.5 kDa can pass through but the channels are closed by calcium and calmodulin (115). Channels formed from truncated MIP, that is MP22, cannot be closed so in older lenses there may be open water channels from cell to cell into the center. This and other evidence (54) indicates that it is the C-terminal region of MIP that is involved in closing the channel and binding calmodulin.

The levels of mRNAs for MIP, MP20 and a rat connexin during development do not reflect the amounts of the proteins present indicating that the mRNAs are unusually stable (136). Notwithstanding the major presence of water channels, diffusion between fiber cells is inhibited relative to diffusion parallel to the cells (103). Lens fiber cell membrane proteins are listed in Table 4.

In addition to phosphorylation, the other major posttranslational modification of MP26 is its slow age-related conversion to MP22 by limited proteolysis (22). The physiological conversion can be demonstrated both in comparisons of old and young human lenses and in analyses of old (nuclear) and young (cortical) regions from a single lens. The cleavage of MP26 to MP22 is accelerated in human and experimental cataracts, and a protein similar in size to MP22 can be produced by a variety of exogenous proteinases. Several possible cleavage sites resulting in the release of a low-molecular-weight peptide from intact MP26 have been suggested (55).

The gene for MP26 appears to be expressed only in the lens, specifically in its fiber cells, not in the epithelial cells (55). Investigations of MP26 expression in normal rat lens using antisense RNA probes, polyclonal antibodies specific for MP26, and in situ hybridization show that the transcription of the *MIP* gene for MP26 and the synthesis of MP26 are directly coupled in cells committed to terminal differentiation (169). The synthesis of MP26 occurs first in presumptive primary fibers and, after little or no time lag, in differentiating secondary fibers in the zone of elongation. The pattern of expression of the *MIP* gene differs sharply from that of the $\beta A_1/A_3$-crystallin gene not only in cellular localization but also in the earlier appearance of the $\beta A_1/A_3$ gene in differentiating cells. Similar findings have been reported in other studies using 3- to 4-week-old rat lenses (13). The *MP26* mRNA transcripts appear first in elongating fibers at the lens equator; concentrations are reduced from the anterior fibers to the nucleus and then increase again in posterior fiber cells. In confirmation of previous studies, no gene transcripts for MP26 mRNA could be detected in epithelial cells.

Table 4 Lens Fiber Cell Plasma Membrane Proteins (MPs)

Component	Function and/or origin
MP26	Possible gap junction protein[a]
MP22	Cleavage product of MP26
MP70	Intrinsic membrane junction protein
MP64	Intrinsic protein closely related to MP70
MP38	Cleavage product of MP70 and MP64
MP19–20	Intrinsic membrane protein
MP17–19	Calmodulin binding membrane protein[b]
MP130, MP140	Glycoproteins
MP33, MP35	EDTA-extractable proteins[c]
MP115	Intrinsic protein[d]
MP90–107	Na^+, K^+-ATPase
MP37	Glyceraldehyde 3-phosphate dehydrogenase
MP200	Spectrin
MP53	Glucose transporter

[a] The main intrinsic protein of lens fiber cells.
[b] Considered second most abundant protein of lens fiber cell membranes, it is a substrate for cAMP-dependent protein kinase (14,104).
[c] Substrate for phosphorylation by Ca^{2+}- and phospholipid-dependent protein kinase C.
[d] Immunologically related to beaded-chain 95 kDa antigen.
Source: Adapted from Refs. 2,58,85.

Other Plasma Membrane Proteins

A total of 20 or more proteins and/or polypeptides are thought to be associated with lens plasma membranes (2,85). In addition to MP26, MP70, and MP64, at least one other protein (MP17) and several glycoproteins have been characterized as intrinsic proteins of lens fiber cell plasma membranes (Table 4). The phosphorylation of a 19- to 20-kDa protein by both cAMP-dependent protein kinase and protein kinase C was just discussed (see preceding section). A plasma membrane polypeptide of similar size, 17 to 19 kDa, has calmodulin binding properties (95). These two peptides probably represent the same protein, which has now been designated MP17 (104). Hydrophobic photolabeling demonstrated that it is the second most abundant lens membrane protein after MP26. The intrinsic membrane protein MP17 is present in several mammalian species but is absent in chickens. Because of its calmodulin binding activity and its ability to act as a substrate for cAMP-dependent protein kinase, MP17 may play an important modulatory role in lens metabolism.

The lens fiber cell membrane fraction contains about 3% to 4% carbohydrate consisting mainly of neutral sugars and amino sugars (1,85) as components of membrane-bound glycolipids and glycoproteins. A prominent 130 kDa concanavalin A binding glycoprotein present in chicken and mammalian lens plasma membranes and other glycoproteins with molecular masses ranging from 35 to 140 kDa have been detected by the use of specific lectins (130).

Another well-characterized component of lens fiber cell plasma membranes, termed EDTA-extractable protein (EEP), consists of two polypeptides of M_r 33,100 and 35,000. These proteins, both of which are glycosylated (85), are bound to the phospholipid bilayer by Ca^{2+} and can be eluted from membranes with chelators of divalent cations. Hence, EEP is an extrinsic protein. It is present in a variety of species and is a substrate for phosphorylation by Ca^{2+}- and phospholipid-dependent protein kinase C in vitro (151). The 35 kDa polypeptide of EEP of bovine lens plasma membranes is immunologically related to calpain I and contains phosphotyrosine residues (131). The 33 kDa protein from EEP may be the core protein of calpain I, a protein known to be associated with actin.

Development of monoclonal and polyclonal antibodies raised to a 115 kDa cytosolic lens antigen has led to the characterization of another extrinsic protein of lens plasma membranes (48). This protein is lens specific and is localized in fiber cell plasma membranes. The 115 kDa polypeptide appears to be immunologically related to a previously described 95 kDa antigen (2), a protein that was thought to be associated with beaded filaments, unusual structural components of chicken and other vertebrate lenses.

Several functional enzymes have been detected in lens plasma membranes using ultrastructural cytochemical and biochemical techniques (Table 4). The most extensively studied, Na^+-K^+-ATPase, is localized mainly in the epithelial cells and in outer cortical fiber cell membranes; as in most other cells, this enzyme is responsible for the energy-dependent inward transport of two K^+ ions and the outward transport of three Na^+ ions. It is barely detectable in lens nucleus where the cation balance depends on activity in the epithelium (21). Fiber cells have a considerable amount of Na^+-K^+-ATPase protein but lack the activity. Another enzyme, a membrane-associated form of glyceraldehyde 3-phosphate dehydrogenase (M_r 37,000), is loosely bound to lens membranes and therefore has been classified as an extrinsic protein. In addition, a Ca^{2+}-stimulated ATPase has been characterized in membrane-enriched fractions isolated from the epithelial and cortical regions of rabbit and bovine lenses (20). Its activity is only about one-fifth of that observed for Na^+-K^+-ATPase.

Lipids

The lens fiber cell plasma membranes, like those of most other cell types, are composed of approximately equal proportions of proteins and lipids (2,177). Cholesterol is the major sterol of lens plasma membranes, accounting for about 50% to 60% (or more in some species) of the total lipids (177). The ratios of cholesterol to phospholipid in chick lens fiber cell membranes and in gap junction membranes are 2.1 and 3.1, respectively, implying a localized accumulation of cholesterol in junctional areas (2). Sphingomyelin is also relatively enriched in gap junctional regions.

Sphingomyelin is the most abundant phospholipid of human and monkey lens plasma membranes (Table 5). Of the other phospholipids, phosphatidylethanolamine (PE) is present at somewhat higher levels than phosphatidylcholine (PC) in most species; human and monkey plasma membranes appear to have a strikingly low PC content. Lens plasma membranes contain mainly long-chain saturated fatty acids; the major species is palmitate (16:0), which accounts for one-third or more of the total saturated fatty acids. Two monounsaturated fatty acids, 18:1 and 24:1, are also prominent in lens plasma membranes. The high concentrations of sphingomyelin and cholesterol and low levels of unsaturated fatty acids contribute to the high rigidity and low fluidity of this lipid bilayer (177). Fluorescence anisotropy measurements show that the lens plasma membrane is the least fluid of any eukaryotic membrane studied.

Most of lens lipid biosynthesis occurs in the epithelium and outer cortex, with relatively little activity detectable in the lens nucleus. Cholesterol synthesis is regulated in part by an active hydroxymethylglutaryl-coenzyme A (CoA) reductase that has been demonstrated in cultured bovine lens epithelial cells (65). There is good correlation between rates of cholesterol synthesis, as measured by incorporation of tritiated water into digitonin-precipitable sterols, and enzyme activity. Both sterol synthesis and enzyme activity increase in cells grown in lipoprotein-depleted medium, a situation that mimics the in vivo state, since the lens is not exposed to significant levels of lipoprotein.

Phosphatidylinositol (PI), although present at only low levels in the lens fiber cell membranes (Table 5), may, as in other tissues, play an important role in receptor-mediated membrane signal

Table 5 Phospholipid Composition of Lens Fiber Cell Membrane

	Phospholipid (% of total)				
Species	**SPH**	**PC**	**PE**	**PS**	**PI**
Human	47–56	2–5	9–18	6–15	1–4
Bovine	18–23	25–32	34	8–13	2
Rabbit	14–32	23–35	28–34	11–13	2
Rat	6–16	31–43	30–33	12–16	2–4
Monkey	46	7	20	9	1
Chicken	29	23–27	25–39	7	3

Abbreviations: PC, phosphatidylcholine; PE, phosphatidylethanolamine; PI, phosphatidylinositol; PS, phosphatidylserine; SPH, sphingomyelin.
Source: Adapted from Ref. 177.

transduction. Half a century ago, Van Heyningen (152) reported unusually high concentrations of inositol in mammalian lenses, with values ranging from about 4 mM in the rat to about 40 mM in the human lens. This important observation remained unexplored for many years, although it was noted that inositol is actively transported into the lens (177). The role of its metabolites as secondary messengers is discussed in the section entitled Messengers.

Lens fiber cell membranes have an unusually high content of sphingomyelin, cholesterol, and saturated fatty acid, resulting in a lipid bilayer of low fluidity and high rigidity. It has long been recognized that the cholesterol-phospholipid (C/PL) ratio is higher in the lens nucleus than in cortical regions, a difference associated with increased rigidity of nuclear fiber membranes (2). Precise changes in the absolute amounts of lipids throughout the lens have been obtained by analyzing consecutive layers of single human lenses (92). The phospholipid content is relatively constant throughout the lens, except in the inner nucleus, where it drops precipitously. The distribution of cholesterol is more complex, however: it is low in the outer cortical region, rises significantly in the inner cortex, and then falls again in the nucleus. Thus, the general increase in C/PL ratio from the epithelium (0.8) to the nucleus (3.5) results from both the low cholesterol content of the outer cortex and the large decrease in phospholipids in the nucleus. Further studies on concentric layers of human lens show a complex age-related disappearance of phosphatidylethanolamine and decrease in phosphatidylserine (PS) in the nucleus (93). Bovine lenses have a lower cholesterol and phospholipid content that human lenses, but analyses of concentric layers show a similar cortex-to-nucleus increase in C/PL ratio from 0.5 to about 2.0 (91). As in human lenses, this is due mainly to a relative decrease in phospholipid content from the cortex to the nucleus. The foregoing studies suggest that in both human and bovine lens, the high C/PL ratio in the nucleus reflects a high membrane rigidity in this older region of the lens.

Cytoskeleton

All three classes of cytoskeletal proteins found in nonocular tissues (microfilaments, intermediate filaments, and microtubules (see Chapter 1) have been identified in the lens. Actin, vimentin, and spectrin, as well as a beaded filamentous cytoskeletal component, are present in crude urea-soluble fractions of lens homogenates (2). Another cytoskeletal component (band 4.1 protein), which is prominent in the lattice network lining the cytoplasmic face of erythrocyte plasma membranes, has also been detected in bovine and chicken lens (14,58). At least six variants are now recognized, and their expression changes significantly during terminal differentiation of lens fiber cells.

Actin microfilaments have been detected by biochemical, morphological and immunocytochemical methods in both epithelial and fiber cells in a wide variety of mammalian lenses (2). The major intermediate filament in lens, vimentin, is localized mainly in epithelial and cortical fiber cells (2); it is not detectable in nuclear fiber cells.

Alpha-crystallin inhibits the assembly of intermediate filaments, and binds to pre-formed filaments (108). A role for α-crystallin as a molecular chaperone aiding correct assembly of filaments in the lens has been postulated, with a parallel role specifically for αB-crystallin in other tissues.

Vimentin filaments are not essential as vimentin knock-out mice do not develop cataracts or any other problem (33). Microtubules have been detected in epithelial and cortical fiber cells, and like vimentin, they are not found in nuclear fiber cells. They may play a role in cell elongation.

Beaded-chain filaments that appear to be unique to the lens have been identified in the fiber cells of chicken and several other vertebrate lenses (2). The name is derived from their characteristic appearance: globular protein particles (about 12 nm in diameter) attached to a filamentous backbone (5 nm diameter). The two major proteins of the beaded filaments have subunit molecular masses of 49 and 115 kDa and are called phakinin and filensin respectively (previously CP49 and CP115). Surprisingly knocking out CP49 disrupted membrane organization without causing cataract (132). Phosphorylation of cytoskeletal proteins plays an important role in their interactions with one another and in their associations with cellular membranes in a variety of nonocular tissues. The functional components for at least two phosphorylating systems have been detected in lens: cAMP-dependent protein kinase (type I) and Ca^{2+}- and phospholipid-dependent protein kinase C (14,58). Incubation of lens homogenates with [^{32}P]orthophosphate results in the rapid phosphorylation of both vimentin and the 47 kDa beaded filament (77). The phosphorylation is stimulated by β-adrenergic drugs, such as isoproterenol and epinephrine; it is also enhanced by forskolin, an agent that directly activates the catalytic site of adenylate cyclase. These observations suggest that phosphorylation of vimentin and the 47 kDa beaded filament is mediated by β-adrenergic receptors coupled to the adenylate cyclase system.

Lens Capsule

The lens capsule was first characterized as a specialized type of collagenous connective tissue more than 50 years ago by Pirie (117); it is now classified as a typical basement membrane secreted by, and tightly attached to, lens epithelial cells. This capsule acts as the primary permeability barrier for substances entering and leaving the lens. Its principal structural component is collagen type IV, and the lens capsule is often used as a model for studying the chemistry and immunology of collagen type IV in other tissues (see Chapter 44) (21). The chemical composition of basement membrane collagen from bovine lens capsule is typical of collagen type IV; glycine comprises approximately one-third of its residues, and it contains about 8% carbohydrate. The structure of lens capsule collagen type IV as determined by rotary shadowing electron microscopy is predominantly that of a triple helix; it also contains nonhelical globular domains (21).

METABOLISM OF NORMAL LENS

Several detailed reviews of lens metabolism are highly recommended for detailed coverage, of this complex field (14,58,59,61,100). In general metabolic pathways in the lens are the same as in other tissues. Fiber cells lack processes based in mitochondria and ribosomes but these systems are active in epithelial cells.

Carbohydrate Metabolism

Glucose is the major source of energy for the lens. Because lens is an avascular tissue, this key metabolite is transported into the lens from the aqueous humor, which also provides oxygen and other essential nutrients. Glucose enters the lens by a passive, facilitated, insulin-independent transport mechanism that is stereo-specific for D-glucose (110). The translocation of glucose is mediated by a transporter (or carrier) that is reversibly inhibited by cytochalasin B (97), an agent that can be made to bind irreversibly by photoaffinity labeling. This unusual property has been exploited to demonstrate that the lens glucose transporter is unexpectedly located primarily in membranes derived from the cortex and nucleus, with very little detectable in capsule epithelium preparations (98). The lens glucose transporter is similar to that of erythrocytes; both are intrinsic membrane glycoproteins that migrate on sodium dodecyl sulfate polyacrylamide gel electrophoresis (SDS-PAGE) as broad 53 kDa bands.

Glycolytic breakdown of glucose provides at least two-thirds of the lens adenosine triphosphate (ATP) (14,17,58); the remainder is generated by oxidative metabolism through the tricarboxylic acid cycle. These metabolic pathways are localized mainly, if not entirely, in the epithelial cells. Oxidative metabolism does not occur in fiber cells since they are devoid of mitochondria.

The major pathways of glucose metabolism in the lens are depicted in Figure 5. All enzymes in this

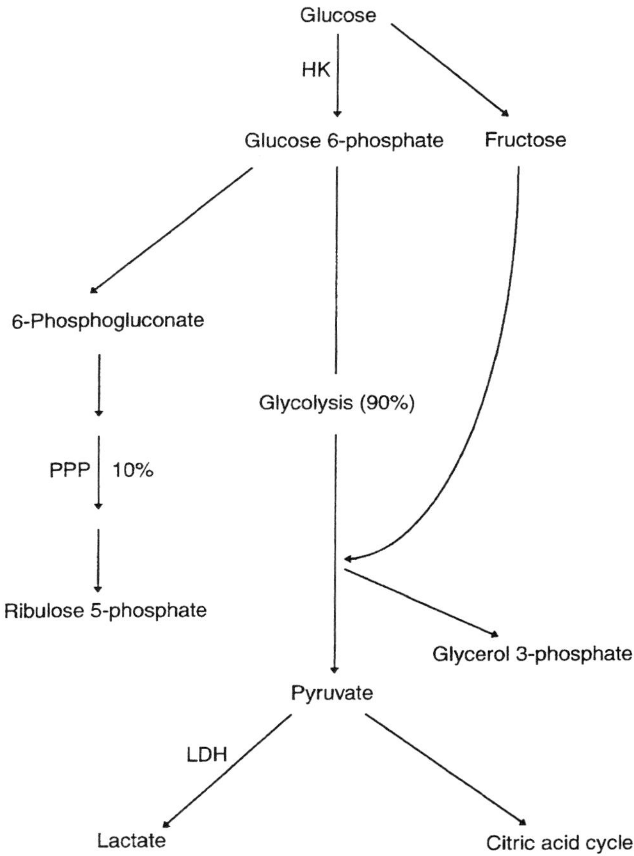

Figure 5 Overview of glucose metabolism in the lens. The major pathways are glycolysis, the pentose phosphate pathway, and the tricarboxylic acid cycle. *Abbreviations*: HK, hexokinase; LDH, lactic dehydrogenase; PPP, pentose phosphate pathway. *Source*: From Ref. 59.

highly coordinated system are present in the lens, and many have been isolated and purified. Some of the salient points may be summarized as follows. Three kinases play key roles in the control of glycolysis and in the generation of ATP in the lens. Initial phosphorylation of free glucose is regulated by hexokinase in a reaction considered a rate-limiting step in glycolysis. Two forms of lens hexokinase, types I and II, are present in most species and differ from one another in kinetic properties and sensitivities to heat inactivation (61). As in other tissues, the two ATP-generating steps in lens glycolysis are mediated by phosphoglycerate kinase and pyruvate kinase.

Most pyruvate produced by glycolysis is converted to lactate by lactic dehydrogenase (LDH). All five known isoenzymic forms of this enzyme are present in lens. The activity of LDH, which uses nicotinamide adenine dinucleotide (NADH) as its cofactor, is regulated in part by the activity of glyceraldehyde 3-phosphate (G3P) dehydrogenase, an enzyme that generates NADH during the glycolytic breakdown of glucose. In the presence of potassium cyanate or excess glucose, the concentration of G3P increases and reaches a new steady-state level in response to changes in the NADH/NAD+ ratio under a particular set of experimental conditions (28). Apart from the availability of NADH, other factors may also control lactate production in the intact lens. For example, increased intracellular concentrations of calcium inhibit lactate production in cultured rabbit lens (64). The effect appears to be specific and is not caused by chelation of ATP by excess calcium. Mitochondria-containing epithelial cells comprise only a small fraction of the total lens mass, yet the tricarboxylic acid cycle operating in this cell layer is thought to supply about one-third of the energy requirements of the lens. All the enzymes necessary for the metabolism of acetyl-CoA, as well as components of electron transport, are present in the lens epithelium and, to a lesser extent, in the outer cortex.

The pentose phosphate pathway (Fig. 5) accounts for about 10% to 20% of the glucose metabolized by the lens. It is not only the major source of CO_2 produced in the tissue but is also important in generating two reducing equivalents of NADPH per mole glucose oxidized. The NADPH is used in several key metabolic systems in the lens, such as the reductive synthesis of fatty acids, the maintenance of GSH in a reduced state, and the supply of pentoses for nucleic acid synthesis. The first two enzymes in the pentose phosphate pathway, glucose 6-phosphate dehydrogenase and 6-phosphogluconate dehydrogenase have been extensively studied in the lens. The pentose phosphate pathway (or hexose monophosphate shunt) can be activated when there is a metabolic demand for NADPH, for example under conditions of oxidative stress when increased intracellular levels of GSH are required.

Other potential sources of NADPH in addition to the pentose phosphate pathway have been detected in capsule-epithelium preparations of rabbit lens (162). The combined activities of two NADP+-dependent cytosolic enzymes, isocitrate dehydrogenase and malic enzyme, are comparable in NADPH-generating potential to glucose 6-phosphate dehydrogenase, suggesting that mitochondria-derived enzymes may be involved in protecting the lens from oxidative stress.

Although the physical basis of lens transparency is well understood, the biochemical basis is still uncertain. There is evidence supporting the view that lens transparency is directly related to the unique and complex nature of its energy metabolism. The interacting pathways of carbohydrate metabolism in the lens are shown in Figure 5. Glycolysis is regulated by two essentially irreversible steps catalyzed by hexokinase and phosphofructokinase; ATP is generated in two steps catalyzed by phosphoglycerate kinase and pyruvate kinase.

The existence of the sorbitol pathway in the lens was first suggested by van Heyningen (153,154) who found an association between the lenticular accumulation of sugar alcohols (polyols) and cataracts following dietary or experimentally induced excesses of xylose, galactose, or glucose in rats (see Chapter 24). The postulated pathway contains two enzymes: aldose reductase (AR), which uses NADPH as its cofactor, and polyol dehydrogenase, an NAD+-dependent enzyme. AR excited much interest as a possible target for anti-therapy but this approach has been undermined as the pure enzyme, recombinant or otherwise seems unable to make sorbitol, which was supposed originally to cause cataract in diabetes mellitus (58,61). Its true role may be to eliminate toxic aldehydes (34,119).

Glutathione

GSH present in relatively high concentration in the lens, especially in the epithelium, is a γ-glutamyl-cysteinyl-glycine tripeptide (Fig. 2). Among its many important functions are (*i*) maintenance of protein sulfhydryl groups in the reduced form, (*ii*) protection from oxidative damage by detoxification of hydrogen peroxide (H_2O_2), (*iii*) removal of xenobiotics by conjugation with hydrophobic compounds with an electrophilic center, a reaction catalyzed by GSH S-transferase, and (*iv*) participation in amino acid transport as a γ-glutamyl donor to the α-amino groups of acceptor amino acids, such as cysteine or glutamine (14,58,61). This last reaction is catalyzed by the membrane-bound enzyme γ-glutamyltranspeptidase. GSH may also play an indirect role in ion transport, particularly of Na^+ and K^+, by protecting the sulfhydryl groups of Na^+-K^+-ATPase from oxidation (27).

Biosynthesis and Degradation

All the enzymes required for the synthesis and degradation of GSH have been detected in the lens (27). Normally, a steady-state concentration of GSH is maintained through operation of the γ-glutamyl cycle (58,61). GSH is synthesized sequentially by two ATP- and Mg^{2+}-requiring enzymes, γ-glutamylcysteine synthetase and GSH synthetase. Synthetic activity declines with age in humans and in several animal species (122); moreover, the levels of GSH are low in most forms of cataract (see Chapter 24) (58). The decline in synthetic activity in aging lenses appears to be caused by a reduction in γ-glutamyl-cysteine synthetase activity. Two enzymes involved in the degradation of GSH in the lens have also been characterized: γ-glutamyltransferase and 5-oxoprolinase.

Other enzymes of GSH metabolism in the lens play important roles in detoxification. One of them, GSH peroxidase, catalyzes the decomposition of H_2O_2 in the presence of GSH, a reaction that is coupled to GSH reductase. The oxidized form of GSH (GSSG) is produced, and GSH is resynthesized by NADPH generated mainly from the pentose phosphate pathway (4,61). There is considerable species variation in the activities of the individual enzymes in this redox cycle, and there are variations with age as well (134). In the monkey lens, GSH peroxidase activity is low at birth, increases until adulthood, and then declines; GSH reductase activity decreases from birth until juvenile life and afterward remains at a rather constant level (123). This enzyme appears to be rate limiting in the GSH redox cycle. Many lines of evidence suggest that this redox cycle plays an important role in H_2O_2 detoxification in the lens.

Protection from Oxidative Damage

In most aerobic cells, univalent reduction of oxygen generates superoxide anion, a free radical that undergoes dismutation by superoxide dismutase, resulting in the formation of H_2O_2. Pirie proposed that H_2O_2 entering the lens is detoxified enzymatically by the GSH redox cycle described earlier, coupled to the pentose phosphate pathway.

Both whole rabbit lenses and cultured epithelial cells (52) are readily able to detoxify exogenous H_2O_2. Exposure to levels of H_2O_2 as high as 50 μM produce neither overt signs of tissue damage nor any decrease in cellular GSH. This absence of H_2O_2 toxicity correlates strongly with a dramatic stimulation of the pentose phosphate pathway, which appears to be a major factor in maintaining adequate supplies of GSH to protect the lens from H_2O_2-induced toxicity. A similar response is demonstrable in lenses of young (4-day-old) rabbits, but cultured lenses from old (8-year-old) animals have considerably less capacity to detoxify H_2O_2, possibly because of their lower GSH reductase activity and diminished pentose phosphate pathway responses (125). Treatment of rabbit lenses with 1,3-bis(chloroethyl)-l-nitrosourea, an inhibitor of GSH reductase, before exposure to normally well-tolerated levels of H_2O_2, results in an accumulation of GSSG and marked disturbances in cation transport (53).

Detoxification of Xenobiotics

Drugs, atmospheric pollutants, and other potentially toxic substances are detoxified in the lens by GSH S-transferases, a group of enzymes that catalyze the conjugation of a diverse group of electrophilic xenobiotics to GSH (Fig. 6). Some forms of GSH S-transferase express selenium-independent GSH peroxidase II activity toward lipid hydroperoxides (6). Multiple forms of GSH S-transferase are found in most tissues, the three major forms being designated α, μ, and π. Their expression is tissue specific. Two isoenzymes of GSH S-transferase in bovine lens, designated GSH S-transferase 7.4 and 5.6, are homodimers composed of 23.5 kDa subunits (1). Although these two enzymatic forms of GSH S-transferase are related chemically and immunologically, they differ in pI values and in peptide fingerprints. Both belong to the μ, class of GSH S-transferases.

Relatively little is known of specific xenobiotics metabolized by the mercapturic acid pathway in lens, but one study has shown that the pathway is operative in rabbits (79). Oral administration of naphthalene to rabbits results in cataract formation, and oxidized derivatives of naphthalene conjugated with GSH were identified in lens extracts. One of the major metabolites, *N*-acetyl-*S*-(1,2-dihydro-2-

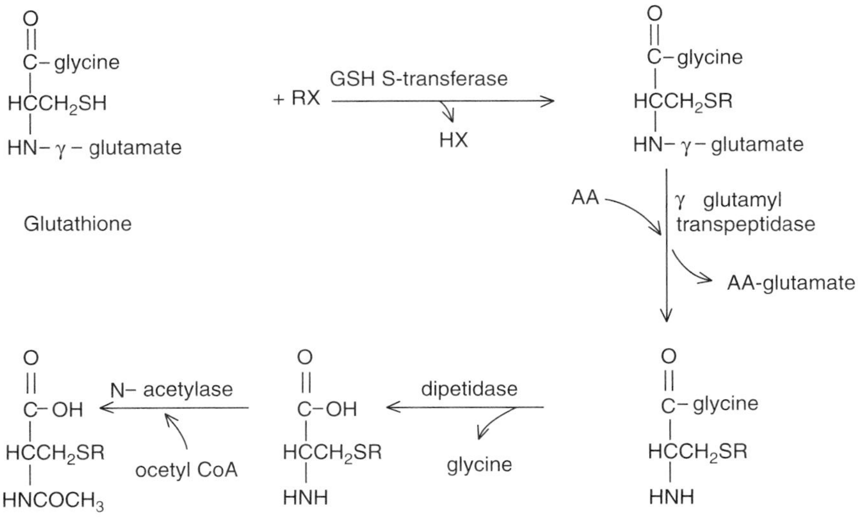

Figure 6 Mechanism for the conjugation of Xenobiotics (RX) with glutathione (GSH) and the formation of mercapturic acid. AA is an amino acid. *Source*: From Ref. 6.

hydroxynaphthyl)-cysteine is an intermediate in the mercapturic acid pathway.

Proteins

Synthesis

Active protein synthesis in the lens occurs principally in the epithelium and peripheral cortex. Little synthesis or turnover occurs in the lens nucleus, since the mature fiber cells in this region are devoid of nuclei and other cytoplasmic organelles. Polyribosomes and mRNA from lenses of calf, chicken, and other species can be translated in several cell-free systems and in oocytes from *Xenopus laevis* (61). Synthesis of the major classes of crystallins, as well as membrane-specific proteins, has been demonstrated using calf lens polyribosomes in a reticulocyte lysate. Not only calf but also fetal human lens mRNAs encoding both crystallin and noncrystallin proteins have been isolated and translated in a heterologous cell-free system (128). In these and other studies, polyribosomes were derived from whole lenses, but the polyribosomes involved in lenticular protein synthesis in the lens are present mainly, if not entirely, in the epithelium and peripheral cortex, where cell differentiation is occurring. These incubation studies were necessarily short-term experiments compared to the life-time of lens proteins. A longer term approach depended on normal protein synthesis. The level of $^{14}CO_2$ in the troposphere doubled as a result of nuclear weapons testing in the 1950s and 1960s. Therefore, biological material synthesized "post-bomb" has higher levels of radioactive carbon than that synthesized "pre-bomb." This was exploited to study protein synthesis by way of radiocarbon levels in protein of monkey lens nucleus (7). The percentage of ^{14}C was very low in the nucleus of a lens of a monkey born in 1950, slightly higher in one born in 1957, but much higher in those born after nuclear testing had produced maximum levels of $^{14}CO_2$ in the atmosphere. The results of this unplanned experiment indicate protein in the lens nucleus of pre-bomb monkeys was synthesized decades before analysis in 1981, providing strong support for the conclusions of the short-term experiments that there is essentially no protein synthesis in lens nucleus. Given that there is no protein synthesis in fiber cells that fill the center of the lens the proteins there must survive for many years as light, metabolites and xenobiotics pass through (159). Even delicate enzymes show some activity in the lens nucleus with the oldest proteins. This leads to questions as to how the proteins survive for so long. The crystallins may be there because they are particularly resilient, but the enzymes and receptor proteins and other specialized proteins are the same as those found in liver where protein molecules are replaced every few days. How is this possible? Part of the answer may lie in the presence of α-crystallin, a molecular chaperone (see above) present at such high levels. No other chaperone is present at the same concentrations in other tissues. There is also GSH and other protection systems working together to maintain all the proteins.

Several studies on crystallin ontogeny in the lens have addressed the complex developmental regulation of these proteins. It has long been recognized that synthesis of the individual polypeptides comprising each class of lens crystallin is temporally and spatially regulated (159). Crystallin synthesis is regulated by differential gene expression, and specific crystallins appear at different times and in different regions throughout development. The primary gene products undergo numerous posttranslational changes whose precise nature is under active investigation. In the rat, protein accumulation, synthesis, and mRNA translation in a reticulocyte lysate show transitions from embryonic to adult crystallin expression that begin 1 week after birth (26). Three β-crystallins are not synthesized in embryonic rat lens, and for at least one of them, a functional mRNA cannot be detected until the first postnatal day. The 27 kDa polypeptide characteristic of adult β-crystallin is detectable only after about postnatal day 5.

Differential regulation of crystallin synthesis with random posttranslational modifications during development occurs in lenses of all species (61). The major protein in neonatal lens is α-crystallin, and β-crystallin is the next most abundant polypeptide; γ-crystallin does not appear to be synthesized in neonatal lenses. Modifications of existing polypeptides, such as deamidation and degradation, occur within each crystallin class, and by birth, at least 20 different modified derivatives are already distinguishable. In a detailed study of the crystallins in cortical and nuclear regions of 33 normal postmortem-obtained human lenses ranging in age from newborn to 70 years of age, McFall-Ngai et al. (102) found a gradual age-related decrease in the 19 and 21 kDa proteins (γ-crystallins), as well as structural changes in nuclear crystallins in 35- to 45-year-old individuals. With modern techniques it has been possible to demonstrate the expression of almost 2000 genes in mouse lens (168).

Posttranslational Modifications

The structural proteins of the lens, both the soluble crystallins and the fiber cell plasma membrane components, undergo major enzymatic and nonenzymatic postsynthetic modifications. One of the most important modifications of primary gene products is the phosphorylation of soluble αA-, αB-, and βB_2-crystallins and plasma membrane proteins (MP26 and others). These topics were discussed in the section entitled Biochemistry of Normal Lens.

Many substances are capable of inducing the formation of aggregates in animal lenses (see Chapter 24). Systems to prevent cataract include the molecular chaperone α-crystallin (see the section entitled The Crystallins) and thioredoxin an enzyme to reduce disulphide bonds (170). Oxidized redoxin is restored by thioredoxin reductase and NADPH.

Proteolysis

There has been renewed interest in recent years on proteolytic breakdown of lens proteins, and it is now recognized that lens contains a number of peptidases and proteinases (Table 6). These enzymes are classified as endopeptidases (neutral proteinases and calpains I and II) and exopeptidases. In addition, an ubiquitin ATP-dependent conjugation system has also been detected in mammalian lenses.

Proteosome/Multicatalytic Proteinase Complex/Neutral Proteinase

A neutral proteinase in bovine and human lenses has been known for many years (61). The purified enzyme from bovine lens has a M_r of about 550,000 in the native state and on SDS-PAGE dissociates into at least eight subunits ranging in size from 24 to 32 kDa (124). The enzyme is not unique to lens, since a similar, if not identical, enzyme has been isolated from bovine pituitary glands which explains the name changes through multicatalytic proteinase complex to the proteosome.

At least three activities were distinguishable from one another by their specificities toward synthetic peptide substrates (157,158). The partially purified enzyme hydrolyzes peptides with nonpolar as well as negatively charged side chains; it also displays trypsin-like activity and hydrolyzes modified proteins at physiological temperatures.

25 kDa Serine Proteinase/Trypsin-Like Proteinase

Another endopeptidase (25 kDa serine proteinase) is found in bovine lens homogenates associated with the α-crystallin fraction (145). Similar to the neutral proteinase just described, it also possesses trypsin-like activity. The purified enzyme has a pH optimum between 7.2 and 8.2 and hydrolyzes synthetic substrates as well as the B-chain extracts owing to the presence of endogenous trypsin inhibitors.

Calpains

Calpains are sulfhydryl (cysteine) Ca^{2+}-dependent neutral endopeptidases ubiquitously distributed in mammalian and avian tissues. Two distinct forms of the enzyme have been characterized: calpain I, activated at a low (approximately 10 μM) concentration of Ca^{2+}, and calpain II, requiring high (1 mM) Ca^{2+} for activity. Endogenous inhibitors of both types of calpain, designated calpastatins, are also found in most tissues. Induction of proteolysis by Ca^{2+} in lens cytoskeletal preparations (75) and in lens homogenates (129) was the first indication that calpain enzymes may be present in the lens. At the same time, Yoshida et al. (171) isolated a highly purified calpain II from the cytosolic fraction of bovine lens; this preparation was active in degrading both the A and B chains of α-crystallin, producing 18 and 19.5 kDa polypeptides, respectively. The chains are cleaved at the C termini, the A chain mainly at the Arg^{163}-Glu^{164} linkage and the B chain principally at the Thr^{170}-Ala^{171} linkage (173). Both calpains, as well as the inhibitor calpastatin, are found mainly in the epithelium and cortex of the lens; no activity is detectable in the lens nucleus (172). Purified calpain II from rat lens is a protein of $M_r \approx 120{,}000$ composed of 80 and 28 kDa subunits (37). Endogenous substrates for calpain include vimentin, intrinsic membrane proteins, and crystallins. Calpain II activity has also been detected in human lens, but the specific activity is only about 3% of that present in rat lens (38). High levels of the inhibitor calpastatin are also present in human lens, especially in the nucleus. Possibly for these reasons no calpain-like cleavage sites have been found in isolated human crystallins (106). Calpain may have a role in

Table 6 Lens Proteinases

	M_r (kDa)	Subunit M_r (kDa)	Activator	Lens substrates
Calpain I	110	80/30	1 μM Ca^{2+}	
Calpain II	110	80/30	1 mM Ca^{2+}	α-Crystallin, β-crystallin, vimentin, actin, MIP26
Multicatalytic proteinase complex	700	21–34	Ca^{2+}	α-Crystallin
Ubiquitin system	Large		ATP, Mg^{2+} ubiquitin	α-Crystallin
Trypsin-like proteinase	25	25	–	α-Crystallin
Membrane-associated proteinase	68	16	–	–
Leucine aminopeptidase	320	54	Zn^{2+}, Mn^{1+}, Mn^{2+}	Proteinase products

differentiation of epithelial cells to lens fibers (59). It cannot attack γ-crystallin.

Ubiquitin ATP-Dependent Conjugation System

Ubiquitin is a small (8.5 kDa) protein present in the cytosol of many types of mammalian cells (80,135). It is an unusual protein in that its carboxy-terminal glycine residues become covalently linked to the ε-amino groups of lysine residues of proteins destined for degradation. The energy for formation of these bonds comes from ATP. At least three enzymes have been characterized that mediate the ATP-dependent conjugation of "damaged" proteins to ubiquitin. The most commonly used source of these conjugating enzymes is reticulocyte lysate. The presence of protein linked to ubiquitin induces hydrolysis through an as yet unknown mechanism. This system is often considered an alternative, or a supplement, to the lysosomal degradation of proteins.

Ubiquitin conjugation systems have been detected in rabbit, bovine, and human lenses; the highest activity is present in the epithelium and the lowest in the lens nucleus (80,81). Like ubiquitin conjugation elsewhere it is ATP dependent in the lens, and the major conjugates formed are with endogenous lens proteins of M_r greater than 150,000. There is a striking difference in the relative distribution of free and conjugated ubiquitin in young (epithelial) and old (nuclear) tissue, with a strong tendency toward diminished proteolytic capabilities in the older tissue.

68 kDa Membrane-Associated Proteinase

A 68 kDa membrane-associated proteinase isolated from bovine lens fiber cell membranes has been purified to homogeneity; it is a tetramer composed of 17 kDa subunits (144). The enzyme displays maximum activity at pH 7.8 and is inhibited by all serine proteinase inhibitors tested. Its substrate specificity toward synthetic peptides and its catalytic properties distinguish it from the other major endopeptidases just described (neutral proteinases, calpains I and II, and 25 kDa trypsin-like proteinase). Its physiological substrates have not yet been examined.

Leucine Aminopeptidase

Proteolysis in most tissues is initiated by endopeptidases, and the final cleavage of peptides to amino acids is carried out by aminopeptidases (exopeptidases). In the lens, the major exopeptidase is leucine aminopeptidase, which catalyzes the hydrolysis of N-terminal amino acids from a wide range of synthetic peptides. This enzyme has been extensively studied in the lens; its structural, kinetic, and catalytic properties are now well understood from studies using highly purified preparations from bovine lens (61). Substrate specificities have been established for both the Mn^{2+}- and Mg^{2+}-activated forms of the enzyme whose pH optima range from 8.5 to 9.0; the physiological significance of this enzyme activity in the lens remains unclear because of its high pH optimum.

Although readily detected in lenses of various animal species, the presence of leucine aminopeptidase in human lens has been less certain. Young animals were used in most early studies, whereas for humans, the lenses analyzed were from elderly individuals who had died. Leucine aminopeptidase activity can be demonstrated in young human lenses by immunological methods, however (148). The purified human lens enzyme has amino acid sequences similar to those isolated from cattle and hog tissues, and the specific activity of leucine aminopeptidase in young human lenses is comparable to that of lenses from young animals. The activity of this enzyme is considerably attenuated in older lenses of all species.

Aminopeptidase HI

Another aminopeptidase has been isolated and characterized in bovine lens (136). Unlike leucine aminopeptidase, this enzyme does not require Mg^{2+} or Mn^{2+} for activation, and its pH optimum is 6.0. Based on substrate specificities and other characteristics, the enzyme has been named aminopeptidase III. This exopeptidase would be more active than leucine aminopeptidase at the physiological pH of the lens (between 7.0 and 7.2) and may have an important functional role in vivo.

Messengers

Lens development, differentiation and growth are influenced by factors from outside the lens that bind at receptors in cell membranes. The receptors pass on the message through the membrane and then via second messengers within the cell. This area has received less attention in the lens than in other ocular tissues possibly because in adult life the lens needs to make relatively few rapid responses to its environment. However, the lens is equipped with at least some of the receptors and messenger systems found elsewhere.

Adrenaline (epinephrine) binds to β-adrenergic receptors in cell membranes to trigger the adenylate cyclase cascade, mediated by a G protein. The α-subunit of the receptor is released on stimulation and activates adenylate cyclase, also in the membrane, to produce cAMP. Isoproterenol can take the place of adrenaline, i.e., it is a β-agonist. When injected into rats isoproterenol decreases mitotic activity in the lens (56). This effect was prevented by a β-blocker, but increased in the presence of theophylline which prevents breakdown of cAMP by phosphodiesterase.

The results of these simple experiments indicate that the entire apparatus from receptor to formation of cAMP is present in the lens epithelial cells. The specific binding of β-adrenergic antagonists to both epithelial and fiber cell membranes has demonstrated the presence of β-adrenergic receptors (45,74).

Most growth factor receptors have an extracellular ligand-binding domain, a transmembrane domain and an intracellular domain with intrinsic tyrosine kinase activity. Chick lens epithelium responds to various growth factors and according to PCR studies has at least eight kinase domains of known growth factors (120). The pool of clones obtained may correspond to the distribution of mRNA present but does not reflect the relative abundance of lens receptors identified in binding studies and the response of lens to various ligands.

cAMP and cGMP occur throughout the lens with the highest levels in epithelial cells and lowest levels in the lens nucleus (174) a finding originally interpreted to mean that the concentrations of the cyclic nucleotides are such that they can function significantly only in the epithelial layer. However it was possible to show increased cAMP levels in whole rat lens homogenates stimulated by isoproterenol and to a lesser extent by salbutanol, a β_2-agonist, indicating the presence of both β_1- and β_2-receptors (114).

Another component of the system, adenylate cyclase, has been identified in lens much more abundantly in the cortex than in the nucleus (17,72). Calmodulin which is required for the activation of adenylate cyclase is abundant in lens epithelium falling to low levels further into the lens (16). Cyclic AMP, the product of adenylate cyclase, is a second messenger mediating the action of various hormones and growth factors. The major function of cAMP is to activate protein kinases which then phosphorylate a variety of proteins modulating their function.

Cyclic AMP-dependent protein kinases occur in both epithelium and cortex (147). Protein phosphatases are also present (150). These could have many substrates but cytoskeletal proteins, including vimentin, fodrin and beaded filament proteins (see the section entitled Cytoskeleton), are prominent targets for phosphorylation (76). Another target is α-crystallin (see the section entitled The Crystallins). The phosphorylation of vimentin and beaded filament proteins in fiber cells is stimulated by adrenergic drugs which also cause the 49 kDa beaded filament protein to become predominantly associated with plasma membranes whereas previously it was found both in cytoplasm and membranes of the fiber cells (77,78).

Inositol is present in the lens at high concentration (152) and the phospholipid components and enzymes for the phosphoinositide cycle (Fig. 7) have now been identified in the lens (155). Phosphatidylinositol (PI) is rapidly synthesized in the differentiating embryonic lens (176). Moreover, formation of phosphatidylinositol 4,5-bisphosphate (PIP_2) from labeled inositol and its hormone-stimulated breakdown to diacylglycerol (DG)

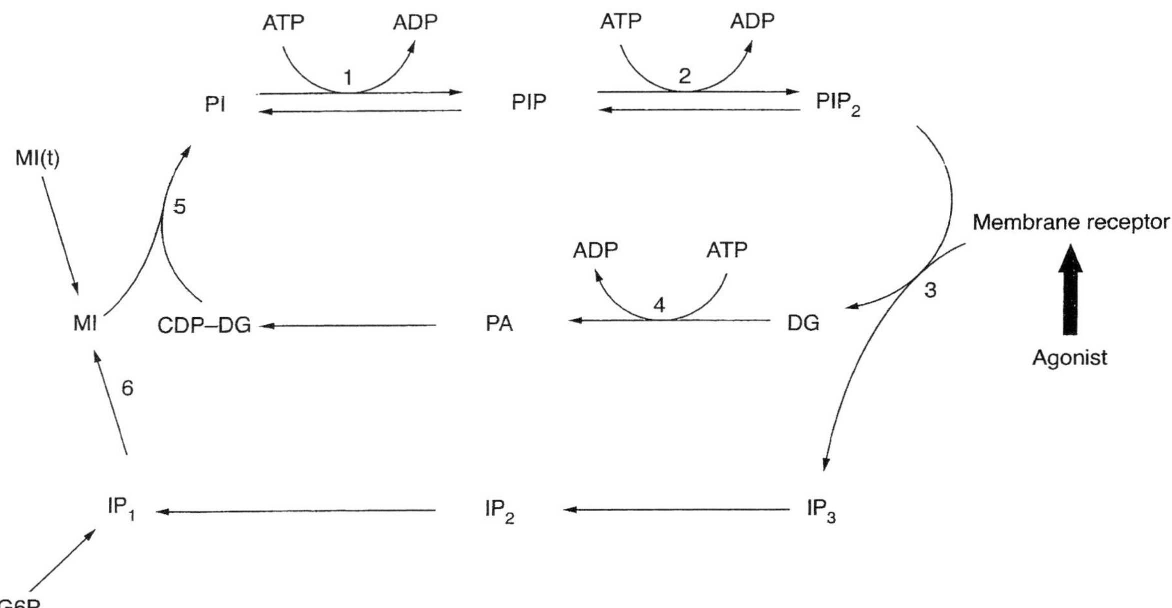

Figure 7 Lens phosphoinositide cycle. *Abbreviations*: ADP, adenosine diphosphate; ATP, adenosine triphosphate; CDP, cytidine diphosphate; DG, diacylglycerol; G6P, glucose-6-phosphate; IP_1, inositol monophosphate; IP_2, inositol biphosphate; IP_3, inositol triphosphate; MI, myoinositol; MI(t), myoinositol transported; PA, phosphatidic acid; PI, phosphatidylinositol; PIP, phosphatidylinositol phosphate; PIP_2, phosphatidylinositol 4,5-bisphosphate. *Source*: From Ref. 155.

and inositol trisphosphate (IP_3) have been demonstrated in rabbit lens epithelial cells (155). The initial product formed is PI, which is rapidly phosphorylated by two phosphoinositide kinases to PIP_2. The breakdown of this key intermediate, presumably mediated by lens phospholipase C activity, is stimulated by a number of physiological agonists, such as glucagon, epidermal growth factor (EGF) and serotonin. Hormone-stimulated PI breakdown correlates with the rate of epithelial cell division in the lens and thus may have important regulatory functions.

Receptor-controlled hydrolysis of phosphatidylinositol 4,5-diphosphate produces two second messengers, DG and IP_3, that control a great range of cellular processes. IP_3 (Fig. 7) is a second messenger that controls many cellular processes by releasing sequestered calcium. Activation of acetylcholine receptors initiates the pathway leading to calcium mobilization (161), and IP_3 itself can cause immediate calcium release (121). The IP_3 treatment causes the actin cytoskeleton to change from a stress fiber pattern to polygonal networks. The IP_3 receptor is probably on the endoplasmic reticulum (ER) (121).

Cyclo-oxygenase (prostaglandin H_2 synthase) catalyses the first step in prostaglandin synthesis. It converts arachidonic acid to prostaglandin G_2 and then through a peroxidase activity to prostaglandin H_2. Pathways of prostaglandin synthesis have been identified in the lens. Synthesis of PGE_2 and $PGF_{2\alpha}$ was demonstrated so the formation of intermediates PGG_2 and PGH_2 can be assumed (49,84,109). The two prostaglandins may serve to stimulate cyclic nucleotide formation as their other major functions in non-lens tissues would not be relevant in the lens. Immunofluorescent studies identified cyclo-oxygenase in the epithelial cells but not further into the rat lens (178), although arachidonic acid can be released from phospholipid in all parts of the lens (8). Lipoxygenases convert arachidonic acid to hydroxyeicosatetraenoic acids which can be synthesized by both epithelial and fiber cells of rat lens (99). Synthesis fell off rapidly with growth and was undetectable in the lens of the 180-day-old rat. Products of both the cyclo-oxygenase and lipoxygenase pathways may play a role in lens cell differentiation (99,178).

It is clear that the lens has a considerable array of messenger systems but as yet their interplay and functions have not been defined.

ACKNOWLEDGMENTS

Portions of this text are based on material prepared by the late Dr. Elaine Berman for the first and second editions of *Pathobiology of Ocular Disease*.

REFERENCES

1. Ahmad H, Singh SV, Medh RD, et al. Differential expression of α, μ and π classes of isozymes of glutathione S-transferase in bovine lens, cornea, and retina. Arch Biochem Biophys 1988; 266:416–26.
2. Alcala J, Maisel H. Biochemistry of lens plasma membranes and cytoskeleton. In: Maisel H, ed. The Ocular Lens Structure, Function, and Pathology. New York: Marcel Dekker, 1985:169–222.
3. Allen DP, Low PS, Dola A. Maisel H. Band 3 and ankyrin homologues are present in eye lens: evidence for all major erythrocyte membrane components in same non-erythroid cell. Biochem Biophys Res Commun 1987; 149: 266–75.
4. Aquilina JA, Benesch JLP, Bateman OA, et al. Polydispersity of a mammalian chaperone: mass spectrometry reveals the population of oligomers in αB-crystallin. Proc Natl Acad Sci USA 100, 2003; 10611–6.
5. Augusteyn RC. Dissociation is not required for alpha-crystallin's chaperone function. Exp Eye Res 2004; 79: 781–4.
6. Awasthi YC, Saneto RP, Srivastava SK. Purification and properties of bovine lens glutathione S-transferase. Exp Eye Res 1980; 30:29–39.
7. Bada JL, Vrolijk CD, Brown S, et al. Bomb radiocarbon in metabolically inert tissues from terrestrial and marine animals. Geophys Res Lett 1987; 14:1065–7.
8. Baghieri S, Garner MH. Na, K-ATPase and phospholipid degradation in bovine and human lenses. Exp Eye Res 1992; 11:459–67.
9. Banh A, Bantseev V, Choh V, Moran KL, Sivak JG. The lens of the eye as a focusing device and its response to stress. Prog Ret Eye Res 2006; 25:189–206.
10. Bassnett S. Lens organelle degradation. Exp Eye Res 2002; 74:1–6.
11. Bax B, Lapatto R, Nalini V, et al. X-ray anlysis of βB2-crystallin and evolution of oligomeric lens proteins. Nature 1990; 347:776–80.
12. Baynes JW, Watkins NJ, Fisher CI. The Amadori product on protein: structure and reactions. In: Baynes JW, Monnier V, eds. The Maillard Reaction in Ageing, Diabetes and Nutrition. New York: Alan Liss, 1989:43–67.
13. Bekhor I. MP26 messenger RNA sequences in normal and cataractous lens. Invest Ophthalmol Vis Sci 1988; 29: 802–13.
14. Berman ER. Biochemistry of the Eye. New York: Plenum Press, 1991.
15. Berman ER. Biochemistry of cataracts. In: Garner A, Klintworth GK, eds. Pathobiology of Ocular Disease. New York: Marcel Dekker, 1994:533–90.
16. Bizec JC, Klethi J, Mandel. P. Calcium-dependent regulation of adenylate cyclase and phosphodiesterase activities in bovine lens: involvement of lens calmodulin. Exp Eye Res 1985; 41:239–47.
17. Bizec JC, Klethi J, Mandel P. Modulation of adenylate cyclase activity in bovine lens epithelial cells. Ophthalmic Res 1989; 21:167–74.
18. Bloemendal H, Piatigorsky T, Spector A. Recommenda-tions for crystallin nomenclature. Exp Eye Res 1989; 48:465–6.
19. Bloemendal H, de Jong W, Jaenicke R, et al. Ageing and vision: structure, stability and function of lens crystallins. Prog Biophys Mol Biol 2004; 86:407–85.
20. Borchman D, Delamere NA, Paterson CA. Ca-ATPase activity in the rabbit and bovine lens. Invest Ophthalmol Vis Sci 1988; 29:982–7.

21. Brinker JM, Pegg MT, Howard PS, Kefalides NA. Immunochemical characterization of type IV procollagen from anterior lens capsule. Collagen 1985; 5:233–44.
22. Broekhuyse RM, Kuhlmann ED. Lens membranes. XI. Some properties of human lens main intrinsic protein (MIP) and its enzymatic conversion into a 22000 dalton polypeptide. Exp Eye Res 1980; 30:305–10.
23. Brown HG, Pappas GD, Ireland ME. Kuszak JR. Ultrastructural, biochemical and immunologic evidence of receptor-mediated endocytosis in the crystalline lens. Invest Ophthal Vis Sci 1990; 31:2579–92.
24. Bruzzone R, White TW, Paul DL. Connections with connexins: the molecular basis of direct intercellular signalling. Eur J Biochem 1996; 238:1–27.
25. Carper D, Nishimura C, Shinohara T, et al. Aldose reductase and β-crystallin belong to the same protein superfamily as aldehyde reductase. FEBS Lett 1987; 220: 209–13.
26. Carper D, Russell F, Shinohara T, Kinoshita JH. Differential synthesis of rat lens proteins during development. Exp Eye Res 1985; 40:85–94.
27. Cheng H-M, Chylack LT Jr. Lens metabolism. In: Maisel H, ed. The Ocular Lens Structure, Function, and Pathology. New York: Marcel Dekker, 1985:223–64.
28. Cheng H-M, Gonzalez RG, von Saltza I, et al. Glucose flux andtheredox state of pyridine dinucleotides in the rat lens. Exp Eye Res 1988; 46:942–52.
29. Chepelinsky AB, Piatigorsky J, Pisano MM, et al. Lens proteins gene expression: α-crystallins and MIP. Lens Eye Toxicity Res 1991; 8:319–44.
30. Chiesa R, Gawinowicz-Kolks MA, Spector A. The phosphorylation of the primary gene products of α-crystallin. J Biol Chem 1987; 262:1438–41.
31. Chiesa R, McDermott MJ, Spector A. Differential synthesis and phosphorylation of the α-crystallin A and B chains during bovine lens fiber cell differentiation. Curr Eye Res 1989; 8:151–8.
32. Colucci-Guyon E, Portier MM, Dunia I, et al. Mice lacking vimentin develop and reproduce without any obvious phenotype. Cell 1994; 79:679–94.
33. Cooper PG. Carver JA, Aquilina JA, et al. A ^{1}H-NMR spectroscopic comparison of γS and γB crystallins. Exp Eye Res 1994; 59:211–20.
34. Crabbe MJC. Aldose reductase and the importance of experimental design. Biochem Soc Trans 2003; 31:1367–71.
35. Craghill J, Cronshaw AD, Harding JJ. The identification of a reaction site of glutathione mixed-disulphide formation on gamma-S-crystallin in human lens. Biochem J 2004; 379:595–600.
36. Croft LR. The amino acid sequence of γ-crystallin (fraction II) from calf lens. Biochem J 1972; 128:961–10.
37. David LL, Shearer TR. Purification of calpain II from rat lens and determination of endogenous substrates. Exp Eye Res 1986; 42:227–38.
38. David LL, Varnum MD, Lampi KJ, Shearer TR. Calpain II in human lens. Invest Ophthalmol Vis Sci 1989; 30:269–15.
39. de Jong WW, Lubsen NH, Kraft HJ. Molecular evolution of the eye lens. Prog Ret Eye Res 1994; 13:391–442.
40. Delamere NA, Tamiya S. Expression, regulation and function of Na,K-ATPase in the lens. Prog Ret Eye Res 2004; 23:593–615.
41. Delaye M, Tardieu A. Short-range order of crystallin proteins accounts for eye lens transparency. Nature 1983; 302:415–7.
42. den Dunnen IT, Jongbloed RJE, Geurts van Kessel AHM, Schoenmakers JGG. Human lens γ-crystallin sequences are located in the pl2-qter region of chromosome 2. Hum Genet 1985; 70:211–21.
43. Derham BK, Harding JJ. α-Crystallin as a molecular chaperone. Prog Ret Eye Res 1999; 18:463–509.
44. Dilley KJ, Harding JJ. Changes in proteins in the human lens in development and aging. Biochim Biophys Acta 1975; 386:391–408.
45. Elena P-P, Kosina-Boix M, Moulin G, Lapalus P. Autoradiographic localization of beta-adrenergic receptors in rabbit eye. Invest Ophthal Vis Sci 1987; 28: 1436–41.
46. Fan J, Donovan AK, Ledee DR, et al. γE-crystallin recruitment to the plasma membrane by specific interaction between lens MIP/aquaporin-0 and γE-crystallin Invest Ophthal Vis Sci 2004; 45:863–71.
47. Farahbakhsh ZT, Huang Q-L, Ding L-L, et al. Interaction of α-crystallin with spin-labelled peptides. Biochemistry 1995; 34:509–16.
48. FitzGerald PG. Immunochemical characterization of a M_r 115 lens fiber cell-specific extrinsic membrane protein. Curr Eye Res 1988; 7:1243–53.
49. Fleisher LN, McGahan MC. Endotoxin-induced ocular inflammation increases prostaglandin E_2 synthesis by rabbit lens. Exp Eye Res 1985; 40:711–9.
50. Garland D, Russell P. Phosphorylation of lens fiber cell membrane proteins. Proc Natl Acad Sci USA 1985; 82: 653–7.
51. Garland D, Zigler JS Jr, Kinoshita J. Structural changes in bovine lens crystallins induced by ascorbate, metal and oxygen. Arch Biochem Biophys 1986; 251:771–6.
52. Giblin FJ, McCready JP, Reddan JR, et al. Detoxification of H_2O, by cultured rabbit lens epithelial cells: participation of the glutathione redox cycle. Exp Eye Res 1985; 40: 827–40.
53. Giblin FJ, McCready JP, Schrimscher L, Reddy VN. Peroxide-induced effects on lens cation transport following inhibition of glutathione reductase activity in vitro. Exp Eye Res 1987; 45:77–91.
54. Gonen T, Sliz P, Kistler J, et al. Aquaporin-0 membrane junctions reveal the structure of a closed water pore. Nature 2004; 429:193–7.
55. Gorin MB, Yancey SB, Cline J, et al. The major intrinsic protein (MIP) of the bovine lens fiber membrane: Characterization and structure based on cDNA cloning. Cell 1984; 39:49–59.
56. Grimes P, von Sallmann L. Possible cyclic adenosine monophosphate mediation in isoproterenol-induced suppression of cell division in rat lens epithelium. Invest Ophthalmol 1972; 11:231–5.
57. Haley DA, Horwitz J, Stewart PL. The small heat-shock protein, αB-Crystallin, has a variable quaternary structure. J Mol Biol 1998; 277:27–35.
58. Harding J. Cataract. Biochemistry, Epidemiology and Pharmacology. London: Chapman and Hall, 1991.
59. Harding JJ. Lens. In: Harding JJ, ed. Biochemistry of the Eye. London, UK: Chapman and Hall, 1997:94–134.
60. Harding JJ. Can drugs or micronutrients prevent cataract? Drugs Ageing 2001; 18:473–86.
61. Harding JJ, Crabbe MJC. The lens: development, proteins, metabolism and cataract. In: Davson H, ed. The Eye. 3rd ed. Vol. lb. Orlando, FL: Academic Press, 1984:207–492.
62. Hayashi S, Goto K, Okada TS, Kondoh H. Lens-specific enhancer in the third intron regulates expression of the chicken δ1-crystallin gene. Genes Dev 1987; 1:818–28.
63. Hightower KR. Cytotoxic effects of internal calcium on lens physiology: a review. Curr Eye Res 1985; 4:453–9.

64. Hightower KR, Harrison SE. The influence of calcium on glucose metabolism in the rabbit lens. Invest Ophthalmol Vis Sci 1987; 28:1433–6.
65. Hill RE, Favor J, Hogan BLM, et al. Mouse small eye results from mutations in a paired-like homeobox-containing gene. Nature 1991; 354:522–5.
66. Hitchener WR, Cenedella RJ. HMG CoA reductase activity of lens epithelial cells: compared with true rates of sterol synthesis. Curr Eye Res 1987; 6:1045–9.
67. Hogg D, Gorin MB, Heinzmann C, et al. Nucleotide sequence for the cDNA of the bovine βB2 crystallin and assignment of the orthologous human locus to chromosome 22. Curr Eye Res 1987; 6:1335–42.
68. Hook DWA, Harding JJ. Protection of enzymes by α-crystallin acting as a molecular chaperone. Int. J Biol Macromols 1998; 22:295–306.
69. Horwitz J. α-Crystallin can function as a molecular chaperone. Proc Natl Acad Sci U S A 1992; 89:10449–53.
70. Horwitz J, Huang Q, Ding L. The native oligomeric organization of alpha-crystallin, is it necessary for its chaperone function? Exp Eye Res 2004; 79:817–21.
71. Hulsebos TJM, Cerosaletti KM, Fournier REK, et al. Identification of the human βA2 crystallin gene (CRYBA2): localization of the gene on human chromosome 2 and of the homologous gene on mouse chromosome 1. Genomics 1995; 28:543–8.
72. Hur KC, Louis CF. Regional distribution of the enzymes and substrates mediating the action of cAMP in the mammalian lens. Biochim Biophys Acta 1989; 1010:56–63.
73. Ingolia TD, Craig EA. Four small *Drosophila* heat shock proteins are related to each other and to mammalian α-crystallin. Proc Natl Acad Sci U S A 1982; 79:2360–4.
74. Ireland M, Maisel H. Evidence for a calcium activated protease specific for lens intermediate filaments. Curr Eye Res 1984; 3:423–9.
75. Ireland M, Maisel H. Phosphorylation of chick lens proteins. Curr Eye Res 1984; 3:961–8.
76. Ireland ME, Jacks LA. Initial characterization of lens beta-adrenergic receptors. Invest Ophthal Vis Sci 1989; 30: 2190–4.
77. Ireland ME, Maisel H. Adrenergic stimulation of lens cytoskeletal phosphorylation. Curr Eye Res 1987; 6: 489–96.
78. Ireland ME, Maisel H. Isoproterenol treatment causes cytoskeletal reorganization in chicken lens fiber cells. Invest Ophthal Vis Sci 1988; 29:1356–60.
79. Iwata S, Maesato T. Studies on the mercapturic acid pathway in the rabbit lens. Exp Eye Res 1988; 47:479–88.
80. Jahngen JH, Eisenhauer D, Taylor A. Lens proteins are substrates for the reticulocyte ubiquitin conjugation system. Curr Eye Res 1986; 5:725–33.
81. Jahngen JH, Haas AL, Ciechanover A, et al. The eye lens has an active ubiquitin-protein conjugation system. J Biol Chem 1986; 261:13760–7.
82. Jarvis LJ, Kumar NM, Louis CF. The developmental expression of three mammalian lens fiber cell membrane proteins. Invest Ophthal Vis Sci 1993; 34:613–20.
83. Johnson KR, Panter SS, Johnson RG. Phosphorylation of lens membranes with a cyclic AMP-dependent protein kinase purified from the bovine lens. Biochim Biophys Acta 1985; 844:367–76.
84. Keeting PE, Lysz TW, Contra M, Fu S-C. Prostaglandin biosynthesis in the rat lens. Invest Ophthal Vis Sci 1985; 26:1083–6.
85. Kistler J, Bullivant S. Structure and molecular biology of the eye lens membranes. CRC Crit Rev Biochem Mol Biol 1989; 24:151–81.
86. Kushmerick C, Rice SJ, Baldo GJ, et al. Ion, water and neutral solute transport in *Xenopus* oocytes expressing frog lens MIP. Exp Eye Res 1995; 61:351–62.
87. Lahm D, Lee LK, Bettelheim FA. Age dependence of freezable and nonfreezable water content of normal human lenses. Invest Ophthalmol Vis Sci 1985; 26: 1162–5.
88. Lampe PD, Bazzi MD, Nelsestuen GL, Johnson RG. Phosphorylation of lens intrinsic membrane proteins by protein kinase C. Eur J Biochem 1986; 156:351–7.
89. Lampi KJ. Shih M, Ueda Y, et al. Lens proteomics: analysis of rat crystallin sequences and two-dimensional electrophoresis. Invest Ophthalmol Vis Sci 2002; 43: 216–24.
90. Lea EJA, Marcantonio JM, Jones SP, Duncan G. Discrete channel activity of lens gap junction protein in planar bilayer membranes. In: Duncan G, ed. The Lens: Transparency and Cataract. Rijswijk: EURAGE, 1986: 153–8.
91. Li L-K, So L. Age dependent lipid and protein changes inindividual bovine lenses. Curr Eye Res 1987; 6: 599–605.
92. Li L-K, So L, Spector A. Membrane cholesterol and phospholipidin consecutive concentric sections of human lenses. J Lipid Res 1985; 26:600–9.
93. Li L-K, So L, Spector A. Age-dependent changes in the distribution and concentration of human lens cholesterol and phospholipids. Biochim Biophys Acta 1987; 917: 112–20.
94. Lindley PF, Narebor ME, Summers LJ, Wistow GJ. The structure of lens proteins. In: Maisel H, ed. The Ocular Lens: Structure, Function, and Pathology. New York: Marcel Dekker, 1985:123–67.
95. Louis CF, Johnson R, Turnquist J. Identification of the calmodulin-binding components in bovine lens plasma membranes. Eur J Biochem 1985; 150:271–278.
96. Lovicu FJ, Chamberlain CG, McAvoy JW. Differential effects of aqueous and vitreous on fiber differentiation and extracellular matrix accumulation in lens epithelial explants. Invest Ophthalmol Vis Sci 1995; 36:1459–69.
97. Lucas VA, Zigler JS Jr. Transmembrane glucose carriers in the monkey lens. Invest Ophthalmol Vis Sci 1987; 28: 1404–12.
98. Lucas VA, Zigler JS Jr. Identification of the monkey lens glucose transporter by photoaffinity labeling with cytochalasin B. Invest Ophthalmol Vis Sci 1988; 29:630–5.
99. Lysz TW, Lin C, Fu SCJ, Wu Y. Temporal and regional production of 12(S)hydroxyeicosatetraenoic acid [12(S)-HETE] in rat lens. Exp Eye Res 1992; 54:769–74.
100. Maisel H, ed. The Ocular Lens: Structure, Function and Pathology. New York: Marcel Dekker, 1985.
101. Mandal K, Bose SK, Chakrabarti B, Siezen RJ. Structure and stability of -y-crystallins. U. Differences in micro-environments and spatial arrangements of cysteine residues. Biochim Biophys Acta 1987; 911:277–84.
102. McFall-Ngai MJ, Ding L-L, Takemoto LJ, Horwitz J. Spatial and temporal mapping of the age-related changes in human lens crystallins. Exp Eye Res 1985; 41:745–58.
103. Moffat BA, Pope JM. Anisotropic water transport in the eye lens studied by diffusion tensor NMR micro-imaging. Exp Eye Res 2002; 74:677–87.
104. Mulders JWM, Voorter CEM, Lamers C, et al. MP17, a fiber-specific intrinsic membrane protein from mammalian eye lens. Curr Eye Res 1988; 7:207–19.
105. Najmudin S, Nalini V, Driessen H. et al. Structure of the eye lens protein γB (γII)-crystallin at 1.47 A. Acta Cryst D 1993; 49:223–33.

106. Nakajima E, Walkup RD, Ma H, et al. Low activity by the calpain system in primate lenses causes resistance to calcium-induced proteolysis. Exp Eye Res 2006; 8: 593–601.
107. Nene V, Dunne DW, Johnson KS, et al. Sequence and expression of a major egg antigen from Schistosoma mansoni: homologies to heat shock proteins and alpha-crystallins. Mol Biochem Parasitol 1986; 21:179–88.
108. Nicholl ID, Quinlan R. Chaperone activity of α-crystallin modulates intermediate filament assembly. EMBO J 1994; 13:945–53.
109. Nishi O, Nishi K, Imanishi M. Synthesis of interleukin-1 and prostaglandin E_2 by lens epithelial cells of human cataracts. Br J Ophthalmol 1992; 76:338–41.
110. Okuda J, Kawamura M, Didelot S. Anomeric preference in uptake of D-glucose and of D-galactose by rat lenses. Curr Eye Res 1987; 6:1223–6.
111. Ortwerth BJ, Feather MS, Olesen PR. The precipitation and cross-linking of lens crystallins by ascorbic acid. Exp Eye Res 1988; 47:155–68.
112. Ortwerth BJ, Olesen PR. Ascorbic acid-induced cross-linking of lens proteins: evidence supporting a Maillard reaction. Biochim Biophys Acta 1988; 956:10–22.
113. Ortwerth BJ, Olesen PR. Glutathione inhibits the glycation and crosslinking of lens proteins by ascorbic acid. Exp Eye Res 1988; 47:737–50.
114. Osborne NN. Agonist-induced stimulation of cAMP in the lens: presence of functional β-receptors. Exp Eye Res 1991; 52:105–6.
115. Peracchia C, Girsch SJ, Bernardini G, Peracchia LL. Lens junctions are communicating junctions. Curr Eye Res 1985; 4:1155–69.
116. Piatigorsky J, O'Brien WE, Norman BL, et al. Gene sharing by δ-crystallin and argininosuccinate lyase. Proc Natl Acad Sci U S A 1988; 85:3479–83.
117. Pirie A. Composition of ox lens capsule. Biochem J 1951; 48:368–71.
118. Pirie A. Glutathione peroxidase in lens and a source of hydrogen peroxide in aqueous humour. Biochem J 1965; 96:244–53.
119. Pladzyk A, Ramana KV, Ansari NH, Srivastava SK. Aldose reductase prevents aldehyde toxicity in culatured human lens epithelial cells. Exp Eye Res 2006; 83:408–16.
120. Potts JD, Haracopos GJ, Beebe DC. Identification of receptor tyrosine kinases in the embryonic chicken lens. Curr Eye Res 1993; 12:759–63.
121. Rafferty NS, Rafferty KA, Ito E. Agonist-induced rise in intraocular calcium of lens epithelial cells: effects on the actin cytoskeleton. Exp Eye Res 1994; 59:191–201.
122. Rathbun WB, Bovis MG, Holleschau AM. Glutathione peroxidase, glutathione reductase and glutathione-S-transferase activities in the rhesus monkey lens as a function of age. Curr Eye Res 1986; 5:195–9.
123. Rathbun WB, Bovis MG. Activity of glutathione peroxidase and glutathione reductase in the human lens related to age. Curr Eye Res 1986; 5:381–5.
124. Ray K, Harris H. Purification of neutral lens endopeptidase: close similarity to a neutral proteinase in pituitary. Proc Natl Acad Sci U S A 1985; 82:7545–9.
125. Reddan JR, Giblin FJ, Dziedzic DC, McCready JP, Schrimscher L, Reddy VN. Influence of the activity of glutathione reductase on the response of cultured lens epithelial cells from young and old rabbits to hydrogen peroxide. Exp Eye Res 1988; 46:209–21.
126. Regini JW, Grossman JG, Timmins, P et al. Alpha-crystallin a fenestrated chaperone. Invest Ophthalmol Vis Sci 2007 (in press).
127. Richardson NA, Chamberlain CG, McAvoy JW. IGF-1 enhancement of FGF-induced lens fibre differentiation in rats of different ages. Invest Ophthal Vis Sci 1993; 34: 3303–12.
128. Ringens PJ, Hoenders HJ, Bloemendal H. Cell-free translation of human lens polyribosomes. Exp Eye Res 1982; 34:831–4.
129. Russell P. In vitro alterations similar to posttranslational modification of lens proteins. Invest Ophthalmol Vis Sci 1984; 25:209–12.
130. Russell P, Sato S. A study of lectin-binding to the water-insoluble proteins of the lens. Exp Eye Res 1986; 42: 95–106.
131. Russell P, Zelenka P, Martensen T, Reid TW. Identification of the EDXA-extractable protein in lens as calpactinl. Curr Eye Res 1987; 6:533–8.
132. Sandilands A, Prescott AR, Wegener A, et al. Knockout of the intermediate filament protein CP49 destabilises the lens fibre cell cytoskeleton and decreases lens optical quality, but does not induce cataract. Exp Eye Res 2003; 76:385–91.
133. Schoenmakers JGG, Den Dunnen JT, Moormann RJM, et al. The crystallin gene families. In: Nugent, Whelan J, eds. Human Cataract Formation, Ciba Foundation Symposium 106,1, London: Pitman, 1984:208–18.
134. Sethna SS, Holleschau AM, Rathbun WB. Activity of glutathione synthesis enzymes in human lens related to age. Curr Eye Res 1982; 2:735–42.
135. Shang F, Taylor A. Function of the ubiquitin proteolytic pathway in the eye. Exp Eye Res 2004; 78:1–14.
136. Sharma KK, Ortwerth BJ. Isolation and characterization of a new aminopeptidase from bovine lens. J Biol Chem 1986; 261:4295–301.
137. Sharma KK, Kumar RS, Kumar GS, Quinn PT. Synthesis and characterization of a peptide identified as a functional element in αA-crystallin. J Biol Chem 2000; 275: 3767–71.
138. Shiloh Y, Donlon T, Bruns G, et al. Assignment of the human γ-crystallin gene cluster (CRYG) to the long arm of chromosome 2, region q33-36. Hum Genet 1986; 73: 17–9.
139. Simpson A, Bateman O, Driessen H, et al. The structure of avian eye lens δ-crystallin reveals a new fold for a super-family of oligomeric enzymes. Nat Struct Biol 1994; 1: 724–34.
140. Slingsby C. Structural variation in lens crystallins. Trends Biochem Sci 1985; 10:281–4.
141. Sparkes RS, Mohandas T, Heinzmann C, et al. The gene for the major intrinsic protein (MLP) of the ocular lens is assigned to human chromosome 12cen-ql4. Invest Ophthalmol Vis Sci 1986; 27:1351–4.
142. Spector A, Chiesa R. Sredy T, Garner W. cAMP-dependent phosphorylation of bovine lens α-crystallin. Proc Natl Acad Sci U S A 1985; 82:4712–6.
143. Srikanthan D, Bateman OA, Purkiss AG, Slingsby C. Sulfur in human crystallins. Exp Eye Res 2004; 79: 823–31.
144. Srivastava OP. Characterization of a highly purified membrane proteinase from bovine lens. Exp Eye Res 1988; 46:269–83.
145. Srivastava OP, Ortwerth BJ. Isolation and characterization of a 25K serine proteinase from bovine lens cortex. Exp Eye Res 1983; 37:597–612.
146. Summers LJ, Slingsby C, Blundell TL, et al. Structural variation in mammalian γ-crystallins based on computer graphics analyses of human, rat and calf sequences. 1. Core packing and surface properties. Exp Eye Res 1986; 45:77–92.

147. Takáts A, Antoni F, Faragó A, Kertész P. Some properties of the cyclic AMP-dependent protein kinase of epithelial cells and cortical fibres of bovine eye lens. Exp Eye Res 1978; 26:389–97.
148. Taylor A, Surgenor T, Thomson DKR, et al. Comparison of leucine aminopeptidase from human lens, beef lens and kidney, and hog lens in kidney. Exp Eye Res 1984; 38: 211–329.
149. Tsonis PA, Fuentes EJ. Focus on molecules: Pax-6, the eye master. Exp Eye Res 2006; 83:233–4.
150. Umeda IO, Nakata H, Nishigori H. Identification of protein phosphatase 2C and confirmation of other protein phosphatases in the ocular lens. Exp Eye Res 2004; 79: 385–92.
151. Van denEijnden-vanRaaij AJM, Feijen A, Snoek GT. EDTA-extractable proteins from calf lens fiber membranes are phosphorylated by Ca^{2+}-phospholipid-dependent protein kinase. Exp Eye Res 1987; 45:215–25.
152. Van Heyningen R. Majolnositol in the lens of mammalian eyes. Biochem J 1957; 65:24–8.
153. Van Heyningen R. Formation of polyols by the lens of the rat with "sugar" cataract. Nature 1959; 184:194–5.
154. Van Heyningen R. The sorbitol pathway in the lens. Exp Eye Res 1962; 1:396–404.
155. Vivekanandan S, Lou MF. Evidence for the presence of phosphoinositide cycle and its involvement in cellular signal transduction in the rabbit lens. Curr Eye Res 1989; 5:101–11.
156. Voorter CEM, Mulders JWM, Bloemendal H, de Jong WW. Some aspects of the phosphorylation of α-crystallin A. Eur J Biochem 1986; 160:203–10.
157. Wagner BJ, Margolis JW, Abramovitz AS. The bovine lens neutral proteinase comprises a family of cysteine-dependent proteolytic activities. Curr Eye Res 1986; 5: 863–8.
158. Wagner BJ, Margolis JW, Garland D, Roseman JE. Bovine lens neutral proteinase preferentially hydrolyses oxidatively modified glutamine synthetase. Exp Eye Res 1986; 43:1141–3.
159. Wang X, Garcia CM, Shui Y-B, Beebe DC. Expression and regulation of γ-, β-, and γ-crystallins in mammalian lens epithelial cells. Invest Ophthalmol Vis Sci 2004; 45: 3608–19.
160. Watanabe K, Fujii Y, Nakayama K, et al. Structural similarity of bovine lung prostaglandin F synthase to lens e-crystallin of the European common frog. Proc Natl Acad Sci U S A 1988; 85:11–5.
161. Williams MR, Duncan G, Riach RA, Webb SF. Acetylcholine receptors are coupled to mobilization of intracellular calcium in cultured human lens cells. Exp Eye Res 1993; 57:381–4.
162. Winkler BS, Solomon E High activities of $NADP^{+}$-dependent isocitrate dehydrogenase and malic enzyme in rabbit lens epithelial cells. Invest Ophthalmol Vis Sci 1988; 29:821–3.
163. Wistow GJ, Mulders JWM, de Jong WW. The enzyme lactate dehydrogenase as a structural protein in avian and crocodilian lenses. Nature 1987; 326:622–4.
164. Wistow G, Piatigorsky J. Recruitment of enzymes as lens structural proteins. Science 1987; 236:1554–6.
165. Wistow G, Turnell B, Summers L, et al. X-ray analysis of the eye lens protein γ-II crystallin at 1.9 A resolution. J Mol Biol 1983; 170:175–202.
166. Wistow G, Wyatt K, David L, et al. γN-crystallin and the evolution of the βγ-crystallin superfamily in vertebrates. FEBS J 2005; 272:2276–91.
167. Wolff SF, Wang G-M, Spector A. Pro-oxidant activation of ocular reductants. 1. Copper and riboflavin stimulate ascorbate oxidation causing lens epithelial cytotoxicity in vitro. Exp Eye Res 1987; 45:777–89.
168. Wride MA, Mansergh FC, Adams S, et al. Expression profiling and gene expression in the mouse lens. Mol Vis 2003; 9:360–96.
169. Yancey SB, Koh K, Chung J, Revel J-P. Expression of the gene for main intrinsic polypeptide (MIP): separate spatial distributions of MIP and pi-crystallin gene transcripts in rat lens development. J Cell Biol 1988; 106:705–14.
170. Yegorova S, Liu A, Lou MF. Human lens thioredoxin: molecular cloning and fuctional characterization. Invest Ophthalmol Vis Sci 2003; 44:3263–71.
171. Yoshida H, Murachi T, Tsukahara I. Limited proteolysis of bovine lens α-crystallin by calpain, a Ca^{2+}-dependent cysteine proteinase, isolated from the same tissue. Biochim Biophys Acta 1984; 798:252–9.
172. Yoshida H, Murachi T, Tsukahara I. Distribution of calpain I, calpain II, and calpastatin in bovine lens. Invest Ophthalmol Vis Sci 1985; 26:953–6.
173. Yoshida H, Yumoto N, Tsukahara I, Murachi T. The degradation of α-crystallin at its carboxylterminal portion by calpain in bovine lens. Invest Ophthalmol Vis Sci 1986; 27:1269–73.
174. Zagrod ME, Whitehart DR. Cyclic nucleotides in anatomical subdivisions of the bovine lens. Curr Eye Res 1981; 1:49–52.
175. Zampighi GA, Hall JE, Kreman M. Purified lens junctional protein forms channels in planar lipid films. Proc Natl Acad Sci U S A. 1985; 82:8468–72.
176. Zelenka PS. Changes inphosphatidylinositol metabolism during differentiation of lens epithelial cells into lens fiber cells in the embryonic chick. J Biol Chem 1980; 255: 1296–1300.
177. Zelenka PS. Lens lipids. Curr Eye Res 1984; 3:1337–59.
178. Zheng D-R, Fu S-CJ, Lysz TW, Leung CCK. Immunocytochemical localization of cyclooxygenase in the rat lens. Invest Ophthal Vis Sci 1992; 33:178–83.

23

The Types, Morphology, and Causes of Cataracts

M. Joseph Costello
Department of Cell and Developmental Biology, University of North Carolina, Chapel Hill, North Carolina, U.S.A.

Jerome R. Kuszak
Department of Ophthalmology, Rush University Medical Center, Chicago, Illinois, U.S.A.

INTRODUCTION

The ocular lens is an isolated epithelial tissue encased by a thick capsule and supported by zonular suspensory ligaments. The primary function of the lens is to aid in the focusing of light onto the retina and, during accommodation with a young deformable lens, to dynamically adjust the focus from distant to near objects. Refraction of the lens is enhanced by its biconvex–oblate–spheroidal shape, transparency, high internal refractive index, and radial gradient of refractive index that reduces spherical aberration (61,104,118). The cortical outer layer, about 1 mm thick in adult human lenses, contains compact highly organized cells and has a refractive index that gradually increases toward the interior. The inner nuclear mass has densely packed cells with high protein concentration and high constant refractive index (118). The lens shape, optical properties, and internal organization are the result of a unique pattern of development and differentiation (95).

LENS CELLULAR ORGANIZATION AND TRANSPARENCY

During embryonic development (see Chapter 51), the lens begins as a hollow spherical vesicle with an inner single layer of cuboidal epithelial cells covered by a basement membrane that will become the lens capsule. At about week 5 of development in humans, the posterior half of the epithelium elongates to fill the vesicle, forming the primary fiber cells. The remaining anterior epithelium is the source of new lens cells that will be added in shells throughout life. In the germinative zone near the equator, epithelial cells divide producing daughter cells that migrate inwardly away from the surface and elongate simultaneously toward the lens poles. These secondary fiber cells are arranged end-to-end to form distinct suture patterns within growth shells (96,102). During the elongation process, production of lens-specific membrane and cytoplasmic proteins enlarges the surface area and volume of the fiber cells by several orders of magnitude. After elongation, the fiber cells further differentiate by the regulated disruption and removal of all internal membranous organelles (12). The final stages of differentiation in the lens cortex involve dissolution of the cytoskeleton, condensation of the cytoplasmic crystallin proteins, redistribution of plasma membrane components, and remodeling of the complex interdigitations linking adjacent cells (140). This pattern confines the organelles, most obviously the cell nuclei, to the equatorial region normally in the shadow of the iris, which helps minimize possible light scattering from the organelles and thus contributes to lens transparency.

Transparency of the lens cortex is also thought to be dependent on the regular packing of fiber cells into radial cell columns with the broad faces of the flattened hexagonal fiber cell cross-sections aligned in a nearly crystalline array (19,145). It is hypothesized that the alternating pattern (creating form birefringence) of the array of membranes and cytoplasm creates destructive interference that helps minimize light scattering (17). Recent evidence suggests that the membranes of the cortex have a higher refractive index than the cytoplasm and this distribution assists in the reduction of scattering from the alternating pattern (110). The same study reports that, in contrast, the nuclear membranes have refractive indices that are similar to the cytoplasm (110). This may be consistent with the observation that the extracellular space (ECS) between membranes is reduced from about 10 to 15 nm in the cortex to nearly zero in the nucleus of human and animal lenses (39,43,96). Such close packing minimizes the ECS that is inherently a low refractive index medium. In addition, the nucleus contains fiber cells with irregular shapes and packing, along with progressively more complex interdigitations and edge processes, particularly in human lenses (95,96,140). A smooth variation in the refractive index across these nuclear membranes may reduce light scattering. Probably the most important factor in lens transparency is the close packing of cytoplasmic crystallins in the nuclear fiber cells. The net light scattering is reduced as crystallin proteins associate more closely so that their scattered light waves interfere destructively (cancel each other) producing an assembly of densely packed proteins with minimal overall scattering (17,18,51). Fiber cell organization and the arrangement of cellular components are critical to lens function and maintenance of lens transparency.

As stated above, the sutures begin as the initial secondary fiber cells are layered onto the embryonic nucleus. The first suture pattern in humans is an anterior upright Y and a posterior inverted Y. After birth, the three-branch suture becomes six branches in a simple star pattern and at the infantile to adolescent transition the pattern becomes a nine-branch suture. In the adult nucleus, the pattern becomes more complex, forming a 12-branch complex star suture and later a complex star with up to 15 branches. Unlike the fetal nucleus and many animal models (such as bovine, rat, mouse, and guinea pig) that have Y sutures, the complex suture planes in humans are distributed away from the optic axis. Based on laser-focusing studies, it has been demonstrated that suture planes, by their intrinsic disordered cellular architecture, lower lens optical quality (99). The spreading of suture planes over a wide volume in human lenses may improve the overall optical quality of the human lens.

It is noteworthy that the maximum accommodative ability occurs about 10 years of age during the adolescent period before any adult fiber cells are deposited. Fiber cell shape is similar in the adolescent zone to adjacent zones except that the ends of the cells are more flared and flattened near the sutures. This recent morphological evidence suggests that accommodation can be explained in part by an interdigitation of the ends of fiber cells at the sutures (98). In the fully accommodated state the fiber cells slightly overlap at their ends. As tension in the zonules increases, the lens flattens and the fibers pull apart just enough to relieve the overlap and to compress the fibers along the optic axis. The three-dimensional shape of the fibers is critical to this process. Because of the opposite end curvature of the fibers, the overall shape is a spiral similar to one turn of a helical coil or spring (101). As the lens flattens the spring compresses slightly. Thus, it is hypothesized that accommodation-induced changes within the lens can be accounted for by minimal movements of the fiber cell ends and very little change in cellular volume.

CATARACT

Definition and Classification of Cataracts

A cataract can be considered to be any opacity within the lens. The opacity is usually recognized by its excess light scattering and its effect on visual performance. In general, the scattered light is white in animal and human lenses. The white scattering is directly a result of the disruption of the highly ordered arrangement of lens cellular organization. The alterations in fiber cell structure produce fluctuations in refractive index that also cause light scattering. Early stages of cataract formation may involve cellular alterations that produce no obvious opacification, but these precataractous changes may subtly affect lens optical quality, which impairs visual acuity or functional vision due to increased glare or reduced contrast sensitivity resulting from forward scattering on the macula (151). An understanding of the alterations in lens cellular organization is critical for distinguishing the morphology of different types of cataracts and for deciphering the underlying causes and disease mechanisms.

Cataracts can be classified by their location and severity; mild through advanced cataracts have been described in nearly every region of the lens. They can be classified by the underlying condition or insult, such as a genetic mutation, developmental defect, metabolic disorder, environmental factor, or advancing age. They are often described by the characteristic pattern of light scattering seen on clinical examination, such as the Christmas tree cataract or lamellar cataract (127,162). They can also be described in terms of a specific cause that results in fluctuations in refractive index of the appropriate size to scatter light, such as the cold cataract displayed by certain young animal model lenses. In this example, lowering the temperature below a critical value produces phase separation of cytoplasmic crystallins into micron-sized spherical particles (50,107). Regardless of the fundamental cause, the alteration of lens structure is the underlying basis for generating increased scattering and an understanding of its mechanism of formation is vital for deciphering cataract pathogenesis. This chapter emphasizes the contributions of modern morphological analyses in describing the basis for lens transparency and the formation of cataracts.

Prevalence of Cataracts and Related Blindness

Cataracts are the leading cause of blindness in the world. More than 20 million people are blind worldwide because of cataracts (144). The most common forms are age-related cortical, posterior subcapsular, and age-related nuclear cataracts. In many advanced cases multiple types or mixed cataracts are present within the same lens. Most of those blind with cataract are afflicted with nuclear cataracts that develop with age and are the primary cause of visual impairment in the elderly. Where medical facilities are readily available, cataracts are surgically removed and replaced with plastic intraocular lens implants before significant visual impairment occurs. Where medical services have not been either accessible or affordable, e.g., in developing countries, the cataracts often progress to maturity accompanied by complete loss of vision. In most countries, cataracts are a significant burden on health-care systems (58,136). In the United States more than 1.5 million cataract surgeries are performed per year. In India the rate of cataract operations has been increased recently to 4.5 million per year and by 2020 it is projected that blindness due to cataract will no longer be a major concern (47,62,120,142). However, as medical care and nutrition improve and, as the world population ages, the number of people developing age-related nuclear cataracts will increase (38). At present, surgery is the only effective treatment. Cataract research aims to provide an understanding of the cellular basis of cataract formation that may suggest alternative methods of treatment to retard the progression of cataracts or to prevent their onset.

Cataracts in Developmental Zones of the Lens

Cataracts form in specific regions that can be identified and described in terms of developmental zones. All fiber cells formed during embryonic and fetal development are defined as the embryonic and fetal nuclei, respectively (Fig. 1). All fibers formed from birth to puberty are designated as the juvenile nucleus (jn). Other terms such as infantile nucleus have been used (53,67) and this region can be subdivided into infantile and adolescent to emphasize specific features, such as the increase in complexity of the sutures during early development (102). After puberty, all the fiber cells added to the nucleus constitute the adult nucleus. As discussed elsewhere, the suture pattern in human lenses becomes more complex throughout life as accretion of fiber cells from the cortex enlarges the adult nucleus. The cortex is the outer layer of differentiating fiber cells and can be subdivided into elongating fiber cells (outer cortex), zone of organelle loss (middle cortex), and the zone of final differentiation (inner cortex), where subtle maturation of fiber cells occurs before cortical fiber cells become part of the nuclear mass of fiber cells. For comparison, a cortical fiber cell is soft and flexible, has a well-developed cytoskeleton and is separated from adjacent cells by a small but well-defined ECS, whereas nuclear fiber cells are characterized by the absence of cytoskeleton, condensed cytoplasm, complex undulating surface topology, and minimal space between adjacent cells (140). Moreover, fiber cells have a characteristic morphology in each developmental zone, in part due to variations in gene expression (89). Because of differences in structure and composition, each developmental zone responds differently to aging and to insults that may result in pathological changes.

An alternative definition states that only fibers of the fetal and embryonic nuclei constitute the nucleus (27). Other secondary fibers, formed after birth, are considered to be part of the cortex, which is divided into numerous layers designated by numbers. These layers have been related to the zones of discontinuity seen in slit-lamp images of transparent lenses and some correlations with transitions in the complexity of suture lines in humans have been noted (27,92). It is clear that the definition of what constitutes the nucleus is somewhat arbitrary. Any

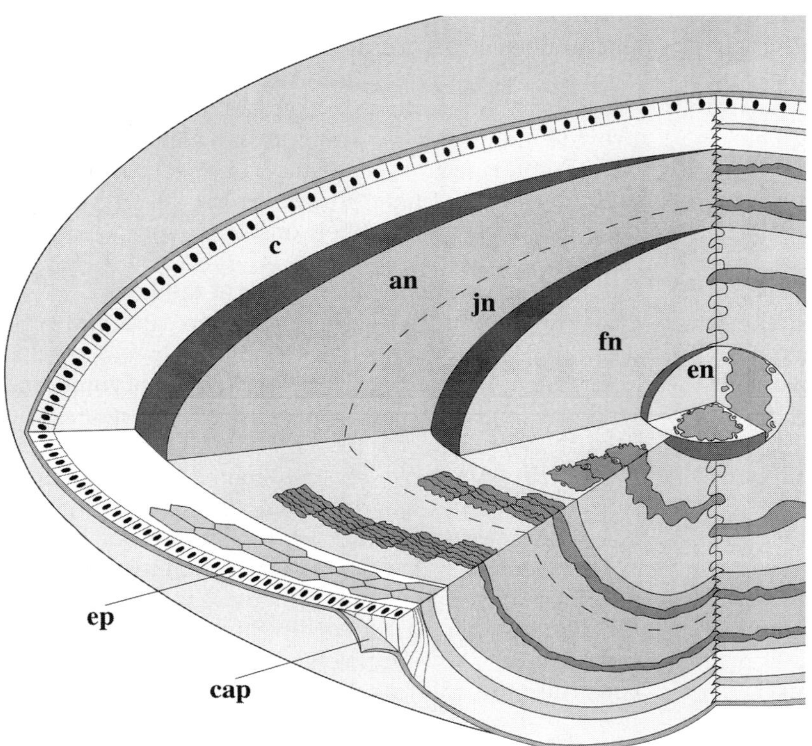

Figure 1 Human lens developmental zones. The embryonic nucleus is enlarged by 4 times for clarity. The cross-sections of fiber cells are roughly sized relative to each other, not the zone. Zone thicknesses are roughly to scale for a 60-year-old human lens. Sutures are not shown. Cell compaction occurs across the cortex–adult nucleus interface. *Abbreviations*: cap, capsule; ep, epithelium; c, cortex; an, adult nucleus; jn, juvenile nucleus; fn, fetal nucleus; en, embryonic nucleus. *Source*: From Ref. 140.

reasonable definition may be useful when landmarks can be related to intrinsic properties of the lens interior. A precise definition avoids incongruous and often confusing terms, such as paranucleus or perinucleus, which have been sometimes employed to emphasize specific layers with high scattering. These terms probably refer to the juvenile nucleus (Fig. 1). Precise terms and locations of a specific growth shell can be specified by noting the distance from the lens center or the capsule and describing the relationship to the optic axis and equator. Reference to a specific nuclear location also depends on the lens species and age because size, growth rate, suture pattern, and mechanical properties of the nucleus are greatly influenced by these factors.

A description of the nucleus based on developmental zones has several advantages. First, the fiber cell morphology is distinctive in each developmental zone. Second, each zone has a different response to injury and aging. For example, aged human lenses display compaction of fiber cells that is most pronounced at the transition from cortex to adult nucleus, about 1 mm from the lens capsule (5,96,140). Third, the fiber cell cytoskeleton is lost before the cells become part of the nucleus. Fourth, the yellow pigmentation of aged human lenses begins and is confined to the nucleus. Fifth, importantly, the hardness of the lens interior begins at the adult nucleus (the 1 mm thick outer layer of cortical cells is always soft compared to the inner nuclear mass) and the hardness increases toward the center. Moreover, the hardness of the nucleus increases with age and nuclear age-related cataract formation (82,155). In younger lenses that actively accommodate, the nucleus is soft and flexible, acting as a dynamic focusing element of nearly constant high refractive index. After the onset of presbyopia in the fourth decade, the nucleus is harder, but still has a relatively constant refractive index and performs its static optical function within the lens, possibly for another four or more decades.

Aging of the Lens in Relation to Cataract Formation

As the human lens ages, the nucleus hardens. This transition begins generally in the fourth decade (82,155), in large part reducing the ability of the lens to change shape and accommodate, and signaling the onset of presbyopia (73,74). The soft cortex that remains is unable to alter the shape of the nucleus as the tension changes in the zonules. In addition, recognition of other aging changes in normal transparent lenses is essential to understand cataract formation. These changes (see Chapter 19) include reduction in oxidative defense mechanisms, association of crystallins (through aggregation, cross-linking, chaperoning, polymerization, loss of water), modification of crystallins (nonenzymatic changes and possibly calcium activated proteases that produce more acidic proteins, protein fragments and reduced osmotic stress compatible with high protein density), and an increase in pigmentation (mostly derivatives of tryptophan). These changes alter the packing of crystallins in the cytoplasm and increase the amount of high-angle scatter or retinal stray light that produces glare visible in slit-lamp images. Understanding of this last factor is critical because increases in nuclear scatter occur in human lenses that are considered to be transparent (no loss in visual acuity and no apparent opacification). These observations suggest that normal aging produces changes that result in small particle scatter seen at high scattering angles without serious loss in visual function. By the age of 75 years, about 50% of human lenses examined with slit-lamp biomicroscopy have nuclear scattering that would qualify as cataract on the current evaluation scales, even though they have normal visual acuity and no other visual deficits. Although cataract can form at any age (including at birth), the majority of cataracts, especially those involving the nucleus, appear in aged lenses after the onset of presbyopia.

Cataract Grading Systems

The Lens Opacity Classification System III (LOCS III) divides nuclear pigmentation and opalescence (white scattering) into six grades using standard photographs from slit-lamp images (35). A slightly different Oxford grading system uses a similar set of scales based on standard photographs (49,133). These systems, which are useful for research and epidemiological studies, have been directly compared and give similar evaluations of cataract progression (77). Clinicians often use simpler 0–4 grading systems, such as that of Pirie (119), described mainly in terms of nuclear color (54,146). This is popular because of its simplicity and because nuclear color and white scattering usually progress together. Nuclear opalescence (sometimes referred to as nuclear sclerosis, which by definition is hardening of the tissue) is superimposed on the yellow pigmentation. Spalton et al. clearly illustrate that in some cases the two properties can be separated by showing a slit-lamp image having the entire nucleus completely opaque due to white scattering compared directly to a similar nucleus with extensive dark yellow pigmentation in addition to the white scattering (116,132). This suggests that, although related perhaps by oxidative damage (10,146), the yellow pigmentation and white scattering do not necessarily increase at the same rate during nuclear cataract formation. This concept is reinforced by the examination of advanced cataracts. The classic picture of a patient with total cataract is the white reflection of ambient light from the pupil, consistent with the original derivation of the term "cataract" as similar to the whiteness of a waterfall. Other blind patients with extensive dark brown or black lens coloration (cataracta nigra) will appear to have a normal black pupil in ambient light, although the cataractous lens will absorb the light needed for image formation. The different causes expected in these forms of advanced (mature, fully opaque) cataracts suggest that different biochemical and cell biological mechanisms can influence pigmentation and scattering.

Slit-lamp images are valuable for the characterization of cataracts but do not necessarily provide critical information about early nuclear cataract formation, such as the influence of large particles that scatter at low angles near the optic axis. Importantly, slit-lamp images detect scattering that has a major component at high angles, specifically small particles or refractive index fluctuations near 100 nm diameter and smaller (148). In the early stages of cataract formation, the slit-lamp image may not correlate with visual acuity loss or poor functional vision. The hyperbaric oxygen (HBO) guinea pig animal model demonstrates that pure nuclear scattering detected by slit-lamp biomicroscopy can be present in otherwise transparent lenses with normal function (20,65,114,129). Thus, increased nuclear high-angle scatter seen in slit-lamp examinations of elderly humans may have minimal affect on image formation or visual acuity and may represent age-related changes rather than nuclear cataract formation (Fig. 2).

SPECIFIC CATARACTS

Nuclear Cataracts

Nuclear cataract includes, in general, congenital cataract, scattering related to a specific nuclear zone (lamellar, Christmas tree, retrodots), specialized types including hypermature and extremely pigmented (brunescent and nigra cataracts), rapidly advancing types, such as postvitrectomy and canine diabetic, animal models with specific defects in crystallins or membrane proteins, or animal models that simulate aging. Congenital and other genetically induced cataracts are discussed in Chapters 33. The most common human nuclear cataract is age-related nuclear cataract, which typically has a fifth decade onset, begins in the oldest cells of the lens core and is slowly progressing. This type of cataract has been thoroughly studied and in its more advanced form causes severe visual disability due to its location along the optic axis.

Age-Related Nuclear Cataract

For age-related nuclear cataract, an increase in light scattering near the inner fetal and embryonic nuclei can be detected as diffuse white scattering that is superimposed on the natural uniform yellow

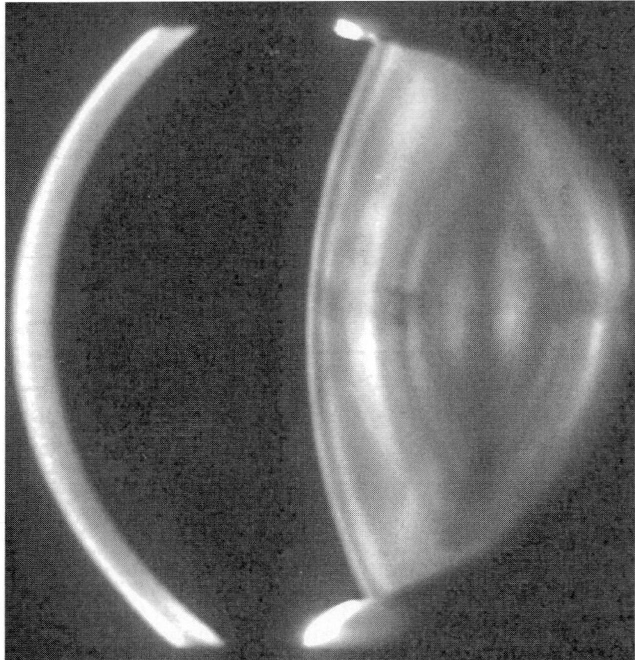

Figure 2 Slit-lamp image of an adult transparent human lens. Note the central sulcus (dark band of low scattering) and various zones of discontinuity where scattering is significant, even though these bands have minimal effect on image formation. *Source*: From Ref. 116.

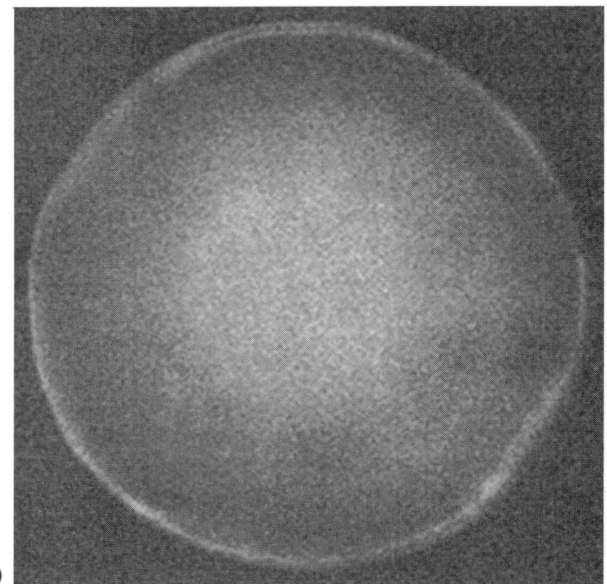

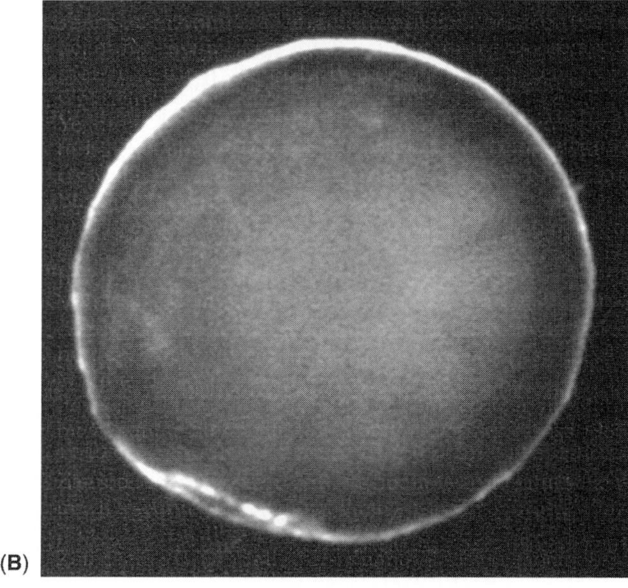

Figure 3 Examples of human age-related nuclear cataract. Darkfield in vitro imaging of two whole lenses removed by intracapsular extraction. (**A**) Pure nuclear cataract with central haze. (**B**) Nuclear cataract mixed with a minor amount of cortical scatter (lamella at 9–11 o'clock). Flattened regions at four o'clock (**A**) and seven o'clock (**B**) are due to the adhesion of a cryoprobe to remove the lenses.

pigmentation of the adult human nucleus (4,34,48, 95,96). At the early stage of cataract development, the visual complaint may be a slight loss of visual acuity, minimally blurred vision in one eye (possibly causing diplopia), and increased glare while driving at night. On a scale of nuclear opalescence, such as LOCS III (35), these early age-related nuclear cataracts would be graded 1–3 for a range of 0–6. Such lenses commonly qualify for cataract extraction; the relatively soft nucleus lends itself to complete emulsification using an ultrasonic probe (phacoemulsification) and extraction. In special cases when medically indicated, the opaque nucleus (extracapsular extraction) or the whole cataractous lens (intracapsular extraction) is removed and becomes available for research analysis (Fig. 3). In the United States, it is rare to have nuclei available from lenses graded 4 or higher in opalescence, or with a deep yellow (brunescent) color. Thus, most nuclear cataractous lenses available in the United States for research represent early stages of age-related nuclear cataracts.

Epidemiology and Risk Factors of Age-Related Nuclear Cataract

Several risk factors for age-related nuclear cataract have been identified. In Western countries, the main risk factors include smoking, diabetes mellitus, ultraviolet (UV) light exposure and age. In developing countries, such as India, the risk factors also include (in addition to the ones previously listed) malnutrition, dehydrating diseases, poverty and possibly other environmental factors as suggested by the early development of cataract, with an onset about 10 to 20 years before Western countries (16,113,142,157). Genetics may play a role in nuclear cataract formation and some studies have suggested a familial link and possibly genetic factors that explain a fraction of the cases (see Chapter 33). However, the prevalence of nuclear cataract over the world, in entirely different environments and cultures, suggests that most cases are caused by modifications in the normal aging process. Age is the strongest and consistently recurring risk factor. The evidence from many approaches suggests that normal aging when accelerated or advanced may be sufficient to trigger cataract formation. Oxidation has been determined to be one of the major factors influencing aging and cataract formation. Some studies link diets high in antioxidants with a reduced risk of nuclear cataract. However, increased intake of antioxidant supplements is not so easily related to reduced risk, and some studies report no protection or even increased risk (11,16,84,123,156). The underlying causes of cataract formation are likely to be in part influenced by lens oxidation; however, it is important to note that oxidation/reduction reactions occur in every cell routinely at the molecular level and are unlikely to be directly responsible for increased light scattering. Accumulation of oxidative damage must result in cellular changes that disrupt the normal uniform refractive index or generate objects that scatter light. Thus, whatever the driving forces are for molecular and cellular damage, analyses of the structural changes within lenses are valuable for understanding the mechanisms of cataract formation.

Etiology and Pathogenesis of Age-Related Nuclear Cataract Formation

Extensive evidence has been presented suggesting that oxidative damage is an important contributing factor in the formation of age-related nuclear cataracts (68,134,146). However, as pointed out previously, oxidative damage, which initially occurs on a small size scale, must accumulate to produce cellular alterations sufficiently large to scatter light (72). Therefore, an examination of the structural changes (whatever their cause) is essential to characterize the physical basis for increased light scattering. The scale of the structural changes has been defined theoretically. For an object to scatter a significant amount of light, it must be about 1/20 of the wavelength, or about 20 nm, in diameter for 400 nm-wavelength light (13,36). These small particles, or more accurately, the fluctuations in refractive index on this small scale, will produce scattering that can be characterized theoretically (14), using modifications of the Rayleigh scattering theory for small particles. Scattering from larger particles can also be predicted (41), employing a scattering theory developed by Mie in 1908 for globular particles of any size (111). When particles are larger than 200 nm there is a significant change in the scattering pattern with increased scattering at low angles (41,71). Thus, the range of 20 to 200 nm diameter (or fluctuations on this size scale) are considered small scattering objects, whereas particles larger than 200 nm diameter, and extending into the visible range, may be considered large particles. These distinctions, although somewhat arbitrary, are helpful for interpreting the sources of excess light scattering within cataractous lenses.

It is widely accepted that nuclear cataracts are caused by the abnormal aggregation of cytoplasmic crystallins into high-molecular-weight particles that scatter light (13,17,85–87). This hypothesis is based on extensive evidence establishing a firm correlation between the presence of protein aggregates and the observed light scattering from objects with predicted dimensions in the range of 20 to 200 nm and above, depending on the interpretation of the scattering data (85). The corresponding molecular weights of the aggregates (assuming protein density of 1.37 g/cc) are from 3×10^6 to 3×10^9 Da, and larger aggregates have been reported (17). It has been proposed that these aggregates precipitate or condense, such that they have higher refractive index than their surroundings, thus producing the fluctuations in refractive index that accounts for the observed scattering. The high-molecular-weight aggregates were first characterized from biochemical assays as the fraction remaining after the whole nucleus was incubated in 8 M urea (85,134). Many studies have shown that the urea-insoluble fraction increased with cataract formation and contained all three classes of crystallins (13,15,146). A common theme is that oxidative damage to the crystallins is the primary cause of posttranslational modifications that result in an enhanced association of crystallins into aggregates (70,78,146). Since the gamma-crystallins have a high sulfur content, it is reasonable to expect that disulfide oxidized forms would be extensive (68,108). Other oxidative modifications have been described and other modes of cross-linking proposed. For example, nonenzymatic glycation was shown to produce pigments and cross-linking (31,112). Moreover, alpha-crystallin was shown to be a chaperone that helped stabilize proteins and prevent their precipitation, presumably through hydrophobic interactions (83,121). It is clear that nearly all the crystallins are modified to some extent in aging and cataract formation and that aggregation is a primary event that occurs over many years (37). A consensus has developed that the cause of nuclear cataracts was the formation protein aggregates that scatter light.

A difficulty with the hypothesis that high-molecular-weight aggregates are the source of scattering in human age-related nuclear cataracts is that these aggregates have never been observed in vivo.

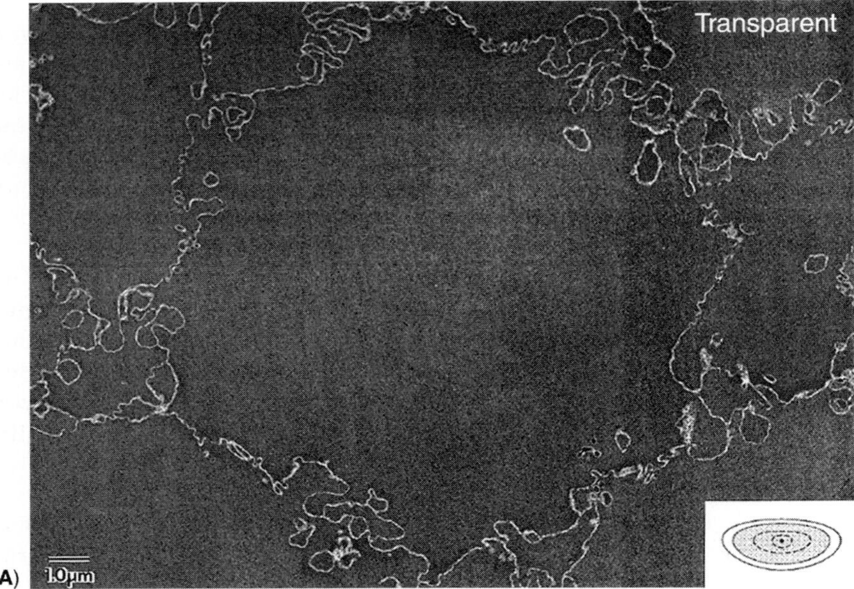

(A)

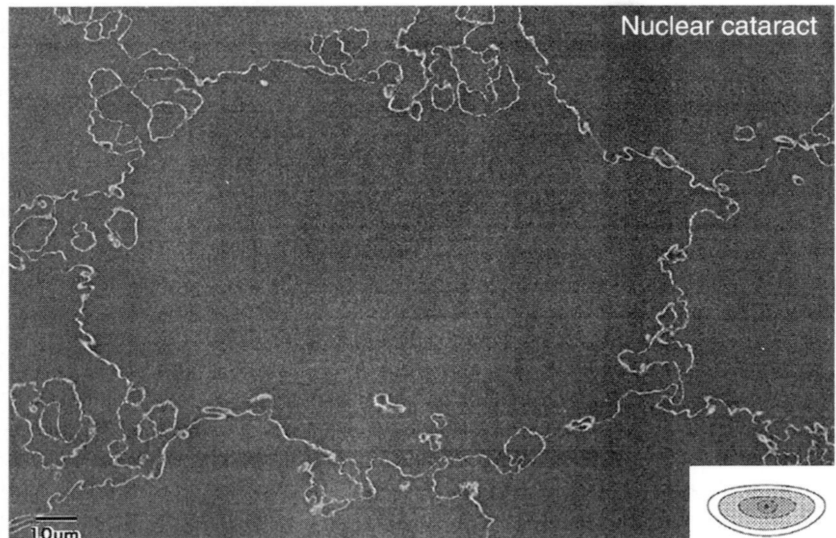

(B)

Figure 4 Fiber cells from the lens core by transmission electron microscopy. (**A**) Image from a 68-year-old transparent lens. (**B**) Image from a 75-year-old age-related nuclear cataract patient. *Source*: From Ref. 4.

Their size (roughly 20–200 nm) makes them ideal for examination using transmission electron microscopy (TEM). The smooth cytoplasm observed in TEM images of aged transparent and age-related nuclear cataracts suggest that other sources of scattering should be considered (Fig. 4) (1,4,66). A few examples of textured cytoplasm in human nuclear cataractous lenses (due to the redistribution of cytoplasmic components) are indicative of age-related changes (1). However, the degree of texturing is similar to that seen in the HBO guinea pig model (70), in which oxidative damage was confirmed by biochemical analysis and nuclear scattering was recorded in slit-lamp images (Fig. 5) (65). It is very important to note that the slit-lamp images clearly show that nuclear scatter increases with oxidative damage in lenses that remained clear and without observable cataracts (69,129). Because guinea pig lenses are still transparent after extended HBO treatment, it was concluded that the observed cytoplasmic texturing in nuclear fiber cells was not sufficient to produce a cataract (64).

The similarity of the nuclear cytoplasmic texture in TEM images of human transparent (noncataractous) and age-related cataractous lenses does not imply that high-molecular-weight aggregates do not exist, only that they do not form discrete particles that scatter light (66). The biochemical evidence for the existence of the aggregates is compelling. In addition the high-molecular-weight aggregates from the urea-insoluble

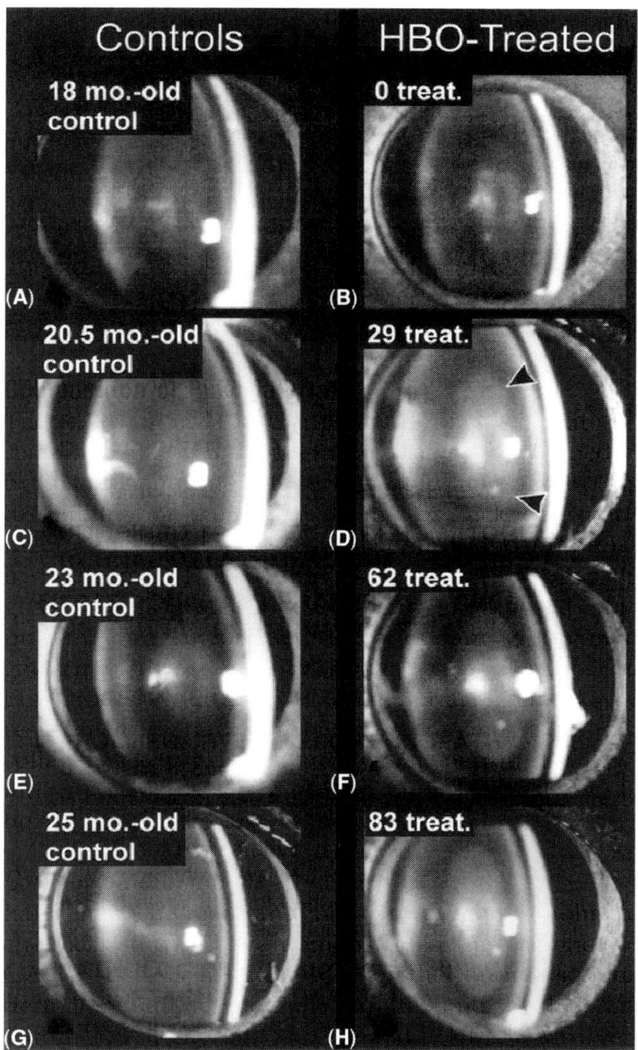

Figure 5 Slit-lamp biomicrographs of control and hyperbaric oxygen (HBO)-treated guinea pig eyes. (**A** and **B**) Controls for 18-month animals. (**C** and **D**) Control and 29 HBO treatments for 20.5-month animals. (**E** and **F**) Control and 62 HBO treatments for 23-month animals. (**G** and **H**) Control and 83 HBO treatments of 25-month animals. Although the scattering in the nucleus increased with HBO treatment, all lenses were clear without cataracts in ambient light. *Source*: From Ref. 65.

fraction have been visualized in vitro from bovine lenses (128) and human lenses (Fig. 6) (40). These aggregates were irregular assemblies of small 16 to 20 nm spheres, similar in size to alpha-crystallins, linked by protein threads. They were not discrete particles. It is reasonable to suggest that these irregular assemblies of proteins (which could be the high-molecular-weight aggregates) pack to form a hydrated network with interior spaces filled by smaller more mobile proteins to produce a uniform cytoplasm. Therefore, the most direct interpretation of the TEM images of cytoplasm in nuclear fiber cells suggests that the high-molecular-weight aggregates are present and form the basis for the close association of crystallins into a smooth and dense network with a high protein concentration and corresponding high refractive index (Fig. 4). The close association of crystallin proteins is fundamental to lens transparency (18,51). The aggregation of proteins reduces the osmotic activity, thus supporting the high protein concentrations found in lens nuclei (90,152).

The most important difference in structure of transparent lenses compared to early nuclear cataracts is the presence of large 1 to 4 μm diameter particles that are more numerous in the nuclear region of cataractous lenses (72). Because these particles are covered by multiple bilayers, they are called multilamellar bodies (MLBs). These rare particles appear to be randomly distributed in the nuclear core (en, fn, and jn; see Fig. 1) of age-related cataracts, and, using Mie scattering theory, it is estimated that they can scatter a significant fraction of the incident light (71). Importantly, the theory predicts that the scattering will be at low angles in the forward direction and thus can affect image formation at the macula of the retina (41,71). It is likely that the MLBs will have an important influence on visual deficits in the early stage of age-related nuclear cataract formation, even if slit-lamp images show relatively little nuclear high-angle scatter (Figs. 7 and 8).

Membranes as Potential Source of Excess Scatter

Membrane vesicles, fragments and multilamellar cell debris have been reported in the cortex of lenses subject to osmotic and other stresses that cause cell swelling and breakdown (2,46,52). These abnormal membrane structures probably account for most of the observed scattering in cortical cataracts. Numerous other studies have suggested a potential role of membranous structures in producing scattering during cataract formation (17,21,110). However, it is very rare in the lens nucleus to find regions of cell disruption containing membrane components sufficiently large to be significant scattering centers (4). The vast majority of membranes are plasma membrane pairs from adjacent cells that form specific patterns and junctional associations. MLBs, which are rare, are exceptional in that their membranes are thin and contain more than two layers (72). Even in regions where the interdigitations between adjacent fiber cells are very complex, the membrane pairs predominate. These pairs have been analyzed extensively using TEM ultrastructural techniques including thin sections, freeze-fracture, and immunogold labeling (42–44,55,160). These membrane pairs are characterized by gap junctions (16 nm thick), square array junctions (14 nm thick) and undulating membrane junctions containing aquaporin 0 (AQP0; 11 nm thick,

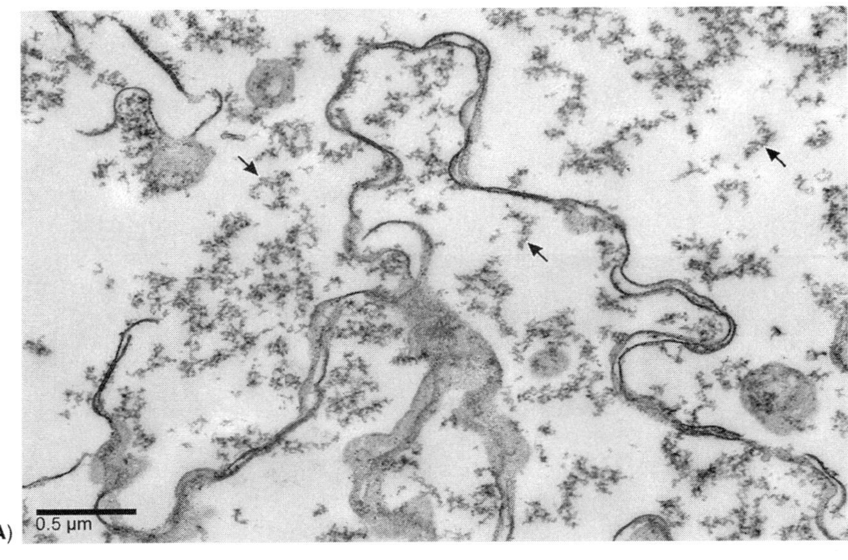

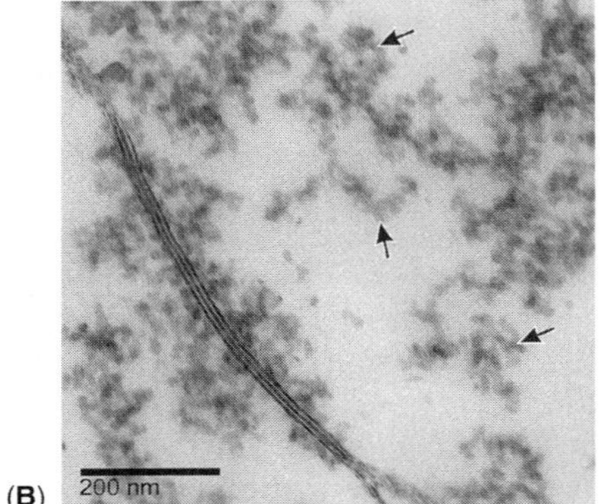

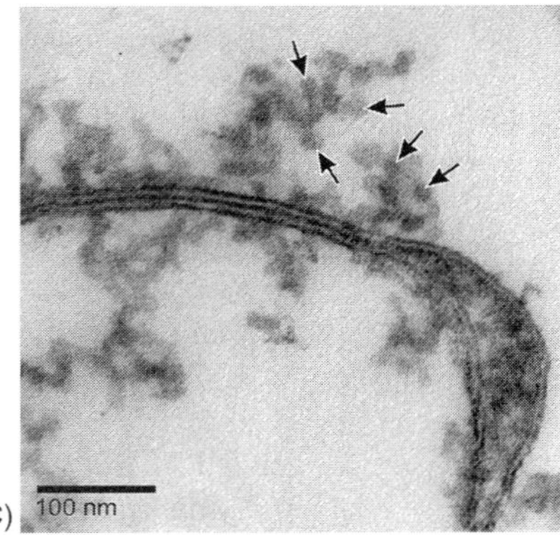

Figure 6 Transmission electron micrographs of the urea-insoluble fraction from the fetal and embryonic nuclei of an age-related nuclear cataract (80-year-old grade 3 on 0–4 scale, dark yellow). (**A**) Low magnification overview. Irregular material (*arrows*) could be high-molecular-weight aggregates. (**B**) Potential high-molecular-weight aggregates (*arrows*) adjacent to a large 16 nm thick gap junction. (**C**) Similar to (**B**) at high enough magnification to compare round profiles of particles (*arrows*) to the adjacent gap junction. It is likely that the particles are alpha-crystallin aggregated with other crystallins.

when both membranes are in contact across the ECS) (95,96). These junctional pairings probably have many functions that change with development and aging. It has been proposed that in early development, the main role of the junctions is in cell–cell communication and movement of water, whereas after differentiation and cell–cell fusion (97,125), the main roles are adhesion and minimization of the ECS (43,63,75,76,80).

It has been suggested that aging and nuclear cataract formation caused disintegration of portions of the membrane pair. Specifically, it was reported that segments of pure lipid bilayers were lost, resulting the direct connections between the cytoplasm and the ECS (Fig. 9) (45). Dense-staining deposits observed within the ECS of immature nuclear cataracts were hypothesized to result from the redistribution of proteins and fragments of posttranslationally modified crystallins and membrane proteins (Fig. 10) (2,4). Recent ultrastructural evidence from totally opaque mature cataractous nuclei from blind patients in India is consistent with these earlier observations. The membranes displayed a similar loss of bilayer segments and formation of ECS protein deposits. These studies also revealed numerous MLBs similar to those observed in less mature cataracts. The cytoplasm and cellular organization of the advanced Indian cataracts were otherwise similar to that of the less advanced cataracts from the United States. These observations support the hypothesis that opacification of advanced nuclear cataracts results from the gradual progression of cellular damage recorded in less mature cataracts. In these nuclear cataracts, it is suggested that high-molecular-weight protein aggregates contribute indirectly to the stability and texturing of the cytoplasm and do not form observable distinct light scattering particles. The excess light scattering and visual impairment are most likely accounted for by small particle (high-angle) scattering from slightly textured cytoplasm, disruption of membranes and ECS deposits, and by large particle (low-angle) scattering from MLBs. The probable cellular events leading to lens nuclear opacification are summarized (Table 1).

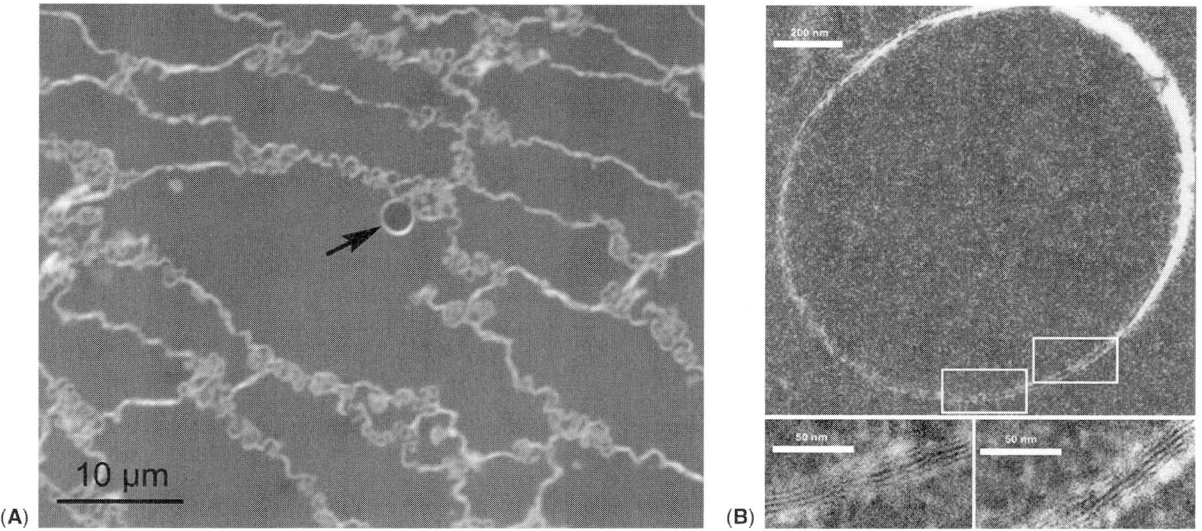

Figure 7 Multilamellar bodies (MLBs) from nuclei of age-related nuclear cataracts. (**A**) Light micrograph of toluidine blue oxide-stained section showing one large round MLB (*arrow*). (**B**) Transmission electron micrographs of an MLB showing multiple thin bilayer membranes in the lipid coat. Typical MLB particles are characterized by their 1 to 4 μm diameter size, spherical shape, lipid-rich coat, and dense protein interior. *Source*: From Ref. 41.

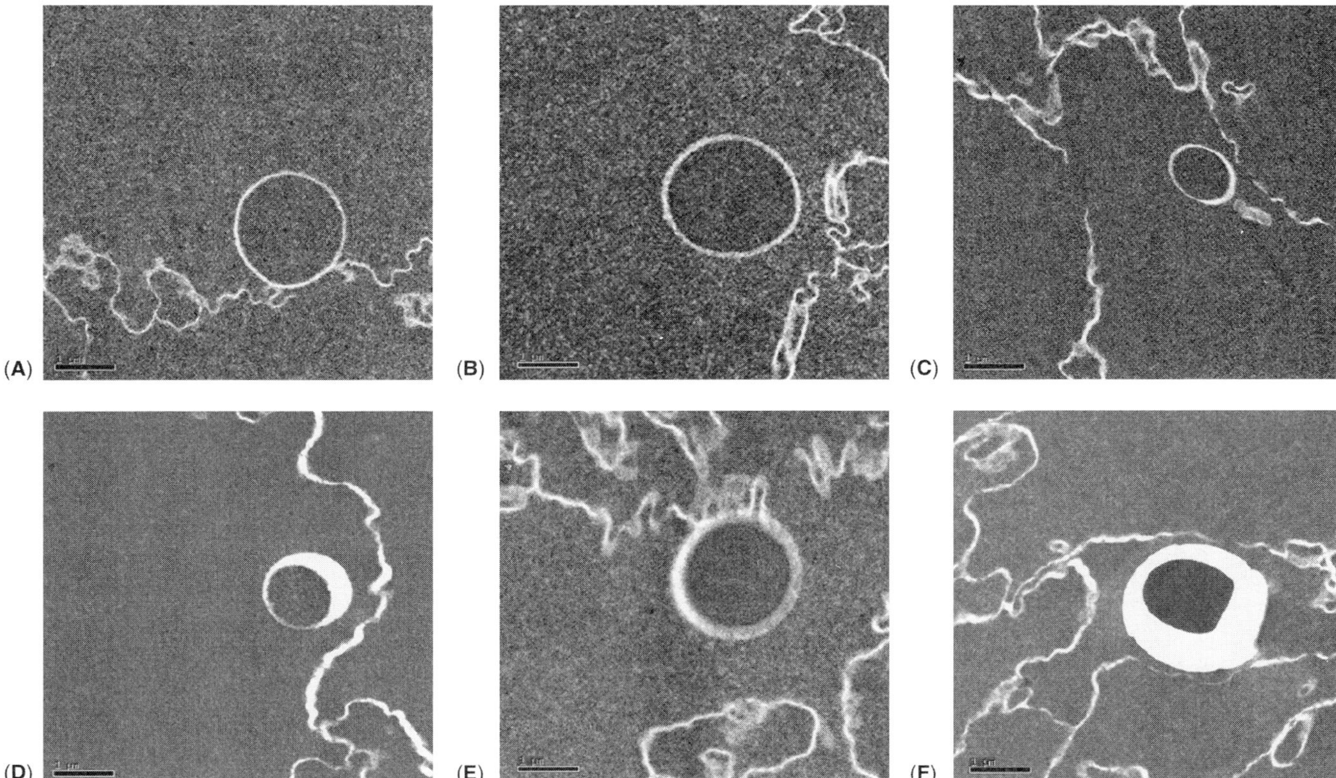

Figure 8 Electron micrographs of multilamellar bodies (MLBs) displaying variable internal protein density. The electron transmission of the MLB cores were compared to the adjacent cytoplasm in minimal dose conditions using en bloc stained samples. Values for internal relative refractive index could be derived from a standard curve. Although there is some variation in the density of the cytoplasm, the images display the key differences from the core to the cytoplasm, which increase in the order A–F. For comparison, if the cytoplasm is assumed to have $n = 1.40$ (97), then the greatest MLB internal densities are equivalent to $n > 1.50$. The scale bars are all 1 μm.

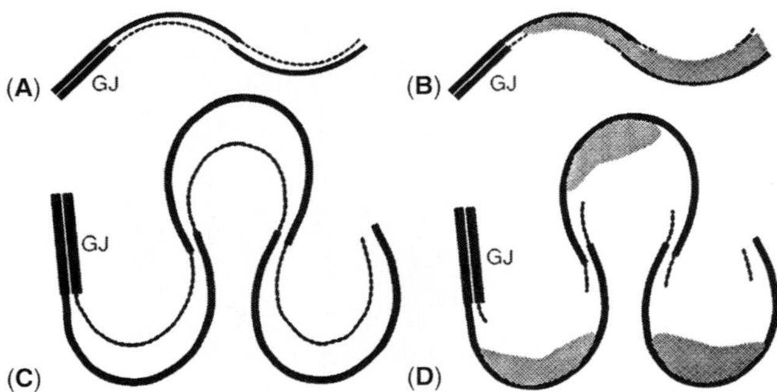

Figure 9 Proposal for membrane damage during age-related nuclear cataract formation. (**A** and **C**) Low- and high-amplitude undulations in normal transparent lenses. (**B** and **D**) Membrane loss at the pure lipid bilayers (*thin-dotted lines*) of junctions, exposing cytoplasm to extracellular space. Gray material represents deposits of protein-like material onto the membranes containing aquaporin 0 (AQP0) (*single thick lines*). *Abbreviation*: GJ, gap junctions (*paired thick lines*). *Source*: From Ref. 45.

Other Noncongenital Nuclear Cataracts

Lamellar (Zonular) Cataract

Lamellar cataract describes a nuclear opacification that occurs usually within one layer or zone (also called zonular). Opacities have been reported in the embryonic and fetal nuclei, but most often they appear in the layer just outside the fetal nucleus, termed the juvenile nucleus here, although terms such as perinucleus have been used. In slit-lamp images the layer can show increased scatter compared to the lower scattering interior (Fig. 11). Rarely, the adult nucleus will display higher scatter than the interior nuclear core (Fig. 12). Although the alteration of lens fiber cell organization creating this distribution of scattering is often unknown, the structural damage in these rare forms of nuclear cataract has been partially characterized (4). Fiber compaction, characteristic of this region, is accompanied by numerous damaged fibers that appear to be broken, producing large variations in protein-staining density and pronounced refractive index fluctuations. The disintegrating fiber cells release protein and membranes forming globular structures and multilamellar focal defects that probably account for the increased scatter (Fig. 13). Typically, lamellar cataract is congenital (8,162) and many specific genetic defects in humans and animal models result in increased scatter in one specific zone (see Chapter 33).

Christmas Tree Cataract

Christmas tree cataracts have been described as rare age-related cataracts comprising needle-shaped, crystalline opacities. They have been so designated because of the glistening, multiple refractile colors observed in these cortical and nuclear opacities. Christmas tree cataract has been thought to be a diffractive phenomenon, since the colors vary according to the angle of incidence and the outline of the opacities is barely visible with retroillumination (Fig. 14) (127).

In the 1967, Burian and Burns (30) described them as one of the ocular changes seen in an autosomal-dominant condition called myotonic dystrophy (MIM #160900; see Chapter 72). However, a later report of a case of Christmas tree cataract did not reveal any systemic associations (139). Therefore, it is likely that the lens changes in myotonic dystrophy are distinct from Christmas tree cataract. Indeed, it has been suggested more recently that the polychromatic granules observed in myotonic dystrophy herald the early stages of posterior subcapsular cataracts (PSCs), which progress to a characteristic stellar pattern at a later stage (116,117,139).

Clinically, Christmas tree cataracts can be unilateral or asymmetrically bilateral and have

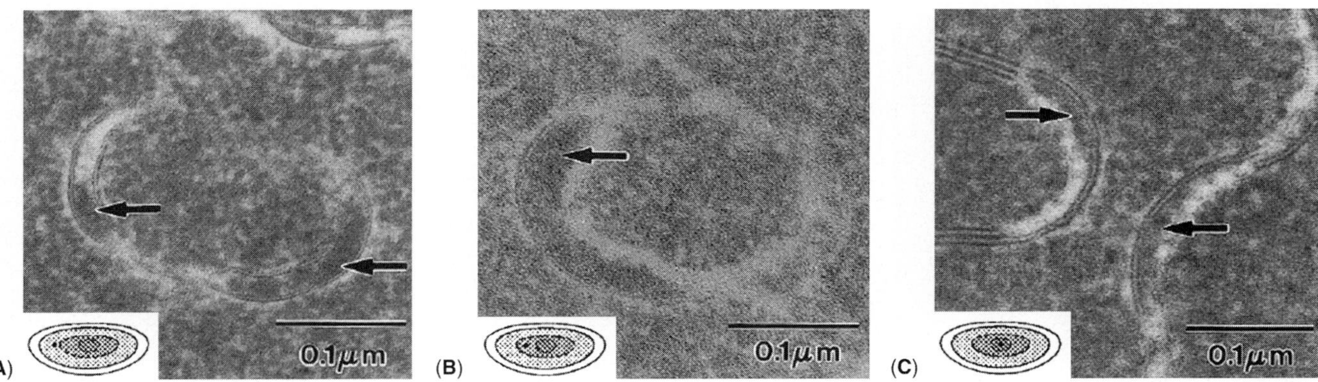

Figure 10 Transmission electron microscopy of protein-like deposits (*arrows*) in extracellular spaces in human nuclear cataracts. (**A**) Oval cross-section of a finger-like projection. (**B**) Curved membrane from fetal nucleus. (**C**) Curved membranes from the embryonic nucleus. Note in (**C**) that gap junctions form at the ends of the single-curved membrane (*left arrow*). *Source*: From Ref. 4.

Table 1 Important Cellular Events Leading to Age-Related Nuclear Cataract Formation

Normal aging produces modifications to cells and components as cortical fiber cells differentiate to become part of the nuclear mass, including loss of cytoskeleton and redistribution of proteins.
Fusion between cells is a key developmental event resulting in the formation of a functional syncytium during early development of the organelle-free zone in the lens nucleus.
Fiber cells respond to aging and outside influences, especially to oxidative stress, osmotic stress, or UV radiation, dependent on their developmental zone.
Cross-linking and association of cytoplasmic crystallins forms a hydrated network, which hardens in the fourth to fifth decade, signaling the onset of presbyopia; loss of water and cell compaction contribute to the lens nuclear hardening up to 1000-fold.
Early nuclear cataract changes include local cell disintegration and damage to membranes and crystallins; whether early changes are due to an extension of normal aging or to cataract abnormalities is unresolved.
Increased scattering usually begins in the lens center and progressively increases in the outer nuclear layers; scattering is white and is superimposed on the yellow coloration from pigments that initially appear in the nucleus, not the cortex, in young adulthood; nuclear color may advance from light yellow to brown to black as cataracts develop; these changes may be due to two separate processes and may or may not advance together; both can affect image formation by increased scattering, as well as light absorption.
Protein modifications result in aggregation and partial disintegration, producing fragments that may redistribute and potentially diffuse out of the lens.
Membranes are modified extensively in topology, in their junctional associations, and in chemical composition caused by lipid peroxidation; the overall membrane composition changes and damage results as segments are lost, thus exposing cytoplasm to extracellular space.
Migration of proteins and fragments into the extracellular space, or even out of the lens, results in deposits, enlargement of the extracellular space, and low-density regions (holes) that together produce refractive index fluctuations on a microscopic scale; these fluctuations are the source of small particle scatter (100 nm and smaller), which contributes to retinal stray light and is detectable by slit-lamp biomicroscopy (high-angle scattering).
High molecular-weight aggregates contribute significantly to the process, even though they are probably not distinct particles, but are most likely complex irregular associations of crystallins that form a stable network and restrict protein movements; the loss of proteins and fragments will thus create small low refractive index regions that are not filled in by mobile proteins, a critical feature that helps relate modern images of fiber cell cytoplasmic texture to biochemical analyses, demonstrating the formation of high-molecular-weight aggregates.
Multilamellar bodies, 1 to 4 μm diameter particles formed early in life, are altered with aging to produce relatively large scattering objects that contribute to low-angle (forward) scattering; although these large objects are not visible by biomicroscopic examination and probably do not contribute significantly to the high-angle scattering seen in slit-lamp images, their forward scattering may account for some of the initial visual deficits of nuclear cataracts.

minimal impact on vision (139). There are several theories as to the composition of these lustrous opacities. They have been thought to be composed of cholesterol, since their double refraction corresponds to that of cholesterol (115). Another group postulated that these opacities were due to parallel-sided stacks of fused cell membranes found at the same depth as the opacities in the slit-lamp (81). Shun-Shin et al. (127) have more recently concluded that cystine may be the most likely candidate for the Christmas tree needles and proposed that age-related aberrant breakdown of crystallins induced by elevated calcium levels resulted in the needles observed in this cataract.

Nuclear Retrodots

Bron and Brown (23) have defined retrodots as small (80–500 μm) round, oval, or oblong birefringent features that can occur in the adult lens after the fifth decade (Fig. 15). They were observed as early as 1914 by Vogt (153,154) and independently by Reese and Wadsworth (122). The term "retrodot" was used by later researchers because of the relative ease with which they could be seen using retroillumination (against the retinal red reflex) as opposed to focal and slit-lamp illumination (22). However, they are also visible using specular illumination (25).

Optically, they have been described as showing a light and a dark region, where the light zone is on the side opposite to the retinal illumination (23), unlike vacuoles which show an "unreversed" pattern (where the light zone is on the same side of the retinal illumination) (28). Consequently, retrodots have been suggested to have a higher refractive index than their surroundings (25,28). They are typically found in the perinuclear zone (juvenile nucleus), although they may also be observed in the superficial layers of the nucleus (23). While their flat "discus" shape and development was initially speculated to be due to the arrangement of lens fibers, a later study suggests they are independent of lens fiber arrangement (29). The lens may show one or two retrodots or up to as many as 400 in a single lens (23).

Lens retrodots may impair visual acuity (23) and contrast sensitivity (56). It has also been suggested that visual function may be more seriously affected when they occur in conjunction with nuclear light scatter (sclerosis) than when either occurs alone (23). Indeed, a statistically significant association has been found between the presence and grade of retrodots and

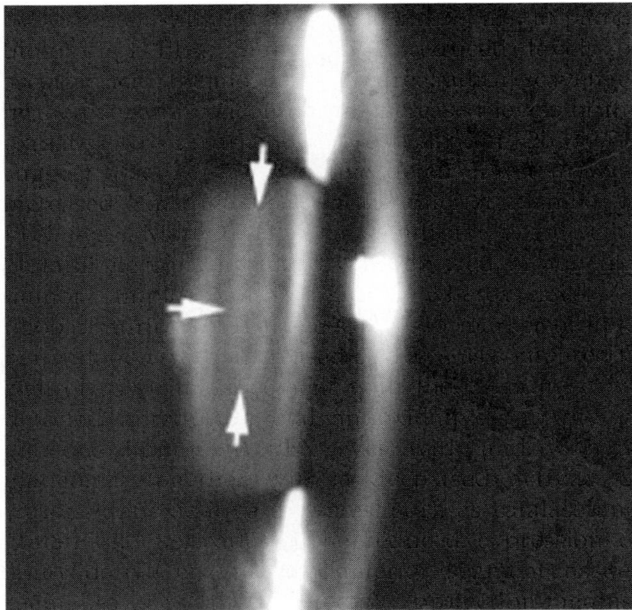

Figure 11 Lamellar or zonular cataract. Slit-lamp image of congenital human cataract shows a faint ring of increased scattering in the fetal nucleus (*arrows*) and a lower scattering interior. The underlying structural damage leading to the diffuse scattering in the ring is unknown. *Source*: Reprinted with permission from Dr. H.D. Riley and http://www.opt.indiana.edu/riley/HomePage/congential_cats/Text_congen_cats.html.

nuclear scatter, suggesting a possible common cause (126,143). It has been suggested that the material within the retrodot, due to its property of birefringence, is most likely calcium oxalate. Bron and Brown (23) have asserted that retrodots are identical to the calcium-containing birefringent bodies observed in vitro using crossed polarizing filters in an earlier study (79). It has been argued the lens containing retrodot opacities has likely suffered oxidative stress, leading to the oxidation of ascorbic acid to oxalate (23). A recent epidemiological multivariable analysis (56) has identified low alcohol consumption and high high-density lipoprotein cholesterol as potential risk factors for retrodot formation.

Hypermature Cataract

Hypermature cataract has been described clinically as an advanced cataract where partial absorption of liquefied cortical material results in a smaller than normal lens with a wrinkled capsule and a dense nucleus (32,158). The nucleus may have been displaced inferiorly due to gravity (Fig. 16) (32,158).

Hypermature cataract appears to have a different cause or pathway to total opacification than other maturing cataract types. Liquefaction of the cortex seems to be involved and these cortical changes may also influence damage in the nucleus, which can appear as a brunescent cataract with white scattering regions that are not symmetric (Fig. 17). The nature of the internal cellular damage is unknown at present, and the exact pathophysiology of hypermature cataract is not clear. Clinical and histopathologic observations suggest that they may follow the formation of a mature cataract, where the lens is either swollen (otherwise called intumescent cataract) principally in the anterior–posterior diameter, or lacks any clear cortex underneath the anterior capsule (32,158). Morgagnian globules consisting of small and large fragments of cortical cells and altered protein material have been suggested to result in a hyperosmolar lens, which leads to the changes seen in the mature

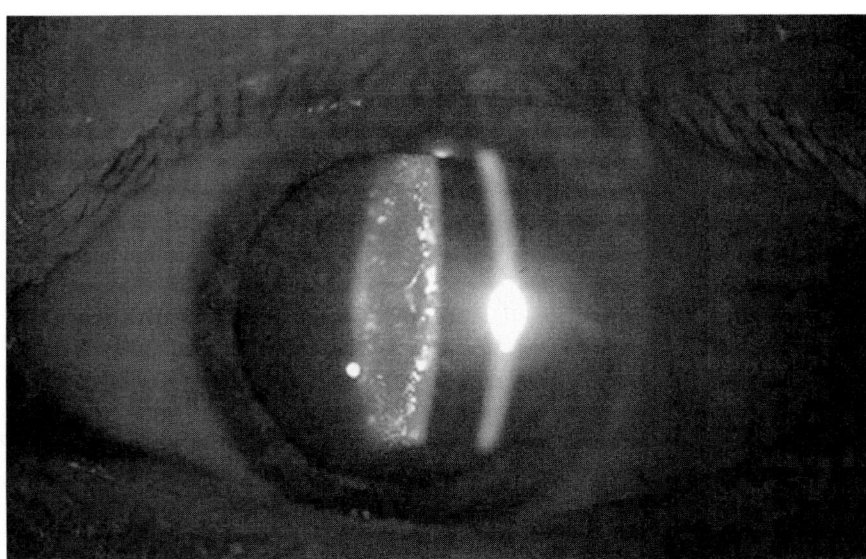

Figure 12 Lamellar cataract showing punctate scattering centers mainly within the adult nucleus. The slit-lamp image reveals large objects at the anterior surface of unknown internal structure. *Source*: Reprinted with permission from P.J. Saine and http://www.pjsaine.com/OphthalmicPhotography/PJSOPAC.html.

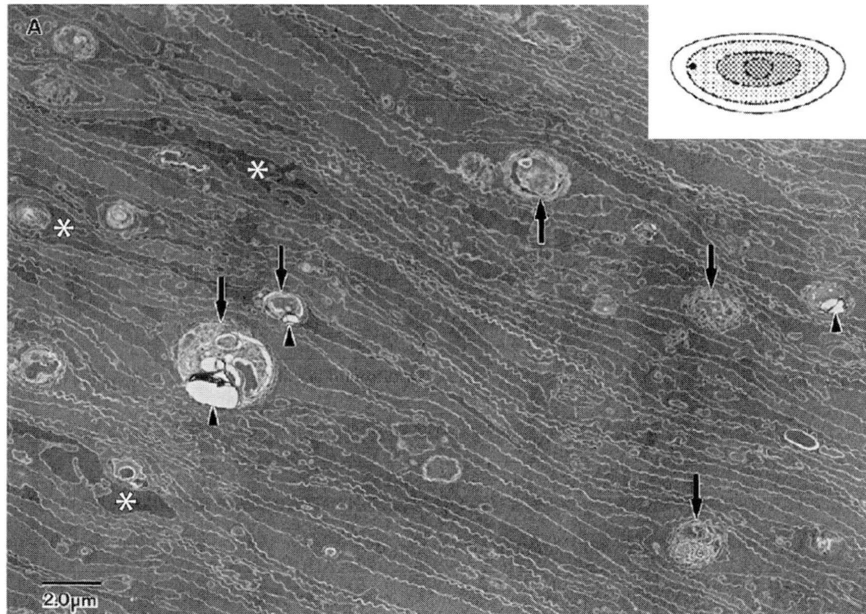

Figure 13 Transmission electron microscopy image of fiber cell damage in a human nuclear cataract (89 years old). As indicated in the diagram (*inset*) the image was taken from the adult nucleus near the equator of the lens. Damage was less severe in the layers on either side of this region, characterized by compacted fiber cells of variable size and density. Some fiber cells were very dense (*asterisks*) probably indicating high protein density and high refractive index compared to adjacent cells. This pattern would increase diffuse light scattering. Many focal defects were observed (*arrows*) that could be punctate scattering objects. Some regions are devoid of material (*arrowheads*) and may indicate low refractive index regions that can also induce strong light scattering. *Source*: From Ref. 4.

cataractous lens described above (158,159). If liquefied material remained intact within the capsule, the lens appears as a bag-containing milky-white fluid no longer able to support the weight of the nucleus (Morgagnian cataract) (158). Liquefied cortical lens material of sufficiently small molecular size has been suggested to be absorbed through the capsule into the anterior chamber resulting in hypermature cataractous changes. Rarely, the thinned capsule in a mature or hypermature cataract may rupture allowing the contents to spill directly into the anterior chamber of the eye. The lens epithelial cells have been reported to be degenerate in mature and hypermature cataracts (158). Also, if allowed to progress further, crystals of calcium oxalate, cholesterol, and insoluble amino acids may become deposited. Additional ultrastructural and biochemical changes in the cortex, as well as reasons for capsular permeability, are presented by Bron and Habgood (24).

Brunescent/Nigra (Black) Cataract

Lens pigmentation is characteristic of any aged primate lens nucleus (54). Most young animals, including those used as models, and the cortex of primate lenses do not display lens coloration. In humans the yellow coloration begins in the second

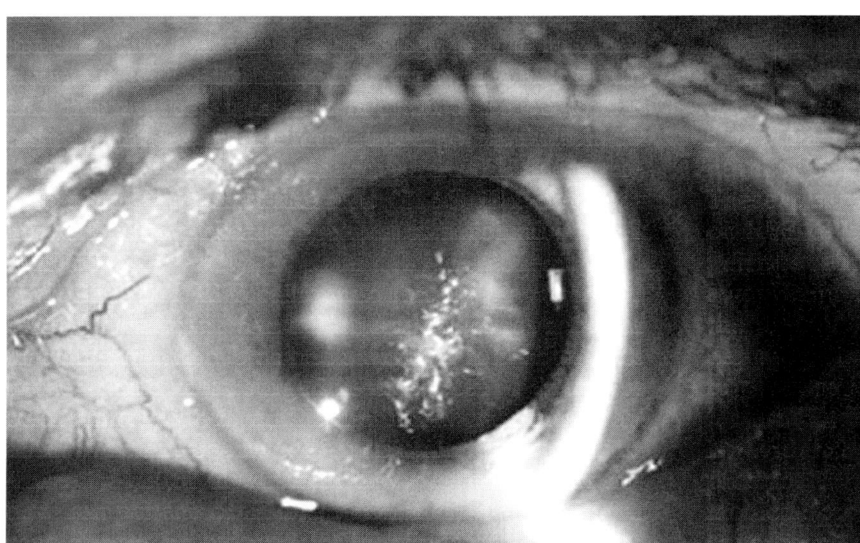

Figure 14 Bright punctate objects of a Christmas tree cataract seen in direct focal illumination. The colors (not seen here) are thought to be a function of the angle of illumination and the crystalline composition. They often have no important influence on visual function. *Source*: From Ref. 139.

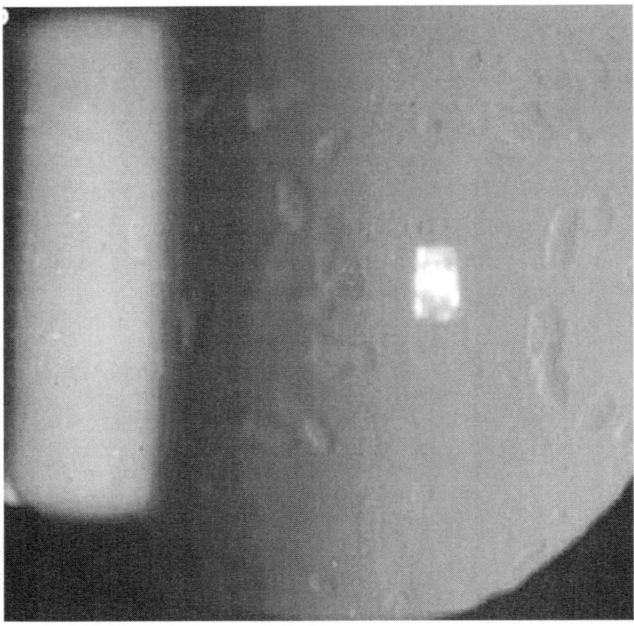

Figure 15 Retrodots seen using retro illumination. *Source*: From Ref. 56.

decade and continues to increase in intensity with age, although at a variable rate. The extent of coloration has been linked to many factors including UV radiation exposure, diabetes mellitus, and nuclear cataract formation (146). The yellow pigments may filter blue light and serve as a protection of the retina (163). Yellow pigmentation has been so closely associated with age-related nuclear cataract that some scales of nuclear opacification have been described in terms of pigmentation intensity (119,146), which can progress through dark yellow-brown (amber or brunescent) to fully black (cataracta nigra). However, because some nuclear cataracts can be totally opaque without significant yellow coloration, this suggests that the white scattering typical of cataractous lenses may in some cases form independently from the build up of yellow pigments. Typically, nuclear opacification and yellow pigmentation progress together and perhaps both are influenced by oxidation (10,146). In extreme cases, the pigmentation can build up without apparent white scattering superimposed and result in totally opaque lenses. In these cases the dark brown-black nucleus causes blindness through the absorption (rather than scattering) of light. The pigmentation has two main sources, modifications of protein-bound tryptophan (93) and glycation of cytoplasmic crystallins (112,161). Therefore, the pigmentation appears mainly to modify crystallins, including the promotion of protein cross-linking.

Cortical Cataracts

Posterior Subcapsular Cataract

PSCs are often described as "complicated cataracts" because they occur secondary to inherited intraocular disease, such as retinitis pigmentosa, gyrate atrophy, Usher syndrome (see Chapter 35), high myopia (see Chapter 26), and aniridia (see Chapter 52), as well as chronic use of pharmaceutical agents (e.g., corticosteroids and phenothiazines), in association with systemic diseases (e.g., diabetes mellitus and myotonic dystrophy), and as a complication of surgery (e.g., vitrectomy and trabeculectomy). Irrespective of their etiopathogenesis, all PSCs are presumed to be the result of dysplastic fiber cells migrating toward,

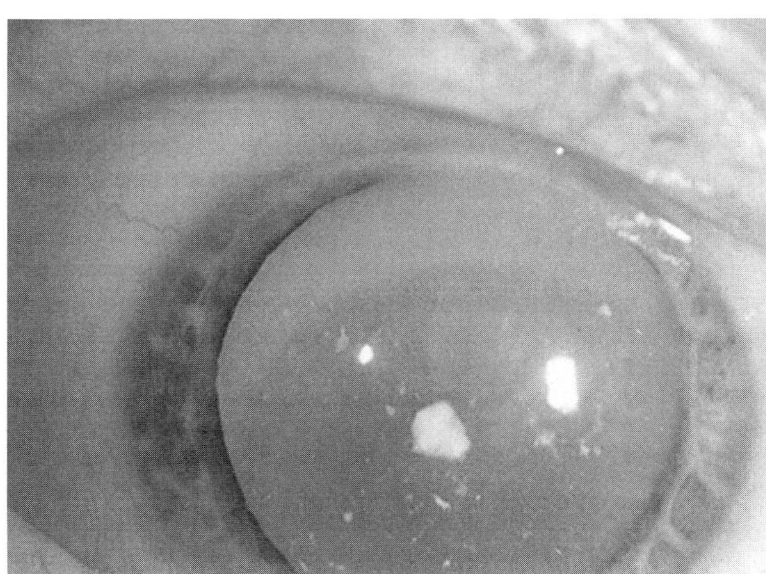

Figure 16 Morgagnian cataract. The cortex has liquefied and become cloudy. The nucleus has descended due to gravity and is opaque. *Source*: From Ref. 116.

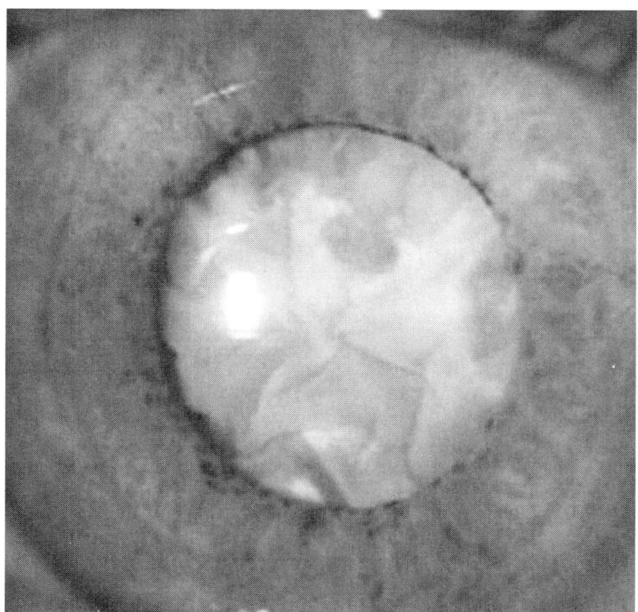

Figure 17 Hypermature cataract. The white scattering of the nucleus is highly irregular and dense. The capsule is wrinkled suggesting major changes in the cortex as well. *Source*: Reprinted with permission from Dr. C.N. Chua and http://www.mrcophth.com/cataract/cataract.html.

and amassing beneath, the lens capsule at the posterior pole to form a dense, opaque plaque. However, correlative structural/optical analysis of PSCs in animal models of retinitis pigmentosa, chronic treatment to mediate long-lasting neural and behavioral plasticity, and long-term use of corticosteroids, strongly suggest that the site of the opacity in most PSCs is primarily a region of abnormal fiber development or malformation of posterior sutures. This principle is best illustrated for a typical PSC from a Royal College of Surgeons Rat, an animal model of human PSC that develops as a consequence of autosomal recessive retinitis pigmentosa (Fig. 18) (6,7). Essentially identical structural compromise has been shown to occur in transgenic animal models, for both autosomal recessive and autosomal-dominant retinitis pigmentosa. The mechanism that induces this type of cataract has been presumed to be lipid peroxidation products released into the vitreous as retinal degeneration occurs. The appearance of these PSCs from animal models is very similar to that seen in human PSCs clinically when observed through a surgical dissecting microscope. But when these same PSCs were examined using a higher resolution scanning electron microscope (SEM), it was apparent that the opaque plaque was a site of enlarged posterior ends of fibers that had turned up and away from the polar axis, rather than abutting and overlapping as paired enantiomeric fibers to form sutures. These micrographs demonstrate the importance of examining cataracts with high-resolution microscopes. The manner in which specimens are prepared and the capabilities of the SEM permit an examination of fibers along their length from the equator to the poles. In sectioned material of such a plaque, the abnormally enlarged and improperly arranged posterior ends of fibers would be cut at a variety of angles that would produce a micrograph of seemingly abnormally enlarged bladder cells of Eshaghian and Streeten (60) gathered at the posterior pole (3). It is noteworthy that these PSCs are internalized by new fiber growth, after retinal degeneration (7). Again, slit-lamp biomicroscopic examination of these lenses suggests that the new growth that internalizes these PSCs is normal. However, correlative low-power helium neon laser scanning analysis of the optical quality in these lenses, followed by ultrastructural examination of their structure, reveals that their optical quality (focusing ability) is significantly compromised, although the lens is not opaque (94). In a similar manner, SEM reveals that the PSCs resulting from long-term use of drugs to treat certain neurological disorders, as well as long-term use of corticosteroids to treat certain diseases, are also likely to be the result of a posterior sutural malformation.

Other Cortical Cataracts

There are numerous types of cortical cataracts with different causes. Sutural cataracts are a common type of cortical cataract that often occurs secondary to certain diseases (e.g., myotonic dystrophy and diabetes mellitus), long-term use of certain drugs (e.g., steroids), and UVB irradiation. The structural compromise at the site of the opacity in these cataracts has been described as being the result of disruption of fiber ends, and a deposition of extraneous cellular material at fiber ends, both of which by definition happen at the sites of sutures. But this information, derived generally from observation of anteroposterior thick- and thin-sectioned material examined at relatively high magnification, is not likely to be accurate for the following reasons. The vast majority of fiber cells has a simple spring or coiled shape. Thus, the entire length of most fibers does not lie within a plane coincident with the lens polar axis. Furthermore, whereas fiber shape is uniform along fiber length, fiber ends are irregular in shape. In addition, since lenses dissected free from the zonules prior to fixation spontaneously assume a more accommodated configuration, the fiber ends are more interfaced. In consideration of all of the above, sectioned material of suture regions reveals a complex field of fiber ends cut at multiple angles that can easily be misinterpreted as being representative of disrupted fiber ends and/or extraneous cellular material. By comparison, the examination of intact, complete

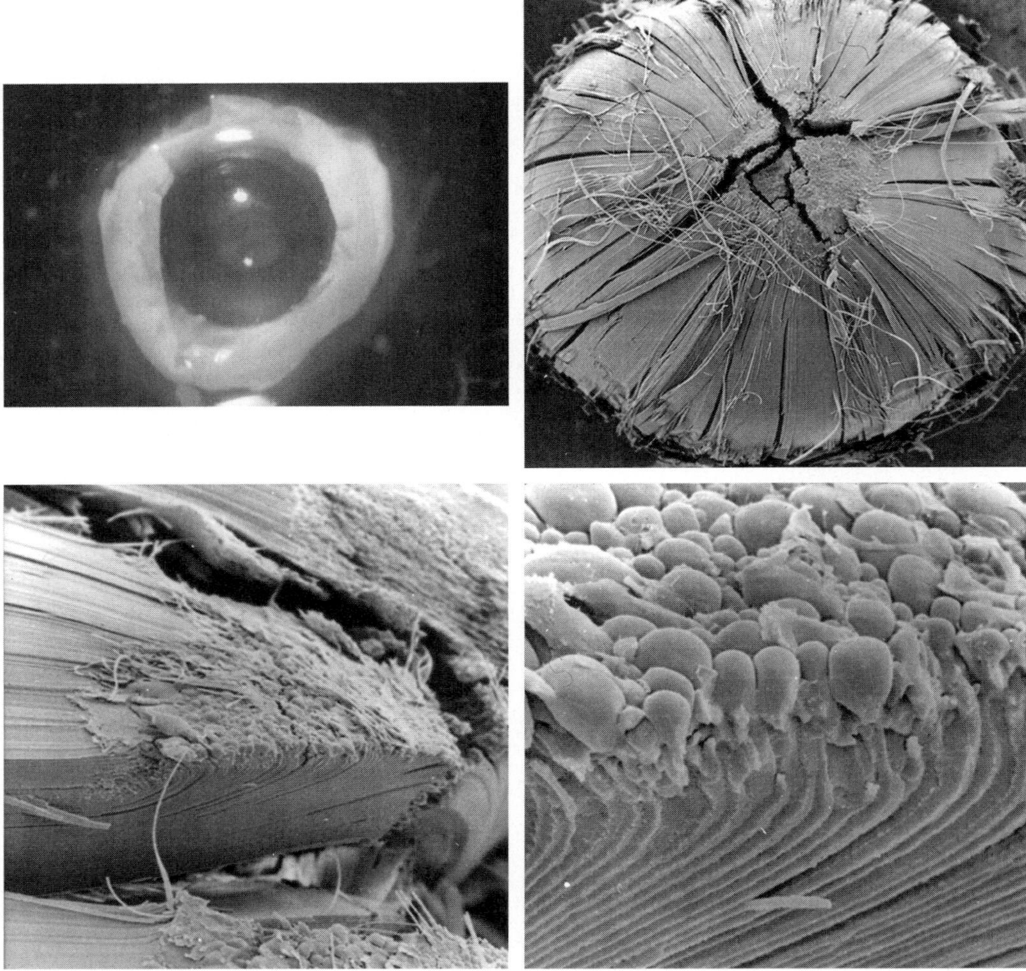

Figure 18 Posterior subcapsular cataract in the Royal College of Surgeons rat model. Low magnification view of posterior lens with polar opacity (*upper left*). Scanning electron microscopy (SEM) image of the posterior pole (*upper right*; × *20*). High magnification SEM images of the posterior pole cell damage showing abnormal orientation of terminal ends of fibers (*lower left*; × *100*) and enlargements of the fiber tips at the posterior suture (*lower right*; × *1000*).

suture patterns at low magnification, and of individual fiber ends from the same suture branches at higher magnification by SEM, reveals that sutural cataracts are characterized by growth malformation. How the diabetic condition or long-term use of steroids causes the normally exact construction of sutures to be so compromised needs to be determined. But as is clearly seen in the micrographs (Figs. 19 and 20) of normal and diabetic human lenses, as well as of rat lenses with experimentally induced diabetes mellitus, the principle structural compromise is clearly abnormal suture development. Again, this abnormal development does not necessarily produce a site of opacity. But rather, such sites can always be quantifiably shown to be indicative of reduced optical quality or focusing ability. If their transition to abnormal image quality can be quantified and proven to be a consistent predictor of nascent cataractogenesis, then such early diagnosis would be invaluable for treatment when restorative treatments for cataracts are developed in the future.

Cuneiform Cortical Cataracts

Similarly, cuneiform cortical cataracts are also the result of suture malformation. This common type of cortical cataract has previously been described as the product of an age-related growth malformation (99). This interpretation is only generally correct. Cuneiform cortical cataracts are typically seen as either early onset, occurring in the third to fourth decade of life, or late onset, occurring in the sixth or seventh decade of life. As the crystalline lens develops and grows throughout life, secondary fiber cells are organized into progressively more intricate iterations of suture patterns: a three-branch Y suture during the

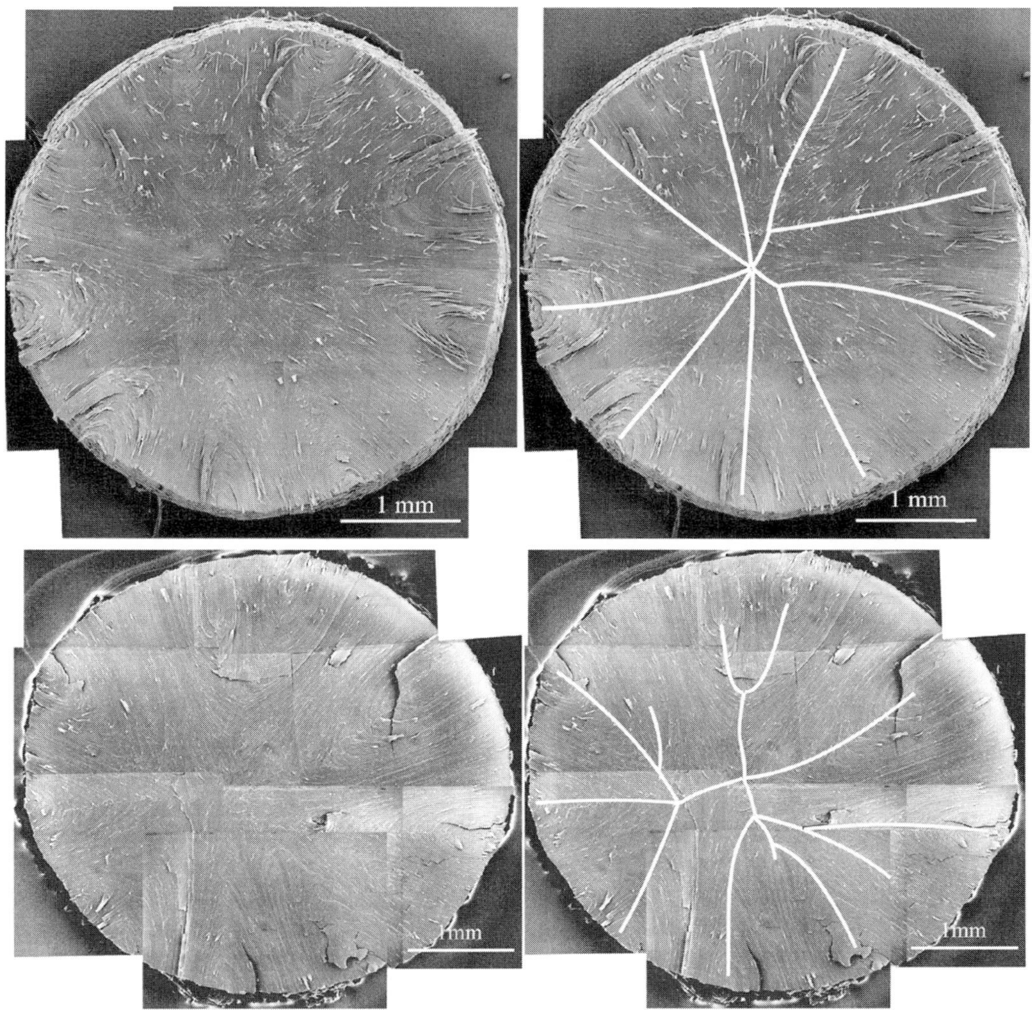

Figure 19 Scanning electron micrographs of suture pattern in a young adult human lens (*upper left*) with the normal suture lines traced (*upper right*). Similar image from an adult patient with diabetes mellitus (*lower left*). The suture pattern is very abnormal (*lower right*). *Source*: From Ref. 95.

fetal period, a six-branch, simple star suture during infancy, the nine-branch star suture throughout childhood and adolescence, the 12-branch complex star suture throughout adulthood, and rarely, the 15-branch most complex star suture from middle- to old-age. SEM examination of early-onset cortical cataracts reveals that the normally orderly and progressive construction of the six- and nine-branch suture patterns were not properly completed during the first three decades of life. Similarly, SEM examination in late onset cortical cataracts, shows that the normally orderly and progressive construction of nine to 12- and 15-branch suture patterns were not properly completed from the fourth through seventh decades. Note that in both cases, it took 30 years before the malformed sutures were manifest as an opacity (99). Thus, while these opacities are age-related, the comparable compromise of the fundamental growth scheme of lenses indicates that this abnormality is not necessarily a direct consequence of age. In addition, it is more accurate to categorize these cortical cataracts as corticonuclear cataracts. That is to say the onset of sutural malformation occurs when these fibers are cortical fibers, but is not manifest as a cuneiform opacity until 30 years later when these same fibers are considered nuclear fibers.

Osmotic Cataracts

Osmotic stress can be created in a lens by the accumulation of sugar alcohols. Following exposure of the lens to excess sugar, as occurs in diabetes, galactosemia or diets rich in sugars, glucose and galactose are metabolized in part by aldose reductase into sorbitol and dulcitol, respectively (33,91,149,150). These polyols do not readily diffuse from the cell

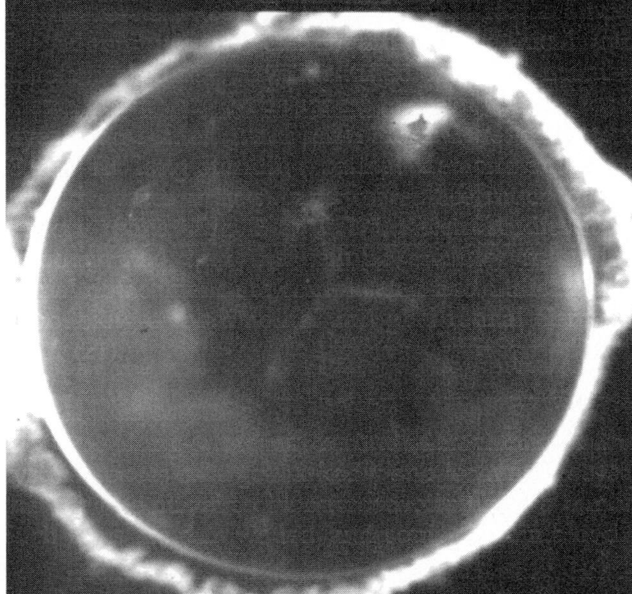

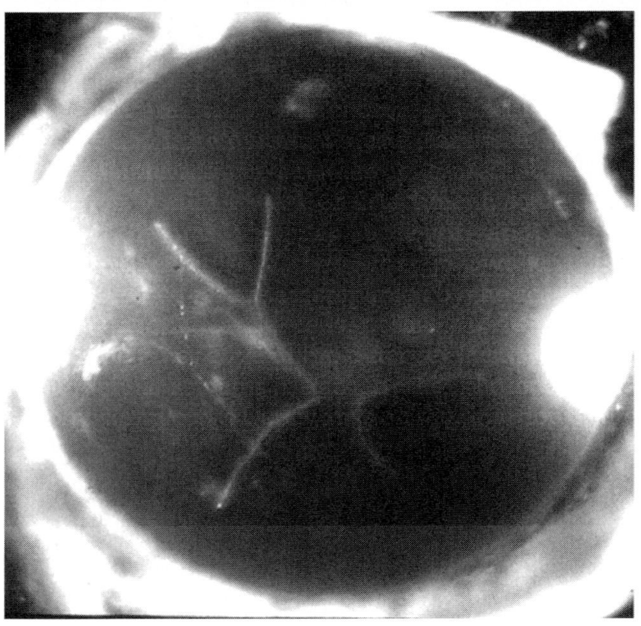

Figure 20 Light micrograph of normal rat lens (*top*) and diabetic rat lens (*bottom*) after streptozotocin treatment.

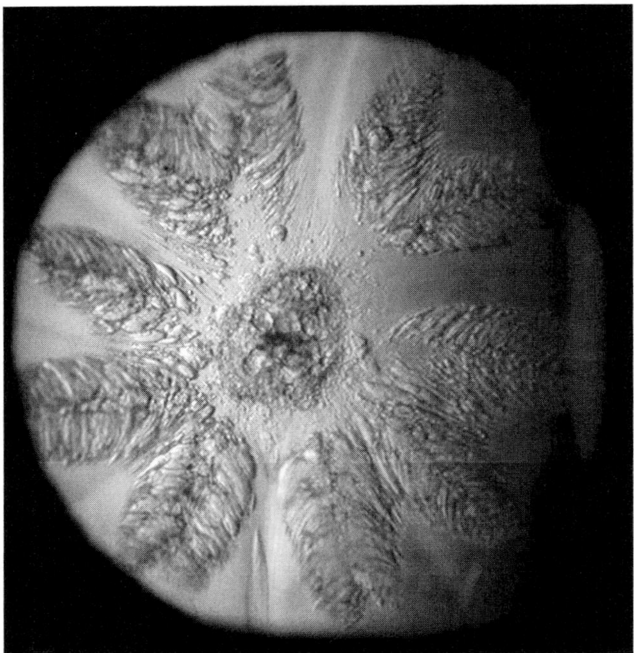

Figure 21 Osmotic cataract light micrograph showing cortical cell swelling aligned with sutures in human lens. *Source*: Reprinted with permission from P.J. Saine and http://www.pjsaine.com/OpthalmicPhotography/PJSOPAC.html.

interior or are not further metabolized efficiently. The accumulation of sugar alcohols creates an osmotic gradient that pulls water from the aqueous humor, causes cell swelling, and possibly cell rupture and cataracts (103). This process has been very well characterized in animal models of induced diabetes and excess galactose feeding (57,141,147). Aldose reductase, the first enzyme in the metabolism of excess sugar, was confirmed to be the critical enzyme based on studies of transgenic mice overexpressing aldose reductase (105). Aldose reductase has been very well characterized structurally (137) and aldose reductase inhibitors have been shown to reduce or eliminate the osmotic-induced opacification in animal models (88,124). Effective aldose reductase inhibitors for humans are being sought to reduce the damage in lenses and other tissues of extended exposure to high levels of glucose in diabetic patients (135). In humans, the initial lens swelling can cause myopia and other visual problems (26). If corrected early or controlled in patients with diabetic mellitus, the swelling can be reversed with no long-term effects (59). Extended exposure or fluctuating high levels of serum glucose can lead to irreversible swelling and cell damage initially in the equatorial region of the cortex and sometimes along the sutures (Fig. 21).

Cortical opacities and PSC are common in patients with diabetes mellitus (26) and extensive cell damage has been reported in human lenses, with the most pronounced damage occurring near the cortex–nucleus interface (2). In a rabbit animal model, it was shown that cell swelling and damage depended on the developmental region examined, with the most severe damage in the cortex and less damage in the nucleus (42). In diabetic humans, it was confirmed that, throughout the nucleus, fiber cell compaction occurred, rather than cell swelling, typical of an aging human lens nucleus (64). Glycation of proteins has been demonstrated in patients with diabetes mellitus and may account for the enhanced yellow coloration of the lens nucleus and rapid advance of nuclear cataracts (138).

Oxidative stress has been shown to contribute to cell damage and cataract formation in osmotic cataracts. Although the source of the oxidative stress in not fully understood, there is evidence that the nucleotide cofactor consumed by aldose reductase is also needed by glutathione reductase to maintain levels of the antioxidant glutathione (106). In an oxidation sensitive (OXYS) rat animal model for oxidative stress, there is an osmotic stress component because fiber cell swelling was observed in the cortex (109). It was hypothesized that glucose uptake was enhanced in these nondiabetic animals and that autoxidation and other sources of oxidative stress may be significant (109). Importantly, lipid peroxidation was shown to be enhanced throughout the lens of OXYS rats and this was associated with several forms of fiber cell damage in different developmental zones, including the formation of multilamellar cell defects in the nucleus (109). Lipid peroxidation has been suggested to be a major factor in human age-related cataracts (9). The oxidative stress may cause damage in different regions of the lens and supports the observation that the initial site of opacification, for example, in the cortex, may lead to classification of the cataract as cortical, even though the damage may be in multiple regions. Moreover, osmotic stress may induce abnormalities in fiber cell development that can adversely affect optical quality even before cataract opacification is observed (see Figs. 19 and 20) (99,130).

Cataracts Secondary to Ocular Surgery

Spaeth (131) has stated that some types of ocular surgery are rarely restorative or curative. Rather, some ocular procedures substitute one problem for another with the result that the new problem is less significant than the old. For example, trabeculectomy, generally considered the standard "filtration" type of surgery for most cases of open-angle glaucoma, very frequently leads to cataract. Thus, while technical success in the treatment of glaucoma (reduction in intraocular pressure) is achieved at satisfactory levels by trabeculectomy, cataract development remains an important issue for glaucoma surgical therapy programs.

Another example of an ocular surgery that often leads to cataract is vitrectomy. The most common indication for vitrectomy is vitreous hemorrhage caused by proliferative diabetic retinopathy. Other indications for vitrectomy are retinal detachment, and as an adjunct treatment for endophthalmitis. Vitrectomy-induced cataractogenesis begins within 24 h following surgery, as a subtle, feathery, PSC centered on posterior suture branches, often with a granular or placoid vacuolar appearance. Although this opacity generally fades over a few days, fine fundus details are unresolvable and thereby compromise diagnostic evaluation of surgical performance. In any case, even though the postvitrectomy PSC is transient, greater than 50% of patients subsequently develop nuclear sclerotic cataract (NSC) within 3 to 5 years following surgery necessitating additional surgery.

Rabbits have been used as an animal model to elucidate the mechanism of cataract formation following the above described surgical procedures, and to test the efficacy of therapeutic drugs designed to prevent the formation of these cataracts (100). The results of these studies are both noteworthy and unexpected. Following either vitrectomy or trabeculectomy, the simple, two branch, horizontal line suture of rabbits is invariably altered by the production of as many as 16 additional, abnormal suture subbranches (Fig. 22). Each of these abnormal subbranches is located either directly at or in close proximity to the surgical site. For example, in the vitrectomy surgery, typically, 3 months postsurgery, one or more abnormal suture branches are seen to be forming. Correlative quantitative optical quality analysis reveals that these structurally compromised posterior sutures are responsible for a significant decrease in focusing ability, though not necessarily a site of opacity. In the case of trabeculectomy surgery, typically 3 months postsurgery, one or more abnormal suture branches are seen at or in close proximity to the surgical site at 11 o'clock. Additional experiments with the surgical procedure performed by a left-handed surgeon, revealed one or more abnormal suture branches in close proximity to the surgical site at the one o'clock position. Again, quantitative optical quality analysis revealed that the compromised posterior sutures were responsible for a significant decrease in focusing ability, although to not necessarily a site of opacity.

The fact that lenses from the above described experimental studies were not opaque might suggest that they are not a good model for studying human cataracts following vitrectomy and trabeculectomy. However, this view fails to account for the potentially precataractous changes detected in the animal models and for the appearance of multiple defects in lenses as cataracts develop. For example, the cuneiform capacities of cortical cataracts are often located far enough on the periphery of the lens so as not to negatively impact vision. It is only when a PSC is formed right along the visual axis or scatter caused by a central nuclear cataract that blindness results, necessitating surgical removal of the lens. It is entirely possible that the compromised posterior sutures in the rabbit lens model for cataract following vitrectomy and/or trabeculectomy would in time have manifested as a PSC. Indeed whereas PSCs are the more predominant type of cataract following vitrectomy in young

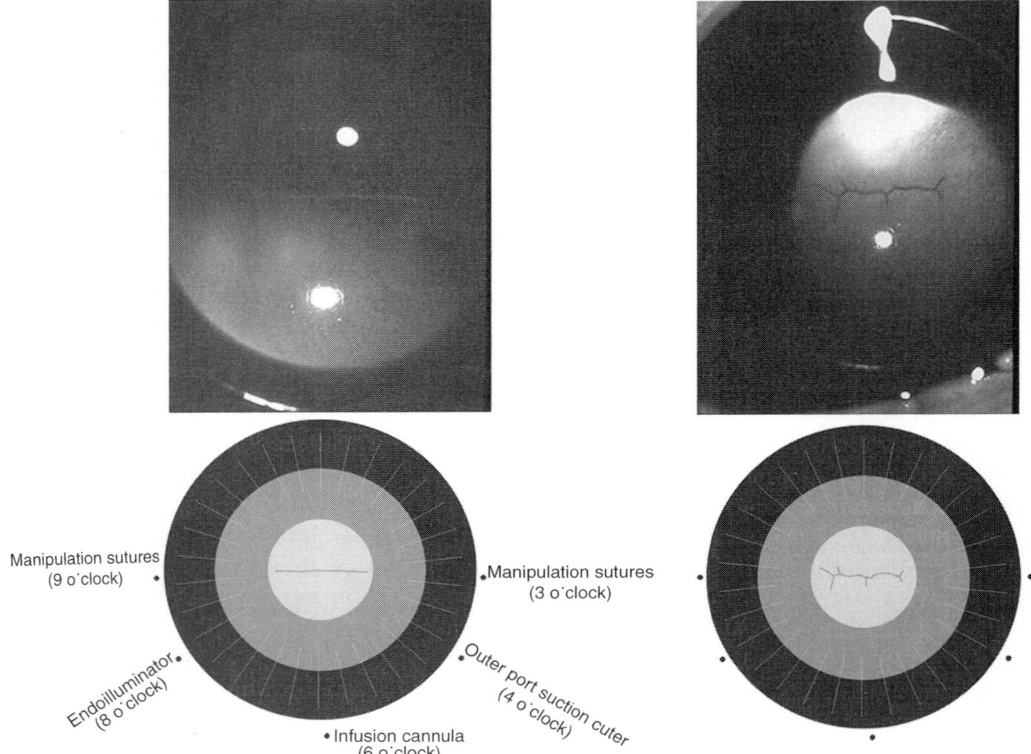

Figure 22 Abnormal suture pattern in rabbit lenses after vitrectomy surgery. Normal lens line suture (*upper left*) and orientation (*lower left*) compared to distorted line suture after vitrectomy (*upper right*) and orientation (*lower right*). *Source*: From Ref. 100.

patients, NSCs are the more predominant type of cataract following the surgical procedure in older patients. In any case, the fact that vitrectomy-induced changes in the suture branches of the rabbit are eliminated by the addition of a specific pharmaceutical drug at a time of surgery, suggests that all of the cataracts described above are formed secondary to other diseases, might be preventable in the future with pharmaceutical intervention.

REFERENCES

1. Al-Ghoul KJ, Costello MJ. Fiber cell morphology and cytoplasmic texture in cataractous and normal human lens nuclei. Curr Eye Res 1996; 15:533–42.
2. Al-Ghoul KJ, Costello MJ. Morphological changes in human nuclear cataracts of late-onset diabetics. Exp Eye Res 1993; 57:469–86.
3. Al-Ghoul KJ, Kuszak JR. Anterior polar cataracts in CS rats: a predictor of mature cataract formation. Invest Ophthalmol Vis Sci 1999; 40:668–79.
4. Al-Ghoul KJ, Lane CW, Taylor VL, et al. Distribution and type of morphological damage in human nuclear age-related cataracts. Exp Eye Res 1996; 62:237–51.
5. Al-Ghoul KJ, Nordgren RK, Kuszak AJ, et al. Structural evidence of human nuclear fiber compaction as a function of ageing and cataractogenesis. Exp Eye Res 2001; 72:199–214.
6. Al-Ghoul KJ, Novak LA, Kuszak JR.. The structure of posterior subcapsular cataracts in the Royal College of Surgeons (RCS) rats. Exp Eye Res 1998; 67:163–77.
7. Al-Ghoul KJ, Peterson KL, Kuszak JR. The internalization of posterior subcapsular cataracts (PSCs) in Royal College of Surgeons (RCS) rats. I. Morphological characterization. Mol Vis 1999; 5:6.
8. Amaya L, Taylor D, Russell-Eggitt I, et al. The morphology and natural history of childhood cataracts. Surv Ophthalmol 2003; 48:125–44.
9. Babizhayev MA. Failure to withstand oxidative stress induced by phospholipid hydroperoxides as a possible cause of the lens opacities in systemic diseases and ageing. Biochim Biophys Acta 1996, 1315:87–99.
10. Balasubramanian D. Photodynamics of cataract: an update on endogenous chromophores and antioxidants. Photochem Photobiol 2005; 81:498–501.
11. Bartlett H, Eperjesi F. An ideal ocular nutritional supplement? Ophthalmic Physiol Opt 2004; 24:339–49.
12. Bassnett S. Lens organelle degradation. Exp Eye Res 2002; 74:1–6.
13. Benedek GB. Theory of transparency of the eye. Appl Opt 1971; 10:459–73.
14. Benedek GB. Cataract as a protein condensation disease: the Proctor lecture. Invest Ophthalmol Vis Sci 1997; 38: 1911–21.
15. Benedek GB, Pande J, Thurston GM, et al. Theoretical and experimental basis for the inhibition of cataract. Prog Retin Eye Res 1999; 18:391–402.
16. Berendschot TT, Broekmans WM, Klopping-Ketelaars IA, et al. Lens aging in relation to nutritional determinants

and possible risk factors for age-related cataract. Arch Ophthalmol 2002; 120:1732–7.
17. Bettelheim FA. Physical basis of lens transparency. In: Maisel E, ed. The Ocular Lens: Structure, Function, and Pathology. New York: Marcel Dekker, 1985:265–300.
18. Bettelheim FA, Siew EL. Effect of change in concentration upon lens turbidity as predicted by the random fluctuation theory. Biophys J 1983; 41:29–33.
19. Bettelheim FA, Vinciguerra MJ, Kaplan D. Dynamic laser diffraction of bovine lenses. Exp Eye Res 1973; 15:149–55.
20. Borchman D, Giblin FJ, Leverenz VR, et al. Impact of aging and hyperbaric oxygen in vivo on guinea pig lens lipids and nuclear light scatter. Invest Ophthalmol Vis Sci 2000; 41:3061–73.
21. Boyle DL, Takemoto LJ. Confocal microscopy of human lens membranes in aged normal and nuclear cataracts. Invest Ophthalmol Vis Sci 1997; 38:2826–32.
22. Bron AJ, Brown NAP. Classification, grading and prevention of cataract. Trans Ophthalmol Soc UK 1983; 4:21–47.
23. Bron AJ, Brown NAP. Perinuclear lens retrodots: a role for ascorbate in cataractogenesis. Br J Ophthalmol 1987; 71: 86–95.
24. Bron AJ, Habgood JO. Morgagnian cataract. Trans Ophthalmol Soc UK 1976; 96:265–77.
25. Bron AJ, Matsuda K. Specular microscopy of the human lens. Trans Ophthalmol Soc UK 1981; 101:163–9.
26. Bron AJ, Sparrow J, Brown NA, et al. The lens in diabetes. Eye 1993; 7:260–75.
27. Bron AJ, Vrensen GF, Koretz J, et al. The ageing lens. Ophthalmologica 2000; 214:86–104.
28. Brown N. Visibility of transparent objects in the eye by retroillumination. Br J Ophthalmol 1971; 55:517–24.
29. Brown N, Shun-Shin GA. Morphological correlations of clinical lens changes: non-opaque lens defects. Prog Retin Eye Res 1995; 14:453–72.
30. Burian HM, Burns CA. Ocular changes in myotonic dystrophy. Am J Ophthalmol 1967; 63:22–34.
31. Cheng R, Lin B, Ortwerth BJ. Rate of formation of AGEs during ascorbate glycation and during aging in human lens tissue. Biochim Biophys Acta 2002; 1587:65–74.
32. Chitkara DK, Colin J. Morphology and visual effects of lens opacities of cataract. In: Yanoff M, Duker JS, eds. Ophthalmology. 2nd ed. St. Louis, MO: Mosby, 2004: 280–2.
33. Chylack LT Jr, Cheng HM. Sugar metabolism in the crystalline lens. Surv Ophthalmol 1978; 23:26–37.
34. Chylack LT Jr, Leske MC, McCarthy D, et al. Lens opacities classification system II (LOCS II). Arch Ophthalmol 1989; 107:991–7.
35. Chylack LT Jr, Wolfe JK, Singer DM, et al. The Lens Opacities Classification System III. The Longitudinal Study of Cataract Study Group. Arch Ophthalmol 1993; 111:831–6.
36. Clark JI. Development and maintenance of lens transparency. In: Albert DM, Jakobiec FA, eds. Principles and Practice of Ophthalmology. Philadelphia, PA: W.B. Saunders, 1994:114–23.
37. Colvis C, Garland D. Posttranslational modification of human alphaA-crystallin: correlation with electrophoretic migration. Arch Biochem Biophys 2002; 397:319–23.
38. Congdon N, Vingerling JR, Klein BE, et al. Prevalence of cataract and pseudophakia/aphakia among adults in the United States. Arch Ophthalmol 2004; 122:487–94.
39. Costello MJ, Al-Ghoul KJ, Oliver TN, et al. Polymorphism of fiber cell junctions in mammalian lens. In: 51st Annual Meeting of the Microscopy Society of America, 1993. Cincinnati, OH: San Francisco Press, 1993:200–1.
40. Costello MJ, Freel CD, Gilliland KO. Identification of multilamellar bodies in the urea insoluble fraction of human age-related nuclear cataracts. Invest Ophthalmol Vis Sci 2003; 44:E Abstract 3502.
41. Costello MJ, Johnsen S, Gilliland KO, et al. Predicted light scattering from particles observed in human age-related nuclear cataracts using Mie scattering theory. Invest Ophthalmol Vis Sci 2007; 48:303–12.
42. Costello MJ, Lane CW, Hatchell DL, et al. Ultrastructure of fiber cells and multilamellar inclusions in experimental diabetes. Invest Ophthalmol Vis Sci 1993; 34:2174–85.
43. Costello MJ, McIntosh TJ, Robertson JD. Distribution of gap junctions and square array junctions in the mammalian lens. Invest Ophthalmol Vis Sci 1989; 30:975–89.
44. Costello MJ, McIntosh TJ, Robertson JD. Membrane specializations in mammalian lens fiber cells: distribution of square arrays. Curr Eye Res 1985; 4:1183–201.
45. Costello MJ, Oliver TN, Cobo LM. Cellular architecture in age-related human nuclear cataracts. Invest Ophthalmol Vis Sci 1992; 33:3209–27.
46. Creighton MO, Trevithick JR, Mousa GY, et al. Globular bodies: a primary cause of the opacity in senile and diabetic posterior cortical subcapsular cataracts? Can J Ophthalmol 1978; 13:166–81.
47. Dandona L, Dandona R, Srinivas M, et al. Blindness in the Indian state of Andhra Pradesh. Invest Ophthalmol Vis Sci 2001; 42:908–16.
48. Datiles MB III, Magno BV. Cataract: clinical types. In: Tasman WT, Jaeger EA, eds. Duane's Clinical Ophthalmology. Philadelphia, PA: Lippincott Williams & Wilkins, 2004: chapter 73: http://80.36.73.149/Libros/Ojos/Actualidad/Duane/pages/v1/v1c073.html (Accessed January 24, 2008).
49. Deane JS, Hall AB, Thompson JR, et al. Prevalence of lenticular abnormalities in a population-based study: Oxford Clinical Cataract Grading in the Melton Eye Study. Ophthalmic Epidemiol 1997; 4:195–206.
50. Delaye M, Clark JI, Benedek GB. Identification of the scattering elements responsible for lens opacification in cold cataracts. Biophys J 1982; 37:647–56.
51. Delaye M, Tardieu A. Short-range order of crystallin proteins accounts for eye lens transparency. Nature 1983; 302:415–7.
52. Dilley KJ, Bron AJ, Habgood JO. Anterior polar and posterior subcapsular cataract in a patient with retinitis pigmentosa: a light-microscopic and ultrastructural study. Exp Eye Res 1976; 22:155–67.
53. Duke-Elder S. Diseases of the lens: General considerations. In: Kimpton H, ed. System of Ophthalmology, vol. XI. St. Louis, MO: C.V. Mosby; 1969:3–18.
54. Duncan G. On classifying human cataractous lenses. In: Duncan G, ed. Mechanisms of Cataract Formation in the Human Lens. London: Academic Press, 1981:1–5.
55. Dunia I, Cibert C, Gong X, et al. Structural and immunocytochemical alterations in eye lens fiber cells from Cx46 and Cx50 knockout mice. Eur J Cell Biol 2006; 85:729–52.
56. Durant JS, Frost NA, Trivella M, et al. Risk factors for cataract subtypes waterclefts and retrodots: two case-control studies. Eye 2006; 20:1254–67.
57. Dvornik E, Simard-Duquesne N, Krami M, et al. Polyol accumulation in galactosemic and diabetic rats: control by an aldose reductase inhibitor. Science 1973; 182:1146–8.
58. Ellwein LB, Urato CJ. Use of eye care and associated charges among the Medicare population: 1991–1998. Arch Ophthalmol 2002; 120:804–11.
59. Epstein DL. Reversible unilateral lens opacities in a diabetic patient. Arch Ophthalmol 1976; 94:461–3.

60. Eshaghian J, Streeten BW. Human posterior subcapsular cataract. An ultrastructural study of the posteriorly migrating cells. Arch Ophthalmol 1980; 98:134–43.
61. Fernald RD, Wright SE. Maintenance of optical quality during crystalline lens growth. Nature 1983; 301:618–20.
62. Foster A. Cataract and "Vision 2020-the right to sight" initiative. Br J Ophthalmol 2001; 85:635–7.
63. Fotiadis D, Hasler L, Muller DJ, et al. Surface tongue-and-groove contours on lens MIP facilitate cell-to-cell adherence. J Mol Biol 2000; 300:779–89.
64. Freel CD, Al-Ghoul KJ, Kuszak JR, et al. Analysis of nuclear fiber cell compaction in transparent and cataractous diabetic human lenses by scanning electron microscopy. BMC Ophthalmol 2003; 3:1–9.
65. Freel CD, Gilliland KO, Mekeel HE, et al. Ultrastructural characterization and Fourier analysis of fiber cell cytoplasm in the hyperbaric oxygen treated guinea pig lens opacification model. Exp Eye Res 2003; 76: 405–15.
66. Freel CD, Gilliland KO, Wesley Lane C, et al. Fourier analysis of cytoplasmic texture in nuclear fiber cells from transparent and cataractous human and animal lenses. Exp Eye Res 2002; 74:689–702.
67. Garner A, Klintoworth GK. The causes, types, and morphology of cataracts. In: Garner A, Klintoworth GK, eds. Pathobiology of Ocular Disease: A Dynamic Approach. 2nd ed. New York, NY: Marcel Dekker, 1994: 481–532.
68. Giblin FJ. Glutathione: a vital lens antioxidant. J Ocul Pharmacol Ther 2000; 16:121–35.
69. Giblin FJ, Leverenz VR, Padgaonkar VA, et al. UVA light in vivo reaches the nucleus of the guinea pig lens and produces deleterious, oxidative effects. Exp Eye Res 2002; 75:445–58.
70. Giblin FJ, Padgaonkar VA, Leverenz VR, et al. Nuclear light scattering, disulfide formation and membrane damage in lenses of older guinea pigs treated with hyperbaric oxygen. Exp Eye Res 1995; 60:219–35.
71. Gilliland KO, Freel CD, Johnsen S, et al. Distribution, spherical structure and predicted Mie scattering of multilamellar bodies in human age-related nuclear cataracts. Exp Eye Res 2004; 79:563–76.
72. Gilliland KO, Freel CD, Lane CW, et al. Multilamellar bodies as potential scattering particles in human age-related nuclear cataracts. Mol Vis 2001; 7:120–30.
73. Glasser A, Campbell MC. Presbyopia and the optical changes in the human crystalline lens with age. Vision Res 1998; 38:209–29.
74. Glasser A, Croft MA, Kaufman PL. Aging of the human crystalline lens and presbyopia. Int Ophthalmol Clin 2001; 41:1–15.
75. Gonen T, Cheng Y, Kistler J, et al. Aquaporin-0 membrane junctions form upon proteolytic cleavage. J Mol Biol 2004; 342:1337–45.
76. Gonen T, Cheng Y, Sliz P, et al. Lipid–protein interactions in double-layered two-dimensional AQP0 crystals. Nature 2005; 438:633–8.
77. Hall AB, Thompson JR, Deane JS, et al. LOCS III versus the Oxford Clinical Cataract Classification and Grading System for the assessment of nuclear, cortical and posterior subcapsular cataract. Ophthalmic Epidemiol 1997; 4:179–94.
78. Hanson SR, Hasan A, Smith DL, et al. The major in vivo modifications of the human water-insoluble lens crystallins are disulfide bonds, deamidation, methionine oxidation and backbone cleavage. Exp Eye Res 2000; 71: 195–207.
79. Harding CV, Chylack LT Jr, Susan SR, et al. Calcium-containing opacities in the human lens. Invest Ophthalmol Vis Sci 1983; 24:1194–202.
80. Harries WE, Akhavan D, Miercke LJ, et al. The channel architecture of aquaporin 0 at a 2.2-A resolution. Proc Natl Acad Sci USA 2004; 101:14045–50.
81. Hayes BP, Fisher RF. Ultrastructural appearances of a lens with marked polychromatic lustre: evidence for diffraction as a cause. Br J Ophthalmol 1984; 68:850–8.
82. Heys KR, Cram SL, Truscott RJ. Massive increase in the stiffness of the human lens nucleus with age: the basis for presbyopia? Mol Vis 2004; 10:956–63.
83. Horwitz J. Alpha-crystallin. Exp Eye Res 2003; 76:145–53.
84. Jacques PF, Taylor A, Moeller S, et al. Long-term nutrient intake and 5-year change in nuclear lens opacities. Arch Ophthalmol 2005; 123:517–26.
85. Jedziniak JA, Kinoshita JH, Yates EM, et al. The concentration and localization of heavy molecular weight aggregates in aging normal and cataractous human lenses. Exp Eye Res 1975; 20:367–9.
86. Jedziniak JA, Kinoshita JH, Yates EM, et al. On the presence and mechanism of formation of heavy molecular weight aggregates in human normal and cataractous lenses. Exp Eye Res 1973; 15:185–92.
87. Jedziniak JA, Nicoli DF, Baram H, et al. Quantitative verification of the existence of high molecular weight protein aggregates in the intact normal human lens by light-scattering spectroscopy. Invest Ophthalmol Vis Sci 1978; 17:51–7.
88. Kador PF, Robison WG Jr, Kinoshita JH. The pharmacology of aldose reductase inhibitors. Ann Rev Pharmacol Toxicol 1985; 25:691–714.
89. Kantorow M, Kays T, Horwitz J, et al. Differential display detects altered gene expression between cataractous and normal human lenses. Invest Ophthalmol Vis Sci 1998; 39:2344–54.
90. Kenworthy AK, Magid AD, Oliver TN, et al. Colloid osmotic pressure of steer alpha- and beta-crystallins: possible functional roles for lens crystallin distribution and structural diversity. Exp Eye Res 1994; 59:11–30.
91. Kinoshita JH, Merola LO, Satoh K, et al. Osmotic changes caused by the accumulation of dulcitol in the lenses of rats fed with galactose. Nature 1962; 194:1085–7.
92. Koretz JF, Cook CA, Kuszak JR. The zones of discontinuity in the human lens: development and distribution with age. Vision Res 1994; 34:2955–62.
93. Korlimbinis A, Truscott RJ. Identification of 3-hydroxykynurenine bound to proteins in the human lens. A possible role in age-related nuclear cataract. Biochemistry 2006; 45:1950–60.
94. Kuszak JR, Al-Ghoul KJ, Novak LA, et al. The internalization of posterior subcapsular cataracts (PSCs) in Royal College of Surgeons (RCS) rats. II. The interrelationship of optical quality and structure as a function of age. Mol Vis 1999; 5:7–17.
95. Kuszak JR, Costello MJ. Embryology and anatomy of human lenses. In: Tasman WT, Jaeger EA, eds. Duane's Clinical Ophthalmology. Philadelphia, PA: Lippincott Williams & Wilkins, 2004: [chapter 71A].
96. Kuszak JR, Costello MJ. The structure of the vertebrate lens. In: Lovicu FJ, Robinson ML, eds. Development of the Ocular Lens. Cambridge, UK: Cambridge University Press, 2004:71–118.
97. Kuszak JR, Macsai MS, Bloom KJ, et al. Cell-to-cell fusion of lens fiber cells in situ: correlative light, scanning electron microscopic, and freeze-fracture studies. J Ultrastruct Res 1985; 93:144–60.

98. Kuszak JR, Mazurkiewicz M, Jison L, et al. Quantitative analysis of animal model lens anatomy: accommodative range is related to fiber structure and organization. Vet Ophthalmol 2006; 9:266–80.
99. Kuszak JR, Peterson KL, Sivak JG, et al. The interrelationship of lens anatomy and optical quality. II. Primate lenses. Exp Eye Res 1994; 59:521–35.
100. Kuszak JR, Sivak JG, Moran KL, et al. Suppression of post-vitrectomy lens changes in the rabbit by novel benzopyranyl esters and amides. Exp Eye Res 2002; 75: 459–73.
101. Kuszak JR, Zoltoski RK. The mechanism of accommodation at the fiber level. In: Ioseliani OR, ed. Focus on Eye Research. New York, NY: Nova Science Publishers, 2006: 117–32.
102. Kuszak JR, Zoltoski RK, Tiedemann CE. Development of lens sutures. Int J Dev Biol 2004; 48:889–902.
103. Kuwabara T, Kinoshita JH, Cogan DG. Electron microscopic study of galactose-induced cataract. Invest Ophthalmol 1969; 8:133–49.
104. Land MF, Fernald RD. The evolution of eyes. Ann Rev Neurosci 1992: 15:1–29.
105. Lee AY, Chung SK, Chung SS. Demonstration that polyol accumulation is responsible for diabetic cataract by the use of transgenic mice expressing the aldose reductase gene in the lens. Proc Natl Acad Sci USA 1995; 92:2780–4.
106. Lee AY, Chung SS. Contributions of polyol pathway to oxidative stress in diabetic cataract. FASEB J 1999; 13: 23–30.
107. Lo WK. Visualization of crystallin droplets associated with cold cataract formation in young intact rat lens. Proc Natl Acad Sci USA 1989; 86:9926–30.
108. Lou MF. Thiol regulation in the lens. J Ocul Pharmacol Ther 2000; 16:137–48.
109. Marsili S, Salganik RI, Albright CD, et al. Cataract formation in a strain of rats selected for high oxidative stress. Exp Eye Res 2004; 79:595–612.
110. Michael R, van Marle J, Vrensen GF, et al. Changes in the refractive index of lens fibre membranes during maturation—impact on lens transparency. Exp Eye Res 2003; 77: 93–9.
111. Mie G. Beitrage zur Optik truber Medien, speziell kolloidalen Metal-losungen. Ann Physik 1908; 25: 377–445.
112. Nagaraj RH, Sell DR, Prabhakaram M, et al. High correlation between pentosidine protein crosslinks and pigmentation implicates ascorbate oxidation in human lens senescence and cataractogenesis. Proc Natl Acad Sci USA 1991; 88:10257–61.
113. Nirmalan PK, Krishnadas R, Ramakrishnan R, et al. Lens opacities in a rural population of southern India: the Aravind Comprehensive Eye Study. Invest Ophthalmol Vis Sci 2003; 44:4639–43.
114. Padgaonkar VA, Lin LR, Leverenz VR, et al. Hyperbaric oxygen in vivo accelerates the loss of cytoskeletal proteins and MIP26 in guinea pig lens nucleus. Exp Eye Res 1999; 68:493–504.
115. Pau H, Forster H. Double refraction of crystals in the lens (spheroliths, "Christmas tree ornaments") and in the vitreous body (scintillatio nivea). Graefes Arch Clin Exp Ophthalmol 1982; 219:295–7.
116. Phelps Brown N. The lens. In: Spalton DJ, Hitchings RA, Hunter PA, eds. Atlas of Clinical Ophthalmology. London: Mosby-Year Book Europe Limited, 1994:11.02–11.26.
117. Phelps Brown N, Bron AJ. Lens Disorders. Oxford: Butterworth-Heinemann, 1996.
118. Pierscionek BK. Refractive index contours in the human lens. Exp Eye Res 1997; 64:887–93.
119. Pirie A. Color and solubility of the proteins of human cataracts. Invest Ophthalmol 1968; 7:634–50.
120. Rao GN. Global Partnerships: A way forward for the control of avoidable blindness. In: ARVO/Alcon Keynote session, April 30, 2006. Fort Lauderdale, FL.
121. Rao PV, Horwitz J, Zigler JS Jr. Chaperone-like activity of alpha-crystallin. The effect of NADPH on its interaction with zeta-crystallin. J Biol Chem 1994; 269: 13266–72.
122. Reese AB, Wadsworth JA. Occurrence of cystoid spaces in the lens. Arch Ophthalmol 1954; 51:315–7.
123. Salganik RI. The benefits and hazards of antioxidants: controlling apoptosis and other protective mechanisms in cancer patients and the human population. J Am Coll Nutr 2001; 20:464S–72 [discussion 473S–5].
124. Sato S, Takahashi Y, Wyman M, et al. Progression of sugar cataract in the dog. Invest Ophthalmol Vis Sci 1991; 32: 1925–31.
125. Shestopalov VI, Bassnett S. Development of a macromolecular diffusion pathway in the lens. J Cell Sci 2003; 116:4191–9.
126. Shun-Shin GA, Bron AJ, Brown NP, et al. The relationship between central nuclear scatter and perinuclear retrodots in the human crystalline lens. Eye 1992; 6: 407–10.
127. Shun-Shin GA, Vrensen GF, Brown NP, et al. Morphologic characteristics and chemical composition of Christmas tree cataract. Invest Ophthalmol Vis Sci 1993; 34: 3489–96.
128. Siezen RJ, Bindels JG, Hoenders HJ. The interrelationship between monomeric, oligomeric and polymeric alpha-crystallin in the calf lens nucleus. Exp Eye Res 1979; 28: 551–67.
129. Simpanya MF, Ansari RR, Suh KI, et al. Aggregation of lens crystallins in an in vivo hyperbaric oxygen guinea pig model of nuclear cataract: dynamic light-scattering and HPLC analysis. Invest Ophthalmol Vis Sci 2005; 46:4641–51.
130. Sivak JG, Herbert KL, Peterson KL, et al. The interrelationship of lens anatomy and optical quality. I. Non-primate lenses. Exp Eye Res 1994; 59:505–20.
131. Spaeth GL. Glaucoma surgery. Methods of Ocular examination. In: Tasman W, Jaeger EA, eds. Duane's Clinical Ophthalmology, vol. 12. Philadelphia, PA: J.B. Lippincott Company, 1991:1–54.
132. Spalton DJ, Hitchings RA, Holder GE. Methods of ocular examination. In: Spalton DJ, Hitchings RA, Hunter PA, eds. Atlas of Clinical Ophthalmology. London: Mosby, 1994:1.02–1.30.
133. Sparrow JM, Bron AJ, Brown NA, et al. The Oxford Clinical Cataract Classification and Grading System. Int Ophthalmol 1986; 9:207–25.
134. Spector A. The search for a solution to senile cataracts. Proctor lecture. Invest Ophthalmol Vis Sci 1984; 25: 130–46.
135. Srivastava SK, Ramana KV, Bhatnagar A. Role of aldose reductase and oxidative damage in diabetes and the consequent potential for therapeutic options. Endocr Rev 2005; 26:380–92.
136. Steinberg EP, Javitt JC, Sharkey PD, et al. The content and cost of cataract surgery. Arch Ophthalmol 1993; 111:1041–9.
137. Steuber H, Zentgraf M, Podjarny A, et al. High-resolution crystal structure of aldose reductase complexed with the novel sulfonyl-pyridazinone inhibitor exhibiting an alternative active site anchoring group. J Mol Biol 2006; 356: 45–56.

138. Stevens A. The contribution of glycation to cataract formation in diabetes. J Am Optom Assoc 1998; 69: 519–30.
139. Stevens P, Swann PG. Christmas tree cataract. Clin Exp Optom 1998; 81:98–9.
140. Taylor VL, Al-Ghoul KJ, Lane CW, et al. Morphology of the normal human lens. Invest Ophthalmol Vis Sci 1996; 37:1396–410.
141. Taylor VL, Peiffer RL, Costello MJ. Ultrastructural analysis of normal and diabetic cataractous canine lenses. Vet Comp Ophthalmol 1997; 7:117–25.
142. Thomas R, Paul P, Rao GN, et al. Present status of eye care in India. Surv Ophthalmol 2005; 50:85–101.
143. Thompson JR, Deane JS, Hall AB, et al. Associations between lens features assessed in the Oxford Clinical Cataract Classification and Grading System. Ophthal Epidemiol 1997; 4:207–12.
144. Thylefors B, Negrel AD, Pararajasegaram R, et al. Global data on blindness. Bull World Health Organ 1995; 73:115–21.
145. Trokel S. The physical basis for transparency of the crystalline lens. Invest Ophthalmol 1962; 1:493–501.
146. Truscott RJ. Age-related nuclear cataract-oxidation is the key. Exp Eye Res 2005; 80:709–25.
147. Unakar NJ, Tsui JY, Johnson MJ. Prefeeding of aldose reductase inhibitor and galactose cataractogenesis. Curr Eye Res 1989; 8:997–1010.
148. van den Berg TJ. Light scattering by donor lenses as a function of depth and wavelength. Invest Ophthalmol Vis Sci 1997; 38:1321–32.
149. van Heyningen R. Formation of polyols by the lens of the rat with sugar cataract. Nature 1959; 184:194–5.
150. van Heyningen R. The sorbitol pathway in the lens. Exp Eye Res 1962; 1:396–404.
151. van Rijn LJ, Nischler C, Gamer D, et al. Measurement of stray light and glare: comparison of Nyktotest, Mesotest, stray light meter, and computer implemented stray light meter. Br J Ophthalmol 2005; 89:345–51.
152. Veretout F, Tardieu A. The protein concentration gradient within eye lens might originate from constant osmotic pressure coupled to differential interactive properties of crystallins. Eur Biophys J 1989; 17:61–8.
153. Vogt A. Klinischer und anatomischer Beitrag zur Kenntis der Cataracta senilis, insbesonderer zur Frage des subcapsularen Beginnes derselben. Graefes Arch Klin Exp Ophthalmol 1914; 88:329–91.
154. Vogt A. Weiterer Ergebnisse der Spaltlampenmikroskopie des vorderen Bulbusabschnittes. IV. Prasenile und senile Linsentrubungen. Graefes Arch Klin Exp Ophthalmol 1922; 108:192–218.
155. Weeber HA, Eckert G, Soergel F, et al. Dynamic mechanical properties of human lenses. Exp Eye Res 2005; 80:425–34.
156. Williams DL. Oxidation, antioxidants and cataract formation: a literature review. Vet Ophthalmol 2006; 9:292–8.
157. Wong TY, Loon SC, Saw SM. The epidemiology of age related eye diseases in Asia. Br J Ophthalmol 2006; 90: 506–11.
158. Yanoff M, Fine BS. Lens. In: Yanoff M, Fine BS, eds. Ocular Pathology: A Text and Atlas. 3rd ed. Philadelphia, PA: J.B. Lippincott Company, 1989:347–76.
159. Yanoff M. Pathology of cataract. In: Bellows JG, ed. Cataract and Abnormalities of the Lens. New York, NY: Grune & Stratton, 1975:155–206.
160. Zampighi GA, Hall JE, Ehring GR, et al. The structural organization and protein composition of lens fiber junctions. J Cell Biol 1989; 108:2255–75.
161. Zarina S, Zhao HR, Abraham EC. Advanced glycation end products in human senile and diabetic cataractous lenses. Mol Cell Biochem 2000; 210:29–34.
162. Zetterstrom C, Lundvall A, Kugelberg M. Cataracts in children. J Cataract Refract Surg 2005; 31:824–40.
163. Zigman S, Paxhia T. The nature and properties of squirrel lens yellow pigment. Exp Eye Res 1988; 47:819–24.

24

Biochemistry of Cataracts

John J. Harding
Nuffield Laboratory of Ophthalmology, University of Oxford, Oxford, U.K.

INTRODUCTION

Cataract is a lenticular opacity, either partial or total, that causes visual impairment. The great variety of metabolic insults that can cause cataracts and the biochemical basis of human senile cataract have been described in detail by Harding (18) and by Chylack and Cheng (9). This chapter is based on the chapter by Elaine Berman in the previous edition (2), and also borrows heavily from my own book on cataract (18). A complete discussion of this vast subject was beyond the scope of Berman's chapter, and only certain topics were selected for inclusion. My book was more comprehensive and covered all the major experimentally induced cataracts as well as human cataract. It was pointed out that many biochemical and other changes were common to many of the experimental cataracts and to human cataract, leading to the conclusion that there are common pathways in cataractogenesis.

ANIMAL MODELS OF CATARACTS AND IN VITRO STUDIES

Cataract may be induced in experimental animals by diabetes, trauma, X-rays, microwave radiation, ultraviolet (UV) radiation, tryptophan deficiency, the administration of galactose, xylose, cyanate, dinitrophenol, selenite, corticosteroids, 4-chlorophenylalanine, naphthalene, dimethylsulfoxide, methionine sulfoximine, and iodoacetate, and is seen in an increasing variety of mutant rodents. Previously I recorded all the changes observed during cataractogenesis in these models in order of their appearance as far as possible and then drew schemes linking the changes to draw out pathways to cataract (18). The schemes were shown for cataract induced by diabetes, galactose, X-irradiation, cyanate, corticosteroids, and selenite. What was striking was that these schemes were almost superimposable. Changes in one type of cataract were the same in another completely different type. The way in which many different authors had measured change at different times made it possible to deduce which were closest to the initiating events.

Some of these common changes can be brought together in a single table (Table 1).

Clearly widely disparate initiating events lead into common pathways toward cataract and a scheme bringing in all the major experimental models and most common changes is summarized in Fig. 1. This draws out the role of major common pathways, in particular one from the chemical modification of proteins leading to their unfolding and thus cataract.

HUMAN CATARACT

A major factor in interpreting laboratory results on human cataract must be the extensive epidemiological research of human populations across the world. Reviewing all such studies in detail is beyond the scope of this chapter, so instead I have compiled tables showing the major risk factors for cataract in Western countries (Table 2) and "Third World countries" (Table 3).

At first sight these data seem rather remote from the laboratory studies. Many of the factors are in fact aspects of relative poverty: black compared with white in the United States, lower social class, lower educational standard (one of the most consistent risk factors), low height, weight, widowhood in India, low caste, low consumption of expensive foods, diarrhea, and so on. Many diseases are associated with poverty but the specific pathways involved are rarely delineated. Could most of these risk factors for cataract be surrogate factors masking the real problem? Most have fairly low relative risks (odds ratios) between 1 and 2 (Table 2 and 3). Diarrhea on the other hand has a high odds ratio: 4.1 for a single episode and 21 for more than one episode (34,35). Could this be the real cause underlying the association of poverty with cataract?

This leaves other risk factors such as glaucoma surgery, which accounts for most of the risk associated with glaucoma, and myopia that may be caused by mechanical effects; and a larger number of factors resulting from diabetes, consumption of various drugs, and plasma factors that are more likely to have purely biochemical origins. Some of these factors can be included in a scheme linking the risk factors to biochemical changes known to occur in human cataract (Fig. 2). The risk factors are arranged around the top of the figure linked to the immediate associated biochemical changes: for example, diabetes, the most important risk factor in Western countries, leads immediately to increased glucose and metabolites of glucose in the lens. These can attack lens proteins, not only the crystallins but also enzymes, membrane proteins, and all other proteins. Chemical modification leads to unfolding of the proteins (4) with loss of function, aggregation leading inexorably toward cataract (Fig. 2). Diarrhea, possibly the most important factor in Third World countries, and renal failure raise urea levels in the lens and this comes to equilibrium with cyanate, which can react with proteins, just as the sugars can, leading to unfolding and all the subsequent changes to cataract. Similarly reactive small molecules produced from alcohol or found in cigarette smoke can react with proteins in the lens and lead to the same common pathway. In fact the impression of a common pathway is more apparent for human cataract than for experimental cataract. So when it is said that cataract is a multifactorial disease we see the truth of this in the many risk factors, but in fact the problem is simpler than it appears to be because the disparate factors feed into a small number of common pathways with the emphasis on nonenzymic modification of proteins followed by unfolding. In this way cataract has become a lead member of a group of

Table 1 Common Changes in Experimental Cataracts

	Lower levels of				Higher levels of	
	GSH	Na^+-K^+-ATPase	PSH	ATP	Na	Modified protein
Diabetes	Y	Y	Y	Y	Y	Y
Galactose	Y	Y	Y	Y	Y	Y
Selenite	Y	ND	Y	ND	ND	Y
Steroids	Y	Y	Y	Y	ND	Y
Naphthalene	Y	ND	Y	ND	ND	Y
X-ray	Y	Y	Y	Y	Y	Y
Microwave	Y	Y	ND	ND	Y	ND
Nakano	Y	Y	Y	Y	Y	Y
Philly	Y	ND	Y	Y	Y	Y
Emory	Y	Y	Y	ND	ND	Y
ICR/1	Y	Y	ND	Y	Y	Y

Abbreviations: ATP, adenosine triphosphate; GSH, glutathione; K, potassium; Na, sodium; ND, not determined; PSH, protein thiol; Y, yes.

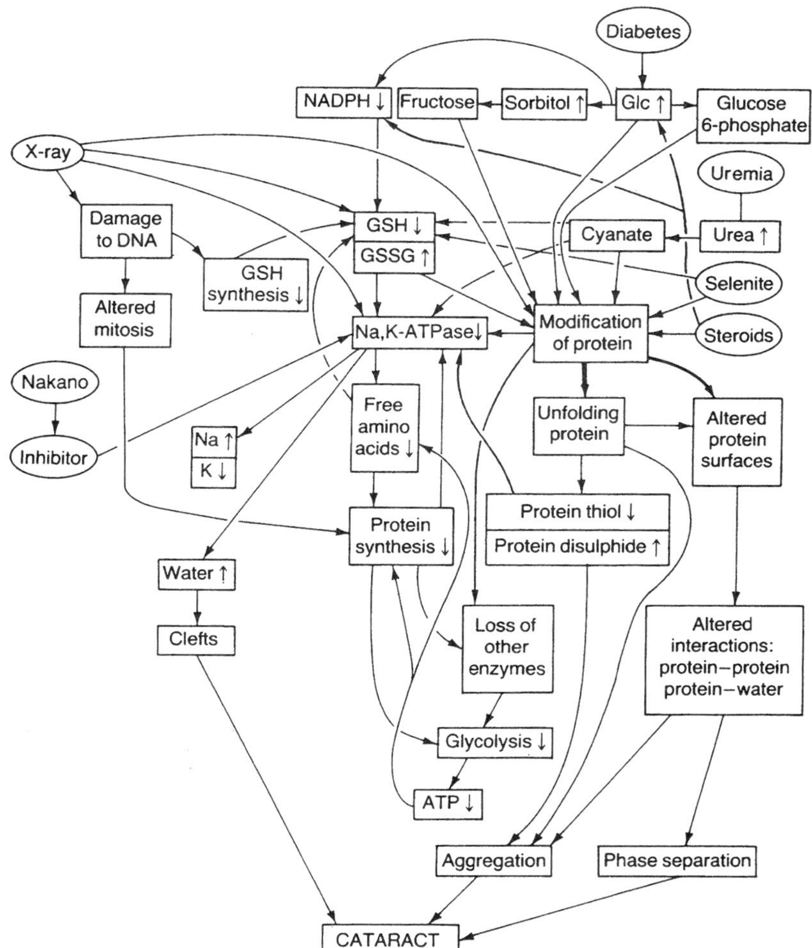

Figure 1 Scheme of common pathways to cataract in experimental animals. *Abbreviations*: ATP, adenosine triphosphate; Glc, glucose; GSH, glutathione; GSSG, oxidized glutathione; K, potassium; Na, sodium; NADPH, nicotinamide adenine dinucleotide phosphate. *Source*: From Ref. 18.

diseases characterized by conformational changes to proteins and now called the conformational diseases (7,21). These include Alzheimer disease and prion diseases (see Chapter 70). Conformational changes that make protein thiols more susceptible to oxidation and disulfide bond formation and lead to the formation of water-insoluble aggregates in human nuclear cataracts have been recognized for years (23,24,46). A generalized scheme (18) outlining some of these changes are depicted in Figure 3.

Can we be sure that unfolding of protein could lead to all the changes seen in experimental and human cataracts? The Philly mouse cataract helps here. In this animal model of congenital cataract the lens epithelial cells fail to differentiate into fiber cells (27). Changes in Philly cataract are similar to those in other experimental cataracts and are shown in Figure 4 (21,51). No functional 27 kDa β-crystallin mRNA was detectable in homozygous Philly mouse lenses (6). The 27 kDa polypeptide (βB_2) is replaced by a protein of somewhat smaller size that is more acid than normal βB_2. The N-terminal amino acid residues of the two proteins are similar, but the Philly mouse lens protein lacks four residues from the C-terminal half of normal βB_2. The protein with four fewer amino acids would be unable to fold normally and in this way results in a cataract. Thus, the pressence of a single protein unable to fold not only causes cataracts but also causes many of the biochemical changes seen in other experimental cataracts, even in human cataracts.

In the following section, we will look more closely at the causes of the unfolding of proteins in cataract.

CAUSES OF UNFOLDING OF LENS PROTEINS IN CATARACT

Unfolding of proteins in cataract was first demonstrated more than 30 years ago (17): before formal demonstrations for most other conformational disorders. The unfolding explained some of the changes to protein thiols seen in cataract formation and some aggregation (Fig. 3) (18). The formation of mixed

Table 2 Some Risk Factors for Cataract in Europe and North America

Risk Factor	Odds ratio (relative risk)
African American vs. Caucasian American	1.3
Lower social class	
Lower educational standard	1.5
Lower height, vital capacity, hand grip strength	
Diabetes	Up to 12
Renal failure	12.4
Glaucoma	5.9 or 2.9
Surgery for glaucoma	14.3
Hypertension	
Cardiovascular disease	
Psychiatric illness	
Severe diarrhea	1.6
Myopia when young	2.0
Military work	2.2
Estimated UV exposure	
Use of:	
Alcohol	2.1
Cigarettes	2.0
Major tranquilizers	
Diuretics	1.6
Steroids	1.8
High plasma:	
Fasting glucose	
Casual glucose	
Phospholipids	
Urea	
Creatinine	
Low plasma:	
Calcium	
Phosphate	
Cholesterol	
Albumin	

Source: From Ref. 18.

disulfides and protein–protein disulfide shown in this figure were explored further over the years but left the intriguing question of what caused the conformation change in the first place. Different authors have subsequently suggested and investigated many possibilities (Table 4). All of these are relatively simple chemical modifications to the proteins, including formation of different adducts (21). Importantly these are not simply theoretical possibilities: all have been identified in human cataracts at levels greater than in normal lens. All are nonenzymic changes and so are neither carefully controlled nor very specific. The different chemical changes correspond to different risk factors. Glycation, the nonenzymic reaction of reducing sugars with proteins, is elevated in diabetes and a powerful risk factor for cataract. Carbamylation is the reaction of cyanate (isocyanate) with proteins. The isocyanate is formed in equilibrium with urea, and therefore is raised in renal failure and severe diarrhea where the circulating level of urea is raised. Corticosteroids are a well-established risk factor for cataract. The notion that disparate risk factors for cataract can be closely linked with chemical changes to proteins in a manner likely to cause conformational change demonstrates how the factors can come together in a multifactorial disease. Different modifications would simply add to the conformational changes until transparency was compromised over the decades leading to cataract.

Table 3 Some Risk Factors for Cataract in India and Nepal

Risk factor	Odds ratio (relative risk)
Living on plain compared to mountain	
Living in slum compared to village	1.8
Low caste	1.9
Widowed	2.2
Less-educated	1.6 to 7.5
Low consumption of protein	2.3
Zero consumption of milk, meat, eggs, curd	1.6 to 2.4
Low height	1.8
Low weight	1.9
Low body mass index (BMI)	1.4
Systolic blood pressure	1.4
Severe diarrhea	4.1 to 21
Heatstroke	1.7

Source: Based on data included in Ref. 18.

CRITERIA FOR CAUSES OF CATARACT

It is possible to draw up at least six criteria for the involvement of factors as initiating factors for a disease (Table 5). These cover epidemiology, key insult, specific damage, and support from in vitro and animal experiments. There may be other criteria that could be applied. On the other hand a convincing case could be established without satisfying all criteria. We can try the criteria against two of the more popular possible causes of cataract: oxidation and glycation as part of diabetes mellitus.

Is Oxidation a Cause of Cataract?

The first criterion asks for an epidemiological relationship and this produces the first problem. The risk factors hardly seem related to oxidation with the possible exception of exposure to UV light (Tables 2 and 3). Epidemiology of the role of sunlight is fraught with difficulty partly because it is impossible to measure exposure to sunlight over many years (19). The oxidation hypothesis was encouraged by many studies of antioxidant vitamins and cataract. Different authors claimed benefits of different vitamins but there was no consistency between the studies (20). The final nail in the coffin came from the age-related eye disease study (AREDS) clinical study where administration of zinc with or without antioxidant vitamins gave no protection against cataract (1). Equally

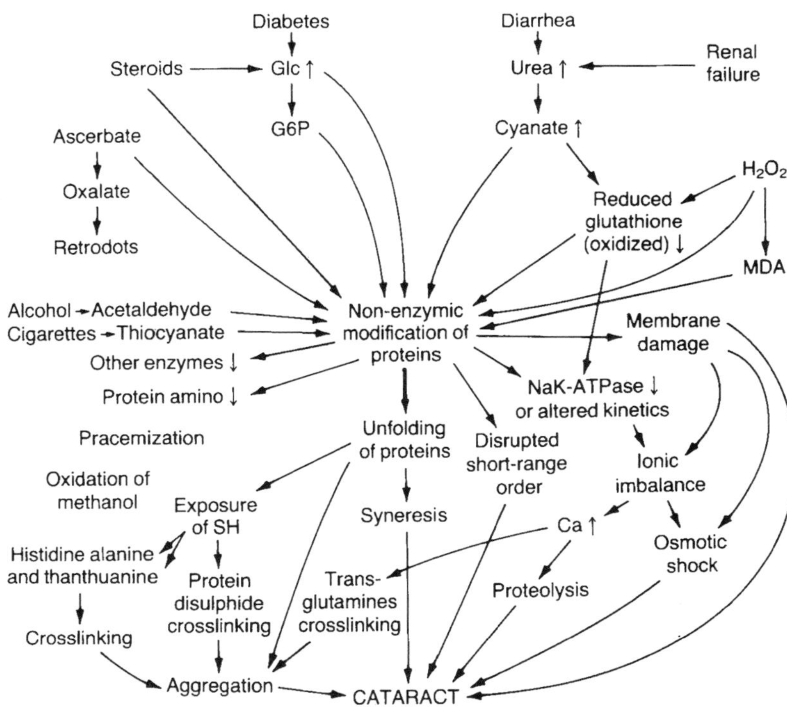

Figure 2 Speculative scheme of common pathways of biochemical and physicochemical changes leading to the formation of human cataracts. A wide variety of (risk) factors or chemical agents that initiate changes in lens crystallins (shown on the periphery of the diagram) lead into a common network of changes (shown at the center of the diagram) that lead to cataract formation. *Abbreviations*: ATP, adenosine triphosphate; Ca, calcium; Glc, glucose; G6P, glucose-6-phosphate; H_2O_2, hydrogen peroxide; K, potassium; MDA, malondialdehyde; Na, sodium; SH, sulfhydryl group. *Source*: From Ref. 18.

negative was the randomized trial of beta-carotene in the United States (8), and administration of vitamin E (32).

What of the "key insult"? If oxidation is an important initiating event in cataractogenesis there must be one or more oxidizing agents. Those discussed at length include oxygen itself, singlet oxygen, superoxide, and hydrogen peroxide (11,16,33,43,44). The more reactive singlet oxygen and superoxide are difficult to measure and the levels of oxygen and hydrogen peroxide are very low. There is no obvious oxidizing agent whereas the lens has both small molecules, glutathione (GSH) and ascorbic acid, etc., and enzymic defenses against oxidation (catalase, superoxide dismutase, GSH peroxidase, GSH reductase, etc.).

Is there specific damage seen in cataractous lens that could only be caused by oxidation? The known products of photooxidation and metal-catalyzed oxidation are oxidation products of tryptophan, histidine, and tyrosine, but these are not found in cataract (18). No loss of these amino acids is reported. Methionine sulfoxide has been reported (18) but only in dark cataracts suggesting it may be a late event, not an initiating factor. On the other hand, there is evidence of disulfide formation both in experimental cataract (3,10,29,36,42) and human cataract (13,18,23,24,26,31,45,46). This is a very limited oxidation, which could be brought about by oxidized GSH (GSSG). This limited evidence for oxidative change in cataract is based on results on bulk proteins. It is possible that the crucial targets of oxidation are minor proteins. Recent evidence in this area comes from the surprising ability from human cataracts to revive enzyme activity that must have been lost decades before during cataractogenesis (40,41). The enzymes evidently lost their activity by a combination of disulfide formation and conformational change. Correlation between marker and disease cannot be established for oxidation as there is no clear marker apart from the disulfides. These increase with the darkness of cataracts (18).

Support from in vitro experiments comes in the observation that photooxidation of lens proteins in the laboratory produces brown cross-linked protein. However, such proteins have lost tryptophan at the earliest stage whereas this is not seen in human cataract. Incubation with hydrogen peroxide at high concentrations can induce lens changes, but at moderate concentrations the lens destroys the peroxide not vice versa. In vivo UV-irradiation can cause cataract, often with associated corneal damage.

In summary, the evidence for oxidation as an initiating factor for human cataract is not good. The epidemiological evidence has become more negative; key insults and specific damage are difficult to discern, and laboratory support is weak. The only role may be for limited oxidation of key targets, but that is perhaps to clutch at straws.

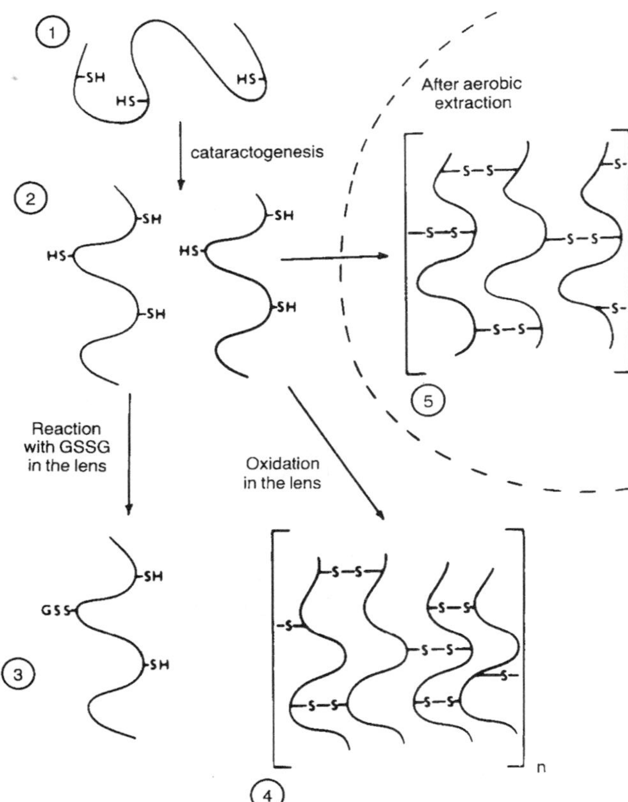

Figure 3 Changes in lens proteins during the development of human senile cataract: (1) native protein; (2) unfolded protein of nuclear cataract; (3) formation of protein-GSH mixed disulfide; (4) disulfide-bonded high-molecular-weight protein; and (5) disulfide-linked urea-insoluble products formed during aerobic extraction of lens proteins. *Source*: From Ref. 18.

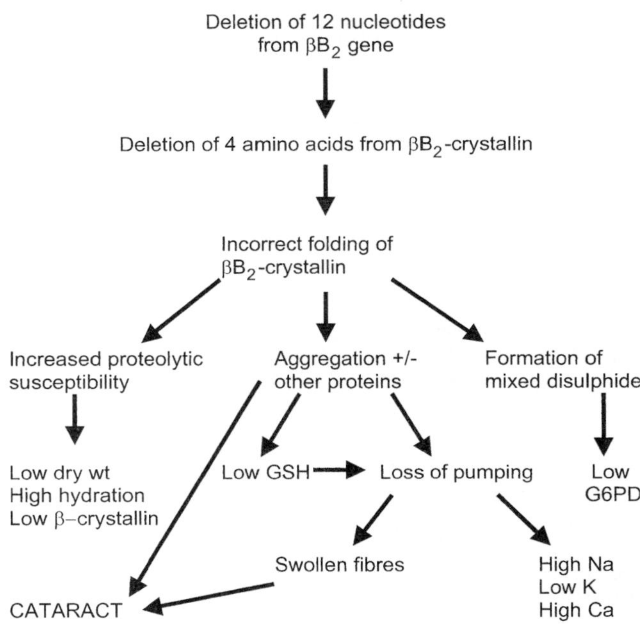

Figure 4 Scheme of changes seen in Philly cataract in mouse. *Abbreviations*: Ca, calcium; GSH, glutathione; G6PD, glucose 6-phosphate dehydrogenase; K, potassium; Na, sodium. *Source*: From Ref. 21.

Is Glycation a Cause of Cataract?

Glycation is the nonenzymic reaction of reducing sugars with proteins (22). It occurs wherever sugars have access to proteins and is uncontrolled depending only on the availability of sugars and their concentrations. Where sugar concentrations are raised glycation will increase.

The key condition with increased sugar concentrations is diabetes, and this is the most important risk factor established for cataract in the West (Table 2) (28,50). Other mechanisms have been proposed for the link between diabetes and cataract but nevertheless the epidemiology supports the idea that glycation is an important initiating factor.

The key insults are attributable to the sugars present in the lens at all times mostly as essential metabolites. They may be elevated in diabetes but are still present in nondiabetic individuals. Glucose is in fact the least reactive sugar so others, especially sugar phosphates, may be more important.

Reaction of sugars with proteins leads to the formation of a number of different glycation products: first Schiff bases and Amadori products and then the late glycation products or advanced glycation end products (22). Thus many key markers of glycation have been identified in human cataract and in experimental cataract.

The next criterion is that there should be a correlation between specific damage, in this case glycation and cataract severity. This has been found in diabetic rats (5,49). It has not been shown clearly in human cataracts beyond the demonstration that patients with diabetes have more glycation than nondiabetic patients. The levels of glycated proteins in human diabetic lenses are approximately twice those of age-matched controls (12). However in major trials to tighten glucose control, lowered glycation was associated with diminished complications (37,48).

Table 4 Some Possible Causes of Conformational Change in Human Cataract

Glycation
Carbamylation
Addition of glutathione
Addition of corticosteroids
Addition of aldehydes
Truncation
Deamidation
Protein–protein disulphide formation
Racemization of aspartic acid
Oxidation of methionine

Table 5 Ideal Criteria to Test Factors as Initiating Factors in a Disease

Epidemiological association
Presence of a key insult
Evidence of specific damage
Correlation between marker (biochemical change) and disease
Relevant animal model support
Relevant in vitro support

In vitro there are many studies demonstrating that glycation occurs whenever sugars come into contact with proteins, including lens proteins. In model systems studied by Stevens et al. (47), incubation of bovine lens crystallins with glucose or glucose 6-phosphate led to the glycation of ϵ-amino groups of lysine residues, the formation of high-molecular-weight aggregates, and the production of opalescence.

Crystallins from diabetic rats express enhanced glycation compared with normal controls (47), and aggregated crystallins linked in part by disulfide bonds have been shown to accumulate in cataractous lenses of both diabetic and galactosemic rats (36). The urea-soluble crystallins in particular become increasingly glycated as hyperglycemia develops (39). Water-soluble γ-crystallins and their reactive thiols decrease as disulfide-linked high-molecular-weight aggregates form. In all, glycation causes conformational changes in lens crystallins, resulting in unfolding of their tertiary structures.

Galactose also forms adducts with lens proteins at a rate somewhat faster than glucose (25). Aspirin as well as the reduced form of GSH at physiological concentrations inhibits galactosylation of lens proteins, possibly by blocking its initial binding and preventing the formation of adducts. Although the mechanisms appear to differ, it is noteworthy that GSH and other reducing agents also inhibit the glycation of lens crystallins by ascorbic acid (38). The rate of adduct formation by galactose and glucose 6-phosphate is substantially decreased by 5-hydroxybendazac, a metabolite of the experimental anticataract drug bendazac (30). Aspirin and similar drugs protect against glycation and the increasing evidence that they can prevent lens opacification in vitro and in vivo adds support to the postulated role of glycation.

The foregoing findings suggest that glycation of lens crystallins leads to major changes in their conformation; resulting in the formation of disulfide-linked high-molecular-weight aggregates, which may be responsible for increased light scattering and opacification. Other lens proteins can also be glycated, however; for example, incubation of bovine lens epithelial cells in a high-glucose-containing medium (30.5 mM) results in the glycation of Na^+-K^+-ATPase (14,15). The Na^+-K^+-ATPase-dependent transport of K^+ is inhibited, and the rate of ATP hydrolysis decreased at nearly saturating substrate concentrations.

In vivo induction of diabetes in a variety of animals leads to cataract and where studied increased glycation has been observed as part of that process. Thus glycation, unlike oxidation, is able to satisfy all the criteria for an initiating cause of cataract (Table 5). It is not only at least part of the causation of cataract in diabetes mellitus, but it also undoubtedly contributes to cataract in nondiabetics.

Other Hypotheses for Cataract Formation

Other initiating factors for human cataract have been discussed over the years and they could all be tested by the same criteria (Table 5). In the previous edition emphasis was placed on the role of aldose reductase in diabetic cataract (1), but as this enzyme cannot make sorbitol from glucose at a significant rate it will not be dealt with again here; earlier discussion can be seen elsewhere (18).

The reaction with cyanate is similar to glycation in that it modifies amino groups on proteins. Rat lenses incubated with cyanate develop opacities that in the early stages may be caused by phase separation resulting from interactions between modified proteins and the surrounding water, as well as with unmodified neighboring proteins (10). This has been considered part of a general phenomenon in which any agent that causes a decrease in positive surface charges or an increase in negative charges, as in deamidation or reaction with GSSG, induces conformational changes leading to cataract formation. Preincubation of lenses with aspirin prevents the cyanate-induced increase in phase separation temperature. Aspirin, which appears to act by transfer of acetyl groups to protein amino groups, prevented the carbamylation and the development of opacities in this model system. Reaction with cyanate causing conformational change also satisfies many criteria of Table 5. The cyanate (isocyanate) is derived from urea which is elevated in renal failure and severe diarrhea, which are risk factors for cataract (Table 2 and 3) (35). Cyanate is the key damaging molecule with carbamylation as the specific evidence of damage. Recent evidence for carbamylation in human cataract came from mass spectrometry studies. Animal and in vitro experiments provide further support (18).

REFERENCES

1. AREDS. A randomized, placebo-controlled, clinical trial of high-dose supplementation with vitamins C and E and beta carotene for age-related cataract and vision loss. Arch Ophthalmol 2001; 119:1439–52.

2. Berman ER. Biochemistry of cataracts. In: Garner A, Klintworth GK, eds. Pathobiology of Ocular Disease. New York: Marcel Dekker, 1994:533–90.
3. Beswick HT, Harding JJ. High-molecular-weight crystallin aggregate formation resulting from non-enzymic carbamylation of lens crystallins: relevance to cataract formation. Exp Eye Res 1987; 45:569–78.
4. Beswick HT, Harding JJ. Conformational changes induced in lens α- and γ-crystallins by modification with glucose 6-phosphate. Biochem J 1987; 246:161–9.
5. Blakytny R, Harding JJ. Prevention of cataract in diabetic rats by aspirin, paracetamol (acetaminophen) and ibuprofen. Exp Eye Res 1992; 54:509–18.
6. Carper D, Shinohara T, Piatigorsky J, Kinoshita JH. Deficiency of functional messenger RNA for a developmentally regulated β-crystallin polypeptide in a hereditary cataract. Science 1982; 217:463–4.
7. Carrell RW, Lomas DA. Conformational disease. Lancet 1997; 350:134–8.
8. Christen WG, Glyn RJ, Sperduto RD, et al. Age-related cataract in a randomized trial of beta-carotene in women. Arch Ophthalmol 2003; 121:372–8.
9. Chylack LT Jr, Cheng H-M. Clinical implications of research on lens and cataract. In: Maisel H, ed. The Ocular Lens. Structure, Function, and Pathology. New York: Marcel Dekker, 1985:439–66.
10. Crompton M, Rixon KC, Harding JJ. Aspirin prevents carbamylation of soluble lens proteins and prevents cyanate-induced phase separation opacities in vitro: a possible mechanism by which aspirin could prevent cataract. Exp Eye Res 1985; 40:291–311.
11. Fecondo JV, Augusteyn RC. Superoxide dismutase, catalase and glutathione peroxidase in the human cataractous lens. Exp Eye Res 1983; 36:15–23.
12. Garlick RL, Mazer JS, Chylack LT Jr, et al. Nonenzymatic glycation of human lens crystallin: effect of aging and diabetes mellitus. J Clin Invest 1984; 74:1742–9.
13. Garner WH, Garner MH, Spector A. Comparison of the 10,000 and 43,000 Dalton polypeptide populations isolated from the water soluble and insoluble fractions of human cataractous lenses. Exp Eye Res 1979; 29:257–76.
14. Garner MH, Spector A. ATP hydrolysis kinetics by Na,K-ATPase in cataract. Exp Eye Res 1986; 42:339–48.
15. Garner MH, Wang G-M, Spector A. Stimulation of glycosylated lens epithelial Na,K-ATPase by an aldose reductase inhibitor. Exp Eye Res 1987; 44:339–45.
16. Goosey JD, Zigler IS Jr, Kinoshita JH. Cross-linking of lens crystallins in a photodynamic system: a process mediated by singlet oxygen. Science 1980; 208:1278–80.
17. Harding JJ. Conformational changes in human lens proteins in cataract. Biochem J 1972; 129:97–100.
18. Harding J. Cataract. Biochemistry, Epidemiology and Pharmacology. London: Chapman & Hall, 1991.
19. Harding JJ. The untenability of the sunlight hypothesis of cataractogenesis. Doc Ophthalmol 1995; 88:345–9.
20. Harding JJ. Can drugs or micronutrients prevent cataract? Drugs Ageing 2001; 18:473–86.
21. Harding JJ. Viewing molecular mechanisms of ageing through a lens. Ageing Res Rev 2002; 1:465–79.
22. Harding JJ. Protein glycation and cataract: a conformational disease. In: Uversky VN, Fink AL, eds. Protein Misfolding, Aggregation and Conformational Disease, Vol. II. In press.
23. Harding JJ, Crabbe MJC. The lens: development, proteins, metabolism and cataract. In: Davson H, ed. The Eye, vol. 1b. 3rd ed. Orlando, FL: Academic Press, 1984:207–492.
24. Harding JJ, Dilley KJ. Structural proteins of the mammalian lens: a review with emphasis on changes in development, aging and cataract. Exp Eye Res 1976; 22:1–73.
25. Huby R, Harding JJ. Non-enzymic glycosylation (glycation) of lens proteins by galactose and protection by aspirin and reduced glutathione. Exp Eye Res 1988; 47:53–9.
26. Hum TE, Augusteyn RC. The state of sulphydryl groups in proteins isolated from normal and cataractous human lenses. Curr Eye Res 1987; 6:1091–101.
27. Kador PF, Fukui HN, Fukushi S, et al. Philly mouse: a new model of hereditary cataract. Exp Eye Res 1980; 30:59–68.
28. Klein BEK, Klein R, Moss SE. Prevalence of cataracts in a population-based study of persons with diabetes mellitus. Ophthalmology 1985; 92:1191–6.
29. Kuck JFR, Kuck KD. The Emory mouse cataract: loss of soluble protein, glutathione, protein sulfhydryl and other changes. Exp Eye Res 1983; 36:351–62.
30. Lewis BS, Harding JJ. The major metabolite of bendazac inhibits the glycosylation of soluble lens proteins: a possible mechanism for a delay in cataractogenesis. Exp Eye Res 1988; 47:217–25.
31. Liang JN, Chylack LT Jr. Spectroscopic study on the effects of nonenzymatic glycation in human α-crystallin. Invest Ophthalmol Vis Sci 1987; 28:790–4.
32. McNamara M, Augusteyn RC. The effects of hydrogen peroxide on lens proteins: a possible model for nuclear cataract. Exp Eye Res 1984; 38:45–56.
33. McNeil J, Robman L, Tikellis G, et al. Vitamin E supplementation and cataract. Randomized controlled trial. Ophthalmology 2004; 111:75–84.
34. Minassian DC, Mehra VJ, Jones BR. Dehydrational crises from severe diarrhoea or heatstroke and risk of cataract. Lancet 1984; 1:751–3.
35. Minassian DC, Mehra VJ, Verrey J-D. Dehydrational crises: a major factor in blinding cataract. Br J Ophthalmol 1989; 73:100–5.
36. Monnier VM, Stevens VJ, Cerami A. Nonenzymatic glycosylation, sulfhydryl oxidation, and aggregation of lens proteins in experimental sugar cataracts. J Exp Med 1979; 150:1098–107.
37. Monnier VM, Bautista O, Kenny D, et al. Skin collagen glycation, glycoxidation, and crosslinking are lower in subjects with long-term intensive versus conventional therapy of type I diabetes. Diabetes 1999; 48:870–80.
38. Ortwerth BJ, Olesen PR. Glutathione inhibits the glycation and crosslinking of lens proteins by ascorbic acid. Exp Eye Res 1988; 47:737–50.
39. Perry RE, Swamy MS, Abraham EC. Progressive changes in lens crystallin glycation and high-molecular-weight aggregate formation leading to cataract development in streptozotocin-diabetic rats. Exp Eye Res 1987; 44: 269–82.
40. Rachdan D, Lou MF, Harding JJ. Revival of inactive glyceraldehyde 3-phosphate dehydrogenase in human cataract lenses by reduction. Exp Eye Res 2004; 79: 105–9.
41. Rachdan D, Lou MF, Harding JJ. Glutathione reductase from human cataract lenses can be revived by reducing agents and by a molecular chaperone, α-crystallin. Curr Eye Res 2005; 30:1–7.
42. Roy D, Garner MH, Spector A, et al. Investigation of Nakano lens proteins. Exp Eye Res 1982; 34:909–20.
43. Siezen RJ, Coppin CM, Kaplan ED, et al. Oxidative modifications to crystallins induced in calf lenses in vitro by hydrogen peroxide. Exp Eye Res 1989; 48:225–35.
44. Spector A, Garner WH. Hydrogen peroxide and human cataract. Exp Eye Res 1981; 33:673–81.

45. Spector A, Garner MH, Garner WH, Roy D, Farnsworth P, Shyne S. An extrinsic membrane polypeptide associated with high-molecular-weight protein aggregates in human cataract. Science 1979; 204:1323–6.
46. Spector A, Roy D. Disulfide-linked high molecular weight protein associated with human cataract. Proc Natl Acad Sci USA 1978; 75:3244–8.
47. Stevens VJ, Rouzer CA, Monnier VM, Cerami A. Diabetic cataract formation: potential role of glycosylation of lens crystallins. Proc Natl Acad Sci USA 1978; 75:2918–22.
48. Stratton IM, Kohner EM, Aldington SJ, et al. UKPDS 50: risk factors for incidence and progression of retinopathy in type II diabetes over 6 years from diagnosis. Diabetologia 2001; 44:156–63.
49. Swamy MS, Abraham EC. Inhibition of lens crystalline glycation and high molecular weight aggregate formation by aspirin in vitro and in vivo. Invest Ophthalmol Vis Sci 1989; 30:1120–6.
50. Van Heyningen R, Harding JJ. A case-control study of cataract in Oxfordshire: some risk factors. Br J Ophthalmol 1988; 72:804–8.
51. Zigler JS Jr, Carper DA, Kinoshita JH. Changes in lens crystallins during cataract development in the Philly mouse. Ophthal Res 1981; 13:237–51.

25

Pseudoexfoliation Syndrome

Ursula Schlötzer-Schrehardt
University of Erlangen-Nürnberg, Erlangen, Germany

Barbara A. W. Streeten
State University of New York Upstate Medical University, Syracuse, New York, U.S.A.

INTRODUCTION

Pseudoexfoliation syndrome (PEX) is a common age-related disorder of the extracellular matrix characterized by an excessive production and progressive accumulation of an abnormal fibrillar material throughout the anterior segment of the eye (105,131). PEX may affect up to 30% of people over the age of 60 across the world and PEX is frequently associated with severe chronic secondary open-angle glaucoma and cataract. It is clinically diagnosed by seeing dandruff-like white flakes deposited on the structures that line the aqueous humor-bathed surfaces of the anterior segment, particularly the anterior lens surface and the pupillary border of the iris. The term PEX has been widely used for this entity, however, the process does not represent a true exfoliation of the lens capsule, like in infrared light-induced true lens exfoliation of its basement membrane.

PEX was recognized as a frequent cause of glaucoma associated with characteristic changes of the anterior lens capsule almost 90 years ago (179). It is presently acknowledged as the most common identifiable cause of open-angle glaucoma, accounting for the majority of glaucoma cases in some countries and for about 25% of all open-angle glaucomas worldwide (129). The characteristic tissue alterations predispose to a broad spectrum of intraocular complications including phacodonesis and lens subluxation, angle-closure glaucoma, melanin dispersion, insufficient mydriasis, blood–aqueous barrier dysfunction, and posterior synechiae as well as corneal endothelial decompensation (105,131). The pathological alterations also explain the wide range of complications associated with intraocular surgery in PEX patients (22).

Recent years have seen a significant increase in our understanding of this disorder (148). Apart from the long-known intraocular manifestations, PEX has been shown to be a systemic process, which appears to be associated with increased cardiovascular and cerebrovascular morbidity. Nevertheless, much remains to be learned about its ocular and systemic manifestations as well as its cause and pathogenesis.

EPIDEMIOLOGY

PEX was first described in Finland by Lindberg in 1917 (94,169), and at one time it was considered to be much more common in Scandinavia than elsewhere. It has, however, become realized, that PEX occurs in all geographic regions worldwide with reported prevalence rates averaging about 10% to 20% of the general population >60 years of age (32,33,123). In all populations, the frequency rises with increasing age, with its incidence doubling every decade after the age of 50 years, and females are more frequently affected in most series (131). There is a clear tendency for PEX to cluster geographically and in certain racial or ethnic subgroups. There is a high prevalence of PEX in Finland, Lapland, Iceland, Norway, and Northern Russia, where it affects from 10% to 13% of persons from 50 to 69 years and 21% to 35% >70 years of age. Similar figures apply to Saudi Arabia, Mediterranean, and Baltic countries and among the Navajo Indians in the United States. In contrast, PEX occurs in only 2–10% of persons >60 years of age in most European populations, in Japan, and in parts of the United States. Even within populations of one country, large variability over short distances has been observed.

The reasons for differences in prevalences between age-matched geographical and ethnic populations remain unknown, but appear to be mainly related to genetic variability. A recent epidemiologic study found no significant influence of climate on the occurrence of PEX (33). PEX was not found in the Inuit, but a prevalence rate of 13% was seen in the Saami, both of whom live in arctic climes. Moreover, populations living in tropical regions had less PEX than those living in temperate zones, despite the fact that they had more climatically induced alterations of the cornea and conjunctiva. These observations support the notion that genetic factors underlie the differences in prevalences between populations.

ETIOLOGY

Besides regional clustering, evidence supporting a genetic basis for PEX includes familial aggregation, transmission in two-generation families, higher concordance rates in monozygous twins, an increased risk of PEX in relatives of affected patients, loss of heterozygosity, and human leukocyte antigen (HLA) studies (23,109). PEX appears to be inherited as an autosomal-dominant trait, the late onset and incomplete penetrance of which pose considerable problems to genetic analyses. Most published two-generation pedigrees showed matrilineal inheritance (2,23), but others provide evidence of paternal transmission (50). Among the three families of the island of Gozo presented in the latter study, the expression of PEX and associated conditions seemed to vary considerably: one family had a high incidence of both cataract and PEX-associated glaucoma, another family had mainly PEX glaucoma, while in the third family all affected individuals had cataract but no evidence of glaucoma. These observations suggest that PEX may be clinically and genetically heterogenous. Indeed PEX has been mapped tentatively to several chromosomal regions. Preliminary linkage analyses have identified two putative gene loci on chromosome 2 (2p16, 2q35-36) and another one on chromosome 3 (3q13-q21) (5,158,181). A recent study has implicated mutations in the *LOXL1* gene (175). In addition, PEX specimens (iris, lens capsule) displayed a high incidence of loss of heterozygosity in microsatellite markers located on chromosome 7 indicating that nearby genes could be affected by the genetic lesions (80,188).

Moreover, nongenetic factors, including dietary factors, autoimmunity, infectious agents, and trauma, have also been hypothesized to be involved in the pathogenesis of PEX (23,121). A significant relation to ultraviolet (UV) light exposure was reported by Taylor (172) in Australian aborigines, but could not be substantiated by more recent studies (33). It is noteworthy that the exceptional diagnosis of PEX in younger patients <40 years old seems to be generally preceded by prior intraocular surgery or trauma to the anterior segment, particularly to the iris (74), or by corneal transplantation with grafts from elderly donors (83). These events may trigger the premature development of PEX in a predisposed individual or even raise the possibility of a transmissible agent.

Altogether, PEX appears to represent a complex, multifactorial, late-onset disease, involving both genetic and nongenetic factors in its etiopathogenesis.

CLINICAL FINDINGS

Established PEX

The most important diagnostic criteria of PEX are the whitish flake-like deposits on anterior segment structures, particularly on the anterior lens surface (Figs. 1A,B) and the pupillary margin (Figs. 1C,D). The material is occasionally also on the posterior surface of the cornea (Fig. 1E), on the anterior surface of intraocular lens implants, and on the anterior vitreous face in aphakic eyes. However, most intraocular PEX deposits cannot be observed by direct biomicroscopy, and the accumulations on zonules (Fig. 1F), ciliary processes (Fig. 1G), and trabecular meshwork (Fig. 1H) may be only detected on gonioscopy, cycloscopy, or by high-resolution ultrasound biomicroscopy.

Lens

The characteristic target-shaped pattern on the lens, consisting of a homogenous central disc resembling

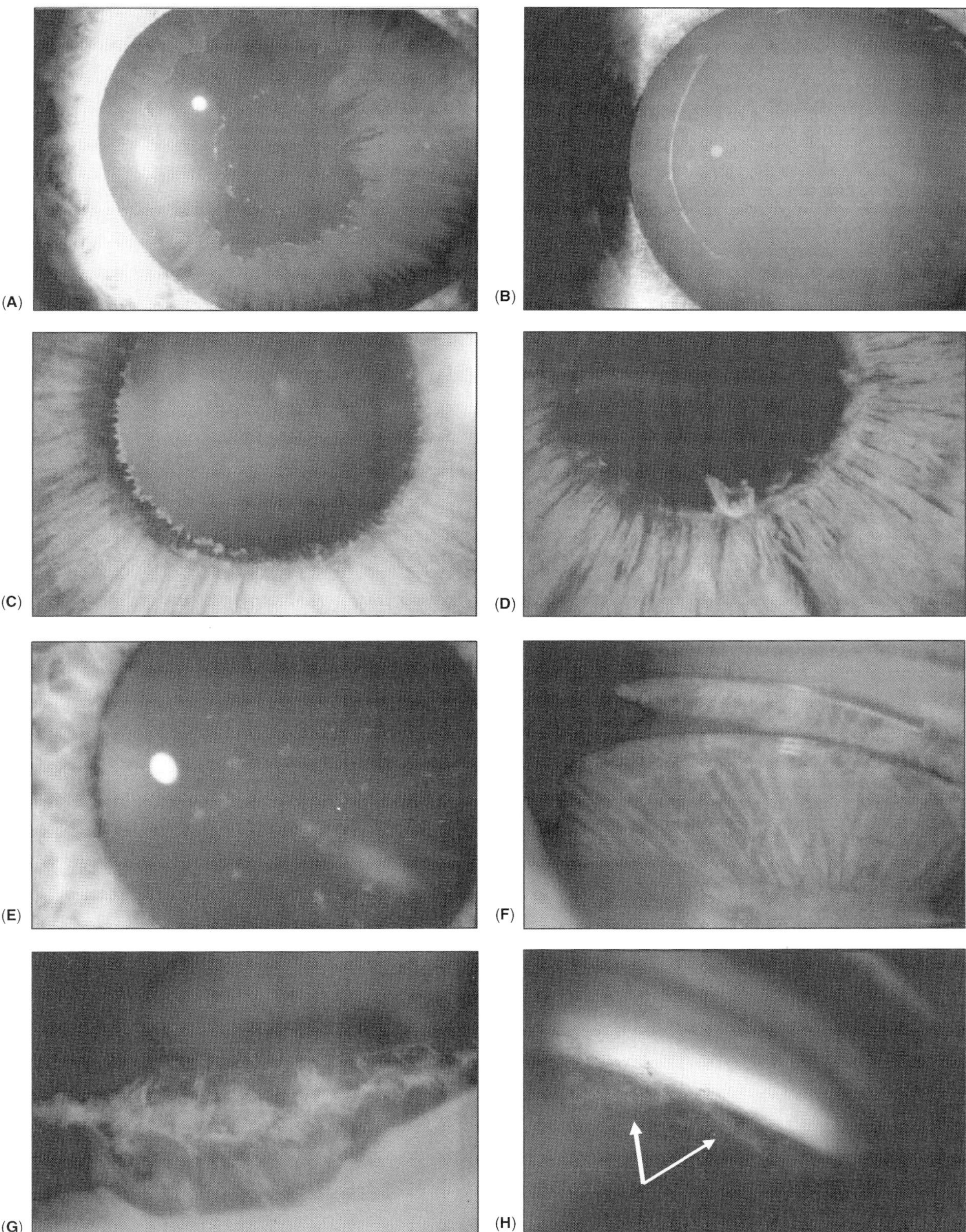

Figure 1 Clinical signs of pseudoexfoliation syndrome (PEX). (**A**) Classic target-shaped pattern of PEX material accumulation on the lens with the central disc and peripheral zone separated by a clear intermediate zone; a few remaining bridges of PEX material span the clear zone. (**B**) The central disc may be absent and the peripheral zone may show curled edges; lenticular PEX deposits can only be seen after pupillary dilation. (**C,D**) PEX material deposits on the pupillary border. (**E**) Retrocorneal PEX deposits. (**F**) Gonioscopically evident accumulations of PEX material on zonules and ciliary processes. (**G**) PEX deposits on ciliary processes and zonules as observed through an iris defect. (**H**) Flakes of PEX material (*arrows*) in the anterior chamber angle. *Source*: Courtesy of G.K. Krieglstein.

a cellophane-like membrane, an intermediate clear zone, and a peripheral granular zone with nodular vegetations, can be only seen after pupillary dilation (Fig. 1A). In routine examinations without pupillary dilation, the diagnosis may be missed, because the central disc, corresponding to the size of the pupil, may be very subtle or even absent in 20% to 50% of cases (Fig. 1B). Many variations of this pattern on the anterior lens surface have been observed, such as bridges of PEX material crossing the intermediate clear zone or evidence of peeling. Sometimes a second or third granular zone with smaller vegetations forms immediately central to the primary granular zone, giving the impression of a later formation after continuous reduction of the pupil size. These variations may relate to the topographical relationship between the lens and the iris or to different stages of development.

Iris

In addition to deposits of PEX material, several other, mostly pigment-related, clinical signs aid in the diagnosis, including melanin dispersion in the anterior chamber after pupillary dilation (Fig. 2A), peripupillary atrophy (Fig. 2B), and loss of pupillary ruff (Fig. 2C) (112,131). Pigment loss from the peripupillary iris pigment epithelium and pigment deposition on the iris surface (Fig. 2D), corneal endothelium (Fig. 2E), and trabecular meshwork (Fig. 2F), are hallmarks of PEX. In particular, a heavily pigmented trabecular meshwork is a constant feature of PEX eyes. Unlike pigment dispersion syndrome (see Chapter 20), the trabecular pigment tends to be uneven or patchy and less well defined. Pigment also deposits on or anterior to Schwalbe line forming one or more undulating lines of pigment in the peripheral cornea (Sampaolesi line). Pigment dispersion is caused by mechanical friction of the peripupillary iris against the rough anterior lens surface during pupillary movement. This manifests clinically in a peripupillary atrophy producing a characteristic "moth-eaten" transillumination pattern (Fig. 2B) and pupillary ruff defects (Fig. 2C).

Further signs that can alert the clinician to PEX include phacodonesis, iris stroma atrophy, iris hemorrhages after pupillary dilation (Fig. 2G), increased aqueous flare values, posterior synechiae (Fig. 2H), elevated intraocular pressure (IOP), and insufficient pupillary dilation, particularly if asymmetric (105,131).

Posing a diagnostic challenge, the deposits on the lens may be obscured by posterior synechiae. PEX predisposes to the formation of adhesions between the iris pigment epithelium and the anterior lens capsule, even in the absence of miotics. Posterior synechiae may hinder an evaluation of the anterior lens surface masking a diagnosis of PEX (96). In these cases, high-resolution ultrasound biomicroscopy may reveal PEX deposits on the lens or zonules (105).

Early Stages of PEX

The classical picture of lens deposits represents, however, a very late stage of the disease, which is preceded by a long preclinical course of several years. By thorough biomicroscopic examination, a diffuse-frosted grayish film on the entire surface of the anterior lens capsule can be observed prior to typical PEX deposits (24,105,173). The layer is thought to represent a precursor of PEX material diffusely deposited on the lens surface from the aqueous humor. This layer is difficult to detect unless it has developed holes or clefts in the parapupillary region or radial striations in the mid-zone. As this precapsular layer becomes thicker, focal defects begin to form in the midperipheral zone by virtue of abrasive movements of the iris, often in the upper nasal quadrant (Fig. 3A), with subsequent enlargement and confluence to form the classical picture of PEX (Figs. 3B,C). Eventually, only small bridges may remain as an indication of the initially continuous layer of PEX material in the intermediate zone. Transmission electron microscopy (TEM) confirms the presence of a precapsular layer composed of microfibrils, which is thought to represent a precursor of typical PEX fibrils on the lens surface (Fig. 3D).

Additional clinical signs of the early stages are peripupillary atrophy of the iris pigment epithelium, anterior chamber melanin dispersion associated with pupillary dilation, melanin deposition on anterior segment structures, particularly the trabecular meshwork, and poor mydriasis (113,173). Because PEX is often asymmetric, comparison with the fellow eye is diagnostically helpful in highlighting the early changes. In addition, the zonules are affected early in PEX. Examination by high-resolution ultrasound biomicroscopy has been shown to be useful for detecting early deposits of PEX material on zonules, particularly in cases with inadequate pupillary dilation or opaque media (64).

Asymmetric Involvement

PEX can present with either unilateral or markedly asymmetric bilateral involvement. In several large series, PEX was unilateral at the time of diagnosis in 50% to 70% of patients and the conversion rates to bilaterality were found to vary from 15% to 40% within 5 years (131). It may take many years for the disorder to become bilateral or this may not occur at all during the patient's lifetime (114). Tarkkanen and Kivelä (170) found after 29 years follow-up that most

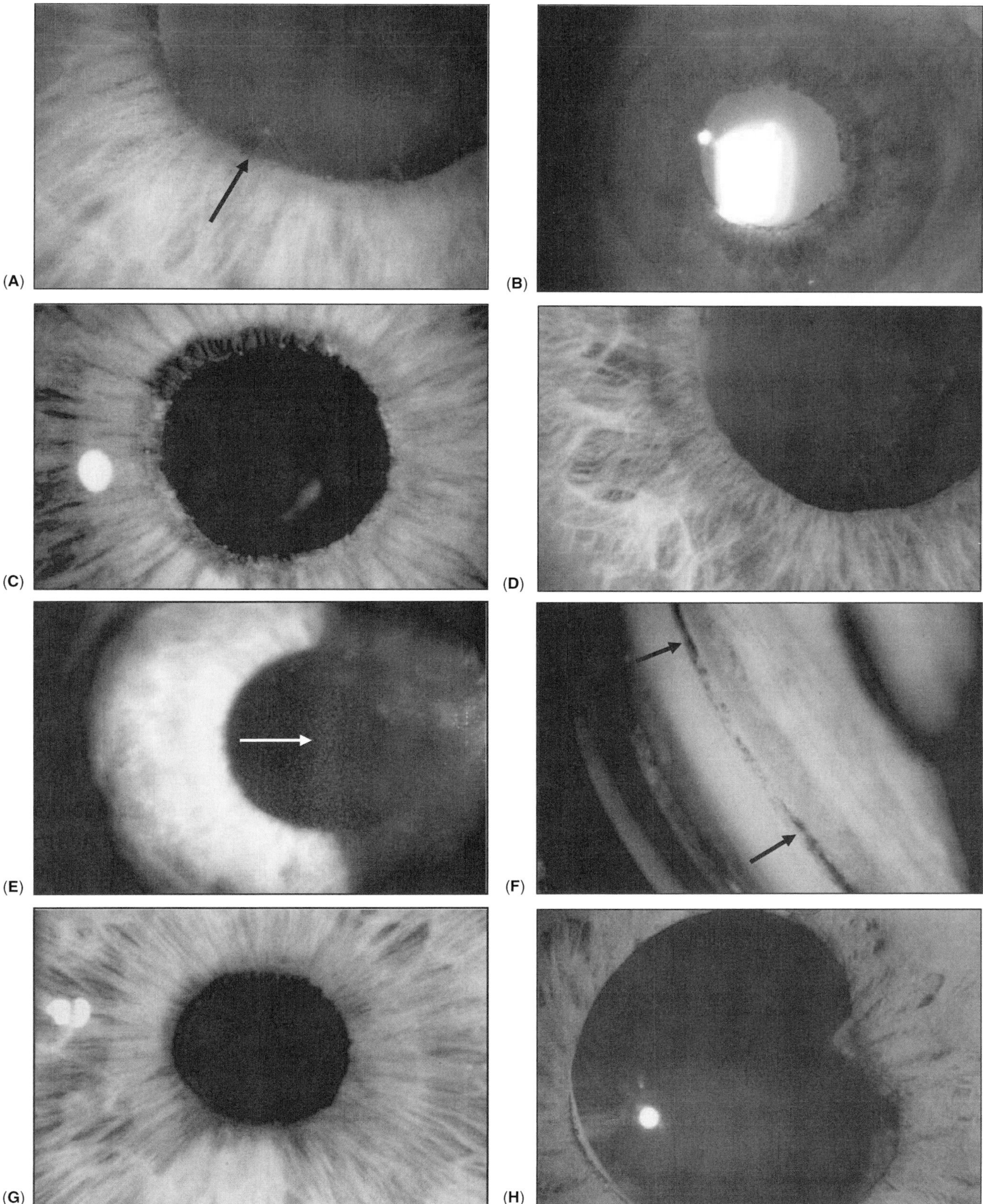

Figure 2 Additional clinical signs in eyes with pseudoexfoliation syndrome (PEX). (**A**) Pigment loss (*arrow*) from the peripupillary iris pigment epithelium. (**B**) Peripupillary atrophy producing a characteristic "moth-eaten" transillumination pattern. (**C**) Pupillary ruff defects. (**D**) Pigment deposition on the iris sphincter region. (**E**) Retrocorneal pigment accumulation (*arrow*). (**F**) Uneven trabecular meshwork pigmentation (*arrows*). (**G**) Spontaneous intrastromal hemorrhages of iridal vessels. (**H**) Formation of posterior synechiae.

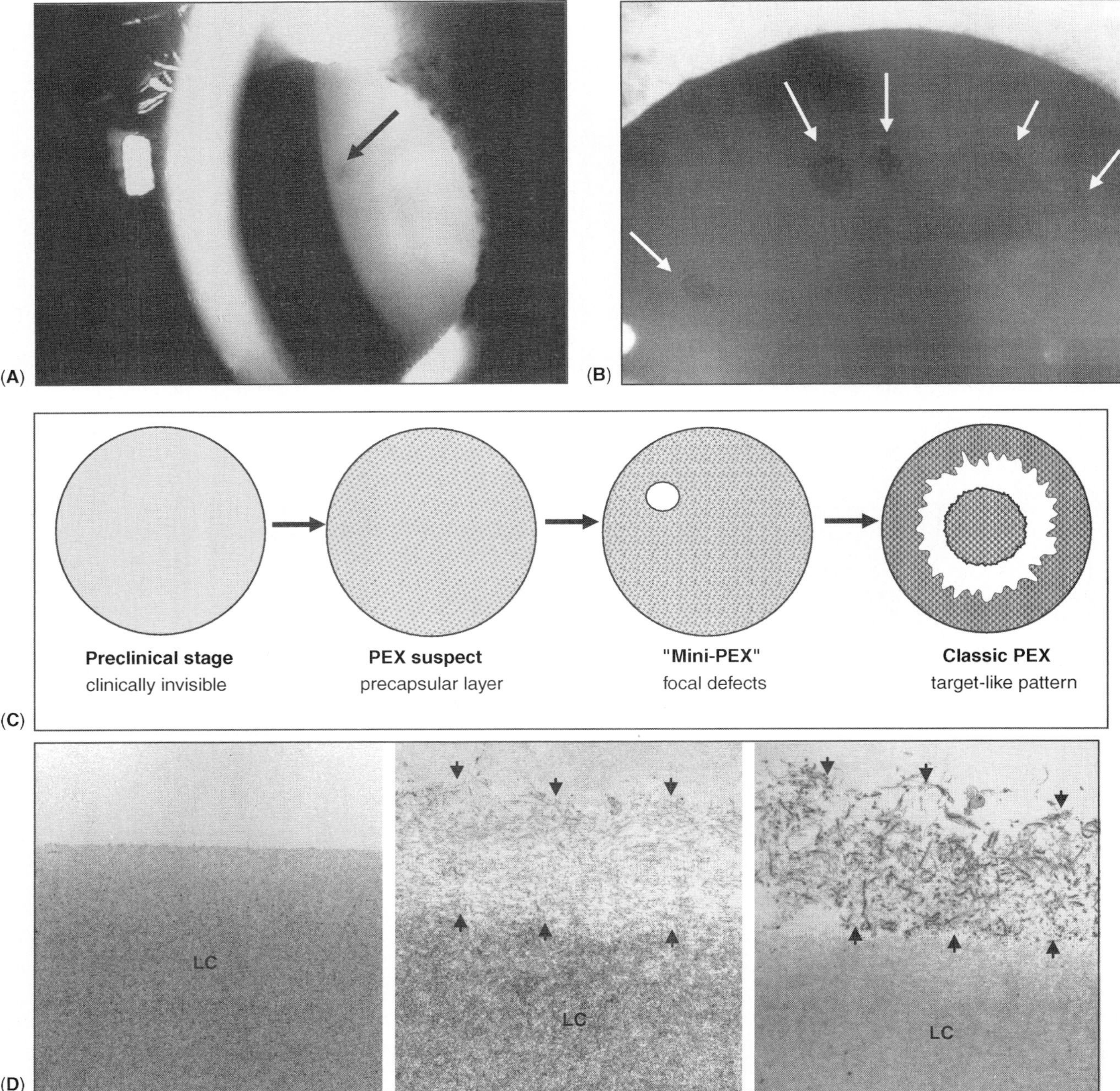

Figure 3 Early stages of pseudoexfoliation syndrome (PEX). (**A**) Clinical appearance of "Mini-PEX" with a focal rub-off defect (*arrow*) in the homogenous precapsular layer in the supranasal mid-zone of the lens. (**B**) An early stage in the formation of the intermediate clear zone with larger clefts (*arrows*) in the precapsular layer created by iris movements. (**C**) Schematic representation of the clinical classification of PEX syndrome based on morphologic alterations of the anterior lens surface. (**D**) Clinical classification of PEX syndrome based on ultrastructural alterations of the anterior lens capsule (LC): *left*, normal capsule with smooth surface; *center*, PEX suspect with a precapsular layer of microfibrils (*arrowheads*); *right*, classic PEX with both microfibrils and mature PEX fibrils in the area of the central disc (*arrowheads*).

patients with unilateral PEX will not convert to clinically apparent bilateral disease. Clinically, the involved eye often has a poorer visual acuity, more advanced lens opacity, higher IOP, a smaller pupil, and a more pronounced trabecular pigmentation than the noninvolved fellow eye.

However, the majority of apparent unilateral cases detected clinically have subtle changes in the fellow eye suggesting that all cases are in fact bilateral. By cycloscopy, Mizuno and Muroi (99) observed that in apparent unilateral cases PEX material encrusting the zonules and ciliary processes can be among the first clinical signs of PEX in the apparently unaffected eye. PEX material has been shown to be almost invariably present by TEM in the conjunctiva (113) and in the iris, particularly in the dilator pupillae and blood vessel walls, of the clinically uninvolved fellow eye (49,68). These changes may account for the clinical signs of early PEX, such as melanin dispersion, peripupillary atrophy, insufficient mydriasis, and blood–aqueous barrier defects leading to increased aqueous flare values. They further support the concept of PEX as being a generalized, basically bilateral disorder with a clinically marked asymmetric presentation. The question of whether subtle differences in ocular blood flow, aqueous humor dynamics, or blood–aqueous humor barrier function are or are not responsible for this asymmetric manifestation, remains to be determined.

PEX and Cataract

Lens opacification, most commonly of a nuclear type, has long been known to be associated with PEX (56) and is the most common reason for PEX patients to require surgical intervention (22). Cataract development may be causally linked to the presence of ocular ischemia, aqueous hypoxia, increased growth factor levels, or reduced protection against ultraviolet radiation by lower levels of ascorbic acid in the aqueous humor of PEX eyes (see section Molecular Pathogenesis).

Cataract surgery in eyes with PEX has been a challenge because of weakened zonules and the reduced pupillary diameter (47,104). Intra- and postoperative surgical complications, such as zonular ruptures, vitreous loss, blood–aqueous barrier breakdown, anterior capsule fibrosis/contraction, secondary cataract, and decentration or dislocation of the lens implant, have been reported to be more common and more serious than in eyes without PEX and are related to the pathological tissue alterations of the anterior segment (53,87,88). Today, the common use of phacoemulsification with anterior capsulorhexis by experienced surgeons has provided significantly better results with a lower rate of intraoperative complications compared with the conventional extracapsular cataract extraction technique (63). However, improvements in intraoperative results may reflect a shift of complications to the postoperative period, as reflected by a growing number of case reports of late intraocular lens displacement/dislocation after uneventful phacoemulsification due to progressive zonular weakening (66). Continued destabilization of the zonules appears to result from ongoing PEX material production by remaining lens epithelial cells and from anterior capsule fibrosis and contraction exerting additional centripetal stress on the compromised zonules.

PEX and Glaucoma

The most serious ocular complication of PEX is secondary open-angle glaucoma, affecting 20% to 60% of patients in different series (see Chapter 20) (131,132). PEX-associated open-angle glaucoma accounts for approximately 25% of all glaucomas and represents the most common identifiably cause of glaucoma overall. In some populations (e.g., Baltic, Mediterranean, Arabian), the frequency of PEX-associated secondary glaucoma may reach a higher percentage of the population than the primary forms of glaucoma. The probability that PEX eyes will develop glaucoma has been reported to vary from 5% to 35% within 5 years and from 15% to 40% within 10 years. Factors associated with conversion to PEX glaucoma were the initial IOP, degree of pupil dilation, and difference in IOP between the two eyes (114). Accordingly, the frequency of PEX syndrome is usually high among glaucoma patients and has been reported to range from 10% to 30% in the United States and from 50% to 60% in Northern Europe.

PEX glaucoma is also believed to be more difficult to manage clinically, with a higher incidence of treatment failure than primary open-angle glaucoma (POAG). The worse prognosis may be related to characteristically higher mean IOP levels, greater diurnal fluctuations in IOP, and marked pressure spikes (75,76). A significant correlation between the IOP level at the time of diagnosis and the mean visual field defect (174) as well as between diurnal IOP fluctuations and retinal nerve fiber layer thickness (46) could be only established in patients with PEX glaucoma, but not with POAG. These findings suggest that glaucomatous damage in PEX patients may be more directly related to IOP than pertains in POAG patients. Correspondingly, reduction and stabilization of mean IOP levels and IOP fluctuations have been shown to improve visual field prognosis much more in PEX glaucoma than in POAG (77).

Patients with PEX are also at increased risk of developing significant but transient IOP rises following diagnostic pupillary dilation due to dispersion of pigment granules and PEX material in the anterior chamber. Pigment liberation and pressure elevation, which can rise to 30 mmHg above baseline IOP, may peak only 2 to 3 h postdilation and go back to normal levels after 10 to 15 h (81). Such pressure peaks can even mimic acute glaucomas including pain, a red eye, corneal edema, and pressure rises over 50 mmHg (105).

Although PEX glaucoma is characteristically a high-pressure disease, pressure-independent risk factors, such as an impaired ocular and retrobulbar perfusion (51,187) and abnormalities of elastic tissue of the lamina cribrosa (106), may be present and further increase the individual risk of glaucomatous damage.

Glaucoma in PEX usually occurs in the presence of an open anterior chamber angle, but an association between PEX and angle-closure glaucoma is not rare (11,45,130). Because eyes with PEX often have narrowed anterior chamber angles and smaller anterior chamber volumes (40,45,183) in the presence of a weak zonular apparatus, a minimal anterior subluxation of the lens predisposes to the development of angle-closure glaucoma via a pupillary block mechanism. Further features of PEX eyes that may predispose to the development of pupillary block angle-closure glaucoma include the formation of posterior synechiae, an increased iris rigidity and decreased iris motility, an impairment of the blood–aqueous barrier, and increased protein concentrations of aqueous humor (105). Miotics may aggravate both pupillary block and forward movement of the lens-iris diaphragm. In extreme and rather rare cases with marked zonular laxity, anterior displacement of the lens may be so pronounced that a ciliary block angle-closure glaucoma (malignant glaucoma) is induced by contraction of the ciliary muscle (180). Secondary angle-closure glaucoma following central retinal vein occlusion with iris neovascularization (neovascular glaucoma) may also occur in PEX eyes, because retinal vein occlusion appears to be more common in patients with PEX with and without glaucoma (43).

Systemic Associations

More than 10 years ago, aggregates of PEX material were identified by TEM in autopsy specimens of heart, lung, liver, kidney, gall bladder, and cerebral meninges in two patients with PEX (138,166). In these extraocular locations, PEX material was primarily found in connective tissue portions of visceral organs, often in the periphery of blood vessels. These findings suggested that the ocular manifestations of PEX are part of a systemic disorder of the extracellular matrix. Subsequently, many studies have examined the potential clinical consequences of these deposits and attempted to determine whether there is an association of PEX syndrome with systemic disease.

In the meantime, a growing number of small-scale studies are part of an emerging clinical spectrum in which PEX appears to be associated with cardiovascular and/or cerebrovascular disease. These include transient ischemic attacks (116), a history of angina pectoris, arterial hypertension, myocardial infarction, or stroke (97), aneurysms of the abdominal aorta (152), asymptomatic myocardial dysfunction (16), ischemic white matter lesions in the brain (187), Alzheimer disease (95), and sensorineural hearing loss (18). A more recent study retrospectively investigating 1150 patients with either PEX glaucoma or POAG found a higher frequency of chronic cerebral disorders and acute cerebrovascular events in the PEX group (133). However, no correlation with cardiovascular or cerebrovascular disease has been found in six Icelandic families (2) and the mortality rate does not appear to be increased in PEX (128,157). Therefore, prospective, randomized multicenter studies are indicated to resolve these issues and determine whether other age-related diseases are coincidental or not.

The prevalence of mild to moderate hyperhomocysteinemia has been suggested as one possible cause for an increased vascular risk in PEX patients. Meanwhile, elevated plasma homocysteine has been found in patients with PEX by several research teams and has been shown to be independent of the presence of glaucoma (14,91,177). The known pathophysiological roles of homocysteine in alterating extracellular matrix metabolism through dysregulation of matrix metalloproteinases (MMPs) and tissue inhibitors of metalloproteinase (TIMPs), in vascular endothelial dysfunction, oxidative stress, neuronal apoptosis, and elastinolysis have been discussed in respect of the pathogenesis of PEX and glaucoma. The most common genetic risk factor for hyperhomocysteinemia, the C677T single nucleotide polymorphism in the 5,10 methylenetetrahydrofolate reductase (*MTHFR*) gene, was not significantly increased in patients with PEX glaucoma (67). However, vitamin B6, vitamin B12, and folate plasma levels were significantly decreased in patients with PEX glaucoma and correlated negatively with total plasma homocysteine levels (J.B. Rödl, 2006, submitted for publication). Since vitamin B6, vitamin B12, and folate are involved in homocysteine metabolism, their deficiency might explain the hyperhomocysteinemia in PEX patients.

HISTOPATHOLOGY

In the eye, all tissues of the anterior segment that are closely associated with the aqueous humor circulation appear to be affected by PEX material accumulations, whereas PEX material has not been found in posterior segment structures.

Lens

In up to 70% of patients with clinically suspected early PEX a precapsular layer (0.5–3.5 μm thick), composed of microfibrils (3–6 and 8–10 nm in diameter) can be detected by TEM on the entire surface of the anterior lens capsule (Fig. 3D) (24,173). Scanning electron microscopy (SEM) reveals a delicate microfibrillar network with rolled-up edges, suggesting a loose attachment. This loosely arranged microfibrillar layer can be immunostained for fibrillin-1, suggesting that it represents a precursor of typical PEX material on the lens surface, which may be diffusely deposited from the aqueous humor.

PEX material typically deposits in a "target-like" pattern on the anterior lens surface (Fig. 4A). It consists of a loosely attached central disc of fibrillar PEX material, which is separated from a peripheral granular zone by a 1 to 2 mm wide clear intermediate zone (105,131). The central disc, corresponding to the size of the undilated pupil, frequently shows rolled-up edges and is composed of a loose layer of mixed microfibrils and mature PEX fibrils that seem to originate by lateral aggregation of the microfibrils (Fig. 4B). The peripheral granular zone consists of abundant nodular PEX aggregates deposited on a continuous fibrillar basal layer, which may detach from the capsular surface as a continuous lamella (Fig. 4C). The underlying lens capsule and lens epithelium appear essentially normal. The central disc and the fibrillar basal lamella of the granular zone may develop from the central and peripheral portions of the precapsular layer of early stages, whereas the nodular PEX aggregates of the granular zone seem to build up by undisturbed production and accumulation by the iris pigment epithelium; the intermediate clear zone is created by abrasive movements of the peripupillary iris during pupillary movement (Fig. 5) (105,131). The diagnostically characteristic distribution pattern is primarily created by the topographic relation to the iris, which deposits granular aggregates in some areas and rubs material off in others. The anatomical relationship between iris and lens may be also responsible for the formation of a second- or even third-granular zone central to the first one due to gradually reduced dilating properties of the iris.

The anterior and posterior lens capsules are morphologically normal with a thickness and elasticity comparable to control eyes (Fig. 6A) (13). In contrast, the preequatorial part of the lens capsule, corresponding to the proliferative zone of the lens epithelium and the zone of zonular anchorage, is significantly altered (Fig. 6B). In this area, abundant nodular PEX aggregates cover the zonules and their attachment to the anterior lens capsule (Fig. 4D). By TEM bundles of PEX fibrils appear to originate from the preequatorial lens epithelial cells, invading the capsule proper and forming an unique deep layer called the fibrogranular zone (Fig. 6B) (7,13,25). It is composed of vertically oriented PEX fibers arising from pit-like surface invaginations of the preequatorial lens epithelial cells and aggregating within the capsule from microfibrils to typical PEX fibrils (Fig. 14A). The lens capsule surrounding these fibrils is more lamellar and not as densely compacted as the remaining capsule. The apparently locally produced PEX fibrils appear to infiltrate and traverse the lens capsule and seem to erupt through its surface, thereby disrupting and separating the zonular lamella from their insertion on the anterior lens capsule (Fig. 4D and Fig. 6B) (145). The deep zone fibrils may extend up through the capsule to join PEX material deposits on the capsular surface.

Thus, regarding the origin of PEX material on the surface of the lens, the clinically obvious PEX deposits in the central and peripheral regions are considered to result from aqueous- and iris-derived passive deposition, whereas the biomicroscopically invisible material in the preequatorial zone of zonular attachment, which is of greatest clinical significance, appears to be actively produced by the lens epithelium (105,131).

Ciliary Body and Zonules

Bush-like, feathery deposits of PEX material cover the crests of the ciliary processes in the pars plicata of the ciliary body, whereas the posterior half of the pars plana is generally devoid of PEX material accumulations. By TEM, the PEX fibrils appear to emanate from focal irregular surface invaginations of the nonpigmented epithelial cells and to be intermixed with microfibrils and fragments of thick redundant basement membrane characteristic of the aging ciliary epithelium (Fig. 14B) (41,154,168). In a later stage of the disease, some epithelial cells seem to degenerate under the progressively accumulating PEX masses. No PEX material has been found in relation to the pigmented ciliary epithelium, in the stroma or blood vessel walls of the ciliary body, except at the junction of the ciliary muscle with the trabecular meshwork.

At the sites of zonular anchorage in the ciliary body, PEX fibers also percolate through the free and attaching zonular bundles. Similar to the impaired zonular attachment on the anterior lens capsule, the zonular bundles are separated from their connection to the disrupted basement membrane of the nonpigmented epithelium by locally produced, intercalating PEX fibers (Fig. 6D) (145).

The zonular fiber bundles passing between the ciliary body and lens are heavily encrusted with and focally infiltrated by PEX material along their course, leading to zonular ruptures (Fig. 6C). Zonular disintegration may be further facilitated by proteolytic mechanisms, because proteolytic enzymes, such as cathepsin B, have been shown to be present within PEX material (145). The zonular fibrils proper may be intact or partially fragmented; however, in cases associated with phacodonesis or lens subluxation, marked degenerative changes of the zonular fibers have been observed (35). A direct transition between zonular fibers and PEX fibrils has also been reported (20,167). The two fibrillar elements are most intimately mixed at the edges of the zonular bundles, where the zonular fibrils appear to become part of complex PEX fibrils (Fig. 12F).

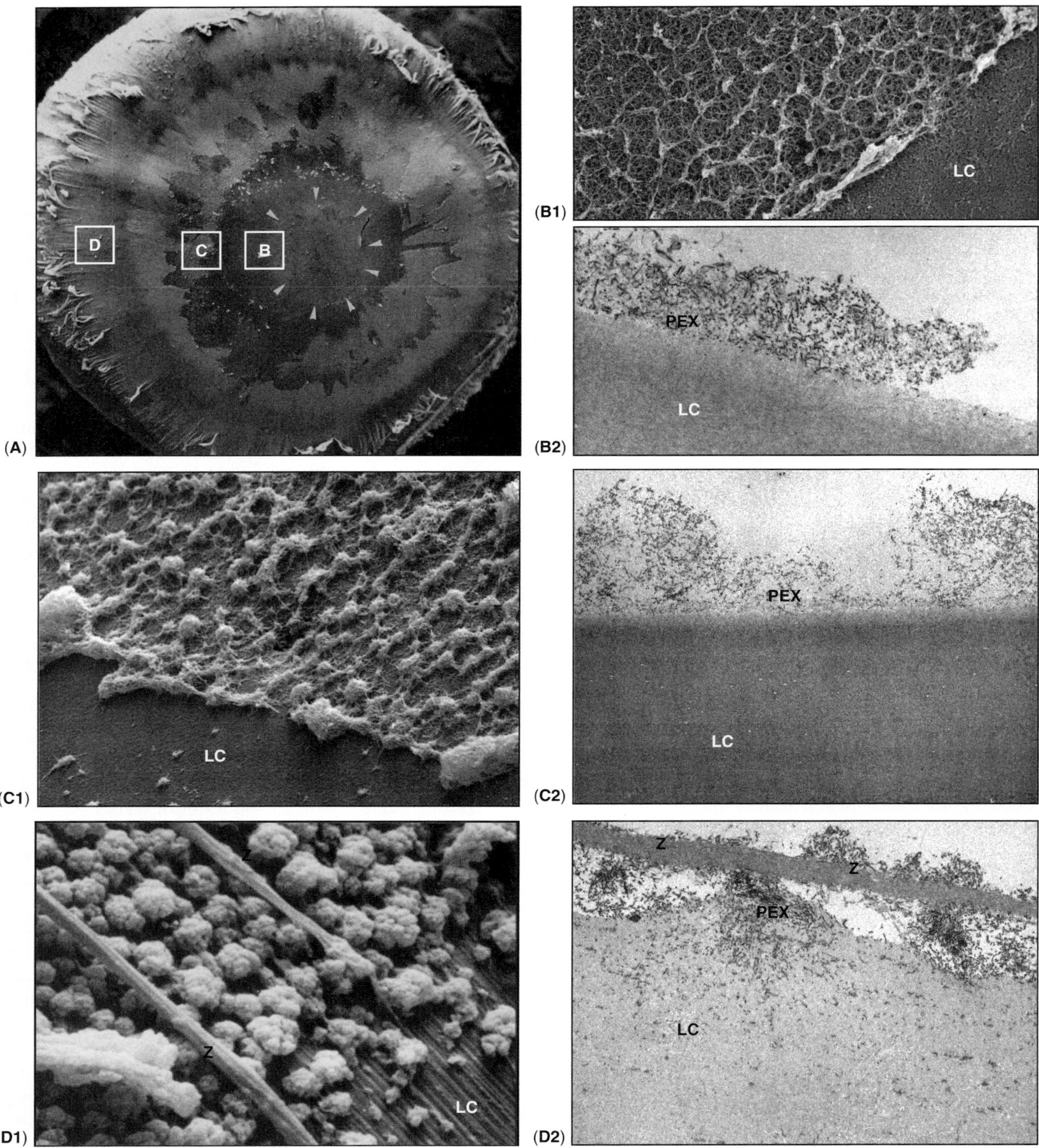

Figure 4 Involvement of the lens in pseudoexfoliation syndrome (PEX). (**A**) Scanning electron micrograph of the anterior lens surface showing signs of classic PEX syndrome with a central disc (*arrowheads*; B), the peripheral granular zone (C), and the preequatorial zone of zonular insertion (D); the boxed areas are shown in higher magnification in Figures (**B**)–(**D**). (**B1**) Scanning and (**B2**) transmission electron micrographs showing the fibrillar deposits of the loosely attached central disc. (**C1**) Scanning and (**C2**) transmission electron microscopic appearance of nodular PEX deposits in the peripheral granular zone. (**D1**) Scanning and (**D2**) transmission electron micrographs of the pre-equatorial zone of the lens capsule showing nodular PEX aggregates separating the zonular lamella from the capsular surface. *Abbreviations*: LC, lens capsule; Z, zonules.

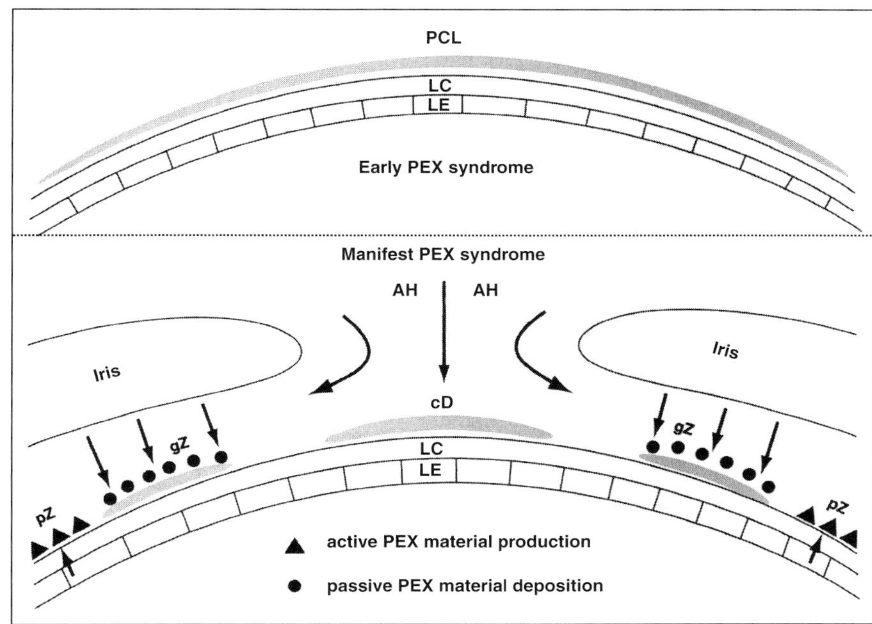

Figure 5 Schematic representation of the presumed origin of lenticular PEX material. *Abbreviations*: AH, aqueous humor; cD, central disc; gZ, granular zone; LC, lens capsule; LE, lens epithelium; PCL, precapsular layer; pZ, pre-equatorial zone.

These alterations are usually not visible on clinical examination, being hidden behind the iris, but give rise to a marked instability of the zonular apparatus and its attachment to the ciliary body and lens. This zonular instability may produce a characteristic phacodonesis or inferior displacement of the lens or predispose to angle-closure glaucoma in PEX patients (9,10,34,130,180).

Iris

PEX has a multitude of clinically important effects on iris tissues. Numerous histopathological studies have demonstrated that virtually all iris cell types are involved in PEX material production and deposition (105).

By light microscopy, bush-shaped aggregates of PEX material cover the surface of the posterior pigment epithelium, which shows a characteristic serrated appearance (Fig. 7A). TEM studies have demonstrated additional accumulations of PEX material within the stromal connective tissue and the anterior border layer, within sphincter pupillae and dilator pupillae, and in the walls of stromal blood vessels (6,42,73,118,154,155). The posterior pigment epithelial cells exhibit degenerative changes with focally ruptured cell membranes and the liberation of melanin granules (Fig. 7B) (156), producing the characteristic peripupillary atrophy with "moth-eaten" transillumination defects and anterior chamber pigment dispersion. PEX fibrils appear to be extruded from irregular membrane infoldings and are intermingled with disorganized basement membrane material (Figs. 14C,D).

Clinically, the iris of PEX patients is characteristically rigid with reduced dilating properties (19), which has been attributed to a combination of PEX fiber deposition in the stroma and muscle tissues (Fig. 7C) along with degenerative changes of the sphincter and dilator muscles (6). Plenty of PEX fibrils are related to the stromal cells in the superficial 20 to 30 μm of the anterior iris surface. Stromal PEX deposits are found in close proximity to fibroblasts and melanocytes and are particularly prominent in the walls of blood vessels. The affected blood vessels show basement membrane abnormalities and a gradual degeneration of vascular wall cells progressing from adventitial (pericytes, smooth muscle cells) to endothelial cells (Fig. 7D) (54,73). Vascular endothelial cells, pericytes, and smooth muscle cells appear to be sites of origin of PEX fibrils. In advanced stages, the vascular wall cells degenerate completely, leaving an acellular vessel wall outlined by a ring of PEX material (ghost vessels). Obliteration of the vessel lumen by PEX material or degenerating endothelial cells has also been observed (Fig. 7E).

Involvement of the iris stromal blood vessels has major functional consequences. Vessel degeneration and obliteration results in iris hypoperfusion and reduced partial pressure of oxygen in the anterior chamber (54). The accompanying tissue hypoxia may contribute to the atrophic changes of the iris stroma and muscle tissues. On fluorescein or indocyanine green angiography, changes including iris vessel dropout and dye leakage may be seen (17,111). Spontaneous intrastromal hemorrhages after mydriasis, without iris neovascularization, indicate significant vascular

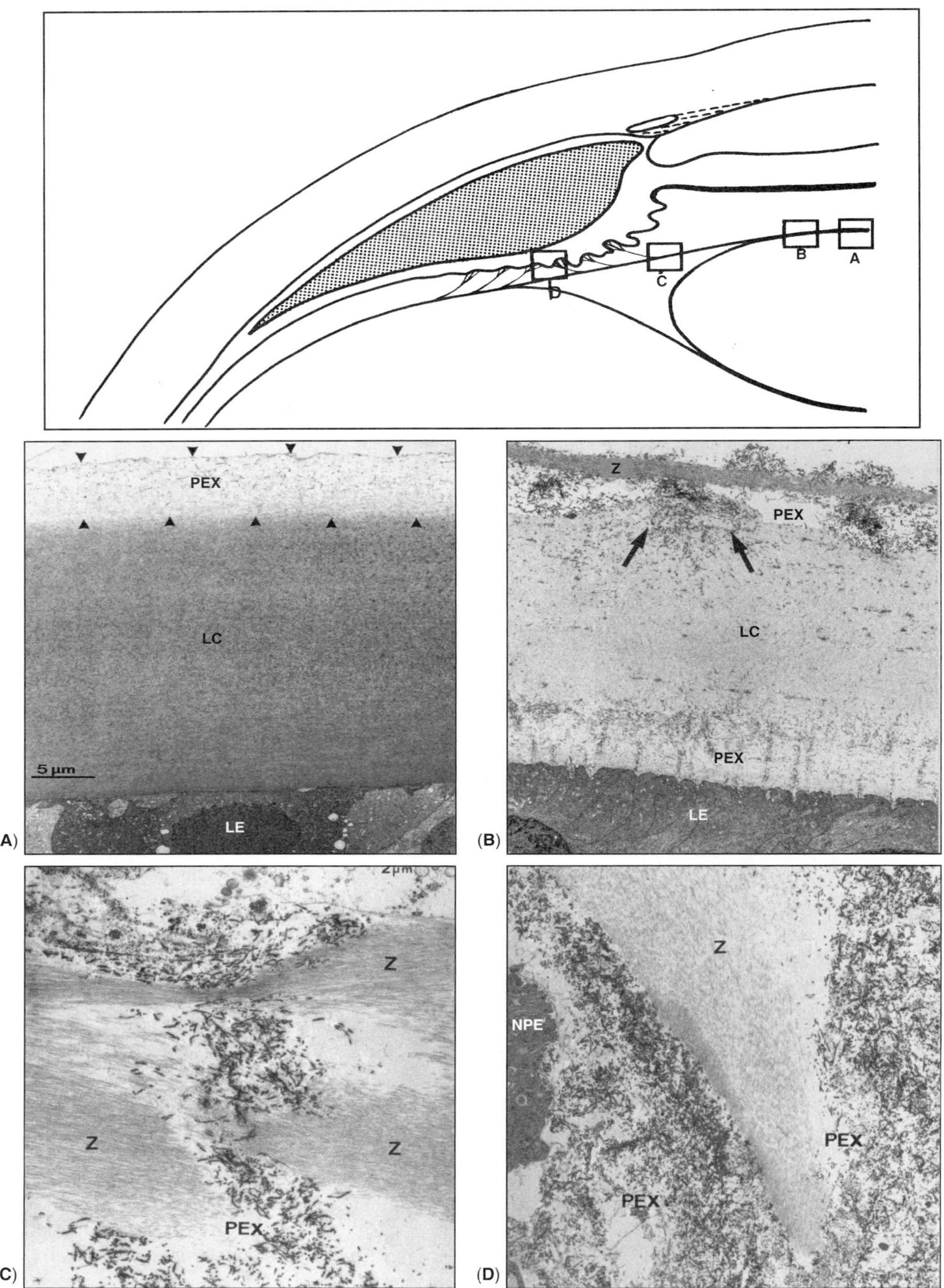

Figure 6 Schematic drawing (*top*) of the lens, zonular apparatus, and ciliary body, with corresponding representative transmission electron micrographs from designated regions of an eye with PEX syndrome. (**A**) Central anterior lens capsule in the area of the central disc; PEX fibrils and microfibrils (*arrowheads*) are homogenously deposited on the surface of the anterior lens capsule; however, the capsule itself appears morphologically normal. (**B**) In contrast to the anterior lens capsule, the lens capsule and zonular attachment in the pre-equatorial region are disrupted due to exuberant production of PEX material by the underlying lens epithelial cells. (**C**) A zonular bundle is seen to be severely disrupted and fragmented by PEX material. (**D**) A zonular bundle at its insertion into the basement membrane of the nonpigmented ciliary epithelium (NPE); the attachment of the zonular fibers is loosened and the anchoring basement membrane of the ciliary epithelium is completely destroyed by intercalating PEX material. *Abbreviations*: LC, lens capsule; LE, lens epithelium; PEX, PEX material; Z, zonules.

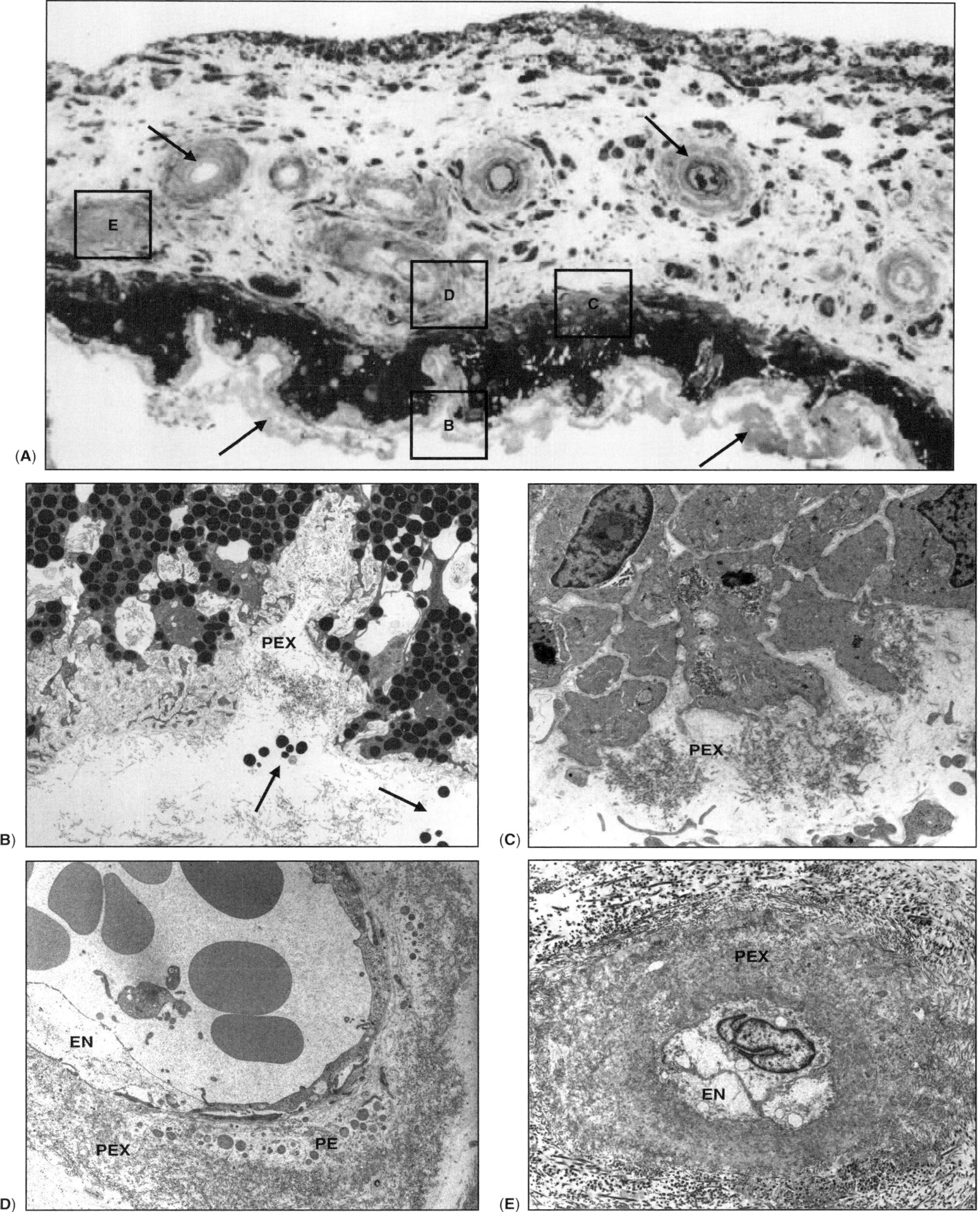

Figure 7 Involvement of the iris in pseudoexfoliation syndrome (PEX). (**A**) Light microscopic appearance and PEX material deposits (*arrows*) on the surface of the posterior pigment epithelium and in the periphery of blood vessels (magnification ×350). (**B**) Transmission electron micrograph of iris pigment epithelial cells; the epithelial cells are involved by thick deposits of PEX material on their surface and display degenerative changes evidenced by the liberation of melanin granules (*arrows*). (**C**) Electron micrograph showing PEX aggregates between sphincter muscle cells. (**D,E**) Ultrastructural alterations of iris blood vessels: perivascular PEX material accumulation and degenerative alterations of vascular endothelial cells (EN) and pericytes (PE) (**D**); degenerative swollen endothelial cells (EN) obstructing the vessel lumen (**E**).

damage (105). Another important consequence of the iris vasculopathy is a chronic breakdown of the blood–aqueous barrier in eyes with PEX syndrome (86). Clinically, this may manifest as a pseudouveitis with elevated aqueous flare and formation of posterior synechiae due to adherence of the posterior pigment epithelium to the PEX material-coated anterior lens capsule. Furthermore, blood–aqueous barrier dysfunction is compromised to a greater extent in eyes with PEX compared to eyes without PEX following intraocular surgery including cataract surgery, trabeculectomy, and laser trabeculoplasty (107,151). Postlaser and postoperative surgical complications, such as inflammatory responses, fibrin reactions, formation of synechiae, and IOP spikes, are more common in PEX eyes and can be directly attributed to the exaggerated and prolonged breakdown of the chronically defective blood–aqueous barrier.

Subtle ultrastructural alterations, such as microfibrillar deposits in the dilator muscle or the periphery of iris vessels, can be observed in virtually all contralateral eyes in clinically unilateral cases (49). These findings support the concept that PEX syndrome is a bilateral disease (68,113).

Trabecular Meshwork

The cause of chronic IOP elevation in PEX eyes is an increased outflow resistance in the trabecular meshwork (40), most probably caused by a blockage of the outflow channels by PEX material. Aggregates of PEX material have been found by TEM in the intertrabecular spaces, within the trabecular beams, and in the periphery of Schlemm canal (124). Most deposits are found in the juxtacanalicular tissue beneath the inner wall endothelium of Schlemm canal and in the uveal meshwork, while the corneoscleral portion of the meshwork appears largely uninvolved (44,117,146). PEX material also accumulates along the outer wall of Schlemm canal, in the periphery of collector channels and scleral aqueous veins. The PEX material accumulation in the trabecular meshwork may derive from both passive deposition from the aqueous humor in the inner uveal meshwork and from local production by trabecular cells in the outer portions.

Pathologic changes appear to affect primarily the juxtacanalicular tissue beneath the inner wall of Schlemm canal, the site of greatest resistance to aqueous humor outflow (Figs. 8A,B) (146). In this critical area, PEX material has been found within surface invaginations of the endothelial cells, suggesting local production by the endothelial cells lining Schlemm canal (Figs. 9A,B). There is no evidence of transport into the lumen of Schlemm canal, resulting in a progressive accumulation of PEX material in the thickened subendothelial space (Fig. 8B and Fig. 9C). In eyes with advanced PEX glaucoma, masses of PEX material accumulate along the whole periphery of Schlemm canal, causing a considerable disorganization of the normal tissue architecture, including narrowing and focal collapse of the canal lumen, disruption of its endothelial lining, and splitting and fragmentation into smaller channels (Figs. 8C and 9D). Collapse of aqueous veins due to perivascular accumulation of PEX material can also occasionally be observed. In the uveal meshwork, clumps of PEX material are found loosely within intertrabecular spaces suggesting passive deposition from the aqueous humor (Figs. 9E,F). Additional changes in glaucomatous eyes, such as thickening of trabecular lamellae, compression of intertrabecular spaces, and accumulation of long-spacing collagen in the trabecular beams (124,135) probably represent nonspecific secondary changes caused by high pressure and antiglaucomatous medications.

The amount of PEX material within the juxtacanalicular region has been shown to correlate with the presence of glaucoma, the average thickness of the juxtacanalicular tissue and the mean cross-sectional area of Schlemm canal (146), and also with the IOP level and the axon count in the optic nerve (44). These findings indicate a direct causative relationship between the build-up of PEX material in the meshwork and IOP level and the presence and severity of glaucomatous optic nerve damage.

Even though obstruction of the trabecular outflow channels by locally produced PEX material appears to be the major mechanism of increased outflow resistance and chronic IOP elevation, contributions due to pigment dispersion and increased aqueous protein concentrations have also been proposed (143,147). Increased trabecular meshwork pigmentation is a prominent and early clinical sign of PEX eyes, the pigment probably deriving from the degenerate iris pigment epithelium. However, the degree of anterior chamber angle pigmentation does not correlate with the degree of glaucomatous disc damage in most studies (21) arguing against a decisive role of pigment dispersion in the chronic rise in IOP rise. By TEM melanin granules are invariably present within trabecular endothelial cells, preferentially in the innermost uveal portions of the meshwork in contrast to the deeper involvement seen in the pigment dispersion syndrome (135,146).

Another observation in some eyes with PEX has been the migration and proliferation of corneal endothelial cells beyond Schwalbe line resulting in a pretrabecular layer of extracellular material including PEX fibrils produced by migrating/proliferating endothelial cells (Fig. 8D) (143,146). This may be a consequence of anterior chamber hypoxia in PEX eyes, stimulating corneal endothelial cell proliferation.

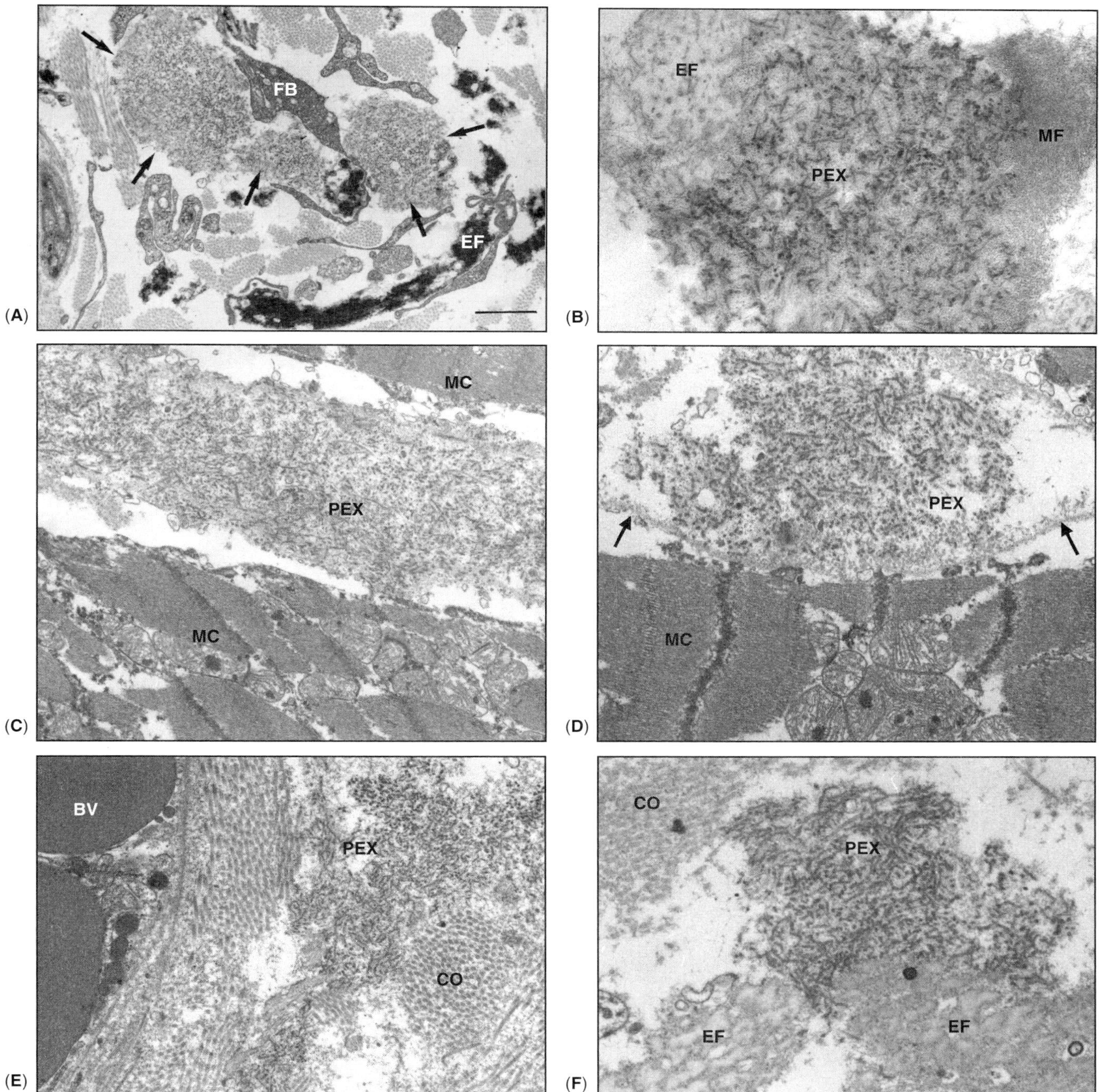

Figure 11 Extraocular manifestations of pseudoexfoliation syndrome (PEX). (**A**) PEX aggregate (*arrows*) in the connective tissue of a skin specimen in association with fibrocytes and elastotic fibers; bar = 2μm. (**B**) Close association of PEX fibrils with elastic fibers (EF) and elastic microfibrils (MF) in dermal connective tissue. (**C,D**) PEX aggregates in myocardial tissue specimens in association with heart muscle cells (MC) and their defective basement membranes (*arrows*). (**E**) PEX material in lung tissue adjacent to a pulmonary blood vessel (BV). (**F**) Close association of PEX fibrils with elastic fibers (EF) in the interstitial connective tissue of a lung specimen (CO, collagen fibers).

electron-dense, fuzzy fibrils that run straight, curved, or bent with occasional ramifications. Generally, two types of PEX fibrils can be distinguished: Type A fibers are thin, 18 to 25 nm in diameter, and up to 1 μm in length, frequently with 20 to 25 or 45 to 50 nm cross banding (Fig. 12C). Type B fibers are more electron-dense, shorter (0.3–0.5 μm), thicker (30–45 nm), and have a less definite cross banding (Fig. 12D). These composite fibers are generally associated with microfibrils, 8 to 10 nm in diameter, with a 12 to 14 nm microperiodicity and a tubular cross-section. These microfibrils, which resemble elastic microfibrils, appear to aggregate laterally into mature PEX fibrils (Fig. 12E). A fibrillar substructure of at least three microfibrils can be occasionally appreciated. However, the microfibrillar core of the complex fibers is usually hidden by an apparent coating of electron-dense amorphous material with lateral excrescences at regular intervals corresponding to the cross-bands of PEX fibrils (27,29). The PEX fibers are embedded in an amorphous interfibrillar ground substance. Most likely, glycosaminoglycans (GAGs) are present on the surface of the PEX fibrils and represent the interfibrillar matrix (26,28).

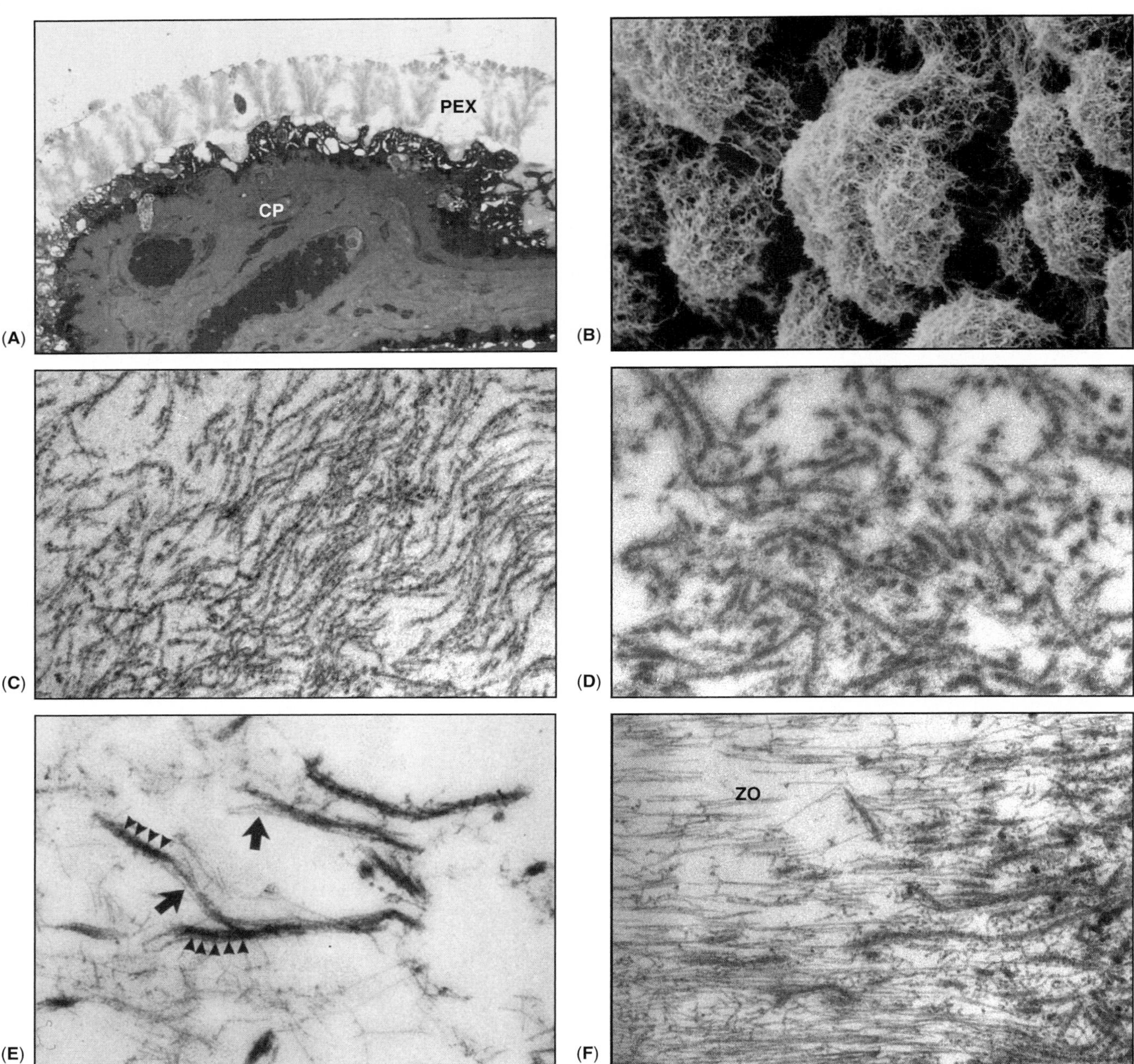

Figure 12 Structure of pseudoexfoliation (PEX) material. (**A**) Bush-like, feathery PEX deposits on a ciliary process (CP) by light microscopy (magnification x400). (**B**) Scanning electron micrograph of PEX deposits showing nodular aggregates of intertwined fibrils. (**C,D**) Transmission electron micrographs of different types of PEX fibrils: thinner type-A fibers with a clear banding pattern (**C**), and thicker, more electron-dense type-B fibers with a less clear banding pattern (**D**). (**E**) Aggregation of pre-lenticular microfibrils (*arrows*) into mature PEX fibrils showing cross-bands at 50 nm (*arrowheads*). (**F**) Transition of zonular microfibrils (ZO) into mature PEX fibrils.

At places, a direct transition of preexisting elastic microfibrils, e.g., zonular fibers, into PEX fibers can be observed. PEX fibers blend with zonular fibrils and zonular fibrils may become incorporated into PEX fibers (Fig. 12F).

Although extraocular PEX fibers often have a less distinct banding pattern and increased amounts of interfibrillar matrix (138,166), the ultrastructural criteria of both intra- and extraocular PEX fibers are highly characteristic making them clearly distinguishable from any other known form of extracellular matrix.

Composition of PEX Material

The exact chemical composition of PEX material remains unknown. Biochemical analyses are impeded by insufficient amounts of available material, by the insolubility of the material, and by lack of experimental models. Indirect histochemical and immunohistochemical evidence suggests a complex glycoprotein/proteoglycan-structure composed of a protein core surrounded by abundant glycoconjugates, probably GAGs, indicating excessive glycosylation processes (26,27,28). PEX material is remarkably resistant to degradation by most enzymes including collagenase, trypsin, chymotrypsin, pepsin, hyaluronidase, amylase, ribonuclease, and papain (12,153), but appears to be dissolved by elastase.

Carbohydrate Components

Early histochemical and more recent immunohistochemical studies have demonstrated the presence of GAGs, such as heparan sulfate, chondroitin sulfate, dermatan sulfate, keratan sulfate, and hyaluronan within PEX material (31,37,52,136,171,182). An overproduction and abnormal metabolism of GAGs have, therefore, been suggested as one of the key changes in PEX (8). This hypothesis is supported by the finding of higher levels of hyaluronan in the aqueous humor of PEX patients (89).

Based on lectin histochemical studies, the carbohydrate component associated with PEX material seems to contain O-linked sialomucin-type and N-linked oligosaccharide chains, and two different galactosamine-containing moieties (3,55,57,58,162). Moreover, the HNK-1 epitope, a 3-sulfoglucoronic acid-containing carbohydrate moiety present on many cell adhesion-related glycoproteins, can be demonstrated in intraocular PEX material (82,115,176). The human natural killer-1 (HNK-1) epitope may be involved in the adhesiveness of PEX material deposits on intraocular surfaces. HNK-1 negativity on extraocular PEX aggregates indicates a difference in composition of intraocular and extraocular PEX material (82,115). While PEX material from the skin and lens had the same lectin-binding characteristics in one study (3), intra- and extraocular deposits appeared to have different carbohydrate composition in others (58,82,115).

Protein Components

The protein components of PEX material bear epitopes of the basement membrane and elastic fiber system and include both noncollagenous basement membrane components, such as nidogen and fibronectin, and elastic fiber components, such as elastin, tropoelastin, amyloid-P, vitronectin, and particularly components of elastic microfibrils, previously termed oxytalan fibrils (92,93,136,140,149,163,178). In view of similar histochemical staining affinities of PEX material and the zonular–elastic microfibrillar system (36,161), it is not surprising that the PEX aggregates contain epitopes for elastic microfibrils (Fig. 13). Antibodies to fibrillin-1, the main component of elastic microfibrils, strongly and consistently immunoreact with PEX material deposits in intra- and extraocular tissues (Figs. 13A,B). Immunoelectron microscopic studies demonstrated fibrillin-1 in association with PEX fibers and their microfibrillar subunits, often in immediate proximity to cell surface invaginations, and suggested an excessive production of fibrillin-containing microfibrils in PEX (Figs. 13E,F) (149,163). Occasionally, an immunochemical marker for fibrillin-1 displays a linear pattern of arrangement with a periodicity of 50 to 55 nm along the PEX fibrils (Fig. 13F). Other components of elastic microfibrils, such as microfibril-associated glycoprotein (MAGP-1) and the latent-transforming growth factor-β binding proteins 1 and 2 (LTBP-1 and LTBP-2), were additionally shown to be associated with all PEX material deposits in intra- and extraocular locations and to colocalize with latent transforming growth factor β1 (TGFβ1) on PEX fibers (141,150). The results suggest dual roles for LTBP-1 and LTBP-2, both as structural components of PEX fibrils and as a means of matrix anchorage of latent TGFβ1 to PEX material. Antibodies to such elastic microfibril components, particularly LTBP-1, have been proven useful as markers for PEX deposits in extraocular tissues (Figs. 13C,D).

Despite slight variations in carbohydrate composition, both intra- and extraocular PEX fibers share epitopes for elastin, vitronectin, fibrillin-1, fibronectin, and amyloid P, indicating basic identity of the protein cores and a common underlying pathogenetic process (4,140,149).

Immunostaining has been negative for lysyl oxidase, an enzyme necessary for the cross-linking of normal elastic fibers, as well as for lysozyme and several protease inhibitors, including alpha-1-antichymotrypsin, that are found in dermal actinic elastosis. Collagen types I, II, III, IV, VI, and VIII are not present either (52,136). Although there was initially a positive labeling of PEX material with a

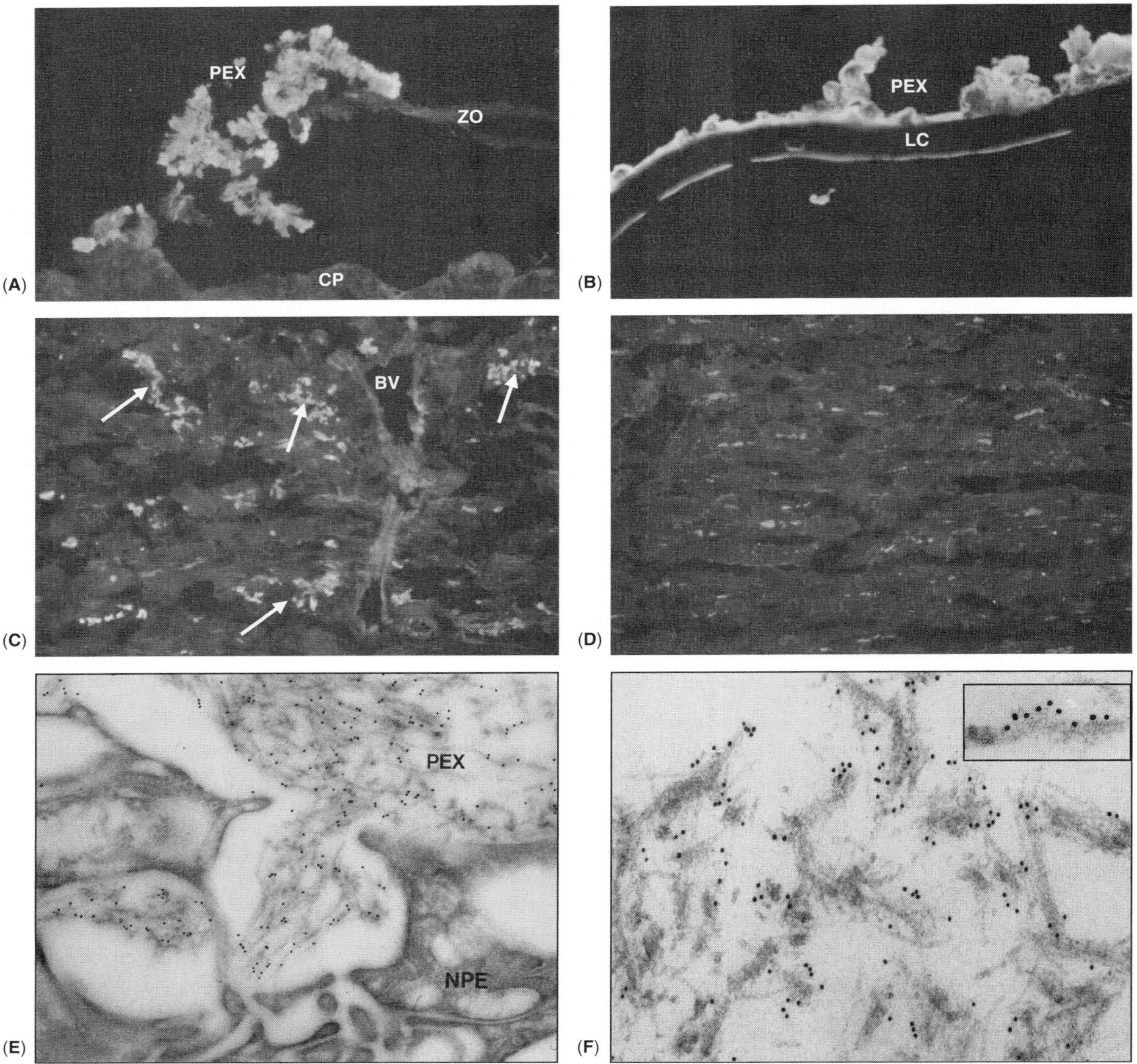

Figure 13 Immunohistochemical labeling of intra- and extraocular pseudoexfoliation (PEX) material with antibodies against elastic microfibril components. (**A**) Positive immunofluorescence staining of PEX deposits on the surface of ciliary processes (CP) and zonules (ZO) using an antibody against LTBP-1 (magnification × 200). (**B**) Strong immunofluorescence of PEX material accumulations on the lens capsule using antibodies against fibrillin-1 (magnification ×300). (**C,D**) LTBP-1 positive systemic PEX deposits in an autopsy specimen of myocardial tissue of a case with ocular PEX (**C**) as compared to the negative control tissue of an age-matched subject without ocular PEX (**D**) (BV, blood vessel; magnification ×125). (**E**) Immunogold labeling with antibodies against fibrillin-1 showing a clear association of the gold marker with PEX fibrils and microfibrils emerging from a nonpigmented ciliary epithelial cell (NPE). (**F**) Gold particles indicating LTBP-1 decorate PEX fibrils and microfibrils, often in a regular pattern (*inset*).

crude antiamyloid A antiserum (125), probably due to contamination with amyloid-P, more significant tests using Congo red staining or monoclonal antibodies against amyloid A, β-amyloid, amyloid precursor protein, transthyretin, or immunoglobulin light chains have yielded negative results (25,122,160). Therefore, the amyloid theory for the pathogenesis of PEX has not been substantiated.

Available immunohistochemical data strongly supports the current belief that the PEX deposits involve elastic microfibrils and that PEX is a type of elastosis affecting elastic microfibrils (160). This theory was originally based on the frequent structural association of PEX fibers with components of the elastic system, such as zonular fibers, oxytalan fibers, elastic fibers, and elastotic material, on ultrastructural indications for the transition of elastic microfibrils into PEX fibrils, and on similar histochemical staining properties of PEX material and zonules (20,36,134,161,164,167). The elastic microfibril theory gains increasing support by recent molecular biologic studies confirming an overexpression of mRNA for fibrillin-1, LTBP-1, and LTBP-2 in most tissues involved (150,189). Although an abnormal aggregation of newly produced or preexisting elastic microfibrils into PEX fibrils appears plausible, other extracellular matrix components, such as basement membrane components and GAGs, may interact and become secondarily incorporated into the composite PEX fibers.

Biochemical Analyses

A preliminary amino acid analysis of PEX material showed an amino acid composition, characterized by a high serine, proline, and glutamic acid content, which was compatible with amyloid, noncollagenous basement membrane components, and elastic microfibrils (120). However, hydroxyproline, the hallmark of collagen, was absent. The additional absence of cysteine is surprising as virtually all components of the PEX-associated fibrillopathy identified to date, e.g., fibrillin-1, are rich in cysteine. Additional amino acid analyses of PEX material are needed.

Biochemical studies using gel electrophoretic analyses of PEX material have been equallly inconclusive. The analysis of extracted lens capsules has disclosed two specific polypeptides with molecular weight (MW) of 14.4 and 16.3 kDa, the latter of which was faintly present in aqueous humor samples as well (127). Electrophoretic analyses of aqueous humor proteins demonstrated a prominent band (12.5 kDa) in 56% of PEX patients (85).

An analysis of the elemental composition of PEX material by energy-filtering TEM disclosed the presence of nitrogen, sulfur, chlorine, and zinc in PEX fibers and calcium in the fiber periphery (139).

Recently, a direct analytical approach by using liquid chromatography coupled with tandem mass spectrometry (LC-MS/MS) has shown that PEX material consists of the elastic microfibril components fibrillin-1, fibulin-2, and vitronectin, the proteoglycans syndecan and versican, the extracellular chaperone clusterin, the cross-linking enzyme lysyl oxidase, and some other proteins, confirming data from many previously reported immunohistochemical studies (110). Together, these findings support the notion that PEX material is an elastotic material arising from abnormal aggregation of elastic microfibril components interacting with multiple ligands.

Origin of PEX Material

The characteristic PEX fibrils appear to be multifocally produced by various intra- and extraocular cell types including epithelial and endothelial cells, pericytes, fibrocytes, and all types of muscle cells. In the eye, typical PEX fibers have been demonstrated by light microscopy and TEM in close association with the preequatorial lens epithelium (Fig. 14A), the nonpigmented ciliary epithelium (Fig. 14B), the iris pigment epithelium (Figs. 14C,D), the trabecular endothelium (Fig. 9B), the corneal endothelium (Fig. 10D), and virtually all cell types in the iris stroma and its vasculature (Fig. 7) (101). Therefore, the abnormal matrix process virtually affects all anterior segment tissues, which appear to be actively involved in the production of PEX material (105,131). Passive distribution of PEX material by the aqueous humor is responsible for PEX material accumulations on the central anterior lens capsule, the zonules, the anterior hyaloid surface, and artificial lenses, if present. In extraocular locations, typical PEX fibers can be identified in close proximity to fibroblasts, vascular wall cells, smooth and striated muscle cells, and heart muscle cells (136,166). All of these cell types show ultrastructural signs of active fibrillogenesis. The cells are characterized by an irregular surface outline, forming extracellular concavities and compartments-containing PEX fibers mixed with fragments of interrupted basement membrane. The PEX fibrils extend out from invaginations of the cell surface, interrupting the continuity of the basement membrane, and frequently show a maturation or aggregation process from microfibrils to thicker composite fibers (Figs. 14A,B). Direct cell-fiber contacts are restricted to minute foci characterized by coated pits of the cell membrane (Fig. 14D). Clusters of such coated vesicles-containing amorphous material fuse with the cell membrane in the region of the concavities and open towards the extracellular space. Finally, the cells involved manifest morphologic evidence of a metabolically activated state by having a prominent rough endoplasmic reticulum (RER) and other cell organelles. Comparable ultrastructural features, such as fiber formation within infoldings of cell surfaces, are known from the secretion of other extracellular matrix elements, e.g., elastic fibers and collagen fibers. PEX fibers have never been observed intracellularly, but appear to form extracellularly close to the cell surface. The pericellularly accumulating PEX material successively disrupts and destroys the normal basement membranes of the cells (Figs. 14C,D), and may eventually result in degeneration of the cells involved.

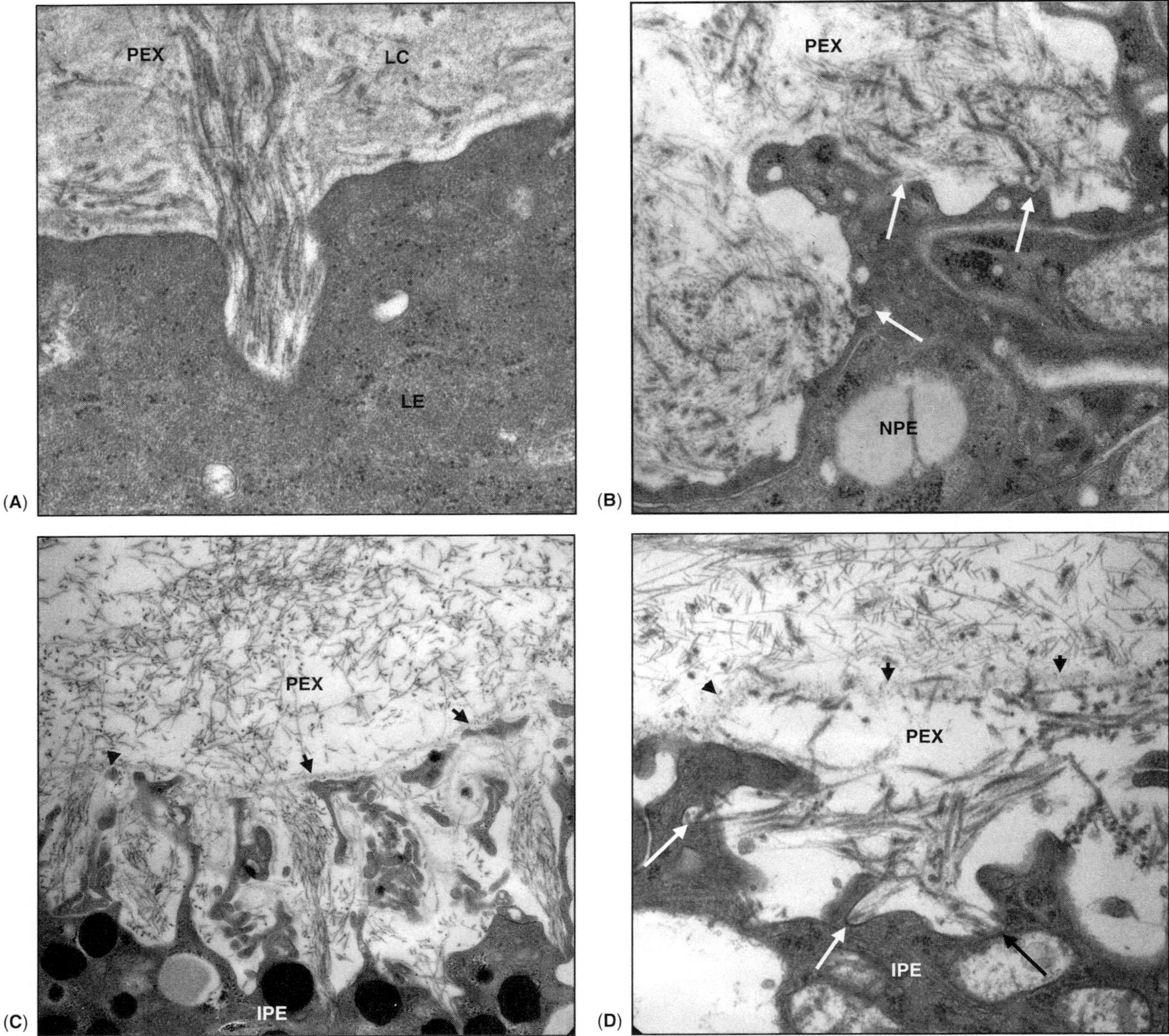

Figure 14 Origin of pseudoexfoliation (PEX) fibrils. (**A**) Origin of PEX fibrils from pit-like membrane invagination of a pre-equatorial lens epithelial cell. *Abbreviations*: LC, lens capsule; LE, lens epithelium. (**B**). Apparent origin of PEX fibers and their microfibrillar subunits from surface invaginations and coated pits (*arrows*) of a nonpigmented ciliary epithelial cell (NPE); the basement membrane of the epithelium is completely destroyed. (**C**) Production of PEX fibrils by the posterior pigment epithelium of the iris (IPE); the basement membrane (*arrowheads*) is lifted off by accumulating PEX material. (**D**) Cell-fiber contact is characterized by coated pits of an iris pigment epithelial cell opening into the extracellular space (*arrows*); detached basement membrane fragments (*arrowheads*) are intermingled with PEX fibrils and microfibrils.

Thus, it appears that a variety of unrelated epithelial and mesenchymal cells may have a common metabolic lesion resulting in the excessive and disordered synthesis of extracellular fibrillar material at multiple sites accompanied by degenerative alterations (degenerative fibrillopathy).

Abnormal fibrils resembling PEX fibers have also been detected in primary cell cultures of iris pigment epithelial cells (62,126). However, cultured conjunctival fibroblasts derived from patients with and without PEX, do not show any differences in morphology and metabolic behavior as indicated by amino acid incorporation (48,108).

It is possible that PEX fibrils are derived from either preformed or newly synthesized elastic microfibrils, because a direct transition between preexisting elastic microfibrils and PEX fibrils has also been reported (Fig. 12F) (20,134,167).

Molecular Pathogenesis

Differential Gene Expression

Differential gene expression analysis using suppression subtractive hybridization (SSH) and differential screening identified and verified more than 20 differentially expressed genes with a high level of reproducibility in PEX tissues, which were mainly involved in extracellular matrix metabolism and in cellular stress (189). One set of genes consistently upregulated in anterior segment tissues from different PEX patients comprised those that encode for the elastic microfibril components fibrillin-1 (*FBN1*), LTBP-1 (*LTBP1*) and LTBP-2 (*LTBP2*), the cross-linking enzyme transglutaminase 2 (*TGM2*), tissue inhibitor of matrix metalloproteinase 2 (*TIMP2*), A-kinase anchor protein 2 (*AKAP2*), apolipoprotein D (*APOD*), and the adenosine receptor A3 (*A3AR*). Genes reproducibly downregulated in PEX tissues included those that code for TIMP1 (*TIMP1*), clusterin (*CLU*), the glutathione-S-transferases mGST-1 (*GSTM1*) and GST-T1 (*GSTT1*), and serum amyloid A1 (*SAA1*).

In addition, cDNA-array hybridization revealed another set of genes differentially expressed in anterior segment tissues of PEX eyes, which partly overlapped with the SSH approach and which were mainly involved in cellular stress (190). The expression of genes for TGFβ1, AdoR-A3 (*A3AR*), several heat shock proteins [HSP 27 (*HSPB1*), HSP 40 (*HSPF1*), HSP 60 (*HSPD1*)], manganese superoxide dismutase (*SOD2*), the proinflammatory cytokines interleukin-1α (*IL1A*), interleukin-1β (*IL1B*), and interleukin-2 (*IL2*), mitogen-activated protein kinase p38 (*MAPK14*), and protein phosphatase 2A (*PPP2CA*) were found to be consistently upregulated in PEX specimens. In contrast, the antioxidant defense enzymes glutaredoxin (*GLRX*) and mGST-1 (*GSTM1*), components of the ubiquitin-proteasome pathway, the ubiquitin conjugating enzymes E2A (*UBE2A*) and E2B (*UBE2B*), several DNA repair proteins (*ERCC1*, hMLH1, GADD153), the transcription factor inhibitor of DNA binding 3 (*ID3*) and clusterin (*CLU*) were downregulated in PEX tissues.

Together, these findings provide evidence that the underlying pathophysiology of PEX is associated with an excessive production of elastic microfibril components, enzymatic cross-linking processes, overexpression of TGFβ1, a proteolytic imbalance between MMPs and TIMPs, low-grade inflammatory processes, increased cellular and oxidative stress, and an impaired cellular stress response, as reflected by the downregulation of antioxidative enzymes, ubiquitin-conjugating enzymes, clusterin, and DNA repair proteins.

Pathogenetic Factors and Key Molecules

Factors which might stimulate the synthesis of abnormal PEX fibers include growth factors turning on aberrant expression of components, failure of normal regulatory or catabolic processes, or genetic abnormalities of any of the molecules involved in the process. Most of the experimental work has been done by analyzing the aqueous humor composition of PEX patients, because aqueous humor can be easily obtained at intraocular surgery, and because all ocular tissues involved are bathed by the aqueous humor and should therefore be influenced by the factors contained therein. The studies showed increased concentrations of basic fibroblast growth factor, hepatocyte growth factor, connective tissue growth factor, and TGFβ1 (37,61,69,150), a dysbalance of MMPs and TIMPs (38,59,144), an increase in oxidative stress markers (8-Isoprostaglandin-F2α) and a concomitant decrease in antioxidative protective factors (ascorbic acid) (70,71), and an increase of the vasoactive peptide endothelin-1 (72) in PEX eyes with and without glaucoma.

TGFβ1, which is a major modulator of matrix formation in many fibrotic diseases, is considered to be a key mediator in the fibrotic PEX process. It is significantly increased in the aqueous humor of PEX patients, both in its latent and active form, it is upregulated and actively produced by anterior segment tissues, it promotes PEX material formation in vitro, and it is known to regulate most of the genes found to be differentially expressed in PEX eyes. Binding of TGFβ1 to PEX material via the TGFβ binding proteins LTBP-1 and LTBP-2 may represent a mechanism of regulation of growth factor activity in PEX eyes (150). In contrast, TGFβ2 levels are significantly higher in the aqueous humor of patients with POAG but not those with PEX.

Excessive matrix accumulation may be due either to increased de novo synthesis or decreased turnover of matrix components or both. Significantly increased concentrations of MMP2, MMP3, TIMP1, and TIMP2 were detected in aqueous humor samples from PEX patients with and without glaucoma compared to control patients with cataract. However, levels of endogenously active MMP2, the major MMP in human aqueous humor, were decreased as was the ratio of MMP2 to TIMP2, resulting in a molar excess of TIMP2 over MMP-2 in PEX samples (144). These findings suggest that complex changes in the local MMP/TIMP balance and reduced MMP activity in the aqueous humor may promote the abnormal matrix accumulation in PEX. TIMPs also bind to PEX material creating so-called cold spots for proteolysis. Moreover, aqueous humor from PEX patients had a higher level of acid phosphatase activity compared to that from cataract patients (100).

There is increasing evidence that cellular stress conditions, such as oxidative stress and ischemia/

hypoxia, constitute major mechanisms in the pathobiology of PEX. Significantly reduced levels of ascorbic acid, the most effective free radical scavenger in the eye, and concomitantly increased levels of the oxidative stress marker 8-isoprostaglandin-F2α (70,71) suggest a faulty antioxidative defense system with increased oxidative stress in the anterior chamber of PEX eyes. More recently, a significant decrease in glutathione concentrations was reported in aqueous humor samples of PEX patients, whereas levels of thiobarbituric acid reactive species, a marker of lipid peroxidation, were increased by 100% as compared to controls (39). In agreement with these findings, we detected a reduced total antioxidative capacity of aqueous humor in PEX eyes with and without glaucoma, together with a decreased activity of various antioxidative enzymes, such as catalase and glutathione peroxidase. The reduced expression of antioxidative enzymes in anterior segment tissues seems to confirm a defective protection against oxidative stress (189,190). Yilmaz et al. (184) analyzed the serum concentrations of oxidative stress markers (such as myeloperoxidase and malondialdehyde), as well as antioxidative factors (such as vitamin A, vitamin C, vitamin E, and catalase), and total antioxidant status in 27 patients with PEX. Whereas serum myeloperoxidase, vitamin A and vitamin E, catalase and total antioxidant parameters were not different among the groups, serum vitamin C concentrations were lower and malondialdehyde concentrations were significantly higher in PEX subjects, reflecting free radical damage to lipid peroxides.

PEX is also associated with ocular ischemia, particularly iris hypoperfusion and anterior chamber hypoxia (54), and with a reduced ocular and retrobulbar micro- and macrovascular blood flow occurring both in patients with and without glaucoma (51,186). Moreover, higher rates of central retinal vein occlusions have been reported in PEX patients (43). Systemically, a lower baseline fingertip capillary perfusion (60) and reduced ipsilateral middle cerebral artery blood flow (1) have been reported and are indicative of generalized ischemic conditions. Endothelin-1, which is known as the most potent vasoconstrictor in the body, is significantly increased in the aqueous humor of normotensive PEX patients compared with that of age-matched controls (72). On the other hand, aqueous humor levels of nitric oxide, which is a potent physiological vasodilator, were decreased in a small number of PEX patients (79). This imbalance may play a role in the obliterative vasculopathy of the iris causing local ischemia early in the disease process. Elevated homocysteine levels in the aqueous humor of patients with PEX (15) may further contribute to ischemic alterations, such as endothelial dysfunction, oxidative stress, enhancement of platelet aggregation, reduction of nitric oxide bioavailability, and abnormal perivascular matrix metabolism.

Pathogenetic Concept of PEX

For more than five decades after its recognition, PEX was considered to be a local phenomenon, such as an "exfoliation" of layers from a degenerative lens capsule or as "deposits" from a local source such as the aqueous humor. The early suggestion that PEX material is a form of amyloid (125) has not been confirmed. PEX material was also thought to represent an abnormal basement membrane material (30). However, an abnormality of basement membrane metabolism may also been inferred from focal interruption of this layer by emerging PEX fibers.

Although not representing a form of amyloidosis, PEX shares common features with amyloid disorders, such as Alzheimer disease, because amyloid-β peptide was found to be present in the aqueous humor of PEX patients (65). Amyloid-associated proteins, which are not part of the fibrils, include P component, GAGs, extracellular matrix components, complement proteins, apolipoproteins, and cytokines, which also occur in association with PEX fibrils. Polymorphism of apolipoprotein E, which is involved in many amyloid disorders promoting the aggregation of amyloidogenic proteins into the beta-pleated sheet conformation, was found to be significantly associated with PEX development (185). These analogies suggest that PEX may be a conformational disorder, like Alzheimer disease, which is characterized by the accumulation of a host protein that undergoes structural changes (190). A common pathogenetic step driving this group of disorders is the accumulation of misfolded proteins in response to external stimuli, e.g., oxidative stress, and dysfunction or overload of the proteasome system. Misfolded proteins accumulating in form of plaques and fibrils escape proteolysis by aggregation, cross-linking, mutations, or posttranslational modifications. Future analysis of proteasome activity and posttranslational protein modifications in PEX tissues might shed some light on these issues and clarify their role in pathogenesis.

Immunohistochemical, biochemical, and molecular biologic data give strong support to the elastic microfibril theory of pathogenesis, which was first proposed by Streeten (160) on the basis of histochemical similarities between PEX and zonular fibers and which explains PEX as a type of elastosis affecting elastic microfibrils. Elastic microfibrils are common elements of connective tissues for attaching the basement membranes of cells to each other and connecting them to the elastic fiber system of the stroma. Often the same cells direct synthesis of both basement membranes and elastic components. Most of the recent evidence suggests that PEX is a fibrillinopathy.

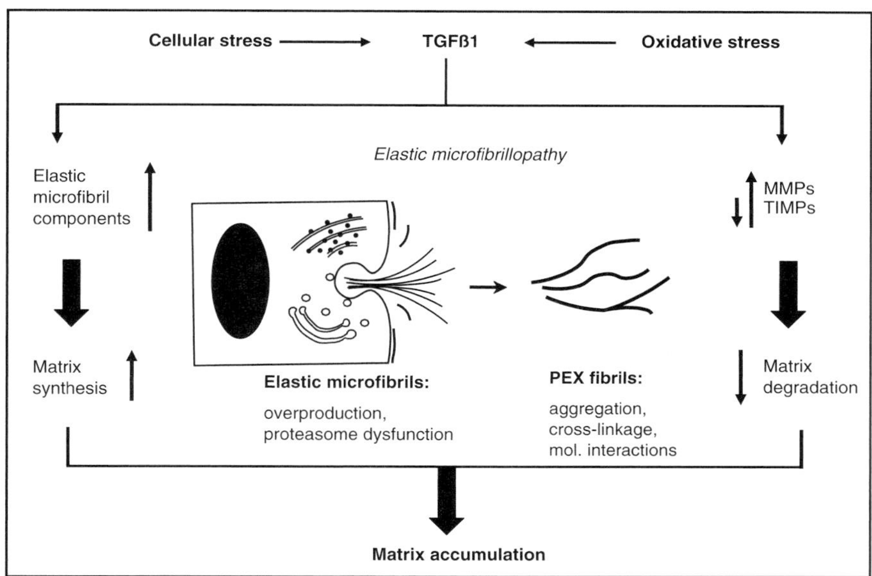

Figure 15 Summary of the current pathogenetic concept of pseudoexfoliation syndrome (PEX). *Abbreviations*: MMP, matrix metalloproteinase; TGFβ1, transforming growth factor β1; TIMP, tissue inhibitor of metalloproteinase.

Fibrillin-1, the main component of elastic microfibrils and presumably also of PEX fibrils, is a large glycoprotein with a high-cysteine content and a mosaic composition of different modules, i.e. epidermal growth factor (EGF)-like motifs with calcium-binding sequences and TGF-binding protein-like motifs. It is capable of multiple molecular interactions with various matrix components, such as fibronectin, fibulin-1/2, versican, and LTBP-1, which are all present in PEX material. In PEX, the excessively synthesized fibrillin molecules may aggregate into normal or abnormal microfibrils cross-linked together to form mature PEX fibrils by secondary molecular interaction with other matrix components and glycoconjugates. Abnormal protein accumulation and aggregation may be promoted by dysfunction of the ubiquitin-proteasome system (see Chapter 36) and by a deficiency of clusterin, which acts as an extracellular chaperone and normally prevents the stress-induced precipitation and aggregation of misfolded proteins (190).

Thus, the currently proposed pathogenetic concept of PEX is that it is a specific type of stress-induced elastosis, an elastic microfibrillopathy, associated with the excessive production of elastic microfibrils and their aggregation into mature PEX fibrils by a variety of potentially elastogenic cells (Fig. 15) (148,188). Growth factors, particularly TGFβ1, increased cellular and oxidative stress, an impaired cellular protection system, and the stable aggregation of misfolded stressed proteins appear to be involved. Due to an imbalance between MMPs and TIMPs and extensive cross-linking in fiber formation, the pathologic material is not properly degraded but progressively accumulates within the tissues over time. Interestingly, similar pathogenetic mechanisms involving oxidative stress, TGFβ1, and MMP dysregulation, have been proposed for a number of systemic fibrotic disorders involving pathologic accumulation of extracellular material (90).

REFERENCES

1. Akarsu C, Ünal B. Cerebral haemodynamics in patients with pseudoexfoliation glaucoma. Eye 2005; 19: 1297–300.
2. Allingham RR, Loftsdottir M, Gottfredsdottir MS, et al. Pseudoexfoliation syndrome in Icelandic families. Br J Ophthalmol 2001; 85:702–7.
3. Amari F, Nagata S, Umihira J, et al. Lectin electron microscopic histochemistry of the pseudoexfoliative material in the skin. Invest Ophthalmol Vis Sci 1994; 35: 3962–6.
4. Amari F, Umihira J, Nohara M. Electron microscopic immunohistochemistry of ocular and extraocular pseudoexfoliative material. Exp Eye Res 1997; 65:51–6.
5. Aragon-Martin JA, Child A, Mercieca F, et al. Genome scan of Maltese families with pseudoexfoliation syndrome (PEX). Annual Meeting of the Association for Research in Vision and Ophthalmology 2005; Abstract 39.
6. Asano N, Schlötzer-Schrehardt U. Naumann GOH: A histopathologic study of iris changes in pseudoexfoliation syndrome. Ophthalmology 1995; 102:1279–90.
7. Ashton N, Shakib M, Collyer R, Blach R. Electron microscopic study of pseudo-exfoliation of the lens capsule. I. Lens capsule and zonular fibers. Invest Ophthalmol 1965; 4:141–53.
8. Baba H. Histochemical and polarization optical investigation for glycosaminoglycans in exfoliation syndrome. Graefes Arch Clin Exp Ophthalmol 1983; 221:106–9.
9. Bartholomew RS. Phakodonesis. A sign of incipient lens displacement. Br J Ophthalmol 1970a; 54:663–6.
10. Bartholomew RS. Lens displacement associated with pseudocapsular exfoliation. A report on 19 cases in the Southern Bantu. Br J Ophthalmol 1970b; 54:744–50.

11. Bartholomew RS. Pseudoexfoliation and angle-closure glaucoma. Glaucoma 1981; 3:213–6.
12. Bertelsen TI, Ehlers N. Morphological and histochemical studies on fibrillopathia epitheliocapsularis. Acta Ophthalmol 1969; 47:476–88.
13. Bertelsen TI, Drablös PA, Flood PR. The so-called senile exfoliation (pseudoexfoliation) of the anterior lens capsule, a product of the lens epithelium. Fibrillopathia epitheliocapsularis. Acta Ophthalmol 1964; 42:1096–113.
14. Bleich S, Jünemann A, von Ahsen N, et al. Homocysteine and risk of open-angle glaucoma. J Neural Transm 2002; 109:499–504.
15. Bleich S, Roedl J, von Ahsen N, Schlötzer-Schrehardt U, et al. Elevated homocysteine levels in aqueous humor of patients with pseudoexfoliation glaucoma. Am J Ophthalmol 2004; 138:162–4.
16. Bojic L, Ermacora R, Polic S, et al. Pseudoexfoliation syndrome and asymptomatic myocardial dysfunction. Graefe's Arch Clin Exp Ophthalmol 2005; 243:446–9.
17. Brooks AMV, Gillies WE. Fluorescein angiography and fluorophotometry of the iris in pseudoexfoliation of the lens capsule. Br J Ophthalmol 1983; 67:249–54.
18. Cahill M, Early A, Stack S, et al. Pseudoexfoliation and sensorineural hearing loss. Eye 2002; 16:261–6.
19. Carpel EF. Pupillary dilation in eyes with pseudoexfoliation syndrome. Am J Ophthalmol 1988; 105:692–4.
20. Chijiiwa T, Araki H, Ishibashi T, Inomata H. Degeneration of zonular fibrils in a case of exfoliation glaucoma. Ophthalmologica 1989; 199:16–23.
21. Cobb CJ, Blanco G, Spaeth GL. Exfoliation syndrome angle characteristics: a lack of correlation with amount of disc damage. Br J Ophthalmol 2004; 88:1002–3.
22. Conway RM, Schlötzer-Schrehardt U, Küchle M, Naumann GOH. Pseudoexfoliation syndrome: pathologic manifestations of relevance to intraocular surgery. Clin Exp Ophthalmol. 2004; 32:199–210.
23. Damji KF, Bains HS, Stefansson E, et al. Is pseudoexfoliation syndrome inherited? A review of genetic and nongenetic factors and a new observation. Ophthal Genet 1998; 19:175–85.
24. Dark AJ, Streeten BW. Precapsular film on the aging human lens: Precursor of pseudoexfoliation? Br J Ophthalmol 1990; 74:717–22.
25. Dark AJ, Streeten BW, Cornwall CC. Pseudoexfoliative disease of the lens: a study in electron microscopy and histochemistry. Br J Ophthalmol 1977; 61:462–72.
26. Davanger M. On the molecular composition and physicochemical properties of the pseudo-exfoliation material. Acta Ophthalmol 1977; 55:621–33.
27. Davanger M. Studies on the pseudo-exfoliation material: A review. Graefes Arch Clin Exp Ophthalmol 1978a; 208: 65–8.
28. Davanger M. On the interfibrillar matrix of the pseudoexfoliation material. Acta Ophthalmol 1978b; 56:233–9.
29. Davanger M. On the ultrastructure and the formation of pseudo-exfoliation material. Acta Ophthalmol 1980; 58: 520–7.
30. Eagle RC, Font RL, Fine BS. The basement membrane exfoliation syndrome. Arch Ophthalmol 1979; 97:510–5.
31. Fitzsimmons TD, Fagerholm P, Wallin Ö. Hyaluronan in the exfoliation syndrome. Acta Ophthalmol 1997; 75: 257–60.
32. Forsius H. Exfoliation syndrome in various ethnic populations. Acta Ophthalmol 1988; 66(Suppl. 184): 71–85.
33. Forsius H, Forsman E, Fellman J, Eriksson AW. Exfoliation syndrome: frequency, gender distribution and association with climatically induced alterations of the cornea and conjunctiva. Acta Ophthalmol Scan 2002; 80:478–84.
34. Freissler K, Küchle M, Naumann GOH. Spontaneous dislocation of the lens in pseudoexfoliation syndrome. Arch Ophthalmol 1995; 113:1095–6.
35. Futa R, Furuyoshi N. Phakodonesis in capsular glaucoma: a clinical and electron microscopic study. Jpn J Ophthalmol 1989; 33:311–7.
36. Garner A, Alexander RA. Pseudoexfoliative disease: histochemical evidence of an affinity with zonular fibres. Br J Ophthalmol 1984; 68:574–80.
37. Gartaganis SP, Georgakopoulos CD, Exarchou AM, et al. Increased aqueous humor basic fibroblast growth factor and hyaluronan levels in relation to the exfoliation syndrome and exfoliative glaucoma. Acta Ophthalmol Scand 2001; 79:572–5.
38. Gartaganis SP, Georgakopoulos CD, Mela EK, et al. Matrix metalloproteinases and their inhibitors in exfoliation syndrome. Ophthalmic Res 2002; 34:165–71.
39. Gartaganis SP, Georgakopoulos CD, Patsoukis NE, et al. Glutathione and lipid peroxide changes in pseudoexfoliation syndrome. Curr Eye Res 2005; 30:647–51.
40. Gharagozloo NZ, Baker RH, Brubaker RF. Aqueous dynamics in exfoliation syndrome. Am J Ophthalmol 1992; 114:473–8.
41. Ghosh M, Speakman JS. The ciliary body in senile exfoliation of the lens. Can J Ophthalmol 1973; 8:394–403.
42. Ghosh M, Speakman JS. The iris in senile exfoliation of the lens. Can J Ophthalmol 1974; 9:289–97.
43. Gillies WE, Brooks AMV. Central retinal vein occlusion in pseudoexfoliation of the lens capsule. Clin Exp Ophthalmol 2002; 30:176–8.
44. Gottanka J, Flügel-Koch C, Martus P. Correlation of pseudoexfoliative material and optic nerve damage in pseudoexfoliation syndrome. Invest Ophthalmol Vis Sci 1997; 38:2435–46.
45. Gross FJ, Tingey D, Epstein DL. Increased prevalence of occludable angles and angle-closure glaucoma in patients with pseudoexfoliation. Am J Ophthalmol 1994; 117: 333–6.
46. Gumus K, Bozkurt B, Sonmez B, et al. Diurnal variation of intraocular pressure and its correlation with retinal nerve fiber analysis in Turkish patients with exfoliation syndrome. Graefe's Arch Clin Exp Ophthalmol 2006; 244: 170–6.
47. Guzek JP, Holm M, Cotter JB, et al. Risk factors for intraoperative complications in 1000 extracapsular cataract cases. Ophthalmology 1987; 94:461–6.
48. Halvorsen F, Nicolaissen B, Ringvold A, Näss O. Invitro studies of conjunctival cells from eyes with and without pseudoexfoliation. Acta Ophthalmol Scand 1995; 73:37–40.
49. Hammer TH, Schlötzer-Schrehardt U, Naumann GOH1. Unilateral or asymmetric pseudoexfoliation syndrome? An ultrastructural study. Arch Ophthalmol 2001; 119: 1023–31.
50. Hardie JG, Mercieca F, Fenech T, Cuschieri A. Familial pseudoexfoliation in Gozo. Eye 2005; 19:1280–5.
51. Harju M, Vesti E. Blood flow of the optic nerve head and peripapillary retina in exfoliation syndrome with unilateral glaucoma or ocular hypertension. Graefe's Arch Clin Exp Ophthalmol 2001; 239:271–7.
52. Harnisch JP, Barrach HJ, Hassell JR, Sinha PK. Identification of a basement membrane proteoglycan in exfoliation material. Graefes Arch Clin Exp Ophthalmol 1981; 215:273–8.
53. Hayashi H, Hayashi K, Nakao F, Hayashi F. Anterior capsule contraction and intraocular lens dislocation in

eyes with pseudoexfoliation syndrome. Br J Ophthalmol 1998; 82:1429–32.

54. Helbig H, Schlötzer-Schrehardt U, Noske W, et al. Anterior chamber hypoxia and iris vasculopathy in pseudoexfoliation syndrome. German J Ophthalmol 1994; 3:148–53.
55. Hietanen J, Tarkkanen A. Glycoconjugates in exfoliation syndrome: a lectin histochemical study of the ciliary body and lens. Acta Ophthalmol 1989; 67:288–94.
56. Hietanen J, Kivelä T, Vesti E, Tarkkanen A. Exfoliation syndrome in patients scheduled for cataract surgery. Acta Ophthalmol 1992; 70:440–6.
57. Hietanen J, Tarkkanen A, Kivelä T. Galactose-containing glycoconjugates of the ciliary body and lens in capsular glaucoma: a lectin histochemical study. Graefes Arch Clin Exp Ophthalmol 1994; 232:575–83.
58. Hietanen J, Uusitalo M, Tarkkanen A, Kivelä T. Lectin and immunohistochemical comparison of glycoconjugates in the conjunctiva of patients with and without exfoliation syndrome. Br J Ophthalmol 1995; 79:467–72.
59. Ho SL, Dogar GF, Wang J, et al. Elevated aqueous humour tissue inhibitor of matrix metalloproteinase-1 and connective tissue growth factor in pseudoexfoliation syndrome. Br J Ophthalmol 2005; 89:169–73.
60. Hollo G, Lakatos P, Farkas K. Cold pressure test and plasma endothelin-1 concentration in primary open-angle and capsular glaucoma. J Glaucoma 1998; 7:105–10.
61. Hu D-N, Ritch R. Hepatocyte growth factor is increased in the aqueous humor of glaucomatous eyes. J Glaucoma 2001; 10:152–7.
62. Hu D-N, McCormick SA, Ritch R. Isolation and culture of iris pigment epithelium from iridectomy specimens of eyes with and without exfoliation syndrome. Arch Ophthalmol 1997; 115:89–94.
63. Hyams M, Mathalone N, Herskovitz M, et al. Intraoperative complications of phacoemulsification in eyes with and without pseudoexfoliation. J Cataract Refract Surg 2005; 31:1002–5.
64. Inazumi K, Takahashi D, Taniguchi T, Yamamoto T. Ultrasound biomicroscopic classification of zonules in exfoliation syndrome. Jpn J Ophthalmol 2002; 46: 502–9.
65. Janciauskiene S, Krakau T. Alzheimer's peptide: a possible link between glaucoma, exfoliation syndrome and Alzheimer's disease. Acta Ophthalmol Scand 2001; 79:328–9.
66. Jehan FS, Mamalis N, Crandall AS. Spontaneous late dislocation of intraocular lens within the capsular bag in pseudoexfoliation patients. Ophthalmology 2001; 108: 1727–31.
67. Jünemann AG, von Ahsen N, Reulbach U, et al. C677T variant in the methylentetrahydrofolate reductase gene is a genetic risk factor for primary open-angle glaucoma. Am J Ophthalmol 2005; 139:721–3.
68. Kivelä T, Hietanen J, Uusitalo M. Autopsy analysis of clinically unilateral exfoliation syndrome. Invest Ophthalmol Vis Sci 1997; 38:2008–15.
69. Koliakos GG, Schlötzer-Schrehardt U, Konstas AGP, et al. Transforming and insulin-like growth factors in the aqueous humor of patients with exfoliation syndrome. Graefe's Arch Clin Exp Ophthalmol 2001; 239:482–7.
70. Koliakos GG, Konstas AGP, Schlötzer-Schrehardt U, et al. Ascorbic acid concentration is reduced in the aqueous humor of patients with exfoliation syndrome. Am J Ophthalmol 2002; 134:879–83.
71. Koliakos GG, Konstas AGP, Schlötzer-Schrehardt U, et al. 8-isoprostaglandin F2α and ascorbic acid concentration in the aqueous humour of patients with exfoliation syndrome. Br J Ophthalmol 2003; 87:353–6.
72. Koliakos GG, Konstas AGP, Schlötzer-Schrehardt U, et al. Endothelin-1 concentration is increased in the aqueous humour of patients with exfoliation syndrome. Br J Ophthalmol 2004; 88:523–7.
73. Konstas AGP, Marshall GE, Cameron SA, Lee WR. Morphology of iris vasculopathy in exfoliation glaucoma. Acta Ophthalmol 1993; 71:751–9.
74. Konstas AG, Ritch R, Bufidis T. Exfoliation syndrome in a 17-year-old girl. Arch Ophthalmol 1997a; 115:1063–7.
75. Konstas AGP, Mantziris DA, Stewart WC. Diurnal intraocular pressure in untreated exfoliation and primary open-angle glaucoma. Arch Ophthalmol 1997b; 115: 182–5.
76. Konstas AGP, Stewart WC, Stromann GA. Clinical presentation and initial treatment patterns in patients with exfoliation glaucoma versus primary open-angle glaucoma. Ophth Surg Lasers 1997c; 28:111–7.
77. Konstas AGP, Hollo G, Astakhov YS, et al. Factors associated with long-term progression or stability in exfoliation glaucoma. Arch Ophthalmol 2004; 122: 29–33.
78. Konstas AGP, Koliakos GG, Liakos P. et al. Latanoprost therapy reduces the levels of TGF beta 1 and gelatinases in the aqueous humor of patients with exfoliative glaucoma. Exp Eye Res. 2006; 82:319–22.
79. Kotikoski H, Moilanen E, Vapaatalo H, Aine E. Biochemical markers of the L-arginine-nitric oxide pathway in the aqueous humour in glaucoma patients. Acta Ophthalmol Scand 2002; 80:191–5.
80. Kozobolis VP, Detorakis ET, Sourvinos G, et al. Loss of heterozygosity in pseudoexfoliation syndrome. Invest Ophthalmol Vis Sci 1999; 40:1255–60.
81. Krause U, Helve J, Forsius H. Pseudoexfoliation of the lens capsule and liberation of iris pigment. Acta Ophthalmol 1973; 51:39–46.
82. Kubota T, Schlötzer-Schrehardt U, Inomata H, Naumann GOH. Immunoelectron microscopic localization of the HNK-1 carbohydrate epitope in the anterior segment of pseudoexfoliation and normal eyes. Curr Eye Res 1997; 16:231–8.
83. Küchle M, Naumann GOH. Occurrence of pseudoexfoliation following penetrating keratoplasty for keratoconus. Br J Ophthalmol 1992; 76:98–100.
84. Küchle M, Schlötzer-Schrehardt U. Naumann GOH: Occurrence of pseudoexfoliative material in parabulbar structures in pseudoexfoliation syndrome. Acta Ophthalmol 1991; 69:124–30.
85. Küchle M, Küchle M, Ho TS, et al. Protein quantification and electrophoresis in aqueous humor of pseudoexfoliation eyes. Invest Ophthalmol Vis Sci 1994; 35:748–52.
86. Küchle M, Nguyen N, Hannappel E. The blood–aqueous barrier in eyes with pseudoexfoliation syndrome. Ophthalmic Res 1995; 27(Suppl. 1):136–42.
87. Küchle M, Amberg A, Martus P, et al. Pseudoexfoliation syndrome and secondary cataract. Br J Ophthalmol 1997; 81:862–6.
88. Küchle M, Viestenz A, Martus P, et al. Anterior chamber depth and complications during cataract surgery in eyes with pseudoexfoliation syndrome. Am J Ophthalmol 2000; 129:281–5.
89. Lamari F, Katsimpris J, Gartaganis S, Karamanos NK. Profiling of the eye aqueous humor in exfoliation syndrome by high-performance liquid chromatographic analysis of hyaluronan and galactosaminoglycans. J Chromatogr B Biomed Sci Appl 1998; 709:173–8.

90. Lee S, Lee S, Sharma K. The pathogenesis of fibrosis and renal disease in scleroderma: recent insights from glomerulosclerosis. Curr Rheumatol Rep 2004; 6:141–8.
91. Leibovitch I, Kurtz S, Shemesh G, et al. Hyperhomocysteinemia in pseudoexfoliation glaucoma. J Glaucoma 2003; 12:36–9.
92. Li Z-Y, Streeten BW, Wallace RN. Association of elastin with pseudoexfoliative material. An immunoelectron microscopic study. Curr Eye Res 1988; 7:1163–72.
93. Li Z-Y, Streeten BW, Yohai N. Amyloid P protein in pseudoexfoliative fibrillopathy. Curr Eye Res 1989; 8: 217–27.
94. Lindberg JG. Clinical investigations on depigmentation of the pupillary border and translucency of the iris. Acta Ophthalmol 1989; 67 (Suppl. 190):1–96.
95. Linner E, Popovic V, Gottfries C-G, et al. The exfoliation syndrome in cognitive impairment of cerebrovascular or Alzheimer's type. Acta Ophthalmol Scand 2001; 79: 283–5.
96. Mardin CY, Schlötzer-Schrehardt U, Naumann GOH. Masked pseudoexfoliation syndrome in unoperated eyes with circular posterior synechiae. Arch Ophthalmol 2001; 119:1500–4.
97. Mitchell P, Wang JJ, Smith W. Association of pseudoexfoliation syndrome with increased vascular risk. Am J Ophthalmol 1997; 124:685–7.
98. Miyake K, Matsuda M, Inaba M. Corneal endothelial changes in pseudoexfoliation syndrome. Am J Ophthalmol 1989; 108:49–52.
99. Mizuno K, Muroi S. Cycloscopy of pseudoexfoliation. Am J Ophthalmol 1979; 87:513–8.
100. Mizuno K, Hara S, Ishiguro S, Takei Y. Acid phosphatase in eyes with pseudoexfoliation. Am J Ophthalmol 1980; 89:482–9.
101. Morrison JC, Green WR. Light microscopy of the exfoliation syndrome. Acta Ophthalmol 1988; 66 (Suppl. 184):5–27.
102. Naumann GOH. The Bowman Lecture. Part II. Corneal transplantation in anterior segment diseases. Eye 1995; 9: 398–421.
103. Naumann GOH, Schlötzer-Schrehardt U. Keratopathy in pseudoexfoliation syndrome as a cause of corneal endothelial decompensation. A clinicopathologic study. Ophthalmology 2000; 107:1111–24.
104. Naumann GOH. Erlanger Augenblätter-Group. Exfoliation syndrome as a risk factor for vitreous loss in extracapsular cataract surgery (preliminary report). Acta Ophthalmol 1988; 66 (Suppl. 184):129–31.
105. Naumann GOH, Schlötzer-Schrehardt U, Küchle M. Pseudoexfoliation syndrome for the comprehensive ophthalmologist. Intraocular and systemic manifestations. Ophthalmology 1998; 105:951–68.
106. Netland PA, Ye H, Streeten BW, Hernandez MR. Elastosis of the lamina cribrosa in pseudoexfoliation syndrome with glaucoma. Ophthalmology 1995; 102: 878–86.
107. Nguyen NX, Küchle M, Martus P, Naumann GOH. Quantification of blood–aqueous barrier breakdown after trabeculectomy: pseudoexfoliation versus primary open-angle glaucoma. J Glaucoma 1999; 8:18–23.
108. Nicolaissen B Jr, Ringvold A, Naess O. Amino acid incorporation in cell cultures from eyes with pseudoexfoliation material. Acta Ophthalmol 1992; 70:371–5.
109. Orr AC, Robitaille JM, Price PA, et al. Exfoliation syndrome: clinical and genetic features. Ophthalmic Genetics 2001; 22:171–85.
110. Ovodenko B, Rostagno A, Neubert TA, et al. Proteomic analysis of exfoliation deposits. Invest Ophthalmol Vis Sc 2006 (in press).
111. Parodi MB, Bondel E, Saviano S, Ravalico G. Iris indocyanine green angiography in pseudoexfoliation syndrome and capsular glaucoma. Acta Ophthalmol Scand 2000; 78:437–42.
112. Prince AM, Ritch R. Clinical signs of the pseudoexfoliation syndrome. Ophthalmology 1986; 93:803–7.
113. Prince AM, Streeten BW, Ritch R. Preclinical diagnosis of pseudoexfoliation syndrome. Arch Ophthalmol 1987; 105: 1076–82.
114. Puska PM. Unilateral exfoliation syndrome: conversion to bilateral exfoliation and to glaucoma: a prospective 10-year follow-up study. J Glaucoma 2002; 11:517–24.
115. Qi Y, Streeten BW, Wallace RN. HNK-1 epitope in the lens-ciliary zonular region in normal and pseudoexfoliative eyes. Arch Ophthalmol 1997; 115:637–44.
116. Repo LP, Teräsvirta ME, Koivisto KJ. Generalized transluminance of the iris and the frequency of the pseudoexfoliation syndrome in the eyes of transient ischemic attack patients. Ophthalmology 1993; 100: 352–5.
117. Richardson TM, Epstein DL. Exfoliation glaucoma. A quantitative perfusion and ultrastructural study. Ophthalmology 1981; 88:968–80.
118. Ringvold A. Light and electron microscopy of the wall of iris vessels in eyes with and without exfoliation syndrome (pseudoexfoliation of the lens capsule). Virchows Arch Abt A Path Anat 1970; 349:1–9.
119. Ringvold A. Electron microscopy of the limbal conjunctiva in eyes with pseudo-exfoliation syndrome (PE Syndrome). Virchows Arch Abt A Path Anat 1972; 355: 275–83.
120. Ringvold A. A preliminary report on the amino acid composition of the pseudo-exfoliation material (PE material). Exp Eye Res 1973; 15:37–42.
121. Ringvold A. Exfoliation syndrome: Immunological aspects. Acta Ophthalmol 1988; 66(Suppl. 184):35–43.
122. Ringvold A. Update on etiology and pathogenesis of the pseudoexfoliation syndrome. New Trends Ophthalmol 1993; 8:177–80.
123. Ringvold A. Epidemiology of the pseudoexfoliation syndrome. Acta Ophthalmol Scand 1999; 77:371–5.
124. Ringvold A, Vegge T. Electron microscopy of the trabecular meshwork in eyes with exfoliation syndrome (pseudoexfoliation of the lens capsule). Virchows Arch A Path Anat 1971; 353:110–27.
125. Ringvold A, Husby G. Pseudoexfoliation material: an amyloid-like substance. Exp Eye Res 1973; 17:289–99.
126. Ringvold A, Nicolaissen B Jr. Culture of iris tissue from human eyes with and without pseudoexfoliation. Acta Ophthalmol 1990; 68:310–6.
127. Ringvold A, Husby G, Pettersen S. Electrophoretic study of proteins associated with pseudoexfoliation syndrome. Acta Ophthalmol 1989; 67:724–6.
128. Ringvold A, Blika S, Sandvik L. Pseudoexfoliation and mortality. Acta Ophthalmol Scand 1997; 75:255–6.
129. Ritch R. Exfoliation syndrome: the most common identifiable cause of open-angle glaucoma. J Glaucoma 1994; 3:176–8.
130. Ritch R. Exfoliation syndrome and occludable angles. Trans Am Ophthalm Soc 1994; 92:845–944.
131. Ritch R, Schlötzer-Schrehardt U. Exfoliation syndrome. Surv Ophthalmol 2001; 45:265–315.
132. Ritch R, Schlötzer-Schrehardt U, Konstas AGP. Why is glaucoma associated with exfoliation syndrome? Progr Ret Eye Res. 2003; 22:253–75.
133. Ritland JS, Egge K, Lydersen S, Juul R, Semb SO. Exfoliative glaucoma and primary open-angle glaucoma:

associations with death causes and comorbidity. Acta Ophthalmol Scand 2004; 82:401–4.

134. Roh YB, Ishibashi T, Ito N, Inomata H. Alteration of microfibrils in the conjunctiva of patients with exfoliation syndrome. Arch Ophthalmol 1987; 105:978–82.
135. Sampaolesi R, Zarate J, Croxato O. The chamber angle in exfoliation syndrome: Clinical and pathological findings. Acta Ophthalmol 1988; 66(Suppl. 184):48–53.
136. Schlötzer-Schrehardt U, Dörfler S, Naumann GOH. Immunohistochemical localization of basement membrane components in pseudoexfoliation material of the lens capsule. Curr Eye Res 1992; 11:343–55.
137. Schlötzer-Schrehardt U, Dörfler S, Naumann GOH. Corneal endothelial involvement in pseudoexfoliation syndrome. Arch Ophthalmol 1993; 111:666–74.
138. Schlötzer-Schrehardt U, Koca M, Naumann GOH, Volkholz H. Pseudoexfoliation syndrome: ocular manifestation of a systemic disorder? Arch Ophthalmol 1992; 110:1752–6.
139. Schlötzer-Schrehardt U, Körtje K-H, Erb C. Energy-filtering transmission electron microscopy (EFTEM) in the elemental analysis of pseudoexfoliative material. Curr Eye Res 2001b; 22:154–62.
140. Schlötzer-Schrehardt U, Küchle M, Dörfler S, Naumann GOH: Pseudoexfoliative material in eyelid skin of pseudoexfoliation suspect patients: a clinico-histopathological correlation. German J Ophthalmol 1993; 2:51–60.
141. Schlötzer-Schrehardt U, Küchle M, Hofmann-Rummelt C, et al. Latent TGF-β1 binding protein (LTBP-1): a new marker for intra- and extraocular PEX deposits. Klin Monatsbl Augenheilkd 2000; 216:412–9.
142. Schlötzer-Schrehardt U, Küchle M, Naumann GOH: Electron microscopic identification of pseudoexfoliative material in extrabulbar tissue. Arch Ophthalmol 1991; 109:565–70.
143. Schlötzer-Schrehardt U, Küchle M, Naumann GOH. Mechanisms of Glaucoma Development in Pseudoexfoliation Syndrome. In: Gramer E, Grehn F, eds. Pathogenesis and Risk Factors of Glaucoma. Heidelberg, Springer. 1999:34–49 [chapter 5].
144. Schlötzer-Schrehardt U, Lommatzsch J, Küchle M, et al. Matrix metalloproteinases and their inhibitors in aqueous humor of patients with pseudoexfoliation syndrome, pseudoexfoliation glaucoma, and primary open-angle glaucoma. Invest Ophthalmol Vis Sci 2003; 44:1117–25.
145. Schlötzer-Schrehardt U, Naumann GOH: A histopathologic study of zonular instability in pseudoexfoliation syndrome. Am J Ophthalmol 1994; 118:730–43.
146. Schlötzer-Schrehardt U, Naumann GOH: Trabecular meshwork in pseudoexfoliation syndrome with and without open-angle glaucoma. A morphometric, ultrastructural study. Invest Ophthalmol Vis Sci 1995; 36:1750–64.
147. Schlötzer-Schrehardt U, Naumann GOH. Pseudoexfoliation Glaucoma. In: Krieglstein GK, Weinreb RN, eds. Essentials in Ophthalmology—Glaucoma. Springer, Heidelberg; 2004: 157–176.
148. Schlötzer-Schrehardt U, Naumann GOH. Ocular and systemic pseudoexfoliation syndrome. Am J Ophthalmol 2006; 141:921–37.
149. Schlötzer-Schrehardt U, von der Mark K, Sakai LY, Naumann GOH. Increased extracellular deposition of fibrillin-containing fibrils in pseudoexfoliation syndrome. Invest Ophthalmol Vis Sci 1997; 38:970–84.
150. Schlötzer-Schrehardt U, Zenkel M, Küchle M, et al. Role of transforming growth factor-β1 and its latent form binding protein in pseudoexfoliation syndrome. Exp Eye Res 2001a; 73:765–80.
151. Schumacher S, Nguyen NX, Küchle M, Naumann GOH. Quantification of aqueous flare after phacoemulsification with intraocular lens implantation in eyes with pseudoexfoliation syndrome. Arch Ophthalmol 1999; 117: 733–5.
152. Schumacher S, Schlötzer-Schrehardt U, Martus P, et al. Pseudoexfoliation syndrome and aneurysms of the abdominal aorta. Lancet 2001; 357:359–60.
153. Seland JH. Histopathology of the lens capsule in fibrillopathia epitheliocapsularis (FEC) or so-called senile exfoliation or pseudoexfoliation. Acta Ophthalmol 1979; 57:477–99.
154. Shakib M, Ashton N, Blach R. Electron microscopic study of pseudoexfoliation of the lens capsule. II. Iris and ciliary body. Invest Ophthalmol 1965; 4:154–61.
155. Shimizu T. Changes of iris vessels in capsular glaucoma: three-dimensional and electron microscopic studies. Jpn J Ophthalmol 1985; 29:434–52.
156. Shimizu T, Futa R. The fine structure of pigment epithelium of the iris in capsular glaucoma. Graefes Arch Clin Exp Ophthalmol 1985; 223:77–82.
157. Shrum KR, Hattenhauer MG, Hodge D. Cardiovascular and cerebrovascular mortality associated with ocular pseudoexfoliation. Am J Ophthalmol 2000; 129:83–6.
158. Sotirova V, Irkec M, Percin EF, et al. Molecular genetic study of families with pseudoexfoliation syndrome (PEX) suggests two putative locations on 2p14-2Cen and 2q35-q36 regions. Annual Meeting of the Association for Research in Vision and Ophthalmology 1999; Abstract 512.
159. Speakman JS, Ghosh M. The conjunctiva in senile lens exfoliation. Arch Ophthalmol 1976; 94:1757–9.
160. Streeten BW. Aberrant synthesis and aggregation of elastic tissue components in pseudoexfoliative fibrillopathy: a unifying concept. New Trends in Ophthalmology 1993; 8:187–96.
161. Streeten BW, Dark AJ, Barnes CW. Pseudoexfoliative material and oxytalan fibers. Exp Eye Res 1984; 38: 523–31.
162. Streeten BW, Gibson SA, Li Z-Y. Lectin binding to pseudoexfoliative material and the ocular zonules. Invest Ophthalmol Vis Sci 1986; 27:1516–21.
163. Streeten BW, Gibson SA, Dark AJ. Pseudoexfoliative material contains an elastic microfibrillar-associated glycoprotein. Trans Am Ophthalmol Soc 1986b; 84: 304–20.
164. Streeten BW, Bookman L, Ritch R, et al. Pseudoexfoliative fibrillopathy in the conjunctiva: a relation to elastic fibers and elastosis. Ophthalmology 1987; 94:1439–49.
165. Streeten BW, Dark AJ, Wallace RN, Li Z-Y, Hoepner JA. Pseudoexfoliative fibrillopathy in the skin of patients with ocular pseudoexfoliation. Am J Ophthalmol 1990; 110:490–9.
166. Streeten BW, Li Z-Y, Wallace RN, et al. Pseudoexfoliative fibrillopathy in visceral organs of a patient with pseudoexfoliation syndrome. Arch Ophthalmol 1992; 110: 1757–62.
167. Takei Y, Mizuno K. Electron-microscopic study of pseudo-exfoliation of the lens capsule. Graefes Arch Klin Ophthalmol 1978; 205:213–20.
168. Tarkkanen A. Pseudoexfoliation of the lens capsule: A clinical study of 418 patients with special reference to glaucoma, cataract, and changes of the vitreous. Acta Ophthalmol 1962; 71(Suppl.):1–98.
169. Tarkkanen A, Kivelä T, John G. Lindberg and the discovery of exfoliation syndrome. Acta Ophthalmol Scand 2002; 80:151–4.

170. Tarkkanen A, Kivelä T. Cumulative incidence of converting from clinically unilateral to bilateral exfoliation syndrome. J Glaucoma 2004; 13:181–4.
171. Tawara A, Fujisawa K, Kiyosawa R, Inomata H. Distribution and characterization of proteoglycans associated with exfoliation materials. Curr Eye Res 1996; 15: 1101–11.
172. Taylor HR. Pseudoexfoliation, an environmental disease? Trans Ophthalmol Soc UK 1979; 99:302–7.
173. Tetsumoto K, Schlötzer-Schrehardt U, Küchle M, et al. Precapsular layer of the anterior lens capsule in early pseudoexfoliation syndrome. Graefe's Arch Clin Exp Ophthalmol 1992; 230:252–7.
174. Teus MA, Castejon MA, Calvo MA. Intraocular pressure as a risk factor for visual field loss in pseudoexfoliative and in primary open-angle glaucoma. Ophthalmology 1998; 105:2225–9.
175. Thorleifson G, Magnusson KP, Sulem P, et al. Common sequence variants in the *LOXL1* gene confer succeptibility to exfoliation glaucoma. Science 2007; 317: 1307–415.
176. Uusitalo M, Kivelä T, Tarkkanen A. Immunoreactivity of exfoliation material for the cell adhesion-related HNK-1 carbohydrate epitope. Arch Ophthalmol 1993; 111: 1419–23.
177. Vessani RM, Ritch R, Liebmann J, Jofe M. Plasma homocysteine is elevated in patients with exfoliation syndrome. Am J Ophthalmol 2003; 136:41–6.
178. Vogiatzis A, Marshall GE, Konstas AG, Lee WR, Immunogold study of non-collagenous matrix components in normal and exfoliative iris. Br J Ophthalmol 1994; 78:850–8.
179. Vogt A. Ein neues Spaltlampenbild des Pupillengebiets: Hellblauer Pupillensaumfilz mit Häutchenbildung auf der Linsenvorderkapsel. Klin Monatsbl Augenheilkd 1925; 75:1–12.
180. von der Lippe I, Küchle M, Naumann GOH. Pseudoexfoliation syndrome as a risk factor for acute ciliary block angle closure glaucoma. Acta Ophthalmol 1993; 71:277–9.
181. Wiggs JL, Andersen JS, Stefansson E, et al. A genomic screen suggests a locus on chromosome 2p16 for pseudoexfoliation syndrome. In: 48th Annual Meeting of the American Society of Human Genetics 1998; Abstract 1818.
182. Winkler J, Lünsdorf H, Wirbelauer C, et al. Immunohistochemical and charge-specific localization of anionic constituents in pseudoexfoliation deposits on the central anterior lens capsule from individuals with pseudoexfoliation syndrome. Graefe's Arch Clin Exp Ophthalmol 2001; 239:952–60.
183. Wishart PK, Spaeth GL, Poryzees EM. Anterior chamber angle in the exfoliation syndrome. Br J Ophthalmol 1985; 69:103–7.
184. Yilmaz A, Adigüzel U, Tamer L, et al. Serum oxidant/antioxidant balance in exfoliation syndrome. Clin Exp Ophthalmol 2005a; 33:63–6.
185. Yilmaz A, Tamer L, Ates NA, et al. Effects of apolipoprotein E genotypes on the development of exfoliation syndrome. Exp Eye Res 2005b; 80:871–5.
186. Yüksel N, Anik Y, Altintas Ö, et al. Magnetic resonance imaging of the brain in patients with pseudoexfoliation syndrome and glaucoma. Ophthalmologica 2006; 220: 125–30.
187. Yüksel N, Karabas VL, Arslan A, et al. Ocular hemodynamics in pseudoexfoliation syndrome and pseudoexfoliation glaucoma. Ophthalmology 2001; 108:1043–9.
188. Zalewska R, Pepinski W, Smolenska-Janica D, et al. Loss of heterozygosity in patients with pseudoexfoliation syndrome. Mol Vis 2003; 9:257–61.
189. Zenkel M, Pöschl E, von der Mark K, et al. Differential gene expression in pseudoexfoliation syndrome. Invest Ophthalmol Vis Sci 2005; 46:3742–52.
190. Zenkel M, Kruse FE, Naumann GOH, Schlötzer-Schrehardt U. Impaired cellular stress response in eyes with pseudoexfoliation syndrome/glaucoma. Annual Meeting of the Association for Research in Vision and Ophthalmology 2005; Abstract 3789.
191. Zenkel M, Kruse FE, Jünemann AG, et al. Clusterin deficiency in eyes with pseudoexfoliation syndrome may be implicated in the aggregation and deposition of pseudoexfoliative material. Invest Ophthalmol Vis Sci 2006; 47:1982–90.

26

Myopia

Thomas T. Norton
Department of Vision Sciences, University of Alabama at Birmingham, Birmingham, Alabama, U.S.A.

Ravikanth Metlapally
Duke Center for Human Genetics and Duke Eye Center, Duke University, Durham, North Carolina, U.S.A.

Terri L. Young
Duke Eye Center and Duke Center for Human Genetics, Duke University, Durham, North Carolina, U.S.A.

INTRODUCTION

This chapter summarizes knowledge about the refractive error, myopia, describes human eye growth patterns, describes how animal models have advanced our understanding of the visually guided mechanism that matches the eye's axial length to its optical power, and discusses the genetic basis of human myopia. Understanding the mechanism that controls axial length in humans is an important step toward the goal of learning how to treat myopia in humans by controlling axial elongation with pharmacological and/or optical therapies.

IMPORTANCE OF MYOPIA

Types and Prevalence

In a myopic eye, the retina is located behind the focal plane so that a concave (negative-power) lens is needed to move the focal plane to the retina, restoring focused images. Myopia is the most common human eye disorder in the world. Definitions of myopia vary, but generally an eye is considered myopic if a negative spherical equivalent correction of at least 0.5 diopters (D) is needed to restore emmetropia, the refractive state in which images are focused on the retina without accommodation. Because of varying definitions, the reported prevalence of myopia varies, but in the adult population of the United States an estimated prevalence of about 25% is supported by multiple studies (2,21,44,77,80,195). Females are reported to have an earlier onset and a slightly higher prevalence than males (44,52,77,160). Comparative prevalence rates from different countries show considerable variability, but confirm that myopia affects a significant proportion of the population in many countries (19,28,80,93,117, 122,195,210,231). Asians and Hispanics have a higher prevalence than Caucasian or African Americans in the

United States (84). Chinese and Japanese populations have very high prevalence rates of >50% to 70% (8,44,160,252). Ashkenazi Jews, especially Orthodox Jewish males, have shown a higher prevalence than other white U.S. and European populations (252). Worldwide, there may be as many as 1 billion myopes (130). Uncorrected myopia is an important cause of correctable low vision (108). That is why, as part of its global initiative, Vision 2020, the World Health Organization has included correction of refractive error as one of its priorities (24).

Myopia is typically divided into two basic types. "juvenile-onset" or moderate myopia (also called "simple" or "school" myopia) most often develops and progresses between the ages of 8 and 16 years and generally does not require a correction stronger than –5 D (21,38,52,73,97). In contrast, "pathologic" or high-grade myopia usually begins to develop in the perinatal period, and is associated with rapid refractive error myopic shifts before 10 to 12 years of age due to axial elongation of the vitreous chamber (19,21,47,52,97).

Whether it occurs from continued progression of juvenile-onset myopia, or from early-onset high-grade myopia, a high level of axial myopia (spherical equivalent refractive correction of –5 D or greater) is a major cause of legal blindness in many developed countries (19,28,77,87,93,210,252). High myopia has a prevalence of 1.7% to 2% in the general population of the United States (2,21) and is especially common in Asia (93,210,231). In Japan, high myopia reportedly affects 6% to 18% of the myopic population and 1% to 2% of the general population (210).

The public health and economic impacts of myopia are considerable (2,8,19,21,38,44,47,52,77,97, 160,195, 252). Costs associated with optical corrections for adults were over US$26 billion in 2005 for glasses, contact lenses, and refractive surgery (from data supplied by Jobson/Vision Council of America, Alexandria, Virginia, U.S.A.) Of this, at least 61% (US$14.6 billion) was for myopia, and did not include costs for correcting myopia in children.

Ocular Morbidity

Many investigators have reported on the association of high myopia with cataract (90), glaucoma (115), retinal detachment (RD), and posterior staphyloma with retinal degenerative changes (7,13,20,21,30,33,46, 56,58,63,72,88,126,140,141,145,199,209) (for a recent review, see Ref. 159). High myopia is associated with progressive and excessive elongation of the globe, which may be accompanied by degenerative changes in the sclera, choroid, Bruch membrane, retinal pigment epithelium (RPE), and neural retina. Various funduscopic changes within the posterior staphyloma develop in highly myopic eyes. These changes include geographic areas of atrophy of the RPE and choroid, lacquer cracks in Bruch membrane, subretinal hemorrhage, and choroidal neovascularization (CNV). Such changes are shown in Figure 1A. Among these fundus lesions, macular CNV is the most common vision-threatening complication of high myopia (7,58,63,72,126,145). Clinical and histopathologic studies have documented CNV in 4% to 11% of highly myopic eyes. Relative to emmetropic eyes, an approximately two-fold increased risk of CNV was estimated for eyes with 1 to 2 D of myopia, a four-fold increase with 3 to 4 D, and a nine-fold increase with 5 to 6 D (7,13,199,221). Poor visual outcome following CNV in myopic eyes is common, and often affects relatively young patients.

The risk of RD is estimated to be 3 to 7 times greater for persons with >5 D of myopia than it is for those with a lesser degree of myopia (13,23,209). Myopia of 5 to 10 D is associated with a 15- to 35-fold greater risk of RD relative to that associated with low levels of hyperopia (13,23,209). The lifetime risk for RD is estimated to be 1.6% for patients with <3 D of myopia and 9.3% for those with >5 D (141,209). A subgroup with lattice degeneration of the retina and >5 D of myopia has an estimated lifetime risk of 35.9% (141). The prevalence of lattice degeneration increases with increasing severity of myopia as measured by axial length (13,23,143,196). Glaucoma is observed in 3% of patients with myopia who have axial lengths of <26.5 mm, in 11% with axial lengths of 26.5 to 33.5 mm, and in 28% of those with lengths >33.5 mm (140).

The high prevalence of myopia, along with the increased risk of blinding complications associated with high myopia, has stimulated many studies aimed at learning why and how myopia develops and whether treatments can be designed to prevent the development or progression of myopia. A fundamental question has been whether myopia is a result of predetermined genetic (200) or environmental factors (17) such as excessive near-work. Both not only appear to play a role in human myopia, but have been suggested to be a major, or even the sole, cause of myopia as described in the following sections.

HUMAN EMMETROPIZATION

Although myopia is highly prevalent, the vast majority of eyes are emmetropic in childhood. The normal postnatal development of emmetropia has been examined for clues about possible underlying mechanisms by which this is achieved. At birth the refractive distribution of human newborns is very broad (Fig. 2A). The mean is approximately 2 D of hyperopia, but the standard deviation is great and nearly 25% of newborns are myopic (18). The major determinants of the focal plane are the cornea and lens, while the axial length (vitreous chamber depth) determines whether the retina is located at the focal plane (216). At birth, the

(A) 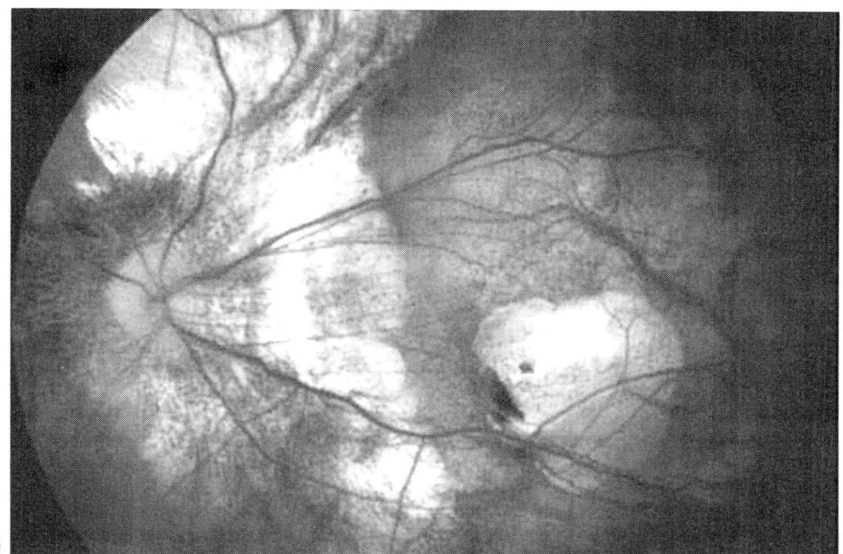

(B) 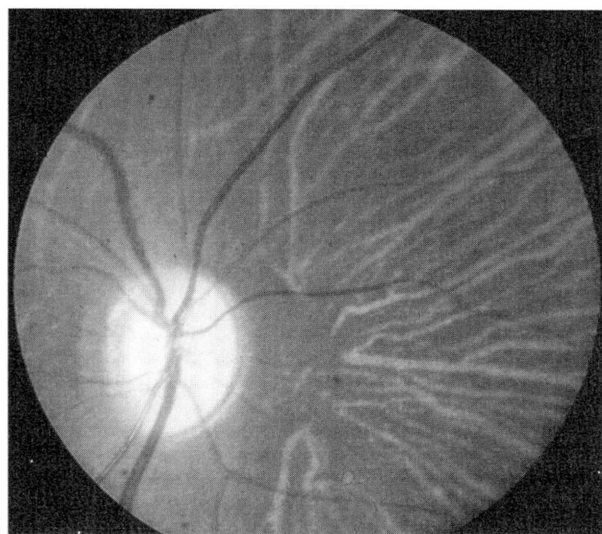

Figure 1 (**A**) A highly myopic human fundus, showing retinal thinning with prominent choroidal vasculature, scleral show, and areas of scleral staphylomatous changes in the posterior pole. (**B**) Myopic fundus of a macaque monkey showing a myopic crescent and tessellation. *Source*: (**B**) Courtesy of Dr. Elio Raviola.

size, shape, and refractive power (RP) of the eye of all are determined largely by inheritance (215), although conformational factors such as intrauterine environment and the bony orbits and eyelids can also influence eye shape and growth (193).

During the first postnatal weeks and months, the ocular components and refractive state undergo rapid changes. The corneal diameter of the infant is 9 to 10 mm compared to the adult size of 12 mm. Due to the steep curvature, corneal RP averages 51 D at birth and flattens to approximately 44 D by 6 weeks of age (41,191). Mutti et al. (118) found the average corneal RP at 3 months of age to be 43.9 D. By 9 months it had decreased to 42.8 D and between 6 and 14 years of age it was stable (244). Lenticular RP averages 34 D at birth and decreases to 28 D by 6 months of age, and to 21 D by adulthood (41). Mutti et al. (121,244) found the average lens RP (Gullstrand–Emsley indices) showed a continual decline with age from 21.5 D at age 6 years to 19.8 D at age 14 years.

In addition to the changes in the RPs of the cornea and lens, the distribution of refractive errors narrows dramatically in the postnatal months (Fig. 2B) (41,52,64,100,118). In the infantile growth period, the eyes grow from around 16-mm axial length at birth (29) to an average of 19 mm at 3 months of age and over 20 mm by 9 months (118). During this time the axial length changes in a manner that moves the retina to the focal plane (29,190). As described by Mutti et al. (118) "modulation in the amount of axial growth in relation to initial refractive error appeared to be the most influential factor in emmetropization of spherical equivalent refractive error." Eyes that are initially hyperopic increase their axial length rapidly to move the retina to the focal plane. Eyes that are initially myopic have a slower axial elongation rate so that, as

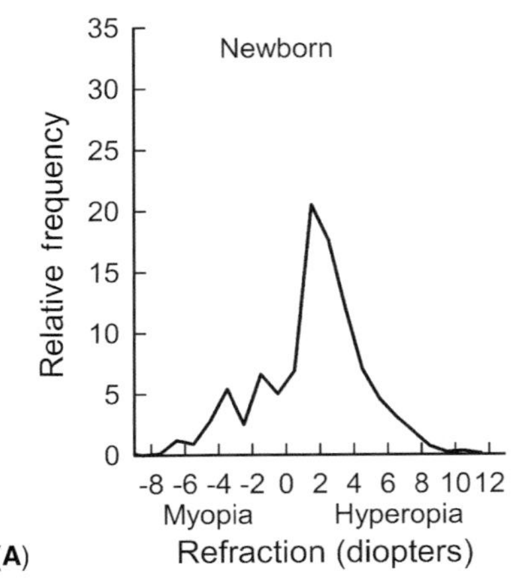

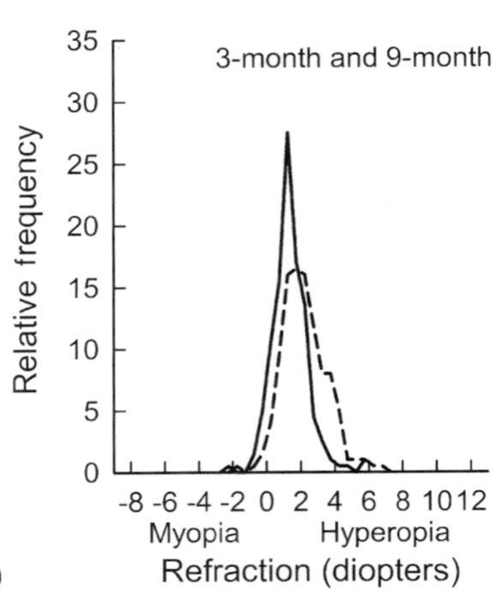

Figure 2 (**A**) Refractive error distribution at birth. (**B**) Refractive error distribution at 3 months (*dashed line*) and 9 months of age. At birth, ~25% of infants are myopic. By 9 months, nearly all children are emmetropic or slightly hyperopic. *Source*: Data from Refs. 18 and 118.

the cornea and lens RPs decrease, the focal plane moves to the retina. The result of the controlled growth of the axial length is that nearly all eyes become emmetropic with the majority being slightly (0.5–1 D) hyperopic when measured with cycloplegia. There is little change in refractive status in most eyes during the rest of childhood, even though there is continued change in anterior chamber depth, lens RP, and axial length. Because of the continued decreases in corneal and lens RP during childhood, control of the axial elongation rate is needed to maintain a match to the focal plane until the eyes are fully mature. The refractive error distribution in the adult population has a narrow shape with most people between emmetropia and +1.0 D. This amount of hyperopia is readily compensated for by accommodation of the crystalline lens, so that most eyes are functionally emmetropic (201,203). The human eye normally maintains an axial length of within 2% of its optimal focal point (21,215,216). In an adult (~24 mm) eye, a deviation from the optimal of 0.2 mm in axial length would produce a refractive error of more than 0.5 D (114).

Although the individual refractive components: corneal and lenticular dioptric powers and anterior chamber depth follow a normal distribution, several studies have shown that the refractive status of the eye is determined primarily by axial length, which does not (21,23,73,193,215). Spherical refractive error usually represents a mismatch between axial length and the combined dioptric powers of the cornea and lens. Moderate myopia results from a "failure of correlation" of these components where all components fall within normal limits but are borderline high or low. For example, an eye with a relatively steep cornea and normal axial length could be myopic even though none of the ocular component dimensions is abnormal. Low myopia (<6 D) is usually the result of this lack of correlation. In children whose myopia is progressing, the amount of progression is closely related to the increase in vitreous chamber length (68). Higher levels of myopia are due to "component ametropia" in which the axial length exceeds normal values (193,216). "Correlational" and "component" myopia may have different genetic causes.

Although some of the narrowing of the distribution of refractive errors during the first postnatal months can be explained by the "passive proportional" growth of the eye (222), more eyes are emmetropic than would be expected from a random combination of the optical elements and the axial length (60,201). This has led to the hypothesis that an active feedback mechanism coordinates the axial length with the optical elements to produce emmetropia (18,60,81,189,201,203,215). However, based on clinical observations, it has not been possible to test this suggestion.

ANIMAL MODELS OF EMMETROPIZATION

In the 1970s studies with animal models, primarily monkeys (213,228), chicks (223), and tree shrews (174), which are small, diurnal, highly visual mammals closely related to primates (94), demonstrated that an emmetropization mechanism exists. It has been shown in animals that this emmetropization mechanism normally controls the axial elongation rate of the eye to achieve and maintain a match of the axial length to the optical power so that the photoreceptors are in focus for distant objects (127,225,229). Vision plays a critical role in this process.

Form-Deprivation Myopia

Animal models of the emmetropization process began with "form-deprivation myopia" (see recent reviews, Refs. 127,166,185,225,229). Form deprivation was initially produced by tarsorrhaphy or by the placement of a translucent diffuser over the eye, held in place by a goggle or mask. This eliminated high spatial frequencies and decreased the contrast of the retinal image, while still allowing limited transmission of light to the retina. It is now recognized that form deprivation removes the visual feedback needed to guide the eye to emmetropia and to maintain emmetropia. Form deprivation during the juvenile postnatal period causes the vitreous chamber of chicks, tree shrews, macaque monkeys, and other species to elongate from a normal, slightly hyperopic state, past the point that would produce emmetropia and become myopic (174,223,228). In monkeys, fundus changes typical of human myopia, including peripapillary atrophy and tesselation have been found (Fig. 1B) (152,153) and tesselation is frequently found in tree shrews with induced myopia (107). A decrease in choroidal thickness also occurs in monkeys (67,214) and tree shrews (104,129), and is prominent in chicks (224). Because the "induced myopia" occurs only in form-deprived eyes and, in the case of monocular treatment, not in the other eye which serves as an untreated within-animal control, the myopia is clearly environmental in origin. The fact that lid-closure myopia could not be induced in dark-reared animals further suggests that visual experience is required (109,151). Form-deprivation myopia occurs consistently across species including the gray squirrel (106), cat (188), and mouse (208).

Compensation for Negative Lenses

Recognition that the emmetropization mechanism uses visual feedback to match the axial length to the focal plane came from studies that used negative-power (and positive-power) lenses to shift the focal plane of the eye (70,164,165). As shown by comparing Figure 3A and 3B, a monocular negative lens moves the focal plane posteriorly, away from the cornea. This has been found to consistently produce a compensatory increase in the axial elongation rate of the growing eye, such that the retinal location is shifted to match the focal plane (Fig. 3C). When measured with the lens in place, the refractive state matches the untreated fellow control eye (164,177,186). Thus, in compensating for the negative lens the eye is, in fact, restoring optical emmetropia. With the lens removed, the eye is myopic (Fig. 3D). Compensation occurs rapidly; full compensation occurs in a few days in chick and tree shrew and a few weeks in monkeys. Compensation can be accurate (66,71,176) and negative lenses of different powers produce different axial elongations that compensate for the lens power. Some strains of mice can develop negative lens-induced myopia even though mice are not strongly dependent on vision (162). Fish (Tilapia), which are more vision-dependent, can also develop this form of myopia (172).

Interestingly, for negative lens compensation to occur in animals, the lens must be worn almost constantly. Removing the negative lens and allowing normal unrestricted vision (or plano-lens wear) for as little as 2 h/day is sufficient to block negative lens compensation in monkeys (78), tree shrews (171), and chicks (167).

Positive Lenses

Positive lenses shift the focal plane anteriorly, making an emmetropic eye myopic. In examining the effect of positive lenses in animal studies, it is noteworthy that they are applied to juvenile eyes that are still undergoing normal axial elongation. If the axial elongation rate is slowed below normal while the optical components continue to mature normally, the eye gradually becomes emmetropic while wearing the positive lens. With the lens removed it is hyperopic.

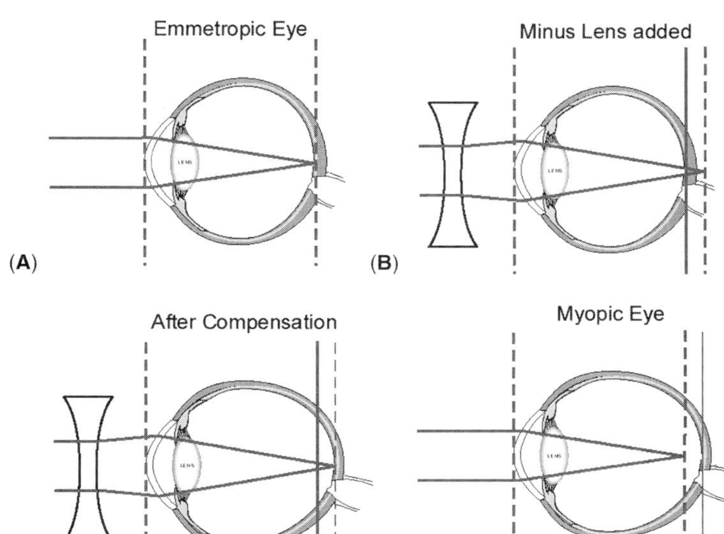

Figure 3 (**A**) Compensation for a negative lens. In an emmetropic eye, the focal plane for distant objects, without accommodation, is coincident with the retina. (**B**) Placing a negative-power lens in front of one eye displaces the focal plane posteriorly, assuming accommodation is set by the control eye. (**C**) The emmetropization mechanism produces elongation that moves the retina to the displaced focal plane so that the eye's refractive state is emmetropic with the lens in place. (**D**) When the lens is removed the eye is myopic.

Thus, to respond to a positive lens, eyes must not only be able to detect that they are myopic, but also be able to slow their elongation rate. In a young, growing chick eye, positive lens wear quickly causes a slowing of the elongation rate so that the eye becomes emmetropic while wearing the lens and hyperopic when the lens is removed (70,164). Even short exposures to myopic defocus have a potent slowing effect (163,167,232,250,251).

The response to positive lenses differs somewhat in monkeys and tree shrews. When positive lenses are applied to tree shrews that have achieved emmetropia, they have little effect (182). However, if positive lenses are applied early in the emmetropization process in younger, hyperopic tree shrews and monkeys, the eyes typically slow their elongation rate and maintain emmetropia while wearing the lens (34,184,186,217). With the lens removed, the eyes are hyperopic. The lack of a response to positive lenses in older tree shrews and monkeys may reflect an inability to slow their axial elongation rate substantially once they have achieved emmetropia. The source of this difference relative to chicks is not yet known, but it may be related to the fact that the chick eye has a sclera with an inner cartilaginous layer in addition to an outer fibrous portion comparable to the sclera of humans, monkeys, and tree shrews. Controlling the growth of the cartilage may be a more powerful way of slowing axial elongation than can be achieved with a fibrous sclera alone.

Recovery from Induced Myopia

Further evidence for active control of the axial length comes from the effect of removing form deprivation or negative lens wear after an induced myopia has developed. In the several species that have been studied, "recovery" from induced myopia occurs. Restoration of unrestricted vision causes the axial elongation rate to decrease below normal. As the focal plane moves posteriorly due to continued corneal flattening and lens maturation the induced myopia dissipates (35,144,176,181,222). It has been suggested that recovery occurs for two reasons: first, the eye is myopic, and second it is elongated relative to normal. These factors together produce a stronger response than what occurs with positive lens wear alone (125). In animals with monocular-induced myopia, the refractive state of the recovering eye eventually matches that of the untreated eye at emmetropia, suggesting active guidance toward a "target" of emmetropia. The process of emmetropization is thus capable of controlling axial elongation to achieve emmetropia from the myopic as well as the hyperopic direction. The consistency of responses to form deprivation, negative lens wear, and recovery provides evidence that an active emmetropization mechanism exists and is conserved across classes of animals. Together with the rapid development in human infants of a very narrow refractive error distribution, these data argue strongly that an emmetropization mechanism exists in humans.

THE EMMETROPIZATION FEEDBACK LOOP

The Signaling Cascade

How does the retina control the axial elongation rate to match itself to the focal plane and maintain that match throughout the juvenile developmental period? A broad outline of a feedback loop has emerged from studies of animal models starting with the visual stimulus ("1" in Fig. 4). Although it is not known precisely what aspect of the images on the retina stimulates ocular elongation there is general agreement that hyperopic defocus (image plane behind the retina) serves as a stimulus for eyes to increase the axial elongation rate (a "go" signal). Myopic defocus, or perhaps clear images on the retina, seems to produce signals that slow axial elongation (a "stop" signal). Defocus, or its absence, of course, is detected by the retina ("2" in Fig. 4), presumably at the level of center-surround bipolar cells or later (9,230). As has been established by single-unit studies of retinal ganglion cells (154), defocused images produce weaker responses from cells with center-surround receptive fields than do sharply focused images. Thus, as the eyes move from target-to-target, changing the images on each part of the retina, focused images will produce large changes in the activity level of retinal cells, and this may be part of the retinal signal.

Recently, in chicks, a class of amacrine cells that contain glucagon have been found to be involved in sending a "stop" signal to slow the eye's elongation rate (27,218,219). Without these cells, eyes elongate and become myopic. With them, and with additional glucagon administered intravitreally (218), eyes resist becoming myopic with form deprivation. It also has been reported that apolipoprotein A1 provides a retinal "stop" signal in chicks (10).

Perhaps surprisingly, the emmetropization mechanism persists after sectioning of the optic nerve (212) or blocking the output from the retina to central visual structures with tetrodotoxin (105,128), leading to the conclusion that there is direct communication across the RPE and choroid ("3" and "4" in Fig. 4) with the sclera. This communication must be spatially local. When form deprivation or negative lens treatment is applied to half of the visual field (either nasal or temporal) using specially designed goggles only the treated half of the eye elongates and becomes myopic (25,61,133,175). More surprisingly, the fovea is neither necessary nor sufficient to establish and maintain emmetropia. Macaque monkeys (*Macaca mulatta*) that have undergone laser destruction of the

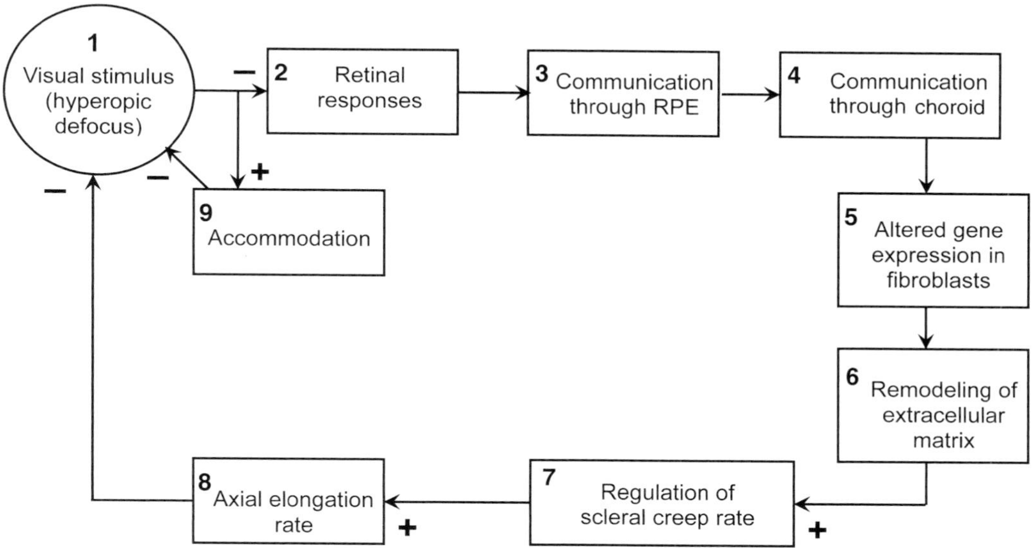

Figure 4 An emmetropization model. When the axial length is shorter than the focal plane, hyperopic defocus (**1**) occurs on the retina unless fully cleared by accommodation (**9**). Hyperopic defocus reduces the amplitude of responses (variability in response) of retinal neurons (**2**), altering the communication of signals (**3**) through the RPE and (**4**) choroid. This is communicated to the sclera where (**5**) gene expression in fibroblasts is altered. Remodeling of the scleral extracellular matrix (ECM) occurs (**6**) increasing the biomechanical property, "creep rate" (increased length under a constant tension) of the sclera (**7**) which increases the axial elongation rate (**8**) of the eye. Axial elongation moves the retina closer to the focal plane, reducing the amount of defocus. As defocus is reduced on the retina, responses in some neurons increase, generating a "stop" signal that is communicated to the sclera. Scleral remodeling is altered such that the creep rate is decreased and axial elongation is slowed. This type of feedback model would produce the gradual normal approach of the axial length to the focal plane from hyperopia. Accurate accommodation (**9**) is important because it reduces defocus (53).

entire macular region maintain emmetropia (187). Monkeys that wear form-depriving diffuser goggles with a clear central 30° to allow foveal vision, develop form-deprivation myopia (79,187).

How the visually derived signals pass through the RPE is unknown. It has been suggested that changes in retinal activity produce changes in ionic concentrations across the RPE that in turn affect the tissues of the choroid (89). Mertz and Wallman (110) suggested that all-trans-retinoic acid in the choroid may serve as a signaling molecule to the sclera. Rada et al. (148) have suggested that ovotransferrin might also serve a similar role.

Visually Guided Remodeling of the Sclera

Composition of the Sclera

As the structural outer coat of the eye, the sclera controls the location of the retina. The sclera in eutherian mammals is a soft, but tough, fibrous viscoelastic connective tissue comprised of an extracellular matrix (ECM) produced by fibroblasts of neural crest origin (103,205,211). It consists of layers, or lamellae, of collagen (85–90% of the scleral total protein), proteoglycans, hyaluronan, and other extracellular proteins produced by the fibroblasts. Collagen type I is the primary subtype (>99%) (131) but collagen types III, V, and VI are present in human and tree shrew sclera (34,98). Unlike cornea, the diameter and spacing of the collagen fibrils varies widely, so that the sclera is not transparent. In addition to collagen, elastic fibrils have been reported in the human sclera (99). The proteoglycans aggrecan, biglycan, and decorin are also present in the adult human sclera (147) and in tree shrew sclera (180). Austin et al. (5) suggested that another proteoglycan, lumican, is important in the formation of scleral collagen fibrils. A simplified scleral structure is depicted in Figure 5.

Glycosaminoglycans (GAGs) constitute a small (~0.2%), but potentially important fraction of the scleral dry weight. Functionally, GAGs are generally attached to proteoglycan core proteins and have been suggested to stabilize the spacing of collagen fibrils (169) and to affect the hydration levels of the ECM (12,112).

In addition to these structural components, the sclera contains several growth factors, including transforming growth factor beta (TGFβ) and basic fibroblast growth factor (FGF2) (36,170) as well as degradative enzymes (matrix metalloproteinases [MMPs] and tissue inhibitors of metalloproteinases [TIMPs]) (101,178).

Scleral Growth and Extensibility

After the infantile growth period is over, there is little evidence in mammals for continued scleral growth

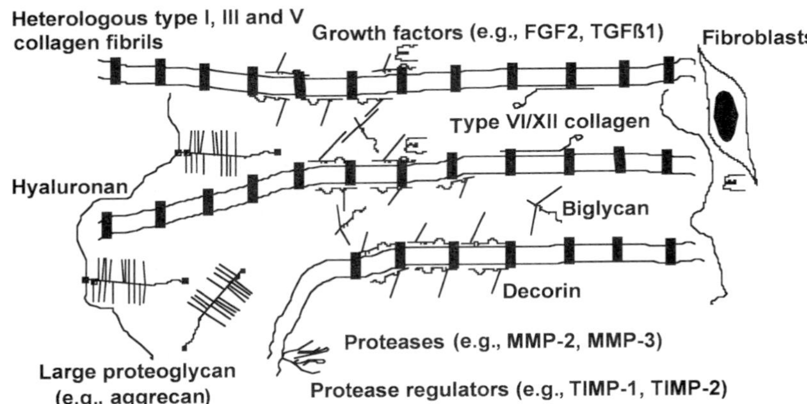

Figure 5 Structure of the mammalian sclera. Model illustrating the likely biochemical structure of the extracellular matrix of the mammalian sclera. *Source*: From Ref. 103.

(131). Rather than modulating cartilage growth as occurs in chicks (16,149), the visual environment controls remodeling of the scleral ECM. This discussion focuses on mammalian sclera, with particular emphasis on tree shrew because it has been the subject of considerable research.

When "go" signals produced by hyperopic defocus or form deprivation reach the sclera, changes in expression for some genes occur ("5" in Fig. 4), along with remodeling ("6" in Fig. 4) of the scleral ECM (132). In tree shrews, and perhaps in mammals generally, these biochemical changes appear to control the extension of the sclera over time when a constant tension is applied (the "creep rate") ("6" in Fig. 4). Normally in juvenile tree shrew eyes scleral extensibility is low. As a result of the remodeling of the sclera, the creep rate rises (177) and the sclera becomes more readily extensible. The changes in creep rate in turn allow normal intraocular pressure (IOP) to increase the axial elongation rate of the eye ("8" in Fig. 4), moving the retina away from the cornea. In a hyperopic eye an increased axial elongation rate reduces the hyperopia, decreasing the defocus on the retina. Through this emmetropization feedback system, a hyperopic eye elongates until the visual signals ("1"in Fig. 4) that drive the feedback loop diminish and the eye stabilizes at emmetropia.

Scleral Changes During Myopia Development and Recovery

Many of the details of how the visual environment controls scleral remodeling summarized in the model shown in Figure 4 emanate from studies using form deprivation or negative lenses to induce myopia. Both interventions produce a visual signal that stimulates the feedback loop, raising the amount of scleral remodeling, increasing the creep, and axial elongation rates. Changes observed during recovery are generally the reverse of ones found during myopia development.

Sclera in Myopia and Recovery

When myopia is induced, the sclera becomes thinner, due in part to a reduction in the amount of collagen type I (102,103,132). Scleral dry weight reduces 3% to 5% after as few as 5 days of form deprivation or negative lens wear in tree shrews (102). Long-term form deprivation in tree shrews leads to a more substantial thinning, as shown in Figure 6, comparable to humans with moderate myopia (15). Humans with pathological myopia have marked scleral thinning, particularly at the posterior pole (6). In addition to scleral thinning, the collagen fibrils often show altered architecture in human high myopia, with a reduction in diameter, loss of longitudinal fibril striations and a derangement of the growth, and organization of the fibrils (22). Following long-term form deprivation in tree shrews, Norton and Rada (132) noted a reduction in hydroxyproline (–11.8%), which suggests a loss of collagen. After months of form deprivation McBrien et al. (101) found a reduction in median fibril diameter and misshapen collagen fibrils in tree shrews.

An advantage of animal models, in contrast to human eyes obtained postmortem (donor eyes) is that it is possible to examine the sclera and other tissues when an induced myopia is developing, rather than only at an endpoint of long-standing myopia. Furthermore, the changes occur after a few days or weeks, rather than years. After short-term form deprivation, the sclera is thinner than normal, but the collagen fibrils possess a normal diameter and interfibril spacing (76,101). During recovery, collagen synthesis and collagen type I mRNA levels increase (34). These findings suggest that more subtle remodeling of the scleral material, rather than destruction of structural elements, occurs and causes axial elongation and myopia development immediately after the onset of form deprivation or negative lens wear.

Considerable attention has been paid to the processes that underlie scleral remodeling. Scleral

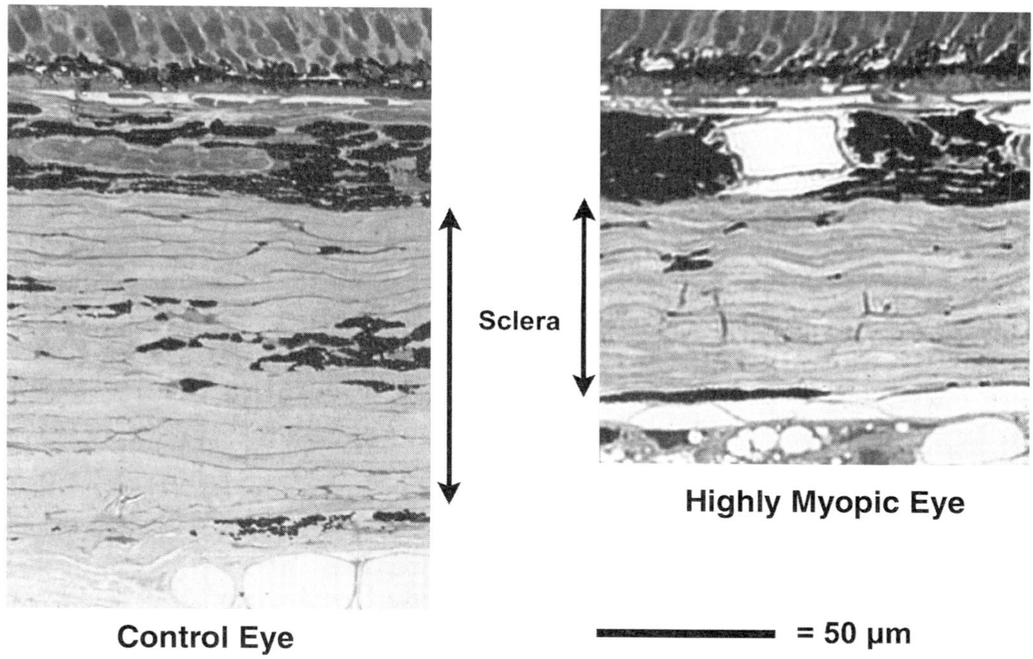

Figure 6 Scleral thickness in myopia. A toluidine blue-stained transverse section of tree shrew sclera at the posterior pole of a control eye and an eye with induced myopia following long-term form deprivation. *Arrows*, thickness of scleral tissue in each eye. *Source*: From Ref. 101.

fibroblasts are a likely cell type to detect and respond to retina-derived signals arriving from the choroid. One possible pathway involves FGF2 which is an inhibitor of collagen synthesis. However, endogenous levels of FGF2 are unchanged in tree shrew sclera during myopia development. The mRNA levels for the high-affinity receptor for FGF2, fibroblast growth factor receptor 1 (FGFR1) are upregulated and return to control levels during recovery (36). The TGFβ modulates the production of ECM, including collagen, as well as MMP-2 (136). Jobling et al. (74) noted a downregulation of the three isoforms of TGFβ during myopia development, and showed that all three isoforms increase collagen synthesis in cultures of scleral fibroblasts. Thus, a reduction in TGFβ during myopia development is consistent with the previously mentioned reduction in collagen levels. Furthermore, integrins, which are cell surface receptors, are present in the tree shrew sclera (111). One function of integrins is activation of TGFβ1, suggesting a possible role for integrin receptors in the observed reduction of this growth factor. Recently, thrombospondin-1, which also promotes TGFβ activation, has been found to be reduced in tree shrew sclera during myopia development (31).

Receipt of the retinally derived "go" signals by the scleral fibroblasts produces selective changes in the sclera. Levels of mRNA for some MMPs (MMP-2 and the membrane type-1 MMP (MT1-MMP) are upregulated (82,181)), while the mRNA levels of MMP-3 (stromelysin) are not different in the treated versus control eye scleras during negative lens-induced myopia development (181). TIMPs are also selectively affected; mRNA for TIMP3 is downregulated in treated eyes but mRNA for TIMP1 and TIMP2 is not differentially altered. In addition to a possible role in directly degrading collagen type I, MT1-MMP has been found to activate MMP-2 (4,204,226). There is evidence that MT1-MMP is the primary agent for cell-surface activation of MMP-2 proenzyme. MT1-MMP forms a trimolecular complex on the fibroblast cell surface with the proenzyme of MMP-2 and with TIMP-2 that activates MMP-2 (116,204,226). MT1-MMP may also play a role by directly degrading collagen (135). In fact, MT1-MMP-deficient mice cannot degrade fibrillar collagen (62). In addition to mRNA changes, higher levels of active form of MMP-2 were found in both equatorial and posterior regions of myopic sclera (51).

Proteoglycans and Glycosaminoglycans

Proteoglycans and their associated GAG chains are also potentially important. Messenger RNA levels for the decorin core protein, which is closely associated with collagen type I fibrils, are unchanged during myopia development (179,183). However, mRNA for aggrecan core protein is downregulated during lens-induced myopia and upregulated during recovery (180). There is little change in mRNA levels for lumican, and only a small downregulation of biglycan during myopia development (180,205).

Some GAGs associated with proteoglycan core proteins are sulfated. Lower levels of sulfated GAGs have been found during myopia development (132). Gentle and McBrien found a significant reduction in GAG synthesis in the posterior sclera of myopic eyes in tree shrews (35). A significant increase in sulfated GAG synthesis (42% in the anterior and 85% in the posterior region of the sclera) has been detected in eyes recovering from form-deprivation myopia (104). Hyaluronan, an unsulfated GAG that is not connected to a proteoglycan core protein, is also reduced during myopia development in tree shrews and returns to normal levels within 1 day in recovery (37).

The end result of the scleral remodeling is an increase in the creep rate, which is significantly higher (200–300%) in eyes that are developing myopia in normal eyes (142,177). When form deprivation or negative lens wear is discontinued, the creep rate decreases to below normal, causing the axial elongation rate to slow during recovery from induced myopia. The relative role of changes in structural collagen versus changes in levels of MMPs, TIMPs, proteoglycans such as aggrecan, and hyaluronan is yet undetermined. Collagen changes clearly are associated with long-standing myopia but the extent to which they are causally involved in the early development of myopia is unclear. It is also possible that the altered levels of enzymes and proteoglycans from the fibroblasts, which are located in between the lamellae of the sclera, may raise the creep rate simply by allowing the scleral lamellae to more readily slip across each other.

It should be noted that changes in gene expression in the sclera of eyes that are developing or recovering from myopia are relatively modest (two-fold) rather than all-or-none. This is consistent with the relatively modest stimulus used to induce myopia, particularly in the case of negative lens wear, which merely shifts the refractive state a small amount. These relatively small changes affect the amount of proteins that are produced but not their nucleotide sequences.

RELATION TO HUMAN MYOPIA

Although animal models have provided information about how environmentally induced myopia can develop, the applicability of animal studies to human myopia has been questioned. For instance, although form-deprivation myopia has been reported in young children with conditions that obstruct the visual axis such as ptosis or cataract (65,134,146) the myopic shift is inconsistent as they do not always develop myopia as a result of such deprivation (220).

However, an important similarity between animals and humans was found by Gwiazda et al. (53) who reported that children with increasing myopia underaccommodate to near visual targets more than emmetropic children. The resulting hyperopic defocus resembles what is produced by negative lens wear, which causes axial elongation in many animal species. This observation led to the "blur hypothesis," which suggests that the eyes of children also elongate in response to the hyperopic defocus that occurs when they underaccommodate to near targets. To the extent that accurate accommodation occurs, the defocus is reduced, which may be why the children with more accurate accommodation remained emmetropic in the Gwiazda et al. study (53). The blur hypothesis is attractive in that it not only relates animal studies to the human experience, but it also is consistent with the many studies that have associated myopia development with near work (2,252). It contrasts with the suggestion, never supported by direct measurement, that accommodation itself is a cause of myopia (236,238) by increasing tension on the sclera, stretching it so the eye elongates (216). According to the blur hypothesis, accommodation is beneficial because it provides clear images on the retina and thereby removes the visual stimuli for increased axial elongation that can lead to myopia ("9" in Fig. 4).

ROLE OF ENVIRONMENT IN HUMAN MYOPIA DEVELOPMENT

A role for the environment in the development and progression of juvenile-onset myopia has been suggested by epidemiological studies that have examined myopia prevalence. In general, myopia is more prevalent among populations living in urban environments, people with higher levels of education or people who engage in occupations involving extensive near work. For instance, myopia is rare in rural or illiterate societies. In adults in rural Mongolia, noncycloplegic measures found 17% of adults were myopic (227). By cycloplegic autorefraction, less than 6% of children aged 7 to 17 years of age were myopic. By contrast, 40% of people in Hong Kong aged 19 to 39 were myopic (39). Among an isolated group in Brazil that has no written language, 2.7% were myopic (>1 D). Lin et al. (93) found higher levels of myopia in school children in metropolitan and provincial cities in comparison with those in villages and "aboriginal" areas of Taiwan. Garner et al. (32) found low levels of myopia among Tibetan Sherpa children educated in the mountain areas and higher levels among Tibetan children going to school in Nepal.

Other studies have found an association between the years of education and myopia prevalence (2). Further, the type of educational experience affects myopia prevalence. Zylbermann et al. (252) found greater amounts of myopia among orthodox Jewish male students, whose education involved many hours of reading each day, than in students educated in standard public schools in Israel. An association between myopia and professions involving near work, such as inspectors in textile mills or microscopists have long been recognized (1,40). In addition, the prevalence of myopia in some populations appears to have increased dramatically from one generation to the next in progressively industrialized settings, or with increased levels of educational achievement (13,92,157,237,239).

Despite the epidemiological data suggesting a role for near work in the environment in myopia development, finding a causal link has been very difficult, possibly for several reasons. One is difficulty in measuring the amount and duration of "near work" (150). Another is that other factors, such as diet, also can vary between rural versus urban populations or even as a function of educational level. Perhaps the most important reason is that there is strong evidence that genetic factors also play a role, both in familial high myopia and for juvenile-onset myopia as will be discussed in the following sections.

A detailed assessment of confounding effects and interactions between hereditary and environmental influences in juvenile-onset myopia (119) reported that near work describes very little of the variance in refractive error compared to the number of myopic parents. Additionally, a measure of near work exerted no confounding influence on the association between parent and child myopia, indicating that children do not become myopic by adopting parental reading habits. More importantly, there was no significant interaction between parental myopia and near work; reading was weakly and equally associated with myopia regardless of the number of myopic parents. Yet, another study (158) found an association between myopia in Singaporean children reading more than two books per week. Recently, the inverse of near work, hours spent outdoors engaged in athletics, has been reported to be protective against myopia (75,156). Thus, although there is epidemiological evidence for a role of near work in the development of myopia, and a basis (hyperopic defocus) from animal studies for near work to play a role, it is yet to be determined precisely how the visual environment may contribute to human myopia, and how environmental factors interact with genetic factors.

HUMAN MOLECULAR GENETICS OF MYOPIA

Genetics of Ocular Refractive Components

As has been described, the refractive state is determined by the relative contributions of the optical components, primarily corneal curvature, anterior chamber depth, and lens curvature and thickness, which determine the location of the focal plane, and the axial length (primarily the vitreous chamber depth), which determines whether the retina is located at the focal plane. Separately these may be assessed as quantitative traits intimately related to the clinical phenotype of myopia. Multiple reports have examined familial aggregation and heritability of ocular components (11,14,49,54,55,95,96,202,206,234).

As expected from the previous sections, axial length is the largest contributor to the determination of refractive error. Several studies have reported a relationship of axial length to refraction (the longer the eye, the more myopic the refractive error) (14,49,96,202,234). Axial length of a myopic adult population may show a bimodal distribution with a second peak of increased axial length relating to high myopia (<6 D of myopia at 24 mm, >6 D at 30 mm) when plotted as a distribution curve (215). This suggests that myopia of 6 D or greater represents a deviation from the normal distribution of axial length and is not physiologic.

Estimates of heritability for axial length range from 40% to 94% (11,55,95,206). A study of three large Sardinian families found modest evidence for linkage on chromosome 2 (2p24) with a logarithm of the odds (LOD) score of 2.64 (11). Overall axial length includes anterior chamber depth, and studies have shown that increased anterior chamber depth has a relationship as well to myopic refractive error (234). The heritability reports for anterior chamber depth range from 70% to 94%, (11,54,95,206) and the same Sardinian study found modest linkage evidence to chromosome 1 (1p32.2) with a LOD score of 2.32 (11).

The steeper the corneal curvature the more likely the resulting refractive error is myopic; eyes with hyperopia are more likely to have flatter corneal curvature readings by keratometry (14,48,173). Heritability estimates for corneal curvature range from 60% to 92% (11,54,95,206). The Sardinian family study noted modest linkage evidence of corneal curvature to chromosomes 2p25, 3p26, and 7q22 with LOD scores ranging from 2.34 to 2.50 (11). Increased lens thickness correlates with increased myopia (234). A di- and monozygotic twin study reported 90% to 93% heritability for lens thickness (95).

Role of Genetics in Myopia Development

Multiple familial aggregation studies report a positive correlation between parental myopia and myopia in their children, indicating a hereditary factor in myopia susceptibility (43,137,235,243,245). Children with a family history of myopia had on average less hyperopia, deeper anterior chambers, and longer vitreous chambers even before becoming myopic. Yap and colleagues noted a prevalence of myopia in 7-year-old children of 7.3% when neither parent was myopic, 26.2% when one parent was myopic, and 45% when both parents were myopic. This implies a strong role for genetics in myopia (235).

Multiple familial studies support a high genetic effect for myopia (3,40,42,207). Naiglin and colleagues performed segregation analysis on 32 French multiplex families with high myopia, and determined an autosomal dominant (AD) mode of inheritance (123). The increase in risk to siblings of a person with myopia compared to the population prevalence (λs) has been estimated to be approximately 4.9 to 19.8 for sibs for high myopia (–6.00 spherical D or greater), and approximately 1.5 to 3 for low or common myopia (approximately –1.00 to –3.00 spherical D), suggesting a definite genetic basis for high myopia, and a strong genetic basis for low myopia (26,50). A high degree of familial aggregation of refraction, particularly myopia, was recently reported in the Beaver Dam Eye Study population after accounting for the effects of age, sex, and education (83). Segregation analysis suggested the involvement of multiple genes, rather than a single major gene effect.

Twin studies provide the most compelling evidence that inheritance plays a significant role in myopia (55,95,192,193,207). Multiple studies note an increased concordance of refractive error as well as refractive components (axial length, corneal curvature, lens power) in monozygotic twins compared to dizygotic twins (95,193,194,207). Sorsby et al. noted a correlation coefficient for myopia of 0 for control pairs, 0.5 for dizygotic twins, and almost 1.0 for monozygotic twins in a study of 78 pairs of monozygotic twins and 40 pairs of dizygotic twins (194). Twin studies estimate a notable high heritability value for myopia (the proportion of the total phenotypic variance that is attributed to genetic variance) of between 0.5 and 0.96. (55,95,192,194,207).

Molecular Genetic Studies of Human Myopia

High Myopia

Much of the current information on the molecular genetics of nonsyndromic human myopia has been drawn from studies of relatively small numbers of families affected by high myopia, usually defined as spherical refractive error >6 D. An X-linked recessive form of myopia, named the Bornholm (Denmark) eye disease (BED), was designated the first myopia locus (MYP1; MIM %310460) on the X chromosome (Xq28) (168). Collaborating with BED researchers, Young and colleagues made comparative molecular genetic haplotype and sequence analyses of a large Minnesota family of Danish descent that showed significant linkage of myopia to the X chromosome (Xq27.3–q28). The phenotype of both families appears to be due to a novel cone dysfunction, and not simple myopia. The genetic basis of each family appears to be distinct, as the haplotypes were different (240). A recent report by Michaelides et al. (113) confirmed the different X-linked cone dysfunction syndromes with associated high myopia phenotype in 4 United Kingdom families. Young et al. (242) identified the first AD locus for nonsyndromic high myopia within a 7.6 centimorgan (cM) region on chromosome 18 (18p11.31) (MYP2, MIM %160700) in 7 U.S. families. This locus was confirmed in Chinese Hong Kong and Italian Sardinian cohorts (59,86). Using the Hong Kong cohort, investigators identified the gene for transforming growth factor beta-induced factor (*TGIF*) as the implicated gene for MYP2 using limited single nucleotide polymorphism (SNP) association studies and exonic sequencing (85). However, Young's group fully sequenced the *TGIF* gene that encodes TGIF in the cohort of original MYP2 families, and found no associations with high myopia affection status (161). A second locus for AD high myopia mapped to a 30.1 cM region on chromosome 12 (12q21-23) (MYP3, MIM %603221) in an American family of German–Italian descent (241). This locus was confirmed in a high myopia Caucasian British cohort (26). A statistically suggestive third locus for AD high myopia was reported on chromosome 7 (7q36) in a Caucasian French cohort (MYP4, MIM %608367) (124). A fourth AD locus on chromosome 17 (17q21-23) (MYP5, MIM %608474) was determined in a large multigenerational English-Canadian family in Young's laboratory (138). Paluru et al. recently identified a locus for AD high myopia on chromosome 2 (2q37) in a large, multigenerational U.S. Caucasian family (139). Loci on the X chromosome (Xq23–25) and chromosome 4 (4q) have also recently been identified by Zhang et al. in ethnic Chinese families (246,247). All loci identified to date for isolated nonsyndromic high myopia are either AD or X-linked and highly penetrant. Table 1 summarizes all myopia loci identified to date.

Juvenile-Onset Myopia

At least two studies have shown nominal or no linkage of juvenile-onset myopia (low to moderate myopia) to many of the known high myopia loci. Mutti et al. (120) genotyped 53 common (low to moderate) myopia families (at least one child with >–0.75D myopia in each meridian) using the highest intra-interval LOD score microsatellite markers for the chromosome 18 (18p) and chromosome 12 (12q) loci

Table 1 Identified Myopia Loci as Approved by the HUGO Gene Nomenclature Committee

Locus	MIM	Chromosomal location	Myopia severity age of onset	References
MYP1	%310460	Xq28	High: −6.75 to −11.25 D Early: 1.5 to 5 years	113,168,240
MYP2	%160700	18p11.31	High: −6 to −21 D Early: 6.8 years (average)	86,242
MYP3	%603221	12q21–q23	High: −6.25 to −15 D Early: 5.9 years (average)	26,241
MYP4	%608367	7q36	High: −13.05 D (average)	124
MYP5	%608474	17q21–q22	High: −5.5 to −50 D Early: 8.9 years (average)	138
MYP6	%608908	22q12	Mild-moderate: −1.00 D or lower	198
MYP7	%609256	11p13	−12.12 to +7.25 D	54
MYP8	%609257	3q26	−12.12 to +7.25 D	54
MYP9	%609258	4q12	−12.12 to +7.25 D	54
MYP10	%609259	8p23	−12.12 to +7.25 D	54,197
MYP11	%609994	4q22–q27	High: −5 to −20 D Early: before school age	246
MYP12	%609995	2q37.1	High: −7.25 D to −27 D Early: before 12 years	139
MYP13	%300613	Xq23–q25	High: −6 to −20 D Early: before school age	247
MYP14	%610320	1p36	Moderate to high: −3.46 D (average)	233

Abbreviations: D, diopters; HGNC, HUGO Gene Nomenclature Committee (www.gene.ucl.ac.uk/cgi-bin/nomenclature/searchgenes); MIM, Mendelian Inheritance in Man (www.ncbi.nlm.nih.gov/entrez/query.fcgi?db=OMIM); MYP, myopia locus; p, short arm of a chromosome; q, long arm of a chromosome.

and did not establish linkage. Ibay et al. (69) found no strong evidence of linkage to the previously identified high myopia loci of MYP2, MYP3, MYP4, and MYP5, on chromosomes 18p, 12q, 7q, and 17q respectively, in a cohort of 38 Ashkenazi Jewish families with mild or moderate myopia (−1 D or more). These studies suggest that different genes may account for mild or moderate myopia susceptibility or development, or that the effect of these genes is too small to be detected with the relatively small sample sizes.

Three whole-genome mapping studies have identified several candidate gene intervals for common, juvenile-onset myopia using spherical refractive error data. The results of these studies demonstrate the potential for determining molecular genetic factors implicated in myopia at all levels of severity. These studies however, used microsatellite genotyping instead of SNP technology and a limited cohort sample size. Two of the studies used homogenous isolated populations, which brings into question the generalizability relative to populations with high admixture. One study was a genome screen of 44 families of Ashkenazi Jewish descent (198). Individuals with at least −1 D of myopic spherical refractive error were classified as affected. Their strongest signal localized to chromosome 22q12 (LOD score = 3.56; nonparametric linkage [NPL] score = 4.62). Eight additional regions (chromosomes 14q, 4q22–q28, 8q22.2, 10q22, 11q23, 13q22, 14q32, and 17qter) showed nominal linkage evidence. Hammond and colleagues evaluated 221 dizygotic twin pairs with moderate myopia and found significant linkage to 4 loci, with a maximum LOD score of 6.1 on chromosome 11 (11p13) (54). Other identified loci mapped to chromosomes 3q26 (LOD 3.7), 4q12 (LOD 3.3), 8p23 (LOD 4.1), and 11q23–24 (LOD 2.9). Hammond et al. found that the PAX6 gene on chromosome 11 (11p13) showed linkage with 5 SNPs, but no association. They suggested that PAX6 (a major eye development gene) may play a role in myopia development, possibly due to genetic variation in an upstream promoter or regulator. A recent report confirmed the myopia locus at chromosome 8 (8p23) in an isolated Pennsylvania Old Order Amish population of 34 families (197).

Another report found significant evidence for linkage of refractive error to a novel quantitative trait locus (QTL) on chromosome 1 (1p36) in an Ashkenazi Jewish population. Wojciechowski et al. (233) performed regression-based QTL linkage analysis on 49 Ashkenazi Jewish families with at least two myopic members. Maximum LOD scores of 9.5 for ocular refraction and 8.7 for log-transformed refraction (LTR) were observed at 49.1 cM on chromosome 1(1p36) between markers D1S552 and D1S1622. The empirical genome-wide significance levels were $p = .065$ for ocular refraction and $p < .005$ for LTR, providing strong evidence for linkage of refraction to this locus.

Factors that regulate the rate and duration of eye growth in mice have revealed two loci (Eye1 and Eye2) that may be responsible for genetic factors influencing myopia (166,248,249). Human homologous regions of synteny are chromosomes 6 (6p), chromosome 16 (16q13.3), and chromosome 19 (19q13) for Eye 2, and chromosome 7 (7q) for Eye1. These human loci have been scrutinized for potential candidate genes in myopia genetic studies.

Two independent groups have recently investigated candidate genes highlighted from animal model studies, and found a statistically significant association of candidate gene SNPs with high myopia in their respective human study cohorts (57,91). Han et al. performed a family-based association analysis of SNPs in the *HGF* gene, which encodes hepatocyte growth factor (HGF) using 128 nuclear Han Chinese families with 133 severely myopic offspring (57). HGF is an important multifunctional cytokine, is expressed in the eye, and maps to chromosome 7 (7q21.1) locus of Eye 1 (45). The HGF5-5b tagged SNP selected for association study was found to be significantly associated with high myopia as a quantitative trait in additive, dominant, and recessive models, as well as with high myopia considered as a dichotomous qualitative trait. Lin et al. performed a case control SNP association analysis of the transforming growth factor-beta 1 (*TGFB1*) gene that encodes TGFβ1 comparing 201 high myopic adult Chinese Taiwanese to 86 nonmyopic controls (91). The *TGFB1* gene maps to chromosome 19 (19q13.1–q13.3) of the Eye 2 locus. As described earlier in this chapter TGFβ1 is a growth factor that modulates the production of ECM (155). It modulates the production of collagen and MMP-2 (136), which in turn influences scleral creep rate and axial length (103). Thus, genetic studies in humans are finding associations with genes whose expression has been shown to change in animals during the development of induced myopia.

In conclusion, the field of myopia research continues to expand with new techniques for both assessing the details of retinal and scleral changes that occur during myopia development and for determining genetic abnormalities. Based on the animal studies that have shown the existence of an active emmetropization mechanism and studies in humans that have shown an important role for genetics in myopia development, it seems safe to conclude that both those who originally argued myopia is caused by the environment and those who argued myopia is inherited were correct. Determining how these two factors interact to produce juvenile-onset myopia is an important task for the future.

REFERENCES

1. Adams DW, McBrien NA. Prevalence of myopia and myopic progression in a population of clinical microscopists. Optom Vis Sci 1992; 69:467–73.
2. Angle J, Wissmann DA. The epidemiology of myopia. Am J Epidemiol 1980; 111:220–8.
3. Ashton GC. Segregation analysis of ocular refraction and myopia. Hum Hered 1985; 35:232–9.
4. Atkinson SJ, Crabbe T, Cowell S, et al. Intermolecular autolytic cleavage can contribute to the activation of progelatinase A by cell membranes. J Biol Chem 1995; 270:30479–85.
5. Austin BA, Coulon C, Liu CY, et al. Altered collagen fibril formation in the sclera of lumican-deficient mice. Invest Ophthalmol Vis Sci 2002; 43:1695–701.
6. Avetisov ES, Savitskaya NF, Vinetskaya MI, et al. A study of biochemical and biomechanical qualities of normal and myopic eye sclera in humans of different age groups. Metab Pediatr Syst Ophthalmol 1983; 7, 183–8.
7. Avila MP, Weiter JJ, Jalkh AE, et al. Natural history of choroidal neovascularization in degenerative myopia. Ophthalmol 1984; 91:1573–81.
8. Baldwin WR. A review of statistical studies of relations between myopia and ethnic, behavioral, and physiological characteristics. Am J Optom Physiol Opt 1981; 58: 516–27.
9. Barrington M, Sattayasai J, Zappia J, et al. Excitatory amino acids interfere with normal eye growth in posthatch chick. Curr Eye Res 1989; 8, 781–92.
10. Bertrand E, Fritsch C, Diether S, et al. Identification of Apolipoprotein A1 as a "STOP" signal for myopia. Mol Cell Proteomics 2006.
11. Biino G, Palmas MA, Corona C, et al. Ocular refraction: heritability and genome-wide search for eye morphometry traits in an isolated Sardinian population. Hum Genet 2005; 116:152–9.
12. Bohlandt S, von Kaisenberg CS, Wewetzer K, et al. Hyaluronan in the nuchal skin of chromosomally abnormal fetuses. Hum Reprod 2000; 15:1155–8.
13. Burton TC. The influence of refractive error and lattice degeneration on the incidence of retinal detachment. Trans Am Ophthalmol Soc 1989; 87:143–55.
14. Carney LG, Mainstone JC, Henderson BA. Corneal topography and myopia: a cross-sectional study. Invest Ophthalmol Vis Sci 1997; 38:311–20.
15. Cheng H, Singh OS, Kwong KK, et al. Shape of the myopic eye as seen with high-resolution magnetic resonance imaging. Optom Vis Sci 1992; 69:698–701.
16. Christensen AM, Wallman J. Evidence that increased scleral growth underlies visual deprivation myopia in chicks. Invest Ophthalmol Vis Sci 1991; 32:2143–21.
17. Cohn H. The Hygiene of the Eye in School, an English Translation. London: Simpkin, Marshall, 1886.
18. Cook RC, Glasscock RE. Refractive and ocular findings in the newborn. Am J Ophthalmol 1951; 34:1407–13.
19. Curtin BJ. Myopia: a review of its etiology, pathogenesis and treatment. Surv Ophthalmol 1970; 15:1–17.
20. Curtin BJ. Posterior staphyloma development in pathologic myopia. Ann Ophthalmol 1982; 14:655–8.
21. Curtin BJ. The Myopias: Basic Science and Clinical Management. Philadelphia, PA: Harper & Row, 1985: 1–495.
22. Curtin BJ, Iwamoto T, Renaldo DP. Normal and staphylomatous sclera of high myopia. Arch Ophthalmol 1979; 97:912–5.
23. Curtin BJ, Karlin DB. Axial length measurements and fundus changes of the myopic eye. Am J Ophthalmol 1971; 71:42–53.
24. Dandona R, Dandona L. Refractive error blindness. Bulletin of the World Health Organization 2001; 79: 237–47.

25. Diether S, Schaeffel F. Local changes in eye growth induced by imposed local refractive error despite active accommodation. Vision Res 1997; 37:659–68.
26. Farbrother JE, Kirov G, Owen MJ, et al. Family aggregation of high myopia: estimation of the sibling recurrence risk ratio. Invest Ophthalmol Vis Sci 2004; 45:2873–8.
27. Fischer AJ, McGuire JJ, Schaeffel F, et al. Light- and focus-dependent expression of the transcription factor ZENK in the chick retina. Nat Neurosci 1999; 2, 706–12.
28. Fledelius HC. Myopia prevalence in Scandinavia. A survey, with emphasis on factors of relevance for epidemiological refraction studies in general. Acta Ophthalmol Suppl 1988; 185:44–50.
29. Fledelius HC, Christensen AC. Reappraisal of the human ocular growth curve in fetal life, infancy, and early childhood. Br J Ophthalmol 1996; 80:918–21.
30. Fried M, Siebert A, Meyer-Schwickerath G. A natural history of Fuchs' spot: a long-term follow up study. Doc Ophthalmol 1981; 28:215–21.
31. Frost MR, Norton TT. Differential protein expression in tree shrew sclera during recovery from lens-induced myopia. Ophthal Physiol Opt 2006; 26(Suppl. 1):52.
32. Garner LF, Owens H, Kinnear RF, et al. Prevalence of myopia in Sherpa and Tibetan children in Nepal. Optom Vis Sci 1999; 76:282–5.
33. Gass JDM. Stereoscopic atlas of macular diseases: diagnosis and treatment, vol. 1. 4th ed. St. Louis: C.V. Mosby, 1997:126–8.
34. Gentle A, Liu Y, Martin JE, et al. Collagen gene expression and the altered accumulation of scleral collagen during the development of high myopia. J Biol Chem 2003; 278: 16587–94.
35. Gentle A, McBrien NA. Modulation of scleral DNA synthesis in development of and recovery from induced axial myopia in the tree shrew. Exp Eye Res 1999; 68: 155–63.
36. Gentle A, McBrien NA. Retinoscleral control of scleral remodelling in refractive development: a role for endogenous FGF-2? Cytokine 2002; 18:344–8.
37. German A, Baker J, Norton TT. Changes in glycosaminoglycan levels in tree shrew sclera during lens-induced myopia and recovery. Invest Ophthalmol Vis Sci 2002; 43: E-Abstract 215.
38. Ghafour IM, Allan D, Foulds WS. Common causes of blindness and visual handicap in the west of Scotland. Br J Ophthalmol 1983; 67:209–13.
39. Goh WSH, Lam CSY. Changes in refractive trends and optical components of Hong Kong Chinese aged 19–39 years. Ophthalmic Physiol Opt 1994; 14:378–82.
40. Goldschmidt E. On the etiology of myopia: an epidemiological study. Acta Ophthalmol Suppl 1968; 98:1–172.
41. Gordon RA, Donzis PB. Refractive development of the human eye. Arch Ophthalmol 1985; 103:785–9.
42. Goss DA, Hampton MJ, Wickham MG. Selected review on genetic factors in myopia. J Am Optom Assoc 1988; 59: 875–84.
43. Goss DA, Jackson TW. Clinical findings before the onset of myopia in youth: parental history of myopia. Optom Vis Sci 1995; 73:279–82.
44. Goss DA, Winkler RL. Progression of myopia in youth: age of cessation. Am J Optom Physiol Opt 1983; 60:651–8.
45. Grierson I, Heathcote L, Hiscott P, et al. Hepatocyte growth factor/scatter factor in the eye. Prog Retin Eye Res 2000; 19:779–802.
46. Grossniklaus HE, Green WR. Pathologic findings in pathologic myopia. Retina 1992; 12:127–33.
47. Grosvenor T. A review and a suggested classification system for myopia on the basis of age-related prevalence and age of onset. Am J Optom Physiol Opt 1987; 64: 545–54.
48. Grosvenor T, Goss DA. Role of the cornea in emmetropia and myopia. Optom Vis Sci 1998; 75:132–45.
49. Grosvenor T, Scott R. Role of the axial length/corneal radius ratio in determining the refractive state of the eye. Optom Vis Sci 1994; 71:573–9.
50. Guggenheim JA, Kirov G, Hodson SA. The heritability of high myopia: a reanalysis of Goldschmidt's data. J Med Genet 2000; 37:227–31.
51. Guggenheim JA, McBrien NA. Form-deprivation myopia induces activation of scleral matrix metalloproteinase-2 in tree shrew. Invest Ophthalmol Vis Sci 1996; 37:1380–95.
52. Gwiazda J, Thorn F, Bauer J, et al. Emmetropization and the progression of manifest refraction in children followed from infancy to puberty. Clin Vision Sci 1993; 8, 337–44.
53. Gwiazda J, Thorn F, Bauer J, et al. Myopic children show insufficient accommodative response to blur. Invest Ophthalmol Vis Sci 1993; 34:690–4.
54. Hammond CJ, Andrew T, Mak YT, et al. A susceptibility locus for myopia in the normal population is linked to the PAX6 gene region on chromosome 11: a genomewide scan of dizygotic twins. Am J Hum Genet 2004; 75: 294–304.
55. Hammond CJ, Snieder H, Gilbert CE, et al. Genes and environment in refractive error: the twin eye study. Invest Ophthalmol Vis Sci 2001; 42:1232–6.
56. Hampton GR, Kohen D, Bird AC. Visual prognosis of disciform degeneration in myopia. Ophthalmol 1983; 90: 923–6.
57. Han W, Yap MK, Wang J, et al. Family-based association analysis of hepatocyte growth factor (HGF) gene polymorphisms in high myopia. Invest Ophthalmol Vis Sci 2006; 47:2291–9.
58. Hayasaka S, Uchida M, Setogawa T. Subretinal hemorrhages with or without choroidal neovascularization in the maculas of patients with pathologic myopia. Graefes Arch Clin Exp Ophthalmol 1990; 228:277–80.
59. Heath S, Robledo R, Beggs W, et al. A novel approach to search for identity by descent in small samples of patients and controls from the same Mendelian breeding unit: a pilot study on myopia. Hum Hered 2001; 52:183–90.
60. Hirsch M, Weymouth F. Notes on ametropia: a further analysis of Stenstrom's data. Am J Optom Arch Am Acad Optom 1947; 24:601–3.
61. Hodos W, Kuenzel WJ. Retinal-image degradation produces ocular enlargement in chicks. Invest Ophthalmol Vis Sci 1984; 25:652–9.
62. Holmbeck K, Bianco P, Caterina J, et al. MT1-MMP-deficient mice develop dwarfism, osteopenia, arthritis, and connective tissue disease due to inadequate collagen turnover. Cell 1999; 99:81–92.
63. Hotchkiss ML, Fine SL. Pathologic myopia and choroidal neovascularization. Am J Ophthalmol 1981; 91:177–83.
64. Howland HC, Waite S, Peck L. Early focusing history predicts later refractive state: a longitudinal photorefractive study. Optical Society of America 1993; 3, 210–3.
65. Hoyt CS, Stone RD, Frommer C, et al. Monocular axial myopia associated with neonatal eyelid closure in human infants. Am J Ophthalmol 1981; 91:197–200.

66. Hung LF, Crawford ML, Smith EL. Spectacle lenses alter eye growth and the refractive status of young monkeys. Nat Med 1995; 1, 761–5.
67. Hung LF, Wallman J, Smith EL III. Vision-dependent changes in the choroidal thickness of macaque monkeys. Invest Ophthalmol Vis Sci 2000; 41:1259–69.
68. Hyman L, Gwiazda J, Hussein M, et al. Relationship of age, sex, and ethnicity with myopia progression and axial elongation in the correction of myopia evaluation trial. Arch Ophthalmol 2005; 123:977–87.
69. Ibay G, Doan B, Reider L, et al. Candidate high myopia loci on chromosomes 18p and 12q do not play a major role in susceptibility to common myopia. BMC Med Genet 2004; 5, 20.
70. Irving EL, Callender MG, Sivak JG. Inducing ametropias in hatchling chicks by defocus—aperture effects and cylindrical lenses. Vision Res 1995; 35:1165–74.
71. Irving EL, Callender MG, Sivak JG. Inducing myopia, hyperopia, and astigmatism in chicks. Optom Vis Sci 1991; 68:364–8.
72. Jalkh AE, Weiter JJ, Trempe CL, et al. Choroidal neovascularization in degenerative myopia: role of laser photocoagulation. Ophthalmic Surg 1987; 18:721–5.
73. Jansson F. Measurements of intraocular distances by ultrasound. Acta Ophthalmol (Copenh) 1963; (Suppl 74):1–51.
74. Jobling AI, Nguyen M, Gentle A, et al. Isoform-specific changes in scleral transforming growth factor-beta expression and the regulation of collagen synthesis during myopia progression. J Biol Chem 2004; 279:18121–6.
75. Jones LA, Sinnott L, Mitchell GL, et al. Parental history of myopia, sports and outdoor activities, and future myopa. Invest Ophthalmol Vis Sci 2007; 48:3524–32.
76. Kang RN, Norton TT. Electronmicroscopic examination of tree shrew sclera during normal development, induced myopia, and recovery [ARVO Abstract]. Invest Ophthalmol Vis Sci 1996; 37:S3241.
77. Katz J, Tielsch JM, Sommer A. Prevalence and risk factors for refractive errors in an adult inner city population. Invest Ophthalmol Vis Sci 1997; 38:334–40.
78. Kee C-S, Hung L-F, Qiao-Grider Y, et al. Temporal constraints on experimental emmetropization in infant monkeys. Invest Ophthalmol Vis Sci 2007; 48:957–62.
79. Kee C-S, Ramamirtham R, Qiao-Grider Y, et al. The role of peripheral vision in the refractive-error development of infant monkeys (*Macaca mulatta*). Invest Ophthalmol Vis Sci 2004; 45: E-Abstract 1157.
80. Kempen JH, Mitchell P, Lee KE, et al. The prevalence of refractive errors among adults in the United States, Western Europe, and Australia. Arch Ophthalmol 2004; 122:495–505.
81. Kempf GA, Collins SD, Jarman BL. Refractive errors in the eyes of children as determined by retinoscopic examination with a cycloplegic—Results of eye examinations of 1,860 white school children in Washington, D.C. In: Treasury Department, ed. United States Public Health Service. Washington: United States Government Printing Office, 1928:1–56.
82. Kenning MS, Gentle A, McBrien NA. Expression and cDNA sequence of matrix metalloproteinase-2 (MMP-2) in a mammalian model of human disease processes: Tupaia belangeri. DNA Seq 2004; 15:332–7.
83. Klein AP, Duggal P, Lee KE, et al. Support for polygenic influences on ocular refractive error. Invest Ophthalmol Vis Sci 2005; 46:442–6.
84. Kleinstein RN, Jones LA, Hullett S, et al. Refractive error and ethnicity in children. Arch Ophthalmol 2003; 121: 1141–7.
85. Lam DS, Lee WS, Leung YF, et al. TGFbeta-induced factor: a candidate gene for high myopia. Invest Ophthalmol Vis Sci 2003; 44:1012–5.
86. Lam DS, Tam PO, Fan DS, et al. Familial high myopia linkage to chromosome 18p. Ophthalmologica 2003; 217: 115–8.
87. Leibowitz HM, Krueger DE, Maunder LR, et al. The Framingham Eye Study monograph: an ophthalmological and epidemiological study of cataract, glaucoma, diabetic retinopathy, macular degeneration, and visual acuity in a general population of 2631 adults, 1973–1975. Surv Ophthalmol 1980; 24:335–610.
88. Levy JH, Pollock HM, Curtin BJ. The Fuchs' spot: an ophthalmoscopic and fluorescein angiographic study. Annals of Ophthalmology 1977; 1433–43.
89. Liang H, Crewther SG, Crewther DP, et al. Structural and elemental evidence for edema in the retina, retinal pigment epithelium, and choroid during recovery from experimentally induced myopia. Invest Ophthalmol Vis Sci 2004; 45:2463–74.
90. Lim R, Mitchell P, Cumming RG. Refractive associations with cataract: the Blue Mountains Eye Study. Invest Ophthalmol Vis Sci 1999; 40:3021–6.
91. Lin HJ, Wan L, Tsai Y, et al. The TGFbeta1 gene codon 10 polymorphism contributes to the genetic predisposition to high myopia. Mol Vis 2006; 12:698–703.
92. Lin LL, Hung PT, Ko LS, et al. Study of myopia among aboriginal school children in Taiwan. Acta Ophthalmol Suppl 1988; 185:34–6.
93. Lin LLK, Chen CJ, Hung PT, et al. Nation-wide survey of myopia among schoolchildren in Taiwan, 1986. Acta Ophthalmol Suppl 1988; 185:29–33.
94. Luckett WP. Comparative Biology and Evolutionary Relationships of Tree Shrews. New York: Plenum Press, 1980:1–314.
95. Lyhne N, Sjolie AK, Kyvik KO, et al. The importance of genes and environment for ocular refraction and its determiners: a population based study among 20–45 year old twins. Br J Ophthalmol 2001; 85:1470–6.
96. Mainstone JC, Carney LG, Anderson CR, et al. Corneal shape in hyperopia. Clin Exp Optom 1998; 81:131–7.
97. Mantyjarvi MI. Changes of refraction in schoolchildren. Arch Ophthalmol 1985; 103:790–2.
98. Marshall GE. Human scleral elastic system: an immunoelectron microscopic study. Br J Ophthalmol 1995; 79: 57–64.
99. Marshall GE, Konstas AG, Lee WR. Collagens in ocular tissues. Br J Ophthalmol 1993; 77:515–24.
100. Mayer DL, Hansen RM, Moore BD, et al. Cycloplegic refractions in healthy children aged 1 through 48 months. Arch Ophthalmol 2001; 119:1625–28.
101. McBrien NA, Cornell LM, Gentle A. Structural and ultrastructural changes to the sclera in a mammalian model of high myopia. Invest Ophthalmol Vis Sci 2001; 42:2179–87.
102. McBrien NA, Gentle A. The role of visual information in the control of scleral matrix biology in myopia. Curr Eye Res 2001; 23:313–9.
103. McBrien NA, Gentle A. Role of the sclera in the development and pathological complications of myopia. Prog Retin Eye Res 2003; 22:307–38.
104. McBrien NA, Lawlor P, Gentle A. Scleral remodeling during the development of and recovery from axial myopia in the tree shrew. Invest Ophthalmol Vis Sci 2000; 41:3713–9.
105. McBrien NA, Moghaddam HO, Cottriall CL, et al. The effects of blockade of retinal cell action potentials on

ocular growth, emmetropization and form deprivation myopia in young chicks. Vision Res 1995; 35:1141–52.

106. McBrien NA, Moghaddam HO, New R, et al. Experimental myopia in a diurnal mammal (*Sciurus carolinensis*) with no accommodative ability. J Physiol 1993; 469: 427–41.
107. McBrien NA, Norton TT. The development of experimental myopia and ocular component dimensions in monocularly lid-sutured tree shrews (*Tupaia belangeri*). Vision Res 1992; 32:843–52.
108. McCarty CA, Taylor HR. Myopia and vision 2020. Am J Ophthalmol 2000; 129:525–7.
109. McKanna JA, Casagrande VA, Norton TT, et al. Dark-reared tree shrews do not develop lid-suture myopia. Invest Ophthalmol Vis Sci 1983; (Suppl. 24), 226.
110. Mertz JR, Wallman J. Choroidal retinoic acid synthesis: a possible mediator between refractive error and compensatory eye growth. Exp Eye Res 2000; 70:519–27.
111. Metlapally R, Jobling AI, Gentle A, et al. Characterization of the integrin receptor subunit profile in the mammalian sclera. Mol Vis 2006; 12:725–34.
112. Meyer LJ, Stern R. Age-dependent changes of hyaluronan in human skin. J Invest Dermatol 1994; 102:385–9.
113. Michaelides M, Johnson S, Bradshaw K, et al. X-linked cone dysfunction syndrome with myopia and protanopia. Ophthalmol 2005; 112:1448–54.
114. Michaels DD. Visual Optics and Refraction: a Clinical Approach. 3rd ed. St. Louis: Mosby, 1985.
115. Mitchell P, Hourihan F, Sandbach J, et al. The relationship between glaucoma and myopia: the Blue Mountains Eye Study. Ophthalmol 1999; 106:2010–5.
116. Murphy G, Willenbrock F, Ward RV, et al. The C-terminal domain of 72 kDa gelatinase A is not required for catalysis, but is essential for membrane activation and modulates interactions with tissue inhibitors of metalloproteinases. Biochem J 1992; 283 (Pt. 3), 637–41.
117. Murthy GV, Gupta SK, Ellwein LB, et al. Refractive error in children in an urban population in New Delhi. Invest Ophthalmol Vis Sci 2002; 43:623–31.
118. Mutti DO, Mitchell GL, Jones LA, et al. Axial growth and changes in lenticular and corneal power during emmetropization in infants. Invest Ophthalmol Vis Sci 2005; 46: 3074–80.
119. Mutti DO, Mitchell GL, Moeschberger ML, et al. Parental myopia, near work, school achievement, and children's refractive error. Invest Ophthalmol Vis Sci 2002; 43: 3633–40.
120. Mutti DO, Semina E, Marazita M, et al. Genetic loci for pathological myopia are not associated with juvenile myopia. Am J Med Genet 2002; 112:355–60.
121. Mutti DO, Zadnik K, Fusaro RE, et al. Optical and structural development of the crystalline lens in childhood. Invest Ophthalmol Vis Sci 1998; 39:120–33.
122. Naidoo KS, Raghunandan A, Mashige KP, et al. Refractive error and visual impairment in African children in South Africa. Invest Ophthalmol Vis Sci 2003; 44:3764–70.
123. Naiglin L, Clayton J, Gazagne C, et al. Familial high myopia: evidence of an autosomal dominant mode of inheritance and genetic heterogeneity. Ann Genet 1999; 42:140–6.
124. Naiglin L, Gazagne C, Dallongeville F, et al. A genome wide scan for familial high myopia suggests a novel locus on chromosome 7q36. J Med Genet 2002; 39: 118–24.
125. Nickla DL, Sharda V, Troilo D. Temporal integration characteristics of the axial and choroidal responses to myopic defocus induced by prior form deprivation versus positive spectacle lens wear in chickens. Optom Vis Sci 2005; 82:318–27.
126. Noble KG, Carr RE. Pathologic myopia. Ophthalmol 1982; 89:1099–100.
127. Norton TT. Animal models of myopia: learning how vision controls the size of the eye. ILAR J 1999; 40: 59–77.
128. Norton TT, Essinger JA, McBrien NA. Lid-suture myopia in tree shrews with retinal ganglion cell blockade. Vis Neurosci 1994; 11:143–53.
129. Norton TT, Kang RN. Morphology of tree shrew sclera and choroid during normal development, induced myopia, and recovery [ARVO Abstract]. Invest Ophthalmol Vis Sci 1996; 37:S324.
130. Norton TT, Manny R, O'Leary DJ. Myopia—global problem, global research. Optom Vis Sci 2005; 82:223–5.
131. Norton TT, Miller EJ. Collagen and protein levels in sclera during normal development, induced myopia, and recovery in tree shrews [ARVO Abstract]. Invest Ophthalmol Vis Sci 1995; 36:S760.
132. Norton TT, Rada JA. Reduced extracellular matrix accumulation in mammalian sclera with induced myopia. Vision Res 1995; 35:1271–81.
133. Norton TT, Siegwart JT. Local myopia produced by partial visual-field deprivation in tree shrew. Soc Neurosci Abstr 1991; 17:558.
134. O'Leary DJ, Millodot M. Eyelid closure causes myopia in humans. Experientia 1979; 35:1478–9.
135. Ohuchi E, Imai K, Fujii Y, et al. Membrane type 1 matrix metalloproteinase digests interstitial collagens and other extracellular matrix macromolecules. J Biol Chem 1997; 272:2446–51.
136. Overall CM, Wrana JL, Sodek J. Independent regulation of collagenase, 72-kDa progelatinase, and metalloendoproteinase inhibitor expression in human fibroblasts by transforming growth factor-beta. J Biol Chem 1989; 264: 1860–9.
137. Pacella R, McLellan J, Grice K, et al. Role of genetic factors in the etiology of juvenile-onset myopia based on a longitudinal study of refractive error. Optom Vis Sci 1999; 76:381–6.
138. Paluru P, Ronan SM, Heon E, et al. New locus for autosomal dominant high myopia maps to the long arm of chromosome 17. Invest Ophthalmol Vis Sci 2003; 44: 1830–6.
139. Paluru PC, Nallasamy S, Devoto M, et al. Identification of a novel locus on 2q for autosomal dominant high-grade myopia. Invest Ophthalmol Vis Sci 2005; 46:2300–7.
140. Perkins ES. Glaucoma in the younger age groups. Arch Ophthalmol 1960; 64:882–91.
141. Perkins ES. Morbidity from myopia. Sight Sav Rev 1979; 49:11–9.
142. Phillips JR, Khalaj M, McBrien NA. Induced myopia associated with increased scleral creep in chick and tree shrew eyes. Invest Ophthalmol Vis Sci 2000; 41:2028–34.
143. Pierro L, Camesasca FI, Mischi M, et al. Peripheral retinal changes and axial myopia. Retina 1992; 12:12–7.
144. Qiao-Grider Y, Hung LF, Kee CS, et al. Recovery from form-deprivation myopia in rhesus monkeys. Invest Ophthalmol Vis Sci 2004; 45:3361–72.
145. Rabb MF, Garoon I, LaFranco FP. Myopic macular degeneration. Int Ophthalmol Clin 1981; 21:51–9.

146. Rabin J, VanSluyters RC, Malach R. Emmetropization: a vision-dependent phenomenon. Invest Ophthalmol Vis Sci 1981; 20:561–4.
147. Rada JA, Achen VR, Perry CA, et al. Proteoglycans in the human sclera: evidence for the presence of aggrecan. Invest Ophthalmol Vis Sci 1997; 38:1740–51.
148. Rada JA, Huang Y, Rada KG. Identification of choroidal ovotransferrin as a potential ocular growth regulator. Curr Eye Res 2001; 22:121–32.
149. Rada JA, Thoft RA, Hassell JR. Increased aggrecan (cartilage proteoglycan) production in the sclera of myopic chicks. Dev Biol 1991; 147:303–12.
150. Rah MJ, Mitchell GL, Mutti DO, et al. Levels of agreement between parents' and children's reports of near work. Ophthalmic Epidemiol 2002; 9, 191–203.
151. Raviola E, Wiesel TN. Effect of dark-rearing on experimental myopia in monkeys. Invest Ophthalmol Vis Sci 1978; 17:485–8.
152. Raviola E, Wiesel TN. An animal model of myopia. New Engl J Med 1985; 312:1609–15.
153. Raviola E, Wiesel TN. Neural control of eye growth and experimental myopia in primates. In: Bock G, Widdows K, eds. Myopia and the Control of Eye Growth. Chichester: Wiley, 1990:22–39.
154. Rodieck RW. The Vertebrate Retina. Principles of Structure and Function. San Francisco: W. H. Freeman and Company, 1973:1–1044.
155. Rohrer B, Stell WK. Basic fibroblast growth factor (bFGF) and transforming growth factor beta (TGF-b) act as stop and go signals to modulate postnatal ocular growth in the chick. Exp Eye Res 1994; 58:553–61.
156. Rose K, Morgan I, Smith W, et al. Myopia: prevalence, risk factors and natural history. Ophthal Physiol Opt 2006; 26:25.
157. Rosner M, Belkin M. Intelligence, education, and myopia in males. Arch Ophthalmol 1987; 105:1508–11.
158. Saw SM, Chua WH, Hong CY, et al. Nearwork in early-onset myopia. Invest Ophthalmol Vis Sci 2002; 43: 332–9.
159. Saw SM, Gazzard G, Shih-Yen EC, et al. Myopia and associated pathological complications. Ophthalmic Physiol Opt 2005; 25:381–91.
160. Saw SM, Katz J, Schein OD, et al. Epidemiology of myopia. Epidemiol Rev 1996; 18:175–87.
161. Scavello GS, Paluru PC, Ganter WR, et al. Sequence variants in the transforming growth beta-induced factor (TGIF) gene are not associated with high myopia. Invest Ophthalmol Vis Sci 2004; 45:2091–7.
162. Schaeffel F, Burkhardt E, Howland HC, et al. Measurement of refractive state and deprivation myopia in two strains of mice. Optom Vis Sci 2004; 81: 99–110.
163. Schaeffel F, Diether S. The growing eye: an autofocus system that works on very poor images. Vision Res 1999; 39:1585–9.
164. Schaeffel F, Glasser A, Howland HC. Accommodation, refractive error and eye growth in chickens. Vision Res 1988; 28:639–57.
165. Schaeffel F, Howland HC. Properties of the feedback loops controlling eye growth and refractive state in the chicken. Vision Res 1991; 31:717–34.
166. Schaeffel F, Simon P, Feldkaemper M, et al. Molecular biology of myopia. Clin Exp Optom 2003; 86:295–307.
167. Schmid KL, Wildsoet CF. Effects on the compensatory responses to positive and negative lenses of intermittent lens wear and ciliary nerve section in chicks. Vision Res 1996; 36:1023–36.
168. Schwartz M, Haim M, Skarsholm D. X-linked myopia: bornholm eye disease—linkage to DNA markers on the distal part of Xq. Clinical Genetics 1990; 38:281–6.
169. Scott JE. Proteoglycan: collagen interactions and subfibrillar structure in collagen fibrils. Implications in the development and ageing of connective tissues. J Anat 1990; 169:23–35.
170. Seko Y, Tanaka Y, Tokoro T. Influence of bFGF as a potent growth stimulator and TGF-beta as a growth regulator on scleral chondrocytes and scleral fibroblasts invitro. Ophthalmic Res 1995; 27:144–52.
171. Shaikh AW, Siegwart JT, Norton TT. Effect of interrupted lens wear on compensation for a minus lens in tree shrews. Optom Vis Sci 1999; 76:308–15.
172. Shen W, Sivak JG. Eyes of lower vertebrates are susceptible to visual environment. Ophthalmic Physiol Opt 2006; 26:11–12.
173. Sheridan M, Douthwaite WA. Corneal asphericity and refractive error. Ophthalmic Physiol Opt 1989; 9, 235–8.
174. Sherman SM, Norton TT, Casagrande VA. Myopia in the lid-sutured tree shrew (*Tupaia glis*). Brain Res 1977; 124:154–7.
175. Siegwart JT, Norton TT. Refractive and ocular changes in tree shrews raised with plus or minus lenses [ARVO Abstract]. Invest Ophthalmol Vis Sci 1993; 34:S1208.
176. Siegwart JT Jr., Norton TT. The susceptible period for deprivation-induced myopia in tree shrew. Vision Res 1998; 38:3505–15.
177. Siegwart JT Jr., Norton TT. Regulation of the mechanical properties of tree shrew sclera by the visual environment. Vision Res 1999; 39:387–407.
178. Siegwart JT Jr., Norton TT. Steady state mRNA levels in tree shrew sclera with form-deprivation myopia and during recovery. Invest Ophthalmol Vis Sci 2001; 42:1153–9.
179. Siegwart JT Jr., Norton TT. The time course of changes in mRNA levels in tree shrew sclera during induced myopia and recovery. Invest Ophthalmol Vis Sci 2002; 43: 2067–75.
180. Siegwart JT Jr., Norton TT. Proteoglycan mRNA Levels in tree shrew sclera during minus lens treatment and during recovery. Invest Ophthalmol Vis Sci 2005; 46: E-Abstract 3335.
181. Siegwart JT Jr., Norton TT. Selective regulation of MMP and TIMP mRNA levels in tree shrew sclera during minus lens compensation and recovery. Invest Ophthalmol Vis Sci 2005; 46:3484–92.
182. Siegwart JT Jr, Norton TT, Robertson JD. Binocular lens treatment in tree shrews. Investigative Ophthalmology & Visual Science 2003; 44: E-abstract 1984.
183. Siegwart JT, Robertson JD, Norton TT. Changes in MMP and TIMP mRNA levels during minus lens treatment and during recovery in tree shrew. Invest Ophthalmol Vis Sci 2004; 45: E-abstract 1232.
184. Siegwart JT Jr., Norton TT. Plus lens wear in young, hyperopic tree shrews halts progression toward emmetropia. Ophthal Physiol Opt 2006; 26(Suppl. 1):12.
185. Smith EL, III. Environmentally induced refractive errors in animals. In: Rosenfield M, Gilmartin B, eds. Myopia and Nearwork. Oxford: Butterworth-Heinemann, 1998:57–90.
186. Smith EL III, Hung LF. The role of optical defocus in regulating refractive development in infant monkeys. Vision Res 1999; 39:1415–35.
187. Smith EL, III, Kee CS, Ramamirtham R, et al. Peripheral vision can influence eye growth and refractive development in infant monkeys. Invest Ophthalmol Vis Sci 2005; 46:3965–72.
188. Sommers D, Kaiser-Kupfer MI, Kupfer C. Increased axial length of the eye following neonatal lid suture as measured

with A-scan ultrasonography. Invest Ophthalmol Vis Sci 1978; (Suppl 17), 295.
189. Sorsby A, Benjamin B, Davey JB, et al. Emmetropia and its aberrations. Med Res Counc Spec Rep Ser 1957; 293: 1–69.
190. Sorsby A, Benjamin B, Sheridan M, et al. Refraction and its components during the growth of the eye from the age of three. Med Res Counc Spec Rep Ser 1961; 301:1–67.
191. Sorsby A, Leary GA. A Longitudinal Study of Refraction and its Components during Growth. 309th ed. London: Her Majesty's Stationery Office, 1970:1–41.
192. Sorsby A, Leary GA, Fraser GR. Family studies on ocular refraction and its components. J Med Genet 1966; 3, 269–73.
193. Sorsby A, Leary GA, Richards MJ. Correlation ametropia and component ametropia. Vision Res 1962; 2, 309–13.
194. Sorsby A, Sheridan M, Leary G. Refraction and its components in twins. Med Res Counc Spec Rep Ser 1962; 303.
195. Sperduto RD, Seigel D, Roberts J, et al. Prevalence of myopia in the United States. Arch Ophthalmol 1983; 101: 405–7.
196. Spitznas M, Boker T. Idiopathic posterior subretinal neovascularization (IPSN) is related to myopia. Graefes Arch Clin Exp Ophthalmol 1991; 229:536–8.
197. Stambolian D, Ciner EB, Reider LC, et al. Genome-wide scan for myopia in the Old Order Amish. Am J Ophthalmol 2005; 140:469–76.
198. Stambolian D, Ibay G, Reider L, et al. Genomewide linkage scan for myopia susceptibility loci among Ashkenazi Jewish families shows evidence of linkage on chromosome 22q12. Am J Hum Genet 2004; 75: 448–59.
199. Steidl SM, Pruett RC. Macular complications associated with posterior staphyloma. Am J Ophthalmol 1997; 123: 181–7.
200. Steiger A. Die Entstehung Der Spharischen Refracktionen Des menschlichen Auges. Berlin: Karger, 1913.
201. Stenstrom S. Investigation of the variation and the correlation of the optical elements of human eyes. Am J Optom Arch Am Acad Optom 1948, Monograph 58, Part I–Part VI.
202. Strang NC, Schmid KL, Carney LG. Hyperopia is predominantly axial in nature. Curr Eye Res 1998; 17: 380–3.
203. Strömberg E. Uber refraktion und achsenlänge des menschlichen auges. Acta Ophthalmol Suppl 1936; 14:281.
204. Strongin AY, Collier I, Bannikov G, et al. Mechanism of cell surface activation of 72-kDa type IV collagenase. Isolation of the activated form of the membrane metalloprotease. J Biol Chem 1995; 270:5331–8.
205. Summers Rada JA, Shelton S, Norton TT. The sclera and myopia. Exp Eye Res 2006; 82:185–200.
206. Teikari J, O'Donnell JJ, Kaprio J, et al. Genetic and environmental effects on oculometric traits. Optom Vis Sci 1989; 66:594–9.
207. Teikari JM, O'Donnell J, Kaprio J, et al. Impact of heredity in myopia. Hum Hered 1991; 41:151–6.
208. Tejedor J, de l V. Refractive changes induced by form deprivation in the mouse eye. Invest Ophthalmol Vis Sci 2003; 44:32–6.
209. The Eye Disease Case-Control Study Group. Risk factors for idiopathic rhegmatogenous retinal detachment. Am J Epidemiol 1993; 137:749–57.
210. Tokoro T, Sato A. Results of investigation of pathologic myopia in Japan. Report of myopic chorioretinal atrophy. Ministry of Health and Welfare 1982; 32–35. Tokyo, Ministry of Health and Welfare.
211. Torczynski E. Sclera. In: Jakobiec FA, ed. Ocular Anatomy, Embryology, and Teratology. Philadelphia, PA: Harper & Row, 1982:587–99.
212. Troilo D, Gottlieb MD, Wallman J. Visual deprivation causes myopia in chicks with optic nerve section. Curr Eye Res 1987; 6, 993–9.
213. Troilo D, Judge SJ. Ocular development and visual deprivation myopia in the common marmoset (*Callithrix jacchus*). Vision Res 1993; 33:1311–24.
214. Troilo D, Nickla DL, Wildsoet CF. Choroidal thickness changes during altered eye growth and refractive state in a primate. Invest Ophthalmol Vis Sci 2000; 41: 1249–58.
215. Tron EJ. The optical elements of the refractive power of the eye. Graefes Arch Ophthalmol 1929; 122:1–33.
216. van Alphen GWHM. On emmetropia and ametropia. Opt Acta (Lond) 1961; (Suppl. 142), 1–92.
217. Venkataraman S, Nguyen L, McBrien NA. Compensatory ocular growth responses to positive lens defocus in the tree shrew. Invest Ophthalmol Vis Sci 2005; 46: E-Abstract 1973.
218. Vessey KA, Lencses KA, Rushforth DA, et al. Glucagon receptor agonists and antagonists affect the growth of the chick eye: a role for glucagonergic regulation of emmetropization? Invest Ophthalmol Vis Sci 2005; 46:3922–31.
219. Vessey KA, Rushforth DA, Stell WK. Glucagon- and secretin-related peptides differentially alter ocular growth and the development of form-deprivation myopia in chicks. Invest Ophthalmol Vis Sci 2005; 46:3932–42.
220. von Noorden GK, Lewis RA. Ocular axial length in unilateral congenital cataracts and blepharoptosis. Invest Ophthalmol Vis Sci 1987; 28:750–2.
221. Vongphanit J, Mitchell P, Wang JJ. Prevalence and progression of myopic retinopathy in an older population. Ophthalmol 2002; 109:704–11.
222. Wallman J, Adams JI. Developmental aspects of experimental myopia in chicks: susceptibility, recovery and relation to emmetropization. Vision Res 1987; 27:1139–63.
223. Wallman J, Turkel J, Trachtman J. Extreme myopia produced by modest change in early visual experience. Science 1978; 201:1249–51.
224. Wallman J, Wildsoet C, Xu A, et al. Moving the retina: choroidal modulation of refractive state. Vision Res 1995; 35:37–50.
225. Wallman J, Winawer J. Homeostasis of eye growth and the question of myopia. Neuron 2004; 43:447–68.
226. Ward RV, Atkinson SJ, Reynolds JJ, et al. Cell surface-mediated activation of progelatinase A: demonstration of the involvement of the C-terminal domain of progelatinase A in cell surface binding and activation of progelatinase A by primary fibroblasts. Biochem J 1994; 304 (Pt. 1), 263–9.
227. Wickremasinghe S, Foster PJ, Uranchimeg D, et al. Ocular biometry and refraction in Mongolian adults. Invest Ophthalmol Vis Sci 2004; 45:776–83.
228. Wiesel TN, Raviola E. Myopia and eye enlargement after neonatal lid fusion in monkeys. Nature 1977; 266: 66–8.
229. Wildsoet CF. Active emmetropization—evidence for its existence and ramifications for clinical practice. Ophthal Physiol Opt 1997; 17:279–90.
230. Wildsoet CF, Pettigrew JD. Kainic acid-induced eye enlargement in chickens: differential effects on anterior and posterior segments. Invest Ophthalmol Vis Sci 1988; 29:311–9.

231. Wilson A, Woo G. A review of the prevalence and causes of myopia. Singapore Medical Journal 1989; 30:479–84.
232. Winawer J, Zhu X, Choi J, et al. Ocular compensation for alternating myopic and hyperopic defocus. Vision Res 2005; 45:1667–77.
233. Wojciechowski R, Moy C, Ciner E, et al. Genomewide scan in Ashkenazi Jewish families demonstrates evidence of linkage of ocular refraction to a QTL on chromosome 1p36. Hum Genet 2006; 119:389–99.
234. Wong TY, Foster PJ, Ng TP, et al. Variations in ocular biometry in an adult Chinese population in Singapore: the Tanjong Pagar Survey. Invest Ophthalmol Vis Sci 2001; 42:73–80.
235. Yap M, Wu M, Liu ZM, et al. Role of heredity in the genesis of myopia. Ophthalmic Physiol Opt 1993; 13: 316–9.
236. Young FA. The effects of nearwork illumination level on monkey refraction. Am J Optom Arch Am Acad Optom 1962; 39:60–7.
237. Young FA. Reading, measures of intelligence and refractive errors. Am J Optom Arch Am Acad Optom 1963; 40: 257–64.
238. Young FA. The effect of restricted visual space on the refractive error of the young monkey eye. Invest Ophthalmol 1963; 2, 571–7.
239. Young FA. Myopia and personality. Am J Optom Arch Am Acad Optom 1967; 44:192–201.
240. Young TL, Deeb SS, Ronan SM, et al. X-linked high myopia associated with cone dysfunction. Arch Ophthalmol 2004; 122:897–908.
241. Young TL, Ronan SM, Alvear AB, et al. A second locus for familial high myopia maps to chromosome 12q. Am J Hum Genet 1998; 63:1419–24.
242. Young TL, Ronan SM, Drahozal LA, et al. Evidence that a locus for familial high myopia maps to chromosome 18p. Am J Hum Genet 1998; 63:109–19.
243. Zadnik K. Myopia development in childhood. Optom Vis Sci 1997; 74:603–8.
244. Zadnik K, Manny RE, Yu JA, et al. Ocular component data in schoolchildren as a function of age and gender. Optom Vis Sci 2003; 80:226–36.
245. Zadnik K, Satariano WA, Mutti DO, et al. The effect of parental history of myopia on children's eye size. JAMA 1994; 271:1323–7.
246. Zhang Q, Guo X, Xiao X, et al. A new locus for autosomal dominant high myopia maps to 4q22-q27 between D4S1578 and D4S1612. Mol Vis 2005; 11:554–60.
247. Zhang Q, Guo X, Xiao X, et al. Novel locus for X linked recessive high myopia maps to Xq23-q25 but outside MYP1. J Med Genet 2006; 43:e20.
248. Zhou G, Williams RW. Eye1 and Eye2: gene loci that modulate eye size, lens weight, and retinal area in the mouse. Invest Ophthalmol Vis Sci 1999; 40:817–25.
249. Zhou G, Williams RW. Mouse models for the analysis of myopia: an analysis of variation in eye size of adult mice. Optom Vis Sci 1999; 76:408–18.
250. Zhu X, Park TW, Winawer J, et al. In a matter of minutes, the eye can know which way to grow. Invest Ophthalmol Vis Sci 2005; 46:2238–41.
251. Zhu X, Winawer JA, Wallman J. Potency of myopic defocus in spectacle lens compensation. Invest Ophthalmol Vis Sci 2003; 44:2818–27.
252. Zylbermann R, Landau D, Berson D. The influence of study habits on myopia in Jewish teenagers. J Pediatr Ophthalmol Strabismus 1993; 30:319–22.

27

Other Degenerative and Related Disorders of the Retina and Choroid

Peter J. Francis and David J. Wilson
Casey Eye Institute, Oregon Health and Science University, Portland, Oregon, U.S.A.

Alec Garner
Institute of Ophthalmology, Moorfields Eye Hospital, London, U.K.

DEGENERATION OF THE NEURAL RETINA

The morphological changes that accompany degenerative processes in the neural retina tend ultimately to assume a common pattern irrespective of their cause. Loss of neurons is followed by a net loss of tissue volume with replacement by a minor reactive proliferation of astrocytes or by cystoid changes within a network formed by the supporting Müller cells. With age there is a gradual nonpathological dropout of retinal ganglion cells at an approximate rate of 5000 per year resulting in a decrease in the fovea of about 16% from the second to the sixth decade (10). Photoreceptors, particularly the rods, are also vulnerable to loss during aging, but the ratio of photoreceptors to retinal pigment epithelium (RPE) cells remains the same, suggesting parallel loss of these closely apposed cells (10). The human macula comprises a cone-dense fovea encircled by a rod-dense parafovea. Throughout adult life, the cone density is maintained in the fovea however in the same time period the rod parafoveal density reduces by 30% (5). Loss of neurons in this way is accompanied by loss of the foveal reflex, due to shallowing of the foveal depression and enlargement of the capillary-free zone at the fovea.

RETINAL EDEMA

Edema results when plasma constituents and water enter the extracellular space of the retina. This space normally represents only a small proportion of retinal volume because the blood–retina barrier restricts water inflow and the RPE pump facilitates outflow. The barrier exists in two parts, an inner and outer, reflecting the dual blood supply of the retina. It is represented by the tight junctions between the endothelial cells lining the retinal capillaries and between the cells of the RPE. However, although these barriers exclude proteinaceous fluid from the retinal and choroidal circulations, water continues to enter the retina and moves toward the choroid. This water is prevented from accumulating in the potential subretinal space by the RPE pump (7).

The RPE pump comprises: (*i*) an active mechanism, wherein the transport of ions across the infolded basal cell membrane of the RPE generates local osmotic gradients, and (*ii*) a passive mechanism, the lack of plasma proteins in the ocular fluids producing a colloidal osmotic pressure gradient. The fenestrated choroidal capillaries leak protein into the extravascular space, and this protein-containing fluid passes through Bruch membrane and between the RPE cells as far as the tight junctions. Here it is separated from water in the subretinal space that has passed through the retina by diffusion from the vitreous or from the retinal capillaries, so that a colloidal osmotic pressure gradient is created. If the plasma proteins fall to below 3 g per 100 g, edema and serous retinal detachments result (18). Figure 1 illustrates the possible sources of fluid accumulating in the retina.

Retinal edema is most visually significant when at the macula and is a frequent outcome of ischemic disorders of the retina, such as diabetic retinopathy or branch retinal vein occlusion, or where inflammatory processes (uveitis) result in increased retinal vascular permeability.

CYSTOID MACULAR EDEMA

General Remarks

Within the sensory retina, fluid has a tendency to collect in the outer plexiform layer of Henle where the fibers are longer and larger spaces can form. This cystoid macular edema (CME) may result because Müller cell processes are fewer than in other parts of the retina and because there are few retinal vessels to resorb any fluid. On pathological examination the retina is swollen by an eosinophilic exudate in the outer plexiform and inner nuclear layers (25). Whether the "edema" represents fluid in the extracellular space constitutes a primary transudative process or degenerative swelling of Müller cells is unresolved. The sensory retina may be detached from the RPE, with a reverse pit or fold in the affected area (Figs. 2–4).

Clinical Features

CME can be hard to detect without fluorescein angiography (FA) and/or optical coherent tomography (OCT). It is mostly suspected on the basis of defective vision. Examination reveals an absent foveal reflex and sometimes a yellow spot. Retinal hemorrhages may arise from capillaries in the outer plexiform layer and spread into the cystoid spaces, where the blood may form a fluid level.

FA demonstrates a characteristic "petaloid" arrangement of the cysts, usually about four larger central cysts surrounded by smaller cysts. Fluorescein pools in these cystoid spaces, which are separated by a dark branching figure, presumably the compressed Henle fibers containing xanthophyll, which also accounts for the central yellow spot. "Pseudocystoid macular edema" refers to cysts occurring without accompanying retinal vascular leakage on FA and is found in nicotinic acid maculopathy and juvenile retinoschisis or when the cysts persist after loss of neural tissue, as after resolution of the increased permeability that produced CME.

CME may resolve spontaneously, when the cause is removed, or with medical treatment (such as topical nonsteroidal medications or oral acetozolamide). If the edema persists, there is progressive atrophy of the retinal layers, although Müller cells are more resistant.

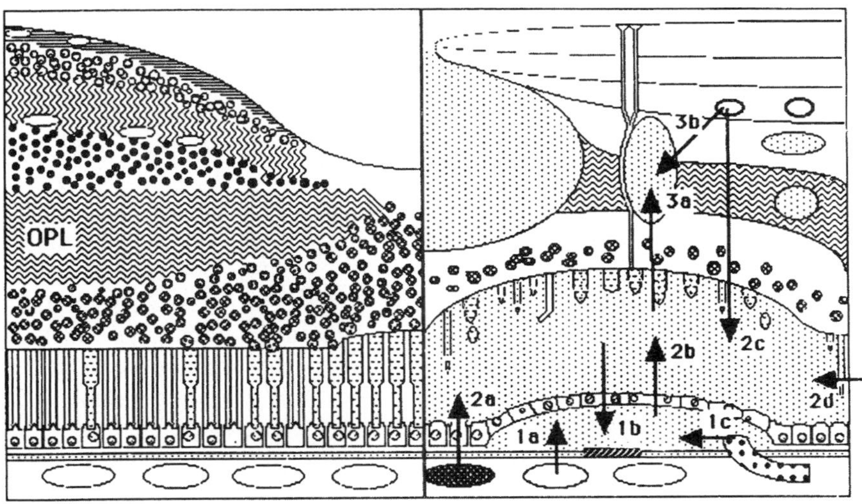

Figure 1 Pathogenesis of macular edema. Fluid may collect: (*i*) beneath the RPE by movement from the choroid (1a) or the neural retina (1b); (*ii*) between the RPE and the sensory retina by movement from the choroid (2a), the sub-RPE space (2b), the retinal vasculature (2c), or from adjacent neural retina (2d); or (*iii*) within the inner retina by movement from the outer retina (3a) or from the retinal vaculature (3b), as described in the text. *Abbreviations*: OPL, outer plexiform layer; RPE, retinal pigment epithelium.

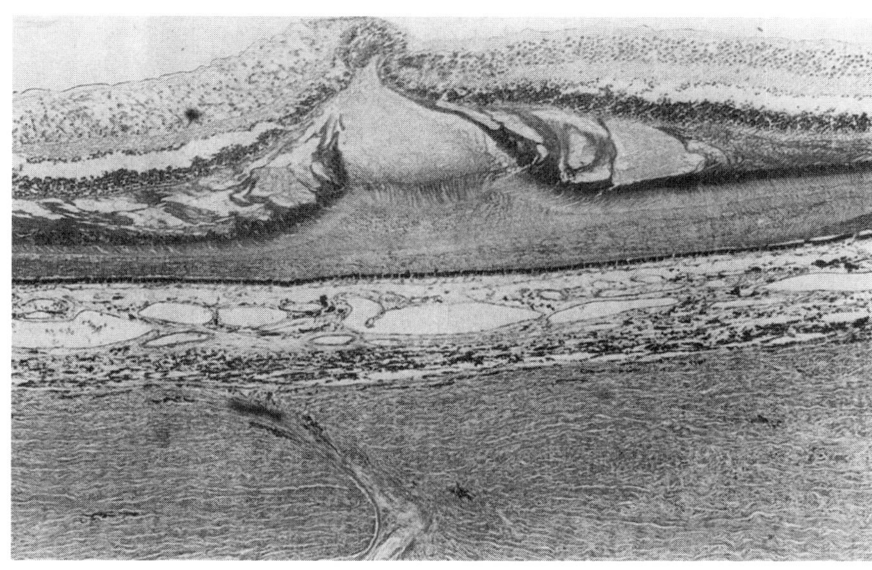

Figure 2 Cystoid macular edema in a diabetic patient. The fluid collected principally in the outer plexiform layer of the retina and, to a lesser extent, in the outer nuclear layer, creating cystoid spaces, the walls of which are provided by the residual neural tissue. There is also slight lifting or folding of the foveal region (hematoxylin and eosin, ×55).

Finally, however, the Müller fibers also atrophy and the cystoid spaces coalesce to form a macrocyst or schisis (Fig. 3).

Pathogenesis

Damage to the Outer Blood–Retina Barrier

From the subsensory retinal space fluid may move into the outer plexiform layer by passing through the external limiting membrane, a series of desmosomal junctions between photoreceptors and Müller cells. CME can thus occur over subretinal neovascular membranes (2) or over old disciform scars, presumably because the RPE pump is no longer operating. CME accompanying subretinal neovascularization indicates significant disruption of the entire blood–retinal barrier so that fluid accumulates in the retina as described previously.

Damage to the Inner Blood–Retina Barrier

In most cases CME results from damage to the retinal capillary endothelium, and the causes are many (24), with more than one factor operative in many cases. Inflammation results in the synthesis of prostaglandins and disruption of the tight junctions of the perifoveal capillaries, and CME can be the main cause for visual loss in long-standing uveitis, such as pars planitis and related intermediate

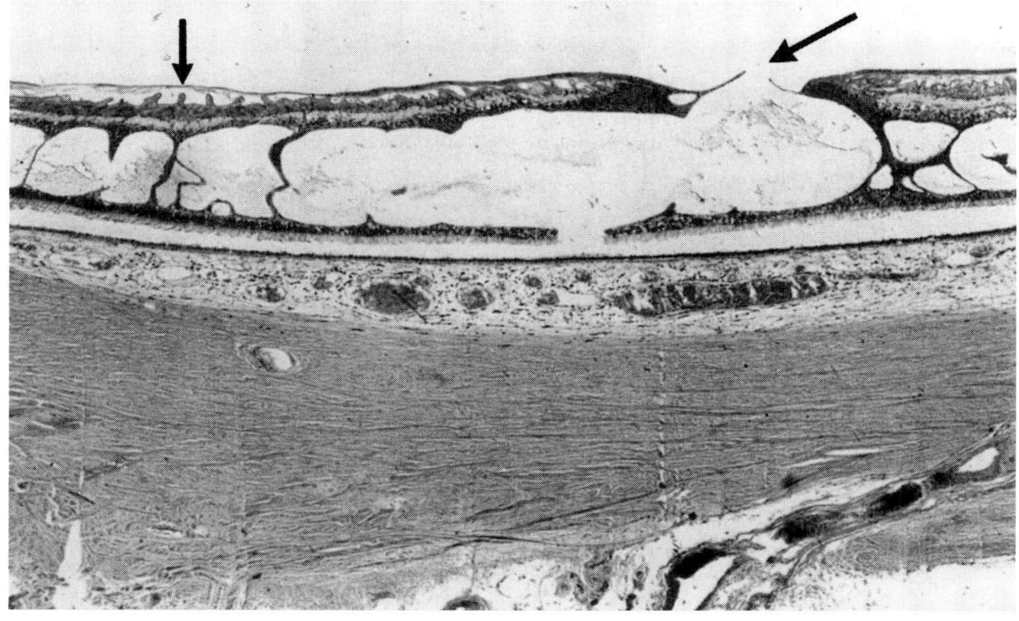

Figure 3 Long-standing cystoid edema. Loss of Müller fibers results in the formation of a central macrocyst or schisis. Rupture of the inner wall (*long arrow at right*) converts the schisis into a lamellar hole, which will still be surrounded by cystoid spaces. The break in the outer wall is an artifact. An epiretinal membrane present at left (*short arrow*) led to folding of the inner limiting membrane. Tangential traction by epiretinal membranes or by the condensed prefoveolar vitreous is believed to be incriminated in the pathogenesis of macular holes (Picro-Mallory stain, ×75).

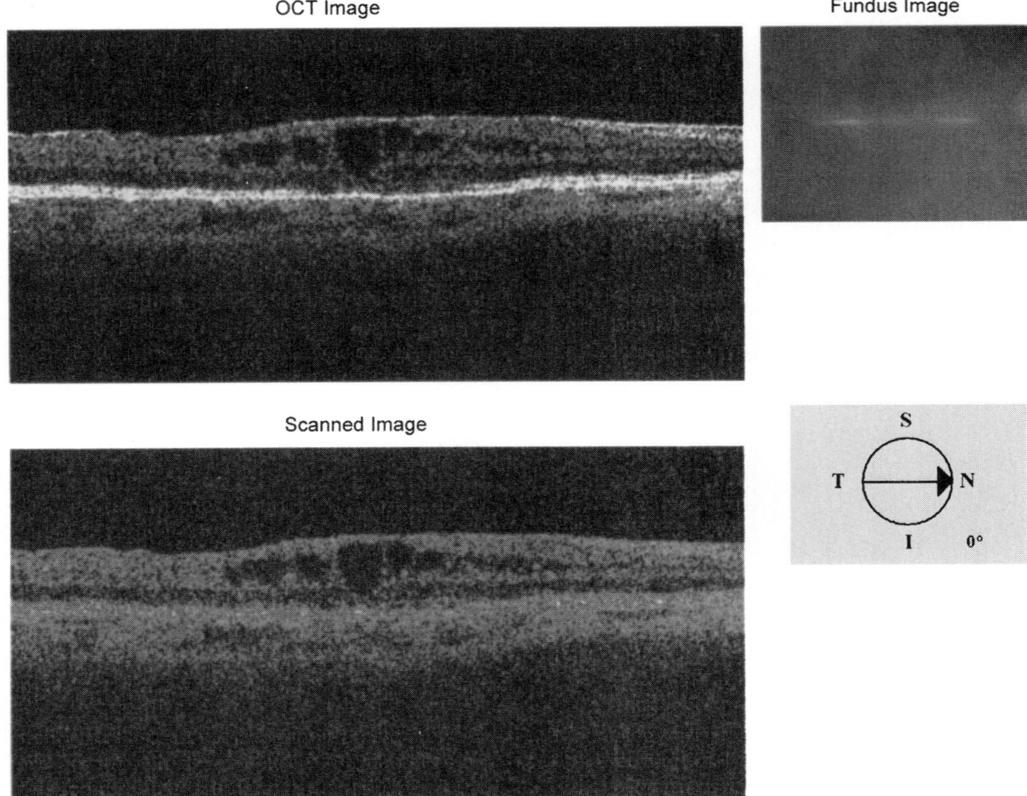

Figure 4 Ocular coherence tomography (OCT) of cystoid macular edema in a diabetic patient showing close correlation with histological appearances.

uveitis. A similar mechanism probably accounts for postsurgical CME.

Other Causes

Other cause of CME may be summarized as follows: (*i*) metabolic damage as in diabetes mellitus, (*ii*) increased intravascular hydrostatic pressure as in retinal vein occlusion or reduced tissue pressure in ocular hypotony, (*iii*) ischemia, occurring as an additional factor in retinal vein occlusion and diabetic retinopathy, (*iv*) distortion of retinal capillaries by epiretinal membranes or osteomas and other hamartomas, (*v*) radiation damage or other causes of weakness of the vessel walls, such as juxtafoveolar or parafoveolar telangiectasia, Coats syndrome, retinal angioma, or arterial macroaneurysm, (*vi*) drugs, such as epinephrine, and (*vii*) hereditary diseases, such as retinitis pigmentosa, in which fluid leaks from dilated retinal capillaries.

A major additional mediator in the development of edema in these three causes of CME appears to vascular endothelial growth factor (VEGF) (see Chapter 68).

Fluid accumulation may be compounded in the pigmentary retinopathies through damage to the pumping function of the RPE.

Complications

Lamellar Macular Hole

The inner wall of large intraretinal cysts in chronic CME may rupture, resulting in a lamellar macular hole (Figs. 5 and 6) usually surrounded by cystoid spaces. In postmortem eyes, apparent traction by an epiretinal membrane is found in about half of the eyes with lamellar holes and may be implicated in the pathogenesis (15).

The base of the lamellar hole shows a sheen or bright reflex due to the remaining retinal tissue, and the underlying RPE is not disturbed as in a full-thickness hole. Fluorescein does not pool in the hole as it leaks into the vitreous, so that the hole appears nonfluorescent and is often surrounded by the petaloid pattern of CME. Progression to a full-thickness macular hole is uncommon.

FLUID IN OTHER RETINAL COMPARTMENTS

Detachment of the RPE

An RPE detachment per se does not constitute macular edema since there is no breakdown of the blood–retina barrier, but fluid leaks inward if the

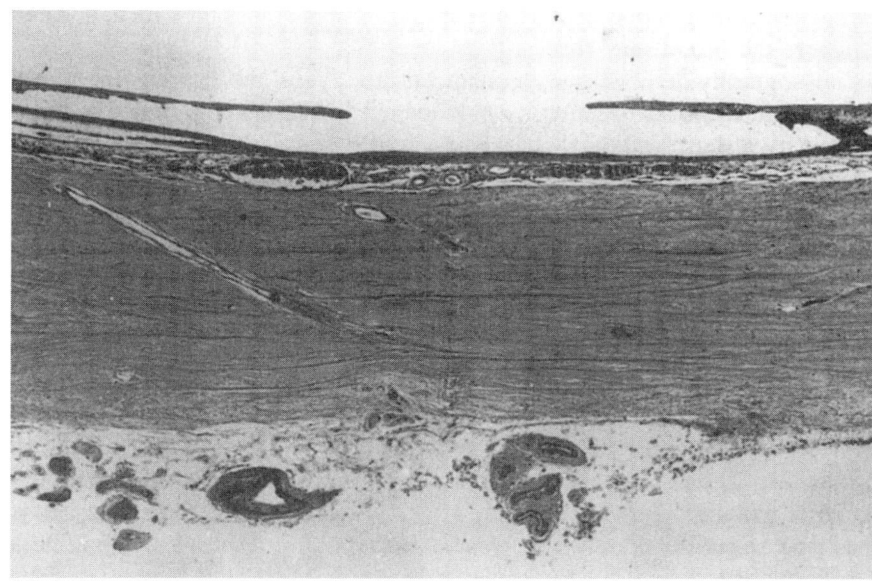

Figure 5 Lamellar macular hole due to loss of the inner retinal layers. The base of the hole is lined by compressed outer retinal layers. The hole was surrounded by cystoid spaces in the outer plexiform layer, just visible at right (Picro-Mallory stain, ×88).

overlying RPE tight junctions are disturbed. This subject is discussed in detail in Chapter 28.

Fluid Under the Sensory Retina

Fluid may enter the potential subsensory retinal space from the choroid when the RPE decompensates any of the following mechanisms: (*i*) inflammations, such as choroiditis including Vogt–Koyanagi–Harada disease, (*ii*) choroidal tumors, notably melanoma or hemangioma, (*iii*) ischemia resulting from occlusion of the precapillary arterioles and choriocapillaris, as occurs in severe hypertension, toxemia of pregnancy, or disseminated intravascular coagulation, (*iv*) traction retinal detachments, and (*v*) hypotony.

In diabetes mellitus, moreover, the macular edema, so often correlated with fluorescein angiographic evidence of leakage from the retinal circulation, may also be due in part to damage to the outer blood–retina barrier. Decompensation of the RPE may also occur over an RPE detachment or over a subretinal neovascular membrane. Outward movement of fluid can occur after breakdown of the inner blood–retina barrier, for example in exudative detachments due to retinal vascular disease. A localized sensory retinal detachment may occur beneath CME. Fluid may track under the sensory retina from outside the macula in rhegmatogenous retinal detachment or from an optic disc pit or a peripheral choroidal tumor.

Central Serous Retinopathy: Central Serous Choroidopathy

In this self-limiting although frequently recurrent condition, serous exudate collects at the posterior pole of the eye and likely represents a functional rather than a structural change in the circulation serving the macula. Young adults (mostly males) aged between 20 and 40 years are affected predominantly and commonly at a competitive stage of their lives, with a history of stress. Often there is evidence of clinical or subclinical involvement in the second eye. Clinically, a rounded blister of fluid lies under the sensory retina, which often has dot-like yellow precipitates on the posterior surface.

The fluid may gravitate inferiorly, leaving an atrophic track of RPE in its wake (9). Commonly there are other residual foci of depigmentation (window defects), indicating previous damage to the RPE. Attacks often resolve spontaneously within a few months but recur in about one-third of patients. When the condition continues to relapse, extensive RPE mottling may result. The fluorescein angiographic appearances are shown in Figure 7. Histopathological studies have shown eosinophilic material beneath the photoreceptors. An RPE detachment, which can be small, may also be found.

The cause of central serous retinopathy (CSR) is unknown but is generally believed to be a focal disturbance of the choriocapillaris (hence the alternative name "central serous choroidopathy"). Focal loss of adhesion of the overlying RPE to Bruch membrane may ensue, the fluid then usually finding its way through the RPE tight junctions to enter the subretinal space. A focal reversal of the RPE pump has also been postulated, with fluid being pumped into the subretinal space in one area and returned to the choroid by the adjacent healthy RPE. Among several possible etiologic factors for CSR, corticosteroids appear the most frequent

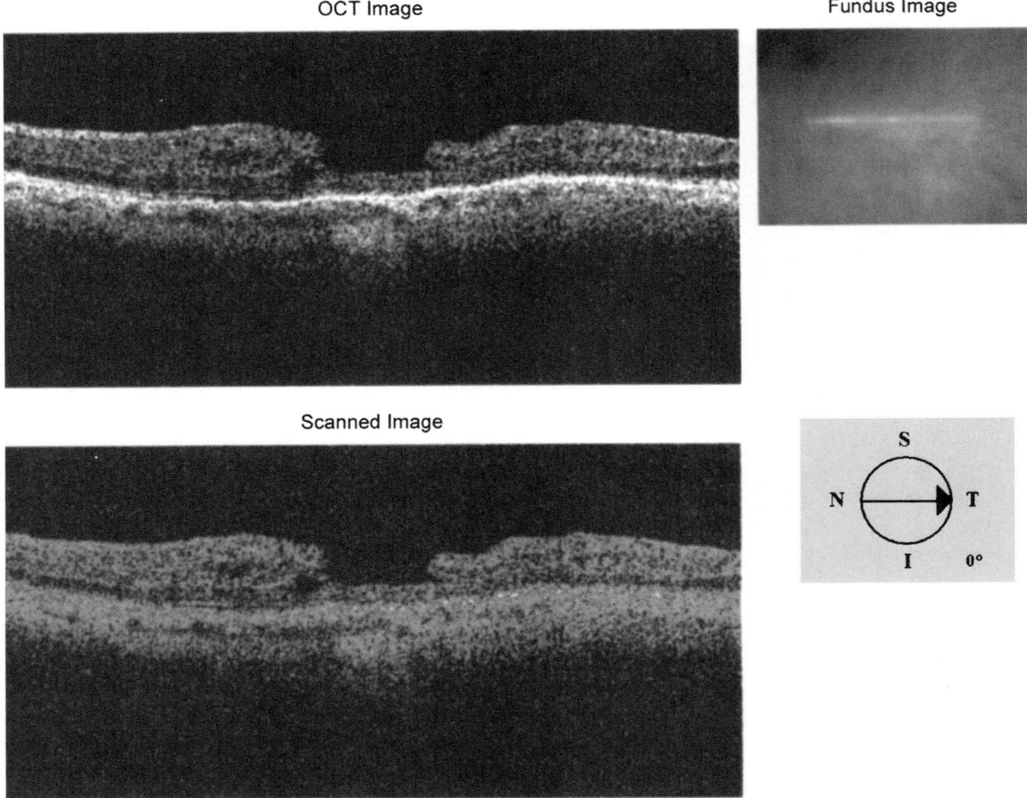

Figure 6 Ocular coherence tomography (OCT) of lamellar macular hole. Note the presence of remnants of retinal tissue at the base of the hole.

association (12). Resolution of the clinical picture with cessation of steroid use has also been reported however reports are limited to small case series. The possible ways in which corticosteroids may mediate increased chorioretinal permeability include an increased alteration in ion and water transport across epithelia, increased capillary fragility and reduced wound healing, leukocyte migration inhibition with release of proteolytic enzymes and other peptides (16).

Optic Disc Pit

An optic disc pit is a congenital anomaly of the optic nerve presenting as a grayish depression within the optic disc. Most frequently the pit is unilateral and single but all combinations have been reported. The pathogenesis is not yet resolved.

Optic disc pits may be associated with serous detachment of the retina adjacent to the optic disc and extending into the macula. Detachment can occur at any age but typically manifests after the second decade of life. In some instances, retinal separation occurs in different layers and can therefore resemble macular retinoschisis. Chronic serous detachment can result in permanent visual loss due to cystic degeneration of the retina and atrophy of the underlying RPE. It seems likely that fluid either enters the optic pit from the vitreous (by a mechanism mimicking rhegmatogenous retinal detachment or by pure hydrostatic pressure) or from the subarachnoid space around the optic nerve. The optic pit offers in some fashion direct access to the macular subretinal space (21).

FULL-THICKNESS MACULAR HOLE

A full-thickness macular hole appears as a round, punched-out defect about one-third of an optic disc diameter in (Fig. 8). It is surrounded by a gray halo of elevated retina, and in the base of the hole there is an RPE disturbance with small drusen. Opercula are found in almost half the eyes, usually applied to the posterior surface of the detached vitreous. The FA demonstrates a mottled window defect, partly due to degeneration of the RPE and partly to the loss of xanthophyll, which normally obstructs the blue light from reaching the dye in the choroid. The OCT typically identifies a full-thickness hole centered on the fovea (Fig. 9).

Most cases are idiopathic and appear to develop spontaneously in the sixth or seventh decade. Ten percent become bilateral. Other causes include trauma,

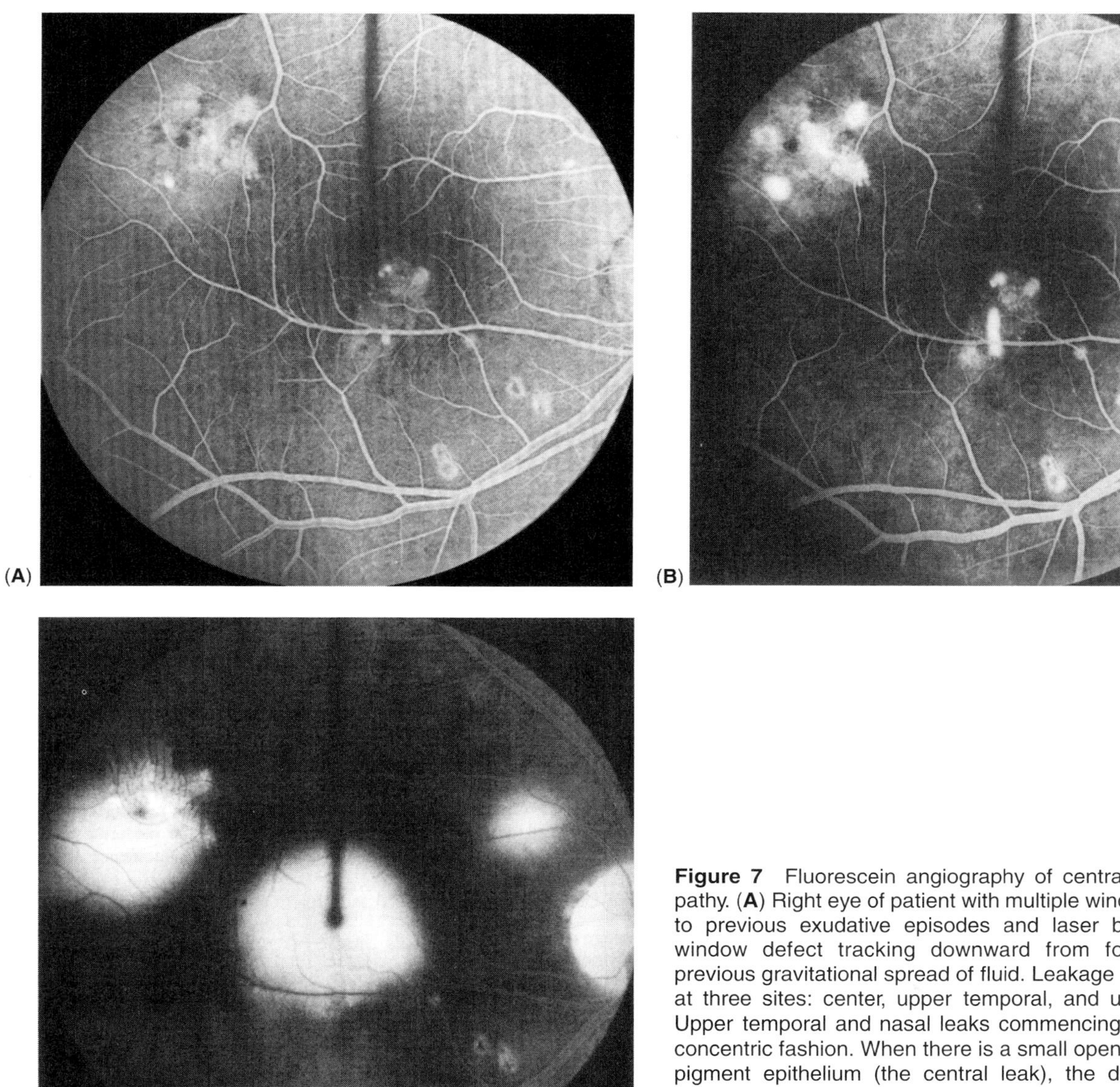

Figure 7 Fluorescein angiography of central serous retinopathy. (**A**) Right eye of patient with multiple window defects due to previous exudative episodes and laser burns. Note the window defect tracking downward from fovea, indicating previous gravitational spread of fluid. Leakage of dye occurring at three sites: center, upper temporal, and upper nasal. (**B**) Upper temporal and nasal leaks commencing to enlarge in a concentric fashion. When there is a small opening in the retinal pigment epithelium (the central leak), the dye may stream upward with a smokestack appearance due to convection currents. (**C**) Late phase, showing filling of three serous detachments. Note gravitational spread of dye downward from central blister.

myopia, inflammation, central retinal vein or artery occlusion, cataract extraction, solar retinopathy, and surgery for retinal detachment.

Vitreous adhesion to the retina is greater at the fovea and optic disc than elsewhere in the fundus, as evidenced by the higher density of hemidesmosomes in these areas, and Gass (11) proposed that tangential traction of the prefoveal vitreous cortex may be implicated in the pathogenesis of the idiopathic macular holes. Release of the vitreous traction may flatten the halo of elevated retina around the hole, leaving a flat reddish lesion. Gaudric et al. (13) studied OCTs of fellow eyes of patients with macular holes and suggested that in these cases, detachment of the vitreous begins around the macula (Fig. 9). However, the hyaloid remains adherent to the foveolar center, resulting in the development of an anteroposterior force leading to an intraretinal split, which evolves into a cystic space. Finally, the outer retinal layer becomes disrupted with opening of the foveal floor and consequent a full-thickness macular hole development.

Associated findings in about 70% of postmortem eyes with full-thickness holes are CME and epiretinal membrane formation (15), even though the membranes do not cause obvious tangential traction. Occasionally, a localized retinal detachment around the hole is present together with a mild phlebitis or choroiditis (14).

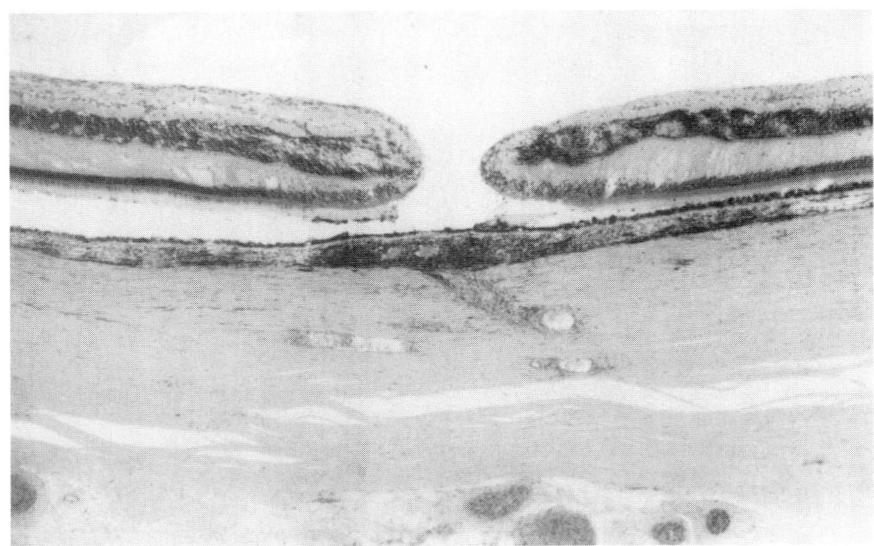

Figure 8 Full-thickness macular hole. The retinal pigment epithelium at the base of the hole is mildly atrophic (hematoxylin and eosin, ×55).

Impending macular hole formation may be recognized by loss of the foveal depression, by the presence of a yellow spot or ring, probably representing displacement of xanthophyll due to traction on the foveola, and by persistent attachment of the vitreous to the foveal retina. Patients usually manifest visual reduction (20/50) and distortion. Most cases then progress to spontaneous vitreous separation or macular hole formation (8).

MASSIVE GLIOSIS OF THE RETINA

Massive gliosis is a benign proliferation of retinal glial cells that entirely replaces and thickens the affected area of the retina (Fig. 10). A review of 38 cases by Yanoff et al. (28) indicates that the condition is a nonspecific reaction to a variety of underlying conditions, including postinflammatory states, Coats disease, retinopathy of prematurity, glaucoma, and intraocular neoplasia (28). A delay of 10 years or more is common between the initial disorder and the glial response. The cells responsible for the massive gliosis are usually regular spindle-shaped astrocytes with well-defined fibrillar processes and generally uniform nuclei devoid of apparent mitotic activity. Dilated and often varicose blood vessels are a constant feature and may be surrounded by a serous exudate and scanty leukocytes. Calcification occurs in about 50% of cases, and bone formation on the part of metaplastic RPE is common.

ANGIOID STREAKS

Angioid streaks are linear red or dark brown strands radiating from the optic disc and bearing a superficial resemblance to blood vessels. The condition is invariably bilateral and may occur as an isolated finding or as part of systemic disorder, most commonly pseudoxanthoma elasticum (MIM #264800) (85% of patients) (Fig. 11), sickle cell disease (MIM #603903) (22%), or Paget disease of bone (MIM #602080) (15%). Other systemic disorders linked with angioid streaks include Ehlers–Danlos syndrome (MIM #130000), Gardner syndrome (MIM +175100) (intestinal polyposis, soft tissue tumors, and benign osteomas), and hemolytic anemias, but the evidence that the association in these conditions is more than coincidental is open to doubt.

Histological examination shows that the streaks represent breaks or dehiscences in a heavily calcified Bruch membrane (Fig. 12). The overlying RPE is atrophic but not necessarily discontinuous and the blood–retinal barrier is intact. Frequently, blood vessels from underlying choriocapillaris invade the break, breach the epithelium, and proliferate in the subretinal space. The consequences are those of subretinal neovascularization with visual compromise should the macula be involved (4).

The propensity for angioid streak formation is attributed to mechanical stresses incurred by extraocular muscle contraction or by rubbing the eyes in the presence of a calcified, brittle Bruch membrane. Even so, it is remarkable that similar streaks are not seen in the elderly eye, in which Bruch membrane also commonly calcifies. More than one factor may cause the calcification, which usually begins in the elastic core of the membrane: a primary abnormality at this level is probably critical in pseudoxanthoma elasticum. Furthermore, the iron deposition in Bruch membrane of some eyes with angioid streaks may

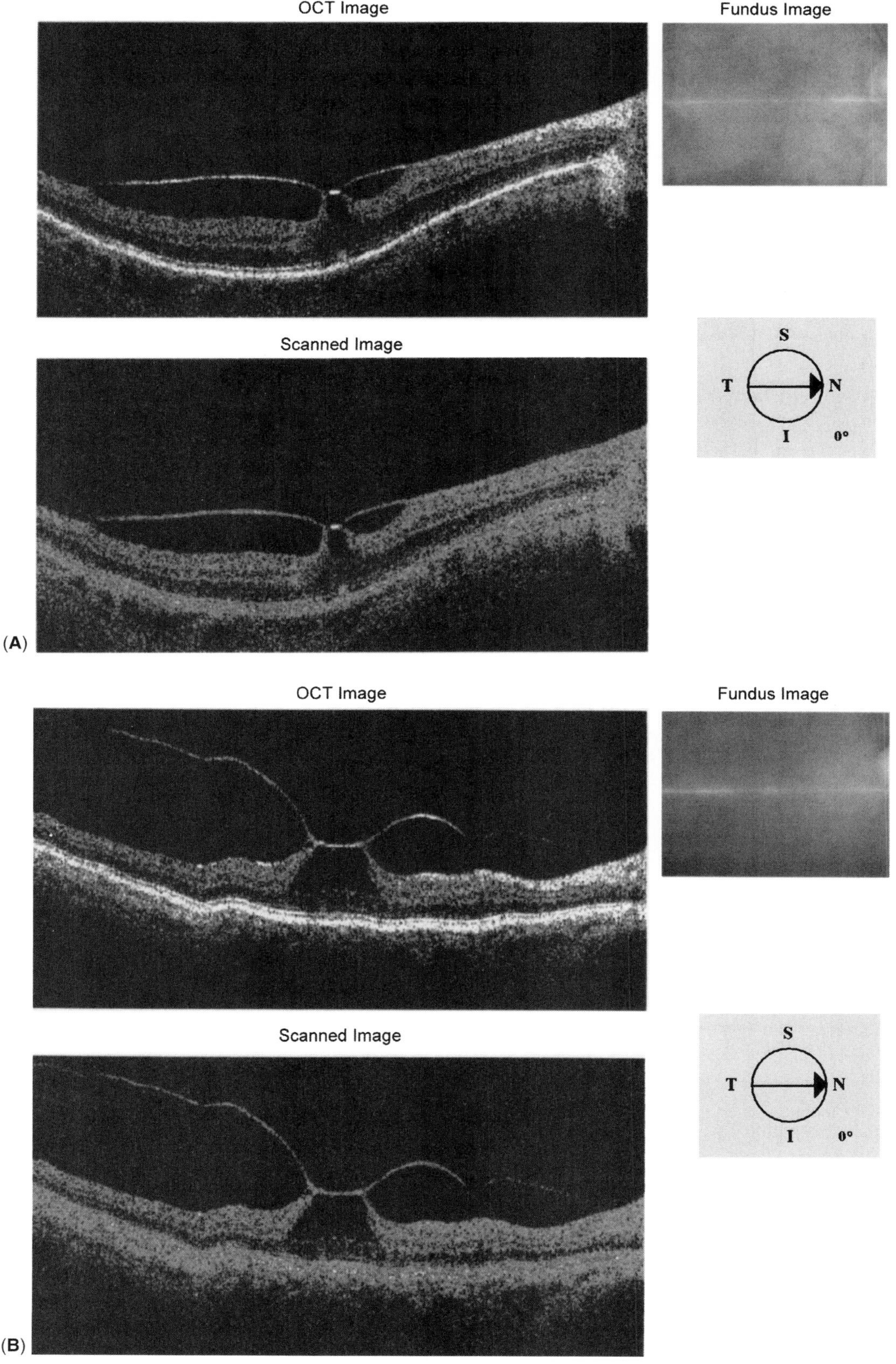

Figure 9 Development of full thickness macular hole. (**A**) Early stage: detachment of the vitreous begins around the macula. However, (**B**) the hyaloid remains adherent to the foveolar center, resulting in the development of an anteroposterior force leading to an intraretinal split which evolves into a cystic space. (*Continued*)

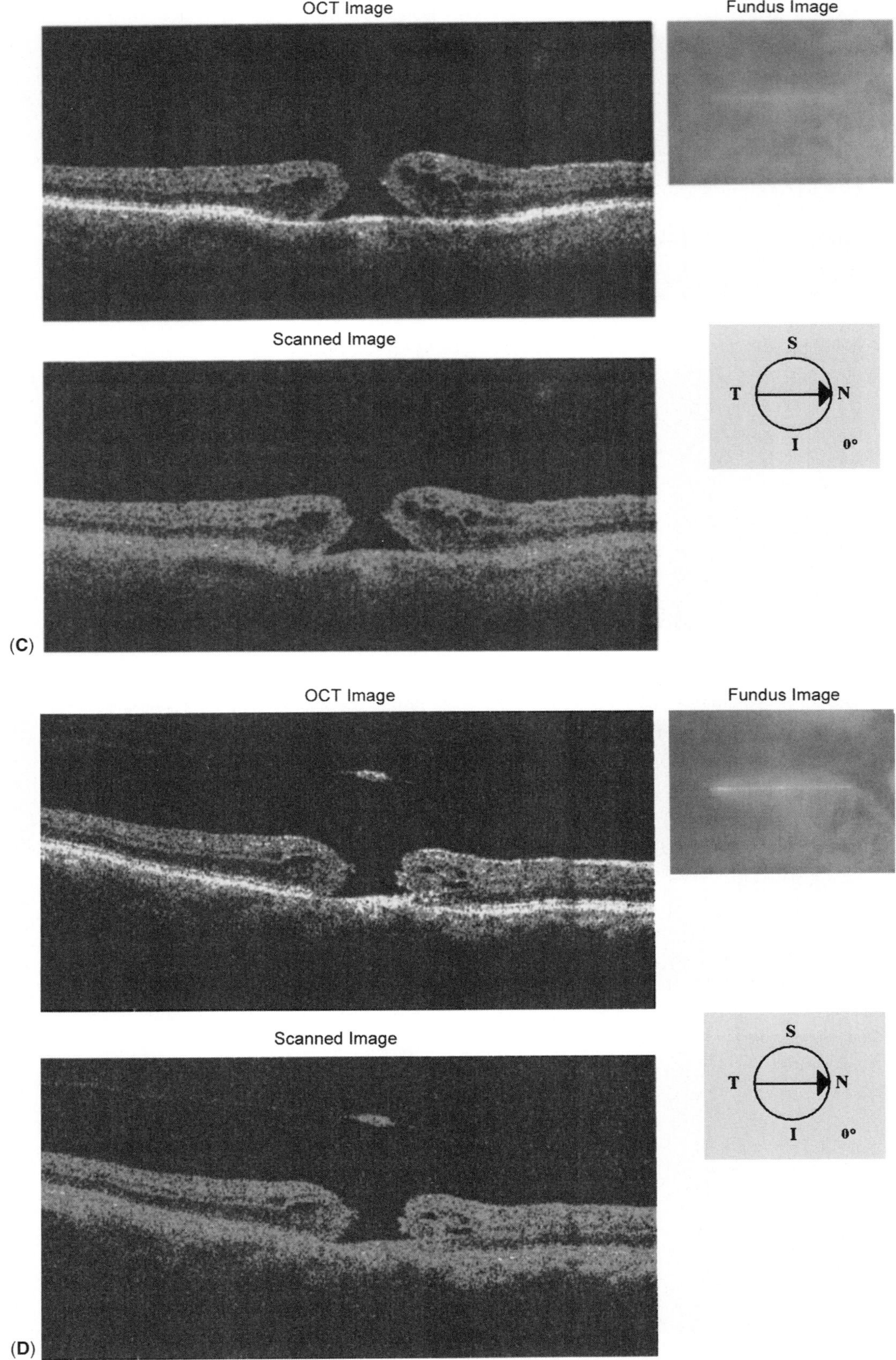

Figure 9 (*Continued*) Finally, (**C**) the outer retinal layer becomes disrupted with opening of the foveal floor and consequent a full-thickness macular hole development. (**D**) full-thickness macular hole with operculum.

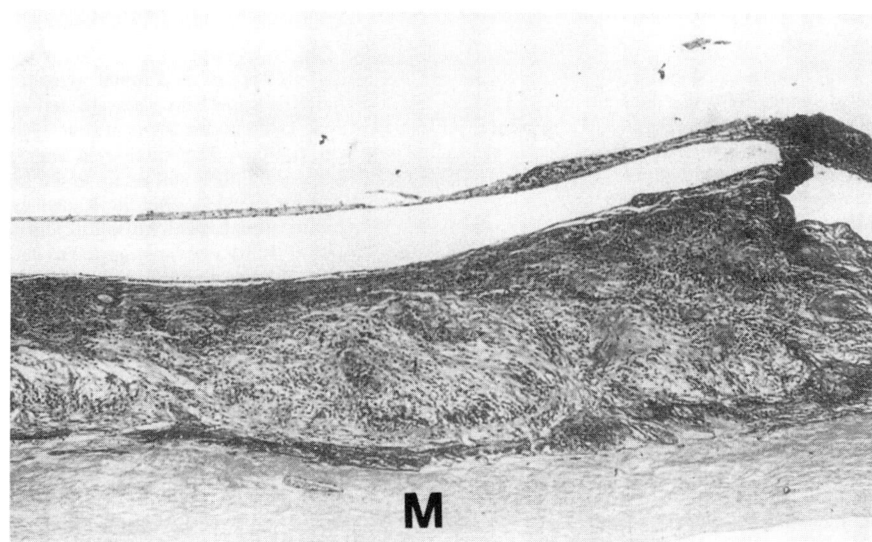

Figure 10 Massive gliosis occurring in an eye with a long-standing retinal detachment. Glial proliferation resulted in a dense membrane (M), which is attached to the degenerate peripheral retina (Picro-Mallory stain, ×40).

be a further factor; especially as the iron salts are deposited before calcification in embryonic bone and at other sites. A predisposing effect of iron provides an explanation for angioid streak development in sickle cell disease and other hematological disorders, especially when the anemia has necessitated repeated blood transfusions, but iron deposition is not a universal finding in these situations.

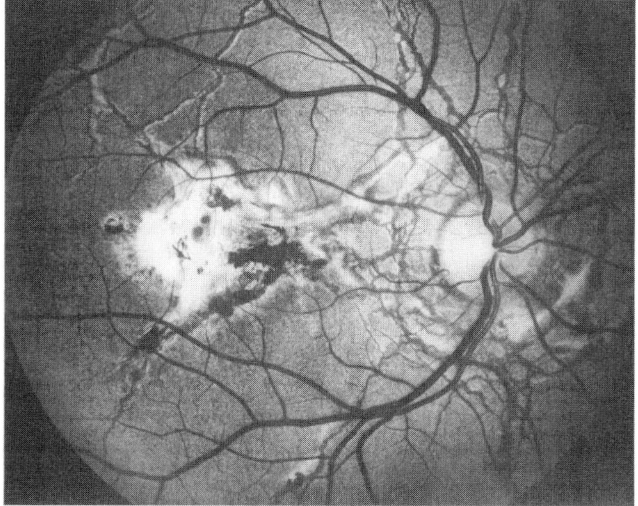

Figure 11 Angioid streaks in a patient with pseudoxanthoma elasticum. The streaks appear as brownish meandering lines communicating in a ringlike manner around the optic disc and from which they when radiate outward. Choroidal neovascularization has occurred through a streak passing through the fovea, resulting in disciform scarring. Lateral to the scar the fundus has a characteristic mottled appearance referred to as peau d'orange, and because this may be noted before streaks develop, such patients should avoid contact sports.

RADIATION RETINOPATHY

The effects of irradiation on the eye in general are reviewed in Chapter 15 and the present discussion relates specifically to the nature and mechanism of retinal damage. As with most tissues formed of nondividing cells, the retina is relatively resistant to radiation-induced damage, and most of the harm incurred by the retina is secondary to vascular injury. The effects are dose related and cumulative, although there is some evidence that the same dose given in small fractions is less damaging than in large fractions. There is considerable variation in the total dose required to cause a clinically significant retinal effect, but it seems that amounts less than 30 gray are usually innocuous to the human retina. Doses of this order primarily injure the microcirculation, and much greater amounts of radiation, approaching 100 gray, are needed to cause direct neuronal degeneration. Most instances of human radiation retinopathy are secondary to treatment of ocular or adjacent tumors.

The initial angiopathy in patients irradiated for therapeutic reasons is rarely evident in less than 6 months (3), although a considerably shorter period of 3–5 weeks was noted in individuals exposed to atomic bomb radiation in Japan (6). Conversely, it can take as long as 3 years before the effects are manifest (3).

As indicated, the initial brunt is borne by the retinal circulation, with degeneration of capillary endothelial cells and pericytes. Involvement of the arterioles, often in the form of an endarteritis with myointimal hyperplasia, and venules follows, with thrombotic occlusions, capillary nonperfusion, and the transient formation of cotton–wool spots. Serous

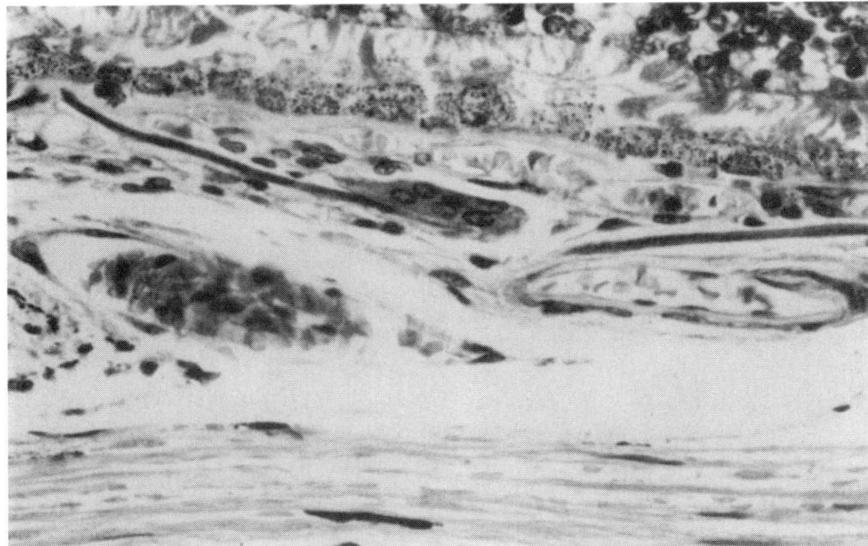

Figure 12 Section showing fractures of Bruch membrane, with multinuclear giant cell and subretinal neovascular membrane. Angioid streaks represent similar fractures of a Bruch membrane rendered brittle by calcification. New vessels from the choroid may then grow through these gaps (Picro-Mallory stain, ×453).

exudation, which may be confused with choroidal infarcts, and intraretinal hemorrhage are common, and subsequently the damaged capillaries may become telangiectatic or form microaneurysms. Furthermore, iris neovascularization, possibly related to the presence of an angiogenic substance in the vitreous, and angle-closure glaucoma developed in a minority of animals some 2 to 3 years after the initial irradiation. Ganglion cell and photoreceptor process loss is common in end-stage radiation retinopathy (Fig. 13) and may be allied with atrophy, dispersion, or reactive hyperplasia of the RPE.

CANCER-ASSOCIATED RETINOPATHY

Occasional cancer patients experience otherwise unexplained loss of vision, which can be both sudden and severe. Known as cancer-associated retinopathy (CAR), it is a paraneoplastic syndrome in that the visual disturbance is not a result of tumor metastasis but likely due to the appearance of antiretinal antibodies such as to recoverin or retinal enolase (1). The pathogenesis is not fully understood, but homology between retinal and tumor antigens may be a key factor and probably the explanation for the restriction of the syndrome to certain tumor types, most commonly, oat cell carcinoma of the lung.

The fundus appearances are variable. Characteristic patterns of electrophysiological abnormality are present (27). Histologically, there is degeneration and loss of photoreceptor cells frequently by apoptosis (19). Secondary changes in the RPE with migration of melanin into the neuroretina may also be seen (22).

OTHER AUTOIMMUNE RETINOPATHIES

Autoimmune retinopathy is the preferred term for an acquired, presumed immunologically mediated retinal degeneration with symptoms resembling

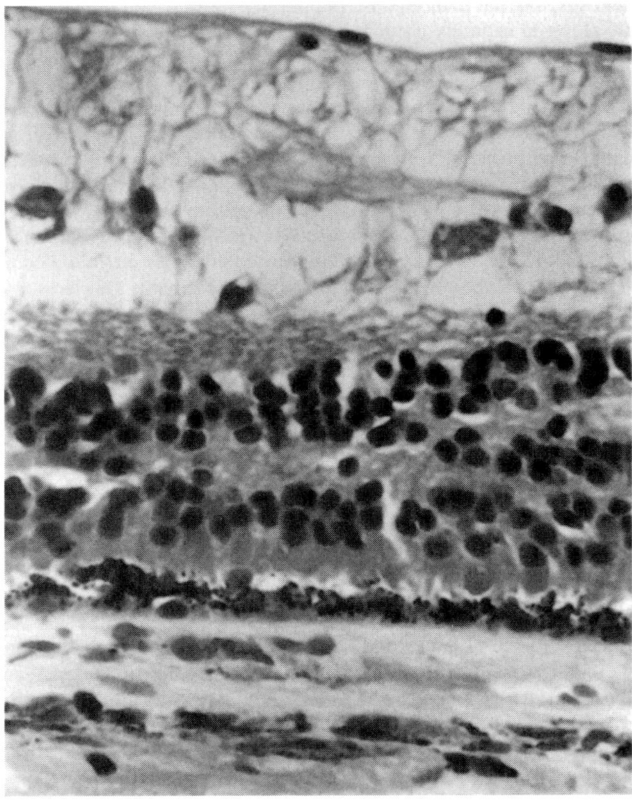

Figure 13 Atrophy of inner retina and stunting of the photoreceptor processes after a tumoricidal dose of irradiation (hematoxylin and eosin, ×388).

paraneoplastic retinopathy but without tumor in association with serum antiretinal autoantibodies. The etiology and source of antigenic stimulation vary but are largely unknown. It is possible that the disease is triggered by molecular mimicry between retinal proteins and presumed viral or bacterial proteins or by the acquired alteration of host tissues or antigens so that autoimmunity is induced against retinal proteins. Multiple retinal proteins have been found to be antigenic, including recoverin, α-enolase, arrestin, transducin, tubby-like protein (TULP1), neurofilament protein, heat-shock protein-70, photoreceptor cell–specific nuclear receptor (PNR), and as yet undefined bipolar cell antigens causing melanoma-associated retinopathy (MAR syndrome) (27).

PERIPHERAL RETINAL DEGENERATION

Peripheral Microcystoid Degeneration

Typical Microcystoid Degeneration (Blessig–Ivanoff Cysts)

The development of cyst-like spaces in the peripheral retina is a universal finding, beginning in adolescence and continuing throughout life until about the seventh or eighth decade. Exceptional instances have been noted in infancy (23). The spaces are formed by the accumulation of hyaluronidase-sensitive glycosaminoglycans (GAGs) in the outer plexiform layer, where increasing size and numbers of the loculi leads to their coalescence (Fig. 14). This can dissect apart the inner and outer layers of the retina, occasionally resulting in clinically significant retinoschisis (Fig. 14). Neuronal loss is a late, secondary event, but in advanced stages the two halves of the retina are often held together only by virtue of residual Müller cells and associated fibrils. Typical cystoid degeneration commences at the ora serrata and gradually extends posteriorly toward the equator of the globe.

The pathogenesis is not entirely clear, but vitreous syneresis with posterior vitreous detachment is a frequent accompaniment. The increased stress that this can be expected to lay on the stronger residual attachments at the vitreous base and resultant traction on the inner limiting membrane may then induce secondary effects within the retina. Foos (26) showed that the inner limiting membrane is thinner at the vitreous base than elsewhere and described a degenerative process in which cellular debris accumulates with a macrophage response and reduced Müller cell attachment to the membrane. The origin of the GAG-rich fluid and fibrils within the cystoid spaces has been attributed to the Müller cells, which corresponds with the postulated Müller cell origin of the secondary vitreous.

Reticular Peripheral Cystoid Degeneration

Reticular peripheral cystoid degeneration occurs in 12% to 18% of eyes (14) and is almost always in continuity with typical cystoid degeneration, developing slightly more posteriorly and showing a predilection for the temporal hemisphere. Whereas the fluid-filled spaces in the more usual form of cystoid degeneration are located in the outer plexiform layer of the retina, those in the reticular form develop in the nerve fiber layer (Fig. 15). The reticular pattern is attributable to a delicate tracery of arborizing blood vessels against a finely stippled opaque background. Light microscopy reveals wide separation between the inner limiting membrane and the inner nuclear layer, ganglion cells being in any case sparse in this region and the inner plexiform layer readily compressed. More extensive splitting to constitute a bullous retinoschisis is said to occur in 1.6% of the adult population (14).

Senescence is not an obvious factor in the pathogenesis of the condition, and movement of the

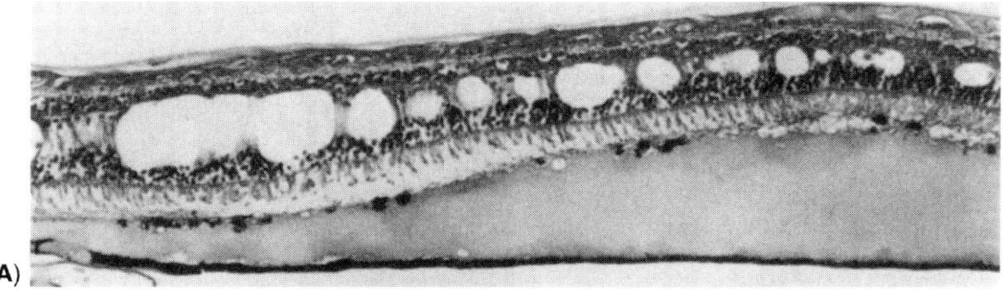

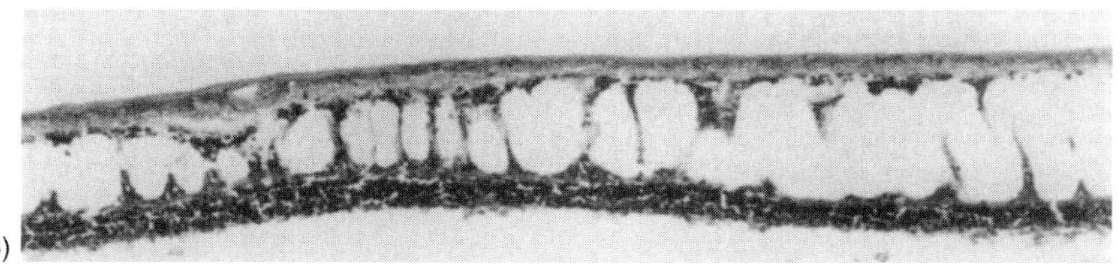

Figure 14 Peripheral microcystoid degeneration. (**A**) Note that the cysts appear in the outer plexiform layer. The retina is detached by exudate. (**B**) The cysts have coalesced to create a retinoschisis (hematoxylin and eosin, ×100).

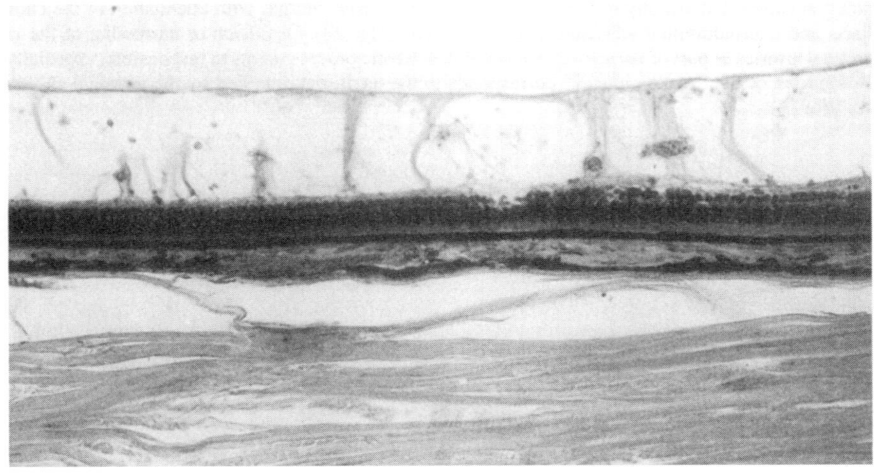

Figure 15 Reticular peripheral cystoid degeneration. The nerve fiber layer of the retina is markedly increased in thickness by the accumulation of clear (hyaluronic acid-rich) fluid, and the inner limiting lamina is attached to the underlying nuclear layers by a few residual Müller cell processes only (hematoxylin and eosin, ×160).

ciliary musculature during accommodation has been considered to exert a shearing stress on the retina through the attachment of the peripheral fibers of the vitreous.

Lattice Degeneration of the Retina

Lattice degeneration occurs anterior to the ocular equator, predominating at the superior and interior meridians, and affects about 10% of the population. The definitive clinical appearance is produced by clearly defined zones of retinal atrophy running parallel to the circumference that expose sclerosed, occluded retinal blood vessels. The overlying vitreous is liquefied, except at the margins of the atrophic area, where it tends to be condensed and reinforced by glial proliferation (14). Microscopic examination indicates neuronal atrophy commencing in the inner layers but extending to involve the entire retina, such that it comes to consist mainly of glial tissue and hyalinized blood vessels partially surrounded by migrated RPE (Fig. 16). Retinal holes within an area of lattice degeneration are a frequent finding but they do not appear to incur a significant risk of retinal detachment, the overall risk of which is of the order of 1% (17). More important in accounting for the well-recognized risk of retinal detachment are the firm vitreoretinal adhesions at the edges of the atrophic zones, since in the presence of posterior vitreous detachment they are subject to traction that can result in retinal tears at the posterior margin. (See Chapter 28 for a fuller discussion of the factors predisposing the rhegmatogenous detachment.)

It is difficult to escape the conclusion that the retinal atrophy in lattice degeneration is related to an impaired vascular supply, although it should be emphasized that the choroidal circulation is not noticeably affected. A familial predisposition has also been noted.

A variant of lattice degeneration referred to as radial perivascular lattice degeneration, in which the foci of thinning are aligned alongside the radially oriented retinal vessels, has also been described (20). The histological features are similar, although RPE changes are often more pronounced, and there is a clear relationship with sclerosis of the underlying capillary circulation. Because of a more posterior location of most atrophic areas, which may also be more extensive, and associated holes the risk of detachment is greater than pertains in the usual form of the degeneration.

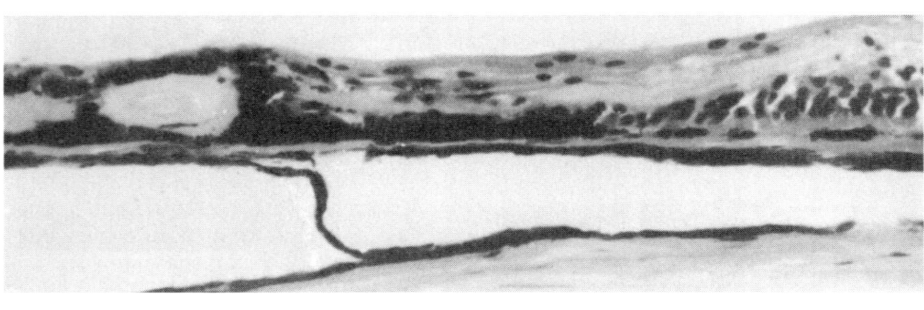

Figure 16 In lattice degeneration there is advanced atrophy of all layers of the retina. Hyalinized blood vessels are also observed (hematoxylin and eosin, ×280).

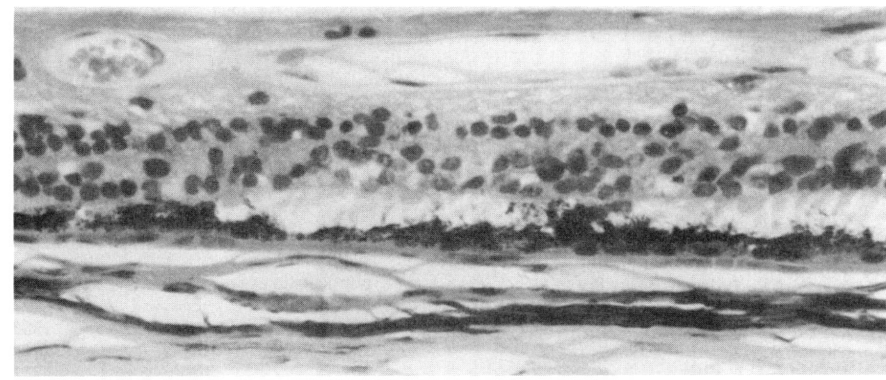

Figure 17 In pavingstone degeneration there is extensive atrophy of the photoreceptors at the center of the lesion associated with proliferation of the pigment epithelium (hematoxylin and eosin, ×270).

Paving Stone Degeneration (Peripheral Choroidoretinal Atrophy)

The essentially asymptomatic and benign degenerative process known as paving stone degeneration presents as sharply demarcated, flat, and whitish areas between the retinal periphery and the equator. They increase in incidence with age from the third decade in about one-quarter of the population, according to autopsy data, and predominate in the inferior half of the globe. Atrophy and loss of the RPE with varying degrees of hyperplasia at the margins is responsible for the clinical appearance, and histological examination shows that atrophy of the outer layers of the sensory retina, with attenuation of the choriocapillaris and choroidoretinal adhesion, is also involved (Fig. 17). Occlusion or narrowing of the choroidoretinal arteries as part of the age-related arteriolosclerotic process seems to responsible, especially as the distribution of the "paving stones" corresponds to the territories supplied by the terminal choroidal blood vessels (26).

REFERENCES

1. Adamus G, Aptsiauri N, Guy J, et al. The occurrence of serum autoantibodies against enolase in cancer-associated retinopathy. Clin Immunol Immunopathol 1996; 78: 120–9.
2. Bressler NM, Bressler SB, Alexander J, et al. The Macular Photocoagulation Study Reading Center. Loculated fluid. A previously undescribed fluorescein angiographic finding in choroidal neovascularization associated with macular degeneration. Arch Ophthalmol 1991; 709:211–5.
3. Brown GC, Shields JA, Sanborn G, et al. Radiation retinopathy. Ophthalmology 1982; 89:1494–504.
4. Clarkson JG, Altman RD. Angioid streaks. Surv Ophthalmol 1982; 26:235–46.
5. Curcio CA, Millican CL, Allen KA, Kalina RE. Aging of the human photoreceptor mosaic: evidence for selective vulnerability of rods in central retina. Invest Ophthalmol Vis Sci 1993; 34:3278–96.
6. Flick JJ. Ocular lesions following the atomic bombing of Hiroshima and Nagasaki. Am J Ophthalmol 1948; 31: 137–54.
7. Foos RY. Vitreoretinal juncture over retinal vessels. Graefes Arch Clin Exp Ophthalmol 1977; 204:223–34.
8. Foulds WS. Is your vitreous really necessary? The role of the vitreous in the eye with particular reference to retinal attachment, detachment and the mode of action of vitreous substitutes. Eye 1987; 1:641–64.
9. Frangich GT, Green WR, Engel HM. A histopathologic study of macular cysts and holes. Retina 2005; (Suppl. 5): 311–36.
10. Gao H, Hollyfield JG. Aging of the human retina. Differential loss of neurons and retinal pigment epithelial cells. Invest Ophthalmol Vis Sci 1992; 33:1–17.
11. Gass JDM. Idiopathic senile macular hole: its early stages and pathogenesis. Arch Ophthalmol 1988; 106: 629–39.
12. Gass JDM, Little H. Bilateral bullous exudative retinal detachment complicating idiopathic central serous chorioretinopathy during systemic corticosteroid therapy. Ophthalmology 1995; 102:737–47.
13. Gaudric A, Haouchine B, Massin P, et al. Macular hole formation: new data provided by optical coherence tomography. Arch Ophthalmol 1999; 117:744–51.
14. Green WR. Retina. In: Spencer WH, ed. Ophthalmic Pathology: An Atlas and Textbook. 3rd ed. Philadelphia, PA: W.B. Saunders, 1985:589–1291.
15. Guyer DR, Green WR, de Bustros S, Fine SL. Histopathologic features of idiopathic macular holes and cysts. Ophthalmology 1990; 97:1045–51.
16. Levy J, Marcus M, Belfair N, et al. Central serous chorioretinopathy in patients receiving systemic corticosteroid therapy. Can J Ophthalmol 2005; 40:217–21.
17. Lewis H. Peripheral retinal degenerations and the risk of retinal detachment. Am J Ophthalmol 2003; 136:155–60.
18. Negi A, Marmor MF. Effects of subretinal and systemic osmolarity on the rate of subretinal fluid resorption. Invest Ophthalmol Vis Sci 1984; 25:616–20.
19. Ohguro H, Yokoi Y, Ohguro I, et al. Clinical and immunologic aspects of cancer-associated retinopathy. Am J Ophthalmol 2004; 137:1117–9.
20. Parelhoff ES, Wood WJ, Green WR, Kenyon KR. Radial perivascular lattice degeneration of the retina. Ann Ophthalmol 1980; 12:25–32.
21. Poulson AV, Snead DR, Jacobs PM, et al. Intraocular surgery for optic nerve disorders. Eye 2004; 18:1056–65.

22. Sawyer RA, Selhorst JB, Zimmerman LE, Hoyt WE. Blindness caused by photoreceptor degeneration as a remote effect of cancer. Am J Ophthalmol 1976; 81:606–13.
23. Straatsma BR, Foos RY, Feman SS. Degenerative diseases of the peripheral retina. In: Duane TD, ed. Clinical Ophthalmology, vol. 3. Hagerstown, MD: Harper & Row, 1979.
24. Tranos PG, Wickremasinghe SS, Stangos NT, et al. Macular edema. Surv Ophthalmol 2004; 49:470–90.
25. Walter JR. The histopathology of cystoid macular edema. Graefes Arch Clin Exp Ophthalmol 1981; 216:85–101.
26. Weiter JJ, Ernest JT. Anatomy of the choroidal vasculature. Am J Ophthalmol 1974; 18:583–90.
27. Weleber RG, Watzke RC, Shults WT, et al. Clinical and electrophysiologic characterization of paraneoplastic and autoimmune retinopathies associated with antienolase antibodies. Am J Ophthalmol 2005; 139: 780–94.
28. Yanoff M, Zimmerman LE, Davis RL. Massive gliosis of the retina. Int Ophthalmol Clin 1971; 11: 211–29.
29. Yannuzzi LA, Shakin JL, Fisher YL, Altomonte MA. Peripheral retinal detachments and retinal pigment epithelial atrophic tracts secondary to central serous pigment epitheliopathy. Ophthalmology 1984; 91:1554–72.

28

Retinal Detachment

Paul Hiscott and Ian Grierson
Unit of Ophthalmology, School of Clinical Sciences, University of Liverpool, Liverpool, U.K.

INTRODUCTION

The inner and outer layers of the embryological optic cup give rise to the adult neuroretina and retinal pigment epithelium (RPE), respectively, and separation of the two structures is termed retinal detachment. Apart from those retinal detachments that occur because of the accumulation of exudate beneath the neuroretina (exudative retinal detachment), as in choroidal tumors and inflammation, retinal detachments are thought to arise as a result of alterations in normal vitreoretinal relations. Our concept of these changes owes much to Gonin, whose work revolutionized the study and management of retinal detachment (29). Key to an understanding of retinal detachment is an appreciation of age-related change in the vitreous (see Chapter 29). The vitreous is a collagen-containing aqueous gel, the gel constituents of which tend to separate as part of the normal aging process (6), to produce a collagen-containing formed vitreous and a fluid vitreous. This syneretic process may be accelerated by a variety of conditions, including myopia and aphakia, and tends to lead to separation of the vitreous cortex from the retinal surface (posterior vitreous detachment [PVD]).

RHEGMATOGENOUS RETINAL DETACHMENT

For the most part, attachments between the vitreous and the posterior neuroretina consist of only a few cortical vitreous fibers passing into the inner limiting lamina (ILL), and most vitreal fibers run parallel to the retinal surface (Fig. 1) (22). Therefore, PVD usually has little effect on the integrity of the retina. However, vitreoretinal contact at the vitreous base (adjacent to the ora serrata) normally persists following PVD. Other exaggerated vitreoretinal adhesions may also occur, located as a rule in the periphery of the retina posterior to the vitreous base, where vitreous fibrils may become incarcerated within clefts between Müller cells (22). Such residual vitreoretinal adhesions are generally considered to transmit and concentrate rotational tractional forces, including the dynamic traction from saccadic eye movements (70), between the retina and vitreous. They may be associated with

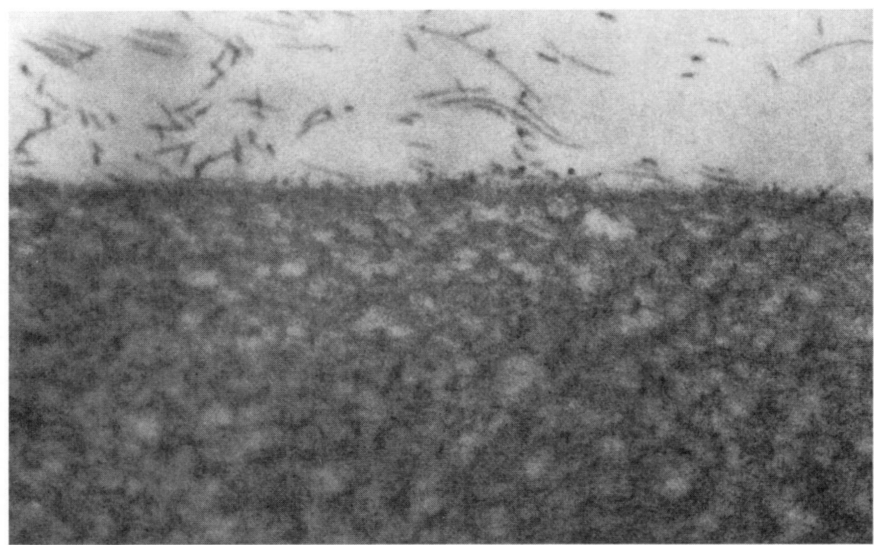

Figure 1 Transmission electron micrograph of the vitreoretinal interface at the posterior pole of the human eye. Most of the cortical vitreous fibers run parallel to the retinal surface, and only a few appear to enter the inner limiting lamina (×87,800).

foci of retinal degeneration, especially in myopia or following trauma. The combination of a weakened retina and dynamic traction is liable to tear the retina. A retinal hole incurred in this way may permit the passage of fluid vitreous (which, if the tear involves a retinal vessel, may contain blood) to the potential space between the two derivatives of the embryological optic cup. The resulting rhegmatogenous retinal detachment is therefore often abrupt in onset, coinciding with the arrival of fluid vitreous in the subretinal space between the sensory retina and the RPE. The distribution of subretinal fluid varies with eye movement and posture, so that the retinal detachment is mobile and convex anteriorly (bullous) and may involve the whole of the retina (total detachment).

TRACTIONAL RETINAL DETACHMENT

Less commonly, vitreoretinal traction may be static in nature and elevate the neuroretina slowly, to produce a localized detachment without tearing the retina. Such detachments differ clinically from rhegmatogenous retinal detachments, the retinal elevation being localized, immobile, and anteriorly concave. These rigid detachments are called tractional retinal detachments and it has long been recognized that they are due to tension generated by cellular or fibrous membranes in the vitreal cavity (75). A wide variety of intraocular disorders cause intravitreal tractional membranes, including the vascular retinopathies (see Chapter 67), inflammatory and degenerative conditions, and trauma. They may also complicate the treatment of rhegmatogenous retinal detachment (17). A localized retinal elevation may also develop over membranes that form beneath the neuroretina (subretinal membranes).

COMBINED TRACTIONAL RHEGMATOGENOUS RETINAL DETACHMENT

Intravitreal membranes may contract and, instead of elevating the retina, may cause one or more retinal holes with subsequent passage of vitreal fluid beneath the retina: combined tractional and rhegmatogenous retinal detachment.

TRACTIONAL MEMBRANES AS A CAUSE OF RETINAL DETACHMENT

Tractional membranes may develop at several locations within the vitreal cavity (70,77). Tractional membranes most frequently occur on the inner retinal surface, however, and a variety of terms have been applied to them, including preretinitis, preretinal membrane, and, depending on the location, epimacular, or epipapillary membrane (34,51,69,78,80–82,98,99). However, the most popular term is probably "epiretinal membrane" (15). Epiretinal membranes are the most important of the intravitreal tractional membranes, and two main types occur: fibrovascular and fibrocellular. Fibrovascular epiretinal membranes typically arise in the ischemic retinopathies, such as proliferative diabetic retinopathy or sickle cell retinopathy (see Chapter 67). Fibrocellular epiretinal membranes, which consist of several different cell types in a variable amount of collagenous tissue, may complicate a variety of conditions, including trauma and inflammation (17,28,35,49,51). Epiretinal membranes

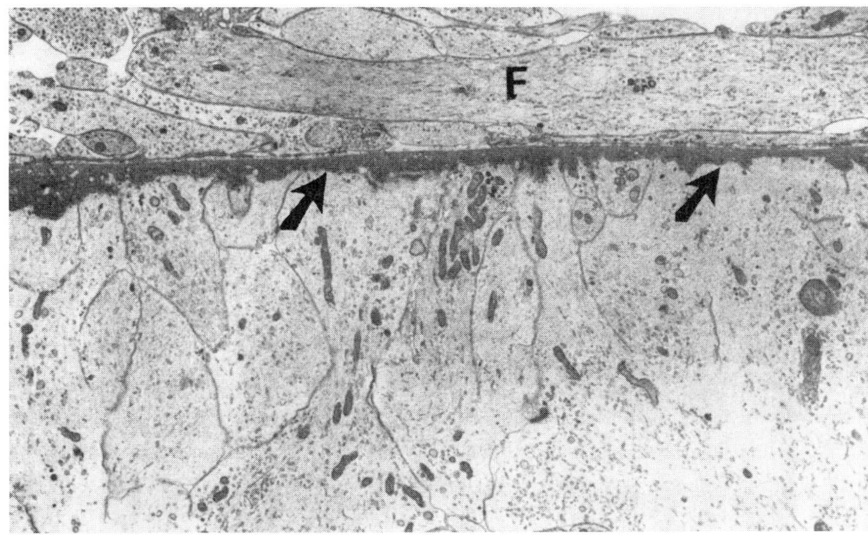

Figure 2 Transmission electron micrograph of a simple epiretinal membrane composed of closely packed cell processes (F). Note that the retinal surface is undistorted (*arrows*, inner limiting lamina) (×2,700). *Source*: Reproduced from McLeod D, Hiscott P, Grierson I. Eye 1987; 1:263–81.

may also arise de novo (idiopathic epiretinal membranes) (80). However, the most important cause of fibrocellular epiretinal membrane formation is rhegmatogenous retinal detachment itself.

TRACTIONAL MEMBRANES AS A RESULT OF RETINAL DETACHMENT

Following rhegmatogenous retinal detachment and its treatment, cells proliferate on the retinal surface in up to 60% of eyes (3). Many of these epiretinal membranes are asymptomatic, and they are often biomicroscopically invisible by virtue of their thinness. Foos (23) termed such asymptomatic membranes simple epiretinal membranes (Fig. 2). However, epiretinal membranes are estimated to be clinically problematical in approximately 10% of eyes with retinal detachment although this figure may reduce with refinements in primary retinal detachment treatment, such as adjuvant therapies (2,7,8,14). The presence of symptom-producing (complex) epiretinal membranes following retinal detachment is a manifestation of the condition known as proliferative vitreoretinopathy (PVR) (89).

PROLIFERATIVE VITREORETINOPATHY

PVR is the currently accepted term for a process that has also been called massive vitreous retraction, massive preretinal fibroplasia, massive preretinal retraction, and massive periretinal proliferation (16,66,83,90). It is characterized by the formation of contractile epiretinal, subretinal, and/or posterior hyaloid membranes as a complication of retinal detachment. Indeed, PVR is the main cause of failure in retinal detachment surgery (2,8), and most often it is marked by epiretinal membranes, although in many eyes with PVR (13.5% of cases), subretinal (or retroretinal) membranes are implicated in the development of the condition (61). Epiretinal membrane contraction causes partial- or full-thickness folds in the sensory retina (52)—that is, focal traction detachment—from tractional forces applied tangentially to the retinal surface. A localized membrane causes a stellate retinal tenting sometimes referred to as a star fold. Several terms have been applied to retinal folds in the macular area produced by an epiretinal (epimacular) membrane. Macular pucker is one of the most popular (62,88). Macular pucker may severely impair vision (69). At the other end of the spectrum, epiretinal membranes may involve a much wider area or even the entire retinal surface, leading to shortening of the retina, the (re)opening of retinal breaks, and, often, a total retinal (re)detachment (Fig. 3), which cannot be reattached unless the

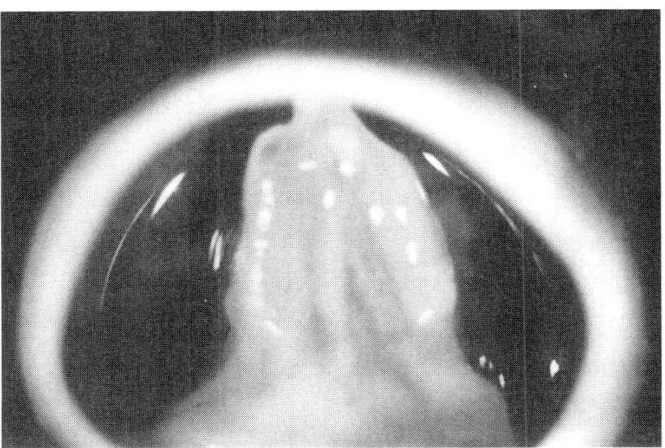

Figure 3 An eye with a completely detached, shortened retina. The retina has assumed a funnel shape, and it contains several cystic degenerative spaces.

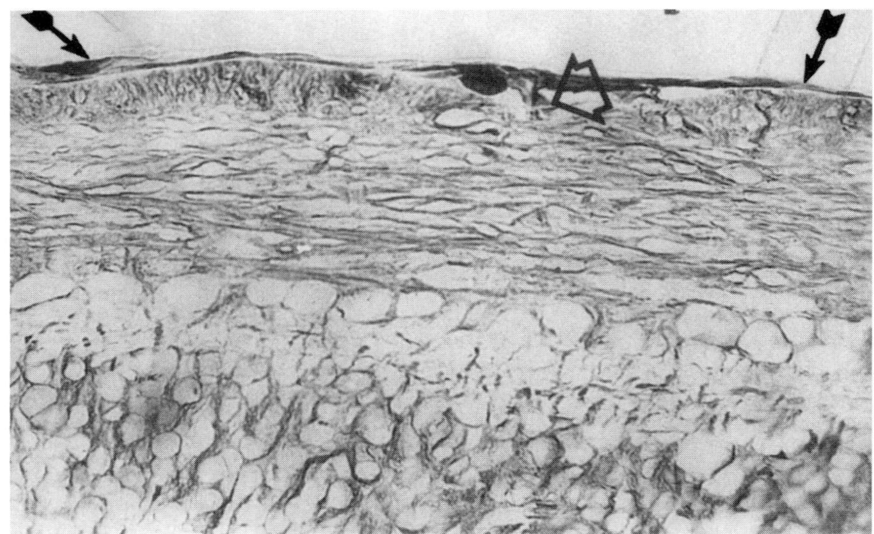

Figure 4 Section of a retina with an overlying simple epiretinal membrane (*closed arrows*) stained with immunoperoxidase for glial fibrillary acid protein (GFAP; no counterstain) and seen by light microscopy. The glial epiretinal membrane is continuous with GFAP-positive retinal elements (*open arrow*) (×480).

tractional membranes are removed, a situation requiring complex microsurgery (15).

Several different classifications of PVR based on the location and extent of membranes and associated detachments have been proposed, although no single system has been universally adopted (76).

Cellular Components

Although early investigators considered that simple epiretinal membranes were formed by endothelial cells (74), transmission electron microscopic (TEM), and immunohistochemical studies have shown that most asymptomatic membranes are composed of glial cells (Figs. 4 and 5) (23,40). By contrast, epiretinal membranes that generate traction usually have a more heterogenous structure (Fig. 6) and often contain a collagenous component (Fig. 7) (44).

The origins of the cells in contractile PVR membranes have long been a source of controversy. Parsons (75) thought that the cells were derived from vascular or perivascular sources. Studies by Machemer and coworkers on PVR membranes in human and owl monkey eyes indicated that both RPE and glial cells are major components of the tissue (67); other authors implicated hyalocytes in the human membranes (50). Most of these investigations were based on light and TEM observations.

Layers of polarized cells with apical microvilli and basal basement membrane-like material (Fig. 8) may be derived from RPE, and epiretinal glial cells

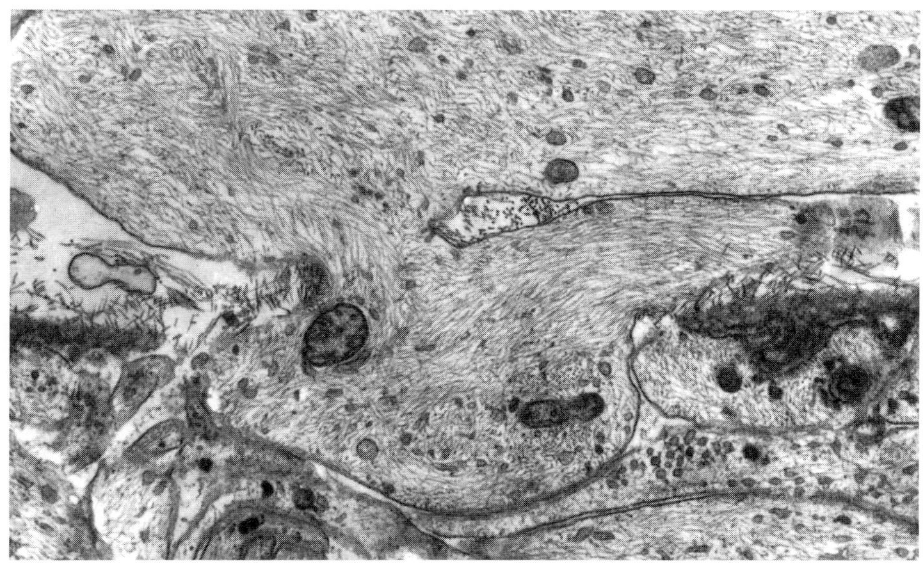

Figure 5 Transmission electron micrograph of a defect in the inner limiting lamina of the retina with an overlying simple epiretinal membrane. The glial cell within the defect has a densely filamentous appearance (×11,900). *Source*: Reproduced from McLeod D, Hiscott P, Grierson I. Eye 1987; 1:263–81.

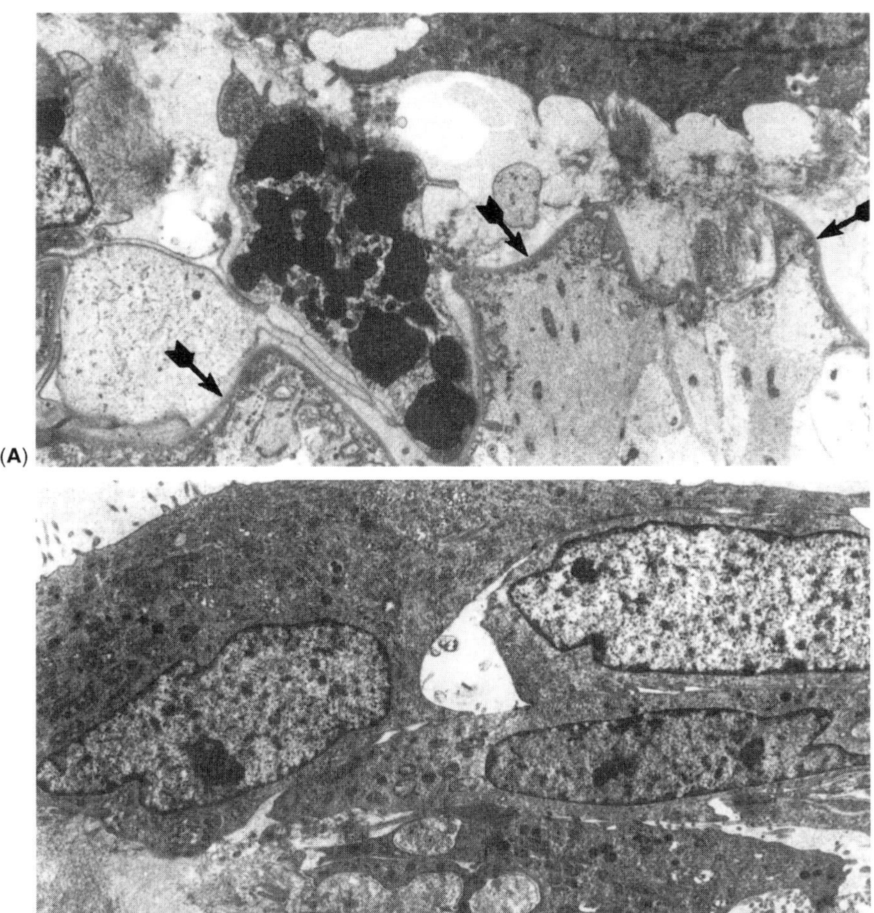

Figure 6 Transmission electron micrographs from the same tractional epiretinal membrane. (**A**) Note the gross folding of the retinal inner limiting lamina, (*arrows*) and (**A** and **B**) the heterogeneous appearance of the membrane cells (×4,500).

can form layers of filamentous cell processes that may also be polarized (30,36,64,80). However, epiretinal neuroglia and RPE often cannot be differentiated on ultrastructural criteria alone (50,95). This is because the cells appear to lose their characteristic ultrastructural features if they dedifferentiate in the membranes or undergo metaplasia and become fibroblast-like (50,73,93,95). A variety of laboratory-based studies have served to resolve the problem of the cellular origins of PVR membranes. Thus, tissue culture and immunohistochemical investigations using human biopsy specimens have highlighted the heterogeneity of cell types found in PVR membranes. Frequently, as many as four or five different cell types may be found in an individual specimen. Nevertheless, despite the use of combined laboratory techniques, it is not always possible to identify the origin of all the cells in individual PVR membranes (94).

Retinal Pigment Epithelial Cells

Analysis of the locomotor characteristics of PVR cells in tissue culture and the cytokeratin immunoreactivity of the cytoskeleton of PVR cells in vivo and in vitro (38,39,48,72) have confirmed earlier ultrastructural findings that RPE cells are present in the majority of human PVR membranes. The cytokeratin-positive cells may form epithelium-like layers in the membranes, similar to the monolayer formed by RPE in situ. Alternatively, the cells may be isolated as rounded or fibroblast-like cells (Fig. 9A). Focal RPE aggregates may also be seen (Fig. 10B). Evidence suggests that the proportion of RPE cells in PVR membranes may decrease with the clinical duration of the membrane (72).

Glial Cells

Cells with the locomotor characteristics of glial cells frequently migrate out of "explanted" PVR membrane biopsies in vitro. The migrating cells also express immunocytochemically detectable glial fibrillary acid protein (GFAP), and GFAP-positive cells are often present in tissue sections of PVR membranes (38,41). Studies of membranes both in situ in enucleated PVR eyes and in surgically excised specimens confirm that glial cells are present in human PVR membranes (Figs. 7, 9B, 10A, and 11). The similar distribution of

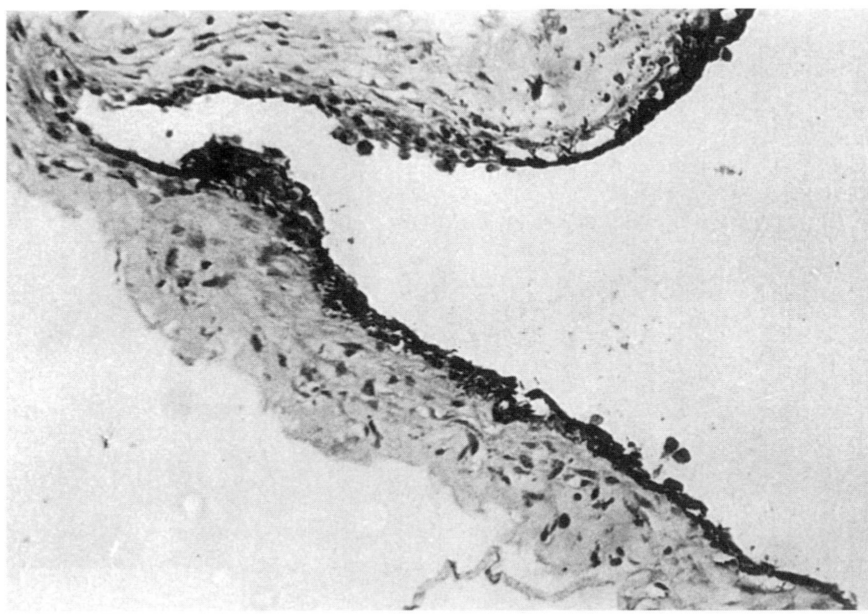

Figure 7 Light micrograph of a surgically excised proliferative vitreoretinopathy (PVR) epiretinal membrane stained with the immunoperoxidase method for glial fibrillary acidic protein (GFAP) and counterstained with hematoxylin. The glial component consists of a layer adjacent to the predominant fibrous portion (×300).

glial elements in excised and in situ membranes makes it unlikely that all the glial cells demonstrated in the former are avulsed from the retina during surgery (41), although it is recognized that portions of the ILL and Müller cell end feet are often present in the biopsies (69). The evidence suggests that both astrocytes and Müller cells contribute to the membranes (22,32,33,41).

Fibroblast-Like Cells

The presence of cytokeratin-positive fibroblast-like cells in PVR membranes (Fig. 9A) (39) is in keeping with the concept that they derive from the RPE (67). Recent investigations have determined that these trans- or dedifferentiated RPE may contain cytokeratin 7 in addition to, or instead of, the types of cytokeratin normally found in simple epithelia such as cytokeratins 8 and 18 (Fig. 12) (86). Other supplementary cytokeratins of the transdifferentiated cells include cytokeratin 19. The use of antibodies to these other cytokeratin subtypes for immunohistochemistry has improved detection of fibroblastic RPE in PVR tissues. Nevertheless, many of the spindle- and kite-shaped cells in the membranes fail to stain with either cytokeratins or GFAP, and the origins of these nonlabeling cells remains obscure (32). It is possible that some of them are derived from vascular pericytes or the advential cells of the larger retinal vessels.

Vascular Endothelial Cells

Vascular endothelial cells lining small blood vessels are found as a minor component in <20% of the epiretinal membranes of PVR. Kampik et al. (50) reported blood vessels in 17% of macular pucker membranes after retinal detachment, but none of their widespread PVR membranes contained vessels. Michels (71) found blood vessels in 8% of epiretinal membranes arising after retinal detachment.

Inflammatory Cells

Inflammatory cells are a constant, though often not prominent, component of PVR membranes. These incorporate lymphocytes (including T cells) and macrophages of hematogenous origin (4,13,38). However, some phagocytic cells in PVR membranes appear to be derived from RPE as judged by cytokeratin staining and/or tyrosinase content, and intriguingly the cells also may express the macrophage marker CD68 (86).

Pathogenesis

Factors involved in the genesis of PVR epiretinal membranes include the presence of a full-thickness break in the neuroretina, with displacement of RPE and glial cells to ectopic sites, such as into fluid vitreous or onto the vitreal surface of the neuroretina, breakdown of the blood–retina barrier, and an influx of blood-borne leukocytes. These factors may be exacerbated by retinal detachment surgery. In addition, several other clinical risk factors have been identified for PVR development, including the number and size or retinal holes, the size and duration of the retinal detachment, failure of previous retinal surgery, fixed posterior edge of retinal tears, liquefied vitreous gel with incomplete PVD, and the presence of vitreous hemorrhage (7,8). The latter are thought to enhance RPE dispersion and/or exacerbate the breakdown of the blood–retina barrier (53).

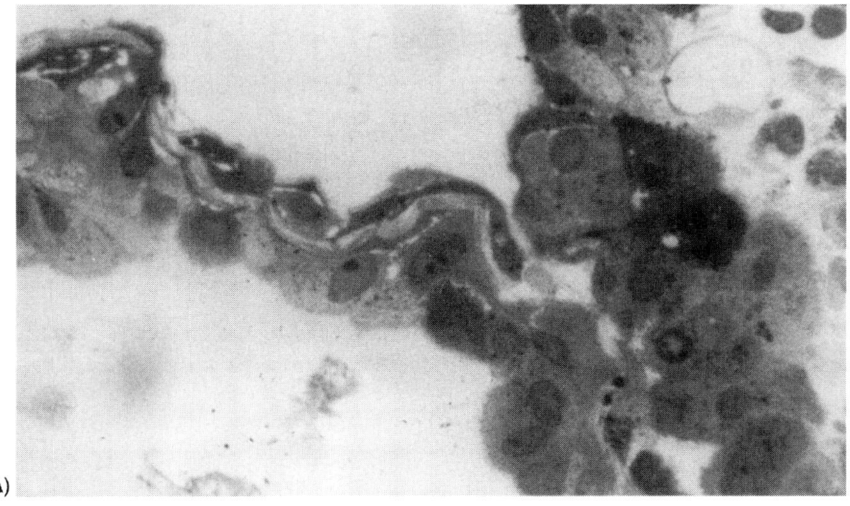

(A)

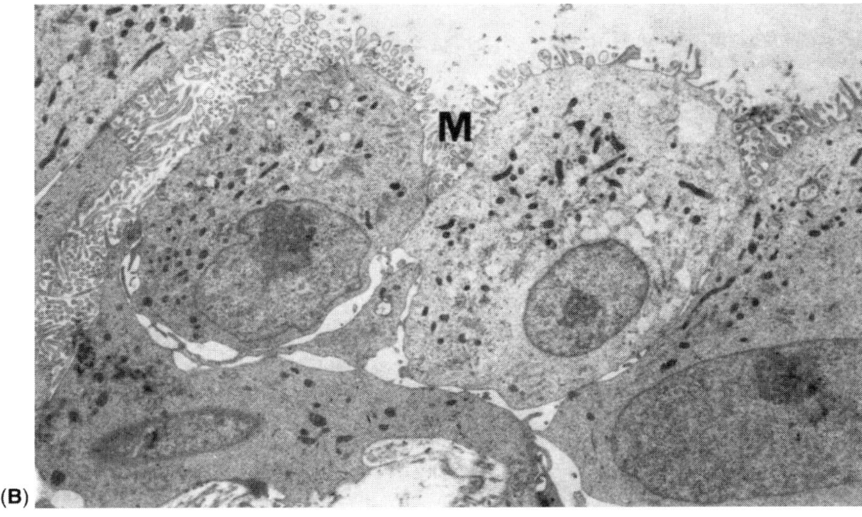

(B)

Figure 8 Sections from a surgically excised PVR membrane (**A**) Light microscopy (toluidine blue, ×900). (**B**) Transmission electron microscopy showing a layer of polarized cells with prominent microvilli (M) (×5,500).

Although the precise mechanisms of PVR formation have yet to be elucidated, a variety of studies in human and in several animal models indicate that following rhegmatogenous retinal detachment, RPE cells detach from their normal location and migrate or are swept in fluid vitreous to the retinal surfaces, where they undergo metaplasia to form several morphologic types, including macrophage- and fibroblast-like cells (21,66). The developing RPE cell membranes are then often joined by glial cells (55,84).

Glial and RPE cells undoubtedly play a major role in membrane formation, and there is evidence that inflammation is also vital in PVR formation (26). Retinal detachment surgery is associated with intraocular inflammation and epiretinal membranes may arise as a consequence of intraocular inflammation alone (7,14,26,31,41). Inflammatory cells are a consistent component of PVR membranes, and PVR-like changes can be induced by injections of agents that cause inflammation in the vitreous of various species (42).

A possible sequence of events is as follows. After rhegmatogenous retinal detachment, there is a breakdown in the blood–retina barrier, with exudation of plasma proteins into the vitreous and subretinal fluid. The plasma proteins include a number of peptide and glycoprotein growth factors. These plasma derivatives have chemotactic effects on RPE cells, and it is possible that these cells, and perhaps retinal glia, are induced to detach or migrate away from their normal locations to the surface of the detached retina (11,12). At the same time, hematogenous mononuclear cells, which are known to produce a wide variety of cytokines and growth factors (53), reach the retinal surface. Moreover, there is evidence that the epiretinal cells themselves produce further molecules with mitogenic or chemotactic properties and a number of growth factors have been identified in PVR membranes (10,24,46).

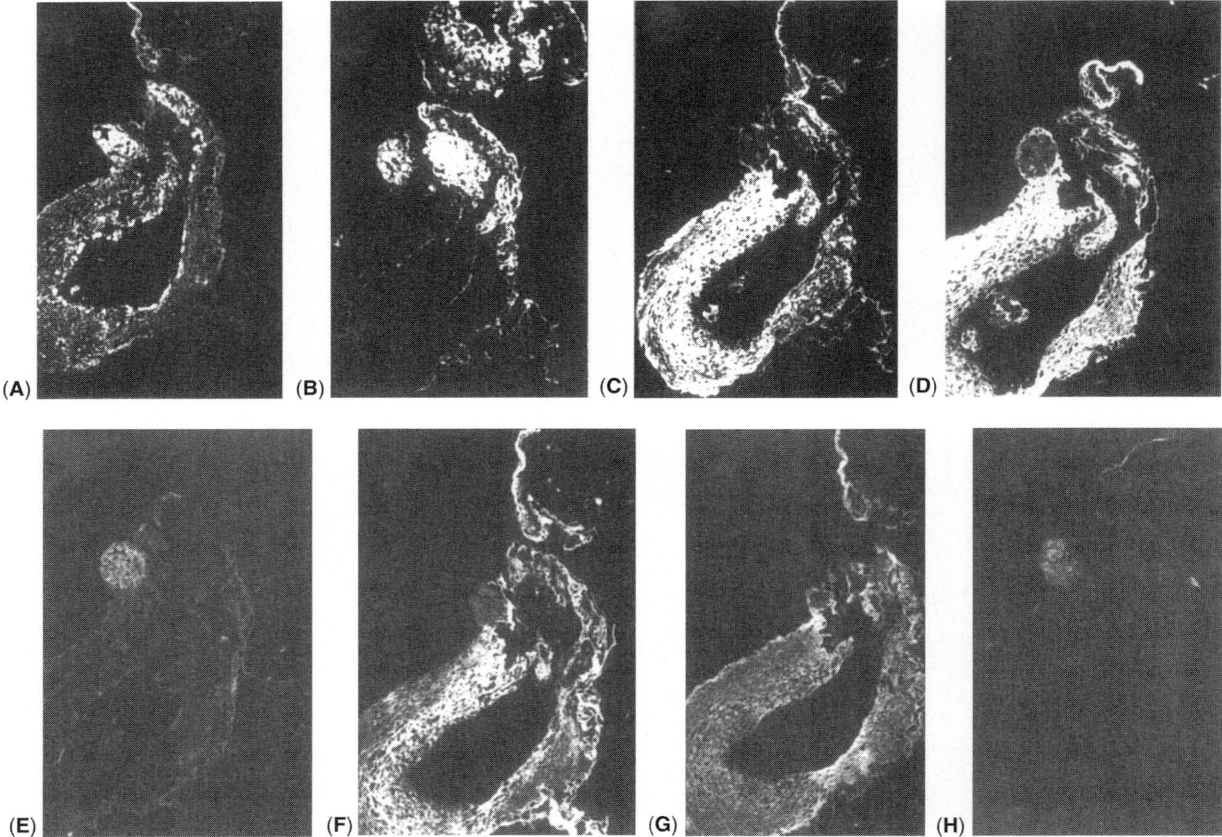

Figure 9 Serial sections from an excised proliferative vitreoretinopathy (PVR) epiretinal membrane stained by the immunofluorescent technique for (**A**) cytokeratins (a retinal pigment epithelial cell marker), (**B**) glial fibrillary corneal dystrophy (GFAP) (a glial cell marker), (**C**) collagen type I, (**D**) collagen type III, (**E**) collagen type II, (**F**) collagen type IV, (**G**) fibronectin, and (**H**) laminin. Note the widespread distribution of pigment epithelial cells; collagen types I, III, and IV; and fibronectin (×80). *Source*: Courtesy of Dr. I. Morino.

Thus inflammatory mediators and autocrine or paracrine growth control factors may collect at the retinal surfaces (46).

These chemical mediators appear to induce the cells involved in epiretinal membrane formation to behave in a fashion resembling the activities of the cells in healing wounds elsewhere in the body (18,77). Indeed, the natural course of healing wounds and PVR membranes is similar.

Natural History

During the development of PVR membranes, several phases of cellular activities can be recognized. These phases overlap to a considerable degree, but include cellular proliferation and contraction and extracellular matrix (ECM) synthesis.

Cellular Proliferation

Experimental evidence indicates that the initial stage of membrane formation is marked by proliferation of RPE cells and neuroglia (45,55,66). These early changes are likely to result from the periretinal accumulation of the mediators alluded to earlier, and at the retinal surface the cells are capable of extended proliferation (Fig. 13). Indeed, cells in the membranes may continue to replicate for several months (41). This is in contrast to the short wave of cell division seen in dermal wound healing. Nevertheless, as with dermal wounds, the hypercellular membranes are contractile (18).

Membrane Contraction

In a clinical context, membrane contraction is a major manifestation of PVR. PVR membrane contraction may result in tractional or combined traction and rhegmatogenous retinal detachment as described earlier in this chapter. If the retina is already detached, the effective shortening of the sensory retina may render conventional reattachment surgery ineffective and necessitate an intraocular approach to reappose the retina.

The mechanism of membrane contraction has elicited much interest. Experimental studies have

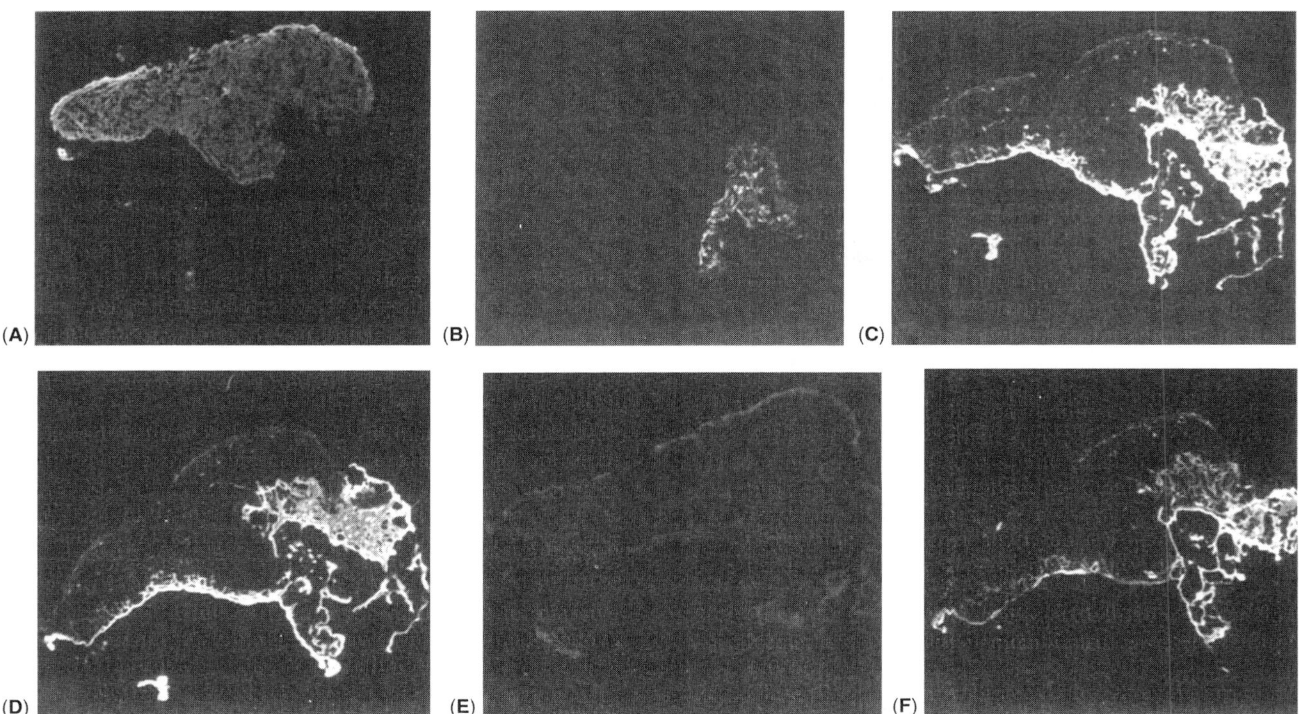

Figure 10 Serial sections from an excised proliferative vitreoretinopathy (PVR) epiretinal membrane stained by the immunofluorescent technique. (**A**) A prominent glial element is seen. (**B**) A smaller retinal pigment epithelial (cytokeratin-positive) focus is present (compare with Fig. 9A). (**C-F**) Collagen types I, III, II, and IV, respectively. Note the paucity of collagen type II immunoreactivity in this specimen (×80). *Source*: Courtesy of Dr. I. Morino.

indicated that membrane contraction is a cellular event. The presence of fibroblasts with some characteristics of smooth muscle cells (myofibroblasts) in human PVR membranes (18,50,71,91) led several authors to suggest that these cells are responsible for membrane contraction in the same way that myofibroblasts might cause contraction of wounds elsewhere in the body (25). PVR membranes may exhibit a dearth of myofibroblasts, however, as judged by the paucity of the characteristic linear actin immunoreactivity of cells in many membranes (41,79). In some instances the relative infrequency of

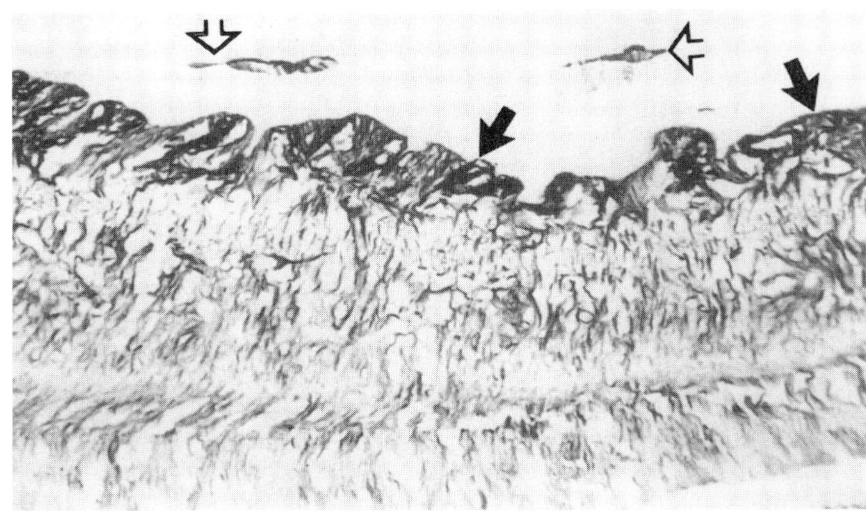

Figure 11 Section through a retinal pucker in proliferative vitreoretinopathy (PVR) stained for glial cells (no counterstain). Most of the epiretinal membrane is not visible, but two foci of glia are seen (*open arrows*). The retina stains strongly. Note the folding in the retinal surface (*solid arrows*) (×450).

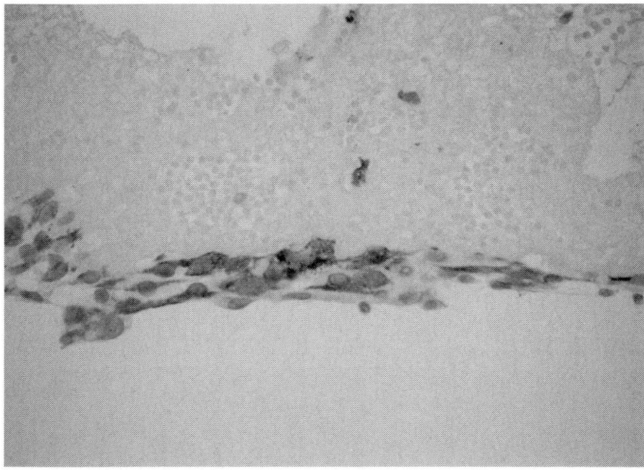

Figure 12 Fibroblastic retinal pigment epithelium (RPE) cells in a proliferative vitreoretinopathy (PVR) membrane (subretinal) labelled for cytokeratin 7 (hematoxylin counterstain). Note that most of the cells are immunoreactive for this cytokeratin subtype (×600).

myofibroblast-like cells in some PVR membranes may reflect the tendency to remove membranes at a postcontractile stage (67). Alternatively, experimental studies show that during the contractile stage of membrane formation, the cells demonstrate an intense diffuse actin staining pattern associated with cell migration (47). It is possible that cellular migration, rather than muscle-like contraction, induces the traction in PVR membranes (47). Another suggestion is that the cells "reel in" ECM components, such as collagen, thus generating tension in the membrane (27). Indeed, there is in vitro evidence that RPE cell: ECM interactions play a key role in RPE-mediated tissue contraction (85). Whatever the mechanism(s) of membrane contraction, even at an early stage in their development they appear to act as a contractile cohesive unit (41). The cohesion within early PVR membranes may relate in part to the constituents of the ECM in the tissue.

ECM Formation

Although early PVR membranes are hypercellular, they still possess some ECM (41). The ECM contains an abundance of glycoproteins such as fibronectin, vitronectin, and thrombospondin 1 (Fig. 9) (44). The glycoproteins have a wide variety of biological roles, including a putative role in cell matrix assembly. The cohesion in early PVR membranes also is conceivably due in part to the adhesive interactions between ECM glycoproteins and cell surface receptors, including those of the integrin family (see Chapter 36) (44). Although the glycoproteins in PVR membranes may be derived at least in part from plasma constituents (11,12), evidence from molecular biological studies suggests that the epiretinal cells themselves are capable of fibronectin production (43).

The epiretinal cells also produce several collagen types, including collagen types I, III, and IV (Figs. 9 and 10) (44). With time, the fibrous component of epiretinal membranes becomes more prominent and their cellularity decreases. The latter may be due to the death of cells entombed in collagen, since cells undergoing lipoidal degeneration are seen within the fibrous tissue and viable cells appear to remain in layers or foci adjacent to the fibrous component (44). Nevertheless, it is possible that some of the cells have migrated out of the collagen, while others probably undergo apoptosis (see Chapter 2) (20). Whatever the reason for the decline in tissue cellularity, the presence of cellular layers adjacent to the fibrous component,

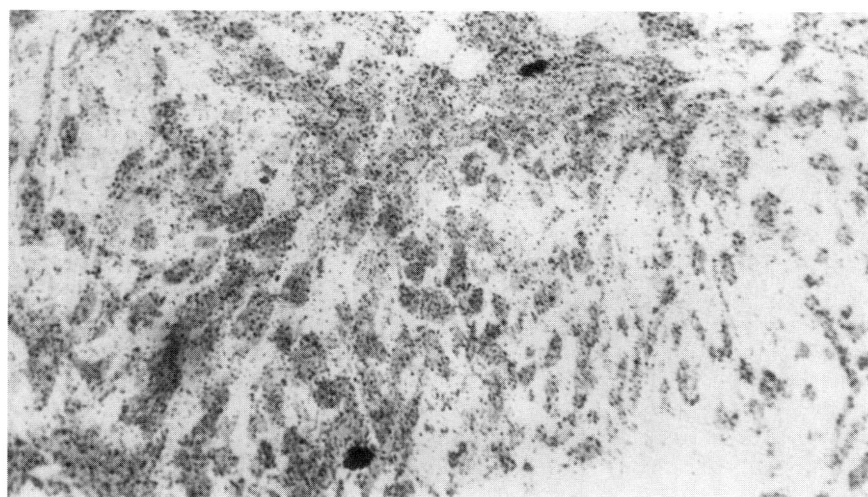

Figure 13 [^{3}H]thymidine autoradiographic section 1 μm thick counterstained with toluidine blue. The proliferative vitreoretinopathy (PVR) epiretinal membrane is hypercellular, and two cells have incorporated the label (×280).

often with strips of ILL from the retinal surface (70), can give the membranes a laminated architecture.

Hence, although the activities of the cells in PVR membranes and the consequent maturation are reminiscent of dermal wounds, profound differences between healing dermal wounds and PVR membranes also exist, not the least of which is the lack of a prominent vascular component and the protracted cellular activities in the latter.

Anterior Proliferative Vitreoretinopathy

Anterior PVR is a variant of PVR in which membranes extend from the peripheral retina to the ciliary body and/or posterior iris (19,60). These membranes may extend as far as the pupillary margin. The cellular components of anterior PVR membranes are similar to those of PVR, although blood vessels are more prominent and cells derived from adjacent structures, such as the ciliary body or perhaps the iris, may also be present (19).

Subretinal Membranes in Proliferative Vitreoretinopathy

Many membranes forming beneath the detached sensory retina consist of diffuse cell sheets, which although associated with photoreceptor loss do not appear to elevate the retina or thwart conventional retinal detachment surgery (65). These membranes are thought to consist principally of glial cells (87,92,96). Conversely, a second type of subretinal membrane composed chiefly of RPE cells is also recognized, and this tends to form bands (sometimes in an annular configuration) that serve to impede retinal reattachment (Figs. 12, 14, and 15) (46). The subretinal bands may be tensile, and, as with the epiretinal membranes of PVR, subretinal membrane tension has been attributed to the presence of myofibroblast-like cells (92). However, such cells are not always found in excised subretinal membranes (96). The cells of subretinal bands are frequently set in ECM that includes glycoproteins and various types of collagen.

PATHOLOGICAL CHANGES WITHIN THE DETACHED RETINA

Apart from the proliferation of cells on the surfaces of the detached retina, a variety of pathological changes occur within the detached retina.

Retinal Edema

Histological evaluations of specimens from monkeys, together with studies in other species including humans, have done much to further our understanding of the effects of retinal detachment (Figs. 16 and 17) (21,63). They demonstrate that the sensory retina may become diffusely edematous within 1 day of detachment, which may reflect metabolic changes in the inner retina secondary to the separation of the sensory retina from the RPE (63). The fluid collects in the extracellular spaces, and by about 3 days cystic spaces form in the inner retina. By 1 week, the edema may throw the outer retina into a series of folds, and by 2 weeks the cystic spaces extend into the outer layers of

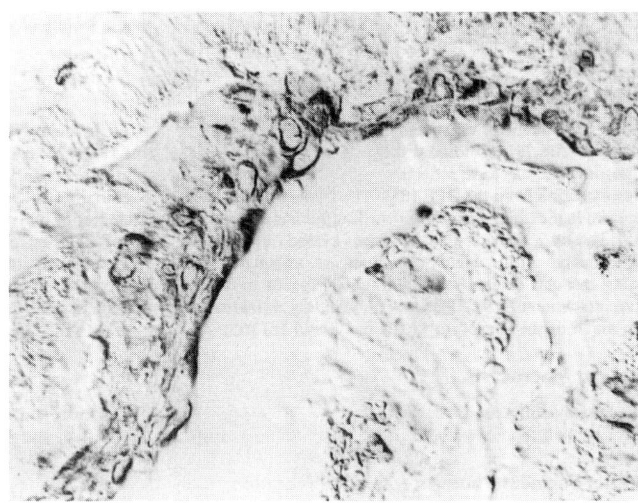

Figure 14 Differential interference contrast micrograph from a section of an excised proliferative vitreoretinopathy (PVR) subretinal membrane stained with the immunoperoxidase technique for cytokeratins (no counterstain). A prominent layer of cytokeratin-positive retinal pigment epithelial cells is seen (×340).

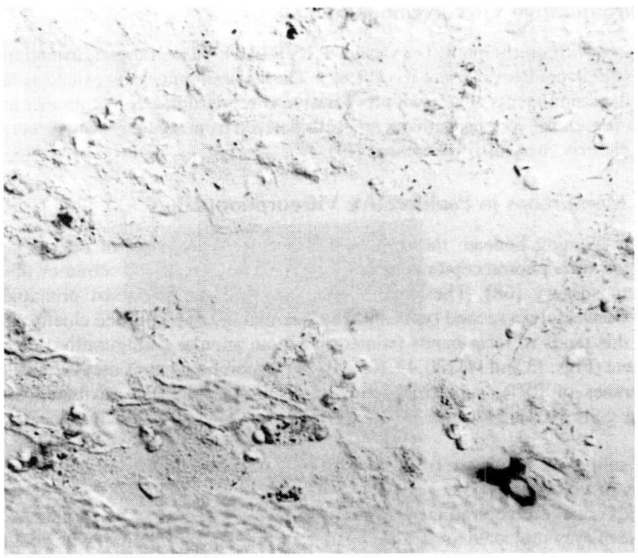

Figure 15 Section of an excised proliferative vitreoretinopathy (PVR) subretinal membrane containing a single glial cell (bottom right: revealed by immunoperoxidase stain for glial fibrillary acidic protein (GFAP) no counterstain) (×450).

the neuroretina (63). Following retinal reattachment the edema usually clears, although clinical and histological studies have identified persistent macular edema, often with cystic spaces in the outer plexiform layer, sometimes years after retinal reattachment (3,97). In long-standing retinal detachments, the cystoid spaces may expand to replace much of the sensory retina (Figs. 3 and 17). Recent studies have demonstrated that the cellular changes following retinal detachment are complicated and indicate that remodeling of both neural and glial retinal elements occur (21).

Retinal Macrocysts

In some long-standing retinal detachments, the cystoid spaces enlarge markedly and form macrocysts that may be mistaken biomicroscopically for a tumor. Such cysts are thin walled, and some contain blood.

Outer-Segment Photoreceptor Degeneration

As with retinal edema, changes in the photoreceptors occur early after retinal detachment and are also thought to reflect the dependence of the outer layers of the neuroretina on the choroidal vasculature for their metabolic requirements and the need for biochemical interactions between photoreceptors and RPE. Thus, within 1 week of detachment, some outer segments become irregular in length and contain fragmented saccules. Others contain swollen discs (54). These changes are accompanied by the accumulation of macrophage-like cells, possibly of RPE origin, around the outer edge of the outer segments (Fig. 18). If the retina remains detached the photoreceptors atrophy completely. Depending on the duration of the

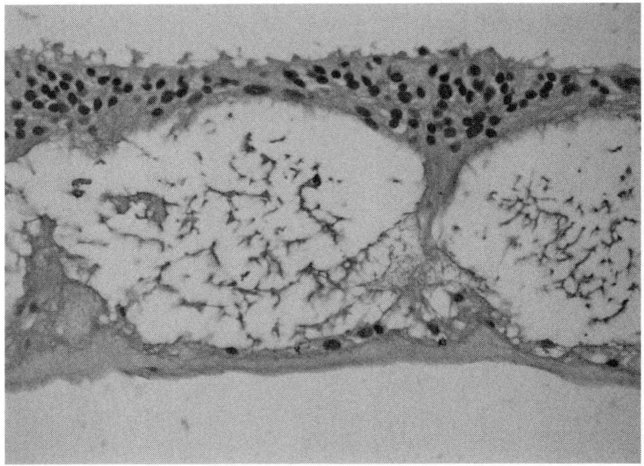

Figure 17 The neuroretina in longstanding human retinal detachment. There are large cystic spaces and widespread photoreceptor atrophy (hematoxylin and eosin, ×300).

retinal detachment, retinal reattachment may permit excellent recovery of the photoreceptors. Rods usually recover more rapidly than cones.

Retinal Pigment Epithelium

The RPE may respond to retinal detachment in several ways. Apart from the changes seen in PVR (the adoption of rounded or fibroblast-like appearances or the formation of monolayers within PVR membranes), the cells may assume a scalloped appearance, with retraction of pigment granules from the cell apices (54). Some RPE cells, particularly in the vicinity of retinal holes, show detachment from the monolayer. Elsewhere, multilayered accumulations of RPE cells,

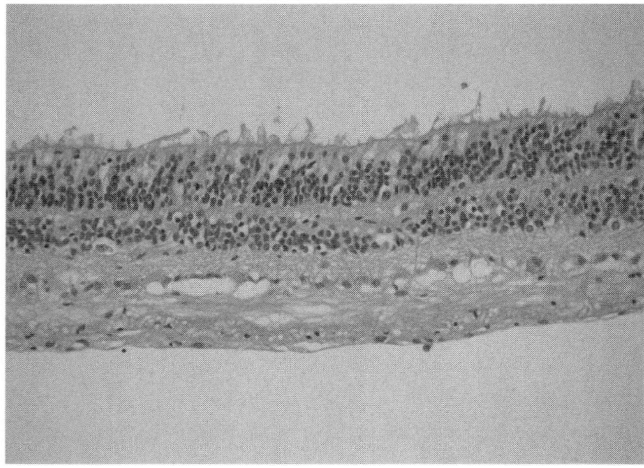

Figure 16 The neuroretina in human retinal detachment. There is retinal edema, early cyst formation, and shortening of photoreceptor outer segments (hematoxylin and eosin, ×200).

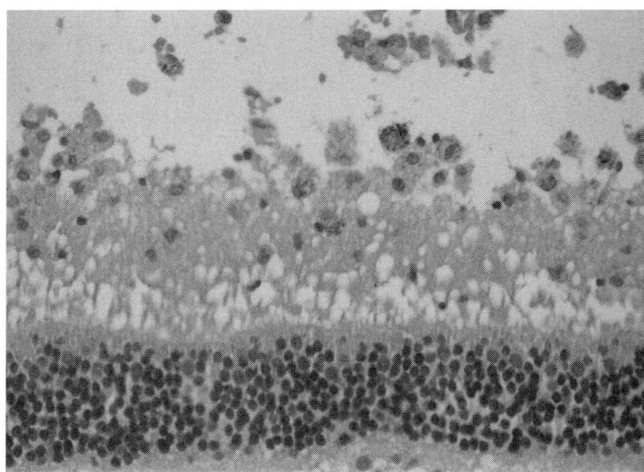

Figure 18 Human retinal detachment. Macrophage-like, variably-pigmented cells beneath and within irregular photoreceptor outer segments (hematoxylin and eosin, ×250).

including cells showing mitotic activity, provide evidence of pigment epithelial proliferation (63). If a long-standing retinal detachment involves the ora serrata, the RPE may proliferate at the ora serrata in an annular configuration along the line of attachment to produce a pigmented ring (*ringschwiele*) (Fig. 19). The RPE may also become hyperplastic at the line of residual retinal attachment and form a biomicroscopically visible, pigmented demarcation line at the site of retinal adhesion.

With successful reattachment, the RPE cells still in the monolayer eventually may regain their normal morphology.

Retinal Neuroglia

Atrophy of the photoreceptor elements is usually accompanied by a gliosis that replaces the lost cells and, possibly, part of the cystoid spaces consequent to the retinal edema.

OTHER SEQUELAE OF RETINAL DETACHMENT

Long-standing retinal detachment may also be accompanied by the formation of extensive, large drusen on Bruch membrane and uveitis. As with the ischemic retinopathies, the relatively hypoxic detached retina may release vasoproliferative factor(s) that diffuse anteriorly and stimulate neovascularization of the iris.

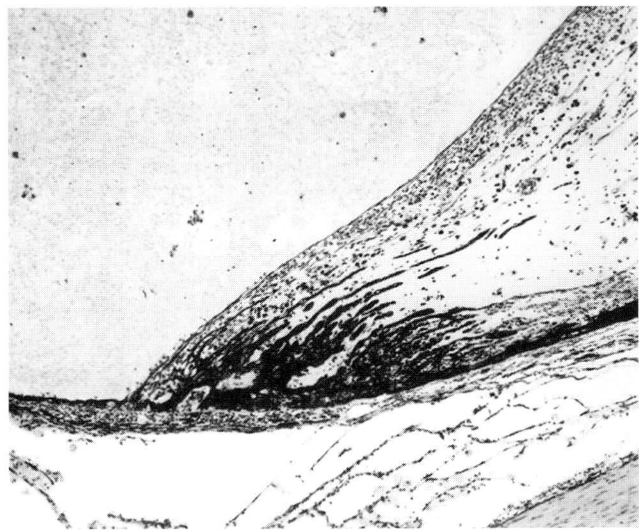

Figure 19 With chronic sensory retinal detachment a zone of retinal pigment epithelium proliferation often encircles the globe at the ora serrata (*ringschwiele*) (hematoxylin and eosin, ×35). *Source*: Reproduced from Klintworth GK, Landers MB II. The Eye. Baltimore, MD: Williams & Wilkins, 1976.

PATHOLOGICAL CHANGES DUE TO RETINAL REATTACHMENT SURGERY

Conventional Surgery

With conventional retinal reattachment surgery, "explants" (such as sponges or bands made from plastic or other synthetic material) are sewn onto the sclera to indent the globe at the site of retinal holes. This procedure is combined with a thermally or light-mediated disruption of the surrounding retina and choroid to stimulate chorioretinal scar formation and thus retinal adhesion. Subretinal fluid is also sometimes drained through a sclerotomy. Hence, eyes that have undergone conventional retinal reattachment surgery manifest a variety of histopathological features secondary to therapeutic interventions. These include changes at the sites of the explants that were sutured onto the globe. Most of the explants dissolve during routine histopathological processing, leaving an empty space surrounded by scar tissue in or adjacent to the sclera. Scleral wounds or scars may also be seen at the sites of drainage of subretinal fluid. Chorioretinal scars most commonly result from cryotherapy or photocoagulation (often produced with a laser), which destroys retinal cells by light absorption and thermal damage. Both methods destroy the RPE and outer retina in the locality of the insult, followed by an inflammatory cell infiltrate and, eventually, a fibrotic scar. RPE cells proliferate around the scar, and the overlying adherent neuroretinal remains become gliotic (68).

Vitrectomy

Some retinal detachments, such as those caused by PVR, a macular hole, or a giant retinal tear, are best treated by removing the vitreous and tamponading the retina flat with a vitreous substitute (15). The vitrectomy is often performed through three small sclerotomies at the pars plana.

A variety of vitreous substitutes have been developed (100), including gases that are gradually absorbed from the vitreous cavity. Silicone oil is sometimes used but should it be left in the globe for a long period of time, it may cause cataract, glaucoma, keratopathy, and possibly alterations in the electroretinogram response (1,16,56–59). It may also travel along the optic nerve (9). If a silicone oil-filled eye is surgically removed, the oil is lost during tissue processing, but rounded vacuoles within or between cells remain as evidence of the oil's presence in tissue sections. Such vacuoles are presumed to have contained silicone oil and are observed in the corneal endothelium, trabecular meshwork, retina, and macrophages (Fig. 20) (56,57).

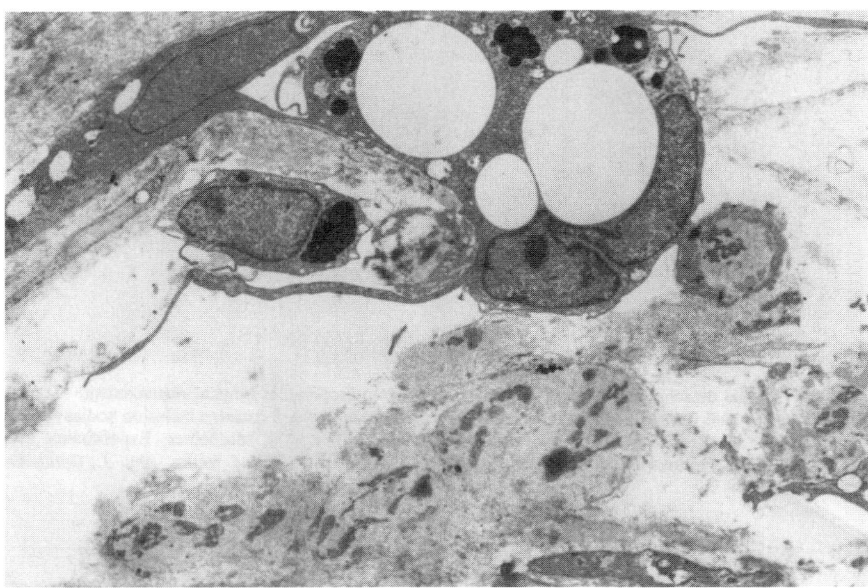

Figure 20 Transmission electron micrograph of a group of macrophage-like cells in the trabecular meshwork in an eye containing silicone oil. Note the rounded vesicle-like structures, which presumably contain silicone oil (×1,800).

Because silicone oil is lighter than water heavier-than-water tamponade agents, such as perfluorocarbon liquids and semifluorinated alkanes (SFAs) are being developed in the hope that they may be useful in the treatment of inferior retinal detachments, which may not be adequately tamponaded by silicone oil because of the its buoyancy (100). One SFA, perfluorohexyloctane (or F_6H_8), can induce a foreign-body type inflammatory response in the vitreous with a severe form of PVR, possibly because of its tendency to emulsify (45) (Fig. 21). Mixtures of silicone oil and F6H8 are being tested to determine whether they will incite less of a reaction. However, it is known that a foreign body type response occasionally complicates silicone oil in the vitreous, especially if silicone oil escapes from the vitreous (5).

Complications of Retinal Surgery

In addition to the effects of vitreous substitutes, as after other intraocular operations, retinal reattachment surgery may be followed by complications that include infection (ranging from infection of an explant site to endophthalmitis), uveitis, sympathetic ophthalmitis (see Chapter 4), and glaucoma (see Chapter 20). Subretinal hemorrhage, internal erosion of encircling bands, extrusion of explants, central retinal artery occlusion, optic atrophy, anterior segment ischemia, and PVR may also complicate surgery for retinal detachments. A rare late but important complication of retinal detachment or its treatment is a benign retinal proliferation of glial cells and blood vessels (37). The blood vessels in these vasoproliferative tumors may exhibit marked mural hyalinization. Their significance lies not only in their ability to impair vision by exudates or hemorrhage, a situation that may be amenable to treatment, but also because the vasoproliferative tumor may be confused clinically with other tumors of the retina or choroid (37). There remains a group of eyes with poor visual recovery despite successful retinal reattachment and no apparent clinical complication or histological abnormality. Barr has suggested that failures in this category may be due in part to irreversible damage at a subcellular level (3).

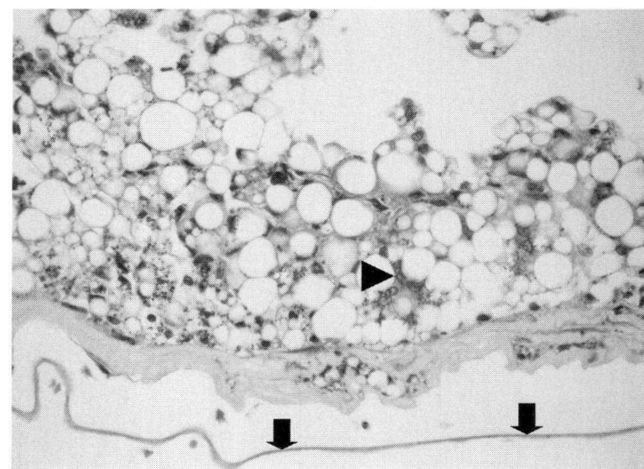

Figure 21 Hematoxylin and eosin stained section (×250) through a surgically excised proliferative vitreoretinopathy (PVR) epiretinal membrane that has arisen in the presence of a heavier-than-water tamponade agent. Numerous vacuolated, partly pigmented, macrophagic cells (including multinucleate forms, *arrowhead*) are observed in the tissue. The retinal inner limiting lamina is present (*arrows*).

REFERENCES

1. Armaly MF. Ocular tolerance to silicones. Arch Ophthalmol 1962; 68:390–5.
2. Asaria RH, Kon CH, Bunce C, et al. Adjuvant 5-fluorouracil and heparin prevents proliferative vitreoretinopathy: results from a randomized, double-blind, controlled clinical trial. Ophthalmology 2001; 108: 1179–83.
3. Barr CC. The histopathology of successful retinal detachment. Retina 1990; 10:189–94.
4. Baudouin C, Fredj-Reygrobellet D, Gordon WC, et al. Immunohistologic study of epiretinal membranes in proliferative vitreoretinopathy. Am J Ophthalmol 1990; 110:593–8.
5. Betis F, Leguay JM, Gastaud P, Hofman P. Multinucleated giant cells in periretinal silicone granulomas are associated with progressive proliferative vitreoretinopathy. Eur J Ophthalmol 2003; 13:634–41.
6. Bishop PN. Structural macromolecules and supramolecular organisation of the vitreous gel. Prog Retin Eye Res 2000; 19:323–44.
7. Bonnet M. Clinical factors predisposing to massive proliferative vitreoretinopathy in rhegmatogenous retinal detachment. Ophthalmologica 1984; 188: 148–58.
8. Bonnet M. Clinical findings associated with the development of postoperative PVR in primary rhegmatogenous retinal detachment. In: Heimann K, Wiedemann P, eds. Proliferative Vitreoretinopathy. Heidelberg, Germany: Kaden, 1989:18–20.
9. Budde M, Cursiefen C, Holbach LM, Naumann GO. Silicone oil-associated optic nerve degeneration. Am J Ophthalmol 2001; 131:392–4.
10. Burke JM. Cell interactions in proliferative vitreoretinopathy: do growth factors play a role? In: Heimann K, Wiedemann R, eds. Proliferative Vitreoretinopathy. Heidelberg, Germany: Kaden, 1989:80–7.
11. Campochiaro PA, Jerdan JA, Glaser BM. Serum contains chemoattractants for human retinal pigment epithelial cells. Arch Ophthalmol 1984; 102:1830–3.
12. Campochiaro RA, Jerdan JA, Glaser BM, et al. Vitreous aspirates from patients with proliferative vitreoretinopathy stimulate retinal pigment epithelial cell migration. Arch Ophthalmol 1985; 103:403–1405.
13. Charteris DG, Hiscott R, Grierson I, Lightman SL. Proliferative vitreoretinopathy: lymphocytes in epiretinal membranes. Ophthalmology 1992; 99:1364–7.
14. Chignell AH, Fison LG, Davies EWG, et al. Failure in retinal detachment surgery. Br J Ophthalmol 1973; 57:525–30.
15. Cibis PA. Recent methods in the surgical treatment of retinal detachment: intravitreal procedures. Trans Ophthalmol Soc UK 1965; 85:111–26.
16. Cibis PA, Becker B, Okun E, Canaan S. The use of liquid silicone in retinal detachment. Arch Ophthalmol 1962; 68: 590–9.
17. Clarkson JG, Green WR, Massof D. A histopathologic view of 168 cases of preretinal membrane. Am J Ophthalmol 1977; 84:1–17.
18. Constable IJ, Tolentino EL, Donovan RH, Schepens CL. Clinico-pathologic correlation of vitreous membranes. In: Pruett RD, Regan DJ, eds. Retinal Congress. New York: Appleton-Century-Crofts, 1974:254–7.
19. Elner SG, Elner VM, Diaz-Rohena R, et al. Anterior proliferative vitreoretinopathy; clinical, light microscopic, and ultrastructural findings. Ophthalmology 1988; 95: 1349–57.
20. Esser P, Bartz-Schmidt KU, Walter P, et al. Apoptotic cell death in proliferative vitreoretinopathy. Ger J Ophthalmol 1996; 5:73–8.
21. Fisher SK, Lewis GP, Linberg KA. Verardo MR. Cellular remodeling in mammalian retina: results from studies of experimental retinal detachment. Prog Retin Eye Res 2005; 24:395–431.
22. Foos RY. Vitreoretinal juncture; topographical variations. Invest Ophthalmol 1972; 11:801–8.
23. Foos RY. Vitreoretinal juncture—simple epiretinal membranes. Graefes Arch Clin Exp Ophthalmol 1974; 189: 231–50.
24. Fredj-Reygrobellet D, Baudouin C, Negre E, et al. Acidic FGF and other growth factors in preretinal membranes from patients with diabetic retinopathy and proliferative vitreoretinopathy. Ophthalmic Res 1991; 25:154–61.
25. Gabbiani G, Hirschel BT, Ryan GB, et al. Granulation tissue as a contractile organ. A study of structure and function. J Exp Med 1972; 135:119–734.
26. Gilbert C, Hiscott P, Unger W, et al. Inflammation and the formation of epiretinal membranes. Eye 1988; 2(Suppl): 140–56.
27. Glaser BM, Cardin A, Biscoe B. Proliferative vitreoretinopathy: the mechanism of development of vitreoretinal traction. Ophthalmology 1987; 94:327–32.
28. Gloor BR, Werner H. Postkoagulation und spontan auftretende internoretinale Fibroplasie mit Macula- degeneration. Klin Monatsbl Augenheilkd 1967; 151:822–45.
29. Gonin J. Detachment of the retina and its treatment. Trans Ophthalmol Soc UK 1930; 50:531–51.
30. Green WR, Kenyon KR, Michels RG, et al. Ultrastructure of epiretinal membranes causing macular pucker after retinal re-attachment surgery. Trans Ophthalmol Soc UK 1979; 99:65–77.
31. Green WR, Kincaid MC, Michels RG, et al. Parsplanitis. Trans Ophthalmol Soc UK 1981; 101:361–7.
32. Grierson I, Hiscott PS, Hitchins CA, et al. Which cells are involved in the formation of epiretinal membranes? Semin Ophthalmol 1987; 2:99–109.
33. Guerin CJ, Wolfshagen RW, Eifrig DE, Anderson DH. Immunocytochemical identification of Mueller's glia as a component of human epiretinal membranes. Invest Ophthalmol Vis Sci 1990; 31:1483–91.
34. Hamilton AM. Pre-retinal traction membranes. Trans Ophthalmol Soc UK 1972; 92:387–93.
35. Hansen RI, Friedman AH, Gartner S, Henkind R. The association of retinitis pigmentosa with preretinal macular gliosis. Br J Ophthalmol 1977; 61:579–600.
36. Harada T, Chauvaud D, Pouliquen Y. An electron microscopic study of the epiretinal membrane of human eyes. Graefes Arch Clin Ophthalmol 1981; 215:327–39.
37. Heimann H, Bornfeld N, Vij O, Coupland SE, et al. Vasoproliferative tumours of the retina. Br J Ophthalmol 2000; 84:1162–9.
38. Hiscott PS, Grierson I, Hitchins CA, et al. Epiretinal membranes in vitro. Trans Ophthalmol Soc UK 1983; 103: 89–102.
39. Hiscott PS, Grierson I, McLeod D. Retinal pigment epithelial cells in epiretinal membranes: an immunohistochemical study. Br J Ophthalmol 1984; 68:708–15.
40. Hiscott PS, Grierson I, Trombetta CJ, et al. Retinal and epiretinal glia: an immunohistochemical study. Br J Ophthalmol 1984; 68:698–707.

41. Hiscott PS, Grierson I, McLeod D. Natural history of fibrocellular epiretinal membranes: a quantitative, autoradiographic and immunohistochemical study. Br J Ophthalmol 1985; 69:810–23.
42. Hiscott PS, Unger WG, Grierson I, McLeod D. The role of inflammation in the development of epiretinal membranes. Curr Eye Res 1988; 7:877–92.
43. Hiscott P, Waller HA, Butler MG, et al. Local production of fibronectin by ectopic human retinal cells. Cell Tissue Res 1992; 267:185–92.
44. Hiscott P, Sheridan C, Magee R Grierson I. Matrix and the retinal pigment epithelium in proliferative retinal disease. Prog Retinal Eye Res 1999; 18:167–90.
45. Hiscott P, Magee RM, Colthurst M, et al. Clinicopathological correlation of epiretinal membranes and posterior lens opacification following perfluorohexyloctane (F6H8) tamponade. Br J Ophthalmol 2001; 85:179–83.
46. Hiscott P, Hagan S, Heathcote L, et al. Pathobiology of epiretinal and subretinal membranes: possible roles for the matricellular proteins thrombospondin 1 and osteonectin (SPARC). Eye 2002; 16:393–403.
47. Hitchins CA, Grierson I, Rahi AHS. Contraction of scar tissue in the rabbit vitreous. Connect Tissue Res 1986; 15: 123–40.
48. Jerdan JA, Pepose JS, Michels RG, et al. Proliferative vitreoretinopathy membranes an immunohistochemical study. Ophthalmology 1988; 96:801–10.
49. Kampik A. Die proliferative vitreoretinale Reaktion. Excerpta Med (Ophthalmol) 1984; 38:75–8.
50. Kampik A, Kenyon KR, Michels RG, et al. Epiretinal and vitreous membranes: Comparative study of 56 cases. Arch Ophthalmol 1981; 99:1445–54.
51. Klein BA. Concerning the pathogenesis of retinal holes. Am J Ophthalmol 1955; 40:512–22.
52. Kleinert H. Primare Netzhautfaltelungim Maculabereich. Graefes Arch Kiln Exp Ophthalmol 1954; 155:350–8.
53. Kon CH, Tranos G, Aylward GW. Risk factors in proliferative vitreoretinopathy. In: Kirchlof B, Wong D, eds. Vitreo-retinal Surgery. Essentials in Ophthalmology. Berlin, Germany: Springer, 2005:120–34.
54. Kroll AJ, Machemer R. Experimental retinal detachment in the owl monkey. III. Electron microscopy of the retina and pigment epithelium. Am J Ophthalmol 1968; 66: 410–27.
55. Laqua H, Machemer R. Glial cell proliferation in retinal detachment (massive periretinal proliferation). Am J Ophthalmol 1975; 80:602–18.
56. Leaver PK, Grey RHB, Garner A. Silicone oil injection in the treatment of massive preretinal retraction. II. Late complications in 93 eyes. Br J Ophthalmol 1979; 63:361–7.
57. Leaver PK, Grey RHB, Garner A. Complications following silicone-oil injection. Mod Probl Ophthalmol 1979; 20: 290–4.
58. Levenson DS, Stocker EW, Georgiade NG. Intracorneal silicone oil. Arch Ophthalmol 1965; 73:90–3.
59. Levine AM, Ellis RA. Intraocular liquid silicone implants. Am J Ophthalmol 1963; 55:939–43.
60. Lewis H, Aaberg TM. Anterior proliferative vitreoretinopathy. Am J Ophthalmol 1988; 105:277–84.
61. Lewis H, Aaberg TM, Abrams GW, et al. Subretinal membranes in proliferative vitreoretinopathy. Ophthalmology 1989; 96:1403–15.
62. Lincoff HA, McLean J. Cryosurgical treatment of retinal detachment, part II. Am J Ophthalmol 1965; 61:287–94.
63. Machemer R. Experimental retinal detachment in the owl monkey. II. Histology of the retina and pigment epithelium. Am J Ophthalmol 1968; 66:396–410.
64. Machemer R. Pathogenesis and classification of massive periretinal proliferation. Br J Ophthalmol 1978; 62:737–47.
65. Machemer R. Discussion of presentation by Federman JL, Foldberg R, Ridley M, Arbizo VA. Subretinal cellular bands. Trans Am Ophthalmol Soc 1983; 81:172–80.
66. Machemer R, Laqua H. Pigment epithelial proliferation in retinal detachment (massive periretinal proliferation). Am J Ophthalmol 1975; 80:1–23.
67. Machemer R, van Horn D, Aaberg TM. Pigment epithelial proliferation in human retinal detachment with massive periretinal proliferation. Am J Ophthalmol 1978; 85: 181–91.
68. Marshall J, Mellerio J. Pathological development of retinal laser photocoagulations. Exp Eye Res 1967; 6: 303–8.
69. McLeod D, Marshall J, Grierson I. Epimacular membrane peeling. Trans Ophthalmol Soc UK 1981; 101:170–80.
70. McLeod D. The vitreous and its disorders. In: Miller S, ed. Clinical Ophthalmology. Bristol, UK: Wright, 1987:258–74.
71. Michels RG. A clinical and histopathological study of epiretinal membranes affecting the macular and removed by vitreous surgery. Trans Am Ophthalmol Soc 1982; 80: 580–656.
72. Morino I, Hiscott R, McKechnie N, Grierson I. Variation in epiretinal membrane components with clinical duration of the proliferative tissue. Br J Ophthalmol 1990; 74:393–9.
73. Müller-Jensen K, Machemer R, Azarnia R. Autotransplantation of retinal pigment epithelium in intravitreal diffusion chamber. Am J Ophthalmol 1975; 80:530–7.
74. Nordenson E. Die netzhautblosung, untersuchung uber deren pathologische anatomie und pathogenese. Wiesbaden, Germany: JF Bergmann, 1887:1–255.
75. Parsons JH. Pathol Eye, Vol. 2. London, UK: Hodder & Stoughton, 1905:542–600.
76. Pastor JC, Rodríguez de la Rúa E, Martín F. Proliferative vitreoretinopathy: risk factors and pathobiology. Prog Retin Eye Res 2002; 21:127–44.
77. Reeser FH, Aaberg TM. Vitreous humor. In: Records RE, ed. The Physiology of the Human Eye and Visual System. Hagerstown, UK: Harper & Row, 1979:261–95.
78. Robertson DM, Buettner H. Pigmented preretinal membranes. Am J Ophthalmol 1977; 83:824–9.
79. Rodrigues MM, Newsome DA, Machemer R. Further characterization of epiretinal membranes in human massive periretinal proliferation. Curr Eye Res 1981; 1: 311–5.
80. Roth AM, Foos RY. Surface wrinkling retinopathy in eyes enucleated at autopsy. Trans Am Acad Ophthalmol Otolaryngol 1971; 75:1047–58.
81. Roth AM, Foos RY. Surface structure of the optic nerve head. I. Epipapillary membranes. Am J Ophthalmol 1972; 74:977–85.
82. Samuels B. Opacities of the vitreous. Arch Ophthalmol 1930; 4:838–57.
83. Schepens CL. Retinal detachment and aphakia. Arch Ophthalmol 1951; 45:1–15.
84. Sethi CS, Lewis GP, Fisher SK, et al. Glial remodeling and neural plasticity in human retinal detachment with proliferative vitreoretinopathy. Invest Ophthalmol Vis Sci 2005; 46:329–42.
85. Sheridan CM, Occleston NL, Hiscott P, et al. Matrix metalloproteinases: a role in the contraction of vitreoretinal scar tissue. Am J Pathol 2001; 159:1555–66.
86. Sheridan C, Hiscott P, Grierson I. Retinal pigment epithelium: differentiation and dedifferentiation. In: Kirchhof B,

Wong D, eds. Vitreo-retinal Surgery. Essentials in Ophthalmology. Berlin, Germany: Springer, 2005:101–19.
87. Sternberg P, Machemer R. Subretinal proliferation. Am J Ophthalmol 1984; 98:456–62.
88. Tanenbaum HL, Schepens CL, Elzenedeiny L, MacKenzie Freeman H. Macular pucker following retinal surgery-a biomicroscopic study. Can J Ophthalmol 1969; 4:20–23.
89. Terminology Committee, Retina Society. The classification of retinal detachment with proliferative vitreoretinopathy. Ophthalmology 1983; 90:121–5.
90. Tolentino EL, Schepens CL, Freeman HM. Massive preretinal retraction: a biomicroscopic study. Arch Ophthalmol 1967; 78:16–22.
91. Trese M, Chandler DB, Machemer R. Macular pucker. II. Ultrastructure. Graefes Arch Clin Exp Ophthalmol 1983; 221:16–26.
92. Trese MT, Chandler DB, Machemer R. Subretinal strands: ultrastructural features. Graefes Arch Clin Exp Ophthalmol 1985; 223:35–40.
93. Vidaurri-Leal J, Hohman R, Glaser BM. Effect of vitreous on morphologic characteristics of retinal pigment epithelial cells: a new approach to the study of proliferative vitreoretinopathy. Arch Ophthalmol 1984; 102:1220–3.
94. Vinores SA, Campochiaro PA, Conway BR Ultrastructural and electron-immunocytochemical characterization of cells in epiretinal membranes. Invest Ophthalmol Vis Sci 1990; 31:14–28.
95. Vinores SA, Conway BP, Campochiaro PA. Comparison of ultrastructural characteristics and intermediate filament protein expression in cells of epiretinal membranes. Invest Ophthalmol Vis Sci 1988; 29 (Suppl):305.
96. Wilkes SR, Mansour AM, Green WR. Proliferative vitreoretinopathy histopathology of retroretinal membranes. Retina 1987; 7:94–101.
97. Wilson DJ, Green WR. Histopathologic study of the effect of retinal detachment surgery on 49 eyes obtained post mortem. Am J Ophthalmol 1987; 103:167–79.
98. Wise GN. Preretinal macular fibrosis. Trans Ophthalmol Soc UK 1972; 92:131–40.
99. Wolter JR. Glia of the human retina. Am J Ophthalmol 1959; 48:310–92.
100. Wong D, Williams R. The tamponade effect. In: Kirchhof B, Wong D, eds. Vitreoretinal surgery. Essentials in Ophthalmology. Berlin, Germany: Springer, 2005: 147–61.

29

Disorders of the Vitreous

Paul N. Bishop
Faculty of Medical and Human Sciences and Wellcome Trust Centre for Cell-Matrix Research, University of Manchester, Manchester, U.K.

COMPOSITION OF THE VITREOUS

The vitreous is a fascinating and unique structure composed of extracellular matrix (ECM) and very few cells. Despite its accessibility and large volume, many aspects of its biochemistry, physiology, and pathobiology have proved difficult to unravel. The vitreous is highly hydrated, composed of approximately 99% water, and its macromolecular components include collagen, glycosaminoglycans (GAGs), proteoglycans, glycoproteins, and other proteins (8).

The fine network of collagen fibrils contained within the vitreous imparts gel-like properties and removal of this network converts the gel into a viscous liquid. Furthermore, it is through this network of collagen fibrils that tractional forces are transmitted in vitreoretinal diseases. The concentration of collagen in the human vitreous is approximately 300 μg/mL (2). The fibrils are unbranched, of uniform diameter and unusually thin (10–20 nm depending upon species). Transmission electron microscopic (TEM) examination of stained fibrils reveals a faint ~ 64 nm D-periodicity typical of fibrillar collagens (Fig. 1A) (12).

The vitreous collagen fibrils are heterotypic (of mixed composition) with three different types of collagen, i.e., collagen type II, collagen type V/XI, and collagen type IX (8); cartilage collagen fibrils have a

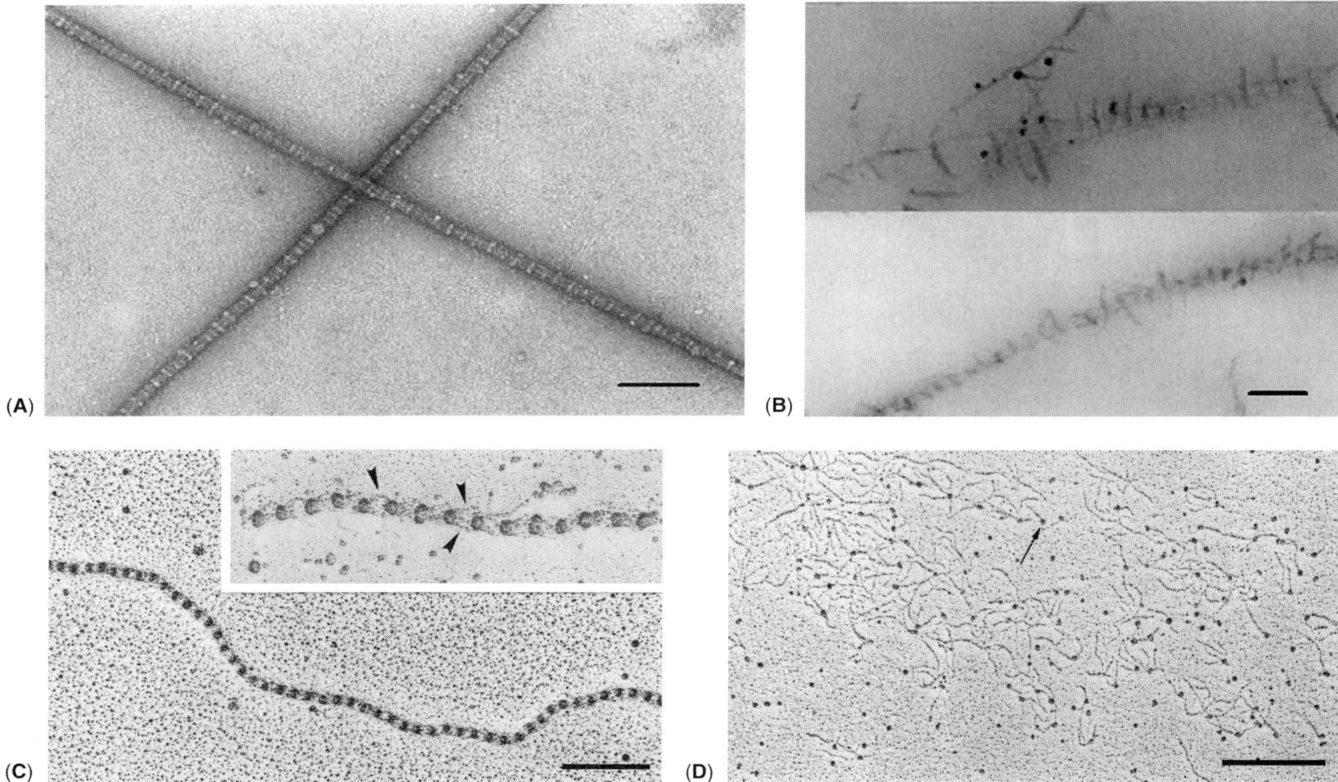

Figure 1 Ultrastructure of vitreous. Transmission electron microscopy of vitreous. (**A**) Two negatively stained vitreous collagen fibrils. They are 15 nm in diameter and show a banding pattern with a 64 nm periodicity (bar = 100 nm). (**B**) Two images of vitreous collagen fibrils stained with cupromeronic blue and uranyl acetate. Cupromeronic blue stains the filaments that extend away from the collagen fibrils and often appear to bridge between adjacent fibrils; these filaments are the chondroitin sulfate chains of collagen type IX proteoglycan (bar = 200 nm). Rotary shadowing electron microscopy. (**C**) A fibrillin-containing microfibril (bar = 300 nm); inset shows the detailed structure of the microfibril with fine filaments (*arrows*) connecting bead-like structures. (**D**) The network of hyaluronan in the vitreous. Globular structures (*arrow*) that are presumed to be proteins associate with the hyaluronan (bar = 300 nm).

very similar composition. The predominant collagen is collagen type II, representing 60% to 75% of the collagen in the fibrils. Collagen type II is a fibrillar collagen composed of three identical polypeptide chains, i.e., $\alpha 1(II)_3$. Fibrillar collagens are synthesized as procollagens with amino- and carboxy-terminal propeptides, that are largely removed during fibril formation (see Chapter 44), but retained amino-propeptides have been demonstrated on mature vitreous collagen fibrils (63). Some, but not all of these amino-propeptides contain an additional domain encoded by exon 2, but due to alternative mRNA splicing this form is absent from cartilage procollagen type II (5). This is a von Willebrand factor type C domain that potentially interacts with transforming growth factor β (TGFβ) and bone morphogenetic protein-2.

Collagen type V/XI is a fibrillar collagen that contains polypeptide chains derived from both collagen type V and collagen type XI (8). This collagen has been estimated to represent between 10% and 25% of the collagen in the vitreous fibrils. It contains the α1(XI) and α2(V) chains, but the identity of the third α-chain is uncertain (50). By contrast, the cartilage form of this collagen contains the α1(XI), α2(XI), and α3(XI) chains. The closely related collagen type V is found in skin and cornea, and there is evidence that collagen type V plays an essential role in the initiation of collagen fibril formation (86); given the similarities between collagen type V and type V/XI it is likely that the collagen type V/XI of vitreous performs a similar role.

The third collagen is collagen type IX and this has been estimated to represent up to 25% of the collagen in the vitreous fibrils. This is not a fibrillar collagen, but rather a fibril-associated collagen with interrupted triple helices (FACIT) that is covalently linked to the surface of the collagen fibrils in a D-periodic manner. It contains three distinct α-chains, namely, α1(IX), α2(IX), and α3(IX). Collagen type IX has three triple-helical domains (COL1–3) and four noncollagenous domains (NC1–4) and also possesses a chondroitin sulfate chain covalently bound to its α2-chain. Its structure varies between different tissues and species. Vitreous collagen type IX lacks the NC4 globular domain that is present in cartilage. In mammalian vitreous collagen type IX has a relatively short chondroitin sulfate chain (Fig. 1B), compared to chick vitreous (6,90).

A number of glycoproteins associate with the surface of vitreous collagen fibrils including vitrin and opticin (51,64). Vitrin is a member of the superfamily that contains von Willebrand type A domains and it is probably the same as akhirin, a molecule expressed by the lens epithelium and ciliary marginal zone during chick eye development (1). Its functions are currently unknown. Opticin was initially identified as the major component of a pool of molecules closely associated with vitreous collagen fibrils (64). It is a homodimeric member of the small leucine-rich repeat protein/proteoglycan family and, uniquely for a member of this family, possesses a cluster of sialylated O-linked oligosaccharides instead of GAG chains (44,64).

The heterotypic collagen fibrils are not the only insoluble fibrillar structures in the vitreous. The ocular zonules are composed of bundles of fibrillin-containing beaded microfibrils; these microfibrils are also present in a low concentration throughout the vitreous (Fig. 1C) (89). In other tissues fibrillin-containing microfibrils typically associate with elastin, but this is not present in the vitreous or zonules. The vitreous also contains small amounts of collagen type VI microfibrils. The developing vitreous contains soluble collagen monomers and various basement membrane components including collagen type IV, collagen type XVIII, laminin-1, perlecan, and agrin (8,30), but their levels decrease markedly after birth.

Filling the spaces between the collagen fibrils is a meshwork of hyaluronan (also called hyaluronic acid or hyaluronate) and this is the major GAG in mammalian vitreous (8). In the concentrations found in vitreous, hyaluronan forms a viscous liquid that contributes to its biomechanical properties. In the human eye the hyaluronan concentration has been estimated to be 65 to 400 μg/mL and its molecular weight to be 2 to 4 million (3). Hyaluronan consists of long chains of repeating units of glucuronic acid and *N*-acetylglucosamine, and a large negative charge allows it to form highly hydrated networks. Biochemical studies have shown that the large proteoglycan versican is present in vitreous and probably binds to the hyaluronan in an interaction stabilized by link protein (62). Rotary shadowing experiments appear to show the hyaluronan network interacting with small globular structures that are presumed to be proteins or glycoproteins (Fig. 1D).

The vitreous also contains other proteins and glycoproteins, some derived from plasma and others are derived locally, with major components being albumin and transferrin. The vitreous contains locally synthesized transthyretin and this is important in familial amyloid polyneuropathy (FAP) (41). Macromolecules with potentially important biological actions include inhibitors of angiogenesis. Conversely, growth factors, some of which are proangiogenic, have been isolated from the vitreous and are found at increased levels in pathological states associated with neovascularization and cellular proliferation in the vitreous cavity. The vitreous also contains high levels of vitamin C, which has antioxidant properties, and contains lipid moieties of uncertain origin.

SUPRAMOLECULAR ORGANIZATION OF THE VITREOUS

The collagen fibrils impart gel-like properties to the vitreous and, as they are nonuniformly distributed, some parts of the gel are more rigid than others. There is a relatively high concentration of collagen in the basal vitreous, the part of the vitreous adjacent to the posterior half of the pars plana and most peripheral retina, and in the ~100 nm thick vitreous cortex adjoining the retina and lens. The concentration of collagen in the central vitreous is lower. The orientation of the collagen fibrils is also variable, with the collagen fibrils in the posterior cortex generally parallel to the inner retinal surface, running in an anterior–posterior direction in the central vitreous and orientated perpendicular to the coats of the eye in the vitreous base.

Freeze-etch rotary shadowing electron microscopy reveals that the collagen fibrils are arranged side-to-side in narrow bundles with fibrils from one bundle branching off and joining other bundles to create an extended interconnecting network (Fig. 2) (11). Within the bundles the individual 15 nm diameter collagen fibrils are closely packed, but not generally fused together. TEM studies using cationic dyes suggest that the spacing between the fibrils in these bundles is maintained by the chondroitin sulfate chains of collagen type IX (Fig. 1B) (8,9). It is also possible that the chondroitin sulfate chains bind to opticin on the surface of adjacent fibrils, thereby linking the fibrils together (33). Hyaluronan fills the spaces between the bundles of collagen fibrils and may be organized in more than one way. Rotary shadowing electron microscopy reveals a network with proteins/glycoproteins often found at nodal points (Fig. 1D), whereas freeze-etch rotary shadowing demonstrates thin fibrillar structures forming interconnections between the collagen fibrils (Fig. 2) (11). These thin fibrillar structures are destroyed when vitreous samples are digested by *Streptomyces* hyaluronan lyase, resulting in the collagen network having a more "relaxed" appearance (11). Therefore it is likely that hyaluronan plays a role in

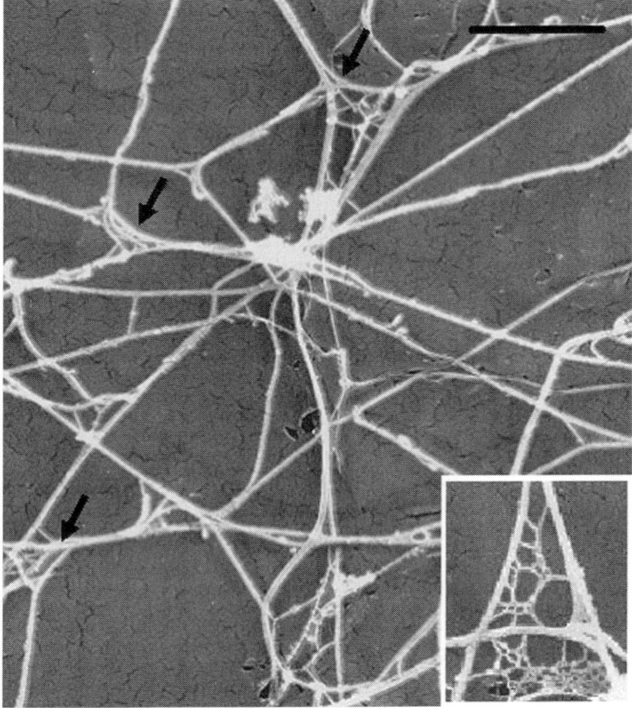

Figure 2 Ultrastructure of the central part of the vitreous visualized by freeze-etch rotary shadowing electron microscopy. A loose network of bundles of collagen fibrils is revealed above the background of ice. Interconnections between the bundles are formed by collagen fibrils running from one bundle to another (*arrows*; bar = 500 nm). Inset is a higher magnification image showing fine filamentous material forming a network between the bundles of collagen fibrils. This fine filamentous network contains hyaluronan.

maintaining the spacing of the collagen fibrillar network and hence the gel structure. However, depolymerization of hyaluronan, while causing some shrinkage of the vitreous gel, does not result in its destruction, at least over a time period of hours (7).

The vitreous base is an annular zone of unbreakable adhesion between the vitreous and the ciliary body and peripheral retina that straddles the ora serrata. Here the vitreous collagen fibrils are orientated perpendicular to the surface of the retina and pars plana and connect through defects in the inner limiting lamina (ILL) with collagen-containing "crypts" in the cellular layers of the peripheral retina and pars plana (Fig. 3A) or blend with a layer of collagen on the cellular side of the ILL (Fig. 3B) (19,85). Most vitreous collagen is synthesized at the vitreous base and then pushed out into the vitreous cavity resulting in this anatomical configuration and an unbreakable vitreoretinal adhesion.

At birth the posterior border of the vitreous base is at the ora serrata, but with age the border moves posteriorly to up to 3 mm behind the ora serrata (85). The posterior extension of the vitreous base is due to the peripheral retina synthesizing new collagen that breaches the ILL and intertwines with the preexisting cortical vitreous collagen. This extension usually produces a smooth posterior border, but

(A)

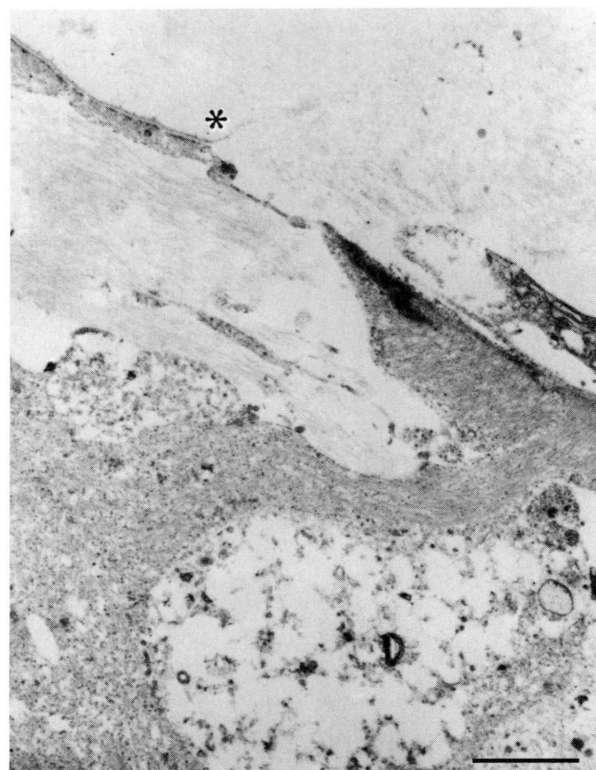

(B)

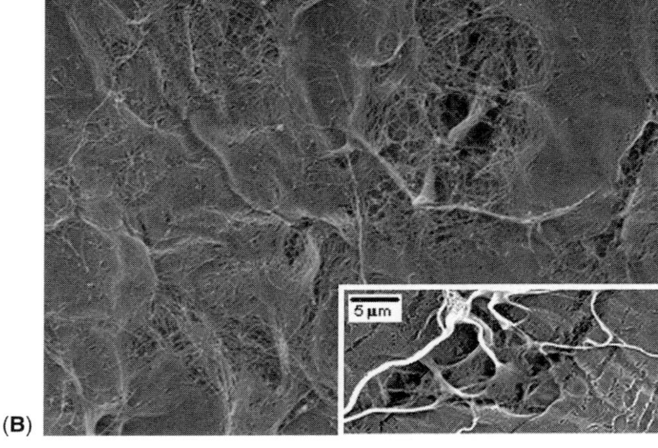

Figure 3 Vitreous base. (**A**) Crypt in the peripheral retina. Collagen fibrils pass from within the crypt through a dehiscence in the inner limiting lamina (ILL) to mingle with the cortical vitreous collagen of the vitreous base (bar = 0.5 μm). *Source*: Courtesy of Dr. B.A.W. Streeten. (**B**) Scanning electron microscopy of the outer (retinal) side of the peripheral ILL, after removal of the retinal cells by trypsin digestion, reveals a dense matting of collagen fibrils in aged eyes. Inset shows bundles of collagen fibrils passing through a defect in the ILL to intertwine with cortical vitreous collagen in the vitreous base.

irregularities may develop predisposing to retinal break formation during posterior vitreous detachment (PVD).

The posterior cortical vitreous (i.e., behind the vitreous base) is more weakly adherent to the ILL, the basement membrane forming the innermost limit of the retina. The cortical vitreous, ILL, and Müller cell footplates form a light microscopic complex called the internal limiting membrane. The ILL varies considerably in thickness, being approximately 50 nm thick in the basal zone but then getting progressively thicker through the equatorial region to the posterior pole where it is approximately 2 μm thick (19). However, there are two areas of abrupt thinning at the fovea and over the optic disc. The ILL is a typical basement membrane composed of collagen type IV, laminin, nidogen and the heparan sulfate proteoglycans type collagen XVIII, perlecan, and agrin (29). Unlike the vitreous base where cortical vitreous collagen fibrils pass into or through the ILL, posteriorly they are orientated parallel with its surface (Fig. 4) (49). The mechanism of adhesion between the cortical vitreous collagen fibrils and the ILL behind the vitreous base is poorly understood, but is likely to involve intermediary molecules. One possibility is that opticin on the surface of collagen fibrils binds heparan sulfate proteoglycans in the ILL thus providing a molecular "glue" at the vitreoretinal interface (33). Vitreoretinal adhesion can be disrupted by proteases and by chondroitinase suggesting that proteins and chondroitin/dermatan sulfate GAGs play a role in vitreoretinal adhesion (68).

Vitreoretinal adhesion shows local variation and is relatively strong in the foveal region and at the margins of the optic disc. Strong perivascular vitreoretinal attachments also occur in the peripheral retina of aging eyes, especially at points of venous confluence. Although such foci of perivascular adhesion exist in fetal eyes, their frequency and distribution is unknown. These perivascular adhesions are formed by Müller cell processes or astrocytes penetrating the ILL and mixing with the adjacent cortical vitreous fibrils (23).

The only cells normally found within the vitreous after the fetal period are a few hyalocytes in the outer part of the vitreous cortex (Fig. 5). These variably rounded or stellate cells are derived from the bone marrow and are of macrophage origin (61). Little is known about their function, but the recent work suggests that they are involved in "vitreous cavity-associated immune deviation" (78).

Macromolecules, including collagen and hyaluronan, contribute to other important characteristics of the vitreous. Hyaluronan and other GAGs interact with water thus imparting osmotic pressure to the vitreous. The vitreous is transparent because it is very highly hydrated and because the collagen fibrils are narrow and at a low concentration. It is also important for transparency that cells are largely excluded from the vitreous and both hyaluronan and collagen impede the movement of cells into the vitreous, as evidenced by the confinement of blood cells to the retrohyaloid space following retrohyaloid hemorrhage. However, the primary block to the ingress of blood cells and large macromolecules into the vitreous is normally the blood–retinal barrier.

VITREOUS SECRETION

The synthesis of secondary (adult) vitreous begins in the sixth week of human embryonic life. A number of recent studies using in situ hybridization to detect specific mRNAs have shed light on the origins of

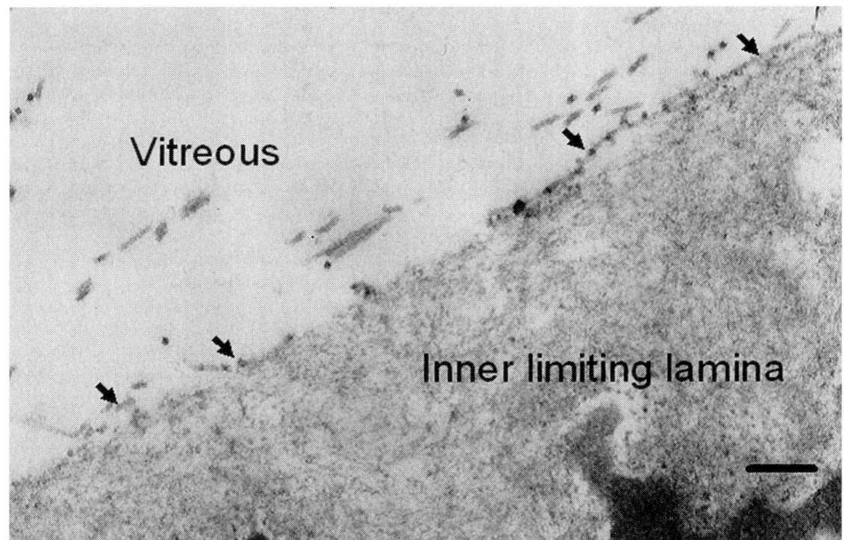

Figure 4 Vitreoretinal interface. Transmission electron microscopy of the postbasal retina showing cortical vitreous collagen fibrils (*arrows*) running parallel with the surface of the inner limiting lamina, but they do not insert into it (bar = 200 nm).

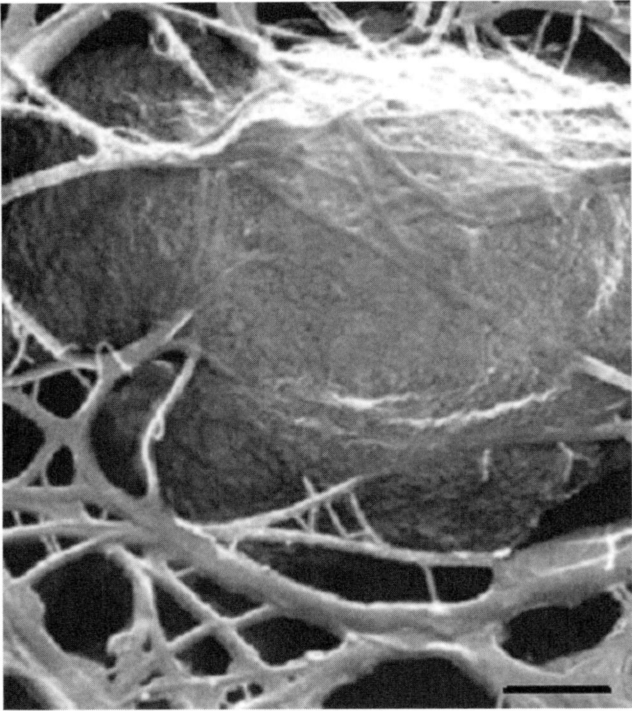

Figure 5 Hyalocyte embedded in bundles of cortical vitreous collagen imaged by freeze-etch rotary shadowing (bar = 200 nm).

vitreous macromolecules. Studies on chick and mouse eyes have shown that collagen type IX and opticin are mainly expressed by the ciliary body and specifically the nonpigmented ciliary epithelium (8,30,81). Collagen type II is expressed throughout the presumptive retina during early development. The collagen type II expression persists in the developing mouse retina, whereas in the chick by embryonic day 14 the mRNA for collagen type II is confined to the presumptive ciliary body (30,36,81). Most components of the ILL in the developing chick eye are secreted by the ciliary body and lens and then traverse the vitreous cavity to assemble on the inner surface of the retina (29).

After birth there is a rapid decline in the synthesis of the structural proteins of the vitreous and ILL in the human and chick eye (30), an exception being opticin that appears to be secreted at high levels throughout life. Balazs and Denlinger (3) showed that the amount of collagen in the vitreous remains constant throughout life and proposed that the prenatally synthesized pool of collagen persists, with little or no turnover. However, Snowdon et al. (77) demonstrated immature collagen cross-links in adult bovine vitreous suggesting recent synthesis and morphological evidence has been found for the postnatal synthesis of collagen by the retina (60,85). Indeed, the switching on of collagen synthesis by the adult peripheral retina, through unknown mechanisms, may explain the age-related posterior extension of the posterior border of the vitreous base (85). Small amounts of procollagen type II found in the vitreous cavity after vitrectomy provide further evidence of postnatal synthesis (37), but a new network of collagen fibrils is not established and the vitreous gel does not reform after vitrectomy.

The distribution of hyaluronan synthases within the eye indicates where hyaluronan is synthesized. The ciliary body and retina express these enzymes (especially hyaluronan synthase 2), and are the presumed sources of vitreous hyaluronan (56,83). Hyaluronan and sulfated GAGs are secreted into the vitreous cavity in adult life (26), suggesting a steady turnover of hyaluronan and some proteoglycans. In human eyes there is an increase in hyaluronan concentration up to the age of 20 years, after which time the concentration remains fairly constant until it starts to increase again after the age of 70 years (3). Hyaluronan is a major component of the fluid in degenerative retinal cysts (acquired retinoschisis) and peripheral cystoid degeneration of the retina, suggesting that continued or aberrant secretion may underlie this pathology.

VITREOUS LIQUEFACTION

Age-Related Syneresis

The human vitreous gel inevitably undergoes age-related liquefaction (syneresis). Balazs and Denlinger (3) observed at least 15% liquefied vitreous in all eyes after the age of 4 years and by the time the eyeball reaches its full size at 14 to 18 years of age approximately 20% of the vitreous cavity is filled with liquid. These early changes may reflect expansion of the vitreous cavity with little new collagen production, resulting in dilution of the collagen network. The vitreous continues to liquefy through adult life until ultimately the vitreous cavity is largely filled with viscous fluid (3,57). Pockets of liquefaction first appear centrally as optically empty areas surrounded by more opaque regions of gel containing "vitreous strands." These liquid pockets gradually become more extensive and coalesce. In advanced liquefaction only a narrow band of residual vitreous cortex remains attached to the posterior retina.

The prominent vitreous strands that are visible by slit-lamp biomicroscopy in the residual vitreous gel are aggregates of collagen fibrils (67). As the half-life of vitreous collagen fibrils is very long, age-related vitreous liquefaction is primarily caused by a gradual process of aggregation of the preexisting collagen fibrils. Aggregation results in a redistribution of the fibrils within the vitreous cavity with the vitreous strands being concentrated in the remaining gel and liquefied areas forming because they are devoid of collagen fibrils (3,9,67). An alternative hypothesis proposed by Los et al. (46) is that syneresis is a result of fragmentation of vitreous collagen. However, there is ample evidence that vitreous collagen fibrils progressively aggregate during aging and that this may be due to an age-related loss of collagen type IX proteoglycan from the surface of the human fibrils (9). In the young eye the chondroitin sulfate chains on the collagen type IX may maintain the short-range spacing between adjacent collagen fibrils, but these are progressively lost resulting in the exposure of "sticky" collagen type II on the fibril surfaces and irreversible aggregation as the fibrils randomly contact each other. This hypothesis is supported by a study showing that digestion of vitreous with an enzyme that removes the chondroitin sulfate chains (chondroitin ABC lyase) results in the aggregation of collagen fibrils (26). Potential reasons for the progressive, age-related loss of collagen type IX proteoglycan from the fibril surfaces include enzymatic degradation and light-induced free radical damage.

Experimental Vitreous Liquefaction

Experimentally, the vitreous gel can be destroyed by collagenase digestion, centrifugation to pellet the vitreous collagen, heating, acidification, alkylation, or dehydration (2). An increase in temperature from diathermy or light coagulation, for example, can cause shrinkage of the collagen fibrillar network and a decrease in gel volume. The vitreous liquefaction induced by metal ions, such as copper and ferrous ions, is due to free radical generation.

High Myopia

High myopia (see Chapter 26) is associated with an increased rate of vitreous liquefaction. In postmortem eyes longer than 26 mm, Berman and Michaelson (22) found the collagen and hyaluronan concentrations to be 20% to 30% lower than in emmetropic eyes, suggesting that the increased volume results in the dilution of key structural macromolecules.

Inflammation

Following an ocular injury or the onset of acute inflammation in tissues bordering the vitreous cavity, constituents of plasma enter the vitreous, followed by polymorphonuclear leukocytes (PMNs) and, later, macrophages, resulting in varying degrees of opacification of the gel. These hematogenous elements enter from the pars plana of the ciliary body, the retina, and the optic disc. The cells then release a variety of enzymes that cause degradation of vitreous macromolecules, collagen fibril aggregation, gel contraction, and liquefaction. Fibrillar aggregates may be visible as retrolental vitreous strands in chronic uveitis (Fig. 6A) with the aggregated collagen fibrils surrounded by macrophages (Fig. 6B).

Vitreous Hemorrhage

Hemorrhage into the vitreous is a common cause of vitreal liquefaction. Conditions that predispose to vitreous hemorrhage include proliferative diabetic retinopathy (PDR), neovascularization after retinal

(A)

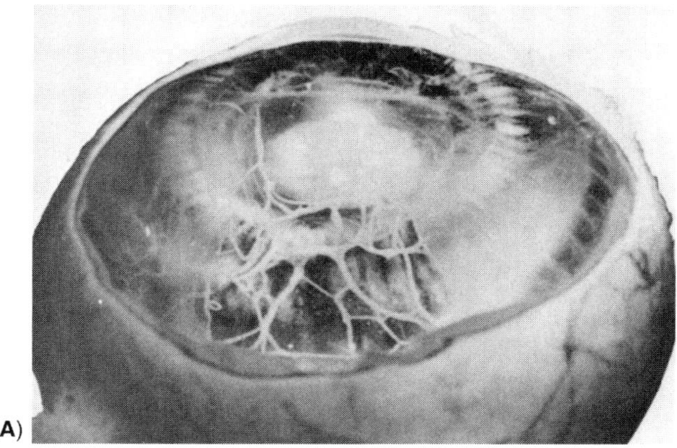

(B)

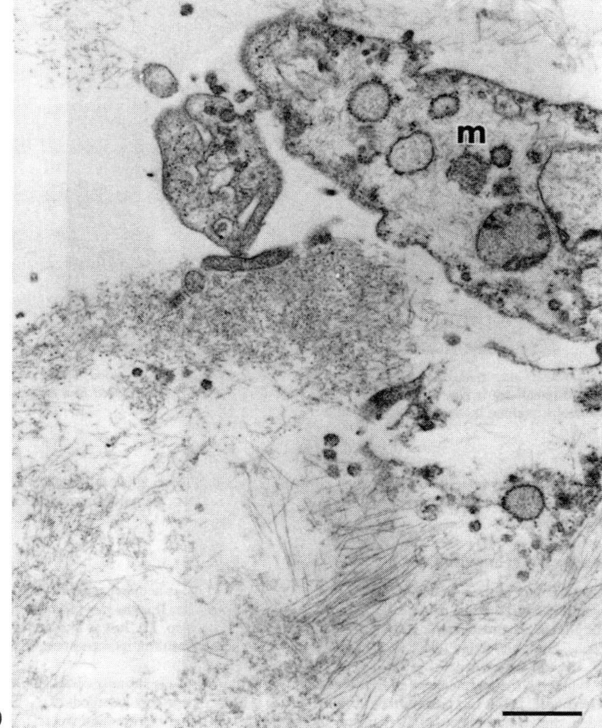

Figure 6 (**A**) Macrophotograph of globe with the anterior segment removed. Aggregates of vitreous collagen fibrils forming thick strands in chronic uveitis. A hypermature morgagnian cataract is also present. (**B**) Transmission electron microscopy shows aggregates of vitreous collagen associated with macrophages (m) from the same eye (bar = 0.5 μm). *Source*: Courtesy of Dr. B.A.W. Streeten.

vein occlusion, retinal tear formation, and PVD without retinal tear formation (79). Hemorrhages can be subdivided into intragel and retrohyaloid varieties. Retrohyaloid hemorrhages can sometimes be difficult to distinguish from intraretinal sub-ILL hemorrhages clinically. The retrohyaloid space is created by PVD and the extent of the hemorrhage depends upon the extent of the detachment. Retrohyaloid hemorrhages clot almost immediately and then undergo fibrinolysis within 24 h to become liquefied (Fig. 7A) the hemorrhage then typically clears over a period of days or weeks. Retrohyaloid hemorrhages can extend through breaks in the posterior hyaloid membrane to become intragel hemorrhages and under these circumstances the intragel hemorrhage remains liquefied. Intragel hemorrhages that initially clot in the vitreous, e.g., after trauma, resolve more slowly because of low fibrinolytic activity and a poor PMN response. As the clot liquefies cells gradually disperse despite their movement being limited by vitreous collagen and hyaluronan. Some erythrocytes undergo hemolysis although others can remain intact for long periods of time. Hemolysis of erythrocytes results in the release of ferrous and ferric ions and consequent free radical generation. These free radicals induce collagen fibril aggregation and vitreous syneresis (24). In a rabbit model of intravitreal hemorrhage giant macrophages were frequently observed and the inflammatory response was likened to a "low-turnover" granuloma (27). Following vitreous hemorrhage an ochre membrane can form consisting of cortical gel stuffed with "ghost cells" or "erythroclasts" (Fig. 7B), which, compared to erythrocytes, are poorly phagocytosed by macrophages. Phagocytosis, hemolysis, and dispersion with exit via the trabecular meshwork contribute toward the clearance of vitreous hemorrhage. The end result of vitreous hemorrhage varies from complete clearing in 1 to 18 months to a persistence of debris, vitreous liquefaction, and ochre membrane formation. Various complications can occur following intragel hemorrhage, including proliferative vitreoretinopathy (PVR) when associated with retinal tears. Synchisis scintillans is caused by cholesterol crystal formation after breakdown of erythroclasts. Hemosiderosis bulbi is a condition whereby ferric ions stain ocular tissues. Ghost cell or hemolytic glaucoma is caused by erythroclasts being more rigid than erythrocytes and less able to pass through the trabecular meshwork (see Chapter 20).

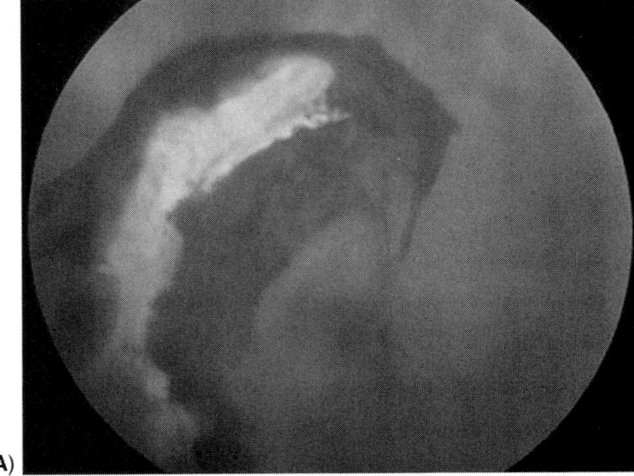
(A)

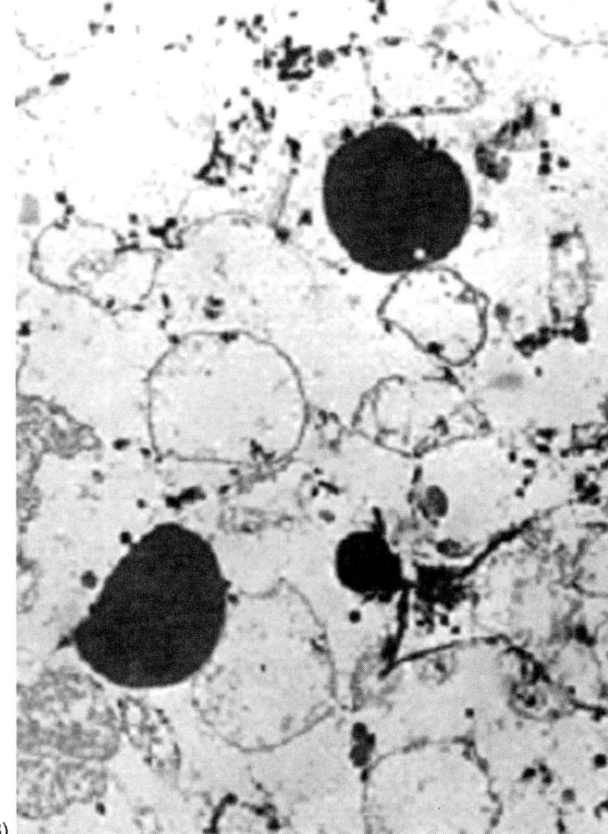
(B)

Figure 7 (**A**) Fundus photograph of a retrohyaloid hemorrhage of 1 h duration; the clotted blood beneath the fibrovascular membrane is beginning to liquefy. (**B**) Electron microscopy of two erythrocytes and numerous erythroclasts, some containing residual hemoglobin (Heinz bodies).

Genetic and Congenital Causes of Vitreous Liquefaction

Vitreous liquefaction is seen developmentally in genetic disorders such as Stickler syndrome type 1 (MIM #108300), Stickler syndrome type 2 (MIM #604841), Wagner syndrome type 1 (MIM %143200), snowflake vitreoretinal degeneration (MIM %193230), and Goldmann–Favre syndrome (enhanced S-cone syndrome, MIM #268100). Premature vitreous syneresis can also be a feature of retinal dystrophies such as X-linked retinoschisis (MIM + 312700) (see Chapter 35). Isolated developmental abnormalities, such as lattice degeneration, are associated with an overlying pocket of vitreous liquefaction.

VITREOUS DETACHMENT

Anterior Detachment of the Vitreous

Separation of the vitreous at its anterior attachment to the posterior lens capsule (Wieger hyaloideocapsular ligament) is almost always secondary to trauma or Marfan syndrome (MIM #154700). The anterior hyaloid membrane may detach completely from the posterior lens surface or may separate partially at its junction with the lens capsule. It is relatively easy to rupture the insertion during the equatorial expansion of the globe and deformation of the lens that occur in blunt ocular trauma. Also the attachment becomes less firm with age and this facilitates peeling of the anterior vitreous from the posterior lens capsule during intracapsular cataract extraction.

Posterior Vitreous Detachment

PVD refers to a separation of the cortical vitreous from the ILL of the retina, which can extend as far anteriorly as the posterior border of the vitreous base. PVD is common in the aging eye, vitreous hemorrhage, vitritis, myopia, diabetes mellitus, vitreoretinal disease, and following surgery or trauma. It is the most significant event in the causation of rhegmatogenous retinal detachment (see Chapter 28). PVD is caused by a combination of vitreous liquefaction and weakening of vitreoretinal adhesion (69). Commonly these two processes are age-related and go hand-in-hand resulting in uncomplicated PVD; this is characterized by symptoms during the acute event with subsequent "floaters," but not usually by sight-threatening complications. However, vitreous liquefaction and partial PVD in the presence of strong residual vitreoretinal adhesion can lead to retinal break formation or complications from chronic vitreoretinal traction (69).

Like vitreous liquefaction, the prevalence of PVD is strongly correlated with age, but has a later onset. In a postmortem study of 786 pairs of eyes using macroscopic methods of examination after fixation, PVDs were uncommon below the middle of the sixth decade, thereafter the incidence increased to 17%, 51%, and 53% in the seventh, eighth, and ninth decades, respectively (20).

PVD usually commences in the macular area where the cortical vitreous is thinner than elsewhere. Fluid within central syneretic cavities enters the retrohyaloid space and dissects the vitreous cortex from the retina. The detached vitreous body then collapses anteriorly, hanging down in a hammock fashion as a result of gravity. PVD can progress rapidly within hours to days, extending to the equator of the globe, the optic disc, and then to the posterior border of the vitreous base. When the PVD reaches the posterior border of the vitreous base it is termed "complete." In the study by Foos (20) partial PVD was relatively uncommon suggesting that in most cases PVD occurs rapidly.

Foos (21) reported that the vitreous separates cleanly in posterior vitreal detachment, leaving "at the most a few fragments of vitreous fibrils," which eventually disappear, so that the basal lamina of the retina has a smooth surface. However, scanning electron microscopy (SEM) studies have demonstrated matted feltworks of vitreous collagen fibrils on the ILL after PVD, particularly in the macular region (42).

A Weiss ring derived from the surface of the optic disc is frequently seen on the back of the detached vitreous (Fig. 8). Usually an annular opacity, although the ring may be incomplete, around a hole in what was the prepapillary vitreous cortex, it is composed of glial cells and cortical vitreous and represents the remnants of the posterior expanded part of Cloquet canal.

Clinical studies have shown that PVD is significantly correlated with female gender and myopia (32). Early PVD in myopic eyes may result from increased vitreous liquefaction and decreased vitreoretinal adhesion secondary to dilution of vitreous macromolecules. PVD may be precipitated by a number of conditions including trauma, inflammation, vitreous hemorrhage, aphakia, pseudophakia, and vitreoretinal disease, but compared with age-related PVD, there is a greater likelihood of strong vitreoretinal adhesion resulting in an increased risk of vitreoretinal traction and its sequelae.

The frequency of PVD in aphakia is high and was found to be approximately 80% following intracapsular cataract surgery in two postmortem series (20,52). Anterior displacement of the vitreous to fill the space previously occupied by the lens, as well as operative vitreous loss, inflammation, and hemorrhage, may play a role in the pathogenesis of aphakic PVD. The marked change in macromolecular composition of the vitreous in aphakic eyes may also be important. In a study of autopsy eyes, Osterlin (58) found 33% to 90% less hyaluronan than in the unoperated fellow eyes. Similarly, he found that intracapsular extraction of the lens in owl monkeys reduced the hyaluronan content of the vitreous by 84% to 91% (59). It appears that the normal diffusion of hyaluronan through the anterior vitreous into the aqueous humor is greatly facilitated by removal of the lens, especially the posterior capsule. This loss of hyaluronan in the aphakic eye contrasts with a normal concentration of hyaluronic acid in age-related vitreous liquefaction.

With the advent of intraocular lens implantation following extracapsular cataract extraction and more

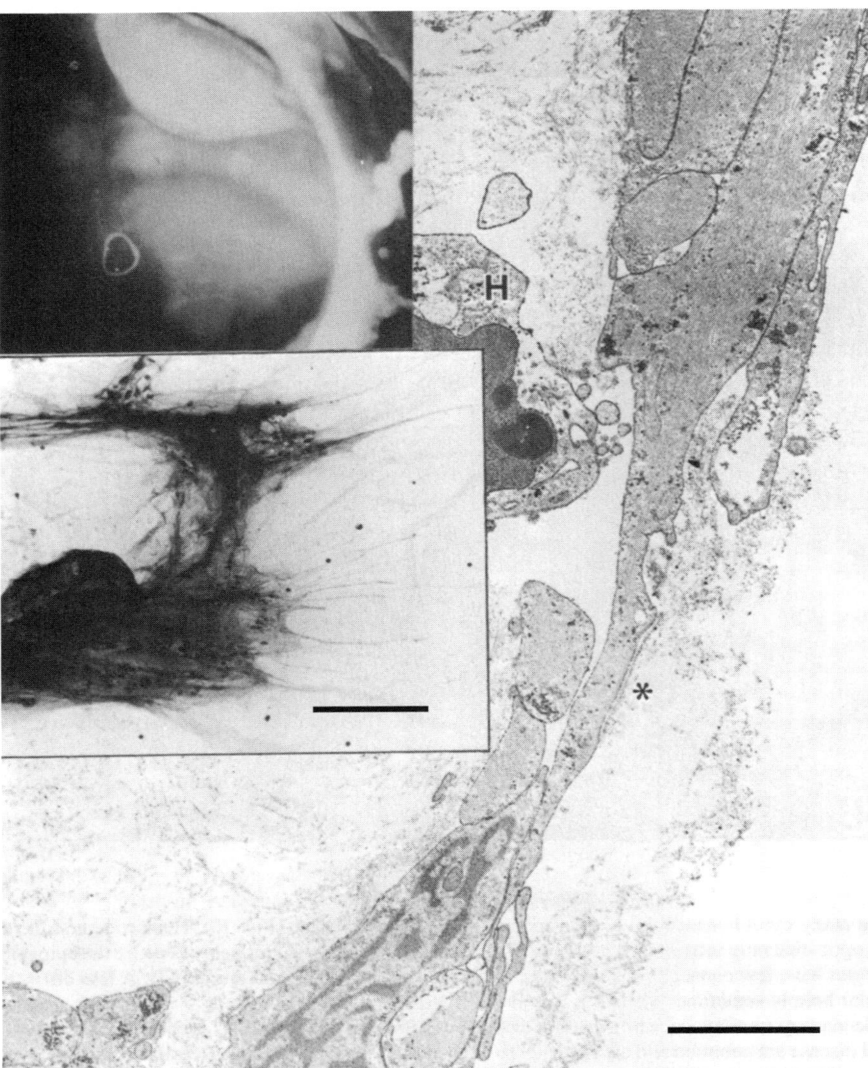

Figure 8 Macrophotograph showing a Weiss ring attached to the posterior hyaloid following posterior vitreous detachment (*upper inset*). Flat preparation of a Weiss ring with long astrocytic processes on the back of the detached hyaloid (stained with periodic acid-Schiff and hematoxylin; bar = 75 μm) (*lower inset*). The main figure shows the edge of a Weiss ring containing astrocytes with scanty basement membrane (*asterisk*). A hyalocyte (H) containing lysosomal dense bodies is also present (bar = 1.5 μm). *Source*: Courtesy of Dr. B.A.W. Streeten.

recently phakoemulsification surgery PVD is less common. This is due to the retention of the posterior lens capsule and an intact anterior hyaloid face. In one autopsy series 40% of eyes had PVDs following extracapsular cataract surgery with an intact posterior capsule, a slightly higher rate of PVD than the 25% to 30% in phakic postmortem eyes, but 76% had PVDs if the posterior capsule was ruptured during the procedure (52). The question has been raised as to whether neodymium-doped yttrium aluminium garnet (Nd:YAG) laser capsulotomy for opacification of the posterior capsule following cataract surgery predisposes to PVD. In one study capsulotomy was not associated with a higher incidence of PVD (71), although capsulotomy has been linked with an increased risk of rhegmatogenous retinal detachment (45). The cause of this increased risk remains uncertain, but it may be due to the induction of PVD, due to disruption of the anterior hyaloid face resulting in retinal traction around the vitreous base, or to direct retinal damage from the laser (45).

Complications of Posterior Vitreous Detachment

Retinal Hemorrhages

Vitreous hemorrhage, arising from disruption of retinal vessels subjected to traction by the detaching vitreous, occurs in approximately 15% of patients presenting with an acute PVD. Vitreous hemorrhage during PVD can be associated with tractional tears, particularly at venous confluences and around lattice degeneration.

Retinal Tears

Studies on autopsy eyes by Foos (20,22) showed that approximately 2% of the eyes had full-thickness retinal tears, and of these eyes 79% had complete PVDs. Retinal tears were behind the ora serrata in 92% of eyes and in the ocular equatorial zone in 95% of

(A) 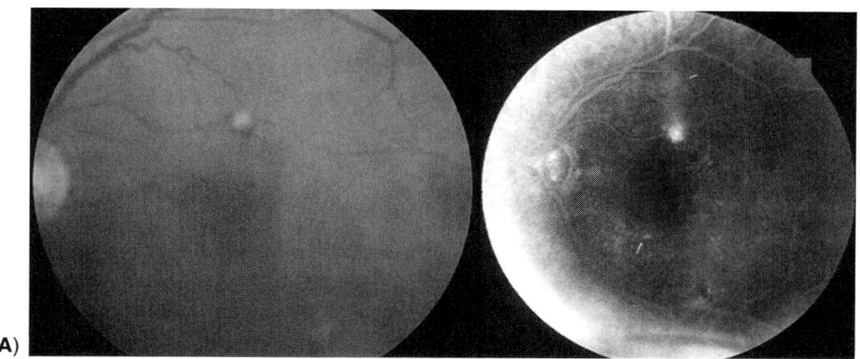

(B) 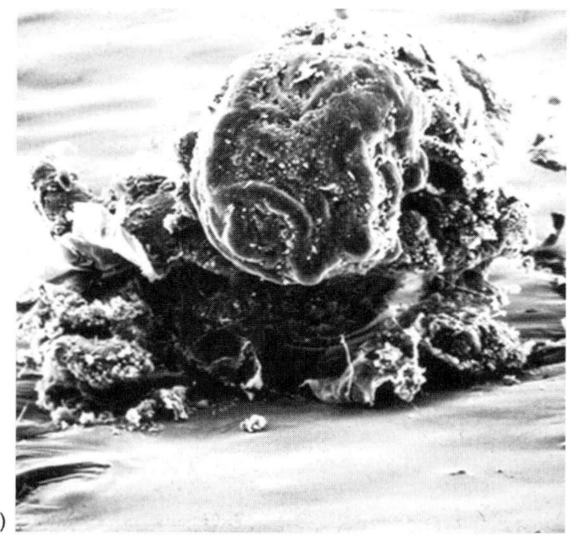

Figure 11 (**A**) Fundus photograph and fluorescein angiogram showing an abortive neovascular outgrowth (ANVO) originating at an arteriovenous crossing in the macula and then breaking through to the inner surface of the retina in an eye that had previously undergone posterior vitreous detachment. The fluorescein angiogram shows a "smoke stack" of fluorescein leakage. (**B**) Scanning electron microscopy of an ANVO on the inner (vitreal) surface of the inner limiting lamina.

effector IGF1, play key roles in preretinal neovascularization induced by ischemia (74,75). Furthermore, placental growth factor and VEGF appear to act synergistically in ischemia-induced preretinal neovascularization (14).

ABNORMAL AGGREGATES WITHIN THE VITREOUS

Vitreous Opacification Due to Collagen, Cells, and Pigment

The most common opacities within the vitreous are aggregates of collagen, the Weiss ring following PVD and hyaloid remnants. In the absence of perforating injury or intraocular surgery, the presence of pigment granules in the vitreous (Shafer sign) is pathognomonic of a rhegmatogenous retinal detachment (70,82). The pigment is thought to arise from RPE migrating through retinal breaks into the vitreous where they reside as intact cells, cell debris, or as remnants within macrophages. The amount of pigment granules correlates with the risk of developing PVR.

Cells derived from the blood may be appreciated by the patient as floaters if they infiltrate the posterior vitreous. Aggregates of inflammatory cells accumulate in the vitreous as a feature of granulomatous inflammations, especially fungal and parasitic disease, sarcoidosis, and pars planitis. Neoplastic cells in the vitreous are uncommon, but when present the usual cause is primary intraocular lymphoma (see Chapter 66). In children, retinoblastomas can seed in the vitreous (see Chapter 60). Vitreous seeding is rare in metastatic tumors (see Chapter 54).

Asteroid Hyalosis

Asteroid hyalosis is a condition in which there are symptomless, cream or yellow particles embedded in aggregates of vitreous fibrils like a "string of pearls" (Fig. 12A). These tend to sway slightly with gel movement but are symptomless. The condition is rare under the age of 40 years. Three large-scale studies (18,53,55) have shown that the overall incidence is approximately 1% in over 45 years population and 2% in autopsy eyes. It is bilateral in 9% of cases. The only other clearly shown associations in these studies are male sex and an inverse relationship with PVD.

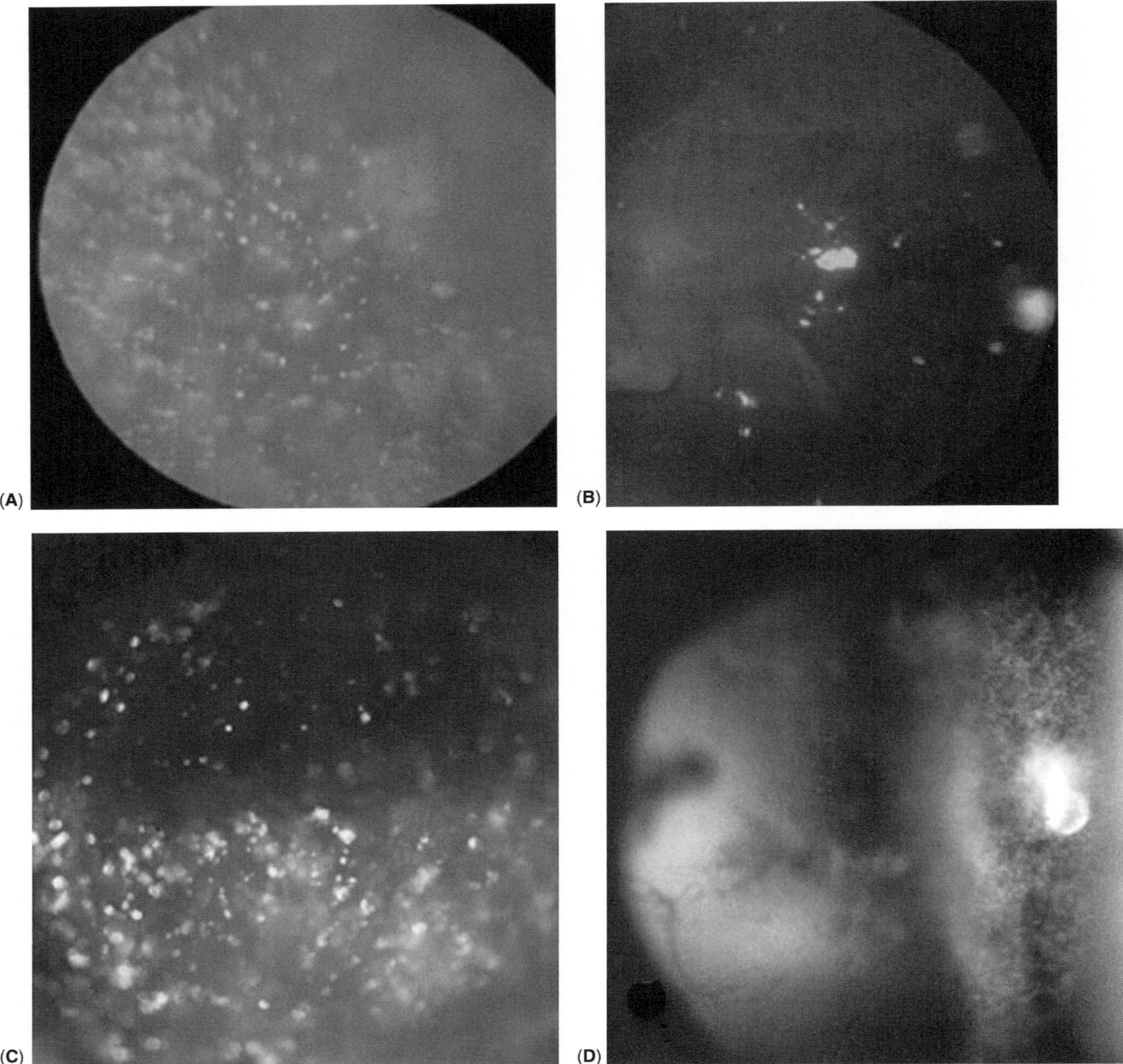

Figure 12 Slit-lamp biomicroscopy of eyes with (**A**) asteroid hyalosis, (**B**) synchysis scintillans, (**C**) synchysis scintillans, with the cholesterol crystals in the anterior chamber emphasizing their crystalline, polychromatic nature, and (**D**) amyloidosis of the vitreous, with the pathognomic "pseudopodia lentis" on the posterior lens surface.

Ultrastructural and compositional analyses of asteroid bodies have shown them to be roughly spherical structures of variable diameter (approximate range 50–200 μm) that have crystalline properties (Fig. 13) (43,87). They contain lipid and hydroxyapatite and can be considered a form of lithiasis. Chondroitin sulfate containing proteoglycans surround the crystalline core, and vitreous collagen is found in close association suggesting an interaction between these macromolecules.

Cholesterolosis Bulbi and Synchysis Scintillans

The term synchysis scintillans refers to the presence of cholesterol crystals in the vitreous, which when viewed "in bulk" have a sparkling (scintillating) yellow appearance (Figs. 12B, 12C). This condition invariably occurs in severely damaged eyes where the gel structure of the vitreous has been destroyed. The movement of the cholesterol crystals in response to gravitational and rotational forces is unimpeded and they settle in the most dependent portion of the eye.

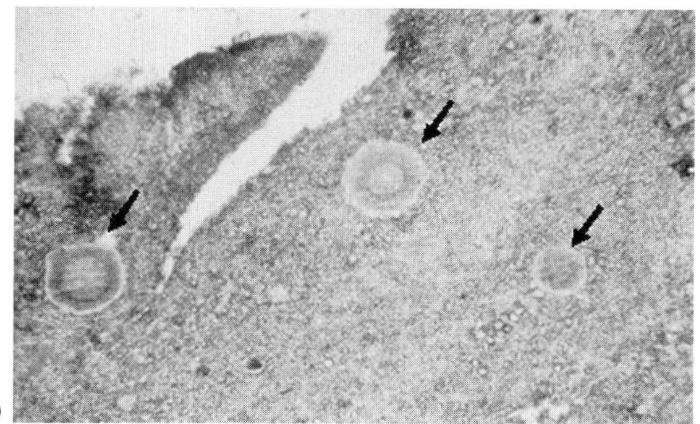

(A)

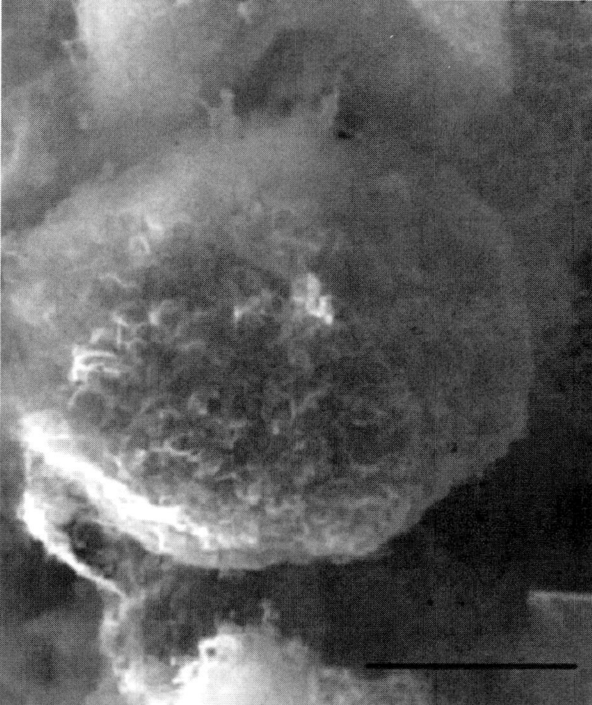

(B)

Figure 13 (**A**) Light microscopy showing three asteroid bodies (*arrows*) that were coincidently present in an ochre membrane with thousands of erythroclasts trapped within the cortical vitreous. (**B**) Scanning electron microscopy of an asteroid body coated with vitreous collagen (bar = 50 μm).

Synchysis scintillans is usually part of a diffuse deposition of cholesterol in the eye (cholesterolosis bulbi). Some degree of cholesterolosis bulbi can occur in eyes with chronic retinal detachments, but the crystals are usually more profuse beneath the neurosensory retina than within the vitreous cavity. Cholesterosis bulbi results from recurrent bleeding, with the formation of "erythroclasts" and eventually their break down to form cholesterol crystals.

Amyloidosis of the Vitreous

The spontaneous development of glass wool-like veils and globules in the vitreous (Fig. 12D), without any cellular component to the infiltration, is highly characteristic of amyloid deposition. This is, in most cases, caused by a FAP with specific mutations in the *TTR* gene that encodes for transthyretin (see Chapter 37) (66). However, vitreous amyloidosis occasionally occurs in familial oculoleptomeningeal amyloidosis (amyloidosis type VII, MIM #10510) or without systemic involvement.

GENETIC DISEASES OF THE VITREOUS

Primary and Secondary Genetic Diseases of the Vitreous

A number of genetic diseases have already been discussed in this chapter where there are secondary or indirect detrimental effects on the vitreous. In axial high myopia (see Chapter 26) there is an enlarged vitreous cavity and vitreous abnormalities, such as premature extensive liquefaction and PVD may be secondary to the dilution of vitreous macromolecules. In Marfan syndrome (MIM #154700; see Chapter 36), there are mutations in the fibrillin-1 that result in globe enlargement and lens subluxation. However, the vitreous also contains some fibrillin-containing microfibrils so it is possible that the mutations directly alter vitreous structure. In other conditions, especially certain "collagenopathies" (see Chapter 44), there are clearly primary defects in vitreous macromolecules.

Empty Vitreous Syndrome and the Vitreoretinal Degenerations

The concept of empty vitreous syndrome is useful for considering genetic diseases directly affecting the vitreous, with or without systemic involvement. It implies that the formation of the vitreous gel is abnormal and usually manifests as an optically empty vitreous cavity, but with retrolental and basal residual collagenous strands. These residual collagenous strands often form an irregular circumferential membrane over the peripheral–equatorial retina. Evidence of retinal involvement varies from lattice degeneration to extensive chorioretinal atrophy, perivascular pigment thinning, visual field constriction, and electroretinogram (ERG) abnormalities. Empty vitreous syndrome is found in Stickler syndrome (MIM #108300, #60841) (76), hyaloideoretinal degeneration of Wagner (MIM %143200) (10,13,54), and Goldmann–Favre syndrome (MIM #268100) (28,40).

Stickler Syndrome

Stickler syndrome is an autosomal-dominant condition characterized by ocular and orofacial features, deafness, and arthritis (76). The main ocular features include congenital vitreous abnormalities, congenital high myopia that is often nonprogressive after the first few years of life, paravascular-pigmented lattice degeneration and rhegmatogenous retinal detachments typically secondary to giant retinal tears. Other ocular features include distinctive "wedge" and "fleck"-like cortical cataracts along with developmental abnormalities of the anterior chamber angle leading to glaucoma. The vitreous changes have been subdivided into type 1 and type 2, which correlate with the underlying genetic locus. The type 1 vitreous anomaly consists of an optically empty vitreous cavity apart from a vestigial gel occupying the immediate retrolental space that is bordered by a distinct-folded membrane. The type 2 phenotype consists of sparse and irregularly thickened bundles of collagen (often with a beaded appearance) running throughout the vitreous cavity.

The orofacial manifestations of Stickler syndrome are midfacial flattening with a depressed nasal bridge, reduced nasal protrusion, anteverted nares, and micrognathia. These features are often most obvious in childhood and may become indistinct in adults. In addition, 25% of Sticker patients have midline orofacial clefting varying in severity from the severe Pierre–Robin sequence, through palatal clefting to a bifid uvula. Approximately 40% of Stickler patients have sensorineural deafness. The joint manifestations include hypermobility in young patients, but then this is replaced in middle age by a degenerative arthropathy especially affecting the hips and knees. A majority of patients with Stickler syndrome have mutations in the *COL2A1* gene that encodes procollagen type II; these patients have the type 1 vitreous anomaly. Most of the mutations described introduce a premature stop codon into the gene and this is presumed to result in haploinsufficiency of procollagen type II. Other mutations have been described that result in amino acid substitutions. Recently there have been reports of premature termination codons in exon 2 of *COL2A1*. Exon 2 encodes a domain in the amino-propeptide of collagen type II that is expressed in the eye, but not in cartilage. Therefore these patients have an "eye-only" or "predominantly ocular" phenotype.

Less commonly Stickler mutations are found in the *COL11A1* gene and this usually, but not always, results in the type 2 vitreous anomaly. In addition there is a form of Stickler syndrome with mutations in the COL11A2 gene, but as the α2(XI) chain is replaced by α2(V) in the vitreous type collagen V/XI, these patients have a nonocular phenotype. In several other pedigrees linkage to collagens II and V/XI have been excluded implying that there is further genetic heterogeneity that has yet to be resolved.

Mutations in *COL2A1* result in a spectrum of conditions and Stickler syndrome is only one manifestation. This spectrum ranges through achondrogenesis type II, hypochondrogenesis, Kniest dysplasia, spondyloepiphyseal dysplasia congenita, forms of spondyloepimetaphyseal dysplasia, and premature osteoarthropathy. Ocular features similar to those of Stickler syndrome have been described in some of these conditions including Kniest dysplasia.

Hyaloideoretinal Degeneration of Wagner

Hyaloideoretinal degeneration of Wagner (Wagner syndrome, erosive vitreoretinopathy, MIM %143200) does not have systemic manifestations (10,13). The most consistent feature is an empty vitreous cavity with avascular strands or veils and chorioretinal atrophy with perivascular sheathing associated with ERG abnormalities. The vitreoretinal changes are sometimes complicated by rhegmatogenous retinal detachment. A variety of ocular developmental abnormalities are associated with this condition including ectopic fovea, congenital cataract, congenital glaucoma, posterior embryotoxon, iris hypoplasia, ectopia lentis, microphthalmia, and persistent hyperplastic primary vitreous. Genetic linkage studies have mapped the disorder to 5q13–q14, and a novel splice site mutation in the *CSPG2* gene that encodes versican has been implicated (10,54).

Goldmann–Favre Syndrome

Goldmann–Favre syndrome (MIM #268100) is part of the spectrum of enhanced S-cone syndrome, which is a recessive retinal degeneration uniquely characterized by a gain of photoreceptor function, resulting in an enhanced sensitivity to blue light (40). However, in the Goldmann–Favre syndrome as well as enhanced S-cone syndrome there is cataract, an empty vitreous, preretinal veils, retinoschisis at the macula, and a progressive retinal degeneration. It is caused by mutations in the nuclear receptor gene *NR2E3* (28).

ACKNOWLEDGMENTS

The author would like to thank Professor David McLeod (University of Manchester, U.K.) and Professors Paul Hiscott and Ian Grierson (University of Liverpool, U.K.) for providing some of the figures used in this chapter.

REFERENCES

1. Ahsan M, Ohta K, Kuriyama S, Tanaka H. Novel soluble molecule, Akhirin, is expressed in the embryonic chick eyes and exhibits heterophilic cell-adhesion activity. Dev Dyn 2005; 233:95–104.
2. Balazs EA. Physiology of the vitreous body. In: Schepens CL, ed. Importance of the Vitreous Body in Retinal Surgery

with Special Emphasis on Re-operation. St. Louis, MO: CV Mosby, 1960:29–57.

3. Balazs EA, Denlinger JL. Aging changes in the vitreous. In: Dismukes N, Sekular R, eds. Aging and Human Visual Function. New York, NY: Alan R Liss, 1982:45–57.
4. Berman ER, Michaelson IC. The chemical composition of the human vitreous body as related to age and myopia. Exp Eye Res 1964; 89:9–15.
5. Bishop PN, Reardon AJ, McLeod D, Ayad S. Identification of alternatively spliced variants of type II procollagen in vitreous. Biochem Biophys Res Commun 1994; 203:289–95.
6. Bishop PN, Crossman MV, McLeod D, Ayad S. Extraction and characterization of the tissue forms of collagen types II and IX from bovine vitreous. Biochem J 1994; 299(Pt 2):497–505.
7. Bishop PN, McLeod D, Reardon A. Effects of hyaluronan lyase, hyaluronidase, and chondroitin ABC lyase on mammalian vitreous gel. Invest Ophthalmol Vis Sci 1999; 40:2173–8.
8. Bishop PN. Structural macromolecules and supramolecular organisation of the vitreous gel. Prog Retin Eye Res 2000; 19:323–44.
9. Bishop PN, Holmes DF, Kadler, et al. Age-related changes on the surface of vitreous collagen fibrils. Invest Ophthalmol Vis Sci 2004; 45:1041–6.
10. Black GC, Perveen R, Wiszniewski, et al. A novel hereditary developmental vitreoretinopathy with multiple ocular abnormalities localizing to a 5-cM region of chromosome 5q13-q14. Ophthalmology 1999; 106:2074–81.
11. Bos KJ, Holmes DF, Meadows, et al. Collagen fibril organisation in mammalian vitreous by freeze etch/rotary shadowing electron microscopy. Micron 2001; 32:301–6.
12. Bos KJ, Holmes DF, Kadler KE, et al. Axial structure of the heterotypic collagen fibrils of vitreous humour and cartilage. J Mol Biol 2001; 306:1011–22.
13. Brown DM, Kimura AE, Weingeist TA, Stone EM. Erosive vitreoretinopathy. A new clinical entity. Ophthalmology 1994; 101:694–704.
14. Carmeliet P, Moons L, Luttun A, et al. Synergism between vascular endothelial growth factor and placental growth factor contributes to angiogenesis and plasma extravasation in pathological conditions. Nat Med 2001; 7:575–83.
15. Chan A, Duker JS, Schuman JS, Fujimoto JG. Stage 0 macular holes: observations by optical coherence tomography. Ophthalmology 2004; 111:2027–32.
16. Charteris DG, Sethi CS, Lewis GP, Fisher SK. Proliferative vitreoretinopathy-developments in adjunctive treatment and retinal pathology. Eye 2002; 16:369–74.
17. Dawson DW, Volpert OV, Gillis P, et al. Pigment epithelium-derived factor: a potent inhibitor of angiogenesis. Science 1999; 285:245–8.
18. Fawzi AA, Vo B, Kriwanek R, et al. Asteroid hyalosis in an autopsy population: The University of California at Los Angeles (UCLA) experience. Arch Ophthalmol 2005; 123: 486–90.
19. Foos RY. Vitreoretinal juncture; topographical variations. Invest Ophthalmol 1972; 11:801–8.
20. Foos RY. Posterior vitreous detachment. Trans Am Acad Ophthalmol Otolaryngol 1972; 76:480–97.
21. Foos RY. Ultrastructural features of posterior vitreous detachment. Albrecht Von Graefes Arch Klin Exp Ophthalmol 1975; 196:103–11.
22. Foos RY. Tears of the peripheral retina; pathogenesis, incidence and classification in autopsy eyes. Mod Probl Ophthalmol 1975; 15:68–81.
23. Foos RY. Vitreoretinal juncture; epiretinal membranes and vitreous. Invest Ophthalmol Vis Sci 1977; 16:416–22.
24. Forrester JV, Grierson I, Lee WR. Vitreous membrane formation after experimental vitreous haemorrhage. Albrecht Von Graefes Arch Klin Exp Ophthalmol 1980; 212:227–42.
25. Fukai N, Eklund L, Marneros AG, et al. Lack of collagen XVIII/endostatin results in eye abnormalities. Embo J 2002; 21:1535–44.
26. Goes RM, Nader HB, Porcionatto MA, et al. Chondroitin sulfate proteoglycans are structural renewable constituents of the rabbit vitreous body. Curr Eye Res 2005; 30: 405–13.
27. Grierson I, Forrester JV. Vitreous haemorrhage and vitreal membranes. Trans Ophthalmol Soc UK 1980; 100: 140–50.
28. Haider NB, Jacobson SG, Cideciyan AV, et al. Mutation of a nuclear receptor gene, NR2E3, causes enhanced S cone syndrome, a disorder of retinal cell fate. Nat Genet 2000; 24:127–31.
29. Halfter W, Dong S, Schurer B, et al. Composition, synthesis, and assembly of the embryonic chick retinal basal lamina. Dev Biol 2000; 220:111–28.
30. Halfter W, Dong S, Schurer B, et al. Embryonic synthesis of the inner limiting membrane and vitreous body. Invest Ophthalmol Vis Sci 2005; 46:2202–9.
31. Harada C, Mitamura Y, Harada T. The role of cytokines and trophic factors in epiretinal membranes: involvement of signal transduction in glial cells. Prog Retin Eye Res 2006; 25:149–64.
32. Hayreh SS, Jonas JB. Posterior vitreous detachment: clinical correlations. Ophthalmologica 2004; 218:333–43.
33. Hindson VJ, Gallagher JT, Halfter W, Bishop PN. Opticin binds to heparan and chondroitin sulfate proteoglycans. Invest Ophthalmol Vis Sci 2005; 46:4417–23.
34. Hiscott P, Cooling RJ, Rosen P, Garner A. The pathology of abortive neovascular outgrowths from the retina. Graefes Arch Clin Exp Ophthalmol 1992; 230:531–6.
35. Hiscott P, Hagan S, Heathcote L, et al. Pathobiology of epiretinal and subretinal membranes: possible roles for the matricellular proteins thrombospondin 1 and osteonectin (SPARC). Eye 2002; 16:393–403.
36. Ihanamaki T, Pelliniemi LJ, Vuorio E. Collagens and collagen-related matrix components in the human and mouse eye. Prog Retin Eye Res 2004; 23:403–34.
37. Itakura H, Kishi S, Kotajima N, Murakami M. Vitreous collagen metabolism before and after vitrectomy. Graefes Arch Clin Exp Ophthalmol 2005; 243:994–8.
38. Jacobson B, Basu PK, Hasany SM. Vascular endothelial cell growth inhibitor of normal and pathologic human vitreous. Arch Ophthalmol 1984; 102:1543–5.
39. Jacobson B, Dorfman T, Basu PK, Hasany SM. Inhibition of vascular endothelial cell growth and trypsin activity by vitreous. Exp Eye Res 1985; 41:581–95.
40. Jacobson SG, Roman AJ, Roman MI, et al. Relatively enhanced S cone function in the Goldmann–Favre syndrome. Am J Ophthalmol 1991; 111:446–53.
41. Kawaji T, Ando Y, Nakamura M, et al. Transthyretin synthesis in rabbit ciliary pigment epithelium. Exp Eye Res 2005; 81:306–12.
42. Kishi S, Demaria C, Shimizu K. Vitreous cortex remnants at the fovea after spontaneous vitreous detachment. Int Ophthalmol 1986; 9:253–60.
43. Komatsu H, Kamura Y, Ishi K, Kashima Y. Fine structure and morphogenesis of asteroid hyalosis. Med Electron Microsc 2003; 36:112–9.
44. Le Goff MM, Hindson VJ, Jowitt TA, et al. Characterization of opticin and evidence of stable dimerization in solution. J Biol Chem 2003; 278:45280–7.
45. Lois N, Wong D. Pseudophakic retinal detachment. Surv Ophthalmol 2003; 48:467–87.

46. Los LI, van der Worp RJ, van Luyn MJ, Hooymans JM. Age-related liquefaction of the human vitreous body: LM and TEM evaluation of the role of proteoglycans and collagen. Invest Ophthalmol Vis Sci 2003; 44:2828–33.
47. Lutty GA, Thompson DC, Gallup JY, et al. Vitreous: an inhibitor of retinal extract-induced neovascularization. Invest Ophthalmol Vis Sci 1983; 24:52–6.
48. Lutty GA, Mello RJ, Chandler C, et al. Regulation of cell growth by vitreous humour. J Cell Sci 1985; 76:53–65.
49. Matsumoto B, Blanks JC, Ryan SJ. Topographic variations in the rabbit and primate internal limiting membrane. Invest Ophthalmol Vis Sci 1984; 25:71–82.
50. Mayne R, Brewton RG, Mayne PM, Baker JR. Isolation and characterization of the chains of type V/type XI collagen present in bovine vitreous. J Biol Chem 1993; 268:9381–6.
51. Mayne R, Ren ZX, Liu J, et al. VIT-1: the second member of a new branch of the von Willebrand factor A domain superfamily. Biochem Soc Trans 1999; 27:832–5.
52. McDonnell PJ, Patel A, Green WR. Comparison of intracapsular and extracapsular cataract surgery. Histopathologic study of eyes obtained postmortem. Ophthalmology 1985; 92:1208–25.
53. Mitchell P, Wang MY, Wang JJ. Asteroid hyalosis in an older population: the Blue Mountains Eye Study. Ophthal Epidemiol 2003; 10:331–5.
54. Miyamoto T, Inoue H, Sakamoto Y, et al. Identification of a novel splice site mutation of the CSPG2 gene in a Japanese family with Wagner syndrome. Invest Ophthalmol Vis Sci 2005; 46:2726–35.
55. Moss SE, Klein R, Klein BE. Asteroid hyalosis in a population: the Beaver Dam eye study. Am J Ophthalmol 2001; 132:70–5.
56. Murata M, Horiuchi S. Hyaluronan synthases, hyaluronan and its CD44 receptors in the posterior segment of rabbit eye. Ophthalmologica 2005; 219:287–91.
57. O'Malley P. The pattern of vitreous syneresis. A study of 800 autopsy eyes. In: Irvine AR, O'Malley C, eds. Advances in Vitreous Surgery. Springfield, IL: Charles C Thomas, 1976:17–33.
58. Osterlin S. Changes in the vitreous with age. Trans Ophthalmol Soc UK 1975; 95:372–7.
59. Osterlin S. Macromolecular composition of the vitreous in the aphakic owl monkey eye. Exp Eye Res 1978; 26: 77–84.
60. Ponsioen TL, van der Worp RJ, van Luyn MJ, et al. Packages of vitreous collagen (type II) in the human retina: an indication of postnatal collagen turnover? Exp Eye Res 2005; 80:643–50.
61. Qiao H, Hisatomi T, Sonoda KH, et al. The characterisation of hyalocytes: the origin, phenotype, and turnover. Br J Ophthalmol 2005; 89:513–7.
62. Reardon A, Heinegard D, McLeod D, et al. The large chondroitin sulphate proteoglycan versican in mammalian vitreous. Matrix Biol 1998; 17:325–33.
63. Reardon A, Sandell L, Jones CJ, et al. Localization of pN-type IIA procollagen on adult bovine vitreous collagen fibrils. Matrix Biol 2000; 19:169–73.
64. Reardon AJ, Le Goff M, Briggs MD, et al. Identification in vitreous and molecular cloning of opticin, a novel member of the family of leucine-rich repeat proteins of the extracellular matrix. J Biol Chem 2000; 275:2123–9.
65. Ryan SJ. Traction retinal detachment. XLIX Edward Jackson Memorial Lecture. Am J Ophthalmol 1993; 115:1–20.
66. Sandgren O. Ocular amyloidosis, with special reference to the hereditary forms with vitreous involvement. Surv Ophthalmol 1995; 40:173–96.
67. Sebag J, Balazs EA. Morphology and ultrastructure of human vitreous fibers. Invest Ophthalmol Vis Sci 1989; 30: 1867–71.
68. Sebag J. Pharmacologic vitreolysis. Retina 1998; 18:1–3.
69. Sebag J. Anomalous posterior vitreous detachment: a unifying concept in vitreo-retinal disease. Graefes Arch Clin Exp Ophthalmol 2004; 242:690–8.
70. Sharma S, Walker R, Brown GC, Cruess AF. The importance of qualitative vitreous examination in patients with acute posterior vitreous detachment. Arch Ophthalmol 1999; 117:343–6.
71. Sheard RM, Goodburn SF, Comer MB, et al. Posterior vitreous detachment after neodymium: YAG laser posterior capsulotomy. J Cataract Refract Surg 2003; 29:930–4.
72. Sheibani N, Sorenson CM, Cornelius LA, et al. Thrombospondin-1, a natural inhibitor of angiogenesis, is present in vitreous and aqueous humor and is modulated by hyperglycemia. Biochem Biophys Res Commun 2000; 267:257–61.
73. Smiddy WE, Flynn HW Jr. Pathogenesis of macular holes and therapeutic implications. Am J Ophthalmol 2004; 137:525–37.
74. Smith LE, Kopchick JJ, Chen W, et al. Essential role of growth hormone in ischemia-induced retinal neovascularization. Science 1997; 276:1706–9.
75. Smith LE, Shen W, Perruzzi C, et al. Regulation of vascular endothelial growth factor-dependent retinal neovascularization by insulin-like growth factor-1 receptor. Nat Med 1999; 5:1390–5.
76. Snead MP, Yates JR. Clinical and molecular genetics of Stickler syndrome. J Med Genet 1999; 36:353–9.
77. Snowden JM, Eyre DR, Swann DA. Vitreous structure. VI. Age-related changes in the thermal stability and crosslinks of vitreous, articular cartilage and tendon collagens. Biochim Biophys Acta 1982; 706:153–7.
78. Sonoda KH, Sakamoto T, Qiao H, et al. The analysis of systemic tolerance elicited by antigen inoculation into the vitreous cavity: vitreous cavity-associated immune deviation. Immunology 2005; 116:390–9.
79. Spraul CW, Grossniklaus HE. Vitreous hemorrhage. Surv Ophthalmol 1997; 42:3–39.
80. Stefansson E. Oxygen and diabetic eye disease. Graefes Arch Clin Exp Ophthalmol 1990; 228:120–3.
81. Takanosu M, Boyd TC, Le Goff M, et al. Structure, chromosomal location, and tissue-specific expression of the mouse opticin gene. Invest Ophthalmol Vis Sci 2001; 42:2202–10.
82. Tanner V, Harle D, Tan J, et al. Acute posterior vitreous detachment: the predictive value of vitreous pigment and symptomatology. Br J Ophthalmol 2000; 84:1264–8.
83. Tien JY, Spicer AP. Three vertebrate hyaluronan synthases are expressed during mouse development in distinct spatial and temporal patterns. Dev Dyn 2005; 233:130–41.
84. Tolentino MJ, McLeod DS, Taomoto M, et al. Pathologic features of vascular endothelial growth factor-induced retinopathy in the nonhuman primate. Am J Ophthalmol 2002; 133:373–85.
85. Wang J, McLeod D, Henson DB, Bishop PN. Age-dependent changes in the basal retinovitreous adhesion. Invest Ophthalmol Vis Sci 2003; 44:1793–800.
86. Wenstrup RJ, Florer JB, Brunskill EW, et al. Type V collagen controls the initiation of collagen fibril assembly. J Biol Chem 2004; 279:53331–7.
87. Winkler J, Lunsdorf H. Ultrastructure and composition of asteroid bodies. Invest Ophthalmol Vis Sci 2001; 42:902–7.
88. Wong HC, Sehmi KS, McLeod D. Abortive neovascular outgrowths discovered during vitrectomy for diabetic

vitreous haemorrhage. Graefes Arch Clin Exp Ophthalmol 1989; 227:237–40.

89. Wright DW, Mayne R. Vitreous humor of chicken contains two fibrillar systems: an analysis of their structure. J Ultrastruct Mol Struct Res 1988; 100:224–34.

90. Yada T, Suzuki S, Kobayashi K, et al. Occurrence in chick embryo vitreous humor of a type IX collagen proteoglycan with an extraordinarily large chondroitin sulfate chain and short alpha 1 polypeptide. J Biol Chem 1990; 265: 6992–9.

30

Degenerations, Depositions, and Miscellaneous Reactions of the Ocular Anterior Segment

Gordon K. Klintworth
Departments of Pathology and Ophthalmology, Duke University, Durham, North Carolina, U.S.A.

PINGUECULAE

Overview

A pinguecula is a localized, slightly elevated yellowish area in the conjunctiva adjacent to the corneoscleral limbus in the interpalpebral fissure (Fig. 1). The designation stems from its yellowish-white fatlike appearance (Greek: *pinguecula,* fat) caused by altered underlying connective tissue.

Clinical Features

This frequently bilateral lesion may be on either or both sides of the globe, but more often it is situated nasally. The color varies with the thickness and degree of pigmentation of the overlying epithelium as well as the vascularity (265). Pingueculae tend to be oval or triangular in shape, with the base on the limbal side. They can appear before the end of the second decade, but pingueculae are predominantly lesions of middle and late life and their incidence increases with age.

Vision is not affected by pingueculae and an associated minor irritation can usually be controlled with artificial tears. Except for cosmetic reasons, these lesions seldom require excision, but following their excision they may recur to a mild degree within 18 months (211).

Epidemiology

Pingueculae are common in tropical and subtropical countries, less frequent in places of greater latitude, and rare in countries like England (27,55) and Finland (87). The prevalence of pingueculae has been determined in several regions including Jordan (90%) (210), Japan (Japanese Mongols in Kyoto) (60%) (212), Maryland, U.S.A. (watermen of Somerset or lower Dorchester County) (76.8%) (271), Greenland (56%) (210), and Denmark (41%) (210). The incidence of pingueculae correlates with outdoor working.

Histopathology

By light microscopy pingueculae are identical to actinic elastosis of the skin (Fig. 2), but have more nonfiber-forming aggregates, perhaps relating to a deficiency of elastic microfibrils, compared with dermal elastoses (179). Characteristically, amorphous hematoxophilic, or weakly eosinophilic, finely granular material accumulates in the immediate subepithelial tissue surrounded by altered collagen. Frequently variably sized and irregular-shaped concretions, which are predominantly basophilic but sometimes eosinophilic, are also present. When viewed by transmission electron microscopy (TEM) these, more or less homogeneously electron-dense structures lack a discernible infrastructure (137). A granular matrix and thickened vermiform, coiled fibers which are often accentuated by stains for elastic tissue are common. The insensitivity of such fibers to elastase digestion (41,281), does not necessarily indicate an absence of elastin, since conformational and other alterations may prevent a substrate from fitting to the active site of the degradative enzyme. Indeed immunoelectron microscopy has disclosed that the abnormal elastic fibers react with antibodies to elastin and microfibrillar protein. They also react with antibodies to amyloid P where these components do not normally colocalize, indicating that the fibers are not just immature but aberrant in composition (179). Other findings by immunoelectron microscopy include a mild positivity at the edges of the abnormal elastic tissue for the serum protease inhibitor α-1

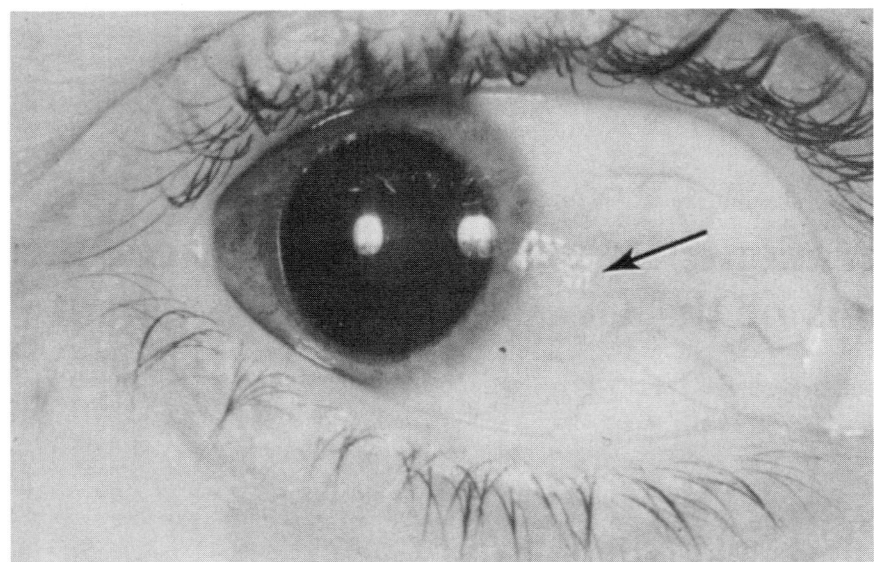

Figure 1 A pinguecula is located at the nasal limbus (*arrow*). *Source*: Reproduced from Klintworth GK, Landers MB III. The Eye: Structure and Function in Disease. Baltimore, MD: Williams and Wilkins, 1976.

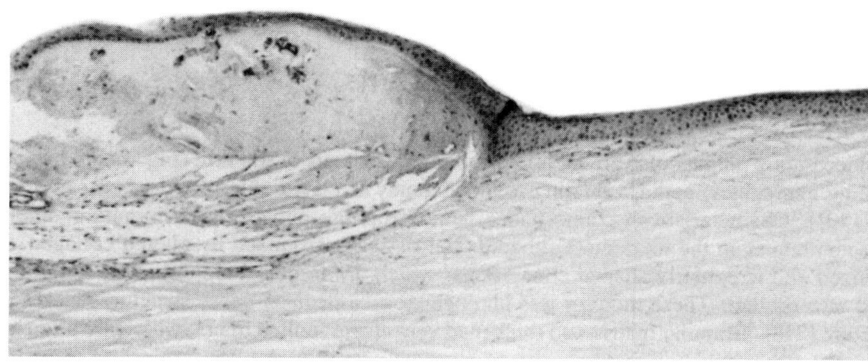

Figure 2 Pinguecula. The subconjunctival connective tissue adjacent to the cornea is thickened and contains degenerated elastotic material (hematoxylin and eosin, × 60).

antitrypsin and marked positivity for lysozyme. Dermal elastosis also contains amyloid P and lysozyme, which are thought to inhibit elastogenesis indirectly. The superficial region of pingueculae contains similar elastic constituents, but no fibers and few elastic microfibrils are present. The subepithelial dense concretions manifest strong staining for lysozyme. Elastic fibers are abnormal and their formation is distorted (7).

By TEM, fibroblasts, other connective tissue cells, and the collagen fibers appear abnormal and have been regarded as "degenerated or degenerating" (137). The tortuous elastotic fibers have been interpreted as enlarged preexisting elastic fibers, as abnormal new elastic fibers, and as a degenerative alteration of collagen (an elastotic or elastoid degeneration).

The subepithelial hyalinized zone of the substantia propria is the only site with morphologic evidence of collagen degeneration (effacement of the longitudinal periodicity and uncurling at the ends of collagen fibers). Material composed of numerous fibroblasts and hollow-centered microfibrils (an elastic fiber precursor), tends to clump centrally in the larger aggregated sheets and to acquire electron-dense inclusions. Focal calcifications and autofluorescent spheroidal bodies [as in chronic actinic keratopathy (CAK)] are frequently detected in pingueculae (161,208).

Fragments of abnormal elastic fibers may be evident within macrophages and a prominent foreign body giant-cell reaction is sometimes associated with the elastotic fibers (actinic granuloma) (81,117,227). A similar reaction, which may cause concern about a possible response to microorganisms or a foreign body, occasionally occurs in sun-damaged skin. The epithelium adjacent to a pinguecula may be normal, atrophic, or hyperplastic and form white plaques. Dysplasia, intraepithelial carcinoma, or even squamous cell carcinoma may develop in the conjunctiva and/or cornea, but the risk of a frank malignancy is extremely low.

Etiology and Pathogenesis

The frequent coexistence of pterygia with the much more common pingueculae has long been recognized and Fuchs (102,103) postulated that most pterygia develop from preexisting pingueculae. The two lesions are, however, distinct and not necessarily related (27,150,209).

In Gaucher disease (see Chapter 41), brown triangular "pingueculae" have been reported during the second decade of life. Such lesions, which are different from the common pingueculae, contain Gaucher cells and are probably extremely rare. The color of these lesions has been attributed to Gaucher cells, but serial light microscopic and TEM observations of yellow pingueculae in persons with Gaucher disease have disclosed the typical morphologic features of typical pinguecula and have not revealed Gaucher cells (33).

The association of ultraviolet (UV) radiation exposure with pinguecula is weaker than with pterygia and CAK (discussed later) (271).

The elastotic fibers appear to represent elastic fibers that are abnormally matured. They are surrounded by microfibrils, but numerous electron-dense inclusions are associated with focal zones of amorphous elastin deposition. Austin and colleagues (7) hypothesize that actinically damaged fibroblasts in the conjunctival substantia propria of pingueculae and pterygia synthesize elastic fiber precursors and abnormal maturational forms of elastic fibers (elastodysplasia) that undergo secondary degeneration (elastodystrophy).

PTERYGIA

Overview

In 1875, Walton (286) introduced the term pterygium (Greek: *pterygion*, wing) into the English literature to signify a flat triangular fold of vascularized bulbar conjunctiva, which encroaches onto the cornea in the horizontal meridian (Fig. 3). Since then the designation has acquired broader use with the introduction of

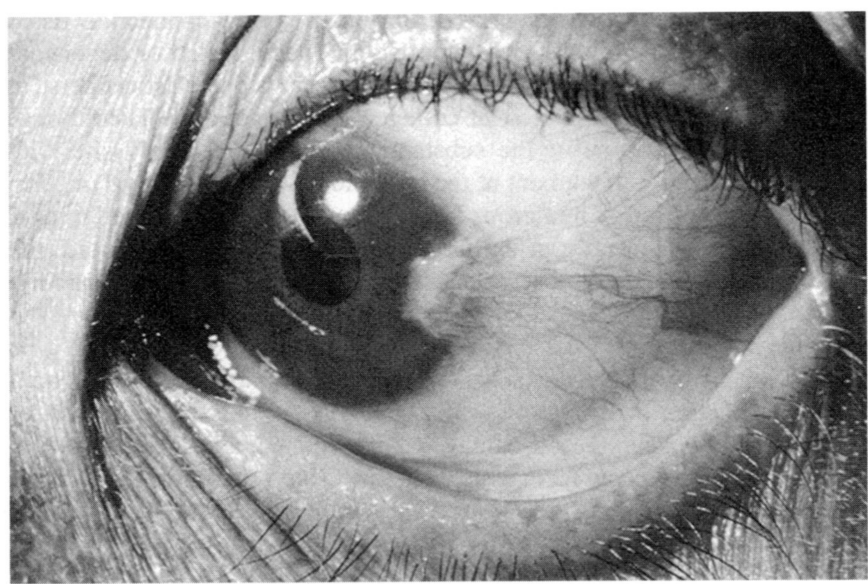

Figure 3 A pterygium has encroached onto the cornea from the temporal limbus. Such lesions commonly overlie an area of actinic elastosis. *Source*: Reproduced from Klintworth GK, Landers MB III. The Eye: Structure and Function in Disease. Baltimore, MD: Williams and Wilkins, 1976.

such terms as pterygium colli, popliteal pterygium, and limb pterygium (57,121,138,233). This has led to some confusion about the term pterygium especially in the genetically determined varieties.

Clinical Features

Epibulbar pterygia may be unilateral or bilateral but usually develop initially in the dominant eye, perhaps because individuals facing the sun keep the dominant eye open, but close the nondominant eye (145). In persons with exotropia a ptergium is found only in the fixing eye (246). Pterygia may occur on either side of the cornea but, like pingueculae with which they are often associated, the nasal corneoscleral limbus is involved much more often (151,157). In one survey 13% of pterygia occurred only on the temporal side of the cornea, despite the traditional belief that they are rare in that location (58).

Focal conjunctivitis at the corneoscleral limbus ("chronic irritative exposure conjunctivitis") frequently precedes a pterygium (150) and pterygia evolve through a conjunctival and a corneal (true pterygial) phase (45). Pterygia induce clinically significant irregular corneal astigmatism due to tractional distortion, the pooling of tears in advance of the pterygium, or both (6,216). Pterygia may encroach upon the visual axis necessitating surgical excision, but following surgical removal ptergyia commonly recur (141) particularly in younger patients and in tropical areas. Most recurrences occur within 2 months of surgery (132) and are more difficult to manage than the primary lesions (141).

Epidemiology

The prevalence of pterygia varies in different countries being highest in tropical and subtropical regions and less common in countries situated further from the equator. They are common in Lima, Peru (31.06%) (244), Australia (184,269), Maryland, U.S.A. (watermen in Somerset or lower Dorchester County) (16.6%) (271), Jordan (12%) (210), Greenland (9%) (210), but uncommon in Japan (1%) (212). Pterygia are common in Hawaii (212), but rare in Britain (27,55), Finland (87), and other places.

Pterygia are common in fishermen (271), Eskimos (253), Canadian Cree Indians (206), and other populations exposed to excessive UV radiation from the sun. In Australian aborigines pterygia correlate positively with lower latitudes and high UV levels (269).

Where pterygia are common their incidence increases with age and surveys in several countries, including Barbados (182), Peru (Lima) (244), Australia (269), Israel (294), Singapore (290), and Greenland (209) have disclosed a predilection of men and outdoor workers for pterygia (87,131). Differences in lifestyle explain discrepancies in the prevalences in the racial groups and between the sexes (199).

Other predisposing occupations include welders in whom there is a close relationship between the incidence and the length of employment. Welders exposed occupationally to excess UV radiation have a significantly high incidence of pterygia (151). In regions where pterygia are endemic, such as the Sahara desert, their presence correlates with the severity and the duration of exposure to predisposing factors (45).

In some populations in which pterygia are frequent putative sun-induced ocular lesions, such as conjunctival spheroidal degeneration and pingeculae, are common (151).

Histopathology

Pterygia possess many histopathologic hallmarks of chronic inflammation (77,153). The lymphocytic infiltration in pterygia consists predominantly of T-cells (132). Eosinophils and basophils are not conspicuous, but the infiltration of small lymphocytes and plasma cells has led some authors to suspect an immunologic mechanism in the pathogenesis of pterygium (223). Neovascularization, which is probably inflammatory in nature, is prominent in the subepithelial connective tissue. These processes, together with actinic damage, are probably responsible for the fibrovascular reaction so characteristic of a growing pterygium (133). At least in some parts of the world almost all pterygia are associated with actinic elastosis (176), but pterygia can apparently develop in the absence of pingueculae (151,266) and elastotic degeneration is reportedly uncommon in pterygia in India (5). A conspicuous feature of the epithelium in pterygia is the increased number of goblet cells. Occasionally as in pingueculae the epithelium may be hyperplastic, dysplastic, or a site of intraepithelial carcinoma.

Myofibroblasts are not a feature of pterygia (216), but the advancing subepithelial connective tissue cap area of pterygia surrounding Bowman layer contains activated fibroblasts. These cells, which probably originate from the pericorneal connective tissue (28), extend into the superficial cornea above and below Bowman layer, destroying the latter and a variable amount of superficial corneal stroma.

Nongoblet epithelial cells of pterygia, but not those of normal conjunctiva react with certain lectins (*Ulex europaeus* agglutinin-1, *Dolichos biflorus* agglutinin and peanut agglutinin), suggesting that pterygia secrete anomalous mucus glycoproteins (153).

Pterygia and normal conjunctival tissue both contain immunohistochemically detectable collagen types I, II, and III (52) and in the epithelial and capillary endothelial basement membranes collagen type IV is also located. In keeping with the conjunctival origin of pterygia their collagens are thought to be derived from conjunctival tissue rather than from the cornea (52) (normal corneal stroma has collagen types I and III, but not collagen type II).

A direct immunofluorescence study of surgically excised pterygia with fluorescein-labeled goat antihuman immunoglobulins has disclosed positive staining for immunoglobulin G (IgG) in 19 of 26 cases (73.1%) and immunoglobulin E (IgE) in all 26 samples (223).

Molecular Biologic Studies

Mutations in the *TP53* gene, which encodes tumor protein p53 (also known by the informal label p53) have been detected in 15.7% of pterygia (267,278,279). A notable protein identified in the nuclei of the epithelium in pterygia is cyclin-dependent kinase inhibitor 2A (p16) (31). Because aberrant methylation of the promoter of the *CDKN2A* gene that encodes p16 has been detected in many human cancers the possibility of this occurring in pterygia has also been investigated and Chen et al. (31) found evidence for this in 21 of 129 pterygia specimens. This hypermethylation was strongly linked to the expression of DNA methyltransferase 3B (*DNMT3B*) proteins and the suppression of cyclin-dependent kinase inhibitor 2A (31). The oncogene *Ki-ras* has been found to be mutated in 10% of pterygia (60).

Etiology and Pathogenesis

Chronic conjunctival irritation due to solar radiation has long been suspected as causing pterygia, as their prevalence, like solar radiation, diminishes with increasing latitude. Both the infrared and UV bands of the solar spectrum have been implicated (270), but because pterygia are not an occupational disease of furnace workers, stokers, and other persons exposed to heat, they are probably not caused by infrared radiation. Conversely, there is ample circumstantial evidence implicating chronic UV light in the pathogenesis of pterygia (27,55,63,75,133,151,155,199,269). Pterygia are associated with a broadband of UV radiation exposure (UVB, 290–320 nm; UVA1, 340–400 nm; and UVA2, 320–340 nm), but UVB seems to be implicated the most (184). As mentioned above under "Epidemiology" section, the frequency of pterygia and the degree of exposure to UV light radiation are positively correlated (63).

It is noteworthy, however, that pterygia are not closely linked to clinically detectable pingueculae, conjunctival spheroidal degeneration and CAK, which are also thought to be effects of chronic UV radiation (133). Also, pterygia are uncommon in Japan (151), whereas conjunctival spheroidal degeneration and pingeculae are common in that country (212).

Consequently UV light is probably not the only environmental factor causing pterygia. Moreover, a survey of ocular disease among Punjabi Indians who immigrated to British Columbia (Canada) (an area with less solar irradiation than India) suggests that sawmill workers may be prone to pterygia. Punjabi Indian workers in sawmills (an indoor occupation) in both British Columbia and New Delhi have a higher prevalence of pterygia than Punjabi farmers (an outdoor occupation) in India. In Canada pterygia are more common in the Indian sawmill workers (12%) than in the white workers (2%) (58). Furthermore, the likelihood of pterygia developing increases with the duration of employment in the mill. A higher prevalence rate in sawmill workers than controls has also been found in Taiwan and Thailand (58).

Pterygia have also been considered a manifestation of chronic conjunctival irritation caused by repeated microtrauma and, to a lesser degree, by other causal factors. In some geographic areas where pterygia are prevalent dust, wind, and excessive desiccation often coexist with the sun-glare but they are not constant features of the external milieu in areas where pterygia are common. Desiccation is not essential since a high incidence of pterygia occurs in some areas of high humidity (63,131). A study of tear function in Australian Aborigines makes it unlikely that pterygia are caused by a flagrant abnormality of the tear film (268). Risk factors for pterygia include previous sun exposure especially during the first 5 years of like, outdoor work and an environment with high service reflectance of UV light (2,62,184,273). Less tenable environmental factors implicated in pterygia are viruses (59). The reported association of pterygia with trachoma and poor housing in Libya (11) has not been confirmed and is probably coincidental. The protection of eyes with regular glasses, sun glasses or the wearing of a hat appears to offer protection against pterygia (184).

Genetics

An inherited susceptibility to ptergyia seems likely in view of twin studies (80) and other investigations. The data in some families are consistent with an autosomal dominant mode of transmission. Unilateral or bilateral pterygia have occurred in two or more generations of several families (102,131,140,296), and some familial cases have lacked a history of unusual exposure to the elements (128). Familial cases are rarely congenital (140,203); others become manifest in early adulthood (128) or midlife (296). Even in persons exposed to apparently similar solar radiation the vulnerability to pterygia is greater in blood relatives of persons with the condition than in the general population (16).

Racial differences in the incidence of pterygia, which may reflect a genetic predisposition, occurs in some geographic areas such as Aruba, an island off the coast of Venezuela (131), and in Canada (58).

The reason why pterygia as well as pingueculae occur more frequently on the nasal side of the eye is uncertain. Mechanical irritation by dust particles enhanced by a tear flow toward the nasally located puncta has been suggested (76,110), but this explanation has serious shortcomings because pterygia occur in relatively dust-free regions and even in sailors (63,131). Others have suggested that the longer temporal eyelashes of the upper eyelid and the greater downward bowing of the upper eyelid protect the outer part of the eye and shade it more from light than the nasal part (27).

Because pterygia are not only growths on the cornea, but also prone to recurrence following excision some investigators regard them as neoplasms rather than degenerative lesions. Moreover, some investigators claim support for this hypothesis with the discovery of p53 protein in the epithelium of pterygia, but this is contrary to the traditional definition of a neoplasm (see Chapter 53).

ELASTOFIBROMA

An elastofibroma-containing islands of adipose tissue, activated fibroblasts, and mature elastic fibers entrenched within thickened clusters of collagen has been documented in the temporal conjunctiva with extension into the lateral fornices and canthus (8). In contradistinction to the considerably commoner pterygium and pinguecula the epibular elastofibroma spares the immediate subepithelial conjunctiva and microfibrillar aggregates and dystrophic elastic fibers are absent.

CHRONIC ACTINIC KERATOPATHY (CLIMATIC DROPLET KERATOPATHY)

Overview

White, grayish, or yellow particles accumulate in the interpalpebral portion of the cornea of both eyes in an entity made notorious by its many names, which include CAK, climatic droplet keratopathy (CDK), Bietti nodular keratopathy, Labrador keratopathy, gelatinous dystrophy, and spheroidal degeneration of the cornea (116,162). The diverse nomenclature reflects the geographic location of the condition, the clinical appearance, histochemical findings, and potential causal factors, with a lack of agreement stemming from the varied backgrounds and viewpoints of different observers, our ignorance of the precise nature of the corneal deposits and the lack of an experimental model of the keratopathy. Many terms are clearly no longer appropriate for reasons considered elsewhere (162). The popular connotation CDK also has serious semantic shortcomings. Firstly, the climate of a region designates the long-term manifestations of weather. It reflects various atmospheric phenomena, such as temperature, wind, moisture, and various atmospheric pollutants. Solar radiation is not part of the climate according to the traditional use of the word, but rather a factor influencing it. Also, "droplet," while descriptive of a solitary clinical feature, not only lacks precision, but ignores many established aspects of the disorder.

Clinical Features

In the absence of overt disease and apparent inflammation, opacities initially become clinically evident in the peripheral cornea in the horizontal meridian, where they commonly appear like oil droplets in the conjunctiva on either side of the cornea. With time the deposits become more numerous, increase in size, and sometimes form a band across the cornea as they extend centrally.

Based on the severity of the condition, which perhaps reflects the evolution of the disorder, CAK can be subdivided into the following grades (116): trace (deposits only in small numbers in one eye or only at the end of the interpalpebral strip in each eye if bilateral), grade 1 (involvement of medial and lateral interpalpebral strips with sparing of central cornea), grade 2 (central cornea affected but not enough to affect visual acuity), grade 3 (central cornea affected and vision reduced), and grade 4 (elevated nodules present in addition to findings of grade 3).

Multiple discrete yellowish spheroidal-shaped globules occasionally gather in the interpalpebral portion of the conjunctiva adjacent to the cornea. The term conjunctival spheroidal degeneration has been coined for this condition (91), which appears to be an earlier and milder manifestation of CAK, but in which the conjunctiva is involved often in the presence of a clinically normal cornea. When present the spheroidal deposits occur more frequently in the conjunctiva alone (74%) than either the cornea (18%), or cornea and conjunctiva combined (8%) (208).

Many of the conjunctival globules manifest autofluorescence when examined by slit-lamp biomicroscopy (208). Like pingueculae and pterygia the nasal conjunctiva is affected more often than the temporal conjunctiva, which is rarely involved in Eskimos perhaps because of their slanting eyes and narrow palpebral fissure (208). Small autofluorescent and colorless spheroids recur in the conjunctiva following excision after an observation period of 18 months (211).

The corneal opacities have been noted to regress spontaneously after cataract surgery (51). This observation is difficult to explain, but a change in corneal curvature, which would affect the degree of indirect scattered or reflected radiation, has been suggested as a possible explanation.

A significant association with pterygium does not exist (94,212,236).

Epidemiology

The prevalence of conjunctival spheroidal degeneration varies in different populations and rises with increasing age. It is high in Jordan (40%) (210), Japan (Mongols in Kyoto) (31%) (212), Southwestern Greenland (Eskimos) (12.3%) (210), and low in Copenhagen Denmark (Caucasians) (4.1%) (208).

A male preponderance has been noted in most (86,91,92,105), but not in all series (208,236).

Surveys of the prevalence of CAK in different countries support the hypothesis that UV light is an important risk factor. The prevalence of CAK is greatest where UV light is at a maximum and it diminishes in proportion to the amount of UV light (210). CAK also has an earlier age of onset in places with the greatest amount of UV light (210).

In regions where conjunctival spheroidal degeneration and CAK are prevalent affected individuals are predominantly men who are, or have been fishermen, divers, trappers, stockman, or other outdoor workers (97,269,293). In Labrador the only affected women have spent a considerable amount of time outdoors (146). In Australia a prevalence of 41% has been detected in aboriginal men who had worked as stockmen for more than 20 years in contrast to 8% for aboriginal women aged 45 years or more (269). Even in Britain where the disease is mild and uncommon, most persons with CAK have spent much of their lives outdoors (105).

CAK appears worldwide, but it is most prevalent and severe in certain geographic areas, such as Labrador (96,146), Dahlak islands in the Red Sea (236). North Cameroon (4), Australia (269), and Saudi Arabia (187), where UV light is unshaded or highly reflected. In watermen working on the Chesapeake Bay in Maryland, U.S.A., the prevalence of CAK was 19.3% (271). Like pterygium CAK is significantly associated with a broadband of UV radiation exposure (290–400 nm). The incidence and severity of CAK are less in the northern than the southern parts of the Arctic region (86). The view that the keratopathy in the Red Sea differs from the one observed in Arctic areas (236) is not accepted by all (210).

Histopathology

Numerous extracellular granules and concretions of variable size constitute a conspicuous finding in CAK (Fig. 4) and are easily identified in unstained tissue secretions viewed by fluorescence microscopy because of their intense yellow autofluorescence (161). The proteinaceous bodies in conjunctival spheroidal degeneration are also strongly autofluorescent and resemble similar bodies in pingueculae (144). They possess a variable electron density with a fine granular structure. The identity of the protein that makes up the bulk of concretions remains unknown. Although not always evident on clinical examination, actinic elastosis (the histopathologic counterpart of pingueculae) is commonly found in tissue sections (162) and these lesions contain identical concretions (161,162). Viewed by TEM the proteinaceous granules occur extracellularly as variably sized round to oval electron densities (Fig. 5) (1,26,106,146,161), and ultrastructural evidence of such material being synthesized by corneal cells has not been observed.

Yellow globules within the cornea in this keratopathy have been likened to oil droplets, but

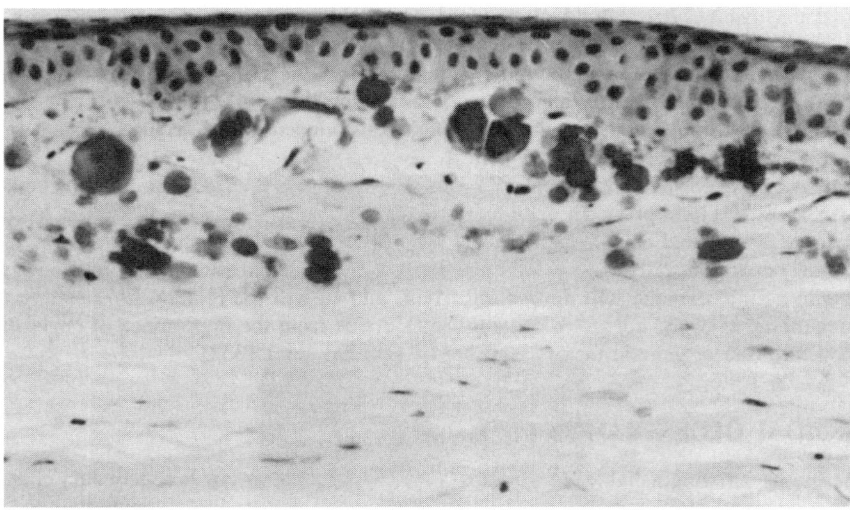

Figure 4 Chronic actinic keratopathy. Numerous rounded concretions are present in the superficial corneal stroma (hematoxylin and eosin, × 250).

lipid is not a significant constituent (26,161). Despite the basophilia of some granules calcification is rarely present by standard histochemical procedures. Although most concretions stain positively with some methods for elastic tissue (such as the Verhoeff–van Gieson technique) (26,32,147,161,241), others lack this affinity (105,147,161). Moreover, unlike normal elastic fibers the accumulations do not stain with orcein or aldehyde fuchsin (105,147). Identical granules are commonly found in pingueculae (161), in actinic (solar) elastosis of the skin (161), and at the corneoscleral limbus of eyes with presumed sun-induced lesions like actinic keratosis, intraepithelial, and invasive squamous carcinoma, and variable degrees of elastotic degeneration (26). In one investigation the deposits were resistant to elastase digestion (26), but this observation indicates nothing about the nature of the material as the cornea had been embedded in paraffin making it an inappropriate substrate to evaluate by enzymatic digestion.

Etiology and Pathogenesis

That CAK is caused by exposure to some environmental factors related to the proportion of time spent outdoors is widely accepted. In some regions where CAK is severe, eyes become exposed to climatic extremes, evaporation, and the traumatic aftermath of windblown sand or ice. For example, in the Dahlak islands, natural or artificial shade does not exist (236). Possible causal factors include evaporation in areas of low humidity, microtrauma from windblown minute particles like snow and ice (in snowbound regions such as Labrador and Newfoundland), or dust and

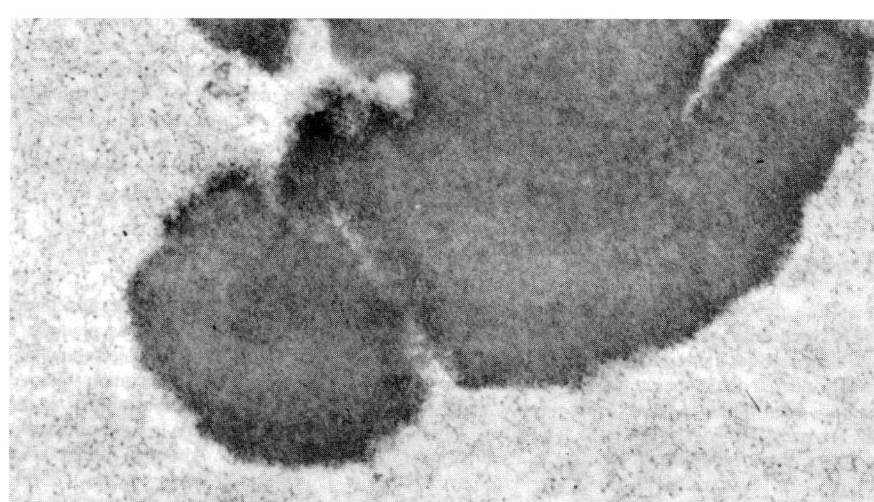

Figure 5 Electron-dense deposits among collagen fibrils in corneal stroma in chronic actinic keratopathy (× 43,900). *Source*: Reproduced from Klintworth GK, McCracken JS. Corneal diseases. In: Johannessen JV, ed. Electron Microscopy in Human Medicine, Vol. 6, Part 3. New York: McGraw-Hill, 1979:239–66.

sand (as in the deserts of North Africa and the Middle East), as well as solar irradiation. The climate varies considerably in geographic areas where CAK is recognized and injurious environmental factors in some regions are absent in other locations with the keratopathy indicating that they are not essential to its development. For instance, CAK can develop where the atmosphere lacks excessive particulate matter. Evaporation could predispose to the precipitation of the proteins in the superficial cornea, as it does in calcific band keratopathy (67), but excessive evaporation from the cornea, does not seem to be important. CAK occurs in some arid areas and in regions like Labrador, where the air contains negligible water vapor (96), but it is also found in regions where the humidity is not low (95). Also, similar stromal deposits are not features of the dry eye syndrome or exposure keratopathy, where excessive evaporation takes place.

UV light from solar irradiation is the prime suspect as the fundamental causal factor of CAK (91,94,98,161,237). The potential for excessive exposure to radiant surgery from the sun is common to all geographic areas where CAK is prevalent. UV light possessing a wavelength of less than 295 nm is almost entirely absorbed by the cornea and this seems to be the most probable form of energy to implicate. The high incidence of CAK in places where sand, snow, and surf predominate is readily accounted for by the fact that most UV light with a wavelength of 295 to 320 nm (UVB) that strikes the ocular surface is indirect, scattered, or reflected radiation (albedo) (46).

Both the prevalence and the gravity of CAK seem to be directly related to the levels of exposure to sunlight. In the extreme northern latitudes, where other adverse climatic factors still exist, the sun does not rise high above the horizon and the effects of UV light are not as pronounced as in more southern areas. In Britain, where the population is to some extent protected from UV irradiation by a blanket of clouds, CAK is less common than in countries with higher levels of sunlight (105). UV light is reflected by snow, desert, and water, which are prominent features of the external milieu in some areas where CAK is severe. Absorption of radiant energy from the sun can account for the predisposition for the exposed interpalpebral portion of the eye, the usual bilaterality of the condition, the male preponderance that reflects outdoor occupations, as well as the increased incidence with advancing years due to an increased time of solar exposure. Further support for the notion that CAK is solar-induced is the finding of an advanced degree of CAK in a 30-year-old black subject with xeroderma pigmentosum (MIM +278700) (discussed in Chapter 56), an inherited disease in individuals who are sensitive to light with a wavelength of 280 to 310 nm (98).

Morphologic observations also support the belief that CAK follows the cumulative effect of chronic solar irradiation. As pointed out above, CAK is associated with conjunctival elastosis in the same eye, and its characteristic concretions are indistinguishable from those found in pingueculae and cutaneous actinic elastosis (solar elastosis) (161). Abundant evidence suggests that that dermal actinic elastosis is a sequel to prolonged exposure to sunlight: (*i*) it is restricted to parts of the skin which are exposed to solar irradiation, (*ii*) it is most severe in areas receiving the most intense and prolonged exposure to sunlight, (*iii*) it is less evident in heavily pigmented skin which protects the dermis from UV light, (*iv*) it can be produced experimentally with UV light, and (*v*) in Caucasians probable sun-induced cutaneous tumors, such as basal cell carcinomas and melanomas, are associated with it.

Aside from the importance of environment as a cause of CAK, the role of genetic factors is raised by familial cases (193).

Excessive ocular exposure to UV light over relatively short time periods produces acute keratoconjunctivitis (AKC). If UV light produces CAK it probably does so at energy levels too low to cause AKC because a history of repeated episodes of AKC is usually lacking in individuals with CAK (94,95).

Unfortunately CAK has neither been detected naturally in any animal nor has it been produced experimentally.

The concretions possess an affinity for certain histochemical and empirical stains, and these properties permit one to deduce that they are predominantly proteinaceous in nature with phenyl, indole, guanidyl, and sulhydryl reactive groups and composed in part of sulfur-containing amino acids, as well as tyrosine, tryptophan, and arginine. Proteins with the latter components are not detectable in the normal cornea by histochemical methods. The claim that the material is of collagenous origin (50) is refuted by histochemical data. Since tryptophan, tyrosine, and sulfur-containing amino acids are absent from collagen or present in insignificant quantities, the denaturation of collagen should not release these reactive moieties. A different source for the concretions must be sought. It is conceivable that they are products of injured corneal and/or conjunctival cells, or that they enter the damaged tissue from the conjunctival blood vessels or elsewhere. Impressed by histochemical similarities to keratin, Garner (104) at one time suggested that the epithelium might be a potential source of the material.

That the concretions appear to be a protein rich in amino acids that are not normally detected in the cornea, combined with the absence of morphologic evidence of their synthesis by corneal cells suggests that the concretions are not formed there by the degradation of normal constituents. If they are synthesized by corneal and other cells, the protein presumably accumulates over time after photochemical reactions that probably results in cross-linkages. A possible site for their origin can be inferred from observations on eyes with the mild forms of the condition. In such instances, which presumably represent early stages in the genesis of the keratopathy, the concretions occur only in the superficial interpalpebral portion of the peripheral cornea. This finding together with the coexistence of the keratopathy with pingueculae containing identical proteinaceous granules suggests that the concretions may form in the conjunctiva. This hypothesis is underscored by the occasional presence of identical concretions in pingueculae of eyes which lack them in the cornea (161). One is led to suspect that a protein, which is synthesized in the conjuctiva, progressively diffuses into the superficial cornea, and accumulates there with time, resulting in larger globules which form by the coalescence of the smaller ones. Clinical findings in individuals with variable degrees of the keratopathy are consistent with this concept. From a clinical standpoint the first detectable droplets are restricted to the medial and lateral parts of the cornea in the interpalpebral fissure, while subsequent progression ensues by centripetal extension across the cornea. The observations that some concretions stain with histochemical procedures which demonstrate elastic fibers and that the corneal concretions coexist with pingueculae raises the possibility of the concretions being derived from constituents of conjunctival elastotic debris. Johnson and Overall (147) have suggested that UV light may act upon plasma proteins in the subconjunctival tissue and as they diffuse through the cornea. An attempt has been made to identify the protein by analyzing specimens by sodium dodecyl sulfate-polyacrylamide gel electrophoresis (SDS-PAGE), but because of the extreme insolubility of the protein it remains uncertain whether extracted high-molecular-weight proteins (molecular mass 20–300 kDa) (263) are identical to those that are evident histologically.

SPHEROIDAL DEGENERATION OF THE CORNEA

Overview

Corneal concretions indistinguishable from those of CAK occasionally occur as a secondary change in eyes with a variety of chronic disorders. Such cases are designated spheroidal degeneration of the cornea, secondary CDK or secondary proteinaceous "droplet" keratopathy for want of a better term (115).

Etiology and Pathogenesis

Spheroidal degeneration has been observed in association with absolute glaucoma, phthisis bulbi, and various chronic corneal conditions including post-traumatic scars, and lattice corneal dystrophy (26,32,50,104,122,161,241). In areas with little actinic radiation, these corneal concretions are almost always associated with an underlying ocular disorder (105). Spheroidal degeneration is clearly relevant to the pathogenesis of CAK. Because actinic elastosis appears to be a unique reaction to irradiation, one might wonder whether the apparently identical corneal concretions in all situations have a common denominator. Subjects with normal vision close their eyes voluntarily in the presence of excessive glare or respond reflex with excessive blinking and blepharospasm. These protective mechanisms are impaired in the blind eye, making it more prone to the effects of solar irradiation than the normal one. Because spheroidal degeneration of the cornea tends to occur in eyes with markedly impaired visual acuity, such eyes may be particularly vulnerable to UV light even in regions with little actinic irradiation. The observation of similar deposits in the peripheral cornea in alkaptonuria (ochronosis) (discussed in Chapter 43), an entity in which a melanin-like pigment derived from polymerized homogentisic acid accumulates in various tissues, including the interpalpebral portion of the sclera, is also relevant since pigment aids in the absorption of UV light. Nevertheless, because it is axiomatic that all tissues, including the cornea, possess limited responses to noxious stimuli multiple pathogenetic mechanisms may culminate in spheroidal degeneration of the cornea.

SENILE SCLERAL PLAQUES

Overview

Discrete slate gray areas immediately in front of the insertions of the horizontal rectus muscles are common in otherwise normal eyes in elderly individuals (Fig. 6). Although often referred to as plaques, the abnormalities are not flattened elevations but part of the sclera.

Clinical Features

Senile scleral plaques are almost always situated about 1.5 to 2 mm anterior to the medial or lateral rectus muscle insertions (39,115,152,160,207,245), but similar "plaques" rarely have been noted in front of the inferior rectus muscles (18,109). The clinical evolution of these lesions has been followed by Norn (207) who found them to begin as grayish bands in front of the rectus muscle insertions and usually to enlarge in all directions with advancing years. Although rare, prior to the seventh decade (39),

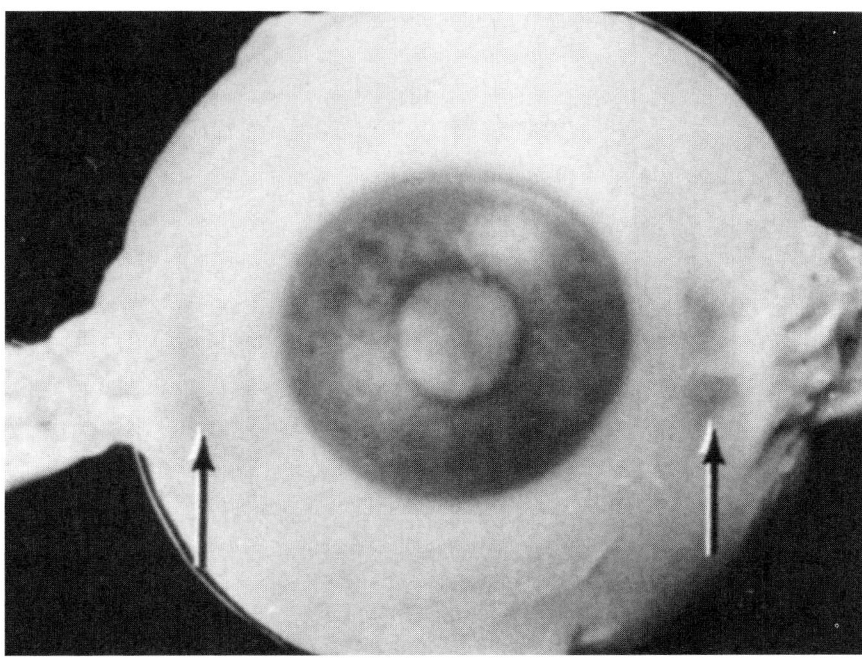

Figure 6 Senile scleral plaques in front of medial and lateral rectus muscles (*arrows*).

scleral plaques increase in incidence with age thereafter. Such patches tend to be bilateral, symmetrical, sharply demarcated, and elliptical in shape, with the vertical and horizontal diameters being about 6 and 2 mm, respectively. The discolored areas have an increased translucency to light, and the dark color results from an enhanced visibility of the underlying ciliary body. The lesion seldom concerns the patient, yet the plaques have clinical significance, since they may be mistaken for transcleral extension of a melanoma or scleromalacia perforans (discussed in Chapter 6).

Histopathology

The scleral thickness at the site of the "plaque" is either normal or slightly increased. Some regard hyalinization of the sclera as a significant abnormality (49), while others stress its absence (170). Microscopic examination of the sclera overlying the pars plana portion of the ciliary body has disclosed a spectrum of histopathologic abnormalities, which include an increased hematoxylinophilia of scleral collagen, decreased cellularity, and the presence of unique corkscrew-shaped fibers (252). Extensive plaques calcify (160) (Fig. 7), probably after the focal loss of scleral cells and alterations in the extracellular matrix of the sclera, predominantly as an apatite (calcium phosphate), although X-ray diffraction disclosed calcium sulfate (gypsum) to be the only calcified salt in an exceptional case (38,39). Rarely, sequestration and expulsion of the calcified "plaque" leaves a crater in the sclera, designated senile scleromalacia (186). Such a scleral defect has well-defined margins and lacks the fibrinoid necrosis and granulomatous inflammatory reaction of scleromalacia perforans, which it mimics clinically.

Etiology and Pathogenesis

Advanced age is the lesion's most consistent association and theories of causation have centered on a poor blood supply, mechanical muscular action, and desiccation. Translucent localized ill-defined spots can form in the sclera due to focal dehydration, as in prolonged surgical procedures on the eye, and in dislocated rabbit eyes treated with topical glycerin (108). Some observers consider these reversible gray patches of desiccation comparable to the senile scleral plaques.

Impaired circulation to the involved portion of the sclera has been implicated (18,229). In the elderly, the scleral plaques often coexist with atherosclerosis, which also increases in incidence with age, but scleral plaques do not accompany atherosclerosis or other occlusive vascular diseases in the young.

Since the plaques occur in front of the insertions of the rectus muscle insertions, some workers suggest that the accumulative stress and strain on the sclera exerted by muscular action over many decades may play a role in the genesis of the lesions (18,160,207). The shape of the plaques and their tendency to enlarge mainly in a vertical plane is in accord with this theory. Several authors have noted the "plaques" to be more common opposite the medial than the lateral rectus muscle (18), and this has been attributed to the excessive use of the medial recti during convergence. Some reports

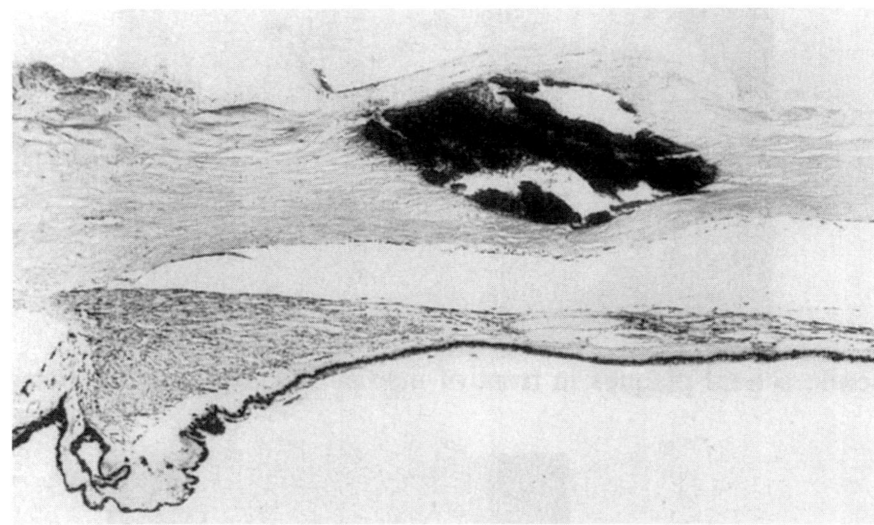

Figure 7 A calcified plaque is present within the sclera adjacent to the pars plana of the ciliary body (hematoxylin and eosin, ×27). *Source*: From Ref. 252.

mention an association with pingueculae (18,217), which may hide the "plaque" from view (18), and although this relationship has received little attention it has also been found in a histologic study of eyes obtained postmortem (252). In view of the putative actinically induced histopathologic connective tissue abnormalities, the possibility that the senile plaques are a culmination of chronic UV light irradiation is the most attractive hypothesis (252).

CORNEAL AND CONJUNCTIVAL CALCIFICATION

Calcific Band Keratopathy

Overview

An opaque band extending across the cornea in the interpalpebral fissure is a common corneal abnormality. Most cases result from a deposition of calcium (calcific band keratopathy); others are caused by an abnormal accumulation of protein presumably as a result of chronic UV irradiation from the sun (CAK) (discussed earlier in this chapter).

Clinical Features

Calcific band keratopathy may occur at any age and has been observed at birth and in early infancy (154,264,272). In this common disorder a slight turbidity usually begins in the peripheral cornea within the interpalpebral fissure. The opacity first appears as numerous gray dots, beneath the corneal epithelium at the level of Bowman layer and they subsequently coalesce and become chalky white. Small round transparent areas remain in the affected cornea and are regarded as pathognomonic for the human condition. The peripheral corneal deposits are well demarcated from the corneoscleral limbus by a clear zone. The opacities, which accumulate from the nasal and temporal sides of the cornea gradually impair vision as they form an opaque band, which may stretch across the cornea. When related to hypercalcemia this process can occur within 8 to 10 weeks (35), but even in the absence of hypercalcemia it can develop within 24 h (93). Less commonly, the condition begins in the central cornea and extends centrifugally. Usually the epithelium and the deeper layers of the cornea, as well as the superior and inferior cornea, are normal. Portions of the incrustation may break-off unexpectedly (69), but the band rarely regresses spontaneously (196). Clearing of the cornea sometimes follows alleviation of hypercalcemia, application of the chelating agent disodium ethylenediaminetetraacetic acid (EDTA) (19,89,231), or the removal of the epithelium but, as after lamellar keratoplasty, the band keratopathy may recur.

Histopathology

Calcific band keratopathy is typified by basophilic extracellular deposits having a predilection for Bowman zone and the adjacent superficial stroma in the interpalpebral portion of the cornea (Fig. 8). The deep stroma may be exclusively involved (93). The overlying corneal epithelium may be thin and the deeper layers of the cornea are unremarkable in the usual case. When band keratopathy complicates hypercalcemia, the sclera calcifies especially adjacent to the ciliary body (35,107). Calcium has been identified in band keratopathy by histochemical methods and energy-dispersive X-ray analysis (50,93), and has been interpreted by X-ray diffraction

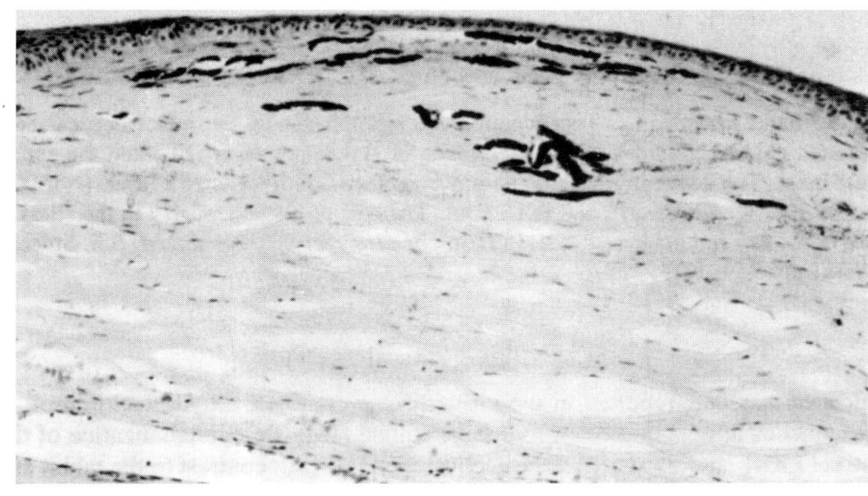

Figure 8 Extracellular calcified deposits in superficial corneal stroma in calcific band keratopathy (Von Kossa stain, × 110). *Source*: Reproduced from Klintworth GK, Landers MB III. The Eye: Structure and Function in Disease. Baltimore, MD: Williams and Wilkins, 1976.

and electron microprobe analysis as hydroxyapatite (13). TEM has disclosed the calcified deposits to be extracellular (Fig. 9), but in hyperparathyroidism and idiopathic hypercalcemia of infancy the calcified precipitates have also been seen in the cytoplasm and nuclei of the corneal epithelium and endothelium, appearing by TEM as multiple needlelike crystals (13,143).

Etiology and Pathogenesis

Calcific band keratopathy usually accompanies other ocular disorders, particularly uveitis, chronic glaucoma, and phthisis bulbi. It may follow chemical injuries (205) and has been described as an occupational hazard of hatters (125). In the absence of an underlying corneal disease, calcific band keratopathy may complicate hypercalcemia (285) as in hyperparathyroidism (13), an excessive ingestion of vitamin D (112), sarcoidosis (48,251), Fanconi syndrome (197), the milk alkali syndrome (70,192,238,261,287,288), and hypophosphatasia (177). In hypercalcemia the keratopathy is usually bilateral and symmetrical and often accompanied by calcification of the bulbar conjunctiva, particularly near the corneoscleral limbus in the interpalpebral fissure; rarely, as discussed later, the entire cornea opacifies.

Band keratopathy occurs in children with uveitis and arthritis (Still disease) (17,56,168,259,296) but rarely with other types of juvenile uveitis.

Calcific band keratopathy has been observed in two successive generations (100,113,272) and with several distinct genetically determined disorders including: (*i*) Norrie disease (MIM + 310600) (272) (see Chapter 52), (*ii*) Hallerman–Doering syndrome (band keratopathy, deafness, and a disordered

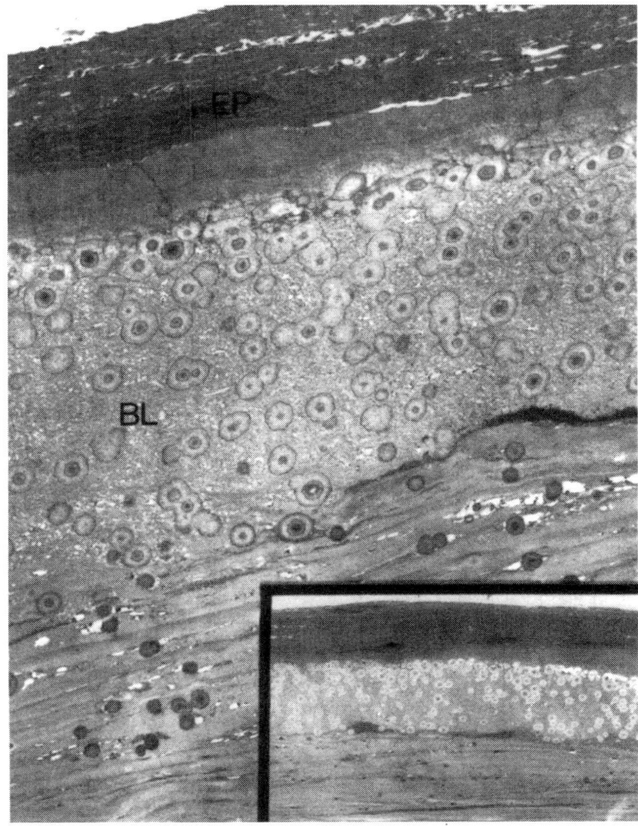

Figure 9 Calcific band keratopathy. This electron micrograph shows the intact corneal epithelium (EP). Numerous laminated calcific granules involve the plane of Bowman layer (BL) and the superficial corneal stroma (× 4,600). *Inset*: The concentration of calcium granules within Bowman layer (× 1,200). *Source*: Reproduced from Klintworth GK, Font RL. The role of histochemistry in the study of normal and pathologic states of the eye and ocular adnexa. In: Spicer SS, ed. Histochemistry for the Pathologist. New York: Marcel Dekker, 1987:959–1018.

calcium metabolism in which the turnover of radioactive calcium is reduced) (120), (*iii*) congenital band keratopathy (264), (*iv*) hypophosphatasia (MIM #146300 and #241500) (177), and (*v*) gelatinous drop-like corneal dystrophy (familial subepithelial corneal amyloidosis) (149) (see Chapter 37).

In the rabbit corneal calcification has followed such diverse conditions as ligation of the vortex veins (282), the intravitreal injection of polyethylene sulfonic acid (67), ocular irradiation with a carbon dioxide laser (82,83), exposure of the cornea to lime and cations (yttrium, lanthanum, samarium, and gadolinium) (114), the intravitreal injection of ovalbumin followed by vitamin D intoxication (112) as well as by the administration of dihydrotachysterol in animals with corneal injuries (213,214). Vitamin D-induced calcific band keratopathy is prevented by suturing the eyelids together and UV irradiation is not necessary for its development, since it occurs even when the vitamin D-treated animals are kept in the dark (67).

Corneal calcification has been elicited in the rat with isoproterenol, dihydrotachysterol, and 5-hydroxytryptamine (254), the subcutaneous administration of morphine sulfate (78), deepithelialization of the cornea plus dihydrotachysterol (214), and by suturing the eyelids open (78). In contrast to the rabbit and rat, corneal calcification is difficult to provoke in guinea pigs (214).

In the rabbit and rat, corneal calcification is subepithelial and similar to human band keratopathy (67,72,82,214), but calcium grains sometimes extend throughout the cornea (67). Doughman and colleagues (66) confirmed the identity of calcium in their experimental model using X-ray microprobe analysis. In experimental corneal calcification the deposits possess the same ultrastructural characteristics as those of human calcific band keratopathy (82).

Hypercalcemia, which often plays a significant role in the pathogenesis of calcific band keratopathy, is not always followed by corneal calcification and is not an essential requirement. The calcium content of the corneal extracellular fluid becomes elevated in hypercalcemia, and certain conditions presumably favor its precipitation or chelation with tissue compounds. Evaporation from the cornea may lead to a supersaturation and precipitation of calcium ions (35) in the superficial cornea, particularly in the interpalpebral region. The importance of evaporation in the genesis of corneal calcification is underscored by experimental studies in which the keratopathy is accentuated by open eyes and prevented by eyelid closure (67,78). The precipitation of the calcium in the superficial cornea may follow a reduced solubility of calcium caused by the rise in pH (35,224) produced by the loss of carbon dioxide.

Despite a predilection for Bowman layer in human calcific band keratopathy, this structure is not essential to its genesis, since it can develop in animals, such as the rabbit, which lack Bowman layer. Experimental evidence implicates the production by fibroblasts of a calcium-binding material (214).

Anterior Crocodile Shagreen (Anterior Mosaic Dystrophy)

Overview

A mosaic of gray opacities in the cornea separated by clear areas and likened to the skin of a crocodile were identified as a nosological entity in 1930 (283) and later recognized by others.

Clinical Features

Usually, unilateral or bilateral opacities are localized to the central third of the cornea, but sometimes the peripheral cornea is affected. The corneal epithelium and stroma are unremarkable, but round or polygonal subepithelial opacities present a pavement-like mosaic when viewed by slit-lamp biomicroscopy. A deep crocodile shagreen (185) or a tear in Bowman layer may be associated. Affected individuals have ranged from 15 to 62 years in age (165,283). Visual loss may be minimal or severe and the condition may have a progressive course.

Histopathology

Corneal tissue has rarely been examined microscopically in this disorder (200,202,225), but like calcific band keratopathy, small basophilic calcified granules appear in Bowman layer. In a posttraumatic case, ruptures were evident in Bowman layer (202).

Etiology and Pathogenesis

Anterior crocodile shagreen has been associated with megalocornea (15,185), calcific band keratopathy (43), multiple ocular malformations (43), and may follow trauma (202). The condition has been documented in the son of a man with bilateral band keratopathy (280). Identical changes have been noted in the cornea of five individuals from two successive generations beginning at approximately the same age (165).

Anterior crocodile shagreen is closely allied to calcific band keratopathy, with which it possesses morphologic similarities. Tripathi and Bron (276) attribute the mosaic pattern to an undulated Bowman layer (a phenomenon common in ocular hypotony), which is irregularly encrusted with calcium. A mosaic pattern can be induced in the normal human cornea by pressure through the eyelids (22). In some individuals the condition has an autosomal dominant mode of inheritance (165,280) and in cases with megalocornea, an X-linked recessive mode of inheritance is evident (185).

Diffuse Corneal Calcification

Rarely, the cornea becomes diffusely calcified. This nonbanded pancorneal calcification may be associated with hypercalcemia (37,167), but sometimes the cause is no apparent. It has been reported in a corneal transplant (68) and in patients with acquired immunodeficiency disease (220). Three cases of acute corneal calcification have been documented after an accidental chemical injury while applying an industrial fire retardant product consisting of a gypsum aggregate of calcium sulfate dihydrate plaster (53). Other cases, which may be recurrent, are associated with an epithelial defect of the cornea (194) that has been treated with topic medications containing calcium or phosphates (9,250). Following bilateral cataract extraction twin sisters with Werner syndrome (MIM #277700) (inherited disorder with juvenile cataracts, premature graying of the hair, premature baldness, bird face and subcutaneous calcification) caused by mutations in the *RECQL2* gene developed bilateral diffuse corneal calcification (167). This calcification was probably secondary to the hypercalcemia and hypophosphatemia and part of metastatic calcification in multiple nonocular sites. However, abnormal corneal tissue in Werner syndrome may contribute to the localization of the calcium deposition. Each of the twins underwent unilateral penetrating keratoplasty and developed metastatic calcification in the corneal grafts.

Conjunctival Calcification

The paralimbal interpalpebral conjunctiva usually calcifies in hypercalcemia, particularly when the product of the inorganic calcium and phosphorus exceeds 3.8 to 4.0 (283). These calcifications are usually asymptomatic but conjunctival inflammation with crystal deposition ("red eyes") can occur in uremic patients, but it has not been documented in individuals undergoing chronic hemodialysis. The calcium deposition is thought to reflect the relatively high alkalinity, resulting from the diffusion of carbon dioxide from the exposed ocular surface. The calcium precipitates in both the basal lamina of the epithelium and in the subepithelial tissue of the conjunctiva (283). The conjunctival calcification in patients with uremia is frequently associated with actinic elastosis suggesting that the local degenerative changes partake in the calcium deposition.

MISCELLANEOUS REACTIONS OF THE CORNEAL EPITHELIUM AND ITS BASEMENT MEMBRANE

Epithelial Erosions and Defective Adherence of the Corneal Epithelium

Foci of corneal epithelium commonly desquamate as a sequel to traumatic abrasions, chemical injuries, several disease processes and rarely, in the absence of any known predisposing factor. Occasionally, epithelial erosions recur episodically, often in the same location, at intervals ranging from weeks to months.

When recurrent corneal erosions are preceded by a corneal abrasion, they are more frequently the sequel to injury with organic objects, such as branches, fingernails, and straws, than trauma from inorganic objects. With nonrecurrent abrasions the reverse is the case (219). Recurrent corneal erosions are a manifestation of several distinct genetically determined disorders, including Fuchs dystrophy, Meesmann dystrophy, Thiel–Benke dystrophy, Reis–Bücklers dystrophy, the lattice corneal dystrophies, granular corneal dystrophies, and familial recurrent corneal erosions (see Chapter 32) (111,247). Recurrent corneal erosions can occur in siblings, and even in two or more successive generations (12,90,172,175,234,284). The largest known pedigree contained 40 affected individuals in six generations (90). In some families corneal erosions may begin at the age of 5 years, with episodes becoming less common later in life and especially unusual after the fifth decade (88,90). Family studies are consistent with some cases having an autosomal dominant mode of inheritance. Perhaps there is an increased susceptibility to corneal desquamation with minor trauma. Bilateral corneal erosions can also occur in Cogan microcystic "dystrophy" and the syndrome of nontraumatic recurrent erosion, and have been observed 10 to 20 years after exposure to nitrogen mustard (dichlorodiethylsulfide) (222).

Recurrent corneal erosions may be associated with dotlike opacities (intraepithelial cysts) (181,239) as well as fingerprint, linear, maplike, and other opacities, but the frequency of these alterations is not known, because detailed clinical observations in individuals with recurrent corneal erosions have not always been recorded.

The normal basal cells of the corneal epithelium possess densities (hemidesmosomes) at irregularly spaced intervals along the posterior cell membrane. Fine anchoring fibrils extend from the hemidesmosomes to a delicate basal lamina and are believed to contribute to the normal adhesion of the corneal epithelium to the underlying tissue (156,228). An inadequate formation of these complexes appears to result in recurrent corneal erosions. Ultrastructural studies in several human conditions with clinically significant erosive symptoms have disclosed an absence or marked diminution of basal epithelial cell hemidesmosome-basement membrane connections (85,274,275).

Disorders of Epithelial Basement Membrane

The basement membrane of the corneal epithelium is particularly well demonstrated in light-microscopic preparations with the periodic acid Schiff (PAS) stain and is readily identified by TEM because of its finely filamentous or granular appearance. Immunohistochemical studies have disclosed the presence of collagen type IV, laminin, bullous pemphigoid antigen, fibronectin, fibrin/fibrinogen and perlecan (heparan sulfate proteoglycan) in the epithelial basement membrane (126,198,201,206). In pathologic conditions the basement membrane of the corneal epithelium may be thickened, sometimes irregularly with occasional duplication, or it may be absent over extensive areas.

Cogan Microcystic "Dystrophy"

Overview

In a clinical paper published in 1950, Guerry (118) documented two cases with a whorl-like contour of extremely fine wavy lines in the corneal epithelium resembling a fingerprint. One of the patients subsequently developed recurrent herpetic keratitis, while the other individual had early bilateral cornea guttae. The fingerprint striae were later found to correspond to intraepithelial basement membrane (20,239,240) and long banded collagen fibers may be present in the aberrant basement membrane (40). Such aberrant basement membrane can follow various corneal diseases including keratitis due to *Herpes simplex* and *Herpes zoster* (21), recurrent corneal erosions (23), trauma, and ulceration in association with bullous keratopathy (61). "Fingerprint lines" may also develop in the superior portion of the cornea of patients after cataract extraction (172,239).

In patients with recurrent epithelial erosions (23) and in persons who are asymptomatic (54), fibrillogranular material between the basement membrane and Bowman zone may form mounds with a clinical appearance of a subepithelial bleb (54). This abnormality, which has been observed in men and women between 39 and 81 years of age, has been designated "bleblike dystrophy" (23). In 1964, Cogan and colleagues (36) drew attention to a common relatively nonprogressive clinicopathologic entity, which has been referred to as epithelial basement membrane dystrophy of the cornea, microcystic dystrophy of the corneal epithelium, Cogan microcystic dystrophy of the corneal epithelium, map-dot-fingerprint dystrophy, and Cogan–Guerry microcystic corneal epithelial dystrophy.

Clinical Features

Small, pleomorphic, lardaceous-appearing grayish white opacities occur predominantly in the pupillary area of the corneal epithelium. They come and go without apparent cause and are characteristically bilateral, although not necessarily symmetrical. The microcysts are associated with an extension of basement membrane into the epithelium, an abnormality that accounts for the associated fingerprint lines (described above) (118).

The epithelial changes are commonly asymptomatic and discovered fortuitously, or accompanied by mild blurring of vision or a foreign body sensation. Associated symptoms are often coincidental, but ocular pain and recurrent epithelial erosions are common (172,277). In some series about one-third of affected individuals have had epithelial erosions (23,277), and in individuals with recurrent epithelial erosions, the keratopathy occurs in most cases.

Most patients have been middle-aged or elderly women, but the condition can occur in children (172). Although usually bilateral, only one eye may be affected in eyes with underlying diseases (20).

Histopathology

The intraepithelial cysts possess an epithelial lining of flattened cells similar to those at the normal corneal surface, and rarely multinucleated cells (20,275) are also present. The microcysts, which appear throughout the depth of the epithelium, contain desquamated cellular debris (Fig. 10). By TEM the lining cells have a corrugated surface due to microprojections (Fig. 11). Pale cells and widening of the extracellular space (spongiosus) in the corneal epithelium have also been noted (275).

Etiology and Pathogenesis

The cause of this keratopathy remains unknown. While sometimes developing spontaneously, other cases have antecedent symptoms related to dry eyes (239), dendritic keratitis (20), trauma (61), bullous keratopathy (61), or zoster keratitis (20). A variety of analyses on the tears in individuals with Cogan microcystic "dystrophy" have not disclosed any notable abnormality (183). The family members of affected individuals have seldom been examined, but a familial pattern of the disease was detected in one study (172). In two families three generations were involved, and in eight families the corneal changes were detected in at least two generations. Some affected individuals in these families were asymptomatic; others had recurrent corneal erosions.

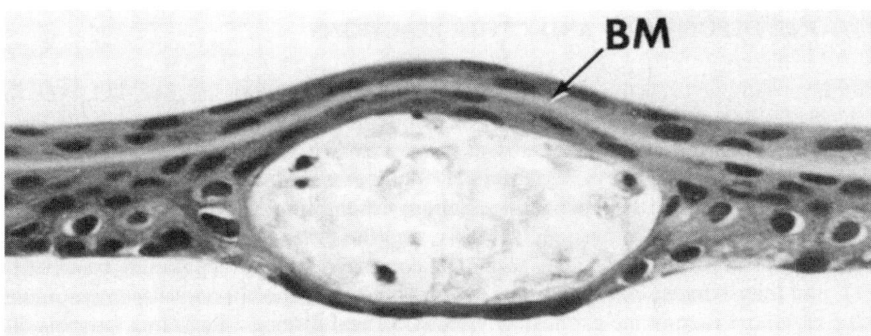

Figure 10 Microcysts in corneal epithelium with ectopic basement membrane (BM) immediately above it (hematoxylin and eosin, × 400). *Source*: From Ref. 40.

Some cysts contain necrotic cellular debris and appear to arise from the gradual intraepithelial desquamation of corneal epithelial cells. The intraepithelial cysts presumably become displaced to the surface, where they rupture and discharge their contents, as the underlying epithelial cells mature. An aberrant insinuation of basement membrane into the epithelium is associated with some intraepithelial cysts (Fig. 10) (40,158,274), and since intraepithelial cysts and degenerating cells are found posterior to ectopic basement membrane (40,158,239), some microcysts may be secondary to malalignment of basal epithelial cells. But the cysts do not necessarily occur beneath aberrant basement membrane and can form in areas without overlying aberrant basement membrane (20,158).

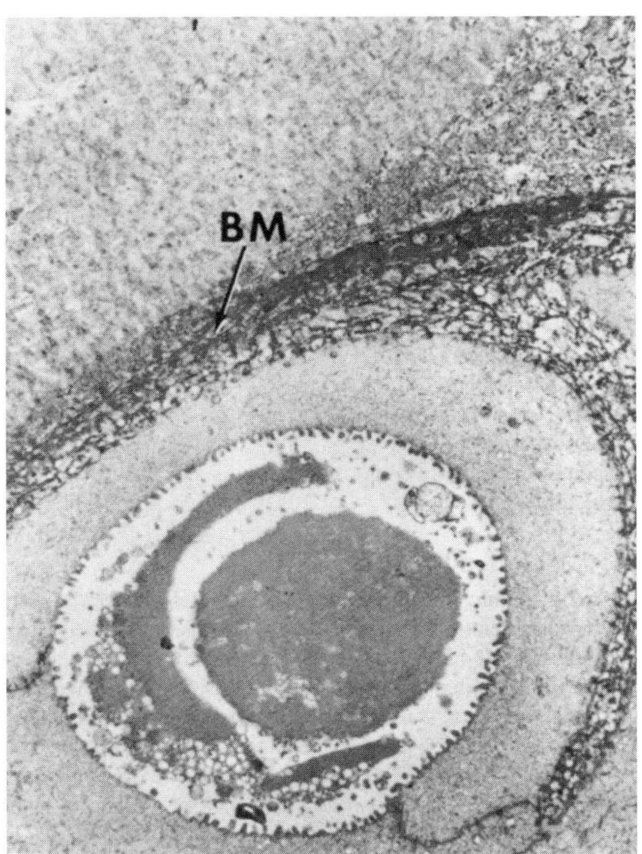

Figure 11 Transmission electron micrograph showing intraepithelial cysts posterior to aberrant basement membrane (BM). The cyst contains cellular debris and is bordered by an intact cell having villous processes (× 6,900). *Source*: From Ref. 40.

This clinicopathologic entity seems to be a nonspecific reaction to a variety of noxious stimuli. Clinical and histopathologic distinctions between map-dot fingerprint keratopathy, Cogan microcystic "dystrophy" and the recurrent erosion syndrome are vague, and the accumulated experience of different observers suggests that these apparently different conditions do not represent separate nosologic entities but perhaps variants of nonspecific reactions.

Other Intraepithelial Microcysts

An extracellular accumulation of fluid between adjacent epithelial cells widens the intercellular space (Fig. 12), which may contain finely granular material and products of cell degeneration (226,275). Eventually, the epithelial cells can separate at their intercellular junctions with the formation of tiny intraepithelial cysts. Such cysts, which follow intracellular edema, have been thoroughly studied by Tripathi and Bron (275) and usually lack cellular debris and appear clear clinically. Most often, subepithelial bullae eventually detach the epithelium from Bowman layer.

Corneal intraepithelial microcysts, with or without corneal lines or maps, form in the corneal epithelium in several disorders: epithelial edema due to corneal endothelial dysfunction, Meesmann corneal dystrophy (169), the recurrent corneal erosion syndrome, Cogan microcystic "dystrophy" (described above), limbal nevi, pannus due to different causes, conditions that affect the integrity of the tear film, various forms of viral keratitis (including *Herpes simplex* and *Herpes zoster*), and other entities (24,171,178,275).

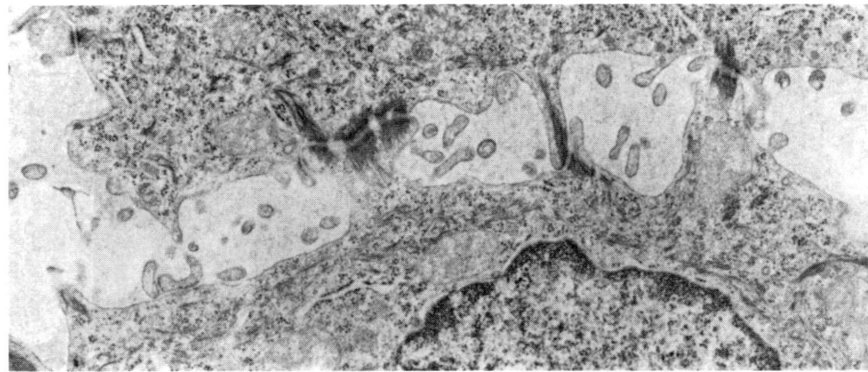

Figure 12 Spongiosus of corneal epithelium. The intercellular space between the corneal epithelial cells is widened (× 15,000) *Source*: Reproduced from Klintworth GK, McCracken JS. Corneal diseases. In: Johannessen JV ed. Electron Microscopy in Human Medicine, Vol. 6, Part 3. New York: McGraw-Hill, 1979:239–66.

INVASION OF THE CORNEA BY FOREIGN CELLS

Aside from the usual cellular infiltrate that accompanies the inflammatory response various other cells invade the cornea under pathologic circumstances. The normal cornea lacks mast cells, lymphatics and capillaries but these cellular elements invade the cornea in certain pathologic states (44,162,163,260). In the dark races and in pigmented animals, melanocytes may infiltrate between individual epithelial cells (Fig. 13) (10,129,142,191). This sharply contrasts with the normal cornea in which the epithelium is nonpigmented even in heavy pigmented individuals. In some animals melanosis of the corneal epithelium complicates keratitis and can be readily reproduced experimentally (129,191). Epithelial pigmentation results from the migration of melanocytes from the pericorneal pigmented conjunctiva into the corneal epithelium and the transfer of melanin granules from these melanocytes into the corneal epithelial cells (Fig. 14). Pigmentation of the corneal epithelium is preceded by a leukocytic infiltration and accompanied by corneal vascularization (129,191). The Langerhans cells, with their dendritic processes and characteristic rod- and racquet-shaped cytoplasmic organelles (Birbeck granules) (see Chapter 1) also invade the corneal epithelium under abnormal circumstances (25,142). These cells are often associated with melanocytes and their function is discussed in Chapter 1.

CORNEAL EDEMA

Corneal edema is a common condition that impairs vision by interfering with corneal transparency (73). Factors that contribute to water content of the cornea include the chemical composition of the cornea, the intraocular pressure, the degree of vascular permeability of pericorneal blood vessels, as well as the structural and functional status of the corneal epithelium and endothelium. The excised cornea of many

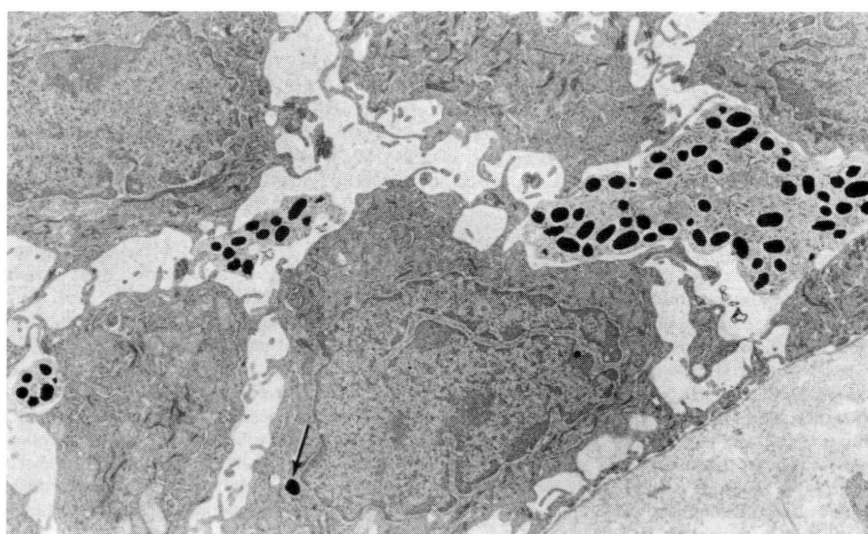

Figure 13 Basal portion of the corneal epithelium showing cytoplasmic processes of melanocytes in the dilated intercellular space. An epithelial cell contains a single melanin granule (*arrow*) (× 5,920). *Source*: From Ref. 191.

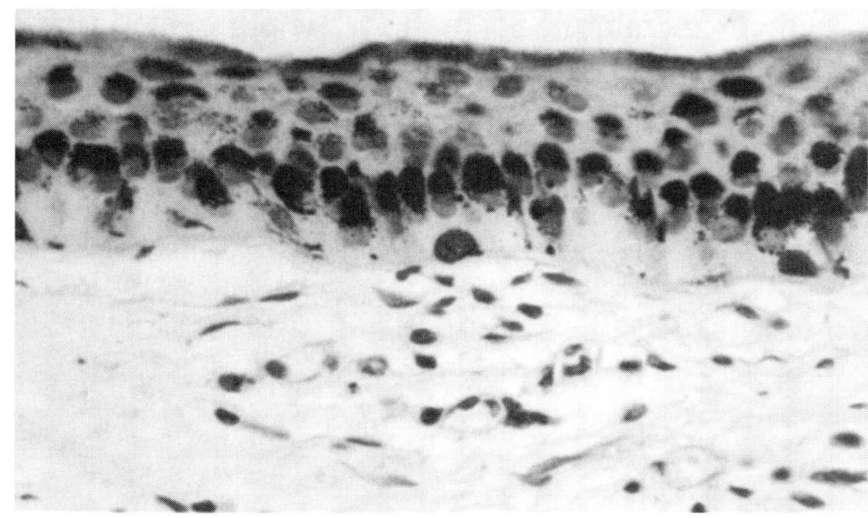

Figure 14 Epithelial melanosis. In contrast to the normal cornea these epithelial cells in the central cornea contain numerous melanin granules. The underlying stroma is vascularized (Fontana stain × 400).

species, including man, is markedly hydrophilic and swells in vitro largely as a result of the marked osmotic force of the stromal proteoglycans (PGs) of which lumican is thought to be the most important. This belief stems from the observation that the cornea of the dogfish, which contains relatively little keratan sulfate (KS) (25%) and much dermatan sulfate (60%), does not swell in distilled water or salt solutions (47).

Water enters the cornea from its anterior and posterior surface by passing through the corneal epithelium and endothelium. Passage through these cells is controlled by aquaporin 5 (epithelium) and aquaporin 1 (endothelium). The cornea is bathed on both surfaces by fluid—tears in front and aqueous humor behind—and the marked hydrophilia of the corneal stroma is counterbalanced and maintained in an ideal state of hydration of about 78% (73) by an active transport of ions (84,123,189). This ability of the normal cornea to maintain a deturgescent state is essential for normal vision since the thickened edematous cornea loses its transparency. The epithelium and, particularly, the endothelium of the cornea both contribute to the maintenance of the normal state of stromal hydration by virtue of their respective barrier and pump functions (64,74,295). The transport of water out of the corneal stroma follows an active ion transport in the corneal endothelium and epithelium (65,124,164,295). Removal of the epithelium from the cornea in the rabbit causes this structure to swell to about 200% of its initial thickness in 24 h, while the fluid inhibition is 500% after removal of the corneal endothelium (188,190). The corneal endothelium was once thought to prevent corneal swelling by an active transport of water, sodium ions, and possibly other electrolytes from the stroma to the aqueous humor. However, this concept lacks experimental confirmation, since only bicarbonate ions have been shown to be pumped into the aqueous humor (136).Corneal edema follows numerous spontaneous, iatrogenic, and experimentally produced abnormalities of the corneal endothelium including Fuchs corneal dystrophy (see Chapter 32), increased intraocular pressure and corneal grafts with defective donor corneal endothelium (34,99,162). A causal relationship between an abnormal corneal endothelium and the accompanying corneal edema was suspected many years ago, and an early hypothesis proposed that the edematous fluid might be derived from aqueous humor percolating through Descemet membrane and a damaged corneal endothelium (69,101,174). Later investigators pointed out that an abnormal corneal endothelium could interfere with a physiologic dehydrating mechanism of the cornea (123,125). Nevertheless, corneal endothelial cell dysfunction does not account for all examples of corneal edema. The pericorneal vascular plexus becomes abnormally permeable to plasma in certain situations, as in the acute inflammatory response, and this may contribute to corneal edema. For instance an increased permeability of the limbal blood vessels to the dye Pontamine sky blue occurs in alloxan-induced corneal edema—a type of edema associated with corneal endothelial lesions (173). Also, inoculation of the surfactant polyoxyethelene sorbitan monooleate into the anterior chamber of rabbit eyes produces pronounced corneal edema, which is accompanied by a marked lysis of corneal endothelial cells, but there is in addition, an increased pericorneal vascular permeability to intravascular markers which diffuse into the cornea (232).

DEPOSITION OF METALS

Iron

Iron commonly accumulates in the corneal epithelium in several situations, producing clinically detectable pigmented lines. The most frequent of these is usually horizontal (Hudson–Stähli line) and occurs particularly after the fifth decade of life. In the Hudson–Stähli line the iron can be readily demonstrated by histochemical methods (108) and has been identified within the corneal epithelium by TEM as ferritin-like particles (262). Iron also deposits in the corneal epithelium in a ring around the abnormal cone (Fleischer ring) in about 50% of individuals with keratoconus. Ferritin particles have been identified by TEM in Fleischer rings in widened intercellular spaces and/or in the cytoplasm of epithelial cells, especially the basal ones (139). An iron-containing pigment line also occurs in the corneal epithelium ahead of a pterygium (Stocker line) or in front of a filtering bleb created in the treatment of glaucoma (Ferry line) (80). The source of the iron and the reason for its deposition in the cornea under these varied circumstances remain speculative.

Copper

Copper deposits within Descemet membrane account for the pigmented ring at the periphery of the cornea in Wilson disease (hepatolenticular degeneration) (MIM #277900) (Kayser–Fleischer ring) (see Chapter 48).

Silver and Gold

Black granules of silver deposit in the basement membrane of the corneal epithelium after the prolonged topical application of silver-containing eyedrops, while granules of gold deposit in the cornea in individuals receiving prolonged gold therapy for rheumatoid arthritis.

KERATOCONJUNCTIVITIS SICCA

The surface of the normal cornea is lubricated by a tear film, composed of mucoid, watery, and oily layers derived from the secretions of conjunctival goblet and nongoblet epithelial cells, major and accessory lacrimal glands, sweat glands (Moll glands), and sebaceous glands (Meibomian glands, Zeis glands). A variety of soluble or membrane bound mucins are derived from the conjunctival and corneal epithelium (215). A defective formation or excessive evaporation of these secretions exposes the cornea to desiccation resulting in a characteristic corneal and conjunctival reaction (keratoconjunctivitis sicca). In numerous ocular and systemic disorders the eye becomes dry because of inadequate moistening causing keratinization and fissures in the corneal and conjunctival epithelia, which lack their normal luster. The damaged cells, which desquamate and form punctate erosions, are readily demonstrated in the living patient by staining with fluorescein or rose bengal. The corneal epithelium may desquamate as filamentous threads (filamentous keratopathy), and secondary infection often ensues. The causes of the dry eye syndrome include the Stevens–Johnson syndrome (see Chapter 5), toxic epidermal necrolysis, benign mucous membrane pemphigoid, avitaminosis A (see Chapter 49), trachoma (see Chapter 10), chemical burns (see Chapter 15), hereditary sensory and autonomic neuropathy type III (Riley–Day syndrome) (MIM #223900), irradiation of the eyelids, and poor approximation of the eyelids to the globe (entropion or ectropion) and the Sjögren syndrome, which may be associated with rheumatoid arthritis, systemic lupus erythematosus, scleroderma or polyarteritis nodosa (see Chapter 6). Ocular surface and lacrimal gland inflammation is prominent in the dry eye and this has led to promising anti-inflammatory therapy (221).

NEUROPATHIC KERATOPATHY

Anesthesia of the cornea, as with lesions of the trigeminal nerve, is associated with a keratopathy, characterized by a diffuse corneal edema, epithelial bullae, and indolent ulceration which may perforate. Since the condition does not invariably follow Gasserian ganglion section and can be prevented by suturing the eyelids together corneal anesthesia is not the direct cause. Rather, the insensitivity of the cornea, which results in a loss of its reflex protective mechanism, predisposes to corneal trauma, desiccation, and secondary infection.

IRIDOCORNEAL–ENDOTHELIAL SYNDROME (ICE SYNDROME)

Overview

In 1978, Campbell and colleagues (29) suggested that an abnormality of the corneal endothelium linked three seemingly different idiopathic degenerative conditions of the cornea and iris previously designated iris nevus syndrome, Chandler syndrome (unilateral corneal edema, broad iridocorneal adhesions, and normal or slightly elevated intraocular pressure) and essential iris atrophy (progressive iris atrophy). These conditions are thought to represent a spectrum of a single entity because they share common features: broad iridocorneal adhesions, iris stromal atrophy, nevus-like nodules on the iris, a dysfunctional corneal endothelium that extends beyond the cornea over the anterior chamber angle and onto the anterior surface of the iris and glaucoma (29,180,255,257,291). In 1979 the term iridocorneal–endothelial (ICE) syndrome was coined by Yanoff (291) to unite these conditions, in which the earliest clinically detectable abnormality seems to involve the corneal endothelium, which is pleomorphic on specular microscopy (130,135).

Clinical Features

The ICE syndrome begins in early or middle adulthood is typically nonfamilial and affects women much more often than men. Most cases are unilateral, but the condition may be bilateral (148). However, some alleged cases that involve both eyes have been found to represent posterior polymorphous corneal dystrophy (PPCD) on further evaluation and cytokeratin may be expressed in the corneal endothelium (166).

The iris nevus syndrome consists of unilateral glaucoma associated with nodules on the anterior surface of the iris that are surrounded by ectopic Descemet membrane, which also covers the anterior chamber angle (42,159,248,289,292).

A mild degree of iris stromal atrophy may be associated with Chandler syndrome (30,258).

The term essential iris atrophy has been applied to an infrequent idiopathic disorder in which the iris degenerates spontaneously producing holes leading to the apparent formation of an abnormally located pupil (corectopia) or multiple pupils (polycoria). Secondary glaucoma with peripheral anterior synechiae eventually ensues.

Histopathology

In Chandler syndrome morphologic studies have been restricted to trabeculectomy specimens and to corneal tissue removed at keratoplasty obtained late in the course of the disorder. The corneal endothelium has been absent or attenuated and sometimes has manifest the ultrastructural and imunohistochemical attributes of squamous epithelium (134,166,230,235). As in PPCD (see Chapter 32) the corneal endothelium may express cytokeratin (166) and when squamous metaplasia is evident the possibility of PPCD needs to be excluded (see Chapter 5). A collagenous layer commonly forms between the endothelium and the posterior surface of Descemet membrane (218,230,235,242,243,257) or on the posterior surface of Descemet membrane (258) (Fig. 15). The corneal endothelium and Descemet membrane-like material may cover the trabecular meshwork and extend onto the anterior iris surface.

Histopathologic evaluations of affected eyes with essential iris atrophy have been performed late in the cause of the disorder after glaucoma has caused blindness. Aside from the morphologic evidence of longstanding glaucoma the abnormalities in such eyes have included the loss of iris stroma, holes extending through all layers of the iris, as well as peripheral anterior synechiae. The latter have not been present in all cases, suggesting that they follow the endothelialization and Descemetization of the iris (71,249). Aggregates of melanocytes (iris nodules) occur at some margins of atrophy and may be clinically evident (256). Other abnormalities have included an attenuated corneal endothelium, a retrocorneal fibrous membrane, the presence corneal endothelium and Descemet membrane on the anterior surface of the iris and over the anterior chamber filtration angle.

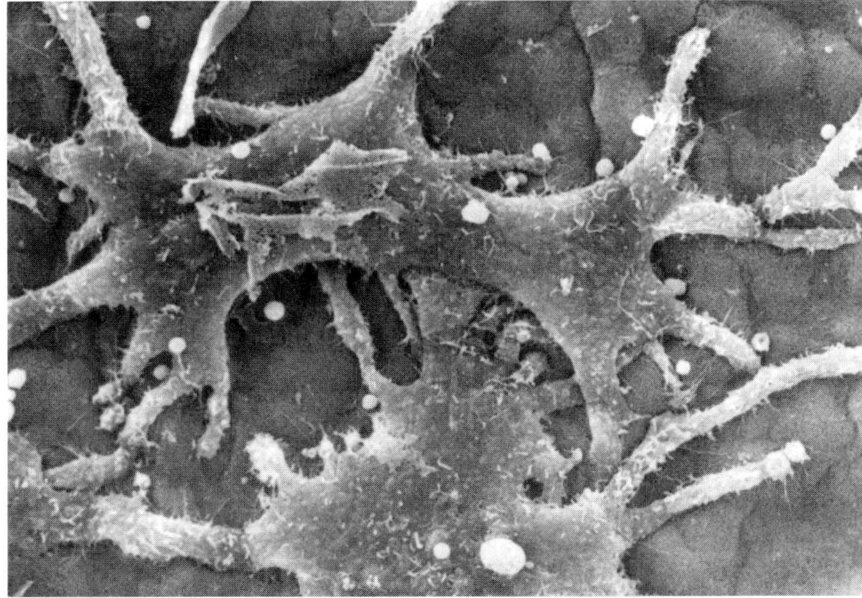

Figure 15 Scanning electron micrograph showing bizarre-shaped cells with dendritic processes and scattered melanin granules on inner surface of cornea from patient with corneal edema and essential iris atrophy (×2,700). *Source*: From Ref. 258.

Etiology and Pathogenesis

The cause of the iris atrophy remains unknown. Ischemia secondary to vascular occlusion has been considered (127) and the pattern of atrophy is consistent with this possibility (249). However, the iris blood vessels have been patent and not abnormal in light microscopic and TEM studies (148,249). That the atrophy may have a neurotrophic basis finds support in the observation of saccular dilatations and terminal swellings of interrupted nerve fibers in the iris (195). On the flimsy evidence of some inflammatory cells in corneal specimens Alvarado and colleagues speculated that a virus may be the etiologic agent (3).

A plausible explanation for some of the manifestations of the ICE syndrome has been offered by Campbell and colleagues (29). They have suggested that the primary defect involves the corneal endothelium and that this not only leads to corneal edema but to other features of the entity as a consequence of the growth of endothelial cells across the anterior chamber angle and onto the surface of the iris, where ectopic Descemet membrane is deposited. According to this theory contracture of the endothelial-derived cellular membrane on the iris causes peripheral anterior synechiae, holes in the iris, corectopia and ectropion uveae. The cellular membrane is also thought to cause the nodules on the anterior surface of the iris ("iris nevi"), by pinching off parts of the iris stroma.

A case of the ICE syndrome has been associated with keratoconus and PPCD (14). Based on this case Blair and colleagues (14) have suggested that the predisposition for the ICE syndrome or for PPCD is inherited as an inactive allele, as in retinoblastoma (the so-called "first hit"). They speculate that inactivation of the second allele, or "second hit", might be the product of the background mutation rate or of an environmental trigger. They suggest that dedifferentiation or an abnormality in normal development follows the first or second hit, resulting in varying clinical patterns. They also believe that PPCD may be part of the spectrum of the ICE syndrome, owing to similarities in their clinical presentations, histopathology, specular microscopy, and natural history.

REFERENCES

1. Ahmad A, Hogan M, Wood I, Ostler HB. Climatic droplet keratopathy in a 16-year-old boy. Arch Ophthalmol 1977; 95:149–51.
2. Al-Bdour M, Al-Layayfeh MM. Risk factors for pterygium in an adult Jordanian population. Acta Ophthalmol Scand 2004; 82:64–7.
3. Alvarado JA, Murphy CG, Maglio M, Hetherington J. Pathogenesis of Chandler's syndrome, essential iris atrophy, and the Cogan Reese syndrome. I. Alterations of the corneal endothelium. Invest Ophthalmol Vis Sci 1986; 27:853–72.
4. Anderson J, Fuglsang H. Droplet degeneration of the cornea in North Cameroon, prevalence and clinical appearance. Br J Ophthalmol 1976; 60:256–62.
5. Ansari MW, Rahi AHS, Shukla BR. Pseudoelastic nature of pterygium. Br J Ophthalmol 1970; 54:473–6.
6. Ashaye AO. Refractive astigmatism and pterygium. Afr J Med Med Sci 1990; 19:225–8.
7. Austin P, Jakobiec FA, Iwamoto T. Elastodysplasia and elastodystrophy as the pathologic bases of ocular pterygia and pinguecula. Ophthalmology 1983; 90:96–109.
8. Austin P, Jakobiec FA, Iwamoto T, Hornblass A. Elastofibroma oculi. Arch Ophthalmol 1983; 101: 1575–9.
9. Barouch FC, Colby KA. Corneal and conjunctival degenerations. In: Foster CS, Azar DT, Dohlman CH, eds. Smolin and Thoft's The Cornea: Scientific Foundations and Clinical Practice, 4th ed. Philadelphia, PA: Lippincott William and Wilkins, 2005:875–87.
10. Bellhorn RW, Henkind P. Superficial pigmentary keratitis in the dog. J Am Vet Med Assoc 1966; 149:173–5.
11. Ben-Amer MI. Pterygium in a Libyan village. Revue Internationale Du Trachome Et De Pathologie Oculaire Tropicale Et Subtropicale Et De Sante Publique 1989; 66: 63–71.
12. Berardi M, Motolese A. Distrofia corneal ereditaria familiare con disepitelizzanioni recidivanti. Boll Ocul 17:711–28.
13. Berkow JW, Fine BS, Zimmerman LE. Unusual ocular calcification in hyperparathyroidism. Am J Ophthalmol 66:812–24.
14. Blair SD, Seabrooks D, Shields WJ, et al. Bilateral progressive essential iris atrophy and keratoconus with coincident features of posterior polymorphous dystrophy: a case report and proposed pathogenesis. Cornea 1992; 11: 255–61.
15. Boles-Carenini B. Juvenile familial mosaic degeneration of the cornea associated with megalocornea. Br J Ophthalmol 1961; 45:64–70.
16. Booth F. Heredity in one hundred patients admitted for excision of pterygia. Austral New Zeal J Ophthalmol 1985; 13:59–61.
17. Bonnet P, Bonnet L. Les Manifestations oculaires dans les rhumatismes chroniques de l'enfance, Lyon. Arch Ophtalmol (Paris) 1953; 13:127–45.
18. Boshoff PH. Hyaline scleral plaques. Arch Ophthalmol 1942; 28:503–6.
19. Breinin GM, DeVoe AG. Chelation of calcium with edathamil calcium-disodium in band keratopathy and corneal calcium affections. Arch Ophthalmol 1954; 52: 846–51.
20. Brodrick JD, Dark AJ, Peace GW. Fingerprint dystrophy of the cornea: a histologic study. Arch Ophthalmol 92: 483–9.
21. Brodrick JD, Dark AJ, Peace GW. Fingerprint striae of the cornea following herpes simplex keratitis. Ann Ophthalmol 1976; 8:481–4.
22. Bron AJ. Anterior corneal mosaic. Br J Ophthalmol 1968; 52:659–69.
23. Bron AJ, Brown JA. Some superficial corneal disorders: preliminary report. Trans Ophthalmol Soc UK 1971; 91: 13–29.
24. Bron AJ, Tripathi RC. Cystic disorders of the corneal epithelium. I. Clinical aspects. Br J Ophthalmol 1973; 57: 361–75.
25. Brown J, Soderstrom CW, Winkelmann RK. Langerhans' cells in guinea pig cornea: response to chemical injury. Invest Ophthalmol 1968; 7:668–71.

26. Brownstein S, Rodrigues M, Fine BS, Albert EN. The elastotic nature of hyaline corneal deposits: a histochemical, fluorescent, and electron microscopic examination. Am J Ophthalmol 1973; 75:799–809.
27. Cameron ME. Pterygium throughout the World. Springfield, Charles C. Thomas, 1965.
28. Cameron ME. Histology of pterygium: an electron microscopic study. Br J Ophthalmol 1983; 67:604–8.
29. Campbell DG, Shields MB, Smith TR. The corneal endothelium and the spectrum of essential iris atrophy. Am J Ophthalmol 1978; 86:317–24.
30. Chandler PA. Atrophy of the stroma of the iris, endothelial dystrophy, corneal edema, and glaucoma. Am J Ophthalmol 1956; 41:607–15.
31. Chen P-L, Cheng Y-W, Chiang C-C, et al. Hypermethylation of the *p16* gene promoter in pterygia and its association with the expression of DNA methyltransferase 3b. Mol Vision 2006; 12:1411–6.
32. Christensen GR. Proteinaceous corneal degeneration: a histochemical study. Arch Ophthalmol 1973; 89:30–2.
33. Chu FC, Rodrigues MM, Cogan DG, Barranger JA. The pathology of pingueculae in Gaucher's disease. Ophthal Paediatr Genet 1984; 4:7–11.
34. Cogan DG. Studies on the clinical physiology of the cornea: the interrelationship of corneal turgescence, epithelial edema, bullous keratopathy, and interstitial vascularization. Am J Ophthalmol 1949; 32:625–33.
35. Cogan DG, Albright F, Bartter FC. Hypercalcemia and band keratopathy: report of nineteen cases. Arch Ophthalmol 1948; 40:624–38.
36. Cogan DG, Donaldson DD, Kuwabara T, Marshall D. Microcystic dystrophy of the corneal epithelium. Trans Am Ophthalmol Soc 1964; 62:213–25.
37. Cogan DG, Henneman PH. Diffuse calcification of the cornea in hypercalcemia. N Engl J Med 1957; 257: 451–3.
38. Cogan DG, Hurlbut CS, Kuwabara T. Crystalline calcium sulfate (gypsum) in scleral plaques of a human eye. J Histochem 1958; 6:142–5.
39. Cogan DG, Kuwabara T. Focal senile translucency of the sclera. Arch Ophthalmol 1959; 62:604–10.
40. Cogan DG, Kuwabara T, Donaldson DD, Collins E. Microcystic dystrophy of the cornea: a partial explanation for its pathogenesis. Arch Ophthalmol 1974; 92:470–4.
41. Cogan DE, Kuwabara T, Howard J. The nonelastic nature of pingueculas. Arch Ophthalmol 1959; 61:388–9.
42. Cogan DG, Reese AB. A syndrome of iris nodules, ectopic Descemet's membrane, and unilateral glaucoma. Doc Ophthalmol 1969; 26:424–33.
43. Collier M. Un nouveau cas unilateral de dégénéerescence en mosaique de la membrane de Bowman associé à une dégénérescence en bandelette sur oeil malformé. Arch Ophtalmol 1966; 26:253–6.
44. Collin HB. Corneal lymphatics in alloxan vascularized rabbit eyes. Invest Ophthalmol 1966; 5:1–13.
45. Cornand, G. Pterygium. Clinical course and treatment. Revue Internationale Du Trachome Et De Pathologie Oculaire Tropicale Et Subtropicale Et De Sante Publique 1989; 66:31–108.
46. Coroneo MT. Albedo concentration in the anterior eye: a phenomenon that locates some solar diseases. Ophthal Surg 1990; 21:60–6.
47. Cremer-Bartels G, Dische Z. Comparison of glycosaminoglycans of elasmobranch and mammalian corneas. Arch Ophtalmol (Paris) 1975; 35:27–32.
48. Crick RP, Hoyle C, Smellie H. The eyes in sarcoidosis. Br J Ophthalmol 1961; 45:461–81.
49. Culler AM. The pathology of sclera plaques: report of five cases of degenerative plaques in the sclera mesially, one studied histologically. Br J Ophthalmol 1939; 23: 44–50.
50. Cursino JW, Fine BS. A histologic study of calcific and noncalcific band keratopathies. Am J Ophthalmol 1976; 82:395–404.
51. Dahan E, Judelson J, Welsh NH. Regression of Labrador keratopathy follows cataract extraction. Br J Ophthalmol 1986; 70:737–41.
52. Dake Y, Mukae R, Soda Y, et al. Immunohistochemical localization of collagen types I, II, III, and IV in pterygium tissues. Acta Histochem 1989; 87:71–4.
53. Daly M, Tuft SJ, Munro PM. Acute corneal calcification following chemical injury. Cornea 2005; 24:761–5.
54. Dark AJ. Bleb dystrophy of the cornea: histochemistry and ultrastructure. Br J Ophthalmol 1977; 61:65–9.
55. Darrell RW, Bachrach CA. Pterygium among veterans: an epidemiologic study showing a correlation between frequency of pterygium and degree of exposure of ultraviolet in sunlight. Arch Ophthalmol 1963; 70:158–69.
56. Davis MD. Endogenous uveitis in children associated with bandshaped keratopathy and rheumatoid arthritis. Arch Ophthalmol 1953; 50:443–54.
57. de Die-Smulders CE, Schrander-Stumpel CT, Fryns JP. The lethal multiple pterygium syndrome: a nosological approach. Genet Counsel 1990; 1:13–23.
58. Detels R, Dhir SP. Pterygium: a geographical study. Arch Ophthalmol 1967; 78:485–91.
59. Detorakis ET, Drakonaki EE, Spandidos DA. Molecular genetic alterations and viral presence in ophthalmic pterygium. Int J Mol Med 2000; 6:35–41.
60. Detorakis ET, Zafiropoulos A, Arvanitis DA, Spandidos DA. Detection of point mutations at codon 12 of KI-ras in ophthalmic pterygia. Eye 2005; 19:210–214.
61. DeVoe AG. Certain abnormalities of Bowman's membrane with particular reference to fingerprint lines in the cornea. Trans Am Ophthalmol Soc 1962; 60:195–201.
62. Dhir SP, Detels R, Alexander ER. Role of environmental factors in cataract pterygium and trachoma. Am J Ophthalmol 1967; 64:128–35.
63. Diponegoro RMA, Mulock-Houwer AW. A statistical contribution to the study of the aetiology of pterygium. Folia Ophthalmol Orient 1936; 2:195–210.
64. Dohlman, CH. The function of the corneal epithelium in health and disease: the Jonas S. Friedenwald memorial lecture. Invest Ophthalmol 1971; 10:383–407.
65. Donn A, Maurice DM, Mills NL. Studies on the living cornea in vitro. 2. The active transport of sodium across the epithelium. Arch Ophthalmol 62:748–57.
66. Doughman D, Ingram JJ, Bourne, WM. Experimental band keratopathy: electron microprobe x-ray analysis of aqueous and corneal calcium concentrations. Invest Ophthalmol 1970; 9:471–271.
67. Doughman D, Olson GA, Nolan S, Hajny RG. Experimental band keratopathy. Arch Ophthalmol 1969; 81:264–71.
68. Duffey R J, LoCasio JA, III. Calcium deposition in a corneal graft. Cornea 1987; 6:212–5.
69. Duke-Elder S, Leigh AG. Diseases of the outer eye. In: Duke-Elder S, ed. System of Ophthalmology, vol. 1, Part 2, St. Louis, Mo: CV Mosby, 1965.
70. Dworetzky M. Milk drinkers syndrome, reversible metastatic calcification. J Am Med Assoc 1954; 155: 830–2.
71. Eagle RC Jr, Font RL, Yanoff M, Fine BS. Proliferative endotheliopathy with iris abnormalities: the iridicorneal endothelial syndrome. Arch Ophthalmol 97:2104–11.

72. Economon JW, Silverstein AM, Zimmerman LE. Band keratopathy in a rabbit colony. Invest Ophthalmol 1963; 2: 361–8.
73. Edelhauser HF. The balance between corneal transparency and edema: the Proctor Lecture. Invest Ophthalmol Vis Sci 2006; 47:1754–67.
74. Edelhauser HF, Van Horn DL, Miller P, Pederson HJ. Effect of thioloxidation of glutathione with diamide on corneal endothelial function, junctional complexes and microfilaments. J Cell Biol 1976; 68:567–78.
75. Elliot R. The etiology of pterygium. Trans Ophthalmol Soc NZ 1961; 13:22–41.
76. Elliot RH. Ophthalmolgie Tropicale. Paris, Masson, 1922.
77. English FP, Yates WH, Kirkwood R, Siu S. The conjunctival goblet cell in pterygium formation. Austral J Ophthalmol 1980; 8:53–4.
78. Fabian FJ, Bond JM, Drobeck HP. Induced corneal opacities in the rat. Br J Ophthalmol 1967; 51:124–9.
79. Faraldi NC, Gracis GP. Pterygium on twins. Ophthalmologica 1976; 172:361–6.
80. Ferry AP. A "new" iron line of the superficial cornea: occurrence in patients with filtering blebs. Arch Ophthalmol 1968; 79:142–5.
81. Ferry AP, Kaltreider SA, Wyatt DB. Actinic granuloma of the conjunctiva. Arch Ophthalmol 1984; 102:1200–2.
82. Fine BS, Berkow JW, Fine S. Corneal calcification. Science 1968; 162:129–30.
83. Fine BS, Fine S, Feigen L, MacKeen D. Corneal injury threshold to carbon dioxide laser irradiation. Am J Ophthalmol 1968; 66:1–15.
84. Fischbarg J. Active and passive properties of rabbit corneal endothelium. Exp Eye Res 1973; 15:615–38.
85. Fogle JA, Kenyon KA, Stark WJ, Green WR. Defective epithelial adhesion in anterior corneal dystrophies. Am J Ophthalmol 1975; 79:925–40.
86. Forsius H. Climatic changes in the eyes of eskimos, lapps and cheremisses. Acta Ophthalmol 1972; 50:532–38.
87. Forsius H, Eriksson A. Die Frequenz von Pinguecula und Pterygium bei Innen-und Aussenarbeitern. Klin Monatsbl Augenheilk 1963; 142:1021–30.
88. Franceschetti A. Hereditäre rezidvierende Erosion der Hornhaut. Z Augenheilkd 1928; 66:309–16.
89. Franceschetti A. Eziologia e tratte mento della degenerazione a cingola della cornea. Atti Soc Oftalmol Lombarda 1956; 11:225–38.
90. Franceschetti A, Klein D. Cornea. In: Waardenburg PJ, Franceschetti A, Klein D, eds. Genetics and Ophthalmology, vol. 1, Oxford, Blackwell, 1961:447–543.
91. Fraunfelder FT, Hanna C. Spheroidal degeneration of cornea and conjunctiva. 3. Incidences, classification, and etiology. Am J Ophthalmol 1973; 76:41–50.
92. Fraunfelder FT, Hanna C, Parker JM. Spheroid degeneration of the cornea and conjunctiva. Am J Ophthalmol 1972; 74:821–8.
93. Freddo TF, Leibowitz HM. Bilateral acute corneal calcification. Ophthalmology 1985; 92:537–42.
94. Freedman A. Labrador keratopathy. Arch Ophthalmol 1965; 74:198–202.
95. Freedman A. Climatic droplet keratopathy. I. Clinical aspects. Arch Ophthalmol 1973; 89:193–7.
96. Freedman A. Labrador keratopathy and related diseases. Can J Ophthalmol 1973; 8:286–90.
97. Freedman J. Nama keratopathy. Br J Ophthalmol 1973; 57: 688–91.
98. Freedman J. Xeroderma pigmentosum and band-shaped nodular corneal dystrophy. Br J Ophthalmol 1977; 61: 96–100.
99. Freeman HM, Hawkins WR, Schepens CL. Anterior segment necrosis: an experiment study. Arch Ophthalmol 1966; 75:644–50.
100. Fuchs A. Über primäre gürtelformige Hornhäuttrubung. Klin Monatsbl Augenheilk 1939; 103:300–9.
101. Fuchs E. Über die Trübung der Hornhaut bei Glaucom. Albrecht von Graefes Arch Ophthalmol 1881; 27: 66–92.
102. Fuchs E. Zur Anatomie der Pinguecula. Albrecht von Graefes Arch Ophthalmol 1891; 37:143–91.
103. Fuchs E. Ueber das Pterygium. Albrecht von Graefes Arch Ophthalmol 1892; 38:1–90.
104. Garner A. Keratinoid corneal degeneration. Br J Ophthalmol 1970; 54:769–80.
105. Garner A, Fraunfelder FT, Barras TC, Hinzpeter EN. Spheroidal degeneration of cornea and conjunctiva. Br J Ophthalmol 1976; 60:437–78.
106. Garner A, Morgan G, Tripathi RC. Climatic droplet keratopathy. II. Pathologic findings. Arch Ophthalmol 1973; 89:198–204.
107. Gartner S, Rubner E. Calcified scleral nodules in hypervitaminosis. Am J Ophthalmol 1955; 39:658–63.
108. Gass JD. The iron lines of the superficial cornea. Arch Ophthalmol 1964; 71:348–58.
109. Gasteiger H. Über senile Entartung der Lederhaut an der Ansatzstellen der geraden Augenmuskein. Klin Monatsbl Augenheilk 1937; 98:767–72.
110. Gerundo M. On the etiology and pathology of pterygium. Am J Ophthalmol 1951; 34:851–6.
111. Gifford SR. Epithelial dystrophy and recurrent erosion of the cornea as seen with the slit-lamp. Arch Ophthalmol 1925; 54:217–32.
112. Gifford ES, Maguire EF. Band keratopathy in vitamin D intoxication. Arch Ophthalmol 1954; 52:106–7.
113. Glees M. Über Familiares Auftreten der Primären bandförmigen Hornhautdegeneration. Klin Monatsbl Augenheilk 1950; 116:185–7.
114. Grant WM, Schuman JS. Toxicology of the Eye: Effects on the Eyes and Visual System from Chemicals, Drugs, Metals and Minerals, Plants, Toxins and Venoms; Also Systemic Side Effects from Eye Medications, 4th ed. Springfield III, Charles C Thomas, 1993.
115. Graves B. Bilateral (mesial) deficiency of the sclera: scleral plaques. Br J Ophthalmol 1941; 25:35–38.
116. Gray RH, Johnson GJ, Freedman A. Climatic droplet keratopathy. Surv Ophthalmol 1992; 36:241–53.
117. Grossniklaus HE, Reinhart WJ, Thomas SW. Giant cell reaction in pterygium: case report. Arch Ophthalmol 106: 312–3.
118. Guerry D, III. Fingerprint lines in the cornea. Am J Ophthalmol 1950; 33:724–6.
119. Guerry D, III. Observations on Cogan's microcystic dystrophy of the corneal epithelium. Trans Am Ophthalmol Soc 1966; 63:320–34. (Also in Am J Ophthalmol 1966; 62:65–73.
120. Hallermann W, Doering P. Stoffwechseluntersuchungenmit Calcium[47] bei einem hereditaren Symptomenkomplex: Primare bandformige Hornhautdegeneration, Schwerhorigkeit und gestorter Calciumsatz. Albrecht von Graefes Arch Ophthalmol 1964; 167:75–88.
121. Hammer J, Kläusler M, Schinzel A. The popliteal pterygium syndrome: distinct phenotypic variation in two families. Helvet Paediatr Acta 1989; 43:507–14.
122. Hanna C, Fraunfelder FT. Spheroid degeneration of the cornea and conjunctiva. II. Pathology. Am J Ophthalmol 1972; 74:829–39.

123. Harris JE. The physiologic control of corneal hydration. The 1st Jonas S. Friedenwald lecture. Am J Ophthalmol 1957; 44:262–80.
124. Harris JE, Nordquist LT. The hydration of the cornea. 1. The transport of water from the cornea. Am J Ophthalmol 1955; 40:100–11.
125. Harrison WJ. Primary zonular opacity of the cornea. Arch Ophthalmol 1936; 16:469-71.
126. Hassell J, Robey PG, Barrach HJ, et al. Isolation of a heparin sulfate-containing proteoglycan from basement membrane. Proc Natl Acad Sci USA 1980; 77:4494–8.
127. Heath P. Essential iris atrophy: a histopathologic study. Trans Am Ophthalmol Soc 1953; 51:167–92.
128. Hecht F, Shoptaugh MG. Winglets of the eye: dominant transmission of early adult pterygium of the conjunctiva. J Med Genet 1990; 27:392–4.
129. Henkind P. Migration of the limbal melanocytes into the corneal epithelium of guinea pigs. Exp Eye Res 1965; 4: 42–7.
130. Hetherington J Jr. The spectrum of Chandler's syndrome. Trans Am Acad Ophthalmol Otolaryngol 1978; 85:240–4.
131. Hilgers JHC. Pterygium: its incidence, heredity, and etiology. Am J Ophthalmol 1960; 50:635–44.
132. Hilgers JHC. Prevention of recurrent pterygium by β–radiation. Ophthalmologica 1960; 140:369–79.
133. Hill JC, Maske R. Pathogenesis of pterygium. Eye 1989; 3: 218–26.
134. Hirst LW, Green WR, Luckenbach M, et al. Epithelial characteristics of the endothelium in Chandler's syndrome. Invest Ophthalmol Vis Sci 1983; 24:603–11.
135. Hirst LW, Quigley HA, Stark WJ, Shields MB. Specular microscopy of iridocorneal endothelial syndrome. Am J Ophthalmol 89:11–21.
136. Hodson S. The endothelial pump of the cornea. Invest Ophthalmol Vis Sci 1977; 16:589–91.
137. Hogan JJ, Alvarado J. Pterygium and pinguecula: electron microscopic study. Arch Ophthalmol 1967; 78:174–86.
138. Hunter A. The popliteal pterygium syndrome: report of a new family and review of the literature. Am J Med Genet 1990; 36:196–208.
139. Iwamoto, T, De Voe, AG. Electron microscopical study of the Fleischer ring. Arch Ophthalmol 1976; 94:1579–84.
140. Jacklin HN. Familial predisposition to pterygium formation: a report of a family. Am J Ophthalmol 1964; 57: 481–2.
141. Jaros PA, DeLuise VP. Pingueculae and pterygia. Surv Ophthalmol 1988; 33:41–9.
142. Jauregui HO, Klintworth GK. Pigmented squamous cell carcinoma of cornea and conjunctiva: a light microscopic histochemical and ultrastructural study. Cancer 38: 778–88.
143. Jensen OA. Ocular calcifications in primary hyperparathyroidism: histochemical and ultrastructural study of a case. Comparison with ocular calcifications in idiopathic hypercalcemia of infancy and in renal failure. Acta Ophthalmol. 1975; 53:173–86.
144. Jensen OA, Norn MS. Spheroid degeneration of the conjunctiva: histochemical and ultrastructural examination. Acta Ophthalmol 1982; 60:79–92.
145. Jensen OL. Pterygium, the dominant eye and the habit of closing one eye in sunlight. Acta Ophthalmol 1982; 60: 568–74.
146. Johnson GJ, Ghosh M. Labrador keratopathy: clinical and pathological findings. Can J Ophthalmol 1975; 10:119–35.
147. Johnson GJ, Overall M. Histology of spheroidal degeneration of the cornea in Labrador. Br J Ophthalmol 1978; 62:53–61.
148. Kaiser-Kupfer M, Kuwabara T, Kupfer C. Progressive bilateral essential iris atrophy. Am J Ophthalmol 1977; 83: 340–6.
149. Kaku K, Suda K. Primary band-shaped and gelatinous drop-shaped degeneration of the cornea in a sister and brother. J Clin Ophthalmol Toyko 1964; 18:807–12 [in Japanese].
150. Kamel S. The pterygium: its etiology and treatment. Am J Ophthalmol 1954; 38:682–8.
151. Karai I, Horiguchi S. Pterygium in welders. Br J Ophthalmol. 1984; 68:347–9.
152. Katz, D. Localized area of calcareous-degeneration in sclera. Arch Ophthalmol 1929; 2:30–8.
153. Kawano K, Uehara F, Ohba N. Lectin-cytochemical study on epithelial mucus glycoprotein of conjunctiva and pterygium. Exp Eye Res 1988; 47:43–51.
154. Kendall AC. Infantile hypercalcaemia with keratopathy and sodium depletion. Br Med J 1957; 2:682–3.
155. Kerkenezov N. A pterygium survey of the far north coast of New South Wales. Trans Ophthalmol Soc Aust 1956; 16:110–9.
156. Khodadoust AA, Silverstein AM, Kenyon KR, Dowling JE. Adhesion of regenerating corneal epithelium: the role of basement membrane. Am J Ophthalmol 1968; 65:339–48.
157. King JH. The pterygium: brief review and evaluation of certain methods of treatment. Arch Ophthalmol 1950; 44: 854–69.
158. King RG Jr, Geeraets R. Cogan-Guerry microcystic corneal epithelial dystrophy: a clinical and electron microscopic study. Med Coll Va Q 1972; 8:241–6.
159. Klein BA. Pseudomelanoma of the iris. Am J Ophthalmol 1941; 24:133–8.
160. Klein-Moncrieff B. Isolated foci of calcification in sclera. Arch Ophthalmol 1932; 7:757–62.
161. Klintworth GK. Chronic actinic keratopathy: a condition associated with conjunctival elastosis (pingueculae) and typified by characteristic extracellular concretions. Am J Pathol 1972; 67:327–48.
162. Klintworth GK. The cornea: structure and macromolecules in health and disease. Am J Pathol 1977; 89:719–808.
163. Klintworth GK. Corneal Angiogenesis: A Comprehensive Critical Review. New York, Springer-Verlag, 1991.
164. Klyce SD, Neufeld AH, Zadunaisky JA. Activation of chloride transport by epinephrine and Db Cyclic-AMP in cornea of rabbit. Invest Ophthalmol 1973; 12:127–39.
165. Kops M, Marusíc K. Contribution à l'étude de la dégénérescence en mosaïque de la membrane de Bowman de la cornée. Ophthalmologica 1958; 136:83–9.
166. Kramer TR, Grossniklaus HE, Vigneswaran N, et al. Cytokeratin expression in corneal endothelium in the iridocorneal endothelial syndrome. Invest Ophthalmol Vis Sci 1992; 33:3581–5.
167. Kremer I, Ingber A, Ben-Sira I. Corneal metastatic calcification in Werner's syndrome. Am J Ophthalmol 1988; 106: 221–6.
168. Kurnick NB. Rare syndrome of band-shaped keratitis and arthritis. Am J Dis Child 1942; 63:742–7.
169. Kuwabara T, Ciccarelli EC. Meesmann's corneal dystrophy: a pathological study. Arch Ophthalmol 1964; 71: 676–82.
170. Kyrieleis, W. Über umschriebenen Lederhautschwund (Skleromalazie) in höherem Lebansalter. Klin Monatsbl Augenheilk 1939; 103:441–52.
171. Laibson PR. Microcystic corneal dystrophy. Trans Am Ophthalmol Soc 1976; 74:488–531.
172. Laibson PR, Krachmer JH. Familial occurrence of dot (microcystic), map, fingerprint dystrophy of the cornea. Invest Ophthalmol 1975; 14:397–9.

173. Langham M. Observations on the growth of blood vessels into the cornea: application of a new experimental technique. Br J Ophthalmol 1953; 37:210–22.
174. Leber T. Studien über den Flüssigkeitswechsel im Auge. Albrecht von Graefes Arch Ophthalmol. 1873; 19:87–185.
175. Legrand J. Dystrophie épithéliale récidivante familiale. Bull Soc Ophtalmol Fr 1963; 63:384–7.
176. Lemercier G, Cornand G, Burckhart M-F. Pinguecula et pterygion: étude histopathologique et ultrastucturale. Virchows Arch. Pathol Anat 1978; 379:321–33.
177. Lessell S, Norton EWD. Band keratopathy and conjunctival calcification and hypophosphatasia. Arch Ophthalmol 1964; 71:497–9.
178. Levitt JM. Microcystic dystrophy of the corneal epithelium. Am J Ophthalmol 1971; 72:381–2.
179. Li ZY, Wallace RN, Streeten BW, et al. Elastic fiber components and protease inhibitors in pinguecula. Invest Ophthalmol Vis Sci 1991; 32:1573–85.
180. Lichter RR. The spectrum of Chandler's syndrome: an often overlooked cause of unilateral glaucoma. Trans Am Acad Ophthalmol Otolarayngol 1978; 74:245–51.
181. Lowe R. Recurrent erosion of the cornea. Br J Ophthalmol 1970; 54:805–9.
182. Luthra R, Nemesure BB, Wu SY, et al. Frequency and risk factors for pterygium in the Barbados Eye Study. ArchOphthalmol 2001; 119:1827–32.
183. Luxenberg MN, Friedland BR, Holder JM. Superficial microcystic corneal dystrophy. Arch Ophthalmol 1975; 93: 107–10.
184. Mackenzie FD, Hirst LW, Battistutta D, Green A. Risk analysis in the development of pterygia. Ophthalmology 1992; 99:1056–61.
185. Malbran E, D'Alessandro C, Valenzuela J. Megalocornea and mosaic dystrophy of the cornea. Ophthalmologica 1965; 149:161–76.
186. Manschot, WA. Senile scleral plaques and senile scleromalacia. Br J Ophthalmol 1978; 62:376–80.
187. Matta CS, Tabbara KF, Cameron JA, et al. Climatic droplet keratopathy with corneal amyloidosis. Ophthalmology 1991; 98:192–5.
188. Maurice DM. The cornea and sclera. In: Davson H, ed. The Eye, vol. 1. 2nd ed. New York, NY: Academic Press, 1969:489–600.
189. Maurice DM. The location of the fluid pump in the cornea. J Physiol (Lond) 1972; 221:43–54.
190. Maurice DM, Giardini AA. Swelling of the cornea in vivo after the destruction of its limiting layers. Br J Ophthalmol 1951; 35:791–7.
191. McCracken JS, Klintworth GK. Ultrastructural observations on experimentally produced melanin pigmentation of the corneal epithelium. Am J Pathol 1976; 85: 167–82.
192. McQueen EG. 'Milk poisoning' and 'calcium gout'. Lancet 1952; 1:67–9.
193. Meisler DM, Tabbara KF, Wood IS, et al. Familial band-shaped nodular keratopathy. Ophthalmology 1985; 92: 217–22.
194. Messmer EM, Hoops JP, Kampik A. Bilateral recurrent calcareous degeneration of the cornea. Cornea 2005; 24: 498–502.
195. Meyran-Garcia J, de Buen S, Babayan I. Essential atrophy of the iris: report of a case. Can J Ophthalmol 10:412–5.
196. Miller JM, Freeman J, Heath WH. Calcinosis due to treatment of duodenal ulcer. J Am Med Assoc 1952; 148: 198–9.
197. Miller S. Band-keratopathy with a report of a case of Fanconi's syndrome with calcium deposits in the cornea. Trans Ophthalmol Soc UK 1958; 78:59–70.
198. Millin JA, Golub BM, Foster CS. Human basement membrane components of keratoconus and normal corneas. Invest Ophthalmol Vis Sci 1986; 27:604–7.
199. Moran DJ, Hollows FC. Pterygium and ultraviolet radiation: a positive correlation. Br J Ophthalmol 1984; 68:343–6.
200. Moro E, Amidei B. Sur rapporti tra degenerazione corneale del tipo a pelle di coccodrillo de Vogt a cheratite a bandetella. G Ital Oftalmol 1953; 6:444–64.
201. Morton K, Hutchinson C, Jeanny JC, et al. Colocalization of fibroblast growth factor binding sites with extracellular matrix components in normal and keratoconus corneas. Curr Eye Res 1989; 8:975–87.
202. Müller P. Dégénérescenceen mosaïque ('Chagrin de Crocodile' Vogt) de la membrane de Bowman à la suite d'une kératite traumatique avec hypopyon. Ann Ocul (Paris) 1949; 182:122–7.
203. Murken JD, Dannheim R. Zur Genetik des Pterygium corneae. Klin Monatsbl Augenheilkd 1965; 147:574–9.
204. Nakayasu K, Tanaka M, Konomi H, Hayashi T. Distribution of types I, II, III, IV and V collagen in normal and keratoconus corneas. Ophthalmic Res 1986; 18:1–10.
205. Nettleship E. On a rare form of primary opacity (transverse calcareous film) of the cornea. Arch Ophthalmol 1879; 8:293–19.
206. Nicholls JVV. A survey of the ophthalmic status of the Cree Indians at Norway house, Manitoba. Can Med Assoc J 1946; 54:344–50.
207. Norn MS. Scleral plaques. II. Follow-up, cause. Acta Ophthalmol 1974; 52:512–20.
208. Norn MS. Spheroid degeneration of cornea and conjunctiva: prevalence among Eskimos in Greenland and Caucasians in Copenhagen. Acta Ophthalmol 1978; 56: 551–62.
209. Norn, MS. Prævalensen af pterygium oculi på Grønland og København. Ugeskr Laeg 1979; 141:214–6.
210. Norn MS. Spheroid degeneration, pinguecula, and pterygium among Arabs in the Red Sea territory, Jordan. Acta Ophthalmol. 60:949–54.
211. Norn MS. Conjunctival spheroid degeneration: recurrence after excision. Acta Ophthalmol 1982; 60:434–8.
212. Norn, M. Spheroid degeneration, keratopathy, pinguecula, and pterygium in Japan (Kyoto). Acta Ophthalmol 1984; 62:54–60.
213. Obenberger J. Calcification in corneas with alloxan-induced vascularization. Am J Ophthalmol 1969; 68: 113–9.
214. Obenberger J, Ocumpaugh DE, Cubberly ME. Experimental corneal calcification in animals treated with dihydrotachysterol. Invest Ophthalmol 1969; 8:467–74.
215. Ohashi Y, Dogru M, Tsubota K. Laboratory findings in tear fluid analysis. Clin Chim Acta 2006; 369:17–28.
216. Oldenburg JB, Garbus J, McDonnell JM, McDonnell PJ. Conjunctival pterygia: mechanism of corneal topographic changes. Cornea 1990; 9:200–4.
217. Parsons JH. The Pathology of the Eye, vol. 1, Part 1. London, Hodder and Stoughton, 1904:279.
218. Patel A, Kenyon KR, Hirst LW, et al. Clinicopathologic studies of nine cases of Chandler's syndrome. Surv Ophthalmol 1983; 27:327–44.
219. Pau H. Aetiologische Betrachtungen zur rezidivierenden Erosion. Klin Monatsbl Augenheilk 1963; 142:388–94.

220. Pecorella I, McCartney AC, Lucas S, et al. Acquired immunodeficiency syndrome and ocular calcification. Cornea 1996; 15:305–11.
221. Pflugfelder SC. Antiinflammatory therapy for dry eye. Am J Ophthalmol 2004; 137:337–42.
222. Phillips TJ. The delayed action of mustard gas and the treatment. Proc R Soc Med 1940; 33:229–32.
223. Pinkerton OD, Hokama Y, Shigemura LA. Immunologic basis for the pathogenesis of pterygium. Am J Ophthalmol 1984; 98:225–8.
224. Porter R, Crombie ALI. Corneal and conjunctival calcification in chronic renal failure. Br J Ophthalmol 1975; 57: 339–43.
225. Pouliquen Y, Dhermy P, Presles D, Tollard MF. Dégénérescence en chagrin de crocodile de Vogt ou dégénérescence en mosaïque de Valerio. Arch Ophtalmol 1976; 36:395–418.
226. Pouliquen Y, Saraux H. Ultrastructure de la cornée d'um buphtalme. Arch Ophtalmol (Paris) 1967; 27:263–72.
227. Proia AD, Browning DJ, Klintworth GK. Actinic granuloma of the conjunctiva. Am J Ophthalmol 1983; 96: 116–8.
228. Pülhorn G, Thiel HJ. Ultrastructural investigations of basement membrane regeneration of corneal epithelium. Albrecht von Graefes Arch Klin Ophthalmol 1974; 189: 21–32.
229. Pur S. Senile hyaline degeneration of the sclera. Cs Ophthalmol 1955; 11:284–8.
230. Quigley HA, Forster RF. Histopathology of cornea and iris in Chandler's syndrome. Arch Ophthalmol 1978; 96: 1878–82.
231. Quinn CA, Crookes GP. Bilateral band-shaped keratopathy associated with endogenous uveitis and rheumatoid arthritis treatment with E.D.T.A. Trans Ophthalmol Soc UK 1955; 75:705–7.
232. Quiroga R, Klintworth GK. The pathogenesis of corneal edema induced by Tween 80. Am J Pathol 1967; 51: 977–99.
233. Ramer JC, Ladda RL, Demuth WW. Multiple pterygium syndrome: an overview. Am J Dis Child 142:1988; 794–8.
234. Remler O. Über familiäres Auftretenvon rezidivierender Hornhauterosion und ihre therapeutische Beeinflussung: Zugleich ein Beitrag zur Entstehung der Cataracta subepithelialis disseminata anterior acuta (Vogt). Klin Monatsbl Augenheilk 1959; 135:263–70.
235. Richardson T M. Corneal decomposition in Chandler's syndrome: a scanning and transmission electron microscopic study. Arch Ophthalmol 97:2112–9.
236. Rodger FC. Clinical findings, course, and progress of Bietti's corneal degeneration in the Dahlak Islands. Br J Ophthalmol 1973; 57:657–64.
237. Rodger FC, Cuthill JA, Fydelor PJ, Lenham AP. Ultraviolet radiation as a possible cause of corneal degenerative changes under certain physiographic conditions. Acta Ophthalmol 1974; 52:777–85.
238. Rodnan G, Johnson H. Chronic renal failure in association with excessive intake of calcium and alkali: report of case and review of pathogenesis. Gastroenterology 1954; 27: 584–97.
239. Rodrigues MM, Fine BS, Laibson PR, Zimmerman LE. Disorders of the corneal epithelium: a clinicopathological study of the dot, geographic and fingerprint patterns. Arch Ophthalmol 1974; 92:475–82.
240. Rodrigues MM, Laibson PR. Recurrent corneal erosions. Trans Pa Acad Ophthalmol Otolaryngol 1976; 29:171–3.
241. Rodrigues MM, Laibson PR, Weinreb S. Corneal elastosis: appearance of band-like keratopathy and spheroidal degeneration. Arch Ophthalmol 1975; 93:111–4.
242. Rodrigues MM, Phelps CD, Krachmer JH, et al. Glaucoma due to endothelialization of the anterior chamber: a comparison of posterior polymorphous dystrophy of cornea and Chandler's syndrome. Arch Ophthalmol 1980; 98:688–96.
243. Rodrigues MM, Streeten BW, Spaeth GL. Chandler's syndrome as a variant of essential iris atrophy. Arch Ophthalmol 1978; 96:643–52.
244. Rojas JR, Málaga H. Pterygium in Lima, Peru. Ann Ophthalmol 1986; 18:147–9.
245. Roper KL. Senile hyaline scleral plaques. Arch. Ophthalmol 1945; 34:283–91.
246. Saad R. Pterygium, pingueculum and visual acuity. Austr J Ophthalmol 5:52–66.
247. Schappert-Kimmijser J. Rezidivierende Hornhauterosion und familiäre Hornhautentartung. Klin Monatsbl Augenheilk 1933; 90:655–61.
248. Scheie HG, Yanoff M. Iris nevus (Cogan-Reese) syndrome. Arch Ophthalmol 1975; 93:963–70.
249. Scheie HG, Yanoff M, Kellogg WT. Essential iris atrophy: report of a case. Arch Ophthalmol 1976; 94:1315–20.
250. Scholzer-Schrehardt U, Zagorski Z, Holbach LM, et al. Corneal stromal calcification after topical steroid-phosphate therapy. Arch Ophthalmol 117:1414–8.
251. Scholz DA, Keating FR, Jr. Renal insufficiency, renal calculi and nephrocalcinosis in sarcoidosis. Am J Med 1956; 21:75–84.
252. Scroggs MW, Klintworth GK. Senile scleral plaques: a histopathologic study using energy-dispersive x-ray microanalysis. Hum Pathol 22:557–62.
253. Seller E. Eye diseases in Greenland. Ugeskr Laeg 1949; 111:529–32.
254. Selye H, Dieudonne JM, Veilleux R. A calciphylactic syndrome affecting the skeletal muscles, the salivary gland and the eyes. Exp Med Surg 1962; 20:185–93.
255. Shields MB. Progressive essential iris atrophy, Chandler's syndrome, and the iris nevus syndrome (Cogan-Reese) syndrome: a spectrum of change. Surv Ophthalmol 1979; 24:3–20.
256. Shields MB, Campbell DG, Simmons RJ, Hutchinson BT. Iris nodules in essential iris atrophy. Arch Ophthalmol 94: 406–10.
257. Shields MB, Campbell DG, Simmons RJ. The essential iris atrophies. Am J Ophthalmol 1978; 85:749–59.
258. Shields MB, McCracken JS, Klintworth GK, Campbell DG. Corneal edema in essential iris atrophy. Ophthalmology 1979; 86:1533–48.
259. Smiley WK, May E, Bywaters EGL. Ocular presentations of Still's disease and their treatment. Iridocyclitis in Still's disease: its complications and treatment. Ann Rheum Dis 1957; 16:371–83.
260. Smith RS. The development of mast cells in the vascularized cornea. Arch Ophthalmol 1961; 66:383–90.
261. Snapper J, Bradley WG, Wilson VE. Metastatic calcification and nephrocalcinosis from medical treatment of peptic ulcer. Arch Intern Med 1954; 93:807–17.
262. Stanka P. Zur Feinstruktur de Pigmentlinie des menschlichen Hornhautepithels (Hudson-Stahlische Linie). Z Mikrosk Anat Forsch 1966; 75:461–73.
263. Tabbara KF. Climatic droplet keratopathy. Int Ophthalmol Clin 1986; 26:63–8.
264. Streiff EB, Zwahlen P. Une famille avec dégénérescence en bandelette de la cornée. Ophthalmologica 1946; 111: 129–34.

265. Sugar S, Kobernick S. Localized irritating lesions involving pingueculae. Am J Ophthalmol 1964; 57:94–8.
266. Talbot G. Pterygium. Trans Ophthalmol Soc NZ 1948; 2: 42–5.
267. Tan DTH, Lim ASM, Goh HS, Smith DR. Abnormal expression of the p53 tumor suppressor gene in the conjunctiva of patients with pterygium. Am J Ophthalmol 1997; 123:404–5.
268. Taylor HR. Studies on the tear film in climatic droplet keratopathy and pterygium. Arch Ophthalmol 1980; 98: 86–8.
269. Taylor HR. Aetiology of climatic droplet keratopathy and pterygium. Br J Ophthalmol 1980; 64:154–63.
270. Taylor HR. Ultraviolet radiation and pterygium (letter). J Am Med Assoc 1982; 247:1698.
271. Taylor HR, West SK, Rosenthal FS, et al. Corneal changes associated with chronic UV irradiation. Arch Ophthalmol 1989; 107:1481–4.
272. Taylor PJ, Coates T, Newhouse ML. Episkopi blindness: hereditary blindness in a Greek cypriot family. Br J Ophthalmol 1959; 43:340–4.
273. Threlfall TJ, English DR. Sun exposure and pterygium of the eye: a dose-response curve. Am J Ophthalmol 1999; 128:280–7.
274. Tripathi RC, Bron AJ. Ultrastructural study of the nontraumatic recurrent corneal erosion. Br J Ophthalmol 1972; 56:73–85.
275. Tripathi RC, Bron AJ. Cystic disorders of the corneal epithelium. II. Pathogenesis. Br J Ophthalmol 1973; 57: 376–90.
276. Tripathi RC, Bron AJ. Secondary anterior crocodile shagreen of Vogt. Br J Ophthalmol 1975; 59:59–63.
277. Trobe JD, Laibson PR. Dystrophic changes in the anterior cornea. Arch Ophthalmol 1972; 87:378–82.
278. Tsai YY, Chang KC, Lee H, et al. Effect of p53 codon 72 polymorphism on p53 expression in ptergium. Clin Experiment Ophthalmol 2005; 33:60–62.
279. Tsai YY, Cheng YW, Lee H, et al. P53 gene mutation spectrum and the relationship between gene mutation and protein levels in pterygium. Mol Vis 2005; 11:50–555.
280. Valerio, M. Di una nouva rara forma di distrofia corneale ereditaria. Arch Ottalmol 1942; 49:76–93.
281. Vass Z, Tapaszto I. The histochemical examination of the fibers of pterygium by elastase. Acta Ophthalmol 1964; 42:849–54.
282. Vignanelli M, Stucchi CA. Les calcifications conjonctivales chez les patients en hémodialyse chronique: etude morphologique, clinique et épidémiologique. J Fr Ophtalmol 1988; 11:483–92.
283. Vogt A. Lehrbuch und Atlas der Spaltlampenmikroskopie des lebenden Auges, vol. 1, 2nd ed. Berlin, Springer, 1930.
284. Wales HJ. A family history of corneal erosions. Trans Ophthalmol Soc NZ 1955; 8:77–8.
285. Walsh FB, Howard JE. Conjunctival and corneal lesions in hypercalcemia. J Clin Endocr 1947; 7:644–52.
286. Walton HH. A Practical Treatise on Diseases of the Eye, 3rd ed. London, J. and A. Churchill, 1875.
287. Werner P, Kuschner M, Riley EA. Reversible metastatic calcification associated with excessive milk and alkali intake. Am J Med 1953; 14:108–15.
288. Wissmer, B. Hypercalcémie et insuffisance rénale après absorption prolongée de lait et d'alcalins dans le traitement de l'ulcère gastroduodénal. Helv Med Acta 1955; 22:509–13.
289. Wolter JR, Makley TA Jr. Cogan-Reese syndrome: formation of a glass membrane on an iris nevus clinically stimulating tumor growth. Pediatr Ophthalmol 9:102–5.
290. Wong TY, Foster PJ, Johnson GJ, et al. The prevalence and risk factors for pterygium in an adult Chinese population in Singapore: The Tanjong Pagar Survey. Am J Ophthalmol 2001; 131:176–83.
291. Yanoff M. Iridocorneal endothelial syndrome: unification of a disease spectrum. Surv Ophthalmol 1979; 24:1–2.
292. Yanoff M, Scheie HG, Allman MI. Endothelialization of filtering bleb in iris nevus syndrome. Arch Ophthalmol 1976; 94:1933–6.
293. Young JDH, Finlay RD. Primary spheroidal degeneration of the cornea in Labrador and northern Newfoundland. Am J Ophthalmol 1975; 79:129–34.
294. Youngson RM. Pterygium in Israel. Am J Ophthalmol 1972; 74:954–9.
295. Zadunaisky JA. Electrophysiology and transparency of the cornea. In: Giebisch G, ed. Electrophysiology of Epithelial Cells. New York, NY: F.K. Schattauer Verlag, 1971:225–50.
296. Zarrabi M, Parhami Y. Un cas de maladie de Still: compliquée de manifestations oculaires. Arch Ophtalmol (Paris) 1956; 16:177–9.
297. Zhang JD. An investigation of aetiology and heredity of pterygium: report of 11 cases in a family. Acta Ophthalmol 1987; 65:413–6.

31

Overview of Genetic Disorders

Janey L. Wiggs
Department of Ophthalmology, Harvard Medical School, and Massachusetts Eye and Ear Infirmary, Boston, Massachusetts, U.S.A.

INTRODUCTION

Deoxyribonucleic acid is the molecule that stores the complex genetic information necessary for normal growth, development, and cell function, and is the site for the mutations responsible for genetic diseases. In humans, DNA is found in the chromosomes of the nucleus and in mitochondria. They are large polymers, with a linear backbone of alternating sugar and phosphate residues. The sugar in DNA is deoxyribose, a 5-carbon sugar, and successive sugar residues are linked by covalent phosphodiester bonds. Covalently attached to carbon atom number 1 of each sugar residue is a nitrogenous base. Four types of base are found: adenine (A), cytosine (C), guanine (G), and thymine (T) and they consist of heterocyclic rings of carbon and nitrogen atoms. They can be divided into two classes: purines (A and G) have two joined heterocyclic rings; pyrimidines (C and T) have a single such ring. RNA is an abbreviation for *r*ibo *n*ucleic *a*cid. The composition of RNA molecules is similar to that of DNA molecules, but differs in that they contain ribose sugar residues in place of deoxyribose and uracil (U) instead of thymine.

GENE STRUCTURE AND EXPRESSION

DNA organized as genes codes for proteins. The sequence of base pairs in DNA is a code directing the synthesis of polypeptide chains that become proteins. There are 64 three-base codons in human DNA, 61 of which code for an amino acid. Three of the codons are stop codons, indicating the position in the sequence where the polypeptide chain should terminate. There is redundancy in the genetic code, with multiple codons for each amino acid. The redundancy is mainly the result of the third base of the codon, which has been called the "wobble base" of the codon (Table 1). For example GCA, GCC, GCG, and GCU are all codons for alanine.

Table 1 The Genetic Code

Amino acid	Symbols	Codons[a]
Alanine	Ala (A)	GCA,GCC,GCG,GCU
Arginine	Arg (R)	AGA,AGG,CGA,CGC,CGG,CGU
Asparagine	Asn (N)	NAAC,AAU
Aspartic acid	Asp (D)	GAC,GAU
Cysteine	Cys (C)	UGC,UGU
Glutamic acid	Glu (E)	GAA,GAG
Glutamine	Gln (Q)	CAA,CAG
Glycine	Gly (G)	GGA,GGC,GGG,GGU
Histidine	His (H)	CAG,CAU
Isoleucine	Ile (I)	AUA,AUC,AUU
Leucine	Leu (L)	CUA,CUC,CUG,CUU,UUA,UUG
Lysine	Lys (K)	AAA,AAG
Methionine	Met (M)	AUG
Phenylalanine	Phe (F)	UUC,UUU
Proline	Pro (P)	CCA,CCC,CCG,CCUv
Serine	Ser (S)	AGC,AGU,UCA,UCC,UCG,UCU
Threonine	Thr (T)	ACA,ACC,ACG,ACU
Tryptophan	Try (W)	UGG
Tyrosine	Tyr (Y)	UAC,UAU
Valine	Val (V)	GUA,GUC,GUG,GUU
Stop		UAA,UAG,UGA

[a] The codons for each amino acid are given in terms of the sequence of bases in messenger RNA with the left- and right-sided symbols being the 5' and 3' ends of the molecule, respectively.
Abbreviations: A, adenine; C, cytosine; G, guanine; U, uracil.

The process of gene expression results in a protein molecule. Human genes (and other eukaryotic genes) are composed of exons (coding sequences) interspersed with introns (noncoding sequences). The gene structure has a specific orientation and direction that begins with a 5′ phosphate and ends with a 3′ hydroxyl. To express a gene, the DNA sequence is first copied into an RNA sequence in a process called transcription and carried out by an enzyme, called RNA polymerase. The promoter sequence is the start site for transcription, and the promoter and other regulatory sequences are located in the 5′ region of DNA called the 5′ untranslated region. Once an RNA copy of the gene is made, the intron sequences are removed during RNA splicing. Specific sequences adjacent to the exons are necessary for accurate splicing. The spliced RNA copy is called the messenger RNA and serves as the template for production of the polypeptide chain, a process performed by ribosomes and transfer RNA (tRNA). The formation of the polypeptide chain is called translation, and begins with an initiation codon, most commonly that for methionine (AUG) but very rarely the codon of valine (GUG). Translation occurs initially in the endoplasmic reticulum in the cell cytoplasm. As the polypeptide chain matures, it proceeds from the rough endoplasmic reticulum to the smooth endoplasmic reticulum and if the protein is secreted it proceeds through the Golgi apparatus. Many proteins undergo posttranslational modifications before they are fully active: the initiating methionine is often removed; some proteins combine with a prosthetic group such as heme; other proteins are activated by an enzymatic removal of part of the polypeptide chain; numerous proteins become modified by methylation, phosphorylation, or acetylation; and carbohydrate chains become attached to glycoproteins and proteoglycans (see Chapter 36). Also, precursors of some molecules, such as collagen, become partially cleaved. In addition, proline and lysine residues become hydroxylated in procollagen, and disulfide bonds and cross-links form (see Chapter 44).

GENETIC DISEASES

Thousands of inherited human disorders have been described, and many of them involve the eye. There are three main types of inherited human diseases, monogenic (single-gene disorders), chromosomal syndromes (often involving multiple genes), and complex polygenic disorders (resulting from multiple gene interactions and environmental effects).

Monogenic Disorders

A single mutation in a gene can result in an inherited disease. These monogenic disorders typically exhibit characteristic inheritance patterns depending on the genetic modes of transmission: autosomal dominant, autosomal recessive, X-linked recessive, or X-linked dominant. Monogenic disorders may result from mutations in genes within the cell nucleus or from mutations in genes within the mitochondria. Mitochondrial mutations create a specific maternal inheritance pattern.

Nuclear Genes

Genes on the autosomes (human chromosomes 1–22) occur in two copies (alleles).

Autosomal recessive disorders develop when both alleles have mutations. If both alleles have the same mutation the individual is homozygous for the disease. Individuals who have one abnormal allele (heterozygous individuals) are carriers of the disease and 50% of their offspring will also be disease gene carriers. If both parents are carriers of an abnormal gene, 25% of their male and female offspring are at risk of having the disease (homozygotes if both alleles have the same mutation, compound heterozygotes if they inherit two different mutations). Autosomal recessive disorders often result from defective enzymes as typified by the glycogen storage diseases (see Chapter 39), mucopolysaccharidoses (see Chapter 40), sphingolipidoses (see Chapter 41), and mucolipidoses (see Chapter 42). Heterozygotes can frequently be detected biochemically when enzymes are involved because they commonly express only half the activity of normal enzyme activity. Occasionally clinical characteristics are also identified in heterozygous carriers.

Autosomal-dominant disorders require that only one allele is abnormal. Usually, one of the parents of the patient is also affected and there is a 50% chance that the disease will be transmitted to the offspring of both sexes. Although it may be easy to separate the dominant from the recessive disorders by pedigree analysis, this traditional classification may breakdown when the molecular basis of the disorder is understood. For example, retinoblastoma (see Chapter 60) was once thought to be a dominantly inherited disorder with incomplete penetrance. At the molecular level, it is now understood to be mainly an autosomal recessive disorder and that reduction to homozygosity in some somatic cells causes the clinical phenotype (26). Based on a two-hit hypothesis the high frequency of the second hit is the cause of the resemblance to a Mendelian-dominant disorder. Another source of confusion may occur when the carrier frequency of mutations causing an autosomal recessive disease is high in a given population. In this case, the likelihood that carriers will produce affected offspring is higher than expected for autosomal recessive disorders and the resulting pedigree structure may resemble a dominant inheritance pattern (pseudodominance).

Many X-linked recessive disorders involve vision and the ocular tissues and affect hemizygous (only one chromosome) males, whereas females infrequently manifest any abnormality. All daughters of an affected male carry the mutant gene (obligate carriers), but the sons who derive their X chromosome only from the mother are not. Half the daughters of obligate carriers become carriers and their sons are 50% at risk for the disease.

Female subjects are occasionally affected in disorders with an X-linked recessive mode of inheritance. In some entities, such as X-linked retinitis pigmentosa (MIM + 312600) (19), Lowe syndrome (MIM # 309000) (62), and Fabry disease (MIM + 301500) (14) clinical evaluation of the female carrier may show subtle abnormalities. This is usually presumed to result from X-chromosome inactivation. Although females have two X chromosomes, only one of these chromosomes is usually active, whereas the other chromosome is inactivated in a random process causing half of the cells of a female carrier to have an active X chromosome with the mutant allele expressing the phenotype (Lyon hypothesis) (42,43). Depending on the ratio of cells having the normal or mutant allele, a carrier may be asymptomatic, show milder clinical signs of the disorder, or be affected as severely as a male.

A female can also develop an X-linked recessive disorder if she is the offspring of a carrier and an affected father. In other instances a translocation of part of the X-chromosome to an autosome is responsible for the transmission of some X-linked disorders to women (20).

X-linked dominant conditions are rare and affected males transmit the entity to all of their daughters, but to none of their sons. Half of the offspring of females with such disorders are at risk. Incontinentia pigmenti (MIM # 308300) is thought to have an X-linked dominant mode of inheritance with males not being affected because the mutation is incompatible with life in hemizygous males who die in utero (45).

Mitochondrial Genes

Human mitochondrial DNA (mtDNA) consists of a 16,569 bp closed circular molecule within the mitochondrial matrix. It contains the genes for 13 subunits of oxidative phosphorylation (7 nicotinamide adenine dinucleotide dehydrogenase genes [NDl, ND2, ND3, ND4L, ND4, ND5, ND6], adenosine triphosphate (ATP) synthetase, ubiquinol: cytochrome *c* oxidoreductase, cytochrome *b*, and 3 cytochrome *c* oxidase genes [COI, COII, COIII]) as well as mitochondrial ribosomal RNAs and tRNAs needed for their expression.

Disorders resulting from mitochondrial gene defects are transmitted from mothers to their children because the mitochondria are inherited from the egg. Point mutations (base substitutions) in mtDNA that affect oxidative phosphorylation cause several neuroophthalmologic-inherited disorders, including Leber hereditary optic neuropathy (MIM # 535000) (82), neurogenic muscle weakness, ataxia and retinitis pigmentosa (MIM # 551500) (missense mutation at nucleotide 8893 in mtDNA ATPase 6 gene) (46), myoclonic epilepsy, lactic acidosis, and stroke-like episodes (MIM # 540000) (mutation in nucleotide 3243 of tRNA Leu (UUR) gene (74) and myoclonic epilepsy with red ragged fibers (MIM # 545000) (mutation at nucleotide 8344 in tRNA Lys gene) (13,63,86) (see Chapter 72). A deletion in mtDNA is responsible for the Kearns–Sayre syndrome (MIM # 530000), which is chronic external ophthalmoplegia and retinal degeneration and can include sensorineural hearing loss (38) and a usually fatal childhood disorder with pancytopenia, pancreatic fibrosis, and splenic atrophy (Pearson syndrome) (MIM # 547000) (68).

The cells of individuals with a mitochondrial mutation contain a mixed population of mitochondria with variable numbers of normal and mutant mtDNA genes (heteroplasmy). The proportion of mutant mitochondrial DNA within an individual shifts markedly across generations and within tissues. Partly because of the variable number of mutant mtDNA molecules the expression of the inherited disorder can vary considerably. Indeed rare individuals who survive the Pearson syndrome develop the Kearns–Sayre syndrome (47).

Polygenic Disorders

Polygenic disorders (complex diseases) are inherited disorders, which do not obey the single-gene dominant or single-gene recessive Mendelian inheritance patterns. Many common adult-onset diseases are inherited as complex traits including adult-onset ocular diseases such as primary open angle glaucoma (POAG) (see Chapters 20 and 34), age-related macular degeneration (AMD) (84) (see Chapter 18), and myopia (32,49) (see Chapter 26). Reduced penetrance, gene–gene interactions, gene–environment interactions, phenotypic heterogeneity, and locus heterogeneity are some of the reasons that a trait may not be inherited according to Mendelian inheritance patterns.

Reduced Penetrance

Reduced penetrance is when the phenotype is not consistently expressed in association with a specified genotype. Stochastic effects may be one cause (49), and the presence of a secondary gene, or modifier gene, which can influence the expression of the phenotype may also be a cause (66).

Gene–Gene Interactions

Gene–gene interactions result when the gene products from two genes interact to create an effect. Examples would be two proteins that form a functional dimer complex; the binding of two transcription factors at a promoter that initiates transcription; and two proteins that participate the same biochemical pathway. The effect of modifier genes on the phenotypic expression of the primary gene is also an example of gene–gene interactions (40). Because more than one gene defect is required for the phenotype, the trait is rarely inherited in a Mendelian fashion. Digenic inheritance is the simplest example of gene–gene interactions and has been observed in patients with retinitis pigmentosa due to mutations in the peripherin gene and the *ROM1* gene (34) (see Chapter 35). Trialleleic inheritance is similar to digenic inheritance except three abnormal alleles are necessary for expression of the phenotype. This type of inheritance has been seen in Bardet–Biedl syndrome (MIM #209900) (17).

Gene–Environment Interactions

Gene–environment interactions cause phenotypes that result from specific gene defects and defined environmental exposures. If an individual inherits the gene defect but does not acquire the environmental exposure the disease does not develop. Since environmental exposures can vary within a pedigree the phenotype is not associated consistently with family members carrying the predisposing gene defects, creating a non-Mendelian inheritance pattern. Age-related disorders, such as AMD, are more likely to demonstrate gene–environmental effects (28).

Phenotypic Heterogeneity

Phenotypic heterogeneity is another reason that a disease or trait does not follow Mendelian inheritance patterns. If the phenotypic definition of a trait is too broad, then the disease may actually be a collection of disorders with different genetic causes. Common disorders, such as glaucoma, many exist within a pedigree as different forms that actually have different predisposing genes. Inheritance of the trait in such families would not be expected to follow a consistent pattern.

Locus Heterogeneity

Locus heterogeneity results when defects in more than one gene can result in the same disease. For common adult disorders, more than one gene may contribute to a phenotype within a single pedigree. Since the gene defects could enter the family from multiple points (i.e., individuals who contribute genetic factors through marriage), the distribution of the trait within the pedigree would not necessarily follow any Mendelian inheritance pattern.

Chromosomal Disorders

Chromosome rearrangements including deletions, insertions, duplications, and translocations can cause an imbalance of the genome, which results in abnormal function of a gene or adjacent genes. For example, a gene responsible for aniridia (MIM #106210) is located on the short arm of chromosome 11 close to the gene encoding for catalase and for the one responsible for Wilms tumor and gonadoblastoma (55). An extensive mutation or deletion in the short arm of chromosome 11 (11p-) can produce both Wilms tumor and aniridia (Wilms tumor–aniridia syndrome) (Miller syndrome) (MIM #194072) and a reduction in the activity of catalase (58). Many chromosomal disorders affect the development of the eye and are frequently associated with other systemic developmental abnormalities (see Chapter 52). Occasionally the chromosome defect can be inherited and can give the appearance of an autosomal dominant or X-linked trait. Detection of chromosome rearrangement by cytogenetic techniques can confirm the origin of the abnormality.

MUTATIONS

Mutations are alterations in the nucleotide sequence of DNA. In humans the two most common types of mutations are point mutations, or changes in a single base pair of DNA and insertion/deletion mutations that may involve larger regions of DNA sequence.

Point Mutations

Point mutations may result from errors in DNA replication replacing a single nucleotide by a different nucleotide to cause a change in the sequence of the base pair and a change in the DNA code. Thirty-two percent of these point mutations have been shown to be C-G to T-G or C-G to C-A. The observed 12-fold higher frequency of these nucleotides in base pair substitutions than expected by chance is thought to result from the hypermutability of the methylated C-G dinucleotide. Deamination of 5-methylcytosine (5mC) to T in this doublet gives rise to C to T or G to A substitutions depending upon which strand the 5mC is mutated (48). Methylation of DNA is one of several postmodifications of DNA that occurs as part of the regulation of gene expression. Methylated cytosines are relatively unstable and can spontaneously deaminate, which leads to the base pair substitutions.

If the point mutation occurs in the coding sequence of a gene, namely in an exon, the change could alter the amino acid sequence of the encoded polypeptide. This case is called a missense mutation. The nucleotide alteration could also cause an inappropriately placed stop codon called a nonsense change. Point mutations can also affect the sequences that regulate exon splicing usually leading to a premature stop codon and a truncated polypeptide chain because of an altered reading frame. They can also affect regulatory sequences that reduce or increase the expression of the gene at either transcriptional or translational levels.

Insertion/Deletion Mutations

Insertion/deletion mutations can be caused by unequal crossing over during recombination during germ cell division. The insertion or deletion may affect a single or may be much larger DNA sequence, sometimes involving hundreds of base pairs. Some mutations that cause color blindness illustrate this principle (53,54). For example, almost all red-green color discrimination defects are due to the deletion of genes or to the generation of red-green or green-red gene hybrids because of unequal crossing over during meiosis (53). Alternatively, blue cone monochromacy (MIM %303700) may follow an unequal chromosomal crossing over and a subsequent point mutation (52).

Causes of Mutations

Mutations may also be caused by radiation. X-rays are capable of producing chromosomal breaks leading to large structural alterations. DNA strongly absorbs UV light with a wavelength of 260 nm and radiation may cause changes in the DNA structure, which lead to a mutation unless repaired properly. In xeroderma pigmentosum (MIM + 278700 and others), and the related Cockayne syndromes (MIM #216400 and #133540) a genetic defect in the repair of DNA damaged by UV light predisposes affected individuals to sun-induced neoplasms (basal and squamous cell carcinomas and melanomas) of the eyelid and other exposed parts of the skin, as a result of a cellular hypersensitivity to UV light-induced damage (31,51,69).

Mutations may also result from exposure to chemical agents such as ethyl-methanesulfonate, which react with bases in DNA, and the insertion of foreign DNA, such as viral DNA, into the human genome, causing a disruption of human genes.

Genetic Heterogeneity

More than one genetic defect can lead to the same clinical phenotype, and a number of different genes can be responsible for the same group of clinical disorders. Such genetic heterogeneity exists for example in the group of disorders collectively designated "retinitis pigmentosa" and which can be inherited as an X-linked, autosomal dominant, or autosomal recessive type (see Chapter 35) (61). Genetic heterogeneity may provide clues to the common cellular mechanisms involved in the pathogenesis of the diseases in question.

Phenotypic Expression of Gene Mutations

Phenotypic expression of genetic mutations is highly variable. DNA sequence changes of all types may cause severe disease (mutations), or no disease at all (polymorphisms). Among individuals sharing a specific mutation there may also be significant variability in the expressed phenotype. Phenotypic variability may even exist among family members sharing a disease-associated mutation. The phenotypic differences between individuals carrying mutations in the same gene may be so extreme that they are classified as different diseases, a situation called allelic heterogeneity. Allelic heterogeneity accounts for the different phenotypes of mucopolysaccharidosis (MPS) types IH (Hurler) (MIM #607014) and IS (Scheie) (MIM #607016), which result from different mutations in the *IDUA* gene encoding for α-L-iduronidase (see Chapter 40) (8).

Variation in the phenotypic expression of a particular mutation may be dependent on modifier genes, which can influence the severity of the biological consequences of the gene defect. Variation in phenotypic expression may also be caused by the location of the mutation in a particular gene and its subsequent effect on a particular part of the protein product. Such variable expressivity based on the location of the mutation is exemplified by mutations in the *rds* gene, which may cause typical autosomal-dominant retinitis pigmentosa (MIM #608133) or a dystrophy of the macula (MIM #608161) (81) depending on the position of the genetic defect (see Chapter 35) (33,38,57,81).

A similar phenomenon is seen in certain inherited corneal disorders in which specific mutations in the transforming growth factor beta-induced protein (*TGFBI*) lead to phenotypically distinct gene entities (see Chapter 32) (37,70).

MOLECULAR MECHANISMS OF GENETIC DISEASE

In humans, there are four main molecular mechanisms for the expression of genetic disease: loss of function, gain of function, dominant negative effects, and an accumulation of the mutant protein.

Loss of Function

Gene mutations that abolish the activity of the protein product are called loss of function mutations. Many different DNA sequence abnormalities can diminish the function of the protein including missense mutations, nonsense mutations, deletions, insertions, and regulatory changes causing a reduction in gene expression. Usually a gene deletion or rearrangement causes a more severe disease than a missense mutation. If a person carrying a mutation that abolishes the protein function is phenotypically normal, then the resultant disease is likely to be inherited as an autosomal recessive condition. Many autosomal recessive conditions result from mutations in genes coding for enzymes, since losing half the normal enzyme activity may be tolerated, however losing all the enzyme activity (resulting from loss of function mutations in both alleles of the gene) produces a disease. Ocular disorders caused by loss of function include one type of Leber congenital amaurosis (MIM #204100) caused by loss of function of RPE65 (see Chapter 35) (50) and congenital glaucoma caused by loss of function of CYP1B1 (MIM #231300) (see Chapter 34) (71).

When both copies of the gene are necessary for normal function, loss of function mutations causes an abnormal phenotype that is inherited as an autosomal-dominant trait. These conditions arise from haploinsufficiency because reduced dosage of the gene product is responsible for the disease. Gene products that are typically sensitive to dosage are those that are part of a quantitative signaling system dependent on a specified amount of a receptor and gene products that compete with each other for a metabolic or developmental switch. Eye diseases that demonstrate haploinsufficiency are mainly developmental and include aniridia caused by mutations in *PAX6*(72), and the Axenfeld–Rieger syndrome caused by mutations in *PITX2* (18) and *FOXC1* (see Chapter 34) (4).

Gain of Function

Mutations may alter a protein so that it acquires a novel function that produces an abnormal phenotype. Such mutations are called gain of function mutations and they typically cause autosomal-dominant disease. Mutations that cause gain of function can create a different disease compared with mutations in the same gene that cause loss of function. For example, loss of function mutations in *PAX3* give rise to Wardenburg syndrome (MIM #148820) (49,73), while an abnormal form of the *PAX3* gene that results from fusion with the *FKHR* gene causes alveolar rhabdomyosarcoma (MIM #268220) due to a gain of function mechanism (see Chapter 64) (35).

Dominant Negative Effects

A dominant negative effect occurs when a mutant polypeptide not only loses its own function, but also interferes with the product of the normal allele in a heterozygote. This type of mutation is found in proteins that form dimers or oligomers. Nonstructural proteins that dimerize or oligomerize also show dominant negative effects. For example, transcription factors of the b-HLH-Zip family bind DNA as dimers. Mutants that cannot dimerize often cause recessive phenotypes, but mutants that are able to sequester functioning molecules into inactive dimers give dominant phenotypes. There is some evidence that the myocilin protein, responsible for some cases of open angle glaucoma (MIM #137750), forms dimers and oligomers, and mutations in this gene can have a dominant negative effect (22,41). Dominant negative effects have also been hypothesized as the mechanism for Stargardt disease type 3 (MIM #600110) resulting from by mutations in the *ELOVL4* gene (23).

Accumulation of Mutant Protein

In some autosomal disease mutant protein accumulates in certain tissues and contributes to the pathologic state. Examples of this phenomenon are mutations in the genes that encode for transforming growth factor beta-induced protein (*TGFBIp*), gelsolin (*GSN*), and transthyretin (*TTR*) (see Chapters 32 and 36).

Molecular Pathology

On a cellular level the effects of gene mutations are diverse, but can be broadly divided into those causing degeneration, specific loss of function, developmental abnormalities, and neoplasia.

Cell Degeneration

Cell degeneration is a frequent outcome of gene mutations and can be the result of loss of function, gain of function, or dominant negative mutations. Missense changes in rhodopsin-causing retinitis pigmentosa (MIM +180380) are an example of a degenerative process produced by a specific gene mutation (76).

Loss of Function

Specific loss of function mutations causes a particular cellular process to be lost without necessarily engendering cell death or loss of other cellular processes. Color vision defects resulting from loss of red-green cone pigment is an example of this type of molecular pathology (9). Mutations causing these phenotypes are loss of function mutations but can be inherited as autosomal recessive or autosomal-dominant traits depending on dosage sensitivity.

Developmental Abnormalities

Mutations in genes affect developmental processes. The encoded proteins of these genes are typically developmentally regulated transcription factors and the resulting developmental defects are usually caused by loss of function mutations that reduce the gene dosage (haploinsufficiency). An example is aniridia (MIM #106210) resulting from loss of function mutations in *PAX6* (25).

Neoplasia

The predisposition to tumor formation may be an inherited trait that is caused by mutations in genes that regulate cell division. Retinoblastoma (MIM + 180200) resulting from mutations in the *RB1* gene is an example of this type of mutation (see Chapter 60). Gene mutations that predispose to neoplasia may be loss of function or gain of function. Loss of both copies of the *RB1* gene results in the development of retinal tumors. Sporadic cases arise when both mutations occur in a somatic cell, while hereditary retinoblastoma occurs when an individual inherits an abnormal copy and develops a second somatic mutation (78) or inherits two mutated alleles. Gain of function mutations causing neoplasia usually result from mutations that cause dysregulation of a protein that participates in cellular growth processes. Transgene fusion proteins resulting from chromosomal translocations may produce this type of gain of function mutation.

Other

Protein accumulations are a feature of mutations involving the *TGFBI*, *TACSTD2* (*M1S1*), *GSN*, and *TTR* genes (see Chapter 36). The mutated protein may be in the form of amyloid (see Chapter 37).

DIAGNOSIS OF GENETIC DISORDERS

Clinical Features

The recognition that a particular disorder is inherited is based on the clinical history, physical examination, as well as knowledge about the condition in question. The family history is especially important. Because some rare inherited disorders affect specific ethnic groups, information in this regard is also crucial. A history of consanguinity supports an autosomal recessive disorder, especially if it is rare, as inbreeding increases the chances that both parents are carriers of the mutant gene in question.

Chromosome Studies

The chromosome composition of a cell can be evaluated during the metaphase stage of the mitotic cell cycle, and is described by a karyotype that states the total number of chromosomes and the sex chromosomes. Normal human females and males are 46,XX and 46,XY, respectively. When a chromosomal abnormality is present the karyotype also describes the type of abnormality and the chromosome bands or subbands affected. Autosomes are numbered according to their length and the location of the centromere with the longest being chromosome 1 and the shortest being chromosome 22. Each chromosome is divided into a short (p) and a long arm (q) by the centromere. Using standard techniques, karyotypes can detect large chromosome rearrangements including translocations, deletions, insertions, and inversions. Some specific gene defects can be identified using fluorescent in situ hybridization mapping techniques. These methods rely on the hybridization of fluorescently labeled probes derived from the gene or chromosome region under investigation to metaphase chromosomes. Once hybridized, the fluorescent-labeled chromosome is visualized using a fluorescent microscope. Recent techniques using whole chromosome oligonucleotide arrays have a much higher resolution and can detect chromosomal amplifications and deletions as small as 1 Mb in size (67).

Mutation Detection

The choice of mutation detection methodology is dependent on the gene responsible for the disease. For genes with a limited number of sites of disease-associated DNA sequence changes, specific mutation tests such as allele specific polymerase chain reaction (PCR) or quantitative PCR (TaqMan®) assays can be developed. For genes with disease-associated mutations distributed throughout the coding and/or regulatory sequences a complete sequencing of the gene is necessary to adequately screen for DNA variants potentially responsible for the disease.

Allele-Specific PCR

Allele specific takes advantage of the specificity of DNA polymerase for recognition of the 3′ OH group of a primed sequence for extension of the newly synthesized DNA strand. If a mismatch occurs at the 3′ end of the oligonucleotide primer used for PCR amplification, DNA polymerase is unable to extend the chain. Oligonucleotide primers are designed to amplify selectively each allele of a single base pair change by placing the variable base at the 3′ end of the primer. This method is inexpensive and provides reliable results for most single nucleotide polymorphisms (SNPs). Use of a restriction enzyme to recognize the altered DNA site is an alternative to primer-based methods. For this assay, primer pairs that flank the sequence of interest are selected and after PCR an appropriate restriction enzyme that recognizes the altered DNA sequence is added and the products evaluated by electrophoresis. These assays are efficient and may be less expensive than direct sequencing, or other methods.

Quantitative PCR (TaqMan Assay)

Quantitative PCR has recently been adapted for assay of SNPs and disease-associated DNA sequence changes (60). The common application of the procedure takes advantage of the 5′-3′ exonuclease activity of Taq DNA polymerase. In the TaqMan assay (Applied BioSystems), a specific probe of 20 to 30 bp is designed to hybridize specifically with the DNA sequence of interest. The TaqMan probe is labeled with both a fluorescent reporter dye and a fluorescent quencher dye and is altered so that it cannot be used as a primer for extension. Two additional unlabeled primers that flank the sequence of interest including the TaqMan probe are used for PCR after hybridization of the TaqMan probe. During PCR, the 5′ exonuclease activity of the Taq DNA polymerase degrades the TaqMan probe from the 5′ end, thus releasing the reporter dye that is now able to fluoresce because the quencher dye is no longer in close proximity. As the PCR reaction continues the fluorescence intensity of the reporter dye increases. To detect single base pair changes two TaqMan probes are developed, one for each allele, with reporters that fluoresce as different colors. This technique is particularly useful when screening for a common recurrent mutation in a population.

Direct Genomic Sequencing

Direct genomic sequencing is used when disease-associated DNA sequence variants can occur throughout the coding/regulatory sequence of a gene. After identification of the intron/exon structure PCR primers flanking individual exons are developed either by inspection or using a specific software program such as primer3 software (http://www-genome.wi.mit.edu/cgi-bin/primer/primer3). Purified amplification products are sequenced directly and size and purity is checked. The finished sequence can be compared with a standard reference sequence to detect sequence variants.

Linkage Analysis

For some inherited disorders the chromosomal location of the disease gene is known, but the gene itself is not yet identified. In this situation, mutations in the gene itself cannot be detected, but the chromosome markers that define the location of the disease gene can be used to identify individuals at risk for the disease in a pedigree demonstrating linkage to the chromosome markers that define the disease region. This approach depends on the fact that in pedigrees, genes that are far apart from each other, such as those located on different chromosomes, sort independently, whereas genes that are physically close to each other tend to be inherited together. Possible linkage between the chromosome marker and the disease gene is determined by calculating the likelihood of linkage versus nonlinkage. In using the method of the logarithm of the odds (LOD), a LOD score of 3 or higher (a chance of 1 in 1000) is accepted as conclusive evidence for linkage (75). Since the chromosomal site of a marker is known, linkage of a gene to this marker discloses the location of the gene.

APPROACHES TO THE IDENTIFICATION OF DISEASE GENES

Identification of a gene responsible for a disease depends on the inheritance of the disease trait, specifically if the disease is inherited as a monogenic disorder with a well-defined inheritance pattern or if the gene is inherited as a complex trait.

Monogenic Disorders

For most single-gene disorders an inheritance pattern can be identified and a model specified for linkage studies. The linkage approaches are similar to those described above and take advantage of the principal that a gene and a genetic marker located near each other on a chromosome will be more likely to be inherited together, while those separated by a large distance will not segregate because of genetic recombination events during meiosis. Many genetic markers have been identified and located for these purposes with the microsatellite repeat marker being the most commonly used. Genetic maps have been constructed that identify a highly informative microsatellite repeat marker every 1 Mb, which approximately corresponds to 1 cM genetic distance. Recently, whole genomes SNPs have been used for this type of genetic mapping. SNPs have the advantage of being the most abundant polymorphism in the human genome, but unfortunately they have only two alleles, which lowers the information content. To compensate for this disadvantage many more SNPs need to be analyzed. Typically an analysis of 300–400 microsatellite repeat markers are required to locate a gene responsible for a monogenic disorder using a pedigree with at least 10 informative meiotic events.

The size of the affected pedigree is an important determinant of the resolution of the mapped chromosome region that contains the responsible gene. The larger the pedigree, the greater the statistical power for linkage. Larger pedigrees also have more recombination events, which help to define the location of the disease gene using haplotype mapping. Once the chromosomal location of the disease gene is satisfactorily defined, candidate genes located within the defined genetic interval are identified and prioritized for screening. The completion of the human genome project has made it easier to identify and prioritize candidate genes. Publicly available Web sites such as that at the University of California, Santa Cruz genome site (http://www.genome.ucsc.edu) provide an excellent annotation of human genes and genetic markers so that many of the genes located within a genetic interval can be listed simply by scanning the human sequence contained between the genetic markers that define the region. Once the genes located in the region are identified they can be prioritized for screening based on expression (also provided by a number of publicly available Web sites) and function.

Candidate genes can be screened using PCR amplification of their exons, followed by methods to detect DNA sequence changes such as single-stranded conformation polymorphism (59) or direct genomic sequencing. Once DNA sequence changes are identified they can be verified as causative of the disorder in question by examining their segregation in affected families and by comparing the distribution of DNA sequence changes in affected individuals and in control individuals without any evidence of the disease.

Polygenic Disorders

The overall approach to the discovery of genes contributing to polygenic disorders is more complex than Mendelian single-gene disorders because an inheritance pattern usually cannot be determined and a genetic model cannot be specified. In addition, defects in multiple genes and exposure to certain environmental factors may be responsible for the full disease phenotype. The lack of a genetic model and the contributions of multiple factors (both genetic and environmental) make gene discovery for polygenic disorders difficult. Approaches to identify the chromosomal location of genes that contribute to these disorders include the identification of Mendelian subtypes, whole genome analyses, case–control association studies, phenotype stratification and qualitative traits.

Mendelian Subtypes

One path to the desired genes is to study simple Mendelian forms of the disease with defined genetic models resulting from defects in a single underlying gene. Mendelian forms of a complex disease are often rare, but the discovery of the responsible gene can provide information applicable to other, more common forms of the disease. Mutant alleles of genes responsible for rare forms of a disease may be one of several factors leading to the development of a more common complex disease, for example some mutations in *MYOC*, which encodes for myocilin, are associated with early onset autosomal-dominant glaucoma while others are associated with the late onset genetically complex adult disease (see Chapter 34) (3).

Whole Genome Analyses

Scanning the entire genome is another approach that has lead to the identification of genes contributing to complex disease. The general approach is to collect affected sibling pairs and compare genetic markers for allele sharing due to identity by descent (IBD). IBD results from inheritance of a common allele from one or both parents, rather than identity by state, which results from spurious inheritance of the same allele. Many families are evaluated and the IBD from all sibling pairs are analyzed to establish evidence of association with the disease trait. A chromosome region shared by the majority of sibling pairs by inheritance indicates that a gene that contributes to the disease trait may be located on the shared segment (27). Because complex disorders are frequently age-related (such as POAG and AMD) the families available for genetic analysis typically comprise only one generation of affected individuals (the grandparents are typically deceased, and the children are too young to be affected). The lack of multiple affected generations significantly reduces the statistical power to detect linkage in single pedigrees. As such, genetic studies designed to identify genes responsible for complex traits usually require a large number of affected sibling pairs from many pedigrees. Genome-wide scans using these methods have been completed for many complex disorders including POAG (56,83). Typically multiple chromosome regions are identified using these approaches, some of which are true positives while others are false positives. Follow-up studies using additional groups of sibpairs, increased marker densities and haplotype analyses are necessary to confirm the true positives and refine the locations of the genes.

Recent approaches for genome-wide scans to identify genes responsible for complex traits have utilized SNPs and information from the HapMap. SNPs are single-letter variations in a DNA-base sequence. There are over 10 million SNPs present in the human genome with a density of one SNP every 100 bases of DNA. Examining every SNP in the genome for disease association would be an overwhelming undertaking, and fortunately this is not necessary, because many SNPs are bound together to form haplotypes, which are blocks of SNPs commonly inherited together. This binding occurs through the phenomenon of linkage disequilibrium. Within a haplotype block, which may extend for 10,000 to 100,000 bases of DNA, the analysis of only a subset of all SNPs may "tag" the entire haplotype. The International HapMap project (30) has developed a rich resource of SNPs and has performed an initial characterization of the linkage disequilibrium patterns between SNPs in multiple different populations. Recently, this approach has successfully led to the identification of complement factor H as a susceptibility gene for AMD (16,24,29,36,87).

Case–Control Association Studies

Case–control association studies have been a productive approach to identify genes that contribute to complex disease. In these studies large numbers of affected and control individuals are collected and used for genotyping of genetic markers to identify chromosome regions harboring genes of interest. Case–control association studies can also be very helpful in evaluating a specific candidate gene located with a defined chromosome region. Case–control allelic/genotypic association studies are particularly powerful because they can measure the magnitude of association between a polymorphism and risk of disease, as well as the impact of that polymorphism on the prevalence of the disease in the population. The usual case–control design involves representative sampling of cases and controls from the same underlying population, minimization of bias (for example by reducing recall bias by using primary sources of data), and matching cases with controls so that confounding variables are eliminated. Case–control studies played an important part in the discovery of the contribution of complement factor H to AMD (16,24,87).

Phenotype Stratification

Identifying a phenotypic subgroup of patients affected with specific features of a complex disease may help reduce the number of genes contributing to the subphenotype, thus making gene identification approaches simpler. For example, stratifying by age of onset made it possible to identify a stronger linkage signal from one chromosome region harboring a gene for POAG (2).

Quantitative Traits

Many complex disorders have precursor states that are quantitative and have strong genetic determinants that are highly heritable (44). For many complex disorders, the heritability of the precursor quantitative trait is greater than the heritability of the complete trait (6). Mapping genes responsible for the precursor quantitative traits, rather than the complete complex phenotype, has several important advantages including objective definitions of the phenotype, the identification of genes that are important risk factors for the disease, and a possible reduction in the underlying molecular heterogeneity. Genome scans mapping ocular quantitative traits, such as intraocular pressure (IOP), have been completed (15).

ANIMAL MODELS

Linkage Approaches Using Mouse Genetics

A tremendous advantage of animal models and mice in particular is that breeding can be experimentally controlled. In mice, litters can be produced every 4 to 5 weeks allowing for the production of multiple generations of affected animals in a relatively short period of time. Given the relatively large size of sibships linkage studies using mice can lead to efficient mapping and identification of a gene responsible for a particular trait. Once the mouse gene is known, the human homolog can be rapidly identified by comparing the human and mouse genomic DNA sequences. The mouse genome is well annotated, and can be accessed through several websites, including the National Center for Biotechnology Information and Jackson Laboratories: (http://www.ncbi.nlm.nih.gov; www.jax.org). It is not surprising that some genes responsible for ocular phenotypes were found in the mouse before being identified in humans. An example is the identification of mutations in the *PITX3* gene as a cause of the human posterior polar cataract after mutations in the *pitx3* gene were shown to cause a developmental defect in the crystalline lens of the mouse (aphakia mouse) (5,65) (see Chapter 33).

Genetically Engineered Mice

Manipulating genes in mice can help determine the function of a gene and can also provide additional evidence that a gene associated with the human genetic disorder is associated with that phenotype in the mouse. Gene function can be determined from cultured cells and cell extracts, but the ability to insert genes into whole animals (transgenic animals) or to selectively delete or alter single predetermined genes in an animal (gene knockout animals) provides an important opportunity to study gene function.

A particular gene can be removed or selectively inhibited in mice by using a variety of techniques. The effects of losing the protein product of the gene can be studied without the gene (gene knock-out mice). These mice are only useful for studies designed to create the human disease phenotype if the responsible gene defect causes a loss of function of the gene product. A knock-out of the mouse *cyp1b1* gene was useful in understanding how this gene causes congenital glaucoma in humans (64).

If the genetically determined human disorder results from the abnormal protein causing a gain of function or a dominant negative effect, then a transgenic animal containing a copy of the abnormal human gene is needed to create the phenotype. To produce a transgenic animal a foreign DNA molecule is artificially introduced into the cells of an animal. The foreign DNA molecule is called a transgene and may contain one or many genes. By inserting a transgene into a fertilized oocyte or cells from the early embryo, the resulting transgenic animal may be able to transmit the foreign DNA stably in its germ line. For studies of human genes, transgenic animals are made by incorporating a copy of the selected human gene into the mouse genome, or by selectively removing the corresponding mouse gene and replacing it with the selected human gene. Transgenic mice have provided insight into a number of genetically determined human ocular disorders including: glaucoma (39), retinal disorders (11), and cataract (85).

In addition to studying the pathobiological effects of a mutant gene, animal models of human diseases provide an important opportunity to evaluate novel therapies that would not be ethically permissible without first testing the efficacy and safety of the treatment in animal models. An example, of this is the recent recreation of the photoreceptor response in a RPE65 deficient dog (1) and mouse (12) after viral delivery of the gene. Since not all animal models of disease are naturally occurring, the creation of the human phenotype in genetically engineered mice can provide an animal model suitable for further study. In addition, animal models can be used to evaluate the efficacy and safety of gene therapy.

In addition to mice (64), rats (80), drosophila (21), zebra fish (79), pigs (7), rabbits (10), and monkeys (77) have all been used for genetic analysis of genes responsible for ocular conditions.

REFERENCES

1. Acland GM, Aguirre GD, Bennett J, et al. Long-term restoration of rod and cone vision by single dose rAAV-mediated gene transfer to the retina in a canine model of childhood blindness. Mol Ther 2005; 12:1072–82.
2. Allingham RR, Wiggs JL, Hauser ER, et al. Early adult-onset POAG linked to 15q11-13 using ordered subset analysis. Invest Ophthalmol Vis Sci 2005; 46:2002–5.
3. Alward WL. The genetics of open-angle glaucoma: the story of GLC1A and myocilin. Eye 2000; 14 (Pt 3B): 429–36.
4. Berry FB, Lines MA, Oas JM, et al. Functional interactions between FOXC1 and PITX2 underlie the sensitivity to FOXC1 gene dose in Axenfeld–Rieger syndrome and anterior segment dysgenesis. Hum Mol Genet 2006; 15: 905–19.
5. Berry V, Yang Z, Addison PK, et al. Recurrent 17 bp duplication in PITX3 is primarily associated with posterior polar cataract (CPP4). J Med Genet 2004; 41:e109.
6. Blangero J. Localization and identification of human quantitative trait loci: king harvest has surely come. Curr Opin Genet Dev 2004; 14:233–40.
7. Bordais A, Bolanos-Jimenez F, Fort P, et al. Molecular cloning and protein expression of Duchenne muscular dystrophy gene products in porcine retina. Neuromuscul Disord 2005; 15:476–87.
8. Brooks DA. Alpha-L-iduronidase and enzyme replacement therapy for mucopolysaccharidosis I. Expert Opin Biol Ther 2002; 2:967–76.
9. Carroll J, Neitz M, Hofer H, et al. Functional photoreceptor loss revealed with adaptive optics: an alternate cause of color blindness. Proc Natl Acad Sci USA 2004; 101:8461–6.
10. Cheng L, Toyoguchi M, Looney DJ, et al. Efficient gene transfer to retinal pigment epithelium cells with long-term expression. Retina 2001; 25:193–201.
11. Dalke C, Graw J. Mouse mutants as models for congenital retinal disorders. Exp Eye Res 2005; 81:503–12.
12. Dejneka NS, Surace EM, Aleman TS, et al. In utero gene therapy rescues vision in a murine model of congenital blindness. Mol Ther 2004; 9:182–8.
13. DiMauro S. Mitochondrial diseases. Biochim Biophys Acta 2004; 1658:80–8.
14. Dobrovolny R, Dvorakova L, Ledvinova J, et al. Relationship between X-inactivation and clinical involvement in Fabry heterozygotes. Eleven novel mutations in the alpha-galactosidase A gene in the Czech and Slovak population. J Mol Med 2005; 83:647–54.
15. Duggal P, Klein AP, Lee KE, et al. A genetic contribution to intraocular pressure: the beaver dam eye study. Invest Ophthalmol Vis Sci 2005; 46:555–60.
16. Edwards AO, Ritter R 3rd, Abel KJ, et al. Complement factor H polymorphism and age-related macular degeneration. Science 2005; 308:421–4.
17. Eichers ER, Lewis RA, Katsanis N, Lupski JR. Triallelic inheritance: a bridge between Mendelian and multifactorial traits. Ann Med 2004; 36:262–72.
18. Evans AL, Gage PJ. Expression of the homeobox gene Pitx2 in neural crest is required for optic stalk and ocular anterior segment development. Hum Mol Genet 2005; 14: 3347–59.
19. Fishman GA, Grover S, Jacobson SG, et al. X-linked retinitis pigmentosa in two families with a missense mutation in the RPGR gene and putative change of glycine to valine at codon 60. Ophthalmology 1998; 105:2286–96.
20. Garcia-Hoyos M, Sanz R, Diego-Alvarez D, et al. New approach for the refinement of the location of the X-chromosome breakpoint in a previously described female patient with choroideremia carrying a X; 4 translocation. Am J Med Genet A 2005; 138:365–8.
21. Gehring WJ. Historical perspective on the development and evolution of eyes and photoreceptors. Int J Dev Biol 2004; 48:707–17.
22. Gobeil S, Rodrigue MA, Moisan S, et al. Intracellular sequestration of hetero-oligomers formed by wild-type and glaucoma-causing myocilin mutants. Invest Ophthalmol Vis Sci 2004; 45:3560–7.
23. Grayson C, Molday RS. Dominant negative mechanism underlies autosomal dominant Stargardt-like macular

dystrophy linked to mutations in ELOVL4. J Biol Chem 2005; 280:32521–30.
24. Haines JL, Hauser MA, Schmidt S, et al. Complement factor H variant increases the risk of age-related macular degeneration. Science 2005; 308:419–21.
25. Hanson IM, Fletcher JM, Jordan T, et al. Mutations at the PAX6 locus are found in heterogeneous anterior segment malformations including Peters' anomaly. Nat Genet 1994; 6:168 – 73.
26. Harbour JW. Molecular basis of low-penetrance retinoblastoma. Arch Ophthalmol 2001; 119:1699–704.
27. Hauser ER, Boehnke M, Guo SW, Risch N. Affected-sib-pair interval mapping and exclusion for complex genetic traits: sampling considerations. Genet Epidemiol 1996; 13: 117–37.
28. Heiba IM, Elston RC, Klein BE, Klein R. Sibling correlations and segregation analysis of age-related maculopathy: the Beaver Dam Eye Study. Genet Epidemiol 1996; 11:51–67.
29. Hyman L, Neborsky R. Risk factors for age-related macular degeneration: an update. Curr Opin Ophthalmol 2002; 13:171–5.
30. The International HapMap Consortium. The International HapMap Project. Nature 2003; 426:789–96.
31. Itoh T. Xeroderma pigmentosum group E and DDB2, a smaller subunit of damage-specific DNA binding protein: Proposed classification of xeroderma pigmentosum, Cockayne syndrome, and ultraviolet-sensitive syndrome. J Dermatol Sci 2006; 41:87–96.
32. Jacobi FK, Zrenner E, Broghammer M, Pusch CM. A genetic perspective on myopia. Cell Mol Life Sci 2005; 62:800–8.
33. Kajiwara K, Sandberg MA, Berson EL, Dryja TP. A null mutation in the human peripherin/RDS gene in a family with autosomal dominant retinitis punctata albescens. Nature Genet 1993; 3:208–12.
34. Kajiwara K, Berson EL, Dryja TP. Digenic retinitis pigmentosa due to mutations at the unlinked peripherin/RDS and ROM1 loci. Science 1994; 264:1604–8.
35. Keller C, Hansen MS, Coffin CM, Capecchi MR. Pax3: Fkhr interferes with embryonic Pax3 and Pax7 function: implications for alveolar rhabdomyosarcoma cell of origin. Genes Dev 2004; 18:2608–13.
36. Klein RJ, Zeiss C, Chew EY, et al. Complement factor H polymorphism in age-related macular degeneration. Science 2005; 308:385–9.
37. Klintworth GK. The molecular genetics of the corneal dystrophies—current status. Front Biosci 2003; 8:d687–713.
38. Kornblum C, Broicher R, Walther E, et al. Sensorineural hearing loss in patients with chronic progressive external ophthalmoplegia or Kearns-Sayre syndrome. J Neurol 2005; 252:1101–7.
39. Kroeber M, Ohlmann A, Russell P, Tamm ER. Transgenic studies on the role of optineurin in the mouse eye. Exp Eye Res 2006; 82:1075–85.
40. Libby RT, Smith RS, Savinova OV, et al. Modification of ocular defects in mouse developmental glaucoma models by tyrosinase. Science 2003; 299:1578–81.
41. Liu Y, Vollrath D. Reversal of mutant myocilin non-secretion and cell killing: implications for glaucoma. Hum Mol Genet 2004; 13:1193–204.
42. Lyon MF. Gene action in the X-chromosome of the mouse (*Mus musculus* L.). Nature 1961; 190:372–3.
43. Lyon MF. X-Chromosome inactivation and developmental patterns in mammals. Biol Rev 1972; 47:1–35.
44. Majumder PP, Ghosh S. Mapping quantitative trait loci in humans: achievements and limitations. J Clin Invest, 2005; 115:1419–24.
45. Martinez-Pomar N, Munoz-Saa I, Heine-Suner D, et al. A new mutation in exon 7 of NEMO gene: late skewed X-chromosome inactivation in an incontinentia pigmenti female patient with immunodeficiency. Hum Genet 2005; 118:458–65.
46. Mattiazzi M, Vijayvergiya C, Gajewski CD, et al. The mtDNA T8993G (NARP) mutation results in an impairment of oxidative phosphorylation that can be improved by antioxidants. Hum Mol Genet 2004; 13:869–79.
47. McShane MA, Hammans SR, Sweeney M, et al. Pearson syndrome and mitochondrial encephalopathy in a patient with a deletion of mtDNA. Am J Hum Genet 1991; 48: 39–42.
48. Millar CB, Guy J, Sansom OJ, et al. Enhanced CpG mutability and tumorigenesis in MBD4-deficient mice. Science 2002; 297:403–5.
49. Morell R, Friedman TB, Asher JH Jr, Robbins LG. The incidence of deafness is non-randomly distributed among families segregating for Wardenburg syndrome type 1 (WS1). J Med Genet 1997; 34:447–52.
50. Morimura H, Fishman GA, Grover SA, et al. Mutations in the RPE65 gene in patients with autosomal recessive retinitis pigmentosa or Leber congenital amaurosis. Proc Natl Acad Sci USA 1988; 95:3088–93.
51. Muftuoglu M, Sharma S, Thorslund T, et al. Cockayne syndrome group B protein has novel strand annealing and exchange activities. Nucleic Acids Res 2006; 34: 295–304.
52. Nathans J, Davenport CM, Maumenee IH, et al. Molecular genetics of human blue cone monochromacy. Science 1989; 245:831–8.
53. Nathans J, Piantanida TP, Eddy RL, et al. Molecular genetics of inherited variation in human color vision. Science 1986; 232:203–10.
54. Nathans J, Thomas D, Hogness DS. Molecular genetics of human color vision: the genes encoding blue, green, and red pigments. Science 1986; 232:193–202.
55. Nelson LB, Spaeth GL, Nowinski TS, et al. Aniridia: a review. Surv Ophthalmol 1984; 28:621–42.
56. Nemesure B, Jiao X, He Q, et al. A genome-wide scan for primary open-angle glaucoma (POAG): the Barbados Family Study of Open-Angle Glaucoma. Hum Genet 2003; 112:600–9.
57. Nichols BE, Sheffield VC, Vandenburgh K, et al. Butterfly-shaped pigment dystrophy of the fovea caused by point mutation in codon 167 of the RDS gene. Nature Genetics 1993; 3:202–7.
58. Niederfuhr A, Hummerich H, Gawin B, et al. A sequence-ready 3-Mb PAC contig covering 16 breakpoints of the Wilms tumor/anirida region of human chromosome 11p13. Genomics 1998; 15:53:155–63.
59. Orita M, Iwahana H, Kanazawa H, et al. Detection of polymorphisms of human DNA by gel electrophoresis as single-strand conformation polymorphisms. Proc Natl Acad Sci USA 1989; 86:2766–70.
60. Ranade K, Chang MS, Ting CT, et al. High-throughput genotyping with single nucleotide polymorphisms. Genome Res 2001; 11:1262–8.
61. Rivolta C, Sharon D, DeAngelis MM, Dryja TP. Retinitis pigmentosa and allied diseases: numerous diseases, genes, and inheritance patterns. Hum Mol Genet 2002; 11:1219–27.
62. Roschinger W, Muntau AC, Rudolph G, et al. Carrier assessment in families with Lowe oculocerebrorenal syndrome: novel mutations in the OCRL1 gene and correlation of direct DNA diagnosis with ocular examination. Mol Genet Metab 2000; 69:213–22.

63. Rossmanith W, Raffelsberger T, Roka J, et al. The expanding mutational spectrum of MERRF substitution G8361A in the mitochondrial tRNA Lys gene. Ann Neurol 2003; 54:820–3.
64. Schweers BA, Dyer MA. Perspective: new genetic tools for studying retinal development and disease. Vis Neurosci 2005; 22:553–60.
65. Semina EV, Murray JC, Reiter R, et al. Deletion in the promoter region and altered expression of Pitx3 homeobox gene in aphakia mice. Hum Mol Genet 2000; 9:1575–85.
66. Silva E, Dharmaraj S, Li YY, et al. A missense mutation in GUCY2D acts as a genetic modifier in RPE65-related Leber Congenital Amaurosis. Ophthalmic Genet 2004; 25:205–17.
67. Slater HR, Bailey DK, Ren H, et al. High-resolution identification of chromosomal abnormalities using oligonucleotide arrays containing 116,204 SNPs. Am J Hum Genet 2005; 77:709–26.
68. Smith OP, Hann IM, Woodward CE, Brockington M. Pearson's marrow/pancreas syndrome: haematological features associated with deletion and duplication of mitochondrial DNA. Br J Haematol 1995; 90:469–72.
69. Spivak G. UV-sensitive syndrome. Mutat Res 2005; 577: 162–9.
70. Stewart HS, Ridgway AE, Dixon MJ, et al. Heterogeneity in granular corneal dystrophy: identification of TGFBI (BIGH3) gene-lessons for corneal amyloidogenesis. Hum Mutat 1999; 14:126–32.
71. Stoilov I, Akarsu AN, Sarfarazi M. Identification of three different truncating mutations in cytochrome P4501B1 (CYP1B1) as the principal cause of primary congenital glaucoma (Buphthalmos) in families linked to the GLC3A locus on chromosome 2p21. Hum Mol Genet 1997; 6:641–7.
72. Tang HK, Chao LY, Saunders GF. Functional analysis of paired box missense mutations in the PAX6 gene. Hum Mol Genet 6:381–6.
73. Tassabehji M, Newton VE, Liu XZ, et al. The mutational spectrum in Waardenburg syndrome. Hum Mol Genet 1995; 4:2131–7.
74. Tay SK, Shanske S, Crowe C, et al. Clinical and genetic features in two families with MELAS and the T3271C mutation in mitochondrial DNA. J Child Neurol 2005; 20: 142–6.
75. Thompson JS, Thompson MW. Genetics in Medicine. 4th ed. Philadelphia, PA: W.B. Saunders, 1986:193–209.
76. To K, Adamian M, Berson EL. Histologic study of retinitis pigmentosa due to a mutation in the RP13 gene (PRPC8): comparison with rhodopsin Pro23His, Cys110Arg, and Glu181Lys. Am J Ophthalmol 2004; 137:946–8.
77. Umeda S, Ayyagari R, Allikmets R, et al. Early-onset macular degeneration with drusen in a cynomolgus monkey (*Macaca fascicularis*) pedigree: exclusion of 13 candidate genes and loci. Invest Ophthalmol Vis Sci 2005; 46:683–91.
78. Valverde JR, Alonso J, Palacios I, Pestana A. RB1 gene mutation up-date, a meta-analysis based on 932 reported mutations available in a searchable database. BMC Genet 2005; 6:53–62.
79. Vihtelic TS, Fadool JM, Gao J, et al. Expressed sequence tag analysis of zebrafish eye tissues for NEIBank. Mol Vis 2005; 11:1083–100.
80. Vollrath D, Feng W, Duncan JL, et al. Correction of the retinal dystrophy phenotype of the RCS rat by viral gene transfer of Mertk. Proc Natl Acad Sci USA 2001; 98: 12584–9.
81. Wells, J, Wroblewski, J, Keen, J, et al. Mutations in the human retinal degeneration slow (RDS) gene can cause either reinitis pigmentosa or macular dystrophy. Nature Genet 1993; 3:213–8.
82. White HE, Durston VJ, Seller A, et al. Accurate detection and quantitation of heteroplasmic mitochondrial point mutations by pyrosequencing. Genet Test 2005; 9:190–9.
83. Wiggs JL, Allingham RR, Hossain A, et al. Genome-wide scan for adult onset primary open angle glaucoma. Hum Mol Genet 2000; 9:1109–17.
84. Wiggs JL. Complex disorders in ophthalmology. Semin Ophthalmol 1995; 10:323–30.
85. Wolf N, Penn P, Pendergrass W, et al. Age-related cataract progression in five mouse models for anti-oxidant protection or hormonal influence. Exp Eye Res 2005; 81: 276–85.
86. Yasukawa T, Kirino Y, Ishii N, et al. Wobble modification deficiency in mutant tRNAs in patients with mitochondrial diseases. FEBS Lett 2005; 579:2948–52.
87. Zareparsi S, Branham KE, Li M, et al. Strong association of the Y402H variant in complement factor H at 1q32 with susceptibility to age-related macular degeneration. Am J Hum Genet 2005; 77:149–53.

32

Genetic Disorders of the Cornea

Gordon K. Klintworth
Departments of Pathology and Ophthalmology, Duke University, Durham, North Carolina, U.S.A.

INTRODUCTION

The timing and sequence of events that follow specific genetic mutations that cause corneal diseases vary considerably. Some become manifest during early corneal development as developmental anomalies; others do not become apparent until later in life. Some genetically determined disorders are restricted to the cornea: others also affect other parts of the eye or are components of a systemic disorder. Some corneal diseases have a simple Mendelian inheritance, others, probably involve more than one gene or an interaction between genetic and environmental factors (see Chapter 31). The affect on vision and the disability created varies with the disorder. During the past decade mutations in more than 38 genes that affect the cornea have been identified and the genes for other corneal disorders have been mapped to specific chromosomal loci (Table 1).

This chapter reviews well-defined inherited corneal disorders and includes keratoconus (KC), which is a multifactorial heterogenous disorder with an indisputable genetic component.

GENETIC DISORDERS AFFECTING THE CORNEA CAUSED BY KNOWN GENETIC DEFECTS

Mutations in the *KRT3* and *KRT12* Genes

General Remarks

The intermediate filaments within the cytoskeleton of the corneal epithelium are composed of pairs of specific cytokeratins that are coexpressed during epithelial differentiation. One member of the duo is an acid cytokeratin with a molecular weight of 40 to 56.5 kDa (cytokeratin 12); the other (cytokeratin 3) has a molecular weight of 53 to 67 kDa. Mutations in the genes for cytokeratin 3 (*KRT3*) and cytokeratin 12 (*KRT12*) cause Meesmann corneal dystrophy (MECD) and Stocker–Holt corneal dystrophy.

Meesmann Corneal Dystrophy

Although first reported clinically in 1935 by Pameijer of the Netherlands (457), MECD (juvenile familial epithelial dystrophy, MIM #122100) was best characterized as a distinct entity by Meesmann and Wilke (412,413).

Table 1 Summary of Genetically Determined Diseases Affecting the Cornea

	Mode of inheritance	Gene locus	Gene	Mutations	OMIM #	Remarks and references
Disorders primarily involving corneal epithelium						
Fabry disease (angiokeratoma corporis diffusum, cornea verticillata)	XR	Xq22-24	*GLA*	More than 62	+301500	(150)
Hereditary benign intraepithelial dyskeratosis	AD	4q35	Unknown	Unknown	%127600	(19,495)
Keratosis follicularis spinulosa decalvans	XR	Xp22.1	*SAT*	Unknown	#308800	Gene not identified with certainty (475)
Lisch epithelial dystrophy	XR	Unknown	Unknown	Unknown	Not listed	(359)
Meesmann dystrophy	AD	12q13	*KRT3*	Glu509Lys	#122100	(244)
Meesmann dystrophy	AD	17q12	*KRT12*	7 known	#122100	(86,244,446)
Stocker–Holt dystrophy	AD	17q12	*KRT12*	Arg19Ile	#122100	(316)
Tyrosine transaminase deficiency (tyrosinemia type II, Richner–Hanhart syndrome)	AR	16q22.1–q22.3	*TAT*	5 known	+276600	(440)
Disorders primarily involving subepithelial corneal tissue						
Gelatinous drop-like corneal dystrophy (familial subepithelial corneal amyloidosis)	AR	1p32	*TACSTD2 (M1S1)*	Multiple	#2004870	(60,500,607,624)
Granular corneal dystrophy type III (Reis–Bücklers dystrophy)	AD	5q31	*TGFBI*	Arg124Leu	#608470	(109,325,390, 452,678)
Grayson–Wilbrant dystrophy	AD	Unknown	Unknown	Unknown	Not listed	(199)
Subepithelial mucinous corneal dystrophy	AD	Unknown	Unknown	Unknown	Not listed	(133)
Thiel–Behnke dystrophy	AD	5q31	*TGFBI*	Arg555Gln	%602082	(109,452,503)
Thiel–Behnke dystrophy	AD	10q23–q24	Unknown	Unknown	%602082	(682)
Disorders primarily involving the corneal stroma						
Bietti crystalline corneoretinal dystrophy	AR	4q35.1	*CYP4V2*	13 known	#210370	(250)
Central cloudy dystrophy	AD	Unknown	Unknown			
Congenital stromal dystrophy	AD	12q13.2	*DCN*	2 known	#610048	(57)
Cystinosis	AR	17p13	*CTNS*	>4 known	#219750	(174)
Fish eye disease	AR	16q22.1	*LCAT*	Unknown	#136120	(172)
Fleck dystrophy	AD	2q35	*PIP5K3*	8 known	#121850	(251)
Galactosialidosis	AR	20q13.1	*PPGB*	>14 known	+256540	(605)
Granular corneal dystrophy type I	AD	5q31	*TGFBI*	Arg555Trp	#121900	(328,433)
Granular corneal dystrophy type II (Avellino dystrophy, combined lattice-granular dystrophy)	AD	5q31	*TGFBI*	Arg124His	#607541	(6,324)
Keratoconus	Not clear	20p11.2	*VSX1*	Leu17Pro Arg116Trp Asp144Glu Leu159Met Gly160Asp Pro247Arg	#148300	Significance of genetic abnormalities is not clear (38,222)
Keratoconus	AD	16q22.3–q23	Unknown	Unknown	%608932	(628)
Keratoconus	AD	3p14–q13	Unknown	Unknown	%608586	(55)
Keratoconus	Not clear	2p24	Unknown	Unknown	%609271	(237)
Keratoconus	AD	5q14.1–q21.3	Unknown	Unknown		(606)
Keratoconus with cataract	AD	15q22.32–24.2	Unknown	Unknown		(98)
Lattice corneal dystrophy type I	AD	5q31	*TGFBI*	Arg124Cys and others	#122000	(297,432)
Lattice corneal dystrophy type II	AD	9q34	*GSN*	Asp187Asn Asp187Tyr	#105120	(103,574)
Lattice corneal dystrophy type III	AR	5q31	*TGFBI*	Homozygous Leu527Arg		(169)
Lattice corneal dystrophy type IIIA	AD	5q31	*TGFBI*	Pro501Thr		(278)
LCAT disease		16q22.1	*LCAT*		#245900	(236)
Macular corneal dystrophy	AR	16q22	*CHST6*	>120 known	#217800	(315)
Disorders primarily involving the corneal stroma (cont.)						
Mucopolysaccharidosis type IH	AR	4p16.3	*IDUA*	Unknown	#607014	(396)
Mucopolysaccharidosis type II	XR	Xq28	*IDS*	>200	+309900	(501)

(Continued)

Table 1 Summary of Genetically Determined Diseases Affecting the Cornea (*Continued*)

	Mode of inheritance	Gene locus	Gene	Mutations	OMIM #	Remarks and references
Mucolipidosis type I (neuraminidase deficiency, sialidosis type II)	AR	6p21.3	*NEU1*	>16 known	#256550	(461)
Mucolipidosis type II (I cell disease)	AR	12q23.3	*GNPTAB*	>10 known	#252500	(456)
Mucolipidossis type IIIA	AR	12q23.3	*GNPTAB*		#252600	(456)
Mucolipidossis type IIIC	AR	16p	*GNPTG*		#252605	(483)
Mucolipidossis type IV	AR	19p13.3–p13.2	*MCOLN1*		#252650	(592)
Niemann–Pick disease type A	AR	11p15.4–p15.1	*SMPD1*	>14 known	#257200	(238)
Posterior amorphous stromal dystrophy	AD	Unknown	Unknown			(525)
Schnyder corneal dystrophy	AD	1p34.1–p36	*UBIAD1*	11 known	%121800	(454)
Disorders primarily involving the deep corneal stroma						
Ichythosis (cornea farinata and XR deep filiform dystrophy)	XR	Xp22.32	*STS*	6 known	+308100	(20,26)
Disorders primarily involving the corneal endothelium and Descemet membrane						
Congenital endothelial dystrophy type 1	AD	20p11.2–q11.2	Unknown		%121700	(70,616)
Congenital endothelial dystrophy type 2 (infantile hereditary endothelial dystrophy)	AR	20p13–p12	*SLC4A11*	47 known	#217700	(634)
Familial corneal guttae	AD	Unknown	Unknown	Unknown	%121390	(112,619)
Fuchs dystrophy (early onset)	AD	1p34.3	*COL8A*	Leu450Lys Gln455Lys	#136800	(39)
Fuchs dystrophy (late onset)		13pTel–13q12.13	Unknown	Unknown		(596)
Fuchs dystrophy (late onset)		18q21.2–q21.32	Unknown	Unknown		(595)
Lisch endothelial dystrophy	XR		Unknown	Unknown	Not listed	
Posterior polymorphous dystrophy type 1	AD	20p11.2	*VSX1*	Leu159Met Gly160Asp	605020	Diagnosis questionable (223)
Posterior polymorphous dystrophy type 2	AD	1p34.3–p32.3	*COL8A2*	Leu450Trp Gln455Lys	#609140	Diagnosis questionable (39)
Posterior polymorphous dystrophy type 3	AD	10p11.2	*TCF8*	17 known	#609141	(333)
Developmental anomalies involving the cornea						
Abnormalities of corneal size						
Microcornea		1q21.1	*GJA8*			
Microcornea		16q22–q23	*MAF*			
Microcornea		21q22.3	*CRYAA*			
Microcornea		11q13	*VMD2*			
Microcornea	XR	Xp22.13	*NHS*		#302350	
Abnormalities of corneal shape						
Cornea plana	AR	12q22	*KERA*		#217300	
Anterior segment dysgenesis						
Peters anomaly		6p25	*FOXC1*		#604229	
Peters anomaly	AD	4q25–q26	*PITX2*		#604229	
Peters anomaly		11p13	*PAX6*		#604229	
Peters anomaly		2p22–p21	*CYP1B1*		#604229	

Abbreviations: AD, autosomal dominant; AR, autosomal recessive; XR, x-linked recessive.

Clinical Features

MECD begins in infancy with symptoms of mild ocular irritation, photophobia, and blurred vision. Distinct bubble-like, round-to-oval punctate opacities are present in the corneal epithelium of both eyes. They affect the central corneal epithelium more than the periphery and occur in the absence of a systemic disorder. The opacities appear as transparent dew drops in retroillumination. The abnormalities are extremely difficult to see without slit-lamp biomicroscopy. Most cysts fail to stain after topically applied fluorescein, because they do not open to the surface, but some cysts take up the dye. MECD which is limited to the corneal epithelium. The disorder often remains asymptomatic until about middle age, when irregular astigmatism and a transient blurring of vision develops at what time the entire corneal epithelium contains the intraepithelial opacities. Breaks through the epithelial surface result in intermittent irritation and photophobia. In severe cases, subepithelial scarring produces a slight grayish central corneal opacification. Corneal sensitivity is normal. Removal of the abnormal corneal epithelium is not curative and the basic defect recurs in the regenerated epithelium.

Histopathology

MECD is characterized histopathologically by intraepithelial cysts at different levels in the corneal epithelium, which is irregular in thickness. Degenerated cellular debris within the intraepithelial microcysts manifests autofluorescence in ultraviolet (UV) light and it stains with the Hale colloidal iron technique for negatively charged substances such as glycosaminoglycans (GAGs) (Fig. 1A). It is also periodic acid Schiff (PAS)-positive and diastase- and neuraminidase-resistant (135). The epithelial basement membrane is variably thickened, but this is a common nonspecific finding in many disorders of the corneal epithelium (135). Bowman layer and the corneal stroma are unremarkable. Transmission electron microscopy (TEM) discloses focal aggregations of keratin within the cytoplasm of the corneal epithelium (67,135,339,436). These characteristic collections of electron-dense fibrillogranular material were termed "peculiar substance" by Kuwabara and Ciccarelli (339) prior to the recognition of the basic molecular defect (Fig. 1B).

Genetics

This autosomal dominant disorder is caused by a mutation in a member of the pair of genes (*KRT3* or *KRT12*) that encode the two units of cytokeratin in the corneal epithelium (82,244,446,597). The mutations have been in extremely conserved keratin boundary motifs. For example, in cytokeratin 12 they involve the helix termination (446) or initiation motif (86,244). Dominant mutations affecting this part of the molecule in other keratins severely impair cytoskeletal function (244).

Pathogenesis

The mutated keratin aggregates within the cytoplasm of the corneal epithelium result in abnormal clumps of cytokeratin, cell death, and intraepithelial cyst formation. At one time, MECD was suspected of being a disorder of glycogen, but despite the finding of excessive intracytoplasmic glycogen within the cytoplasm of epithelial cells of a single case (339), an

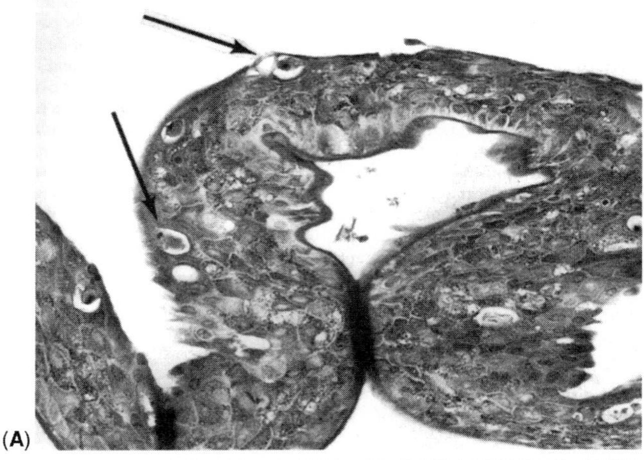

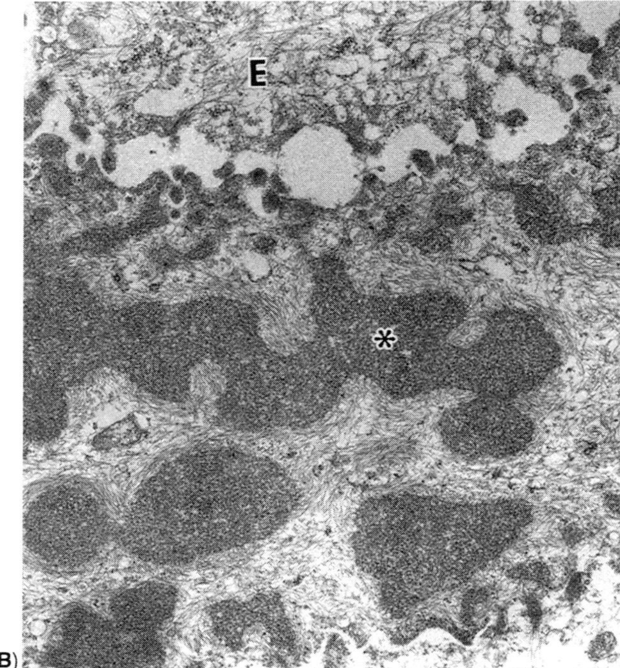

Figure 1 Meesmann dystrophy. (**A**) Numerous epithelial microcysts (*arrows*) are present (periodic acid Schiff, × 250). (**B**) Transmission electron micrograph showing electron-dense "peculiar substance" (*) in the cytoplasm of epithelial cells (E) (× 22,600). *Source*: Courtesy of M.M. Rodrigues, S. Rajagopalan, and K.A. Jones.

ultramicrofluorimetric assay failed to detect increased glycogen compared with normal corneas with a regenerating epithelium (67).

Stocker–Holt Dystrophy

Stocker and Holt (580,581) drew attention to unusual corneal opacities in descendants of Moravians from Dresden in Saxony between the ages of 7 months to 70 years. Affected individuals have numerous small, clear, or whitish-gray, closely packed punctate opacities within the epithelium that are usually not discernible with the naked eye, but they are noted on slit-lamp biomicroscopy, especially in the interpalpebral zone. The corneal spots, which represent microcysts, are uniform in size and shape. They are usually bilaterally symmetrical and most often become apparent during the first two years of life. In neonates asymptomatic epithelial opacities can be detected. By the end of the first decade of life visual impairment, as well as episodic photophobia and lacrimation may develop. Older individuals complain of a foreign body sensation and mildly decreased visual acuity. A specific mutation in the *KRT12* gene (Arg19Ile) has been detected in affected members of the family documented by Stocker and Holt (316).

Mutations in the *TGFB1* Gene

General Remarks

In 1992, Skonier et al. discovered a novel gene that was induced in cultured human adenocarcinoma cells by beta transforming growth factor (557). Because the gene was detected in human clone 3 they named the gene *BIGH3* (Beta transforming growth factor Induced Gene in Human clone 3). As it is expressed in several species, the label *BIGH3* became inappropriate and other terms were proposed. The alternative designation of *TGFB1* (transforming growth factor beta induced) gene is preferable, because it is applicable to all species. Following its discovery the *TGFBI* gene was mapped to the long arm of human chromosome 5 (5q31) (556) and three independent laboratories found the protein product or the gene to be expressed in the cornea (129,304,494). Because three autosomal dominant corneal dystrophies had been mapped to this same locus (583), *TGFBI* became a strong candidate as the gene responsible for these dystrophies and Munier et al. (328) identified four specific mutations in *TGFBI* that corresponded with specific phenotypes. Since then numerous investigators have confirmed that specific mutations in *TGFBI*, which codes for transforming growth factor beta induced protein (TGFBIp) (see Chapter 36), are responsible for several phenotypically distinct corneal disorders. At least 33 mutations in *TGFB1* have been found in clinically and histopathologically distinct phenotypes (274).

Based on the histopathology the *TGFBI* disorders can be divided into the granular corneal dystrophies (GCDs), corneal amyloidoses/lattice corneal dystrophies (LCDs), and Thiel–Behnke dystrophy (TBD) and the phenotypes correlate with the specific mutations in *TGFBI*. In all *TGFBI* inherited disorders the basic defects are specific mutations in the *TGFBI* gene leading to mutant TGFBIp. The particular mutations influence the sites where the mutated protein accumulates. It also influences the configuration of the proteins within the corneal deposits. The entire mutated protein, or fragments of it, deposit in the cornea in these different entities (278,318,325,327,587,600), but a molecular explanation for the different phenotypes remains to be determined. The variable appearance of the opacities depends on the location and nature of the corneal deposits and this is presumably influenced by the three-dimensional structure of the mutant protein.

Granular Corneal Dystrophies

General Remarks

In the GCDs mutant TGFBIp accumulates in the corneal stroma and produces characteristic irregularly lobulated granules with distinct morphologic and staining attributes (Fig. 2) (176,260). Over time it has gradually become apparent that at least three phenotypic variants of GCD exist (GCD type I, GCD type II, and GCD type III) and each of them correlates with specific *TGFBI* mutations.

Clinical Features

In GCD multiple small white discrete sharply demarcated ground glass spots that resemble bread crumbs or snowflakes become apparent in the central cornea beneath Bowman zone within the first decade of life and may be identified by 3 years of age (56). The lesions gradually enlarge and become more numerous with time. By puberty the opacities are obvious, and at the end of a second decade many are perceptible, particularly in the central and superficial cornea (272), but rarely in the deep stroma (161,246). Intervening tissue between the opacities and in the peripheral cornea usually remains clear. The opacities sometimes coalesce and accumulate beneath, or within, the corneal epithelium (176,209,547). Later the opaque spots extend throughout almost two-thirds of the corneal diameter, while the peripheral 2 to 3 mm remains clear. Clinical observations indicate that convectional currents within the corneal stroma do not move the stromal deposits once they form. In adult patients the external corneal surface is often uneven. In most cases visual acuity is usually not sufficiently impaired to justify corneal grafting, but in one pedigree 14 patients were treated with corneal grafting and all grafts remained free of recurrence for at least 30 months (427). In some cases visual impairment may be marked and multiple therapeutic procedures may be necessary because the opacities recur within a year after keratoplasty (234) or are delayed for 10 to 15 years (62,272,350,426,465,517,531,546,589,622). Recurrences are superficial to the donor tissue, even with lamellar grafts, or at the host–graft interface.

Histopathology

The corneal opacities consist predominantly of an extracellular deposition of mutant TGFBIp, which stains red with the Masson trichrome stain. With the

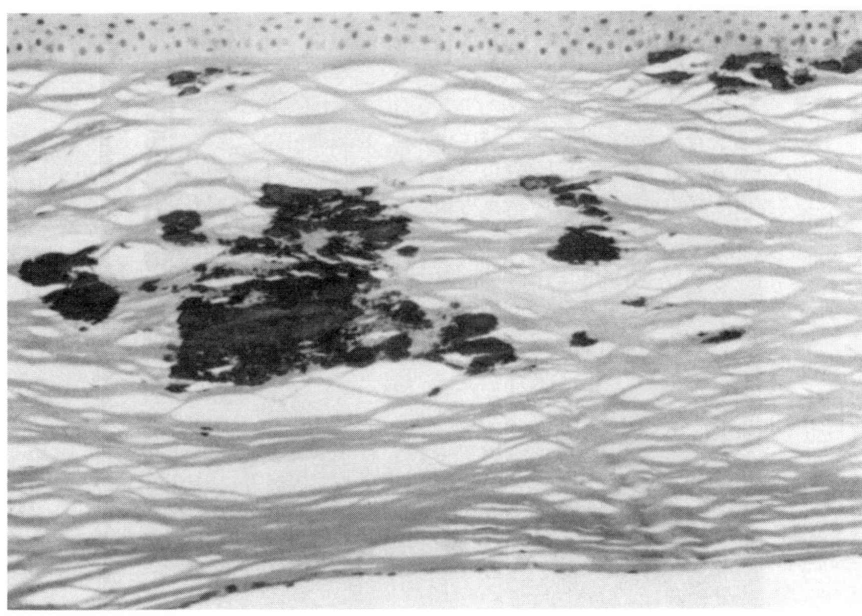

Figure 2 Corneal stromal deposits in granular corneal dystrophy type I. Note the tendency for the superficial stroma to be more extensively involved than the deep stroma (Masson trichrome, × 17).

Wilder reticulin stain the accumulations contain tangles of argyrophilic fibers (260). The deposits react with histochemical methods for protein (176,193,546, 547) as well as with antibodies to TGFBIp (318,587). The granules stain positively with luxol fast blue and are reported to stain positively with antibodies to microfibrillar protein (519).

By TEM characteristic electron-dense, discrete, rod-shaped, or trapezoid bodies are evident (Fig. 3) (7,62,212,247,272,296,300,302,340,341,395,451,589,601). Cross-sectional profiles of the corneal deposits are usually irregularly shaped, but sometimes hexagonal measuring 100 to 500 nm in diameter (7,247,270). Clusters of these elongated bodies occur particularly in the superficial corneal stroma and they may be present in the epithelial intercellular space (601) or within degenerated basal epithelial cells (270). Some rod-shaped structures appear homogenous without a discernible inner structure; others, however, are composed of an orderly array of closely packed filaments (70–100 nm in width) orientated parallel to their long axis, while others appear moth-eaten with variable-shaped cavities containing fine filaments (Figs. 4 and 5) (62). Some superficial and most deep stromal deposits do not all possess the rod-shaped configuration (62). Descemet membrane and the corneal endothelium are unremarkable, and so is the cornea between the deposits.

Most histopathologically confirmed recurrences have been superficial to Bowman layer in subepithelial nonvascularized fibrocollagenous tissue (62,270,350, 517,546,589,622).

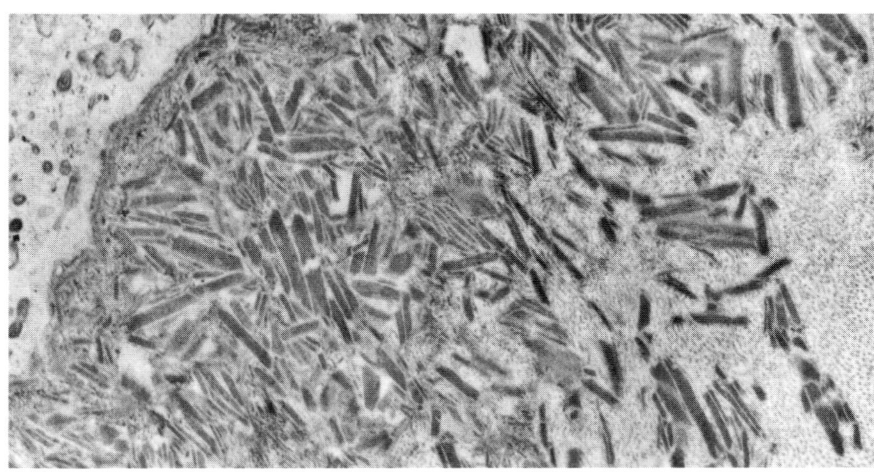

Figure 3 Transmission electron micrograph in granular corneal dystrophy showing characteristic rod-shaped crystalloid bodies in superficial corneal stroma (× 14,950).

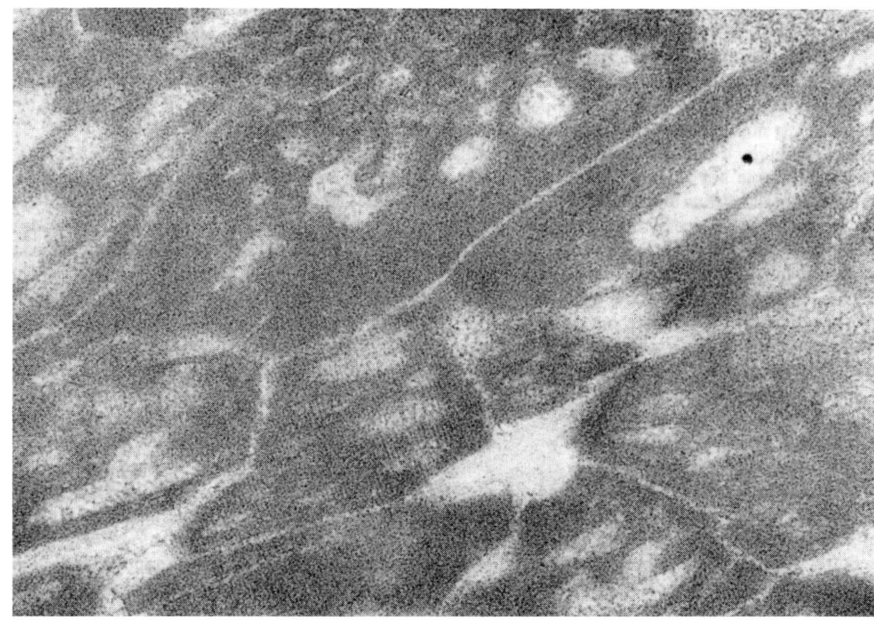

Figure 4 Transmission electron micrograph showing moth-eaten appearance of corneal deposits in deep corneal stroma from patient with granular corneal dystrophy (× 109,000).

Amyloid is uncommon in GCD, but was noted by Garner (176) by light microscopy and by Akiya and Brown (7) by TEM in selected cases suggesting a relationship between GCD and LCD. Subsequently the combination of GCD with stromal amyloid deposition became recognized as Avellino corneal dystrophy (GCD type II) (62,247,395,609), which bridges the phenotypic gap between LCD and GCD (212,589).

Genetics

GCD usually has an autosomal dominant mode of inheritance, but rarely occurs sporadically (209) due to new mutations. In some families the mutant gene is completely penetrant (589), but in others the penetrance is incomplete (91). The mutation rate has been estimated to be about 0.3/1,000,000 in the Danish population (425). Interfamilial differences and intrafamilial similarities occur (424), and while the cornea of some patients have only a few granules, others become markedly opaque.

When both parents have GCD their offspring may be homozygous for the *TGFBI* mutation and develop an unusually severe corneal dystrophy with larger corneal opacities and an earlier onset than heterozygous cases (106,428,453). One family study suggests that persons heterozygous and homozygous for the *TGFBI* gene are phenotypically identical, but genetic mutations were not performed in this instance (91).

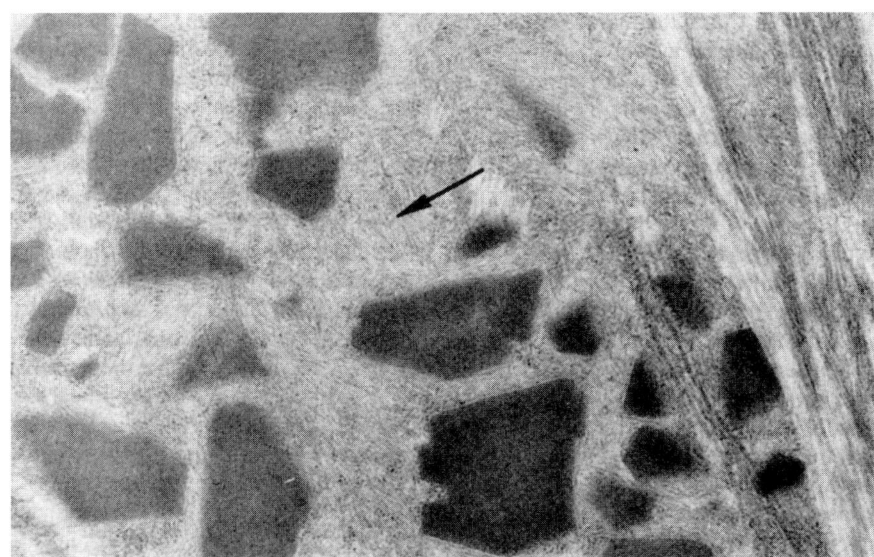

Figure 5 Transmission electron micrograph showing delicate filaments (*arrow*) in corneal stroma with granular corneal dystrophy. Such filaments are frequently associated with larger, variably shaped electron densities (× 50,700).

Pathogenesis

A defective codon in *TGFBI* results in the synthesis and secretion of mutant TGFBIp, which accumulates in the cornea. Because comparable deposits have not been found elsewhere in the body, the mutated TGFBIp may be generated in the cornea. Both the corneal epithelium and keratocytes have been implicated as the source of the extracellular material (7,176), because of the proximity of these cells to the characteristic abnormal accumulations, but convincing morphologic testimony to support this possibility is lacking. Corneal cells containing material with the same morphology as the extracellular deposits has not been observed unequivocally. Nevertheless an epithelial source warrants consideration because corneal epithelium is known to synthesize TGFBIp (176), yet, if the mutant TGFBIp is derived from the corneal epithelium recurrences in grafts should be the rule, rather than the exception as host epithelium soon replaces that of the donor. Also, if the deposits reach the cornea by diffusion from a noncorneal origin, one might expect a high recurrence rate after corneal grafting, and an inconstant relationship of recurrences to host tissue, but as mentioned above this is not the case.

Granular Corneal Dystrophy Type I

GCD type I (classic GCD, Arg555Trp mutant *TGFBI*, MIM #121900) is characterized by multiple discrete crumb-like corneal opacities. GCD type I is slowly progressive and usually becomes apparent during the first decade of life. Visual acuity gradually decreases and painful epithelial erosions are common.

GCD type I, which almost always has the Arg555Trp mutation in *TGFBI* (328,433), is rare in Japan (323). Another mutation (Arg124Ser) in *TGFBI* has been found in a single Asian patient with GCD type I (575). A noteworthy aspect of this case was the lack of amyloid in the corneal stroma, particularly since Arg124Cys and Arg124His mutations in *TGFBI* are accompanied by amyloid deposition.

Granular Corneal Dystrophy Type II

Another variant of GCD called GCD type II by Weidel (648) is also known under other connotations (Avellino corneal dystrophy, GCD with amyloid, combined lattice-granular corneal dystrophy, Arg124His mutant *TGFBI*). It is characterized clinically by corneal opacities that are shaped like rings, discs, stars, and snowflakes. Linear opacities may be present, but the typical lines of LCD are usually absent. Onset is during the second decade. A distinction from GCD type I can be made clinically and histopathologically.

The ancestry of some affected families has been traced to the Avellino region of Italy (139) giving rise to the earlier term Avellino dystrophy, which is no longer justifiable, as other families have been traced to other countries. Moreover, most families have been identified in Japan (164,269,323,324,391) and Korea (289), where this variant of GCD is the most common type of GCD (323,391).

Tissue sections of the corneal stroma contain the same deposits as those found in GCD types I and III and often amyloid, which may be present in only small, insignificant amounts (7,62,176,212,247,395, 589,609). Most amyloid in GCD type II probably does not cause lattice lines.

To date almost all cases of GCD type II have had a heterozygous Arg124His mutation in *TGFBI* and the phenotype of affected individuals varies markedly in severity from family to family (6,324). Visual acuity often becomes severely impaired during childhood in persons with a homozygous mutation, and a corneal graft is often needed before 25 years of age. Individuals homozygous for Arg124His are particularly prone to recurrent disease after a penetrating keratoplasty (269,389). Two different clinical phenotypes have been observed in Japanese patients homozygous for Arg124His depending on the part of Japan to which they trace their ancestry, suggesting that the phenotype is influenced by modifier genes (646). In one variant a discrete grayish white opacity covers the anterior stroma and it is confluent in the central and paracentral cornea; in the other type reticular grayish white diffuse opacity in the anterior stroma of the cornea. In Japan Arg124His has been associated with significantly more corneal guttae than controls (6). In corneal tissue from patients with Arg124His Korvatska et al. (326) found the nonamyloid accumulations to consist of a combination of the 66 and 68 kDa forms of TGFBIp.

Granular Corneal Dystrophy Type III

Corneal deposits morphologically and histochemically indistinguishable from those of typical GCD accumulate mainly in Bowman layer and immediately beneath the corneal epithelium in the subepithelial region (7,193,209,303,423,515,546,663) or in the epithelium (176) in GCD type III (Reis–Bücklers corneal dystrophy, superficial GCD, corneal dystrophy of Bowman layer type I, and geographic corneal dystrophy, Arg124Leu mutant of TGFBI, OMIM #121900). The opacities assume an irregularly ring-shaped pattern of discrete spots and lines that focally elevate the corneal epithelium, producing an irregular surface. This bilateral symmetrical disorder of the superficial cornea was reported in 1917 by Reis (497) and demonstrated three decades later by Bücklers (64) to have an autosomal dominant mode of inheritance. A study of the original pedigree described by Reis and Bücklers had rod-shaped bodies identical to those in the other varieties of GCD (423,663) hence the recommended designation of GCD type III.

The literature on this entity is extremely confusing mainly because the designation of Reis–Bücklers dystrophy has been used for at least two distinct autosomal dominant entities, which cannot always be differentiated from each other clinically. The diagnosis in some reports has really been Thiel–Behnke corneal dystrophy, which is characterized by subepithelial "curly fibers" that can only be identified by TEM (202,259,502). To confuse the subject further, individuals in families with LCD may manifest corneal opacities that are similar to those of Reis–Bücklers dystrophy (292).

GCD type III usually remains asymptomatic until bilateral epithelial erosions precipitate acute episodes of ocular hyperemia, pain, and photophobia at about 4 to 5 years of age. Visual acuity gradually becomes reduced during the second and third decades of life following a progressive diffuse, asymmetric corneal opacification, and an irregular astigmatism. Rings and disc-shaped opacities form within the superficial cornea and stellate figures spread into the deeper stroma. The anterior cornea becomes scarred and acquires an uneven, irregular, and roughened surface. Corneal sensitivity is nearly always diminished or absent (632). The deep corneal stroma and endothelium as well as Descemet membrane are not affected. Opacities consisting of innumerable delicate, cotton-like strands appear in the axial cornea and progressively evolves into a central reticulated ring or geographic-shaped pattern (64,497). The opacification eventually extends into the midperiphery of the cornea with a thinly distributed external stromal haze. Sometimes the clinical appearance lacks these characteristics. GCD type III becomes symptomatic earlier and with a higher frequency of recurrent erosions than patients with other variants of GCD. In advanced cases a superficial keratectomy, phototherapeutic keratectomy or lamellar keratoplasty, may improve vision, but a penetrating keratoplasty is rarely necessary because the pathologic changes only involve the superficial cornea.

The phenotype of this inherited corneal disorder seems to be caused by a specific mutation in *TGFBI* (Arg124Leu) (109,325,390,452,678). Haplotype analyses of different families have provided evidence of multiple origins of this mutation (329). A similar clinical phenotype has been detected in Sardinians with a ΔF540 mutation in *TGFBI* (528) without histopathologic studies. Reports of an Arg555Gln mutation in *TGFBI* in patients alleged to have Reis–Bücklers dystrophy (165,328,433,603,678) are unacceptable, because these individuals were not characterized by appropriate typical light and TEM findings. Korvatska et al. found that the Arg124Leu nonamyloid deposits were all of the 68 kDa form of TGFBIp (326).

Other Variants of GCD

Dighiero et al. (107,109) documented a family with a novel phenotype of GCD intermediate between GCD type I and GCD type III. Affected members of the family had round snowflake-shaped opacities in the subepithelial and most anterior corneal stroma. Recurrent painful corneal erosions began early in childhood. The affected persons were heterozygous for the Arg124Leu mutation in *TGFBI*, but they were also heterozygous for another mutation in the same gene that predicted the deletion of two amino acid residues at codons 125 and 126 (Δ125–ΔE126) (108).

TGFBI-Related Lattice Corneal Dystrophies

General Remarks

LCD type I (MIM #122200) was first described by Biber (34) and its autosomal dominant mode of inheritance was later established by Haab (208) and Dimmer (110). In this disorder foci of amyloid are scattered throughout the corneal stroma and sometimes immediately beneath the epithelium. The corneal endothelium and Descemet membrane are not involved.

Clinical Features

LCD type I usually starts in both eyes toward the end of the first decade of life, but occasionally it begins in middle life and rarely by 2 years of age (569). Delicate interdigitating branching filamentous opacities form a network with the cornea (491,680). These and other shaped opaque areas accumulate particularly within the central corneal stroma producing a superficial haze, while the peripheral cornea remains relatively transparent. The linear opacities may be difficult to identify clinically (138) and are not manifest in all affected members of families with LCD type I (491,492). The opaque interwoven filaments resemble nerves on casual scrutiny and corneal sensation is frequently diminished. Some affected family members may develop a clinical phenotype that resembles GCD type III (292). Recurrent epithelial erosions are common and usually begin during the first decade of life. In some families recurrent epithelial erosions antecede the corneal opacities and appear in individuals lacking recognizable stromal disease (97,224,538). The corneas may be asymmetrically involved, and sometimes one cornea is clear or has discrete rather than linear opacities (347,484). The clinical course varies even within the same family, but the condition is slowly progressive and usually leads to substantial discomfort and visual impairment before the sixth decade.

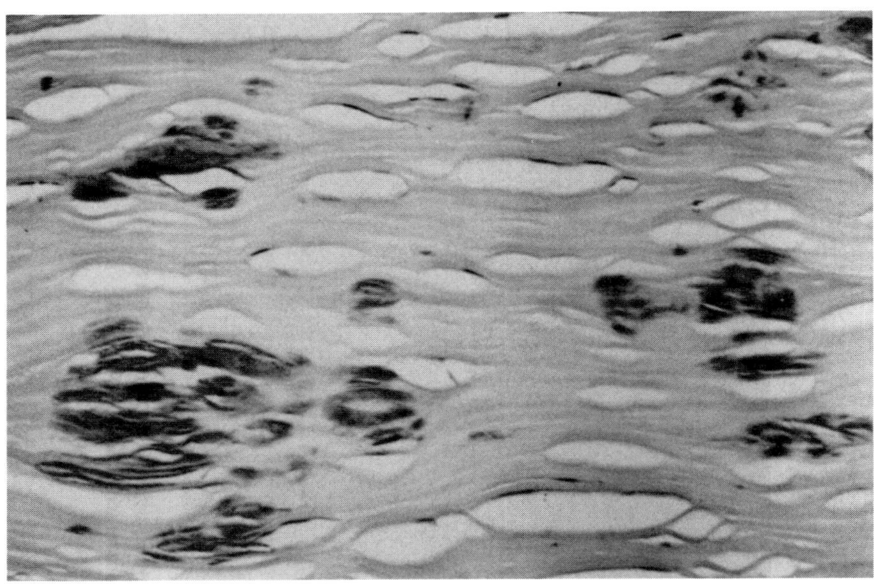

Figure 6 Histologic section of cornea with lattice corneal dystrophy type I showing deposits of amyloid (Congo red, × 210).

A corneal graft may be necessary by 20 years of age, but one is usually not indicated until after the fourth decade (347). The outcome of penetrating keratoplasty is excellent, but amyloid may deposit in the grafted donor tissue some 2 to 14 years later (159,347,371,414).

Histopathology

Like nerves the linear deposits are argyrophilic in silver impregnated preparations and can be mistaken for nerves (671), but nerves have not been identified in relation to the deposits. Amyloid with its usual tinctorial and ultrastructural attributes deposits throughout the corneal stroma (Figs. 6 and 7) and coincides with the lattice pattern of lines and other opacities. The amyloid seems to react mainly with antibodies to the N-terminal sequence of TGFBIp and not with those to the C-terminal portion (325). Korvatska et al. (326) and Takacs et al. (600) have provided evidence that the amyloid in LCD type I results from an accumulation of a 44 kDa N-terminal part of the mutated TGFBIp.

Genetics

The majority of cases of LCD type I throughout the world have been associated with a C→T transition at nucleotide 417 (417 C→T) in exon 4 of the *TGFBI* gene. This causes a Arg124Cys mutation in the affected codon.

Other Variants of LCD

One variant of late onset LCD that is characterized by extremely thick linear deposits of amyloid and an apparent autosomal recessive mode of inheritance has been designated LCD type III (226,227). In keeping with the negative family history this disorder is caused by a homozygous Leu527Arg mutation in *TGFBI* (169). Late in life radially orientated lattice lines, much thicker than those in LCD types I and II, become apparent in the anterior and midstroma (226,227). Usually both eyes are affected, but sporadic unilateral examples have been documented (545). Recurrent epithelial erosions were absent in the first reports (226,227), but present in two sporadic cases

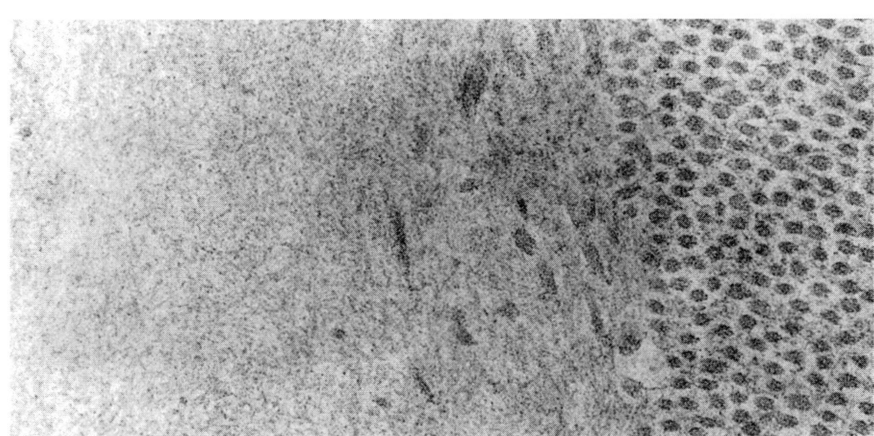

Figure 7 Transmission electron micrograph of amyloid deposit in corneal stroma of lattice corneal dystrophy type I. The amyloid fibrils are adjacent to wider collagen fibers (*right side*) (× 58,000).

that were later recognized (545). A few years after the documentation of these cases a similar phenotype was reported, but with corneal erosions and an autosomal dominant mode of inheritance (LCD type IIIA) (577). Some patients with LCD type IIIA had a Pro501Thr mutation in *TGFBI* and the mutated TGFBIp colocalized with the amyloid (278). Persons with the Pro501Thr mutation may be unaffected by 85 years of age (207).

Nakamura et al. (435) reported five unrelated Japanese individuals with an unusual phenotype, which they called "gelatino-lattice corneal dystrophy." Clinically the disorder resembled a combination of LCD type I and gelatinous drop-like corneal dystrophy (GDLD) (familial subepithelial corneal amyloidosis) (see Mutations in the *TACSTD2* Gene). Painful recurrent corneal erosions occurred during adolescence. The authors claimed that the subepithelial deposits were amyloid, but histopathologic findings were not documented. The only exon of *TGFBI* (exon 4) to be sequenced contained an Arg124Cys mutation. In contrast to Japanese patients with GDLD no mutation was detected in the entire coding region of *TACSTD2* (*M1S1*). Stewart et al. (573) drew attention to three families with LCD that resembled LCD type IIIA, but which was associated with mutations in codon 622 or 626 of exon 14 in *TGFBI*. This disorder had an onset in middle age (fourth to fifth decade) and hence began later than in LCD type I.

An atypical form of LCD with large, nodular lattice shaped, deep stromal opacities in the pupillary zone and a late onset has been found in seven unrelated Japanese patients without a positive family history. The phenotypic variation in the size and shape of the deposits among affected persons is substantial and the disorder is associated with a heterozygous Leu527Arg mutation in *TGFBI* (166, 229,678).

Another variant of LCD is associated with an Ala546Thr mutation in *TGFBI* (109). Schmitt-Bernard et al. documented two families with a type of LCD intermediate between LCD types I and IIIA (541). This variant was associated with two mutations in exon 14 of *TGFBI* (a 9 base pair insertion in position 1885–1886 or a missense mutation at position 1887).

Dighiero et al. (109) found a *TGFBI* His626Arg mutation in an asymmetric variant of LCD in three individuals from two apparently unrelated families.

Thiel and Behnke Corneal Dystrophy

General Remarks

In 1967 Thiel and Behnke (612) drew attention to honeycomb-like opacities at the level of Bowman layer in association with recurrent erosions and a moderately decreased visual acuity in a large 11 generation pedigree containing 234 members with 26 affected persons. This report did not document light microscopic or TEM observations. The slowly progressive disorder, which has become known as TBD ("curly" fiber corneal dystrophy, corneal dystrophy of Bowman layer type II, honeycomb corneal dystrophy, MIM #602082) is a slowly progressive autosomal dominant disorder characterized clinically by the onset of painful corneal erosions during childhood (650). Much of the literature related to GCD type III (discussed above) and TBD is incomprehensible because these two entities have been confused with each other (336,368,468,650). The confusion stems from several sources: (*i*) the original description of TBD was published in German and illustrated with black and white clinical photographs and not accompanied by light or TEM observations on corneal tissue, (*ii*) the clinical features of TBD and GCD type III overlap, (*iii*) families with the ultrastructural hallmarks of TBD had been reported as Reis–Bücklers dystrophy (GCD type III) (468,559), (*iv*) many cases of Reis–Bücklers dystrophy and TBD in the literature have either not been accompanied by acceptable documentation of the diagnostic characteristics. A diagnosis of TBD can be suspected by the clinical phenotype, but the pathognomonic curly fibers should be identified by TEM within the cornea in at least some affected family members to establish a precise diagnosis (649). Because of the confusing nomenclature, the term "corneal dystrophy of Bowman layer and superficial stroma" (CDB) was proposed for both these dystrophies: CDB type 1 for GCD type III and CDB type 2 for TBD (336).

In 1961, Waardenburg and Jonkers (637) documented an autosomal dominant corneal dystrophy characterized by a superficial corneal granularity with clinical features of GCD, but with several clinical differences. Some authors considered it to be a specific corneal dystrophy (the corneal dystrophy of Waardenburg and Jonkers), but in a follow-up study of the original pedigree Wittebol-Post and colleagues (664) found that affected corneas have the characteristic "curly" fibers of TBD.

Clinical Features

Subepithelial corneal opacities with a clear zone at the corneoscleral limbus form a honeycomb-shaped pattern in the superficial cornea. The disorder has a similar, but perhaps a less severe clinical course than GCD type III (612). Like many other inherited corneal disorders the condition may recur in the graft following penetrating keratoplasty (69,650). Without a tissue examination TBD is commonly misdiagnosed as GCD type III (Reis–Bücklers dystrophy).

Histopathology

The corneal epithelium varies in thickness and contains nonspecific degenerative changes. The epithelial basal lamina and Bowman layer display variable degenerative changes and with irregular subepithelial collagenous tissue (Fig. 8A). TEM of this tissue discloses the pathognomonic short, curled filaments (Fig. 8B) measuring (about 8–10 nm in diameter) in a superficial cornea interspersed among normal collagen fibrils in Bowman zone and the contiguous superficial corneal stroma (468,643). The precise molecular composition of the curly filaments remains unknown. In advanced stages of TBD, the anterior stromal collagen and Bowman layer may be markedly disorganized and replaced by numerous aggregates of these filaments. Histopathologically subepithelial fibrous tissue accumulates in a wave-like configuration. Authors of the early morphologic studies of what was probably the same condition (8,202) did not recognize the diagnostic ultrastructural hallmark of TBD. The subepithelial "curly" fibers, which can only be identified by TEM, were elegantly illustrated in 1979 by Perry et al. (468), who unfortunately designated the disorder Reis–Bücklers dystrophy. TEM evaluations of the family originally reported by Thiel and Behnke indicated that these "curly" fibers were a feature of that dystrophy (664). Laminin and bullous pemphigoid antigen have been localized in a piebald mosaic distribution within the aberrant subepithelial fibrous tissue suggesting a primarily epithelial disease with the peculiar curly material paralleling the distribution of attachment proteins (368). Except for abnormalities in the superficial cornea the remainder of the cornea is unremarkable.

Genetics

TBD has an autosomal dominant mode of inheritance and was mapped to chromosome 5 (5q31) (559). It was later found to be associated with a Arg555Gln mutation in *TGFBI*, which may be diagnostic (109,452,503), but more families with the characteristic ultrastructural abnormalities need to be documented to establish this with certainty. Many reports

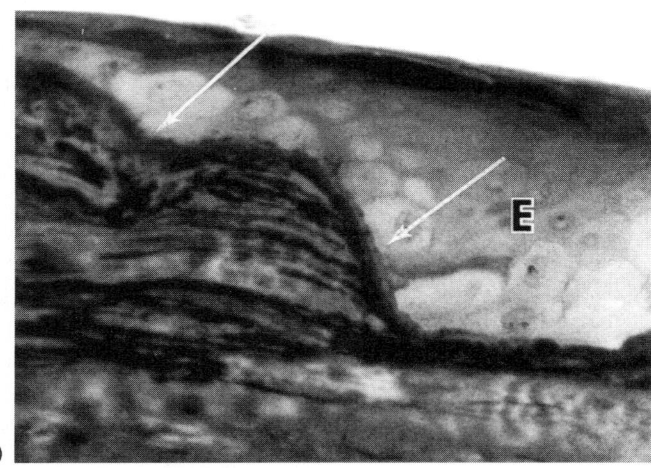

(**A**)

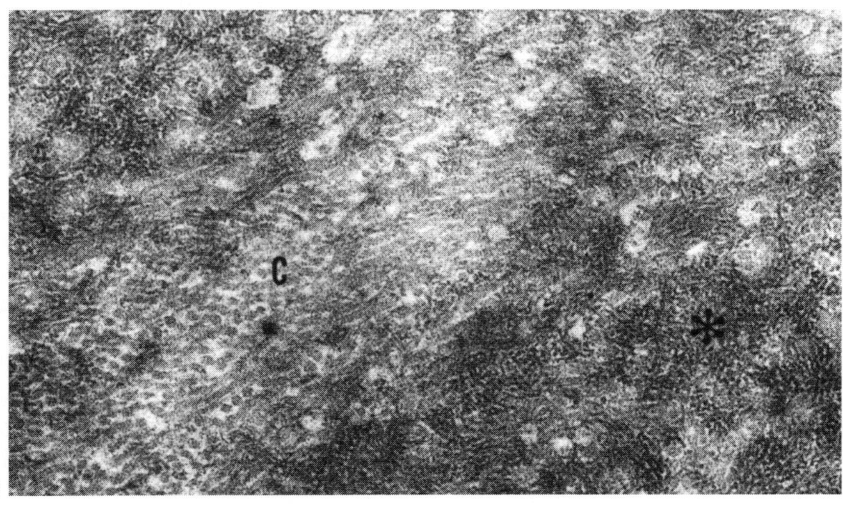

(**B**)

Figure 8 Theil–Behnke dystrophy. (**A**) Irregular dense filamentous aggregates (*arrows*) are present beneath the epithelium (E) (toluidine blue, ×400). (**B**) Electron micrograph showing short, curly, filamentous structures (*) between the collagen fibrils (C) (× 23,800). *Source*: Courtesy of Dr. M.M. Rodrigues, Dr. S. Rajagopalan, and Dr. K.A. Jones.

documenting this mutation have based the diagnosis solely on the clinical phenotype and have not taken into account the necessary requirement of a tissue diagnosis (165,452,678). Genetic heterogeneity seems to exist and another locus for TBD has also been identified on chromosome 10 (10q23–q24) (682).

Mutations in the *CHST6* Gene

Macular Corneal Dystrophy

General Remarks

"Macula" is Latin for a spot and the adjective "macular" was introduced as the name for a specific corneal dystrophy characterized by white spots within a cloudy cornea. Unfortunately, the designation macular corneal dystrophy (MCD) (MIM 217800) has lead to misunderstanding because the adjective "macular" is also applicable to disorders of the macula in the retina, such as macular degenerations and retinal macular dystrophies. A vast body of information has accumulated on MCD. Landmarks in the study of MCD were: (*i*) the recognition that the corneal accumulations were a GAG and most likely keratan sulfate (KS) the major corneal GAG (320); (*ii*) that MCD differed from the systemic mucopolysaccharidoses (MPS) in cell culture (305); (*iii*) that organ cultures of corneas with MCD do not synthesize KS (311) or normal KS-containing proteoglycans (PGs) because of defective sulfation (219,438); (*iv*) the recognition that the absence or paucity of sulfate in KS and KS-containing PGs in corneas with MCD pointed to a deficiency in a carbohydrate sulfotransferase (ST) that catalyses the transfer of sulfate groups to KS (307,438,615); (*v*) the mapping of the gene for MCD type I, and probably MCD type II, to chromosome 16 (16q22) (631) in patients from Iceland; and (*vi*) the eventual identification of *CHST6* as the responsible gene (5).

Clinical Features

Irregular ill-defined cloudy regions usually first appear within a hazy stroma of both corneas during adolescence, but may become apparent in early infancy or even as late as the sixth decade. The nontransparent areas progressively merge over time as the entire corneal stroma gradually becomes cloudy causing severe visual impairment usually before the fifth decade. Vision can be restored by corneal grafting, but the disease may recur in the graft after many years (10,225,309,371,512). The corneal stroma is thinner than normal (113,123,481).

Epidemiology

MCD has been identified throughout the world, but in most populations it is rare. It is most prevalent in India (590,591,645), Saudi Arabia (12,308), Iceland (257,258,366,631), and parts of the United States (301). At one time MCD was the most frequent indication for penetrating keratoplasty in Iceland (257).

Histopathology

In tissue sections the lesions in MCD are characteristic. The corneal epithelium is spared but intracytoplasmic accumulations, identified histochemically as GAGs, occur within the fibroblasts (keratocytes) and endothelium of the cornea (177,183,260,298,301,320,564). The accumulations stain positively with PAS, alcian blue, metachromatic dyes, and possess an affinity for colloidal iron (Fig. 9). By TEM intracytoplasmic vacuoles are a distinct feature of the corneal fibroblasts and with appropriate fixation delicate fibrillogranular material can be discerned within the vesicles (Fig. 10 and Fig. 11) (196). Some corneal endothelial cells frequently contain similar material (Fig. 12) (564,620). For ultrastructural observation the accumulations stain with the PAS/thiocarbohydrazide/silver proteinate (196) and the periodic acid-silver methenamine techniques (Fig. 13) (306). In contrast to the systemic MPS, abnormal material also deposits between the collagen fibers in the corneal stroma. Numerous electron-lucent lacunae are randomly distributed throughout corneas and some lacunae are filled with clusters of abnormal sulfated chondroitinase ABC susceptible PG filaments (411).

The endoplasmic reticulum (ER) within keratocytes and some corneal endothelial cells is dilated and filled with delicate fibrillogranular material (177,183,196,260,298,320,564,620).

The collagen fibrils have a normal diameter, but the interfibrillar spacing of collagen fibrils in affected corneas is less than that in the normal cornea (211,229). This close packing of collagen fibrils seems to be responsible for the reduced corneal thickness in MCD (481).

The anterior-banded portion of Descemet membrane which forms in utero is of normal thickness and has an unremarkable ultrastructure, whereas the posterior layer usually contains numerous excrescences (corneal guttae) (153). The latter, together with intervening parts of the posterior layer of Descemet membrane, are studded with numerous vacuoles giving a honeycombed appearance (Fig. 14) (183,564,620). The electron-lucent areas presumably contained extracellular deposits of GAGs, which dissolved during tissue processing.

Staining with cuprolinic blue reveals an unusual distribution of PGs in some parts of the interfibrillar matrix with "small" PGs running exclusively parallel to the collagen fibrils. Furthermore some lacunae are filled with clusters of abnormal sulfated chondroitinase ABC susceptible PG filaments (of various sizes). Clearly defined regions, both within the lacunae

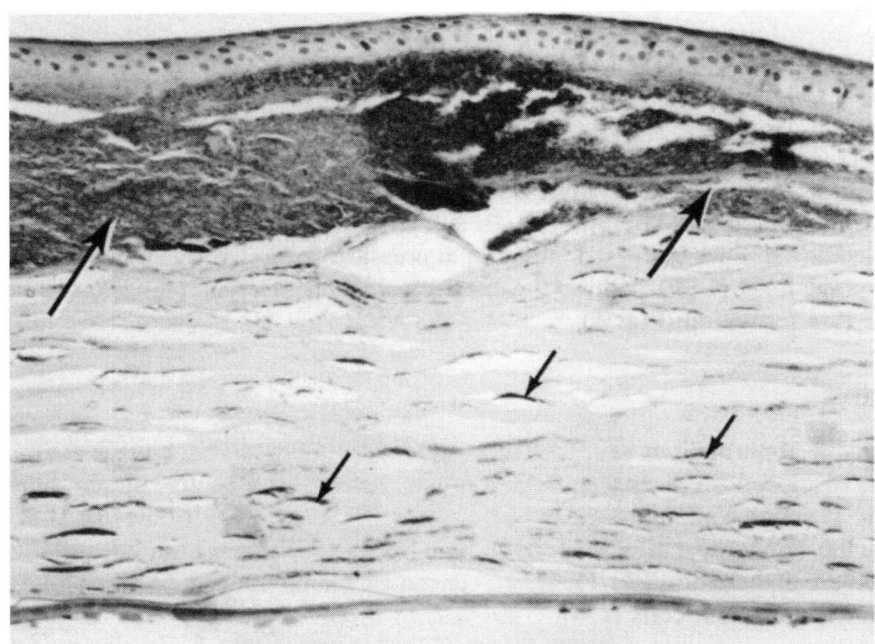

Figure 9 Macular corneal dystrophy. A large extracellular lake of abnormal material is situated beneath the corneal epithelium (*large arrows*). Individual corneal fibroblasts contain a similar substance (Hale colloidal iron technique, × 200).

and elsewhere, fail to stain with cuprolinic blue suggesting an absence of sulfated PGs within these areas. The stroma of MCD corneas contains congregations of various sized cuprolinic blue-stained filaments, which vary both in size and in electron density (411).

Cell and Organ Culture Studies

In an attempt to elucidate the pathogenesis of this disease cell culture techniques have been employed (96,157,305,311). Danes (96) found the uronic acid content in cultured fibroblasts from the cornea, conjunctiva, and skin of six patients with MCD to be normal. In studies employing the vital dye acridine orange Francois and colleagues (157) reported lysosomal abnormalities in cultured corneal fibroblasts from a patient with MCD, but their observations were not confirmed in another investigation of cultured corneal fibroblasts from three patients with MCD (305). Moreover, when stained vitally with acridine

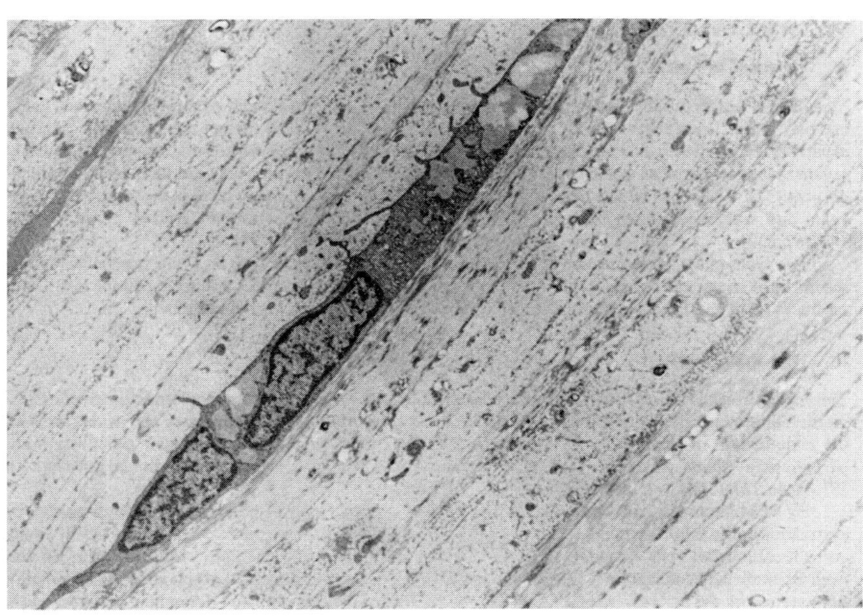

Figure 10 Macular corneal dystrophy. A corneal fibroblast containing fibrillogranular material lies adjacent to collagen fibrils and extracellular electron-lucent and electron-dense material (× 8,600)

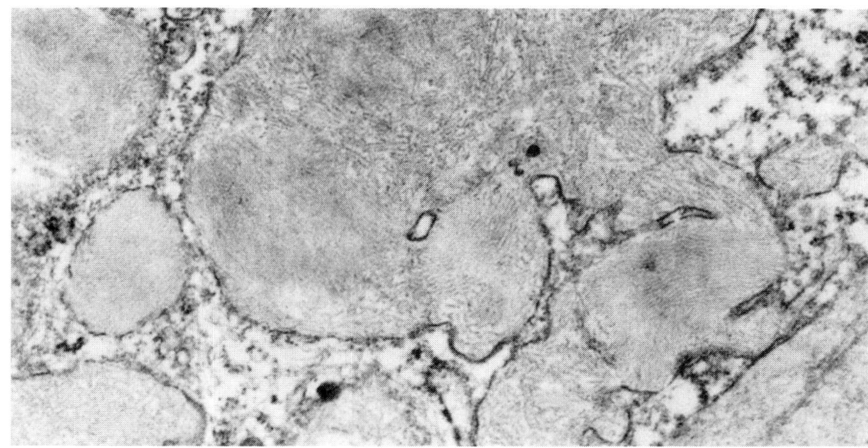

Figure 11 Macular corneal dystrophy. Distended smooth endoplasmic reticulum of fibroblast in cornea with macular corneal dystrophy containing fibrillogranular material (× 40,000).

orange, corneal fibroblasts in MCD do not behave like cultured fibroblasts from individuals with the MPS, such as MPS IH and MPS II (305).

Assuming that MCD might be a localized MPS, Klintworth and Smith (311) studied cultured corneal fibroblasts from patients with MCD by methods yielding valuable data on MPSs. Many cultured MCD corneal fibroblasts contain material with the cytochemical characteristics of GAGs, but they are susceptible to testicular hyaluronidase and chondroitin ABC lyase in contrast to the accumulations in excised corneal tissue. Moreover, unlike the inherited systemic disorders of GAG metabolism, MPS IH and MPS II, corneal fibroblasts from patients with MCD do not accumulate abnormal quantities of ^{35}S-sulfate or ^{3}H-glucosamine labeled GAGs (311). Nevertheless, at the time of these studies the data remained consistent with the hypothesis that MCD is a disorder of KS catabolism, because the synthesis of KS by corneal fibroblasts decreases markedly in culture (310,313).

In 1977 it became recognized that organ cultures of MCD corneas synthesize considerably less KS than normal corneas (311), and a few years later when it was found that MCD corneas produce excessive amounts of a novel glycoprotein (219,312). It became apparent based mainly on biochemical studies, in which corneal organ cultures were incubated in medium containing radioactive isotopes, that a fundamental defect in at least one type of MCD (MCD type I) involved the sulfation of KS in the biosynthesis of corneal KS-containing PGs (220,311,419) and that MCD corneas fail to synthesize normal KS-containing PGs (314,438). This led to the belief that a basic defect involved a specific ST that attaches sulfate moieties to lactosaminoglycan (nonsulfated KS) (307,438,615). Subsequent to their recognition are different immunophenotypes MCD type I and MCD type II corneas

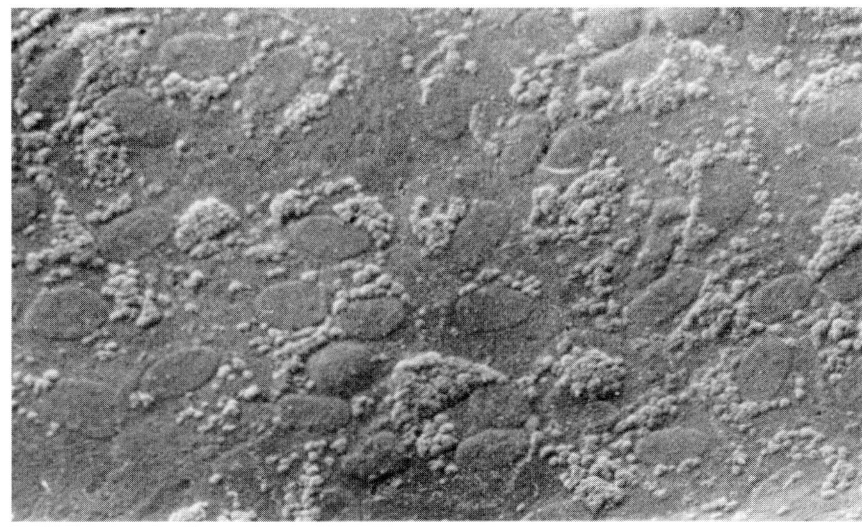

Figure 12 Scanning electron micrograph of corneal endothelium in macular corneal dystrophy, showing profile of endothelial cells created by intracytoplasmic storage vacuoles (× 1,580).

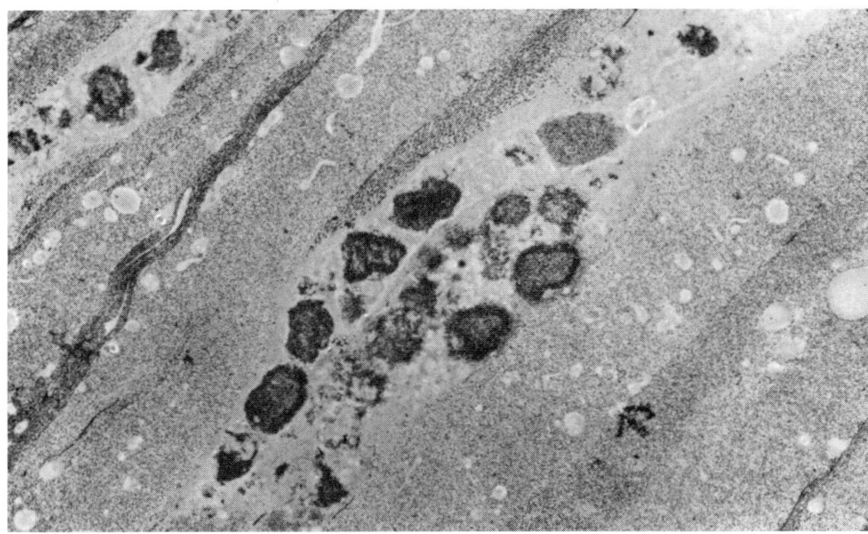

Figure 13 Corneal stroma in macular corneal dystrophy. Silver methenamine periodic acid stain (× 6,700). *Source*: From Ref. 306.

were found to synthesize dissimilar PGs and lactosaminoglycan-glycoproteins (L-GPs) (419). MCD type I corneas produce a normal decorin (previously called dermatan sulfate-PG), but an abnormal lumican and L-GP (419). The core protein of this L-GP possesses a similar hydrophobicity and nearly similar mass to the core protein of lumican and, with the exception of a lack of sulfate, its glycoconjugates as identical to those of lumican. Organ cultures of MCD type I corneas fail to synthesize KS or lumican presumably as a consequence of a defect in a specific ST needed for sulfating lactosaminoglycans. A MCD type II corneal organ culture synthesized less PGs than normal, but the lumican/decorin ratio was normal. The lumican appeared normal whereas the decorin had shorter than normal sulfated dermatan sulfate (DS) chains (419). Later, fluorochrome-assisted carbohydrate electrophoresis disclosed that the KS chain size within the cornea and cartilage in MCD type I was reduced and chain sulfation was absent (472). In a cornea with MCD type II the sulfation of N-acetylglucoamine and galactose was significantly reduced and the chain size was also reduced, but to a lesser degree than in MCD type I (472).

Immunochemical Studies

Heterogeneity among cases of MCD was detected based on the reactivity of corneal tissue with an antibody that recognizes antigenic KS (AgKS) (679). Significant advances in our understanding of MCD came following immunochemical studies with the anti-KS antibody (5D4). The epitope of 5D4 is linear pentasulfated sequences of N-acetylgalactosamine (GalNAc) disaccharides of KS PGs in which the GalNAc and galactose (Gal) are sulfated. These studies led to the discovery that the serum AgKS levels correlate positively with the presence or absence of immunohistochemically detectable AgKS in the cornea. The observation led to the recognition of three immunophenotypes of MCD (MCD type I, MCD type IA, and MCD type II) differ in the reactivity of serum and corneas with an monoclonal antibody that

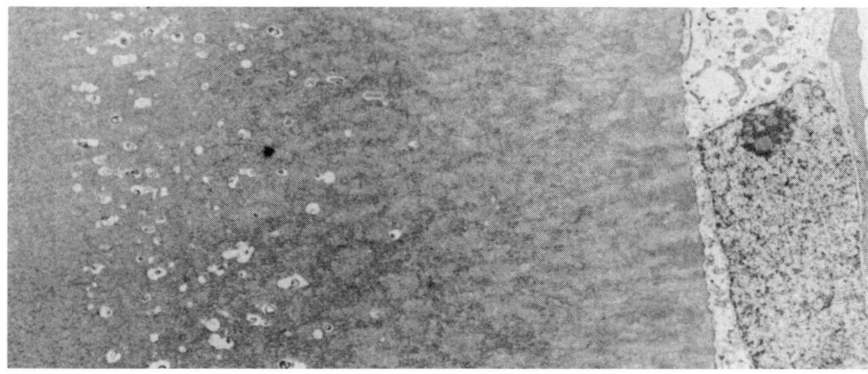

Figure 14 Macular corneal dystrophy. Part of a normal corneal endothelial cell rests on Descemet membrane. Note the abnormal honeycombed appearance of the deeper portion of Descemet membrane (× 6,250). *Source*: From Ref. 306.

recognizes sulfated KS. Most patients with MCD lack AgKS in the cornea and serum (307,614,615) (MCD type I), but rarely AgKS is absent in the corneal stroma and the serum, but detectable in the keratocytes (MCD type IA). The third immunophenotype (MCD type II) is characterized by the presence of AgKS in the corneal tissue and detectable serum levels of AgKS that are often present in normal amounts. (308,679). A determination of the serum KS levels is not helpful in carrier detection.

Serum and Cartilage Studies

Significant headway in our comprehension of MCD followed the discovery that patients with MCD lack AgKS in the serum (615). MCD was thought to be restricted to the cornea, but because of the absence of AgKS in the serum of patients with MCD type I we predicted a lack AgKS in the cartilage of such individuals (307,615). Because cartilage is considered to be the source of serum KS, undetectable levels of AgKS in the serum of individuals with MCD type I suggested that the KS ST deficiency was not restricted to the cornea. Later direct evidence of cartilage involvement in the nose and ear was obtained in MCD type I (121,472). While deposits similar to those in the cornea have not been noted in cartilage, the chondrocytes and extracellular matrix (ECM) of the nasal cartilage do not react with a monoclonal antibody against a sulfated epitope on KS and the KS content of the cartilage is at least 800 times lower than normal (244).

Biochemical Studies

The serum from patients with MCD type I were found to have normal levels of enzymatic activity for sulfating at least one of the two sugars present in KS and an enzyme deficient for sulfating N-acetylglucosamine was thought to be present (218). The observation that patients with MCD have normal serum values for STs (217,218) suggested that the responsible ST was not secreted into the serum. Analyses of ST activities in extracts of corneas with MCD disclosed normal levels of galactose-6-sulfotransferase (Gal6ST), but lower than normal levels of N-acetylglucosamine 6-O-sulfotransferase (GlyNAc6ST) thus providing a biochemical basis for MCD at an enzymatic level (216).

Synchrotron X-ray Diffraction

Synchrotron X-ray diffraction revealed that the interfibrillar spacing of collagen fibrils in fresh corneas with either MCD type I or MCD type II is significantly lower than comparable spacings across a normal adult human cornea (411,481). This close-packing of collagen fibrils seems to be responsible for the reduced thickness of the central cornea in MCD (481). The intermolecular spacing of collagen increases similarly in normal human and MCD type I and type II corneas with hydration from the dry state. The high angle X-ray diffraction MCD corneas differ from normal and other pathologic corneas in having two extra "extra reflections" presumably caused by the abnormal GAG structure (482).

Genetics

The gene responsible for MCD was linked to human chromosome 16 (631) and the relevant region was fine mapped (362,365). By finding ST motifs in expressed tags (ESTs) two adjacent ST genes (*CHST5* and *CHST6*) were discovered within the region of human chromosome 16 to which the MCD gene had been fine mapped (5). Knowing that an enzyme for transferring sulfate moieties to KS was suspected of being deficient in MCD type I (307,438,615) *CHST5* and *CHST6* became obvious candidates as the MCD disease gene. In 2000, Akama et al. (5) discovered mutations in *CHST6* in MCD and also found insertional or deletional defects in the region between *CHST5* and *CHST6* in some cases. Subsequently, these observations were confirmed in numerous laboratories (1,4,5,15,25,127,128,203,204,206,242,297,364,366, 444,590,591,645).

While it was initially uncertain whether the immunophenotypes were genetically different, it later became evident that they were allelic. In addition, different immunophenotypes were detected in the same families (258,308) and even in the same sibship (363). In some families with MCD type II major nucleotide insertions or rearrangements were found upstream of the *CHST6* gene by Akama et al. (5), suggesting a defect in a regulatory element of *CHST6*. Other patients with MCD type II have had nucleotide changes in *CHST6* in the coding region of *CHST6*. Even if MCD types I, IA, and II are allelic and caused by mutations in *CHST6*, or in upstream regulatory elements, an adequate explanation for the differences between the various immunophenotypes is still needed.

More than 125 *CHST6* mutations have been identified in subjects with MCD from different countries [United Kingdom (128), United States (15,297,364), France (444), Iceland (366), India (590,591,645), Italy (1), Japan (5,242), Saudi Arabia (25), and Vietnam (204,206)]. The most frequent abnormalities are single nucleotide polymorphisms (SNPs) in *CHST6* that altered a coded amino acid. Heterozygous mutations have been detected in exon 3 of *CHST6* in most families and almost all of them were in association with another heterozygous mutation in the coding region of *CHST6* on the other chromosome The vast majority of patients with MCD have missense and nonsense mutations in CHST6 that involve a single nucleotide change that is predicted to alter a conserved amino acid (315). Other MCD causing mutations are nucleotide insertions or deletions in the coding region of CHST6 that cause frameshift changes as well as a few deletions or substitutions upstream of CHST6.

A defect in the promoter region of *CHST6* might be expected to control corneal ST activity and cause the milder immunophenotype of MCD and indeed Akama et al. (5) provided evidence that at least some cases of MCD type II (characterized by AgKS in the serum and cornea) are caused by genetic abnormalities upstream of *CHST6*. But other cases of MCD type II have not only had other mutations in the coding region of *CHST6*, but have lacked evidence of a defect upstream of *CHST6*. The molecular basis for the different immunophenotypes remains to be explained as identical *CHST6* mutations have been found in Saudi families with MCD type I, IA, and II (25).

Despite the importance of *CHST6* mutations in MCD mutations in this gene as well as deletions or insertions in the upstream region, and splice site mutations which create or destroy signals for exon--intron splicing (84) have not been found in all affected persons. Numerous other questions remain unanswered. For example, why does a defective ST involved in the biosynthesis of a normal component of the cornea lead to an intracytoplasmic accumulation of GAGs within keratocytes and the corneal endothelium? Why can the normal degradative enzymes not degrade the storage material? Why do GAGs accumulate in the corneal endothelium of a corneal graft many years later apparently within donor tissue as documented by Klintworth et al. (309)?

Pathogenesis

The basic defect in MCD is now known to be a mutation in the *CHST6* gene and this presumably results in lumican, keratocan, mesican, and perhaps other less abundant PGs and glycoproteins, with considerably less sulfation than normal and the absence of this negative charge undoubtedly has a profound affect on these proteins. The defective ST in MCD results in a failure of lactosaminoglycan sulfation and an intracellular storage of the GAGs and their PGs within the Golgi apparatus and probably the ER. The characteristic extracellular deposits in Descemet membrane; however, remains to be explained.

Because of features analogous to the systemic MPS, Klintworth and Vogel (320) proposed in 1964 that MCD was a comparable metabolic disorder restricted to the cornea due to a defective enzyme needed for the degradation of certain corneal GAGs. This concept took into account the mode of inheritance as well as the histochemical and morphologic characteristics of the disease as revealed by light and electron microscopy (Fig. 15). The assumption that the intra- and extracellular deposits in the cornea in MCD were GAGs was in conformity with the ability of the stromal and endothelial cells of the cornea to synthesize GAGs (310,683). Several polysaccharides are synthesized by the cornea and justified investigation: KS, chondroitin-4-sulfate (C4S), chondroitin-6-sulfate (C6S), and low-sulfated GAGs (299). The persistence of the staining qualities of the accumulations after testicular hyaluronidase digestion (177,320) argued against hyaluronic acid (HA) or C4S being significant components, whereas their resistance to chondroitin ABC lyase digestion attested against DS (299,320). By exclusion, KS, the major corneal-sulfated GAG, seemed most likely to be the accumulated substance, and this thesis was supported by the affinity of both the material and KS for alcian blue at low pH with magnesium chloride concentrations with a molarity of up to 0.8 (177,299). Moreover, of the aforementioned methods, which aid in the

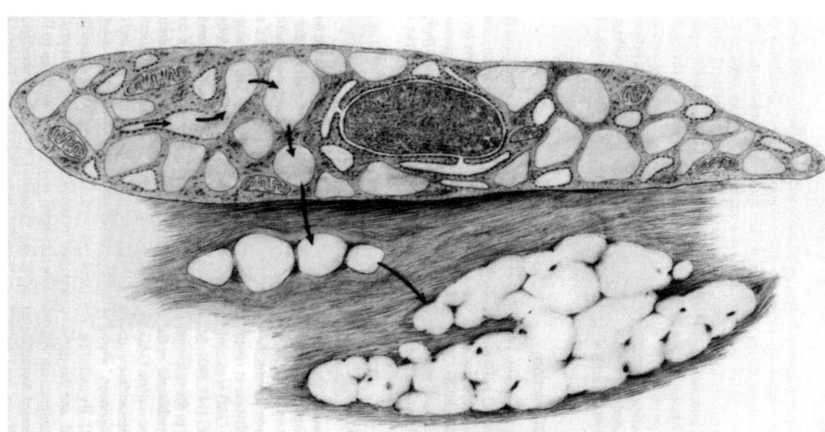

Figure 15 Postulated sequence of ultrastructural events within corneal fibroblast in macular corneal dystrophy. *Source*: Reproduced from Klintworth GK. Current concepts of the ultrastructural pathogenesis of macular and lattice corneal dystrophies. In: Bergsma D, ed. Proceedings of Second Conference on the Clinical Delineation of Birth Defects, Johns Hopkins Medical Institutions, Baltimore, Maryland, May 26–31, 1969. Baltimore: Williams & Wilkins, 1971:27–31.

visualization of the accumulations in tissue sections, PAS may react with KS, whereas, chondroitin sulfates, HA, and other GAGs usually do not (311). Further studies revealed that in contrast to the systemic MPS, MCD was not a lysosomal storage disease (LSD) due to an impaired degradation of corneal GAGs. Lysosomal abnormalities were reported in cultured MCD keratocytes (157), but this observation was not confirmed (305). Surprisingly organ cultures of MCD corneas synthesized considerably less KS than normal corneas (311) and failed to synthesize lumican presumably as a consequence of a defect in an enzyme needed for sulfating lactosaminoglycans (311,438). Corneas with MCD synthesized dissimilar PGs and L-GPs (419), but produced excessive amounts of variably sulfated glycopeptides (219,312). Cartilage and cornea contain reduced KS side chains (472).

Mutations in the *PIP5K3* Gene

Fleck Corneal Dystrophy

General Remarks

In 1956, François and Neetens (152,155) drew attention to an inherited disorder having two different types of corneal opacities. (dystrophie mouchetée and dystrophie nuageuse) (central cloudy and fleck dystrophy) (MIM #121850), which are now known as fleck corneal dystrophy and other terms (24,83, 134,151,152,155,443,568,584,586,617).

Clinical Features

Fleck corneal dystrophy is an autosomal dominant disorder characterized by multiple, nonprogressive symmetric asymptomatic minute opacities disseminated throughout the corneal stroma. One type of opacity consists of numerous small, oval, round, wreath-like, or semicircular-shaped flattened opacities with distinct borders ("flecks") in the central and peripheral cornea with intervening portions of this structure being normal (134,184,460,586). In the central cloudy phenotype asymptomatic opacities resemble snowflakes, or clouds and consist of small grayish aggregations with ill-defined margins and occur particularly in the central third of the cornea, being less numerous in the anterior and peripheral stroma. They are sometimes most dense in the deeper stroma near Descemet membrane, on which they are occasionally localized (54,584). These seemingly different opacities, which usually involve both corneas symmetrically, have been observed in the same family (155) and even in the same individual (83). Both corneas are usually affected, but there are reports of unilateral cases (586). The disorder affects males and females equally and has been observed throughout life and even in children as young as 2 years (11). The corneal epithelium, Bowman layer, and Descemet membrane are unremarkable. This nonprogressive condition is asymptomatic and does not affect vision, and the same characteristics are maintained even after the age of 70 years. Corneal sensation is usually normal, but it was diminished in two members of one family (32). Cases have been associated with angioid streaks and pseudoxanthoma elasticum (MIM #264800) KC, and a limbal dermoid (480). Rarely, mild photophobia is present. Fleck dystrophy does not require specific treatment, but the disorder did not recur in a corneal graft within 10 years of a patient who underwent a penetrating keratoplasty for an associated KC (480). In one patient who underwent a penetrating keratoplasty for KC, there was no clinical evidence of recurrent fleck dystrophy within the donor tissue after a 10 year follow-up (480).

Histopathology

Tissue has rarely been examined (295,443,480). In a single patient in whom both eyes were studied postmortem, related abnormalities were restricted to the cornea (443). By light microscopy and TEM the epithelium, Bowman layer, Descemet membrane and the corneal endothelium are normal and abnormalities are restricted to fibroblasts, which are variably affected throughout the corneal stroma. It is noteworthy that only some fibroblasts scattered throughout the corneal stroma contain large cytoplasmic vacuoles, paralleling the clinically detectable small opacities. Morphologically, normal keratocytes exist between affected areas (295,480), and although extracellular alterations are not conspicuous features, occasional foci of broad spaced collagen have been noted (295,443). By TEM single membrane-limited inclusions containing fine granular material are evident in the affected cells and presumably correspond to those having an affinity for alcian blue (295,443,480). Some keratocytes contain pleomorphic electron-dense and membranous intracytoplasmic inclusions (295,443). The nature of the pathologic material remains unknown, as histochemical investigations have been limited. Nicholson and colleagues (443) found the material in swollen corneal fibroblasts to react positively with Sudan Black B and oil red O stains for lipid and also noted a partial sensitivity to hyaluronidase (type not stated) and β-galactosidase. The evidence for a MPS is limited to an affinity for alcian blue and colloidal iron techniques, and although the possibility of a storage disease of GAGs has been raised (480), an accumulation of lipids also appears to be a manifestation (443).

In fleck dystrophy some corneal fibroblasts contain fibrillogranular material within intracytoplasmic vacuoles or pleomorphic electron-dense and membranous intracytoplasmic inclusions. The stored material has the histochemical attributes of GAGs and lipids and a storage disease involving these compounds is suspected. Extracellular alterations are rare, but foci of broad spaced collagen have been observed. Comparable abnormalities have not been found in other tissues.

Genetics

The condition has been mapped to the long arm of human chromosome 2 (2q35) and is due to a mutation in the *PIP5K3* gene (251).

Mutations in the *TACSTD2* gene

Gelatinous Drop-Like Corneal Dystrophy

General Remarks

The designation GDLD (MIM #204870) is used for a specific serious inherited autosomal recessive disorder characterized by an accumulation of mounds of amyloid primarily in the central subepithelial cornea and in Bowman layer (352,493). Because the entity has a distinct tissue abnormality the term primary familial amyloidosis of the cornea has been recommended as a preferable connotation (293,578) and GDLD.

Clinical Features

During the first decades of life multiple prominent milky-white gelatinous nodules that resemble a mulberry in shape form beneath the corneal epithelium. Hence the clinical designation GDLD. Fusiform deposits similar to those in LCD may also form in the deeper stroma (647). Other features are severe photophobia, tearing, a corneal foreign body sensation and a severe progressive loss of vision. The response to both lamellar and penetrating keratoplasty as well as to a superficial keratectomy is unsatisfactory as amyloid recurs in the graft within about 5 years (63,348).

Histopathology

Multiple nodules of amyloid deposit in the subepithelial corneal tissue of both corneas (Fig. 16) (9,340,394,434,532). The amyloid within the cornea contains lactoferrin (319), but the disease is not linked to the lactoferrin gene (317).

Epidemiology

GDLD is found worldwide but most cases seem to be in Japan where the disorder is estimated to effect in 30,000 to 300,000 persons (625). Other cases have been reported in patients from India (354,499), Tunisia (499), Vietnam (205), Turkey (387), and other countries.

Genetics

This dystrophy has been mapped to the short arm of human chromosome 1 (390) and more than 20 mutations in the *TACSTD2* (formerly *M1S1*, *TROP2*, *GA733-1*) gene that encodes tumor-associated calcium signal transducer 2 (gastrointestinal tumor-associated antigen 1) have been found to cause this disorder (207,387). The Gln118Stop mutation has been detected most often (624,626). Some affected individuals have been found not to have mutations in *TACSTD2* (115), suggesting the existence of genetic heterogeneity.

Mutations in the *GSN* Gene

Lattice Corneal Dystrophy Type II

A second type of LCD with systemic amyloidosis was discovered in Finland (415–418) (familial amyloid polyneuropathy type IV, Finnish or Meretoja type; FAP type IV; Meretoja syndrome, MIM #105120). In this disorder both corneas contain randomly scattered short fine glassy lines, which are less numerous, more delicate and more radially oriented than those in LCD type I. The peripheral cornea is chiefly affected and the central cornea is almost spared. Corneal sensitivity is reduced and there is a reduction in the long nerve bundles in the subepithelial nerve plexus (523). The cornea has fewer amorphous deposits than LCD type I and epithelial erosions are not a feature. The condition first becomes apparent after 20 years of age. In persons homozygous for the relevant mutant gene the disorder begins earlier. Vision does not usually become significantly impaired before the age of 65 years. A corneal graft is rarely indicated, but when performed a neurotrophic persistent epithelial defect may develop (570) LCD type II can be mistaken for LCD type I both clinically and histopathologically.

The corneal abnormalities are accompanied by a progressive bilateral neuropathy involving cranial and peripheral nerves, dysarthria, a dry and extremely lax itchy skin with amyloid deposits. A characteristic "mask-like" facial expression, protruding lips with impaired movement, pendulous ears, and blepharochalasis are also features.

The amyloid in LCD type II is composed of a mutated 71 amino acid long fragment of gelsolin and it accumulates in the corneal stroma and between the epithelium and Bowman layer. It also deposits in scleral, choroidal, and adnexal blood vessels as well as in the lacrimal gland and perineurium of ciliary nerves. The amyloid is also found in the heart, kidney, skin, nerves, wall of arteries, and other tissues (416). The amyloid within the cornea in LCD type II reacts with the antigelsolin antibody (191), but not with the antibodies produced to the amino and carboxy terminals of gelsolin (518).

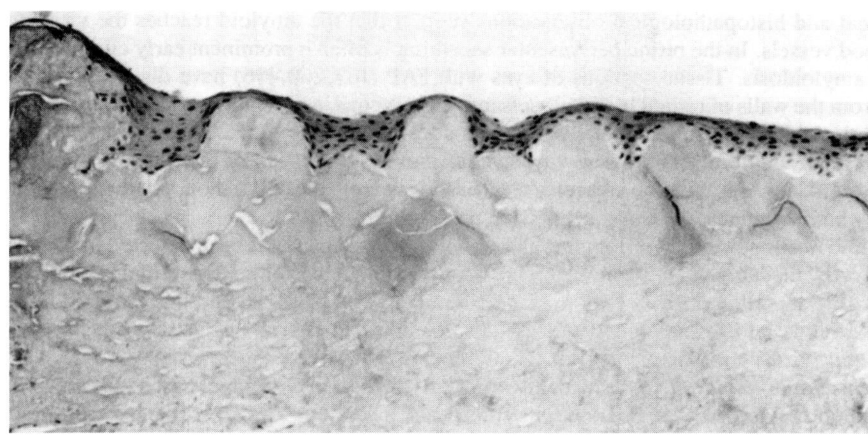

Figure 16 Nodular deposits of amyloid in the superficial cornea of in gelatinous drop-like dystrophy of the cornea (hematoxylin and eosin, × 100).

Genetics

Two single base substitutions in the *GSN* gene, located on human chromosome 9 (9q34), which encodes the actin-modulating protein gelsolin are known to cause LCD type II (Asp187Asn, Asp187Tyr). The mutation in many Finnish (464), three American (3,102,190), one Japanese (594), and one English (574) families involves a G to A substitution at nucleotide 654 (codon 187), resulting in an asparagine-187 variant of gelsolin (593). In one Danish and one Czech family a G to T transversion in position 654 at codon 187 results in the substitution of tyrosine for aspartic acid (103,302).

Mutations in the *SLC4A11* Gene

Congenital Hereditary Endothelial Dystrophy Type 2

General Remarks

Congenital hereditary endothelial dystrophy (CHED) type 2 (CHED2, MIM #217700) is a nonprogressive autosomal recessive corneal disorder in which both corneas are two to three times thicker than normal. There are some similarities to CHED1 (MIM #121700) (see Congenital Hereditary Endothelial Dystrophy Type I).

Clinical Features

CHED2 becomes apparent at or shortly after birth. Affected individuals are born with corneas having a diffuse ground-glass appearance. The condition is asymptomatic and is accompanied by nystagmus.

Histopathology

Marked stromal edema associated with thickened collagen fibrils have been observed (271) together with the decreased fibril density. The keratocytes and Bowman layer are usually unremarkable. The endothelial cells are scant or degenerated when present (642). The abnormal endothelium synthesizes a homogenous, posterior, nonbanded Descemet membrane. Descemet membrane has a normal anterior 110 nm banded portion and a narrow zone of posterior nonbanded material zone. A fibrous connective tissue layer composed of an admixture of fibrils measuring 20 to 40 nm in diameter and small foci of basement membrane-like material has been found posterior to Descemet membrane sometimes resembling an additional layer of Descemet membrane (Fig. 16) (287). The entire multilaminar zone ranges from 2.0 to 35.0 μm in thickness.

Genetics

CHED2 was mapped to human chromosome 20 (20p13) (70,211) and the responsible gene has recently been identified as *SLC4A11* (252,634).

Pathogenesis

The genetic mutation in CHED2 affects the encoded bicarbonate transporter-related protein 1, which reportedly regulates the intracellular boron concentration, and affected corneal endothelial cells presumably function normally in utero as evidenced by the thin embryonic portion of Descemet membrane. The overall thickened Descemet membrane probably follows the synthesis of a posterior collagenous layer later during development. In CHED2 clinical disease is restricted to the cornea, but the reason remains to be determined as *SLC4A11* is strongly expressed in the numerous parts of the body (including kidney, salivary gland, thyroid gland, testis, and trachea).

Mutations in the *DCN* Gene

Congenital Stromal Corneal Dystrophy

Congenital stromal corneal dystrophy (MIM #610048) is an autosomal dominant corneal disease having numerous opaque flakes and spots throughout the corneal stroma. Affected individuals have been extensively studied in large French and Norwegian families (57,105,662).

Clinical Features

The stromal opacities increase with age and prevent a clinical evaluation of corneal endothelium. Corneal erosions, photophobia, and corneal vascularization are absent. Some affected individuals have strabismus or primary open angle glaucoma. Systemic abnormalities are not apparent.

Histopathology

Genetics

The Norwegian family with congenital stromal corneal dystrophy has a 1 bp deletion in the *DCN* gene, which encodes for core protein of decorin (see Chapter 40) (57).

Mutations in the *UBIAD1* Gene

Schnyder Corneal Dystrophy

General Remarks

The presence of crystalline opacities in the anterior central portion of both corneas was described by van Went and Wibaut in 1924 (630). Five years later Schnyder (542,543) established this autosomal dominant condition as a distinct entity, which is now known as Schnyder corneal dystrophy (SCD) (central crystalline dystrophy, MIM # 121800).

Clinical Features

SCD usually becomes apparent early in life, but has not been observed at birth. The condition presents with corneal clouding or the appearance of crystals within the corneal stroma. Because the disorder usually stabilizes with time, only occasional patients with severe impairment require corneal grafting. Over time an initially unremarkable corneal stroma acquires small white opacities and a diffuse haze. Occasionally crystals are not evident clinically and only parts of the central corneal opacity may contain crystals (104). Typically a ring-shaped yellow-white opacity composed of innumerable fine needle-shaped crystals forms beneath the epithelium and Bowman layer and the adjacent anterior stroma of the central cornea. The crystals usually remain in the anterior third of the cornea. The remaining stroma is unremarkable initially, but with time it may acquire small white opacities and a diffuse haze (377). While sometimes appearing dull white, the crystals are frequently scintillating with variegated red and green hues. The epithelium, Descemet membrane, and the endothelium are spared. In some cases crystals are only seen in parts of the central corneal opacity (104). The condition is usually bilateral, but one eye may become affected earlier than the other. Visual acuity is usually good and although usually stationary after childhood, the corneal opacification may progress over time and form a dense, disc of corneal crystals that diminish vision sufficiently in both eyes to require a corneal graft (104,243,384). Most cases lack an apparent systemic disorder (28), but hypercholesterolemia is common (46,185,400,463,544,598), and so is an arcus lipoides (162,377,384,543,630), xanthelasma (905,786,907), familial hypercholesterolemia (60,361), familial dysbetalipoproteinemia (60), or hypertriglyceridemia (126) and other manifestations of hypercholesterolemia (60) have been reported.

Histopathology

Birefringent cholesterol crystals and associated neutral fats accumulate within keratocytes and extracellularly and correspond to the crystals observed clinically. The lipid is also present in Bowman layer, between the superficial corneal lamellae and dispersed within the stroma midst the collagen fibrils. The lipid deposits in SCD comprise mainly multilamellar vesicles containing unesterified cholesterol and phospholipids, with a lesser contribution of cholesteryl ester lipid droplets (401). The lipid deposits within the cornea are predominantly phospholipid and cholesterol (esterified and unesterified) (401,677) probably reflect defective lipid metabolism. The predominant phospholipid is sphingomyelin (677). Apolipoproteins A-I, A-II, and E are present, but not apolipoprotein B (182). An ultrastructural study of a skin biopsy and cultured fibroblasts from an affected person has disclosed lipid containing membrane-bound spherical vacuoles (28). Moreover, skin fibroblasts from one patient showed abnormal cytoplasmic deposits that were fluorescent after staining with filipin, a reagent specific for unesterified cholesterol.

Genetics

SCD has autosomal dominant mode of inheritance and the responsible gene has been mapped to a 2.32 Mbp region of chromosome 1 (1p34.1–p36) (552). The *ARID1A* (*B120*) gene, which is involved in lipid transport and metabolism was a strong candidate (604). After fifteen of the 31 putative genes in the mapped region were ruled out (13), the responsible gene was identified as *UBIAD1* (454).

Pathogenesis

The abovementioned observations on skin fibroblasts taken together with a frequent finding of hyperlipidemia in patients with SCD suggests that a systemic disorder of lipid metabolism is present.

Mutations in Other Genes

The cornea is affected together with other tissues by numerous other identified genes.

COL8A

Collagen type VIII is a major constituent of Descemet membrane and it is noteworthy that mutations in the *COL8A2* gene, which encodes the alpha 2 chain of this collagen, have been detected in two different corneal disorders that affect the corneal endothelium, which synthesizes Descemet membrane. A Gly455Lys missense mutation in *COL8A2* has been found in two families with a rare autosomal dominant early onset variant of Fuchs corneal dystrophy (FCD) (see section on Fuchs corneal dystrophy) (39). The same mutation has been reported in a single poorly documented family with posterior polymorphous corneal dystrophy (PPCD) (39). A Leu450Trp mutant in *COL8A2* has also been found in early onset FCD (195).

CTNS

Adult nonnephropathic cystinosis (MIM #219750) is a LSD (see Chapter 43) caused by one severe and one mild mutation in the *CTNS* gene that encodes for cystinosin. The phenotype is relatively mild in a mutation with some functional cystinosin (174). Crystals in the corneal stroma are prominent in both eyes.

CYP4V2

Bietti marginal crystalline corneoretinal dystrophy (MIM #210370) is a rare autosomal recessive condition characterized by multiple delicate glistening crystals in the peripheral cornea and retina. It was first recognized in Italy by Bietti (35). The disorder is relatively common in China and most reported cases have been in persons of Oriental extraction. Very fine crystals that are difficult to see even by slit-lamp biomicroscopy gather in the peripheral paralimbal anterior corneal stroma in persons with areas of retinal pigment epithelial atrophy. Similar crystals are present in all layers of the retina, especially at the posterior pole. This condition has a slowly progressive loss of visual function resulting in night blindness and a constriction of the visual field. The retina undergoes degeneration and the choroidal blood vessels become sclerotic (268). Many cases retain good vision, but become symptomatic because of poor dark adaptation and paracentral scotomas (656). Corneal (652,656) and conjunctival fibroblasts contain crystals and complex osmiophilic inclusions indicating that the disorder is not limited to the cornea (656). The nature of the crystals and inclusions has not been identified with certainty. The condition, which has been associated with abnormalities in fatty acid metabolism and the absence of fatty acid binding by two cytosolic proteins (349), has been mapped to human chromosome 4 (4q35–4qtel) (250) and is caused by mutations in the *CYP4V2* gene (see Chapter 35 for more details particularly with respect to the retina).

GLA

The designation vortex corneal dystrophy (corneal verticillata) was applied to a corneal disorder characterized by the presence of innumerable tiny brown spots arranged in curved whirlpool-like lines in the superficial cornea (150,154). An autosomal dominant mode of transmission was initially suspected, but later it was realized that these individuals were affected hemizygous males and asymptomatic female carriers of an X-linked systemic metabolic disease caused by a deficiency of α-galactosidase (150) (Fabry disease, Anderson–Fabry disease, ceramide trihexosidase deficiency, hereditary dystopic lipidosis, α-galactosidase deficiency, GLA deficiency, MIM #301500) (see Chapter 41). Some, but not all cases of cornea verticillata are due to mutations in the *GLA* gene. Nonfamilial whorl-like corneal opacities also form in individuals on chloroquine, amiodarone phenothiazines, or indomethacin therapy and striate melanokeratosis.

GNPTAB

Corneal opacification is a feature of mucolipidosis type II (MIM #252500) and MPS type IIIA (MIM #252600), which are both caused by mutations in the *GNPTAB* gene (see Chapter 40).

GNPTG

Corneal opacification is a feature of mucolipidosis type IIIC caused by mutations in the *GNPTG* gene (see Chapter 42).

KERA

The *KERA* gene that encodes the core protein of the proteoglycan keratocan is mutated in autosomal recessive cornea plana (MIM #217300) (see Chapter 40) (185).

NEU1

Fine punctuate corneal opacities occur in mucolipidosis type I (neuraminidase deficiency, MIM #256550) (see Chapter 42) caused by mutations in the *NEU1* gene that encodes for neuraminidase.

MCOLN1

Patients with mucolipidosis type IV (MIM #252650) resulting from mutations in *MCOLN1* have corneal clouding (see Chapter 42).

SMPD1

Corneal opacification is one of several ocular manifestations of Niemann–Pick disease type A (MIM #257200) (see Chapter 41). This disorder is caused by mutations in the *SMPD1* gene that encodes for acid sphingomyelinase (sphingomyelin phosphodiesterase-1). The epithelium and endothelium of the cornea as well as the keratocytes contain multilamellar intracytoplasmic inclusions (508).

STS

Small gray punctate opacities accumulate in the central deep corneal stroma immediately anterior to Descemet membrane in entities known as deep filiform dystrophy and cornea farinata (93,200,381,462,471,576). They are common X-linked ichthyosis (steroid sulfatase deficiency, MIM # 308100) (149,197), but have also been noted in the elderly and in association with KC (381). The phenotype of deep filiform dystrophy can also result from immunoglobulin (Ig) deposition in hypergammaglobulinemia (420,681).

The opacities are of variable shape and may resemble commas, circles, lines, threads (filiform), flour (farina), or dots. They affect the entire width of the cornea except for the perilimbal region (381) or in a ring around the middle of the cornea. The corneal subepithelial and anterior stromal layers may contain white-gray granular opacities associated with irregular overlying corneal epithelium and a thickened basement membrane including irregular extensions into Bowman layer (379). Visual acuity is not usually deceased.

In X-linked ichthyosis abnormal depositions of basement membrane protein have been identified in the anterior stroma (197). Keratocytes anterior to Descemet membrane contain membrane-bound intracytoplasmic vacuoles that include fibrillogranular material and electron-dense lamellar bodies (93).

At least 6 mutations in the steroid sulfatase gene (*STS*) have been identified, but specific mutations have not been correlated with the presence or absence of corneal abnormalities.

Other

Corneal clouding occurs in almost all MPSs (see Chapter 40) and is typically diffuse with fine punctate opacities. In diseases due to mutations in the *IDUA* gene (MPS IH, MIM # 607014; MPS IS, MIM # 607016) and *ARSB* gene (MPS VI, MIM + 253200) it is a significant and clinical feature, while in MPS II (MIM + 309900) caused by a mutation in the *IDS* gene it is a late manifestation.

Numerous genes are involved in corneal development and mutations in them cause abnormalities in the size, shape, and other attributes of the cornea (see Chapter 52). Microcornea occurs with mutations in the *GJA8, MAF, CRYAA, VMD2, HNS* genes and anterior segment dysgenesis, which is associated with corneal abnormalities and has been attributed to *FOXC1, PITX2, PAX6,* and *CYPIB1* mutations.

GENETIC DISORDERS AFFECTING THE CORNEA THAT ARE MAPPED TO SPECIFIC CHROMOSOMES BUT WITHOUT GENE IDENTIFICATION

Congenital Hereditary Endothelial Dystrophy Type 1

General Remarks

CHED type 1 (CHED1) (MIM # 121700) is an autosomal dominant corneal disorder in which both corneas are two to three times thicker than normal and have a diffuse ground-glass appearance.

Clinical Features

CHED1 becomes manifest during the first 2 years of life with photophobia and tearing. It slowly progresses over 5 to 10 years and in contrast to the more common CHED2 nystagmus is absent (264). A diffuse corneal edema in PPCD may simulate CHED1, but the corneas are thicker in the latter condition (642).

Histopathology

The histopathology is similar to CHED2, but a subtle difference in the thickness of collagen in Descemet membrane have been described (294). A posterior collagenous layer of fibrillary collagen contributes to the thickened Descemet membrane (294). In contrast to posterior polymophous corneal dystrophy (PPCD) corneas with CHED1 do not manifest epithelialization of the endothelial cells on the posterior surface of Descemet membrane.

Genetics

The gene responsible for CHED1 has been mapped to the pericentromeric region of chromosome 20 (20p11.2–q11.2) (616) in an area overlapping a gene for autosomal dominant PPCD (223).

Pathogenesis

The spectrum of changes in PPCD and CHED1 remains questionable. Despite distinct light microscopical, ultrastructural, and immunohistochemical differences, some investigators have proposed a common mechanistic process (74,402).

Lisch Corneal Dystrophy

General Remarks

Lisch corneal dystrophy (band-shaped whorled microcystic dystrophy of the corneal epithelium) is a rare inherited disorder of the cornea that was first described by Lisch et al. in 1992 (360).

Clinical Features

Lisch corneal dystrophy is characterized by the presence of feather-shaped opacities and microcysts in the corneal epithelium that are arranged in a band-shaped and sometimes whorled pattern (75,360,513). Painless blurred vision that begins after 60 years of life may be present. There are clinical similarities to MECD and the condition recurs after cellular debridement.

Histopathology

The corneal epithelium has a bubbly vacuolization with optically empty spaces. By TEM the cytoplasmic vacuoles are mainly empty but contain scant nonspecific osmophilic material.

Genetics

The gene has been mapped to the short arm of the X chromosome (Xp22.3) at a maximum likelihood of odds (LOD) score of 2.93 (359). As expected because of the mode of inheritance it is not linked to the *KRT3* and *KRT12* genes.

Keratosis Follicularis Spinulosa Decalvans

General Remarks

Keratosis follicularis spinulosa decalvans (MIM #308800) is a rare disorder that affects the skin and cornea. It was first described by Siemens in 1926 in the Netherlands (554,629).

Clinical Features

Keratosis follicularis spinulosa decalvans is characterized by cutaneous follicular papules and alopecia (especially involving scalp, eyebrows, and eyelashes). Numerous punctate opacities are found beneath the corneal epithelium. Marked photophobia is common. Female carriers may manifest the disorder usually in a mild form.

Histopathology

One report documents the findings on a corneal biopsy (146).

Genetics

This X-linked disorder has been mapped to Xp22.1–p22.13 (475).

X-Linked Endothelial Corneal Dystrophy

General Remarks

Schmid et al. (540) recently drew attention to family of patients with a corneal endothelial dystrophy that affected 35 individuals over four generations.

Clinical Features

Males are affected more severely than females and corneal opacification may be severe in male patients. A congenital ground glass corneal clouding may be present and advanced cases have a subepithelial band keratopathy associated with endothelial changes that resemble moon craters. Penetrating keratoplasty is sometimes indicated and the graft may remain clear for as long as 30 years.

Histopathology

Focal discontinuities and degenerative changes have been noted in the corneal endothelial cells by light microscopy and TEM and Descemet membrane is thickened. Epithelial cells have not been observed lining Descemet membrane.

Genetics

In keeping with an X-linked mode of inheritance affected males transmit the disorder to their daughters, but not to their sons. The condition has been mapped to the long arm of the X-chromosome (Xq25). The critical interval contains 72 genes of which 7 code for putative transcription factors.

GENETICALLY HETEROGENOUS DISORDERS OF THE CORNEA

Fuchs Corneal Dystrophy

General Remarks

FCD (late hereditary endothelial dystrophy) (MIM #136800) is a common bilateral progressive corneal disorder of the corneal endothelium of aging named after Ernst Fuchs the ophthalmologist, who first described epithelial edema, stromal clouding, and impaired corneal sensitivity in elderly individuals in 1910 (163).

Clinical Features

This debilitating disorder leads to corneal edema with a loss of corneal clarity, painful episodes of recurrent corneal erosions, and a severe impairment of visual acuity and sometimes even blindness in the elderly population. Descemet membrane becomes thickened (2,50) due to an excessive accumulation of ECM and excrescences on Descemet membrane (corneal guttae) (50,255). Corneal guttae are common and are not specific for FCD. They may be a sequel to interstitial keratitis (80,668,669,672), aging (372), and as mentioned elsewhere in this chapter, MCD. In Japan patients with the Arg24His mutation in *TGFBI* have been found to have significantly more corneal guttae than controls (6). They have been detected clinically in as many as 70% of individuals over the age of 40 years in one part of the United States (Gainesville, Florida) (372). They are most often observed after the age of 50 years and are most extensive in the elderly. Corneal guttae are more common in females than males in some reviews (79,111), but not in others

(372). They rarely form at an early age, but have been noted at birth when they are associated with an anterior polar cataract and seem to be nonprogressive with an autosomal dominant inheritance (112,322,334,611,619). Even some guttae that are not apparent early in life have an autosomal dominant mode of inheritance. Corneal guttae have been described in monozygotic twins, in siblings, and in two or more successive generations (101,367,636). FCD affects females three times more often than males (332). FCD is characterized by a progressive, stromal, and epithelial edema with subepithelial fibrosis, and the clinical course usually spans 10 to 20 years. Initially the disorder is asymptomatic, but corneal guttae form in the central cornea and they are associated with a fine dusting of pigment. The corneal guttae have a glittering golden brown appearance on slit-lamp biomicroscopy and in retroillumination they appear as small dew drops. Gradually, Descemet membrane thickens and the guttae are frequently ringed by pigment dots.

Subsequently vision becomes hazy and glare begins as the corneal stroma and epithelium become edematous. Stromal edema initially produces a blue-gray haze anterior to Descemet membrane and in the anterior stroma and the entire stroma eventually thickens and acquires a ground-glass appearance, while Descemet membrane wrinkles. Epithelial edema develops resulting in a characteristic fine pigskin texture, commonly designated "bedewing." Fluid accumulated between the epithelial cells and in a subepithelial location (bullous keratopathy) and it bursts through the epithelium causing painful corneal erosions. Eventually the subepithelial edema and discomfort diminishes, but visual acuity continues to deteriorate as connective tissue replaces it. The corneal abnormalities, which started centrally, spread toward the corneoscleral limbus. Microbial keratitis and corneal neovascularization are extremely rare manifestations.

FCD typically becomes symptomatic during the fifth or sixth decade of life and seldom earlier (111,232,332,579), but corneal endothelial abnormalities can be detected clinically several years before the patient becomes symptomatic (47).

Most patients ultimately require penetrating keratoplasty (2) or the more recent Descemet stripping endothelial keratoplasty (DESK). The corneal endothelial cells play a crucial role in maintaining corneal clarity by preventing it from excessive hydration. The endothelial abnormality may be associated with defects in the endothelium in the final differentiation during perinatal period (50). It may also be linked to hormonal changes during aging (256). Altered mitochondrial ionic metabolism, inflammation, and chromosome changes in keratocytes have also been considered (2,469). No significant differences have been found in the endothelial permeability or the aqueous humor components and flow rate between healthy patients and those with FCD (658,659).

Epidemiology

FCD predominantly affects women more often than men, as demonstrated in numerous studies (163,273,382,524,553). Women comprise about 75% of the cases (111) and females tend to express a more severe phenotype than males (163,273,524,553). Population studies have shown a marked difference in the prevalence of FCD in different parts of the world. FCD is common in the United States (52,332,356,369,560), uncommon in Saudi Arabia (12), and extremely rare in Japan (232,532). The incidence and prevalence of FCD have not been reported, but this disease is one of the leading indications for penetrating keratoplasty in the United States and some other developed countries (18,52,356,369,560). In different series it accounts for 10% to 25% of all corneal transplants (2,18,52,273,332, 356,382,524,560). This is a significant number considering that the annual number of corneal transplants in the United States is >32,000. Cataracts are common in individuals with FCD and cataract extraction accelerates the corneal decompensation.

Genetics

Although most patients with FCD lack a positive family history the belief that this condition has a genetic basis stems from several observations: (*i*) the prevalence of FCD varies markedly in different populations; (*ii*) blood relatives of patients with FCD sometimes manifest corneal guttae (131); (*iii*) siblings (81,266) or two or more successive generations (90,131,332,372,382,430,524) are involved in some families with FCD; and (*iv*) in some families FCD appears to be an autosomal dominant disorder with incomplete penetrance and greater expressivity in the female (131,524). Krachmer et al. noted that 38% of relatives of patients with confluent guttae who were >40 years old also were affected with guttae (332). Although FCD is sometimes familial, its exact mode of inheritance is uncertain (332). A simple autosomal dominant pattern is unlikely (332). In an attempt to detect potential candidate genes for FCD Gottsch et al. used serial analysis of gene expression technology to identify RNA gene transcripts in corneas of patients with FCD versus normal human controls (194). Rare young onset cases of FCD have been associated with mutations in the *COL8A2* gene on chromosome 1p34.3 (195). Other cases of FCD have been mapped to chromosome 13 (13pTe1–3q12.13) (596) and chromosome 18q21.2–q21.32 (595).

Histopathology

Histopathologic findings include subepithelial bullae. Aside from the guttae, Descemet membrane is multilayered and often irregularly thickened (two to four times normal) due to an excessive accumulation of collagen especially where the guttae are most abundant. Because of abnormal ECM deposits within Descemet membrane in FCD, an immunohistochemical study on selected cases of FCD was performed, as well as in situ hybridization using labeled sense and antisense *TGFBI* oligonucleotide probes (230). TGFBIp is present in the subepithelial corneal matrix and in the posterior collagenous layer of corneas with FCD. In FCD, the guttae are typically more confluent and more centrally located than the guttae of aging, which characteristically involve predominantly the peripheral cornea (Hassall–Henle warts).

The specific characteristics of FCD involve the corneal endothelium and the posterior part of Descemet membrane where multiple guttae of variable size and shape are evident (Fig. 17). Abnormal endothelial cells generate a multilaminar collagenous layer, which stains with variable intensity with the PAS stain. The new collagenous tissue forms excrescences of differing morphologic types that correspond to the clinically detectable corneal guttae (232). Tissue specimens in advanced cases of FCD contain a layer consisting of loosely packed thin collagen fibrils (20–30 nm in diameter) with a 64 nm banding scattered within basement membrane-like material. The abnormal endothelial cells have widened intercellular spaces, swollen mitochondria, dilated rough ER, and melanin pigment. Some cells adherent to the posterior surface of Descemet membrane possesses morphological features of fibroblasts (474). Some are mushroom- or anvil-shaped and protrude into the anterior chamber (Fig. 17A). Others are multilaminar warts or buried in the multilaminar ECM (Fig. 17A). Some subjects with FCD have multilaminar connective tissue posterior to Descemet membrane, but without corneal guttae. The distribution of the guttae can be visualized in flat preparations of Descemet membrane using phase-contrast microscopy or scanning electron microscopy (SEM) (Fig. 17B). The corneal endothelium is attenuated over the guttae excresences (Fig. 17C) (232). Corneal edema is usually most marked in the central and paracentral cornea (516,519) and this overlies the abnormal corneal endothelium. Oxytalan, a component of the elastic fiber, has been identified histochemically around but not within the guttae excrescences of FCD (17).

When viewed by TEM Descemet membrane has a normal 3-μm-thick anterior-banded layer and a normal nonbanded portion, but posteriorly this product of the corneal endothelium contains fusiform bundles and sheets of wide-spacing (100 nm) collagen with a macroperiodicity of 55 or 100 nm within amorphous material and manifests subbands with a periodicity of about 30 to 40 nm. Horizontal fibrils (Fig. 17C) run perpendicular to the vertical bands Iwamoto and DeVoe (245). The wide-spacing collagen forms a hexagonal pattern, which is evident in tangential sections. This pattern is identical to that observed in horizontal sections of the normal anterior-banded Descemet membrane. Groups of 10- to 20-nm-diameter collagen fibrils are found next to the wide-spacing collagen and may fuse with the horizontal fibrils of the wide-spacing collagen.

The fissures within some guttae are penetrated by cellular debris. The guttae of FCD resemble those that normally form on the periphery of Descemet membrane with aging (Hassall–Henle bodies). The dome-shaped, fissured appearance, and lack of a multilaminar pattern of Hassall–Henle bodies usually distinguish them from the guttae of FCD (245). Fissures similar to those in Hassall–Henle bodies are occasionally found in the guttae of FCD, but they are less plentiful and not as prominent.

Initially edema of the corneal epithelium is restricted to the basal epithelial layer, but the more superficial layers are also involved in more advanced cases and the epithelium becomes separated from its basal lamina, which is fragmented, and the Bowman layer (bullous keratopathy). This is associated with a loss of hemidesmosomes. Bowman layer usually remains intact, but focal breaks become traversed by subepithelial connective tissue.

Corneal endothelial dysfunction becomes manifest much earlier than the symptomatic disorder, which becomes deferred until middle age.

A histochemical analysis of cytochrome oxidase activity in corneal endothelium from patients with FCD disclosed that regional differences that may relate to diminished numbers of mitochondria in the diseased cells.

In FCD Descemet membrane and its adjacent posterior collagenous contain similar collagen types to age-matched controls (53,285) and immunohistochemical studies have disclosed fibrinogen/fibrin in the posterior collagenous layer in FCD, but not in normal Descemet membrane.

Pathogenesis

FCD seems to be a complex inherited disorder caused by the interaction of genetic and other factors. Initially FCD dystrophy was thought to be a disease of the corneal epithelium, but sequential observations on numerous patients disclosed that pleomorphic-attenuated corneal endothelium, premature degenerative alterations of the corneal endothelium in association with the production of excessive amounts of an

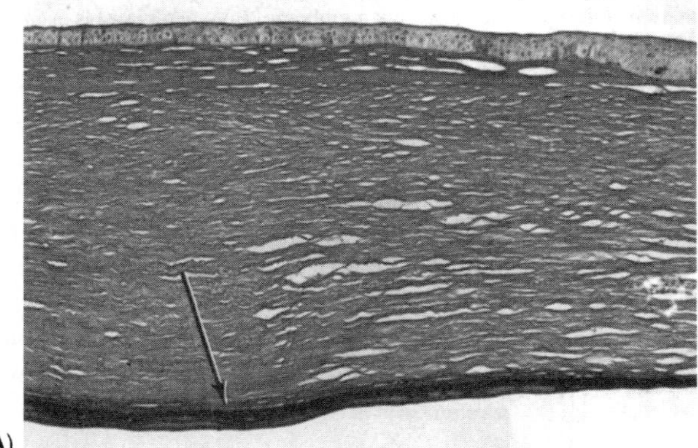
(A)

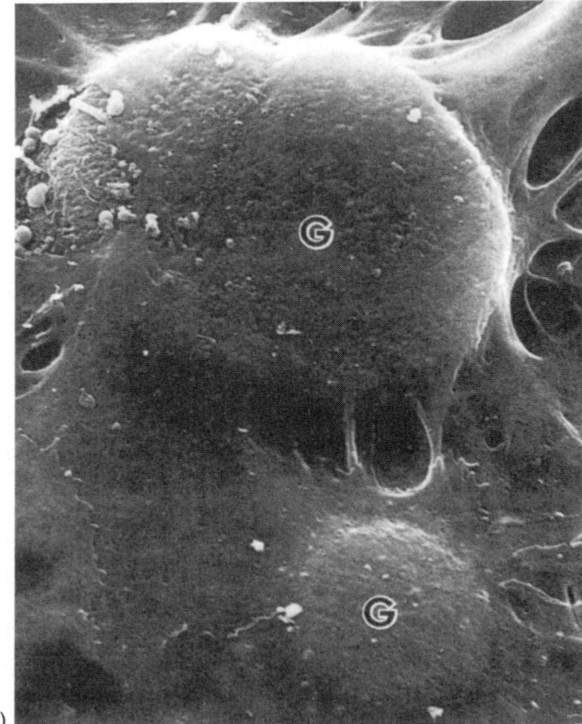

(B)

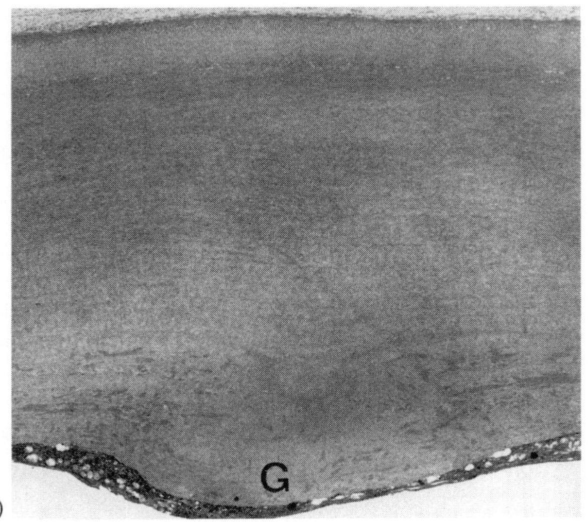

(C)

abnormal Descemet membrane precede the epithelial changes.

Later it became recognized that hyaline corneal guttae form centrally on Descemet membrane in this condition. As a rule FCD presents clinically during the fifth or sixth decade of life and seldom before the sixth decade of life (90,232,286, 332,473). While the molecular defect in most cases of FCD has yet to be determined, the underlying abnormality results in a decline in the number of functional endothelial cells (47,657). Sequential observations on numerous patients have disclosed that the endothelial alterations precede the epithelial changes. The cardinal defect affects the corneal endothelium, which degenerates prematurely and produces excessive amounts of an abnormal Descemet membrane of a type analogous to that assembled in utero. Apoptosis is a feature of FCD (353) and it may be triggered by DNA damage caused by the accumulation of toxic photooxidation products caused by light that enters the eye. Increased levels of intracellular oxidants and DNA damage from ultraviolet (UV) light are known stimulants of apoptosis. Guttae are not specific for FCD and may arise as part of corneal aging or as a response to interstitial keratitis (640).

Based on the level of the initial ultrastructural abnormalities in Descemet membrane, which reflect the timing or the first changes it is apparent the corneal endothelium is expressing dysfunction much earlier than when symptoms begin (657). Normally corneal endothelial cells regulate the transport of fluids in and out of the cornea via Na^+-K^+-ATPase pumps and aquaporins. Aquaporin 1 is normally expressed in the human corneal endothelium and is an important water channel for that cell (378). Previous research indicates that the Na^+-K^+-ATPase pump site density in endothelial cells is decreased in FCD (403–406,533). This defect in the corneal endothelium could account for the corneal edema that characterizes FCD. The barrier function of the endothelium breaks down with resultant stromal and epithelial edema sufficient to reduce visual acuity. The normal corneal endothelium appears capable of pumping water and electrolytes out of the stroma toward the anterior chamber (399). This active fluid transport prevents edema of the normal corneal

Figure 17 (*Left*) Fuchs dystrophy. (**A**) Corneal changes are related to the degree of corneal edema. Thickened Descemet membrane shows interlaminar guttae most pronounced in the most edematous area (*arrow*) (periodic acid Schiff, × 280). (**B**) Scanning electron micrograph with attenuated endothelial cells overlying guttae (G) (× 1,950). (**C**) Transmission electron micrograph showing guttate excrescence (G) with abnormal 110 nm long-spacing collagen covered by attenuated corneal endothelial cells (× 3,400). *Source*: Courtesy of Drs. M.M. Rodrigues, S. Rajagopalan, and K.A. Jones.

stroma (399), and in the endothelial corneal dystrophies this physiological activity is presumably impaired (644). The basic defect in most cases of FCD remains unknown but a primary target of the disorder involves the corneal endothelium, which dies prematurely and produces an abnormal basal lamina. As in other disorders of the corneal endothelium the corneal endothelial cells may undergo fibroblastic transformation leading to the production of collagenous tissue posterior to Descemet membrane (641,642). The effect of this is an accumulation of multilaminar ECM containing loosely arranged fibrillary tissue. This extra layer of material behind Descemet membrane accounts in part for the clinically evident thickened Descemet membrane. Impaired endothelial cell function allows aqueous humor penetration of the endothelial barrier resulting in stromal and epithelial edema. The fibrinolytic system is suspected of perhaps being involved in FCD, because the antifibrinolytic agent, tranexamic acid, diminishes corneal edema in FCD and the aqueous humor in FCD patients, contains elevated levels of substances associated with the fibrinolytic system (53,285). The collagen molecules are thought to not be normally assembled in FCD. Several years ago a virus was suspected of being the causal agent of FCD because intracytoplasmic particles were identified within the corneal endothelium of a single patient by TEM (526). These structures, however, resemble distorted mitochondria and have been observed in other corneal disorders (235). The banded posterior collagenous layer of Descemet membrane starts appearing within the first two decades of life. The corneal edema of FCD results from the progressive loss and functional impairment of the corneal endothelium. The latter is caused by a decrease in the barrier formed by the adjacent endothelial cells and the inability of the corneal endothelium to pump water from the hydrophilic corneal stroma.

Posterior Polymorphous Corneal Dystrophy

General Remarks

The autosomal dominant disorder known as PPCD (MIM #122000) is a genetically heterogenous entity with exceptionally variable expression. The cells lining the posterior surface of the cornea possess the morphologic attributes of epithelial cells, and this is evident clinically by a varied appearance of the corneal endothelial cells.

Clinical Features

PPCD is usually asymptomatic and hence most cases do not require treatment. However, in those that do PPCD can recur in the graft following perforating keratoplasty (49,610). Both corneas are usually affected, but the abnormalities may be asymmetrical and sometimes only one cornea is apparently uninvolved. Most patients remain asymptomatic, but cornea edema is sometimes evident at birth indicating a congenital disorder. Clinically various configurations appear at the level of Descemet membrane. They include the presence of small aggregates of apparent vesicles bordered by a gray haze and gray geographic areas, which occasionally appear nodular and contain round or elliptical vesicular zones creating a pattern that resembles Swiss cheese. Broad bands with more or less parallel edges and gray sheets appear as thickenings of Descemet membrane. These abnormalities exhibit a refractile quality on retroillumination. Adhesions sometimes unite the iris with the posterior surface of the peripheral cornea giving rise to glaucoma. These adhesions differ in appearance from the fine strands that attach iris to a prominent Schwalbe ring in the Axenfeld and Rieger anomalies.

Sometimes edema of the corneal epithelium and stroma occur and anterior cornea may become scarred and develop calcific band keratopathy. Another corneal disorder characterized by a moderately diffuse corneal opacification has been designated hereditary corneal edema (67). This congenital condition is distinguished from CHED1 and CHED2 because the cloudy corneal stroma is minimally thickened.

PPCD needs to be differentiated from an acquired posterior corneal opacification that follows recurrent uveitis and keratitis and which was unfortunately designated posterior polymorphous keratopathy (355).

Histopathology

Corneal tissue has only been examined in cases severe enough to require penetrating keratoplasty. Instead of an endothelial monolayer the posterior cornea is lined by variable numbers of stratified squamous epithelial cells having tonofilaments, cytokeratin, and desmosomes (Fig. 18) (48,254,521,621). It is noteworthy that this abnormality is not specific for PPCD as corneal endothelial cells may be replaced by squamous epithelium in the ICE syndrome (see Chapter 30). The epithelial cells have numerous microvilli (198,642), but unlike normal corneal epithelium, microplicae are not a feature. Cells on the posterior corneal surface of Descemet membrane may also have a fibroblast-like appearance (254).

In corneal specimens obtained at penetrating keratoplasty, Descemet membrane has been multilaminar and irregularly thickened and occasionally with focal nodular excrescences, but they differ from the corneal guttae that characterize FCD (198,254). TEM of Descemet membrane has disclosed an anterior 3 μm thick, 110 nm banded layer, and an extremely thin posterior nonbanded layer (Fig. 18A). Loosely packed collagen fibrils (10–20 nm in diameter) are interspersed with basement membrane-like material

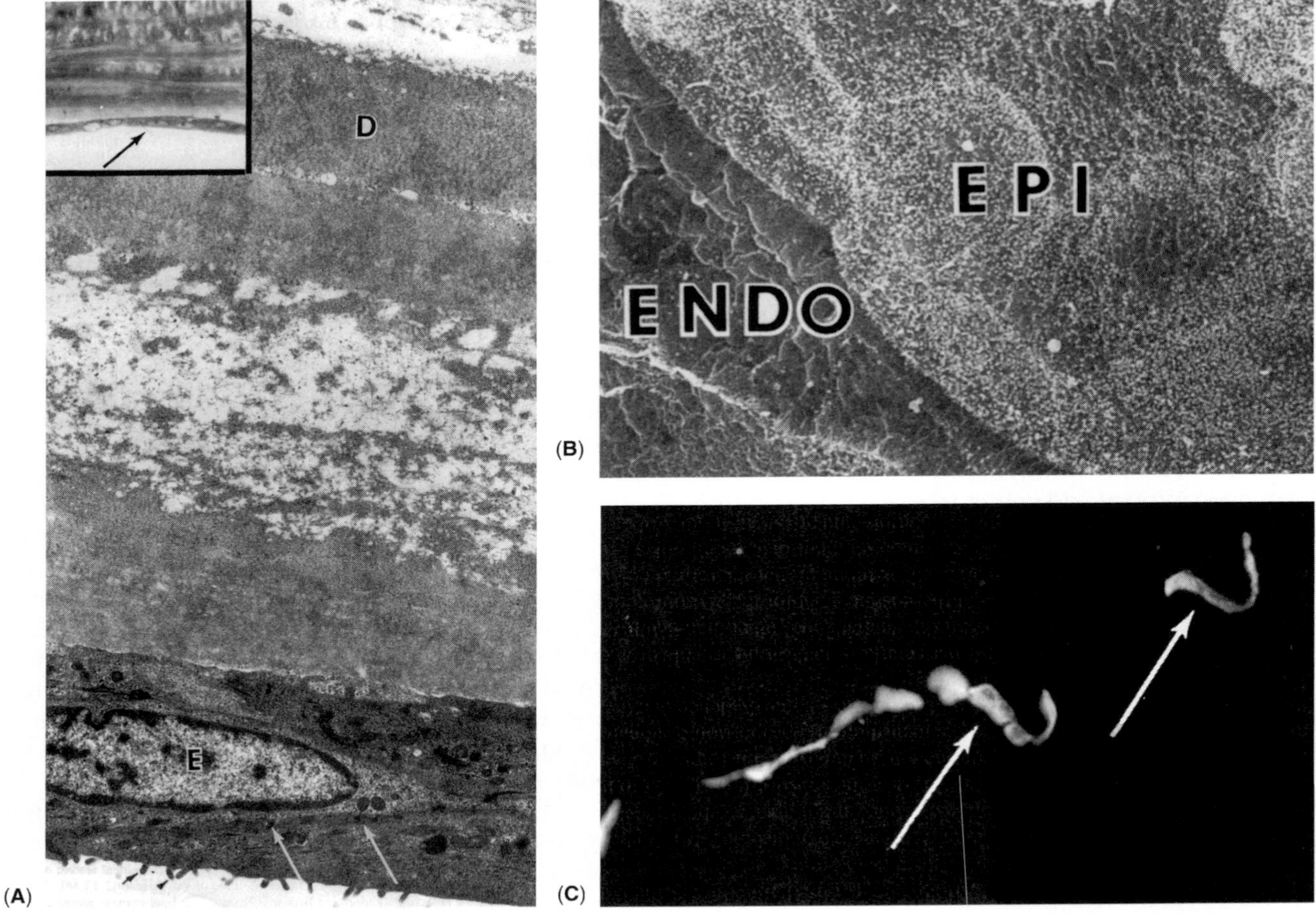

Figure 18 Posterior polymorphous dystrophy. (**A**) Inset shows irregular double layered corneal endothelium (*arrow*) (toluidine blue, × 295). Transmission electron micrograph shows multilaminar Descemet membrane (D) with abnormal "endothelium" (E) showing epithelial-like features, including multiple desmosomal attachments (*arrows*) and microvillous projections (× 7,600). (**B**) Scanning electron micrograph of the posterior cornea showing abnormal "epithelial-like" cells (EPI) with myriad microvilli adjacent to endothelial (ENDO) cells (× 2,600). (**C**) Abnormal expression of keratin by some of the endothelial cells with epithelial-like features (*arrows*) (immunofluorescent stain for keratin AE3, × 470). *Source*: Courtesy of Drs. M.M. Rodrigues, S. Rajagopalan, and K.A. Jones.

and fusiform bundles of 55 to 110 nm banded wide-spacing collagen. Some cells lining the posterior cornea possess epithelial features, such as desmosomes, microvilli, and abundant tonofilaments (keratofibrils) (Fig. 18A and Fig. 18B) (48,198,254,621), and in contrast to the normal corneal endothelium these cells express cytokeratin (Fig. 18C) (521,522). Keratin is normally expressed in the corneal epithelium, the intermediate filament of the endothelium and keratocytes is vimentin (507). Aside from these transformed cells, other cells lining Descemet membrane have the attributes of fibroblasts (254).

Bowman layer is unremarkable but edema of the epithelium and stroma of the cornea may be present in advanced cases. The epithelial transformation of the cells lining the posterior cornea is a prominent feature of advanced cases with corneal edema (48,198,621), but both corneal edema and posterior epithelial cells may be absent (254).

Genetics

Three genes have been implicated in PPCD (*VSX1*, *COL8A2*, *TCF8*). A missense Gln455Lys mutation in the gene encoding the alpha2 chain of collagen type VIII (*COL8A2*) located on human chromosome 1 (1p34.3–p32) has been identified in some patients with PPCD, which a tissue diagnosis in that family has not been documented (39). Leu159Met and Gly160Asp mutations in *VSX1* have also been reported, but the significance of this association is debatable. Evidence for *TCF8* is more convincing (333) and the proband had prominent retrocorneal membrane. *TCF8* encodes transcription factor 8, which has abinding site in the promoter of the *COL4A3* gene.

A yet to be identified gene for autosomal dominant PPCD has also been mapped to the pericentromeric region of human chromosome 20 (20q) (223), where a gene for CHED1 is also located (616). More than one gene in this region could be responsible for both PPCD and CHED1, conceivably because of a cluster of genes with related function; alternatively, the two phenotypes may be allelic (616). However, because blood relatives of individuals with PPCD may have CHED1 (271,351) it seems more likely that one variant of PPCD and CHED1 are due to a mutation in the same gene. PPCD shares developmental, morphological, and clinical similarities with CHED1 and one variant of PPCD is probably related to CHED1 especially since both disorders have been identified in the same family (271,351).

Pathogenesis

The abnormalities of the corneal endothelium presumably represent anomalous development secondary to a genetic mutation. Failure to produce a continuous anterior-banded zone indicates that the cornea is affected before the 12 week of gestation (548). In other cases the morphologically unremarkable anterior-banded portion of Descemet membrane indicates that the corneal endothelium synthesizes normal basement membrane until late in gestation. Because PPCD is usually not associated with corneal edema, the corneal endothelium presumably maintains a normal state of corneal hydration in most affected individuals. Although the morphologically abnormal cells may have been displaced during ocular development, it seems more likely that they underwent metaplasia after lining the posterior surface of the cornea. Other pathologic mesothelial cells sometimes possess epithelial or fibroblastic features.

A major morphologic feature of PPCD is the conversion of the corneal endothelium into cells with epithelial or fibroblastic attributes. The timing of this change remains uncertain, but the observation that Descemet membrane possesses an anterior layer of normal thickness indicates that the corneal endothelium does not manifest functional abnormalities until late in gestation. It also remains to be established whether the corneal endothelial cells undergo a cellular transformation (520,521), because of basic genetic mechanisms, or whether the corneal endothelium gradually gets replaced by embryonally displaced cells of unknown origin (48). Infrequently, desmosomes have been observed in normal human corneal endothelium and this cell presumably may become transformed into a cell with even more epithelial attributes as documented in cell culture studies of rabbit corneal endothelium (375).

Keratoconus

General Remarks

KC, the commonest ectatic disorder of the cornea, was first described more than a quarter of a millennium ago by Mauchart (397) and was differentiated from other aberrations of corneal curvature by Nottingham in 1854 (448). Despite the efforts of numerous individuals knowledge about the basic mechanism whereby the cornea acquires a conical shape with thinning of the stroma remains unknown. However taking into account all available evidence it is apparent that KC is a heterogenous disorder in which there is a genetic predisposition and in which eye rubbing plays an important role in thinning the eye. Perhaps eye rubbing separates the collagen lamellae because of defective glue that keeps the bundles of collagen together. Despite the use of keratoplasty specimens by numerous individuals using a wide variety of techniques most reported findings have been inconsistent.

Clinical Features

KC usually has its onset in youth or adolescence and in about a quarter of the cases, the deformity becomes progressively more severe, particularly during the second decade (21). Myopia and astigmatism are early clinical manifestations (407,566). The earliest sign of KC is a steepening of the corneal curvature. The corneal ectasia most often involves the inferotemporal paracentral cornea (527,688) and the cone extends toward the corneoscleral limbus (660). Some cones are oval sagging; others are nipple-shaped (round) (467). Topographic alterations that develop in the central cornea in a small group of individuals rarely affect the entire corneal surface. Some central conical corneas resemble a bow tie as in astigmatism, but in contrast to the latter the gradient of cones is usually asymmetric (660).

When fully developed, the apex of the cone seldom protrudes more than 10 mm but, in severe cases it may achieve 19 mm. Coinciding with the area of pronounced corneal protrusion corneal hypoesthesia in KC is most marked in the inferior cornea (688). The corneal nerves in KC do not differ from controls despite past claims that they were more prominent.

At an early stage the entire cornea becomes thinner than normal, especially at the cone, and this gradually progresses with time (673). KC is usually bilateral even at the time of diagnosis. Sometimes one eye is minimally involved or appears to be spared but in such cases the conical deformity is often mild and accompanied by asymmetric astigmatism. Computerized video keratography provides a sophisticated method for analyzing the topography of the anterior corneal surface and can detect corneal irregularities in early stages of KC (383,660) before the disorder is evident by slit-lamp biomicroscopy as a slightly relucent anterior corneal stroma.

Irregular superficial linear and often branching defects are frequently evident on slit-lamp biomicroscopy in Bowman layer at the conical apex, and in long-standing cases, a prominent yellow or olive-green ring (Fleischer ring) frequently forms in the epithelium at the base of the cone, which it sometimes encircles.

A progressive visual impairment follows the irregular myopic astigmatism and sometimes opacification of the cone.

The axial length of the eye, which is a major determinant of ocular refractive power, is not significantly different from emmetropic eyes, but shortens after penetrating keratoplasty if the donor tissue is 0.3 mm smaller in diameter than the excised recipient cornea and is a major factor in determining postoperative refractive error (346).

The radius of the central curvature and the central corneal thickness are decreased, whereas the coefficient of radius variation (an expression of the variation radius of curvature) and the coefficient of thickness variation (an expression of the corneal central-peripheral variation) are increased (119).

Specular microscopy has disclosed elongated corneal endothelial cells with their long axes parallel to the lines of stress (343), increased variation in the area (polymegathism) and shape (pleomorphism) of corneal endothelial cells and a decreased number of hexagonal cells (210,393). The possibility of these changes being due to contact lens wear has been raised (210,330).

Striations within the posterior stroma and Descemet membrane are frequently detected early in the course of KC and tears commonly develop in Descemet membrane and the contiguous endothelium (582). If extensive these tears can lead to acute hydrops (discussed below).

Complications

Corneal Opacification

Tears in Bowman layer and the adjacent underlying corneal stroma result in opaque superficial corneal scars. Unusual central corneal opacities may also form in KC due to amyloid deposition (408,409,572).

Acute Hydrops

Posterior corneal tears may produce an abrupt turbid swelling of the central corneal stroma (acute hydrops) in the region of the cone, particularly common in Down syndrome (158,345,539) and sometimes after vigorous eye rubbing, especially in the mentally retarded (45). It has also followed trauma (33) or bathing in a hot, humid Finnish sauna (530).

Acute hydrops may lead to unresponsive glaucoma (malignant glaucoma) (248). Following acute hydrops the cornea can regain its transparency, while the defects in Descemet membrane become scarred. If severe the ruptured Descemet membrane detaches and forms extensive ledges and new endothelium may resurface the exposed posterior stroma and the anterior aspect of the ledges (582). Rarely, a stromal pseudocyst in continuity with the anterior chamber develops through breaks in Descemet membrane and simulates severe corneal ectasia (386).

Corneal Perforation

Corneal perforation in KC is extremely rare (342,529) and pregnancy and topical corticosteroids may have contributed to it in one case (342).

Postoperative Complications

After visual loss is no longer correctable with glasses or contact lenses KC is commonly treated by keratoplasty. Despite the donor material being usually thicker than the adjacent recipient tissue the current success rate of corneal grafting is >80% (429,479,551). After penetrating keratoplasty the graft steadily becomes thinner reaching a subnormal thickness about 6 months postoperatively, but it then gradually thickens and retains a normal compactness within 6 years of corneal grafting (124). KC rarely develops in the graft after many years and in such cases the possibility of the primary defect being in the donor material can not be excluded (125).

Epidemiology

Some reports have documented a female preponderance of KC (21,613), but this sex difference has not been apparent in other reviews (144,281) and in some series males have predominated (68,551,675). In one county (Olmsted County, Minnesota) in the United States the incidence rates of KC have not changed over time, the overall average annual rate being 2.0 per 100,000 population. The overall prevalence rate in that population is 54.5 per 100,000 (281). At the time of their birth 150 patients with KC had an excess of significantly older mothers than the general population (674), perhaps because of age-related chromosomal abnormalities. This observation has not been confirmed (239).

Genetics

Since its recognition as an entity it has become apparent that KC is a heterogenous disorder with a genetic component despite a negative family history in most cases of KC (122,485). KC undoubtedly involves more than one gene and an interaction between genetic and environmental factors probably exists. The frequency of familial KC varies between

6% and 19% (210,281) and numerous cases have apparent or possible autosomal dominant or recessive modes of inheritance (132,140,281,385,487,633). An analysis of other pedigrees with KC suggests a multifactorial mode of inheritance (210) and this may account for the variable expressivity of KC among family members and the occurrence of KC in different syndromes. KC has been reported in monozygotic twins (665), but also in only one identical twin (51). Some members of families with KC only develop myopic asymmetrical astigmatism. Blood relatives of affected individuals may have preconical stages of KC, with the initial discernible abnormality usually being a lack of normal parallelism of the reflected concentric images detected by keratoscopy. Because of this variable expressivity in pedigrees with KC, evaluations of the cornea in family members require sophisticated methods. Investigations using computer-assisted topographic analysis have been started and will hopefully lead to a better understanding of inherited factors in the pathogenesis of KC (488). Also, convincing evidence in support of a genetic role in the commonly associated atopic disease may implicate a genetic component in the causation of KC.

Linkage Studies

Loci for autosomal dominant KC have been mapped to chromosome 2 (2p24) (237), chromosome 3 (3p14–q13) (55), chromosome 5 (5q14.1–q21.3) (606), and chromosome 16 (16q22.3–q23) (628). A form of KC with cataract has been mapped to chromosome 15 (15q) (98).

Candidate Genes

A nucleotide change in the *VSX1* gene have been identified in 4.7% of patients with KC (222), but others have failed to find *VSX1* mutations in KC (14). The frequent association with Down syndrome points to chromosome 21, which also contains the gene *COL6A1* encoding for the α-1 chain of collagen type VI. However, using a probe for this candidate gene linkage was not found in one KC family (487). The finding of KC in a single case of the Angelman syndrome (MIM #105830) (includes ocular and general depigmentation) (376) raises the possibility of a role for genes on chromosome 15 as approximately 50% of individuals with this syndrome have a cytogenetically visible deletion of the long arm of chromosome 15 (15q11–q13).

Rare associations of KC with other inherited diseases may simply be due to chance, but reports of this nature can not be brushed aside as irrelevant as KC may be part of the expression of the mutant gene that causes the accompanying disorder. Regardless it can potentially provide clues for future linkage studies. In this regard it is noteworthy that KC has been documented with Alagille syndrome (MIM #118450 and #610205) (arteriohepatic dysplasia, growth retardation, hypothyroidism, typical facies, brachydactylia, and skin lichenification) (344,618), Bardet–Biedl syndrome (MIM #209900) (156), Leber congenital amaurosis (137,186), retinitis pigmentosa (148,588,635), bilateral macular coloboma and retinitis pigmentosa (160), macular atrophy-Jadassohn type of anetoderma and bilateral subcapsular cataracts (58), gyrate atrophy and hyperornithinemia (76), deep filiform corneal dystrophy (381), FCD (357,358), LCD type I (231), GCD type II (561), fleck corneal dystrophy (480), PPCD with or without progressive essential iris atrophy (30,41,181,345,651), Turner syndrome (450), ectodermal and mesodermal anomalies (335), Crouzon syndrome (MIM #123500) (670), congenital hip dysplasia (449), and false chordae tendineae in the left ventricle (32).

KC has been reported in association with retinopathy of prematurity (373), aniridia, iridoschisis, persistent pupillary membrane, ectopia lentis, congenital cataracts, microcornea, blue sclerae, and Chandler syndrome (180).

Histocompatibility Antigens

Most investigations have not detected an association between a susceptibility to KC and any specific HLA antigen (312,485,493), but three independent studies found an increase in HLA-B5 among Caucasians with KC (40,276,321). In two studies (26,251) a high frequency of HLA-B5 was also present in the controls, but in the other series (321) the frequency of HLA-B5 in KC was statistically significant. HLA-B7 has been significantly less frequent in KC than in controls (2113). One investigation found HLA-B15 to be increased in KC (95). HLA-B27 has been noted in the mother and two siblings with KC (179).

KC patients with HLA-B12 and HLA-B27 and avascular corneas seem to have a high risk of late graft rejection, with reactions triggered by nasopharyngeal infections (210).

Associations

Atopy and Other Allergic Conditions

Since Ridley (504) first drew attention to the association of KC with atopy, many observers have confirmed this observation (99,175,213,228,277,288,370, 490,504,506,567,585). Despite flaws in various studies the belief that atopy is more common in individuals with KC than in general ophthalmic patients remains entrenched in the literature. KC patients with and without atopy do not differ with regard to sex, age of onset, or rate of keratoplasty (213). The serum IgE is significantly elevated in a high percentage of patients with KC in keeping with the associated atopy (280,490).

The atopic conditions associated with KC have included vernal keratoconjunctivitis (VKC), bronchial asthma, hay fever, and atopic dermatitis (eczema) (see Chapter 5) (189,192,288,370,447,537,555,599). Bronchial asthma affects 0.4% to 1% of the general population, but is found in 16% (585) of individuals with KC. Hayfever occurs in about 20% of the general population but is more prevalent in KC (32.6%) (277) and 36% (585). Eczema has been reported in 9% (585) and 32% (85) of cases of KC compared to 3% in the general population. One study of 182 cases of KC detected a history of atopy in 35% compared with 12% in the matched control group (490). Others have found allergies in 30% to 50% of patients with KC (36,85). In 31 patients with KC and unmatched controls, Lowell and Carroll (374) failed to detect an increased incidence of atopy. Aside from atopic dermatitis numerous individuals with KC have had other cutaneous lesions (42,145).

When associated with atopy KC is usually bilateral and the abnormal cornea occurs more frequently on the side of the dominant hand suggesting that the eye on that side may be rubbed more extensively (213). In several unilateral cases of VKC the KC only involved the eye on the side as the VKC (599).

Ocular Massage

In 1961, Ridley (505) first drew attention to the possibility that eye rubbing might be important in the pathogenesis of KC. Since then the relationship between excessive eye rubbing and KC has become well established and one report considered excessive eye rubbing the dominant etiological factor in two-thirds of patients with KC who progress to contact lens wear (277). Eye rubbing is a feature of several conditions with which KC is associated including atopic disease, contact lens wearing, Down syndrome and other causes of mental retardation and miscellaneous ocular disorders. Repeated or vigorous eye rubbing is particularly prominent in the mentally retarded (45).

Two unique case studies add weight to the argument that eye rubbing may contribute to the development of KC. One individual was a celibate priest who achieved orgasms by ocular masturbation (277), the other patient developed unilateral KC after massaging his left eye to terminate many daily episodes of paroxymal atrial tachycardia (88).

Pressure on the Globe

KC has been associated with direct mechanical pressure on the globe as in the floppy eyelid syndrome (114,441,459). This syndrome, which is characterized by a soft rubbery tarsus that allows the upper eyelid to be readily everted and papillary conjunctivitis, typically occurs in obese individuals and is thought to result from eyelid eversion during sleep. Most examples of KC associated with the floppy eyelid syndrome have been unilateral and on the side of the more severely affected eyelid. Unilateral cases have slept with their head facing predominantly on the side with the floppy eyelid and KC. Bilateral KC has accompanied bilateral symmetric floppy eyelids in patients who sleep face down (568). Isolated case reports have documented KC with somnambulism and eye pressing (638) or an ipsilateral chronic slowly progressive eyelid and orbital cavernous hemangioma (233).

Connective Tissue Disorders

KC is seldom associated with obvious connective tissue disorders, but a few reports suggest that some cases may be a manifestation of an inherited disorder of collagen. KC is rarely associated with Ehlers–Danlos syndrome, especially type II (mitis type) (MIM #130010), but also Ehlers–Danlos syndrome type IV (ecchymotic type) (MIM #130050) and Ehlers–Danlos syndrome type VI (ocular Ehlers–Danlos syndrome)(MIM #235400) (173,265,338,422,511). Mitral valve prolapse, a feature of numerous systemic disorders was detected by two-dimensional echocardiography in 12 of 32 (38%) patients with KC and in only 3 of 23 (13%) patients without KC (29), but this increased prevalence was not confirmed in another study of 95 cases patients with KC (585). Robertson (511) reported hypermobile joints in 50% of 44 patients with KC. Another study, however, found trunk or knee joint hypermobility among patients with KC to be as frequent as controls, but noted that patients with KC are five times more likely than normal to show hypermobility of the metacarpophalyngeal and wrist joints (676). An additional review failed to detect a significant difference in the prevalence of hypermobile joints in patients with KC and controls (585). A few reports have described KC or keratoglobus in persons with blue sclerae, hyperextensible joints, and deafness (37,71,201). Rare cases have been associated with Marfan syndrome (MIM #154700) (27) or osteogenesis imperfecta type I (MIM #166200) (690).

Mental Retardation

KC is common in Down syndrome (92,158,277,337, 345,514,539,549,558) and it has been found in in 0.5% (514), 3.5% to 8% (92,277,331,558), and 15% (549) of persons with this chromosomal trisomy. KC is also common in other mentally retarded individuals, including the congenital rubella syndrome (45). A review of 212 institutionalized mentally retarded individuals disclosed 16 with KC (7.5%) and 8 cases were unilateral (221).

Contact Lens Wear

Many individuals with KC have been contact lenses wearers (179,214,380,571). Because contact lenses are commonly used for myopia, astigmatism and for treating the early symptoms of KC (179,566) the association of KC with contact lens wear may be coincidental. However, do they contribute to the expression of KC in a predisposed individual or cause KC? This issue, which is of medicolegal importance, remains unanswered and would require a cohort (prospective) or randomized clinical trial to be resolved (118).

In one retrospective case-control study of 199 patients with KC (398 eyes) 53 patients (106 eyes) developed KC after wearing contact lenses for many years (mean 12.2 years) (380). This group was older at the time of diagnosis than individuals who developed KC spontaneously (380). Moreover they had central rather than decentered cones, and tended toward flatter corneal curvatures (380). As pointed out by Ederer and Ferris (118) case-control studies are unable to establish whether contact lens wear preceded the onset of KC, because contact lenses are often used to treat the early symptoms of KC. Nevertheless, rigid contact lenses frequently produce photokeratoscopic images that simulate early KC (661) and these changes may not resolve until at least 5 months after discontinuing contact lens wear (661).

Thyroid Dysfunction

Individuals with KC may be hypothyroidic, euthyroidic, or hyperthyroidic (267), but several observations have led to the hypothesis that thyroid dysfunction may play a role in the pathogenesis of KC: (*i*) hypothyroidism occurs with greater frequency in Down syndrome than in the general population (94,141); (*ii*) KC may follow thyroidectomy (23,291); (*iii*) thyroid hormones are important in corneal development (87,392); (*iv*) KC usually begins at puberty when thyroxine-binding globulin is at its lowest level during life (136); (*v*) KC has occurred in a patient with the Alagille syndrome and hypothyroidism (344); (*vi*) thyroxine is important in collagen synthesis (116); and (*vii*) irrespective of their thyroid function the tear thyroxine levels in patients with KC are 2 to 50 times higher than normal and that these levels are higher during the progression of KC and decline once corneal curvature reaches a new steady value (267).

Histopathology

Abnormalities have been documented in all layers of the cornea.

Corneal Epithelium and Its Basement Membrane

The corneal epithelium is frequently of irregular thickness and iron deposits occur in areas corresponding to Fleischer ring (178,408). The epithelial cells are relatively normal, but increased ribosomes have been noted (168). SEM of the corneal surface has disclosed nonspecific degenerative changes, such as cell membrane degradation, irregularly shaped cells, sometimes swollen and in other cases shrunken (59,261,263). When viewed by TEM the Fleischer ring contains accumulations of ferritin in widened intercellular spaces and/or in cytoplasmic vacuoles of the corneal epithelium. In a TEM study of the central cone area of 14 KC corneal buttons Iwamoto and DeVoe (246) observed peculiar enveloped particles surrounded by electron-dense finely filamentous zones. These structures were located within a thickened epithelial basement membrane, in Bowman zone and in connective tissue replacing portions of it, as well as within and between corneal epithelial cells. The nature of the particles, which have not been reported by other investigators, remains unknown, but probably represent an artifact of tissue processing.

The basement membrane on which the epithelium rests may be abnormally thickened, fragmented, or disrupted. Bundles of oxytalan fibers (see Chapter 36), which are absent in normal corneas, have been identified in the cornea in early and acute KC as well as in scarred corneas (16). Electron-dense fine fibrils have been noted beneath the basement membrane (168).

Bowman Layer

Multiple fractures of Bowman zone are a prominent morphologic hallmark of KC (Fig. 19) (78) and correspond to the linear and often branching clear spaces, which are frequently evident on slit-lamp biomicroscopy (550). These breaks in Bowman layer are often filled by collagenous tissue, fibroblasts, or epithelium (410).

Stroma

The structural basis for the corneal thinning in KC, which is a paucity of collagen fibers within the corneal stroma (Fig. 19), is the most striking and consistent finding in KC especially in the thin ectatic portion. Jakus maintained that the individual lamellae were thinned (249), but others have found the collagen lamellae in KC to be of normal thickness (602), but with fewer than normal collagen lamellae within the affected cornea (477,602). In contrast to the normal cornea, which contains approximately 40 collagen lamellae in its central portion and about 60 in its periphery, the number of lamellae is markedly reduced in KC (477). The individual collagen fibers

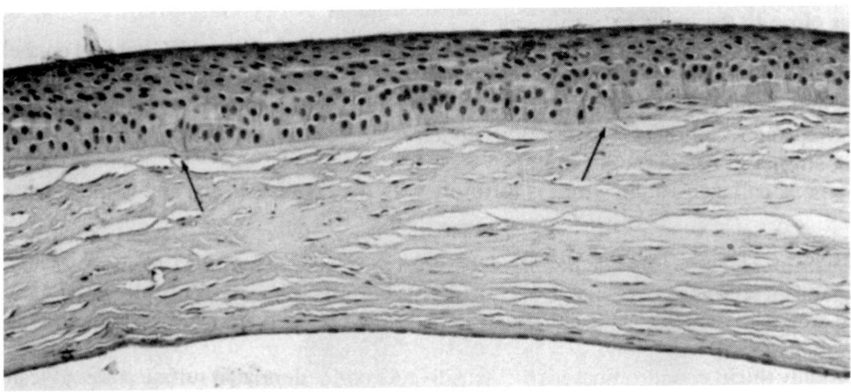

Figure 19 Keratoconus. The corneal stroma is thinner than normal so that the corneal epithelium constitutes more than one-third of the corneal thickness. Bowman zone is also defective in some regions (*arrows*) (hematoxylin and eosin, × 150).

are of normal thickness (25–30 nm) and possess their usual cross-striational periodicity.

In KC the density of corneal fibroblasts (keratocytes) in the central corneal stroma is similar to normal corneas indicating that KC corneas contain fewer fibroblasts than controls, because the stroma of KC corneas is thinner than normal (602). Some observers have been impressed by excessive morphologic variation of the corneal stromal cells (477). Corneal fibroblasts may manifest a variety of ultrastructural abnormalities, such as an apparent increase in the number of cytoplasmic organelles and pseudopodia, cytoplasmic vacuolization, and nuclear indentations. Keratocyte apoptosis has been noted in the anterior corneal stroma (290) in an area where keratocytes may normally contain more mitochondria than in the posterior stroma (136,565).

Disorganized collagen fibers and electron-dense material is often evident in the superficial corneal stroma, but morphologic evidence of collagen degeneration as found in corneal ulcers is conspicuously absent. A noticeable accumulation of fibrillogranular material in the corneal stroma, sometimes surrounds abnormal corneal fibroblasts and separates individual collagen fibers more than usual (477,478). Even amyloid sometimes deposits in the corneal stroma in KC (408,572).

Although the corneal stroma is usually thinner than normal, it may be thickened late in the course of the disease from edema.

Descemet Membrane and the Corneal Endothelium

In advanced KC undulations and even ruptures may develop in Descemet membrane (*Kammerwassereinbruch*). Defects in Descemet membrane and the corneal endothelium are repaired by an extension of neighboring flattened endothelial cells and their secretion of new basement membrane (476). Because of inadequate endothelial cell junctions corneal edema may persist (476). Ultrastructural studies of the cornea after severe hydrops have disclosed basement membrane-like material adjacent to the curled end of the ruptured Descemet membrane and between and around individual corneal endothelial cells (582). Other abnormalities of the corneal endothelium that have been noted include severe degradation of endothelial cells and fibroblastic transformation (261,262,582).

Histochemistry, Immunohistochemistry, and Biochemical Analyses

Biochemical analyses have been performed on KC corneas over many years by many investigators (65,89,455,489,505,666), but these studies have usually lacked adequate controls and have not taken into account the usual accompanying corneal scarring, prior treatment with contact lenses, or the associated clinical conditions. The significance of many of the observations remains uncertain as most investigations do not meet contemporary state-of-the-art analytical standards.

Protein

Corneas with KC contain less total protein/mg dry weight than normal corneas (89,685), decreased protein glycosylation (509), an increased glycoprotein/collagen ratio (509). Some analyses of the extactable corneal proteins have disclosed apparent alterations in the relative amounts of particular proteins or the presence of proteins in KC specimens that are absent in normal corneas. Critchfield and colleagues (89) using sodium dodecyl sulfate-polyacrylamide gel electrophoresis detected a distinctive 75 kDa band in KC corneal extracts that stained with silver, but not with Coomassie blue or Schiff reagent. The patterns of two-dimensional electrophoretic maps of extracts of KC corneas have also differed from normal (458). In such a study KC corneas contained two abnormal components; elevated amounts of three normal corneal components and reduced amounts of three normal corneal proteins (458). One normal corneal protein found in reduced amounts in KC corneas had a molecular weight and isoelectric point suggestive of a subunit of prolyl-4-hydroxylase, an enzyme required for the hydroxylation of proline residues of collagen (458). The significance of these yet to be confirmed observations remains unknown. Based on the ability of their total cellular RNA to produce protein in a cell-free system Yue and colleagues have separated cultured KC cells into those containing normal amounts of total RNA with normal activity and a normal rate of protein synthesis and those consisting of more RNA than normal, but with a markedly reduced protein translational efficiency (686). Some strains of cells derived from KC corneas synthesize protein at the normal rate; other strains produce protein at a decreased rate (685,686).

Protease Inhibitors

α1-proteinase inhibitor (α1-antitrypsin) is normally detectable in the epithelium, stroma, and endothelium of the normal human cornea with the immunoperoxidase technique (627). The staining intensity in the epithelium and stromal lamellae of KC corneas, appears to be markedly reduced but not in scarred or otherwise diseased corneas (534).

Collagen

As expected chemical analyses on KC corneas have disclosed, less collagen than usual (65,89,509,666). Compared to controls some KC corneas have contained decreased total hydroxyproline content (240), but other KC corneas have contained normal amounts of this amino acid, which reflects total collagen content (685).

In keeping with the immunohistochemical findings discussed earlier, soluble collagens of KC corneas consist of 90% collagen type I (normal 85%), 5% type III (normal <10%), and 5% collagen type V (normal 5%) (398).

Except in osteogenesis imperfecta type I (690), the collagen in KC corneas has not differed from normal (489,690). Organ cultures of KC corneas synthesize slightly different ratios of collagen type I: collagen type III than normal (9:1 in KC; 10:1 in normal corneas) (442). Higher than normal levels of collagenolytic activity have been detected in the medium surrounding organ cultures of KC corneas (275,445,496).

The amino acid composition of collagen in KC is normal, but the amino acid sequence of corneal collagen in KC has not been determined. High- and low-angle X-ray diffraction patterns obtained with synchrotron radiation indicate that the interfibrillar spacing between collagen fibrils within KC and control corneas is the same over a range of hydrations. The intermolecular spacings are lower in KC corneas at normal physiological hydration and over a range of hydrations (167).

Collagen cross-linking, which is important in the maintenance of the mechanical properties of the cornea, involves the formation of covalent cross-links within and between collagen molecules (see Chapter 44). The cross-linking pattern of collagen and of reducible collagen cross-linking in KC corneas is normal (89).

The hydroxylysine levels in KS corneas were decreased in some reports (89,509), but have been normal in others (72,275,455). One study detected higher levels of lysinonorleucine, a cross-linking amino acid, in five KC corneas than in normal age-matched corneas (72). The procollagen in the medium surrounding cultured KC corneal stromal cells differs from that of normal cells, but also among cells from various KC patients (684). In culture certain strains of KC cells synthesize normal amounts of collagen in culture, whereas others produce reduced amounts (685).

Cells derived from the stroma of KC corneas have been found to: (*i*) synthesize a normal ratio of collagens types I and III and a normal α1/α2 ratio in collagen type I (241), (*ii*) produce an abnormal relative proportion of collagen type I and A and B collagen chains (684).

In a study of fibroblasts isolated from KC corneas the main structural cross-links were found to be the dihydroxy (hydroxylysinohydroxynorleucine), the monohydroxy (hydroxylysinonorleucine), and the lysinonorleucine cross-links. The levels of individual intermolecular lysine derived cross-links in collagen synthesized from normal and KC corneas did not differ significantly (279).

One study found the activity of prolyl-4-hydroxylase, an enzyme involved in the posttranslational modification of collagen, to be elevated in KC corneas (240), suggesting that the synthesis of collagen by KC corneas may be enhanced.

Because γ interferon (IFNγ), tumor necrosis factor (TNF), and interleukin 1 (IL1) influence the synthesis of collagen by fibroblasts, the number of membrane-binding sites for these cytokines, and the dissociation constant for each ligand were determined on cultured corneal fibroblasts from normal human and KC corneas (130). The IFNγ and TNF-binding sites in normal and KC corneas did not differ, but fibroblasts from KC corneas had fourfold more IL1-binding sites than normal fibroblasts.

An analysis of corneas stained with the collagen dye Sirius red has shown normal stained collagen in some KC corneas, but reduced collagen staining per surface area than controls in others (687).

Based on immunohistochemical studies on tissue sections using specific antibodies, collagen types I, III, IV, V, VI, and VII generally have a normal distribution in corneas with KC (437,442,690), the exception being in scar tissue in Bowman layer of some specimens (442,690). Immunohistochemical evidence supports the biochemical finding that collagen type I is normally the major type of collagen in the human corneal stroma (437). Collagen type I is also present in corneal scars in KC (442). Collagen type III, an attribute of scar tissue, has been detected in KC corneas (398,442) in scarred regions and at the host–graft juncture. Collagen types I and III are located among the collagen fibrils, while collagen type V is either on or close to the collagen fibrils (437). Collagen type IV is found in the basement membrane of the normal and KC corneal epithelium (437), but appears to overexpressed in KC epithelium (431). It is present particularly in Bowman layer and Descemet membrane in KC specimens (437,442). The distribution of collagen type IV is essentially the same in normal and KC corneas, but this ECM component is also abnormally distributed in the anterior stroma in KC corneas (623). Antitype collagen type V antibody reacts diffusely with the corneal stroma and with Bowman layer in KC (437).

Lysosomal and Proteolytic Enzymes

Acid phosphatase, acid esterase, and acid lipase activity has been demonstrated in the epithelium, stroma, and endothelium of KC and normal human corneas (536). The epithelium, especially the basal part, of KC corneas appears to have higher levels of these markers of lysosomal activity than normal or scarred corneas or corneas with FCD (536). The possibility that degradative enzymes might be upregulated or that protease inhibitors might be downregulated has been investigated with some support (689). Enhanced collagenase type I (240) and collagenase type IV (gelatinase) (matrix metalloproteinase 2) activities have been detected in the media of KC corneal fibroblast cultures (284). Elevated gelatinase activity, which is detectable only after proteolytic activation (240), occurs despite lower amounts of total protein being produced by the KC corneal fibroblast cultures (284).

Other Extracellular Matrix Components

The distribution of fibronectin is essentially the same in normal and KC corneas, but it may also be abnormally distributed in the anterior stroma in KC corneas (623). Fibronectin is present in Descemet membrane and in the corneal stroma (437), where more than normal seems to be present (431). The epithelial basement membrane of normal and KC corneas contain laminin, bullous pemphigoid antigen, fibronectin, and fibrin/fibrinogen (421,431,623). Fibronectin is abundant in Descemet membrane in KC. Laminin is abundant in the corneal epithelial basement membrane and Descemet membrane in KC, but KC corneal stroma has less laminin than normal corneas. In KC corneas immunohistochemical staining for fibrin/fibrinogen is weaker than normal (421).

In agreement with immunohistochemical findings, discussed earlier, extracts of the corneal epithelium and stroma in KC contain less α1-proteinase inhibitor than normal (534).

In some studies, the GAGs have been essentially normal (65). Other investigations have, however, reported a relative increase in the glucosaminoglycan (KS) fraction and a decrease in the galactosaminoglycan (chondroitin sulfate) fraction. But with more recent immunochemical methods much less KS has been found in KC than normal corneas (171). The amount of extractable lumican core protein in KC is normal (171), but the lumican in KC corneas seems to contain fewer KS chains than normal, or KS with a modified structure (171). Both lowered total hexosamine sulfate (65,666) and increased extractable hexosamines (509) have been documented. Compared with controls KC corneas have increased hexoses (509) and an increased affinity for the castor-bean agglutinin (89). The uronic acid content has been reported as increased (89) and decreased (509). Using safranin O to measure the polyanion content in paraffin sections (687) many, but not all, KC corneas show markedly higher polyanion staining per surface area than the controls suggesting that KC corneas may contain increased amounts of GAGs and other polyanions (687).

Abnormally thick decorin filaments apparently accumulate especially in scarred areas of KC corneas (535). Lumican (KS proteoglycan) filaments appear to be less abundant than in normal control corneas (535).

Synchrotron X-ray diffraction studies indicate that KC corneas differ from controls after staining collagen-associated PGs with cupromeronic blue. The KC corneal stroma has a specific, ordered PG that is present in lower numbers along the collagen fibrils, and it stains less with cupromeronic blue or is in a more disordered arrangement than in the controls (159,167).

Immunohistochemical studies using monoclonal antibodies have disclosed increased chondroitin and DS and decreased sulfated KS in the stroma of scarred corneas with KC, in common with nonspecific scarred corneas (535). Decorin and lumican synthesized by organ cultures of KC corneas are of normal size, but the decorin/lumican ratio is increased in KC and the KS chains of two lumicans from KC corneas are considerably shorter (Mr 44 and 33 kDa) than normal (667). GAG metabolism of cultured fibroblasts from human KC corneas have disclosed nothing relevant to the pathogenesis of KC. Yue and colleagues (683) found that after incubating corneal stroma in the presence of appropriate radioactive precursors most newly synthesized GAGs produced by KC cells in culture were in the surrounding medium as opposed to the cell layer, which also has markedly reduced heparan sulfate (HS) (683). This was in contrast to what was observed with normal corneal fibroblasts.

However, these observations were not confirmed by other investigators (43,44). KC fibroblasts have been found to produce a higher proportion of HS than controls (43).

The plasma membranes of most strains of cultured KC corneal stromal cells contain more binding sites for concanavalin A, *Ricinus communis* agglutinin I, and soybean agglutinin than controls suggesting that they may contain elevated amounts. Certain lectins bind normally to the epithelium, endothelium, and Descemet membrane of KC corneas (470), but in contrast to normal corneas, some lectins (peanut agglutinin, *Phaseolus vulgaris* erythroagglutinin, *R. communis* agglutinin I, and *Lens culinaris* agglutinin) bind to KC corneal tissue where breaks occur in Bowman layer, in scar tissue and in the adjacent stroma, suggesting that scarred regions of the anterior stroma in KC corneas may contain oligosaccharides with terminal D-galactose (β1-3)-D-N-acetylgalactosamine disaccharides, increased amounts of glycoconjugates with terminal β-galactose residues, increased amounts of glycoconjugates with glucose/mannose residues, as well as biantennary complex-type glycopeptides containing two outer galactose residues and a residue of N-acetylglucosamine (470). These altered lectin-binding sites in KC probably result from scar tissue as corneal scars in other conditions have similar attributes (470).

Other Studies

Cytotoxic byproducts of oxidative stress from pathways involving nitric oxide, lipid peroxidation (66,282), and abnormal enzymes with antioxidant properties (31,187,188,283) have been detected in KC. A gene expression profile study of human corneas found a novel cornea-expressed gene and the absence of transcripts for aquaporin 5 (486).

Transcription factors regulate gene transcription and the expression of one transcription factor (Sp1) has been found to be elevated in KC corneas (77,388,653,654). Another enzyme with reported enhanced expression in KC corneas and cultures of them is a transmembrane phosphotyrosine phosphatase (252). Abnormally low serum magnesium levels have been reported in KC and because this metal is an important cofactor in more than 300 enzymatic reactions a relationship between KC and magnesium deficiency has been postulated (610).

Biomechanics

Because of the reduced mechanical stability of KC corneas the biomechanical properties of the cornea have been evaluated in an attempt to understand the pathogenesis of KC. However, methods for measuring ocular rigidity and the viscoelastic properties of the cornea leave much to be desired. The distensibility of KC corneal tissue is increased (119). Ocular rigidity is decreased in some cases of KC (100,120,215), but one study did not find a significant difference between normal eyes and those with KC (142). An increased elasticity has been detected in strips of KC corneas (22,439), but not in the physiological range of pressure (439).

Animal Models

A satisfactory animal model of KC has not been identified, but lesions resembling some aspects of KC have been documented in several species. Bilaterally thinned and prominently curved corneas with clinical features consistent with KC have been observed in a 15-year-old female rhesus monkey (466). A condition with some features of human KC has been studied in chicken (655).

Pathogenesis

General Remarks

Structural elements of the cornea are lost early and are evident clinically as corneal thinning, while stretching of the cornea increases its curvature. Despite extensive clinical, morphological, histochemical, immunohistochemical, biochemical, and biomechanical observations on KC by many investigators many questions about the pathogenesis remain unanswered. Little is known about the fundamental defect(s) that lead to the corneal thinning or why KC becomes arrested as an abortive form in certain members of affected families.

A major difficulty in understanding KC stems for the considerable disagreement among investigators in various apparently comparable studies and the lack of confirmation of many observations. Observations that have been confirmed by more than one research group are the presence of thin corneas usually with numerous breaks in Bowman layer and a decreased collagen content at the time of corneal grafting (65,89).

Many rare associations of KC are probably coincidental, but some such as atopy, contact lens wearing, Down syndrome, and eye rubbing have occurred sufficiently often to warrant serious consideration in the pathogenesis of KC. KC may share undetermined causal factors with associated multifactorial disorders.

Heterogeneity

In view of the varied associations with KC, several different pathogenetic sequences may culminate in KC. Although there are many plausible explanations for disagreements among investigators one of the more cogent is that KC is not a single condition, but a reaction to different fundamental disorders. Evidence for heterogeneity includes: the wide range of associated conditions; joint hypermobility in some cases

(510), but not in others (142); low ocular rigidity in some cases (100,120), but not in others (142); differences in collagen staining (687); differences in hydroxyproline content of KC corneas in biochemical analyses, as well as differences in protein and total collagen synthesized by KC corneal stromal cells (685); discrepancies in RNA activity of cultured corneal fibroblasts (686); discrepancies in the production of GAGs in culture (43,44,683); two subgroups of KC based on analyses of total protein produced by cultured KC corneal cells (685).

While heterogeneity may explain some contradictory data in the literature, other possibilities include vagaries of cell culture systems, the state of activation of the cultured corneal fibroblasts derived from the cornea, and the degree of associated corneal scarring.

Abnormalities Secondary to Corneal Scarring

Because corneal grafting is performed late in the course of the disease some abnormalities in KC corneas are probably secondary to scarring or to previous treatment, including contact lens wear. The cellular activity varies in different specimens. Studies using cell and organ culture systems have particularly failed to take into account the difficulty, if not impossible ability to control for the variable status of the population of activated corneal cells associated with the inevitable scarring of variable degree and duration.

Structural Basis for Corneal Thinning

Seeing that KC usually develops in apparently normal eyes corneal thinning presumably occurs as a sequel to a flaw in the mechanisms controlling the maintenance of normal corneal curvature. The cornea could become thinner because of fewer collagen lamellae, less collagen fibrils per lamella, closer packing of collagen fibrils, or various combinations of these possibilities. However, the individual collagen lamellae in KC corneas seem to be of normal thickness, but reduced in number (477,602). Also, the individual collagen fibers are of normal diameter and the thinning of the stroma in KC is not a result of closer packing of the collagen fibrils (167).

In theory, the corneal thinning of KC may result from: (*i*) a defective formation of extracellular constituents of corneal tissue, (*ii*) a destruction of previously formed components, (*iii*) an increased distensibility of corneal tissue with sliding of the collagen fibers and/or collagen lamellae, or (*iv*) combinations of these mechanisms.

Defective Formation of Extracellular Constituents of Cornea

Because the mechanical strength of the cornea depends primarily on collagen, abnormalities in this component of the ECM, and especially of its cross-linking, warrant serious consideration in an evaluation of the pathogenesis of KC. But evidence to support this possibility is tenuous, and convincing evidence for defective collagen cross-linking is lacking despite appraisals by several groups of investigators.

From a study combining TEM, biosynthetic and biochemical analytical techniques an interruption in collagen synthesis in KC has been suggested (509). A diminished synthesis of collagen and a relative increase in the synthesis of structural glycoprotein (509) can account for the diminution of collagen fibers, the presence of excessive amounts of fibrillogranular material in the stroma, and the biochemical findings. Evidence of an impaired synthesis of corneal matrix is lacking.

Comparative studies of several collagen types indicate that KC is not directly related to alterations in collagen composition and distribution (690). No abnormality in the molecular structure of collagen has been found that explains the markedly reduced mechanical stability of KC corneas.

An abnormality of corneal growth or a developmental defect in the formation of the collagen lamellae could result in corneal thinning, but evidence for such a possibility is lacking in KC. However, it could account for some rare forms of KC associated with ocular developmental anomalies.

Destruction of Previously Formed Components

An alternative hypothesis attributes the progressive corneal thinning in KC to increased degradative activities by matrix metalloproteinases which destroy corneal stroma (61,275,562,563). The strongest evidence in favor of this view is the finding of enhanced collagenase activity by KC corneas in organ culture (275,496) and by stromal cells from KC corneas in culture (240,284). However, against collagenolysis being the cause of corneal thinning in KC is the observation that KC corneas lack the morphologic features of stromal destruction that one would expect from excessive enzymatic digestion of collagen.

Decreased levels of α1-proteinase inhibitor in both biochemical assays and immunohistochemical studies of KC corneas could account for why stromal loss occurs in KC (534).

Both the corneal epithelium and stroma have been proposed as the source of proteolytic activity. The above mentioned increased collagenase activity in KC corneas in both organ cultures and cultures of stromal cells suggests that the corneal stroma may be the source of collagenolytic activity.

Based on his TEM observations, Teng (608) suggested that the fundamental defect in KC may reside in the corneal epithelium. This hypothesis is supported by an apparent increase in the activity of lysosomal acid hydrolases within the corneal epithelium (536). Also, since the initial digestion from an epithelial source would be expected in the underlying basement membrane a weaker than normal immunohistochemical staining of the epithelial basement membrane for fibrin/fibrinogen in KC corneas suggests that lysis of fibrin or impeded elaboration of fibrin may be involved in KC (421).

An Increased Distensibility of the Corneal Tissue

An increased distensibility of corneal tissue may be important in the pathogenesis of KC (119). The corneal deformity in KC possibly results from an abnormal low coefficient of ocular rigidity (215) and an abnormally low ocular rigidity has been reported in KC (100,120), but this has not been confirmed by other studies (142). Ocular rigidity is lower in eyes with KC than normal controls (120). Since the central cornea in KC becomes thin and weak the mechanical instability of the cornea in KC could in theory result from a deficiency or weakness of collagen the major structural protein of the cornea.

In KC stretching of the cornea clearly takes place and causes tears in Bowman layer and often ruptures in Descemet membrane. The tensile forces that results in these tears are clearly different from those caused by elevated intraocular pressure as these ruptures are not features of glaucomatous eyes.

As discussed earlier KC is associated with ocular massage, entities that predispose to eye rubbing (such as atopic keratoconjunctivitis, skin diseases, and miscellaneous eye diseases) and pressure on the globe. If these associations are more than coincidental one cannot but speculate that excessive eye rubbing or tension on the globe might lead to KC in the presence of a genetically determined thinned and weakened cornea (277). Mechanical pressure on the eye could perhaps cause collagen lamellae to slide over each other and become displaced peripherally and in doing so thin the corneal stroma. Such sliding could be facilitated by a genetically defective glue that normally keeps collagen lamellae compacted together.

GENETIC DISORDERS AFFECTING THE CORNEA THAT HAVE NOT BEEN MAPPED TO A CHROMOSOMAL LOCUS

Congenital Hereditary Stromal Dystrophy

General Remarks

One large family with descendants in Germany and France is known to have congenital hereditary stromal dystrophy (662).

Clinical Features

This nonprogressive disorder is limited to the corneal stroma and it is characterized by flaky or feathery clouding of the corneal stroma.

Histopathology

The abnormalities consist of a peculiar arrangement of tightly packed lamellae having highly aligned collagen fibrils of unusually small diameter (662). The cornea is of normal thickness and both Descemet membrane and the corneal endothelium are relatively normal.

Genetics

The disorder has an autosomal dominant mode of inheritance. The responsible gene remains to be identified and has not been mapped to a specific chromosome.

Pathogenesis

Nothing is known about the biochemical alterations, but the abnormally small stromal collagen fibrils and disordered lamellae suggest a disturbance in collagen fibrogenesis.

Posterior Amorphous Stromal Dystrophy

General Remarks

Carpel et al. (73) reported a family with irregular symmetric gray-white, sheet-like opacities in the deep central posterior corneal stroma that spread peripherally toward the corneoscleral limbus. They coined the term posterior amorphous stromal dystrophy for this autosomal dominant disorder. Posterior amorphous corneal dystrophy is apparently limited to the cornea.

Clinical Features

The condition is characterized clinically by irregular sheet-like opacities in the deep corneal stroma and Descemet membrane. It is distinct from pre-Descemet dystrophy, PPCD, CHED1, and CHED2 (73,117,253).

Histopathology

A tissue study on corneal tissue removed at penetrating keratoplasty from a single patient has disclosed disorganized posterior stromal collagen lamellae, and an attenuated corneal endothelium. A zone of collagen fibers was found interrupting Descemet membrane beneath the anterior-banded layer (253).

Epidemiology

Families with this condition have apparently only been detected in the United States (73,117,253).

Genetics

This rare disorder has an autosomal dominant mode of inheritance. The chromosomal location of the responsible gene has not been mapped.

Pathogenesis

A developmental abnormality is likely as the abnormalities in affected corneas have been observed in infancy and childhood. Transparent stroma may intervene between the corneal opacities, which sometimes indent Descemet membrane and the endothelium, which may have focal endothelial abnormalities. Both centroperipheral and peripheral forms are recognized (117). Visual acuity is usually minimally impaired, but may be severe enough to warrant a penetrating keratoplasty (253).

MISCELLANEOUS PUTATIVE INHERITED DISORDERS AFFECTING THE CORNEA

Several corneal disorders that were described before the era of molecular genetics still attract attention, but their precise nature remains uncertain or speculative. Recurrent corneal erosions in the absence of a well-defined corneal dystrophy are sometimes familial and may be a specific entity (143,498,639).

The term subepithelial mucinous corneal dystrophy was coined by Feder et al. (133) for a unique autosomal dominant corneal disorder in which subepithelial mucinous material accumulates in the cornea. This condition characterized by frequent recurrent corneal erosions in the first decade has only been recognized in one family of Slovak descent. A subepithelial band of GAGs is present in Bowman layer.

The condition referred to as Grayson–Wilbrandt corneal dystrophy (199) may be a variant of GCD type III or TBD.

REFERENCES

1. Abbruzzese C, Kuhn U, Molina F, et al. Novel mutations in the CHST6 gene causing macular corneal dystrophy. Clin Genet 2004; 65:120–5.
2. Adamis AP, Filatov V, Tripathi BJ, Tripathi RC. Fuchs' endothelial dystrophy of the cornea. Surv Ophthalmol 1993; 38:149–68.
3. Afshari NA, Mullally JE, Afshari MA, et al. Survey of patients with granular, lattice, Avellino, and Reis–Bucklers corneal dystrophies for mutations in the BIGH3 and gelsolin genes. Arch Ophthalmol 2001; 119: 16–22.
4. Akama TO, Nakayama J, Nishida K, et al. Human corneal GlcNac 6-*O*-sulfotransferase and mouse intestinal GlcNac 6-*O*-sulfotransferase both produce keratan sulfate. J Biol Chem 2001; 276:16271–8.
5. Akama TO, Nishida K, Nakayama J, et al. Macular corneal dystrophy type I and type II are caused by distinct mutations in a new sulphotransferase gene. Nat Genet 2000; 26:237–41.
6. Akimune C, Watanabe H, Maeda N, et al. Corneal guttata associated with the corneal dystrophy resulting from a betaig-h3 R124H mutation. Br J Ophthalmol 2000; 84: 67–71.
7. Akiya S, Brown SI. Granular dystrophy of the cornea. Characteristic electron microscopic lesion. Arch Ophthalmol 1970; 84:179–92.
8. Akiya S, Brown SI. The ultrastructure of Reis–Bucklers' dystrophy. Am J Ophthalmol 1971; 72:549–54.
9. Akiya S, Ho K, Matsui M. Gelatinous drop-like dystrophy of the cornea: light and electron microscopy study of superficial stromal lesion. Jpn J Clin Ophthalmol 1972; 26: 815–26.
10. Akova YA, Kirkness CM, McCartney AC, et al. Recurrent macular corneal dystrophy following penetrating keratoplasty. Eye 1990; 4:698–705.
11. Akova YA, Unlu N, Duman S. Fleck dystrophy of the cornea; a report of cases from three generations of a family. Eur J Ophthalmol 1994; 4:123–5.
12. al Faran MF, Tabbara KF. Corneal dystrophies among patients undergoing keratoplasty in Saudi Arabia. Cornea 1991; 10:13–6.
13. Aldave AJ, Yellore VS, Salem AK, et al. NoVSX1 gene mutations associated with keratoconus. Invest Ophthalmol Vis Sci 2006; 47:2820–2.
14. Aldave AJ, Rayner SA, Principe AH, et al. Analysis of fifteen positional candidate genes for Schnyder crystalline corneal dystrophy. Molecular Vision 2005; 11:713–6.
15. Aldave AJ, Yellore VS, Thonar EJ, et al. Novel mutations in the carbohydrate sulfotransferase gene (CHST6) in American patients with macular corneal dystrophy. Am J Ophthalmol 2004; 137:465–73.
16. Alexander RA, Garner A. Oxytalan fibre formation in the cornea: a light and electron microscopical study. Histopathology 1977; 1:189–99.
17. Alexander RA, Grierson I, Garner A. Oxytalan fibers in Fuch's endothelial dystrophy. Arch Ophthalmol 1981; 99: 1622–7.
18. Alldredge OC, Krachmer JH. Clinical types of corneal transplant rejection. Their manifestations, frequency, preoperative correlates, and treatment. Arch Ophthalmol 1981; 99:599–604.
19. Allingham RR, Klintworth GK, Bembe M, et al. Hereditary benign intraepithelial dyskeratosis links to a duplication on chromosome 4q34–q35. Proc Internat Soc Eye Res 2000; 71:S113P [abstract].
20. Alperin ES, Shapiro LJ. Characterization of point mutations in patients with X-linked ichthyosis. Effects on the structure and function of the steroid sulfatase protein. J Biol Chem 1997; 272:20756–63.
21. Amsler M. Quelques données du problème du kératocône. Bull Belge Ophtalmol 1961; 129:331–54.
22. Andreassen TT, Simonsen AH, Oxlund H. Biomechanical properties of keratoconus and normal corneas. Exp Eye Res 1980; 31:435–41.
23. Appelbaum A. Keratoconus. Arch Ophthalmol 1936; 15: 900–21.
24. Aracena T. Hereditary fleck dystrophy of the cornea. Report of a family. J Pediatr Ophthalmol 1975; 12:223.
25. Bao W, Smith CF, al-Rajhi A, et al. Novel mutations in the CHST6 gene in Saudi Arabic patients with macular corneal dystrophy. Invest Ophthalmol Vis Sci (Suppl) 2001; 42:S483.
26. Basler E, Grompe M, Parenti G, et al. Identification of point mutations in the steroid sulfatase gene of three

patients with X-linked ichthyosis. Am J Hum Genet 1992; 50:483–91.
27. Bass HN, Sparkes RS, Crandall BF, Marcy SM. Congenital contractural arachnodactyly, keratoconus, and probable Marfan syndrome in the same pedigree. J Pediatr 1981; 98:591–3.
28. Battisti C, Dotti MT, Malandrini A, et al. Schnyder corneal crystalline dystrophy: description of a new family with evidence of abnormal lipid storage in skin fibroblasts. Am J Med Genet 1998; 75:35–9.
29. Beardsley TL, Foulks GN. An association of keratoconus and mitral valve prolapse. Ophthalmology 1982; 89:35–7.
30. Bechara SJ, Grossniklaus HE, Waring GO III, Wells JA III. Keratoconus associated with posterior polymorphous dystrophy [letter]. Am J Ophthalmol 1991; 112:729–31.
31. Behndig A, Karlsson K, Johansson BO, et al. Superoxide dismutase isoenzymes in the normal and diseased human cornea. Invest Ophthalmol Vis Sci 2001; 42:2293–6.
32. Bermudez FJ, Ruiz C, Carreras B, Aneiros J. Association of keratoconus and false chordae tendineae in the left ventricle. Am J Ophthalmol 1989; 108:93–4.
33. Beuchat L, Metzger P. Acquired postcontusion keratoconus. J Fr Ophtalmol 1987; 10:501–3 [in French].
34. Biber H. Ueber einige seltene Hornhauterkrankugen: die oberflachliche gittrige Keratitis. Inaugural Dissertation 35–42. 1890. Zurich.
35. Bietti G. Ueber familäres vorkommen von retinitis punctata albescens (verbunden mit Dystrophia marginalis cristallinea cornea). Glitzern des Glaskörpers und anderen degenerativen Augenveranderungen. Klin Monatsbl Augenheilkd 1937; 99:737–56.
36. Bietti GB, Ferraboschi C. Sur L'association du kèratocône avec le catarrhe printanier et sur son èvidence statistique. Bull Mem Soc Fr Ophtalmol 1958; 185–98.
37. Biglan AW, Brown SI, Johnson BL. Keratoglobus and blue sclera. Am J Ophthalmol 1977; 83:225–33.
38. Bisceglia L, Ciaschetti M, De Bonis P, et al. VSX1 mutational analysis in a series of Italian patients affected by keratoconus: detection of a novel mutation. Invest Ophthalmol Vis Sci 2005; 46:39–45.
39. Biswas S, Munier FL, Yardley J, et al. Missense mutations in COL8A2, the gene encoding the alpha2 chain of type VIII collagen, cause two forms of corneal endothelial dystrophy. Human Mol Genet 2001; 10:2415–23.
40. Blagojevic M, Szanojevic-Paovic A, Susakovic N, Orlic M. HLA antigens 40, 937. 1979. Academic Press, The Cornea in Health and Disease, Royal Society of Medicine International Congress and Symposium.
41. Blair SD, Seabrooks D, Shields WJ, et al. Bilateral progressive essential iris atrophy and keratoconus with coincident features of posterior polymorphous dystrophy: a case report and proposed pathogenesis. Cornea 1992; 11:255–61.
42. Blanksma LJ, Donders PC, van Voorst Vader PC. Xeroderma pigmentosum and keratoconus. Doc Ophthalmol 1986; 64:97–103.
43. Bleckmann H. Influence of dextran macromolecules on the glycosaminoglycan metabolism of cultured corneal stroma and keratoconus fibroblast. Graefe's Arch Clin Exp Ophthalmol 1983; 221:70–2.
44. Bleckmann H, Kresse H. Studies on the glycosaminoglycan metabolism of cultured fibroblasts from human keratoconus corneas. Exp Eye Res 1980; 30:215–9.
45. Boger WP3, Petersen RA, Robb RM. Keratoconus and acute hydrops in mentally retarded patients with congenital rubella syndrome. Am J Ophthalmol 1981; 91:231–3.
46. Bonnet P, Paufique L, Bonamour G. Cristaux de cholestérine au centre de la cornée avec gérontoxon. Bull Soc Ophthalmol (Paris) 1934; 46:225–8.
47. Borboli S, Colby K. Mechanisms of disease: Fuchs' endothelial dystrophy. Ophthalmol Clin North Am 2002; 15:17–25.
48. Boruchoff SA, Kuwabara T. Electron microscopy of posterior polymorphous degeneration. Am J Ophthalmol 1971; 72:879–87.
49. Boruchoff SA, Weiner MJ, Albert DM. Recurrence of posterior polymorphous corneal dystrophy after penetrating keratoplasty [published erratum appears in Am J Ophthalmol 1990 May 15; 109(5):622]. Am J Ophthalmol 1990; 109:323–8.
50. Bourne WM, Johnson DH, Campbell RJ. The ultrastructure of Descemet's membrane. III. Fuchs' dystrophy. Arch Ophthalmol 1982; 100:1952–5.
51. Bourne WM, Michels VV. Keratoconus in one identical twin. Cornea 1982; 1:35–7.
52. Brady SE, Rapuano CJ, Arentsen JJ, et al. Clinical indications for and procedures associated with penetrating keratoplasty, 1983–1988. Am J Ophthalmol 1989; 108: 118–22.
53. Bramsen T, Ehlers N. Bullous keratopathy (Fuchs' endothelial dystrophy) treated systemically with 4-trans-amino-cyclohexano-carboxylic acid. Acta Ophthalmol (Copenh) 1977; 55:665–73.
54. Bramsen T, Ehlers N, Baggesen LH. Central cloudy corneal dystrophy of Francois. Acta Ophthalmol (Copenh) 1976; 54:p):221–6.
55. Brancati F, Valente EM, Sarkozy A, et al. A locus for autosomal dominant keratoconus maps to human chromosome 3p14–q13. J Med Genet 2004; 41:188–92.
56. Brav A. Familial nodular degeneration of the cornea. Arch Ophthalmol 1935; 14:985–6.
57. Bredrup C, Knappskog PM, Majewski J, et al. Congenital stromal dystrophy of the cornea caused by a mutation in the decorin gene. Invest Ophthalmol Vis Sci 2005; 46: 420–6.
58. Brenner S, Nemet P, Legum C. Jadassohn-type anetoderma in association with keratoconus and cataract. Ophthalmologica 1977; 174:181–4.
59. Brewitt H. [Light microscope and scanning electron microscope findings in acute keratoconus (author's transl)]. Klin Monatsbl Augenheilkd 1979; 174:605–13 [German].
60. Bron AJ, Williams HP, Carruthers ME. Hereditary crystalline stromal dystrophy of Schnyder. I. Clinical features of a family with hyperlipoproteinaemia. Br J Ophthalmol 1972; 56:383–99.
61. Brown D, Chwa MM, Opbroek A, Kenney MC. Keratoconus corneas: increased gelatinolytic activity appears after modification of inhibitors. Curr Eye Res 1993; 12:571–81.
62. Brownstein S, Fine BS, Sherman ME, Zimmerman LE. Granular dystrophy of the cornea. Light and electron microscopic confirmation of recurrence in a graft. Am J Ophthalmol 1974; 77:701–10.
63. Buchi ER, Daicker B, Uffer S, Gudat F. Primary gelatinous drop-like corneal dystrophy in a white woman. A pathologic, ultrastructural, and immunohistochemical study. Cornea 1994; 13:190–4.
64. Bücklers M. Über eine weitere familiare Hornhautdystrophie (Reis). Klin Monatsbl Augenheilkd 1949; 114:386–97.
65. Buddecke E, Wollensak J. [Acid mucopolysaccharides and glycoproteins in the human cornea in relationship to age and keratoconus]. Albrecht von Graefes Arch Klin Exp Ophthalmol 1966; 171:105–20 [German].

66. Buddi R, Lin B, Atilano SR, et al. Evidence of oxidative stress in human corneal diseases. Journal of Histochemistry & Cytochemistry 2002; 50:341–51.
67. Burns RP. Meesman's corneal dystrophy. Trans Am Ophthalmol Soc 1968; 66:530–635.
68. Buxton JN. Keratoconus. New Orleans, New Orleans Acad Ophthalmol 1973; 3:88–100 [Symposium on Contact Lenses].
69. Caldwell DR. Reis–Bückler's corneal dystrophy. A case report of a postoperative recurrence. Am J Ophthalmol 1978; 85:4.
70. Callaghan M, Hand CK, Kennedy SM, et al. Homozygosity mapping and linkage analysis demonstrate that autosomal recessive congenital hereditary endothelial dystrophy (CHED) and autosomal dominant CHED are genetically distinct. Br J Ophthalmol 1999; 83: 115–9.
71. Cameron JA, Cotter JB, Risco JM, Alvarez H. Epikeratoplasty for keratoglobus associated with blue sclera. Ophthalmology 1991; 98:446–52.
72. Cannon DJ, Foster CS. Collagen crosslinking in keratoconus. Invest Ophthalmol Vis Sci 1978; 17:63–5.
73. Carpel EF, Sigelman RJ, Doughman DJ. Posterior amorphous corneal dystrophy. Am J Ophthalmol 1977; 83: 629–32.
74. Chan CC, Green WR, Barraquer J, et al. Similarities between posterior polymorphous and congenital hereditary endothelial dystrophies: a study of 14 buttons of 11 cases. Cornea 1982; 1:155–72.
75. Charles NC, Young JA, Kumar A, et al. Band-shaped and whorled microcystic dystrophy of the corneal epithelium. Ophthalmology 2000; 107:1761–4.
76. Chen CJ, Furr P. Bilateral keratoconus in a patient with gyrate atrophy and hyperornithinemia [letter]. Am J Ophthalmol 1983; 95:705–6.
77. Cheng EL, Li Y, Sugar J, Yue BY. Cell density regulated expression of transcription factor Sp1 in corneal stromal cultures. Exp Eye Res 2001; 73:17–24.
78. Chi HH, Katzin HM, Teng CC. Histopathology of keratoconus. Am J Ophthalmol 1956; 42:847–60.
79. Chi HH, Teng CC, Katzin HM. Histopathology of primary endothelial-epithelial dystrophy of the cornea. Am J Ophthalmol 1958; 45:518–35.
80. Chi HH, Teng CC, Katzin HM. Histopathology of corneal endothelium. A study of 176 pathologic discs removed at keratoplasty. Am J Ophthalmol 1962; 53: 215–35.
81. Clegg JG. Remarks on dystrophies of the cornea and glaucoma, with especial reference to a familial variety of the former. Trans Ophthalmol Soc (UK) 1915; 35:245–53.
82. Coleman CM, Hannush S, Covello SP, et al. A novel mutation in the helix termination motif of keratin K12 in a US family with Meesmann corneal dystrophy. Am J Ophthalmol 1999; 128:687–91.
83. Collier M. Dystrophie mouchetée du paranchyme cornéen avec dystrophie nuageuse centrale. Bull Soc Ophtalmol Fr 1964; 64:608–11.
84. Cooper TA, Mattox W. The regulation of splice-site selection, and its role in human disease. Am J Hum Genet 1997; 61:259–66.
85. Copeman PWM. Eczema and keratoconus. Br Med J 1965; 2:977–9.
86. Corden LD, Swensson O, Swensson B, et al. Molecular genetics of Meesmann's corneal dystrophy: ancestral and novel mutations in keratin 12 (K12) and complete sequence of the human KRT12 gene. Exp Eye Res 2000; 70:41–9.
87. Coulombre A, Coulombre J. Corneal development. III. The role of the thyroid in dehydration and the development of transparency. Exp Eye Res 1964; 3: 105–9.
88. Coyle JT. Keratoconus and eye rubbing. Am J Ophthalmol 1984; 97:527–8.
89. Critchfield JW, Calandra AJ, Nesburn AB, Kenney MC. Keratoconus: I. Biochemical studies. Exp Eye Res 1988; 46:953–63.
90. Cross HE, Maumenee AE, Cantolino SJ. Inheritance of Fuchs' endothelial dystrophy. Arch Ophthalmol 1971; 85: 268–72.
91. Cuendet JF, Beuret-Niedzielsky A, Zografos L. Hérédité de la dystrophie granuleuse de la cornée (Groenouw I)]. Oftalmol 1989; 3:265–6 [French].
92. Cullen JT, Butler HG. Mongolism (Down's syndrome) and keratoconus. Br J Ophthalmol 1963; 47:321–30.
93. Curran RE, Kenyon KR, Green WR. Pre-Descemet's membrane corneal dystrophy. Am J Ophthalmol 1974; 77:711–6.
94. Cutler AT, Benezra-Obeiter R, Brink SJ. Thyroid function in young children with Down syndrome. Am J Dis Child 1986; 140:479–83.
95. Damgaard-Jensen L, Ehlers N, Kissmeyer-Nielsen F. HLA types in corneal diseases. Acta Ophthalmol (Copenh) 1979; 57:982–5.
96. Danes BS. Corneal clouding in the genetic mucopolysaccharidoses: a cell culture study. Clin Genet 1973; 4: 1–7.
97. Dark AJ, Thompson DS. Lattice dystrophy of the cornea: a clinical and microscopic study. Br J Ophthalmol 1960; 44:257–79.
98. Dash DP, Silvestri G, Hughes AE. Fine mapping of the keratoconus with catarct locus on chromosome 15q and candidate gene analysis. Mol Vis 2006; 12:499–505.
99. Davies PD, Lobascher D, Menon JA, et al. Immunological studies in keratoconus. Trans Ophthalmol Soc (UK) 1976; 96:173–8.
100. Davies PD, Ruben M. The paretic pupil: its incidence and aetiology after keratoplasty in keratoconus. Br J Ophthalmol 1975; 59:223–8.
101. de Haas HL. Familiarir voorkomende cornea guttata. Ned Tijdschr Geneeskd 1942; 86:3182.
102. de la Chapelle A, Kere J, Sack GH Jr, et al. Familial amyloidosis, Finnish type: G654-a mutation of the gelsolin gene in Finnish families and an unrelated American family. Genomics 1992; 13:898–901.
103. de la Chapelle A, Tolvanen R, Boysen G, et al. Gelsolin-derived familial amyloidosis caused by asparagine or tyrosine substitution for aspartic acid at residue 187. Nat Genet 1992; 2:157–60.
104. Delleman JW, Winkelman JE. Degeneratio corneae cristallinea hereditaria. A clinical, genetical and histological study. Ophthalmologica 1968; 155:409–26.
105. Desvignes P, Vigo (NI). A case of corneal and parencymal dystrophy of dominant type. Bull Soc Fr Ophtalmol 1955; 4:220–5.
106. Diaper CJ. Severe granular dystrophy: a pedigree with presumed homozygotes. Eye 1994; 8:448–52.
107. Dighiero P, Drunat S, D'Hermies F, et al. A novel variant of granular corneal dystrophy caused by association of 2 mutations in the TGFBI gene-R124L and DeltaT125-DeltaE126. Arch Ophthalmol 2000; 118:814–8.
108. Dighiero P, Drunat S, Ellies P, et al. A new mutation (A546T) of the betaig-h3 gene responsible for a French lattice corneal dystrophy type IIIA. Am J Ophthalmol 2000; 129:248–51.

109. Dighiero P, Niel F, Ellies P, et al. Histologic phenotype-genotype correlation of corneal dystrophies associated with eight distinct mutations in the TGFBI gene. Ophthalmology 2001; 108:818–23.
110. Dimmer F. Ueber oberflächliche gittrige Hornhauttrübung. Z Augenheilkd 1899; 2:354–61.
111. Doggart JH. Fuchs's epithelial dystrophy of the cornea. Brit J Ophthalmol 1957; 41:533–40.
112. Dohlman CH. Familial congenital cornea guttata in association with anterior polar cataract. Acta Ophthalmol (Copenh) 1951; 29:445–73.
113. Donnenfeld ED, Cohen EJ, Ingraham HJ, et al. Corneal thinning in macular corneal dystrophy. Am J Ophthalmol 1986; 101:112–3.
114. Donnenfeld ED, Perry HD, Gibralter RP, et al. Keratoconus associated with floppy eyelid syndrome. Ophthalmology 1991; 98:1674–8.
115. Dota A, Nishida K, Honma Y, et al. Gelatinous drop-like corneal dystrophy is not one of the beta ig-h3-mutated corneal amyloidoses. Am J Ophthalmol 1998; 126:832–3.
116. Drozdz M, Kucharz E, Gruckamamczar E. Influence of thyroid-hormones on collagen content in tissues of guinea-pigs. Endokrinologie 1979; 73:105–11.
117. Dunn SP, Krachmer JH, Ching SS. New findings in posterior amorphous corneal dystrophy. Arch Ophthalmol 1984; 102:236–9.
118. Ederer F, Ferris FL. Studying the role of an environmental factor in disease etiology. Am J Ophthalmol 1979; 87:434–5.
119. Edmund C. Assessment of an elastic model in the pathogenesis of keratoconus. Acta Ophthalmol (Copenh) 1987; 65:545–50.
120. Edmund C. Corneal elasticity and ocular rigidity in normal and keratoconic eyes. Acta Ophthalmol (Copenh) 1988; 66:134–40.
121. Edward DP, Thonar EJ, Srinivasan M, et al. Macular dystrophy of the cornea. A systemic disorder of keratan sulfate metabolism. Ophthalmology 1990; 97:1194–200.
122. Edwards M, McGhee C, Dean S. The genetics of keratoconus. Clin Exper Ophthalmol 2007; 29:345–51.
123. Ehlers N, Bramsen T. Central thickness in corneal disorders. Acta Ophthalmol (Copenh) 1978; 56:412–6.
124. Ehlers N, Olsen T. Long term results of corneal grafting in keratoconus. Acta Ophthalmol (Copenh) 1983; 61:918–26.
125. Eiferman RA. Recurrence of keratoconus. Br J Ophthalmol 1984; 68:289–90 [letter].
126. Eiferman RA, Rodrigues MM, Laibson PP, Arentsen JJ. Schnyder's crystalline dystrophy associated with amyloid deposition. Metab Pediatr Ophthalmol 1979; 3: 15–20.
127. El Ashry MF, El Aziz MM, Shalaby O, et al. Novel CHST6 nonsense and missense mutations responsible for macular corneal dystrophy. Am J Ophthalmol 2005; 139:192–3.
128. El Ashry MF, El Aziz MM, Wilkins S, et al. Identification of novel mutations in the carbohydrate sulfotransferase gene (CHST6) causing macular corneal dystrophy. Invest Ophthalmol Vis Sci 2002; 43:377–82.
129. Escribano J, Hernando N, Ghosh S, et al. cDNA from human ocular ciliary epithelium homologous to beta ig-h3 is preferentially expressed as an extracellular protein in the corneal epithelium. J Cell Physiol 1994; 160:511–21.
130. Fabre EJ, Bureau J, Pouliquen Y, Lorans G. Binding sites for human interleukin 1 alpha, gamma interferon and tumor necrosis factor on cultured fibroblasts of normal cornea and keratoconus. Curr Eye Res 1991; 10: 585–92.
131. Falls HF. Detection of the carrier state of genetically determined eye diseases. In New Orleans Academy of Ophthalmology: Symposium on Surgical and Medical Management of Congenital Anomalies of the Eye. St. Louis, MO: C.V. Mosby, 1968.
132. Falls HF, Allen AW. Dominantly inherited keratoconus: report of a family. J Genet Hum 1969; 17:317–24.
133. Feder RS, Jay M, Yue BY, et al. Subepithelial mucinous corneal dystrophy. Clinical and pathological correlations. Arch Ophthalmol 1993; 111:1106–14.
134. Feuvrier Y-M, Bellegro A, Ledu J. Dystrophie mouchetée héréditaire du parenchyme cornéen. A propos du quatre observations familiales. Bull Soc Ophtalmol Fr 1964; 64: 735–7.
135. Fine BS, Yanoff M, Pitts E, Slaughter FD. Meesmann's epithelial dystrophy of the cornea. Am J Ophthalmol 1977; 83:633–42.
136. Fisher DA, Sack J, Oddie TH, et al. Serum T4, TBG, T3 uptake, T3, reverse T3, and TSH concentrations in children 1 to 15 years of age. Journal of Clinical Endocrinology and Metabolism 1977; 45:191–8.
137. Flanders M, Lapointe ML, Brownstein S, Little JM. Keratoconus and Leber's congenital amaurosis: a clinicopathological correlation. Can J Ophthalmol 1984; 19: 310–4.
138. Fogle JA, Kenyon KR, Stark WJ, Green WR. Defective epithelial adhesion in anterior corneal dystrophies. Am J Ophthalmol 1975; 79:925–40.
139. Folberg R, Alfonso E, Croxatto JO, et al. Clinically atypical granular corneal dystrophy with pathologic features of lattice-like amyloid deposits. A study of these families. Ophthalmology 1988; 95:46–51.
140. Forstot SL, Goldstein JH, Damiano RE, Dukes DK. Familial keratoconus. Am J Ophthalmol 1988; 105:92–3.
141. Fort P, Lifshitz F, Bellisario R, et al. Abnormalities of thyroid function in infants with down syndrome. J Pediatr 1984; 104:545–9.
142. Foster CS, Yamamoto GK. Ocular rigidity in keratoconus. Am J Ophthalmol 1978; 86:802–6.
143. Franceschetti A. Hereditäre rezidvierende Erosion der Hornhaut. Z Augenheilkd 1928; 66:309–16.
144. Franceschetti A. Keratoconus. In The Cornea. Washington: Butterworths, 1965.
145. Franceschetti A, Carones AV. Su un caso di cheratocono familiare con nuvrodermite disseminata, cataratta associato a dei sintomi tra cheratocono e nevrodermite disseminata. G Ital Oftalmol 1960; 13:143–60.
146. Franceschetti A, Jaccottet M, Jadassohn W. Manifestations cornéenes dans la keratosis follicularis spinulosa decalvans (Siemens). Ophthalmologica 1957; 133:259–63.
147. Franceschetti A, Klein D. Cornea. In: Waardenburg PJ, Franceschetti A, Klein D, eds. Genetics and Ophthalmology. Oxford: Blackwell, 1961:447–543.
148. Franceschetti A, Linder A. Osservazioni sul lavoro di D. Santino: Esiste effectivamente una correlazione tra cheratocono e retinite pigmentoas? Apparso in questa rivista. G Ital Oftalmol 1960; 13:3–6.
149. Franceschetti A, Maeder G. Dystrophie profonde de la cornee dans un cas d'itchtyose congenitale. Bull Soc Ophtalmol Fr 1954; 67:146.
150. Franceschetti AT. La cornea verticillata (Gruber) et ses relations avec la maladie de Fabry (Angiokeratoma corporis diffusum). Ophthalmologica 1968; 156:232–8.
151. Francois J. Une nouvelle dystrophie heredo-familiale de la cornee USE 892 not 990. J Genet Hum 1956; 5:189–96.
152. François J. Une nouvelle dystrophie hérédo-familiale de la cornée. J Genet Hum 1956; 5:189–96.

153. François J. Heredo-familial corneal dystrophies. Trans Ophthalmol Soc (UK) 1966; 86:367–416.
154. François J. Glycolipid lipoidosis. In Symposium on Surgical and Medical Management of Congenital Anomalies of the Eye: Transactions of the New Orleans Academy of Ophthalmology. St. Louis, MO: C V. Mosby, 1968.
155. François J, Neetens A. Nouvelle dystrophie hérédofamiliale de parenchyme cornée (hérédodystrophie mouchetée). Bull Soc Belge Ophtalmol 1956; 114:641–6.
156. François J, Neetens A, Smets RM. Bardet–Biedl syndrome and keratoconus. Bull Soc Belge Ophtalmol 1982; 203: 117–21.
157. François J, Victoria-Troncoso V, Maudgal PC, Victoria-Ihler A. Study of the lysosomes by vital stains in normal keratocytes and in keratocytes from macular dystrophy of the cornea. Invest Ophthalmol Vis Sci 1976; 15:599–605.
158. Frantz JM, Insler MS, Hagenah M, et al. Penetrating keratoplasty for keratoconus in Down's syndrome. Am J Ophthalmol 1990; 109:143–7.
159. Frayer WC, Blodi FC. The lattice type of familial corneal degeneration. Arch Ophthalmol 1959; 61:712.
160. Freedman J, Gombos GM. Bilateral macular coloboma, keratoconus, and retinitis pigmentosa. Ann Ophthalmol 1971; 3:664–5.
161. Freiberger M. Corneal dystrophy in three generations; with genealogical chart. Arch Ophthalmol 1936; 16: 257–70.
162. Fry WE, Pickett WE. Crystalline dystrophy of the cornea. Trans Am Ophthalmol Soc 1950; 58:220–7.
163. Fuchs E. Dystrophia epithelialis corneae. Albrecht von Graefes Arch Klin Exp Ophthalmol 1910; 76:478–508.
164. Fujiki K, Hotta Y, Nakayasu K, Kanai A. Homozygotic patient with betaig-h3 gene mutation in granular dystrophy. Cornea 1998; 17:288–92.
165. Fujiki K, Hotta Y, Nakayasu K, et al. Six different mutations of TGFBI (betaig-h3, keratoepithelin) gene found in Japanese corneal dystrophies. Cornea 2000; 19: 842–5.
166. Fujiki K, Hotta Y, Nakayasu K, et al. A new L527R mutation of the betaIGH3 gene in patients with lattice corneal dystrophy with deep stromal opacities. Hum Genet 1998; 103:286–9.
167. Fullwood NJ, Tuft SJ, Malik NS, et al. Synchrotron x-ray diffraction studies of keratoconus corneal stroma. Invest Ophthalmol Vis Sci 1992; 33:1734–41.
168. Funahashi M. [Pathological changes in Bowman's layer: light and electron microscopic study of keratoconus and pterygium]. [Japanese]. Nippon Ganka Gakkai Zasshi 1979; 83:1089–108.
169. Funayama T, Mashima Y, Kawashima M, Yamada M. Lattice corneal dystrophy type III in patients with a homozygous L527R mutation in the TGFBI gene. Jpn J Ophthalmol 2006; 50:62–4.
170. Funderburgh JL. Keratan sulfate: structure, biosynthesis, and function. Glycobiology 2000; 10:951–8.
171. Funderburgh JL, Panjwani N, Conrad GW, Baum J. Altered keratan sulfate epitopes in keratoconus. Invest Ophthalmol Vis Sci 1989; 30:2278–81.
172. Funke H, Voneckardstein A, Pritchard PH, et al. A molecular defect causing fish eye disease—an amino-acid exchange in lecithin-cholesterol acyltransferase (LCAT) leads to the selective loss of alpha-LCAT activity. Proc Natl Acad Sci USA 1991; 88:4855–9.
173. Fuxa G, Brandt HP. Beitrag zum Ehlers–Danlos syndrome. Klin Monatsbl Augenheilkd 1975; 166:247–51.
174. Gahl WA, Thoene JG, Schneider JA. Cystinosis. N Engl J Med 2002; 347:111–21.
175. Galin MA, Berger R. Atopy and keratoconus. Am J Ophthalmol 1958; 45:904–6.
176. Garner A. Histochemistry of corneal granular dystrophy. Br J Ophthalmol 1969; 53:799–807.
177. Garner A. Histochemistry of corneal macular dystrophy. Invest Ophthalmol Vis Sci 1969; 8:475–83.
178. Gass JDM. The iron lines of the superficial cornea. Hudson-Stahli line, Stocker's line and Fleischer's ring. Arch Ophthalmol 1964; 71:348–58.
179. Gasset AR, Houde WL, Garcia-Bengochea M. Hard contact lens wear as an environmental risk in keratoconus. Am J Ophthalmol 1978; 85:339–41.
180. Gasset AR, Worthen DM. Keratoconus and Chandler's syndrome. Ann Ophthalmol 1974; 6:819–20.
181. Gasset AR, Zimmerman TJ. Posterior polymorphous dystrophy associated with keratoconus. Am J Ophthalmol 1974; 78:535–7.
182. Gaynor PM, Zhang WY, Weiss JS, et al. Accumulation of HDL apolipoproteins accompanies abnormal cholesterol accumulation in Schnyder's corneal dystrophy. Arteriosclerosis Thrombosis and Vascular Biology 1996; 16:992–9.
183. Ghosh M, McCulloch C. Macular corneal dystrophy. Can J Ophthalmol 1973; 8:515–26.
184. Gillespie F, Covelli B. Fleck (mouchetée) dystrophy of the cornea. Report of a family. South Med J 1963; 56:1265–7.
185. Gillespie FD, Covelli B. Crystalline corneal dystrophy. Report of a case. Am J Ophthalmol 1963; 56:465–7.
186. Godel V, Blumenthal M, Iaina A. Congenital Leber amaurosis, keratoconus, and mental retardation in familial juvenile nephronophtisis. J Pediatr Ophthalmol Strabismus 1978; 15:89–91.
187. Gondhowiardjo TD, van Haeringen NJ. Corneal aldehyde dehydrogenase, glutathione reductase, and glutathione S-transferase in pathologic corneas. Cornea 1993; 12:310–4.
188. Gondhowiardjo TD, van Haeringen NJ, Volker-Dieben HJ, et al. Analysis of corneal aldehyde dehydrogenase patterns in pathologic corneas. Cornea 1993; 12:146–54.
189. Gonzales J de J. Keratoconus consecutive to vernal conjunctivitis. Am J Ophthalmol 1920; 3:127–8.
190. Gorevic PD, Munoz PC, Gorgone G, et al. Amyloidosis due to a mutation of the gelsolin gene in an American family with lattice corneal dystrophy type II. N Engl J Med 1991; 325:1780–5.
191. Gorevic PD, Munoz PC, Rodrigues MM, et al. Shared gelsolin antigenicity between familial amyloidosis Finnish type (FAF) and one form of familial lattice corneal dystrophy (LCD) with polyneuropathy from the United States. In: Natvig JB, Førre Ø, Husby G, et al. eds. Amyloid and Amyloidosis 1990. Springer, 1991:423–35.
192. Gormaz A, Eggers C. Vernal keratoconjunctivitis and keratoconus. Am J Ophthalmol 1983; 96:555–6 [letter].
193. Goslar HG, Seltz R. Das histochemische Bild von Hornhautdegenerationen and dystrophien in Beziehung zum ophthalmoskopischen Befund. Acta Gusti 1961; 12: 289–304.
194. Gottsch JD, Bowers AL, Margulies EH, et al. Serial analysis of gene expression in the corneal endothelium of Fuchs' dystrophy. Invest Ophthalmol Vis Sci 2003; 44: 594–9.
195. Gottsch JD, Zhang C, Sundin OH, et al. Fuchs corneal dystrophy: aberrant collagen distribution in an L450W mutant of the COL8A2 gene. Invest Ophthalmol Vis Sci 2005; 46:4504–11.

196. Graf B, Pouliquen Y, Frouin M-A, et al. Cytochemical study of macular dystrophy of the cornea (Groenouw II): An ultrastructural study. Exp Eye Res 1974; 18:163–9.
197. Grandon SC, Weber RA. Radial keratotomy in patients with atypical inferior steepening. J Cataract Refract Surg 1994; 20:381–6.
198. Grayson M. The nature of hereditary deep polymorphous dystrophy of the cornea: its association with iris and anterior chamber dygenesis. Trans Am Ophthalmol Soc 1974; 72:516–59.
199. Grayson M, Wilbrandt H. Dystrophy of the anterior limiting membrane of the cornea. (Reis–Buckler type). Am J Ophthalmol 1966; 61:345–9.
200. Grayson M, Wilbrandt H. Pre-descemet dystrophy. Am J Ophthalmol 1967; 64:276–82.
201. Greenfield G, Romano A, Stein R, Goodman RM. Blue sclerae and keratoconus: key features of a distinct heritable disorder of connective tissue. Clin Genet 1973; 4:8–16.
202. Griffith DG, Fine BS. Light and electron microscopic observations in a superficial corneal dystrophy probable early Reis–Bucklers' type. Am J Ophthalmol 1967; 63: 1659–66.
203. Gruenauer-Kloevekorn C, Braeutigam S, Froster U, Duncker GIW. Molecular genetic findings and therapeutical options in a well examined German family with macular corneal dystrophy. Invest Ophthalmol Vis Sci 2005; 46:4931.
204. Ha NT, Chau HM, Cung LX, et al. Mutation analysis of the carbohydrate sulfotransferase gene in Vietnamese with macular corneal dystrophy. Invest Ophthalmol Vis Sci 2003; 44:3310–6.
205. Ha NT, Chau HM, Cung LX, et al. A novel mutation of M1S1 gene found in a Vietnamese patient with gelatinous droplike corneal dystrophy. Am J Ophthalmol 2003; 135: 390–3.
206. Ha NT, Chau HMC, Thanh TK, et al. Identification of novel mutations of the CHST6 gene in Vietnamese families affected with macular corneal dystrophy in two generations. Cornea 2003; 22:508–11.
207. Ha NT, Fujiki K, Hotta Y, et al. Q118X mutation of M1S1 gene caused gelatinous drop-like corneal dystrophy: the P501T of BIGH3 gene found in a family with gelatinous drop-like corneal dystrophy. Am J Ophthalmol 2000; 130: 119–20.
208. Haab O. Die gittrige Keratitis. Z Augenheilkd 1899; 2: 235–46.
209. Haddad R, Font RL, Fine BS. Unusual superficial variant of granular dystrophy of the cornea. Am J Ophthalmol 1977; 83:213–8.
210. Hallermann W, Wilson EJ. Genetische Betachtungen über den Keratoconus. Klin Monatsbl Augenheilkd 1977; 170: 906–8.
211. Hand CK, Harmon DL, Kennedy SM, et al. Localization of the gene for autosomal recessive congenital hereditary endothelial dystrophy (CHED2) to chromosome 20 by homozygosity mapping. Genomics 1999; 61:1–4.
212. Harada T, Kojima K, Hoshino M, Murakami M. [A light and electromicroscopic study of heredo-familial corneal dystrophy (Groenouw I)]. Nippon Ganka Gakkai Zasshi 1977; 81:48–61 [Japanese].
213. Harrison RJ, Klouda PT, Easty DL, et al. Association between keratoconus and atopy. Br J Ophthalmol 1989; 73:816–22.
214. Hartstein J. Keratoconus that developed in patients wearing corneal contact lenses. Report of four cases. Arch Ophthalmol 1968; 80:345–6.
215. Hartstein J, Becker B. Research into the pathogenesis of keratoconus. A new syndrome: low ocular rigidity, contact lenses, and keratoconus. Arch Ophthalmol 1970; 84:728–9.
216. Hasegawa N, Torii T, Kato T, et al. Decreased GlcNAc 6-*O*-sulfotransferase activity in the cornea with macular corneal dystrophy. Invest Ophthalmol Vis Sci 2000; 41: 3670–7.
217. Hasegawa N, Torii T, Nagaoka I, et al. Measurement of activities of human serum sulfotransferases which transfer sulfate to the galactose residues of keratan sulfate and to the nonreducing end N-acetylglucosamine residues of N-acetyllactosamine trisaccharide: comparison between normal controls and patients with macular corneal dystrophy. J Biochem 1999; 125:245–52.
218. Hassell JR, Klintworth GK. Serum sulfotransferase levels in patients with macular corneal dystrophy type I. Arch Ophthalmol 1997; 115:1419–21.
219. Hassell JR, Newsome DA, Krachmer JH, Rodrigues MM. Macular corneal dystrophy: failure to synthesize a mature keratan sulfate proteoglycan. Proc Natl Acad Sci USA 1980; 77:3705–9.
220. Hassell JR, SundarRaj N, Cintron C, et al. Alteration in the synthesis of healing and in macular corneal dystrophy. In: Greiling H, Scott JE, eds. Keratan Sulfate: Chemistry, Biology and Chemical Pathology. London: The Biochemical Society, 1988:215–25.
221. Haugen OH. Keratoconus in the mentally retarded. Acta Ophthalmol (Copenh) 1992; 70:111–4.
222. Heon E, Greenberg A, Kopp KK, et al. VSX1: A gene for posterior polymorphous dystrophy and keratoconus. Hum Mol Genet 2002; 11:1029–36.
223. Heon E, Mathers WD, Alward WL, et al. Linkage of posterior polymorphous corneal dystrophy to 20q11. Human Mol Genet 1995; 4:485–8.
224. Herman C. La Dystrophie grillagée de la cornée. Ophthalmologica 1946; 112:350–63.
225. Herman SJ, Hughes WF. Recurrence of hereditary corneal dystrophy following keratoplasty. Am J Ophthalmol 1973; 75:689–94.
226. Hida T, Proia AD, Kigasawa K, et al. Histopathologic and immunochemical features of lattice corneal dystrophy type III. Am J Ophthalmol 1987; 104:249–54.
227. Hida T, Tsubota K, Kigasawa K, et al. Clinical features of a newly recognized type of lattice corneal dystrophy. Am J Ophthalmol 1987; 104:241–8.
228. Hilgartner HL, Hilgartner HL Jr, Gilbert JT. A preliminary report of a case of keratoconus successfully treated with organotherapy, radium and shortwave diathermy. Am J Ophthalmol 1937; 20:1032–9.
229. Hirano K, Hotta Y, Nakamura M, et al. Late-onset form of lattice corneal dystrophy caused by Leu527Arg mutation of the TGFBI gene. Cornea 2001; 20:525–9.
230. Hirano K, Klintworth GK, Zhan Q, et al. ig-h3 is synthesized by corneal epithelium and perhaps endotheliumin Fuchs' dystrophic corneas. Curr Eye Res 1996; 15: 965–72.
231. Hoang-Xuan T, Elmaleh C, Dhermy P, et al. Association d'une dystrophie grillagée et d'un kératocone: étude anatomic-clinique à propos d'une cas. Bull Soc Ophtalmol Fr 1989; 89:35–8.
232. Hogan MJ, Wood I, Fine M. Fuchs' endothelial dystrophy of the cornea 29th Sanford Gifford Memorial lecture. Am J Ophthalmol 1974; 78:363–83.
233. Hornblass A, Sabates WI. Eyelid and orbital cavernous hemangioma associated with keratoconus. Am J Ophthalmol 1980; 89:396–400.

234. Hughes WF. Discussion of Rodrigues MM, McGavic JS (Reference #386). Trans Am Ophthalmol Soc 1975; 73: 315–6.
235. Humayun MS, Pepose JS. A viral etiology in Fuchs' corneal dystrophy. Hum Pathol 1988; 19:245.
236. Humphries SE, Chaves ME, Tata F, et al. A study of the structure of the gene for lecithin—cholesterol acyltransferase in 4 unrelated individuals with familial lecithin—cholesterol acyltransferase deficiency. Clinical Science 1988; 74:91–6.
237. Hutchings H, Ginisty H, Le Gallo M, et al. Identification of a new locus for isolated familail keatoconus at 2p24. J Med Genet 2005; 42:88–94.
238. Ida H, Rennert OM, Maekawa K, E to Y. Identification of three novel mutations in the acid sphingomyelinase gene of Japanese patients with Niemann–Pick disease type A and B. Hum Mutat 1996; 7:65–7.
239. Ihalainen A. Clinical and epidemiological features of keratoconus: genetic and external factors in the pathogenesis of the disease. Acta Ophthalmol Suppl 1986; 64: 5–64.
240. Ihalainen A, Salo T, Forsius H, Peltonen L. Increase in type I and type IV collagenolytic activity in primary cultures of keratoconus cornea. Eur J Clin Invest 1986; 16: 78–84.
241. Ihme A, Krieg T, Muller RK, Wollensak J. Biochemical investigation of cells from keratoconus and normal cornea. Exp Eye Res 1983; 36:625–31.
242. Iida-Hasegawa N, Furuhata A, Hayatsu H, et al. Mutations in the CHST6 gene in patients with macular corneal dystrophy: immunohistochemical evidence of heterogeneity. Invest Ophthalmol Vis Sci 2003; 44: 3272–7.
243. Ingraham HJ, Perry HD, Donnenfeld ED, Donaldson DD. Progressive Schnyder's corneal dystrophy. Ophthalmology 1993; 100:1824–7.
244. Irvine AD, Corden LD, Swensson O, et al. Mutations in cornea-specific keratin K3 or K12 genes cause Meesmann's corneal dystrophy. Nat Genet 1997; 16: 184–7.
245. Iwamoto T, DeVoe AG. Electron microscopic studies on Fuchs' combined dystrophy. I. Posterior portion of the cornea. Invest Ophthalmol Vis Sci 1971; 10:9–28.
246. Iwamoto T, DeVoe AG. Particulate structures in keratoconus. Arch Ophtalmol Rev Gen Ophtalmol 1975; 35: 65–76.
247. Iwamoto T, Stuart JC, Srinivasan BD, et al. Ultrastructural variation in granular dystrophy of the cornea. Albrecht von Graefes Arch Klin Exp Ophthalmol 1975; 194:1–9.
248. Jacoby B, Reed JW, Cashwell LF. Malignant glaucoma in a patient with Down's syndrome and corneal hydrops. Am J Ophthalmol 1990; 110:434–5.
249. Jakus MA. In: Jakus MA, ed. Ocular Fine Structures: Selected Electron Micrographs. Boston: Little Brown, 1964.
250. Jiao X, Munier FL, Iwata F, et al. Genetic linkage of Bietti crystallin corneoretinal dystrophy to chromosome 4q35. Am J Hum Genet 2000; 67:1309–13.
251. Jiao X, Munier FL, Scorderet DF, et al. Genetic linkage of Francois-Neetens fleck (mouchetée) corneal dystrophy to chromosome 2q35. Am J Hum Genet 2002; 71:446.
252. Jiao X, Sultana A, Garg P, et al. Autosomal recessive corneal endothelial dystrophy (CHED2) is associated with mutations in SLC4A11. J Med Genet 2007; 44:64–8.
253. Johnson AT, Folberg R, Vrabec MP, et al. The pathology of posterior amorphous corneal dystrophy. Ophthalmology 1990; 97:104–9.
254. Johnson BL, Brown SI. Posterior polymorphous dystrophy: a light and electron microscopic study. Br J Ophthalmol 1978; 62:89–96.
255. Johnson DH, Bourne WM, Campbell RJ. The ultrastructure of Descemet's membrane. I. Changes with age in normal corneas. Arch Ophthalmol 1982; 100:1942–7.
256. Johnson DH, Bourne WM, Campbell RJ. The ultrastructure of Descemet's membrane. II. Aphakic bullous keratopathy. Arch Ophthalmol 1982; 100:1948–51.
257. Jonasson F, Johannsson JH, Garner A, Rice NS. Macular corneal dystrophy in Iceland. Eye 1989; 3:446–54.
258. Jonasson F, Oshima E, Thonar EJ, et al. Macular corneal dystrophy in Iceland. A clinical, genealogic, and immunohistochemical study of 28 patients. Ophthalmology 1996; 103:1111–7.
259. Jones ST, Stauffer LK. Reis–Bucklers' corneal dystrophy. A clinicopathologic study. Trans Am Acad Ophthalmol Otolaryngol 1970; 74:417–26.
260. Jones ST, Zimmerman LE. Histopathologic differentiation of granular, macular and lattice dystrophies of the cornea. Am J Ophthalmol 1961; 51:394–410.
261. Jongebloed WL, Dijk F, Worst JG. Keratoconus morphology and cell dystrophy: a SEM study. Doc Ophthalmol 1989; 72:403–9.
262. Jongebloed WL, Humalda D, van Andel P, Worst JF. A SEM-study of a keratoconus and an artificially aged human cornea. Doc Ophthalmol 1986; 64:129–42.
263. Jongebloed WL, Worst JF. The keratoconus epithelium studied by SEM. Doc Ophthalmol 1987; 67:171–81.
264. Judisch GF, Maumenee IH. Clinical differentiation of recessive congenital hereditary endothelial dystrophy and dominant hereditary endothelial dystrophy. Am J Ophthalmol 1978; 85:(Pt 1):606–12.
265. Judisch GF, Waziri M, Krachmer JH. Ocular Ehlers–Danlos syndrome with normal lysyl hydroxylase activity. Arch Ophthalmol 1976; 94:1489–91.
266. Juler F. Diseases of the cornea. III. Some cases of damage to Descemet's endothelium. Trans Ophthalmol Soc (UK) 1930; 50:118–27.
267. Kahán IL, Varsányi-Nagy M, Tóth M, Nádrai A. The possible role of tear fluid thyroxine in keratoconus development. Exp Eye Res 1990; 50:339–43.
268. Kaiser-Kupfer MI, Chan CC, Markello TC, et al. Clinical biochemical and pathologic correlations in Bietti's crystalline dystrophy. Am J Ophthalmol 1994; 118:569–82.
269. Kaji Y, Amano S, Oshika T, et al. Chronic clinical course of two patients with severe corneal dystrophy caused by homozygous R124H mutations in the betaig-h3 gene. Am J Ophthalmol 2000; 129:663–5.
270. Kanai A. Electron microscopic studies of keratoconus. Nippon Ganka Gakkai Zasshi 1968; 72:902–18 [Japanese].
271. Kanai A, Waltman S, Polack FM, Kaufman HE. Electron microscopic study of hereditary corneal edema. Invest Ophthalmol Vis Sci 1971; 10:89–99.
272. Kanai A, Yamaguchi T, Nakajima A. [The histochemical and analytical electron microscopy studies of the corneal granular dystrophy (author's transl)]. Nippon Ganka Gakkai Zasshi 1977; 81:145–54 [Japanese].
273. Kang PC, Klintworth GK, Carlson A, et al. Trends in the indications for penetrating keratoplasty, 1980–2001. Invest Ophthalmol Vis Sci (Suppl) 2002; 1738.
274. Kannabiran C, Klintworth GK. TGFBI gene mutations in corneal dystrophies. Mutat Res 2006.
275. Kao WW, Vergnes JP, Ebert J, et al. Increased collagenase and gelatinase activities in keratoconus. Biochem Biophys Res Commun 1982; 107:929–36.

276. Karantinos D, Louletzoglu M, Stavropoulou K, et al. Histocompatibility antigens (HLA) in keratoconus 933–6. 1979. The Cornea in Health and Disease, Royal Society of Medicine International Congress and Symposium Series, Academic Press. Ref Type: Conference Proceeding.
277. Karseras AG, Ruben M. Aetiology of keratoconus. Br J Ophthalmol 1976; 60:522–5.
278. Kawasaki S, Nishida K, Quantock AJ, et al. Amyloid and Pro501 Thr-mutated (beta)ig-h3 gene product colocalize in lattice corneal dystrophy type IIIA. Am J Ophthalmol 1999; 127:456–8.
279. Kelleher MJ, Lindberg KA, Pinnell SR, Klintworth GK. A study of lysine derived crosslinks in corneas with keratoconus. Invest Ophthalmol Vis Sci (Suppl) 1983; 24:123.
280. Kemp EG, Lewis CJ. Immunoglobulin patterns in keratoconus with particular reference to total and specific IgE levels. Br J Ophthalmol 1982; 66:717–20.
281. Kennedy RH, Bourne WM, Dyer JA. A 48-year clinical and epidemiologic study of keratoconus. Am J Ophthalmol 1986; 101:267–73.
282. Kenney MC, Brown DJ, Rajeev B. Everett Kinsey lecture. The elusive causes of keratoconus: a working hypothesis. CLAO J 2000; 26:10–3.
283. Kenney MC, Chwa M, Atilano SR, et al. Increased levels of catalase and cathepsin V/L2 but decreased TIMP-1 in keratoconus corneas: evidence that oxidative stress plays a role in this disorder. Invest Ophthalmol Vis Sci 2005; 46: 823–32.
284. Kenney MC, Chwa M, Escobar M, Brown D. Altered gelatinolytic activity by keratoconus corneal cells. Biochem Biophys Res Commun 1989; 161:353–7.
285. Kenney MC, Labermeier U, Hinds D, Waring GO. Characterization of the Descemet's membrane/posterior collagenous layer isolated from Fuchs' endothelial dystrophy corneas. Exp Eye Res 1984; 39:267–77.
286. Kenyon KR. The synthesis of basement membrane by the corneal epithelium in bullous keratopathy. Invest Ophthalmol Vis Sci 1969; 8:156–68.
287. Kenyon KR, Maumenee AE. Further studies of congenital hereditary endothelial dystrophy of the cornea. Am J Ophthalmol 1973; 76:419–39.
288. Khan MD, Kundi N, Saeed N, et al. Incidence of keratoconus in spring catarrh. Br J Ophthalmol 1988; 72:41–3.
289. Kim HS, Yoon SK, Cho BJ, et al. BIGH3 gene mutations and rapid detection in Korean patients with corneal dystrophy. Cornea 2001; 20:844–9.
290. Kim WJ, Rabinowitz Y, Meisler DM, Wilson SE. Keratocyte apoptosis associated with keratoconus. Invest Ophthalmol Vis Sci 1999; 40:S330.
291. King ET. Keratoconus following thyroidectomy. Trans Ophthalmol Soc (UK) 1953; 73:31–9.
292. King RG Jr, Geeraets WJ. Lattice or Reis–Bücklers corneal dystrophy. A question of stromal pathology. South Med J 1969; 62:1163–9.
293. Kirk HQ, Rabb M, Hattenhauer J, Smith R. Primary familial amyloidosis of the cornea. Trans Am Acad Ophthalmol Otolaryngol 1973; 77:OP411–7.
294. Kirkness CM, McCartney A, Rice NS, et al. Congenital hereditary corneal oedema of Maumenee: its clinical features, management, and pathology. Br J Ophthalmol 1987; 71:130–44.
295. Kiskaddon BM, Campbell RJ, Waller RR, Bourne WM. Fleck dystrophy of the cornea: case report. Ann Ophthalmol 1980; 12:700–4.
296. Klaus E, Freyberger E, Kavka G, Vokcka F. Familiä Vorkommen von bulbärparalytischer Form der amyotrophischen Lateralskerose mit gittriger Hornhautdystrophie und Cutis hyperelastica bei drei Schwestern. Psychiat Neurol Basel 1959; 138:79–97.
297. Klintworth GK. The molecular genetics of the corneal dystrophies—current status. Frontiers in Bioscience 2002; 8:687–713.
298. Klintworth GK. Current concepts on the ultrastructural pathogenesis of macular and lattice corneal dystrophies. Birth Defects Org Art Series 1971; 7:27–31.
299. Klintworth GK. The cornea: structure and macromolecules in health and disease. A review. Am J Pathol 1977; 89:718–808.
300. Klintworth GK. Corneal dystrophies. In: Nicholson DH, ed. Ocular Pathology Update. New York: Masson, 1980:23–54.
301. Klintworth GK. Macular corneal dystrophy—a localized disorder of mucopolysaccharide metabolism? In: Daentl D, ed. Clinical, Structural and Biochemical Advances in Hereditary Eye Disorders. New York: Alan R. Liss, Inc., 1982:69–81.
302. Klintworth GK. Proteins in ocular disease. In: Garner A, Klintworth GK, eds, Pathobiology of Ocular Disease: A Dynamic Approach. 2nd ed. New York: Marcel Dekker, 1994:973–1031.
303. Klintworth GK. Advances in the molecular genetics of corneal dystrophies. Am J Ophthalmol 1999; 128: 747–54.
304. Klintworth GK, Enghild JJ, Valnickova Z. Discovery of a novel protein (βig-h3) in normal human cornea. Invest Ophthalmol Vis Sci (Suppl) 1994; 35:S1938.
305. Klintworth GK, Hawkins HK, Smith CF. Acridine orange particles in cultured fibroblasts. A comparative study of macular corneal dystrophy, systemic mucopolysaccharidoses types I-H and II, and normal controls. Arch Pathol Lab Med 1979; 103:297–9.
306. Klintworth GK, McCracken JS. Corneal diseases. In: Johannessen JV, ed. Electron Microscopy in Human Medicine. New York: McGraw-Hill, 1979:239–66.
307. Klintworth GK, Meyer R, Dennis R, et al. Macular corneal dystrophy. Lack of keratan sulfate in serum and cornea. Ophthal Paediatr Genet 1986; 7:139–43.
308. Klintworth GK, Oshima E, al-Rajhi A, et al. Macular corneal dystrophy in Saudi Arabia: a study of 56 cases and recognition of a new immunophenotype. Am J Ophthalmol 1997; 124:9–18.
309. Klintworth GK, Reed J, Stainer GA, Binder PS. Recurrence of macular corneal dystrophy within grafts. Am J Ophthalmol 1983; 95:60–72.
310. Klintworth GK, Smith CF. A comparative study of extracellular sulfated glycosaminoglycans synthesized by rabbit corneal fibroblasts in organ and confluent cultures. Lab Invest 1976; 35:258–63.
311. Klintworth GK, Smith CF. Macular corneal dystrophy. Studies of sulfated glycosaminoglycans in corneal explant and confluent stromal cell cultures. Am J Pathol 1977; 89: 167–82.
312. Klintworth GK, Smith CF. Abnormal product of corneal explants from patients with macular corneal dystrophy. Am J Pathol 1980; 101:143–58.
313. Klintworth GK, Smith CF. Difference between the glycosaminoglycans synthetized by corneal and cutaneous fibroblasts in culture. Lab Invest 1981; 44:553–9.
314. Klintworth GK, Smith CF. Abnormalities of proteoglycans and glycoproteins synthesized by corneal organ cultures derived from patients with macular corneal dystrophy. Lab Invest 1983; 48:603–12.
315. Klintworth GK, Smith CF, Bowling BL. CHST6 mutations in North American subjects with macular corneal

dystrophy: a comprehensive molecular genetic review. Molecular Vision 2006; 12:159–76.
316. Klintworth GK, Sommer JR, Karolak LA, Reed JW. Identification of a new keratin K12 mutations associated with Stocker–Holt corneal dystrophy that differs from mutations found in Meesmann corneal dystrophy. Invest Ophthalmol Vis Sci 1999; 40:S563.
317. Klintworth GK, Sommer JR, O'Brian G, et al. Familial subepithelial corneal amyloidosis (gelatinous drop-like corneal dystrophy). Mol Vis 1998; 4:31–8.
318. Klintworth GK, Valnickova Z, Enghild JJ. Accumulation of βig-h3 gene product in corneas with granular dystrophy. Am J Pathol 1998; 152:743–8.
319. Klintworth GK, Valnickova Z, Kielar RA, et al. Familial subepithelial corneal amyloidosis-a lactoferrin- related amyloidosis. Invest Ophthalmol Vis Sci 1997; 38:2756–63.
320. Klintworth GK, Vogel FS. Macular corneal dystrophy: an inherited acid mucopolysaccharide storage disease of the corneal fibroblast. Am J Pathol 1964; 45:565.
321. Klouda PT, Syrbopoulos EK, Entwistle CC, et al. HLA and keratoconus. Tiss Antigens 1983; 21:397–9.
322. Koeppe L. Beobachtungen mit der Nernstspaltlampe und dem Hornhautmikroskop. Albrecht von Graefes Arch Klin Exp Ophthalmol 1916; 91:363–79.
323. Konishi M, Mashima Y, Yamada M, et al. The classic form of granular corneal dystrophy associated with R555W mutation in the BIGH3 gene is rare in Japanese patients. Am J Ophthalmol 1998; 126:450–2.
324. Konishi M, Yamada M, Nakamura Y, Mashima Y. Varied appearance of cornea of patients with corneal dystrophy associated with R124H mutation in the BIGH3 gene. Cornea 1999; 18:424–9.
325. Konishi M, Yamada M, Nakamura Y, Mashima Y. Immunohistology of kerato-epithelin in corneal stromal dystrophies associated with R124 mutations of the BIGH3 gene. Curr Eye Res 2000; 21:891–6.
326. Korvatska E, Henry H, Mashima Y, et al. Amyloid and non-amyloid forms of 5q31-linked corneal dystrophy resulting from kerato-epithelin mutations at Arg-124 are associated with abnormal turnover of the protein. J Biol Chem 2000; 275:11465–9.
327. Korvatska E, Munier FL, Chaubert P, et al. On the role of kerato-epithelin in the pathogenesis of 5q31-linked corneal dystrophies. Invest Ophthalmol Vis Sci 1999; 40:2213–9.
328. Korvatska E, Munier FL, Djemai A, et al. Mutation hot spots in 5q31-linked corneal dystrophies. Am J Hum Genet 1998; 62:320–4.
329. Korvatska E, Yamada M, Yamamoto S, et al. Haplotype analysis of Japanese families with a superficial variant of granular corneal dystrohy: evidence for multiple origins of R124L mutation of keratoepithelin. Ophthal Genet 2000; 21:63–5.
330. Kowk LS, Lydon DP, Ho A. Polymethyl methacrylate (PMMA) contact lens wear may explain some of the increase in corneal endothelial polymegethism (variation in cell area) reported in keratoconic eyes. Am J Optom Physiol Opt 1987; 64:871–3.
331. Krachmer JH, Feder RS, Belin MW. Keratoconus and related noninflammatory corneal thinning disorders. Surv Ophthalmol 1984; 28:293–322.
332. Krachmer JH, Purcell JJ Jr, Young CW, Bucher KD. Corneal endothelial dystrophy. A study of 64 families. Arch Ophthalmol 1978; 96:2036–9.
333. Krafchak CM, Pawar H, Moroi SE, et al. Mutations in TCF8 cause posterior polymorphous corneal dystrophy and ectopic expression of COL4A3 by corneal endothelial cells. Am J Hum Genet 2005; 77:694–708.
334. Kraupa A. Ueber Epithel-und Endotheldystrophien. Z Augenheilkd 1934; 83:179–89.
335. Kremer I, Martini AM, Cohen EJ. Keratoconus associated with ectodermal and mesodermal anomalies. CLAO J 1992; 18:141.
336. Kuchle M, Green WR, Volcker HE, Barraquer J. Reevaluation of corneal dystrophies of Bowman's layer and the anterior stroma (Reis–Bucklers and Thiel–Behnke types): a light and electron microscopic study of eight corneas and a review of the literature. Cornea 1995; 14: 333–54.
337. Kuchle M, Naumann GO. Perforierende Keratoplastik wegen Keratokonus bei Trisomie 21. Klin Monatsbl Augenheilkd 1992; 200:228–30.
338. Kuming BS, Joffe L. Ehlers–Danlos syndrome associated with keratoconus. A case report. S Afr Med J 1977; 52: 403–5.
339. Kuwabara T, Ciccarelli EC. Meesmann's corneal dystrophy: a pathological study. Arch Ophthalmol 1964; 71: 676–82.
340. Kuwahara Y, Akiya S, Obazawa H. Electron microscopic study on granular dystrophy, macular dystrophy and gelatinous drop-like dystrophy of the cornea. Nippon Ganka Kiyo 1967; 18:434–5 [Japanese].
341. Kuwahara Y, Akiya S, Obazawa H. Electron microscopic study on the stromal lesion in granular dystrophy of the cornea. Nippon Ganka Gakkai Zasshi 1970; 74:1468–78 [Japanese].
342. Lahoud S, Brownstein S, Laflamme MY, Poleski SA. Keratoconus with spontaneous perforation of the cornea. Can J Ophthalmol 1987; 22:230–3.
343. Laing RA, Sandstrom MM, Berrospi AR, Leibowitz HM. The human corneal endothelium in keratoconus: a specular microscopic study. Arch Ophthalmol 1979; 97: 1867–9.
344. Lang GE, Naumann GO. Keratoconus in Alagille Lembach, R G. Keratoconus. Int Ophthalmol Clin 1991; 31:71–82.
345. Lang GK, Holbach L, Schlotzer U. Pseudokeratoconus bei Trisomie und hinterer polymorpher Hornhautdystrophi (HPHD). Klin Monatsbl Augenheilkd 1989; 195:95–9.
346. Lanier JD, Bullington RH Jr, Prager TC. Axial length in keratoconus. Cornea 1992; 11:250–4.
347. Lanier JD, Fine M, Togni B. Lattice corneal dystrophy. Arch Ophthalmol 1976; 94:921–4.
348. Lasram L, Rais C, el Euch M, Ouertani A. Dystrophie gelatineuse de la cornee. A propos de 5 observations. J Fr Ophtalmol 1994; 17:24–8.
349. Lee J, Jiao X, Hejtmancik JF, et al. The metabolism of fatty acids in human Bietti crystalline dystrophy. Invest Ophthalmol Vis Sci 2001; 42:1707–14.
350. Lempert SL, Jenkins MS, Johnson BL, Brown SI. A simple technique for removal of recurring granular dystrophy in corneal grafts. Am J Ophthalmol 1978; 86:89–91.
351. Levenson JE, Chandler JW, Kaufman HE. Affected asymptomatic relatives in congenital hereditary endothelial dystrophy. Am J Ophthalmol 1973; 76:967–71.
352. Lewkojewa EF. Ueber einen Fall primärer Degenerationamyloidose der Kornea. Klin Monatsbl Augenheilkd 1930; 85:117–37.
353. Li QJ, Ashraf MF, Shen DF, et al. The role of apoptosis in the pathogenesis of Fuchs endothelial dystrophy of the cornea. Arch Ophthalmol 2001; 119:1597–604.
354. Li SH, Edward DP, Ratnakar KS, et al. Clinicohistopathological findings of gelatinous droplike corneal dystrophy among Asians. Cornea 1996; 15:355–62.
355. Liakos GM, Casey TA. Posterior polymorphous keratopathy. Br J Ophthalmol 1978; 62:39–45.

356. Lindquist TD, McGlothan JS, Rotkis WM, Chandler JW. Indications for penetrating keratoplasty: 1980–1988. Cornea 1991; 10:210–6.
357. Lipman RM, Rubenstein JB, Torczynski E. Keratoconus and Fuchs' corneal endothelial dystrophy in a patient and her family. Arch Ophthalmol 1990; 108:993–4.
358. Lipman RM, Rubenstein JB, Torczynski E. Keratoconus and Fuchs' endothelial dystrophy. Cornea 1991; 10:368.
359. Lisch W, Buttner A, Oeffner F, et al. Lisch corneal dystrophy is genetically distinct from Meesmann corneal dystrophy and maps to Xp22.3. Am J Ophthalmol 2000; 130:461–8.
360. Lisch W, Steuhl KP, Lisch C, et al. A new, band-shaped and whorled microcystic dystrophy of the corneal epithelium. Am J Ophthalmol 1992; 114:35–44.
361. Lisch W, Weidle EG, Lisch C, et al. Utermann G. Schnyder's dystrophy. Progression and metabolism. Ophthal Paediatr Genet 1986; 7:45–56.
362. Liu NP, Baldwin J, Jonasson F, et al. Haplotype analysis in Icelandic families defines a minimal interval for the macular corneal dystrophy type I gene. Am J Hum Genet 1998; 63:912–7.
363. Liu NP, Baldwin J, Lennon F, et al. Coexistence of macular corneal dystrophy types I and II in a single sibship. Br J Ophthalmol 1998; 82:241–44.
364. Liu NP, Bao W, Smith CF, et al. Different mutations in carbohydrate sulfotransferase 6 (CHST6) gene cause macular corneal dystrophy types I and II in a single sibship. Am J Ophthalmol 2005; 139:1118–20.
365. Liu NP, Dew-Knight S, Jonasson F, et al. Physical and genetic mapping of the macular corneal dystrophy locus on chromosome 16q and exclusion of TAT and LCAT as candidate genes. Mol Vis 2000; 6:95–100.
366. Liu NP, Dew-Knight S, Rayner M, et al. Mutations in corneal carbohydrate sulfotransferase 6 gene (CHST6) cause macular corneal dystrophy in Iceland. Mol Vis 2000; 6:261–4.
367. Lloyd RI, Levitt JM. Congential and familial endothelial defects. Trans Am Ophthalmol Soc 1950; 48:48–61.
368. Lohse E, Stock EL, Jones JC, et al. Reis–Bucklers' corneal dystrophy. Immunofluorescent and electron microscopic studies. Cornea 1989; 8:200–9.
369. Lois N, Kowal VO, Cohen EJ, et al. Laibson PR. Indications for penetrating keratoplasty and associated procedures, 1989–1995. Cornea 1997; 16:623–9.
370. Longmore L. Atopic dermatitis cataract and keratoconus. Australas J Dermatol 1970; 11:139–41.
371. Lorenzetti DW, Kaufman HE. Macular and lattice dystrophies and their recurrences after keratoplasty. Trans Am Acad Ophthalmol Otolaryngol 1967; 71: 112–8.
372. Lorenzetti DWC, Uotila MH, Parikh H, Kaufman HE. Central cornea guttata. Incidence in general population. Am J Ophthalmol 1967; 64:1155–8.
373. Lorfel RS, Sugar HS. Keratoconus associated with retrolental fibroplasia. Ann Ophthalmol 1976; 8:449–50.
374. Lowell FC, Carroll JM. A study of the occurrence of atopic traits in patients with keratoconus. J Allergy 1970; 46: 32–9.
375. Lowry GM. Corneal endothelium in vitro: characterization by ultrastructure and histochemistry. Invest Ophthalmol 1966; 5:355–66.
376. Lund AM. [The Angelman syndrome. Does the phenotype depend on maternal inheritance?]. [Danish]. Ugeskr Laeger 1991; 153:1993–8.
377. Luxenberg M. Hereditary crystalline dystrophy of the cornea. Am J Ophthalmol 1967; 63:507–11.
378. Macnamara E, Sams GW, Smith K, et al. Aquaporin-1 expression is decreased in human and mouse corneal endothelial dysfunction. Molecular Vision 2004; 10:51–6.
379. Macsai MS, Doshi H. Clinical pathologic correlation of superficial corneal opacities in X-linked ichthyosis. Am J Ophthalmol 1994; 118:477–84.
380. Macsai MS, Varley GA, Krachmer JH. Development of keratoconus after contact lens wear. Patient characteristics. Arch Ophthalmol 1990; 108:534–8.
381. Maeder G, Danis P. Sur une nouvelle forme de dystrophie cornéenne (dystrophia filiformis profunda corneae) associée à un kératocône. Ophthalmologica 1947; 114:246–8.
382. Magovern M, Beauchamp GR, McTigue JW, et al. Inheritance of Fuchs' combined dystrophy. Ophthalmology 1979; 86: 1897–923.
383. Maguire LJ, Bourne WM. Corneal topography of early keratoconus. Am J Ophthalmol 1989; 108:107–12 [see comments].
384. Malbran JL, Paunessa JM, Vidal F. Hereditary crystalline degeneration of the cornea. Ophthalmologica 1953; 126: 369–78.
385. Malbrel PH, Monbrun C, Puech B. Deux nouveaux cas de kératocône familial. Bull Soc Ophtalmol Fr 1984; 84: 1155–7.
386. Margo CE, Mosteller MW. Corneal pseudocyst following acute hydrops. Br J Ophthalmol 1987; 71:359–60.
387. Markoff A, Bogdanova N, Uhlig CE, et al.: A novel TACSTD2 gene mutation in a Turkish family with a gelatinous drop-like corneal dystrophy. Mol Vis 2007; 12: 1473–6.
388. Maruyama Y, Wang XP, Li YH, et al. Involvement of Sp1 elements in the promoter activity of genes affected in keratoconus. Invest Ophthalmol Vis Sci 2001; 42:1980–5.
389. Mashima Y, Konishi M, Nakamura Y, et al. Severe form of juvenile corneal stromal dystrophy with homozygous R124H mutation in the keratoepithelin gene in five Japanese patients. Br J Ophthalmol 1998; 82:1280–4.
390. Mashima Y, Nakamura Y, Noda K, et al. A novel mutation at codon 124 (R124L) in the BIGH3 gene is associated with a superficial variant of granular corneal dystrophy. Arch Ophthalmol 1999; 117:90–3.
391. Mashima Y, Yamamoto S, Inoue Y, et al. Association of autosomal dominantly inherited corneal dystrophies with BIGH3 gene mutations in Japan. Am J Ophthalmol 2000; 130:516–7.
392. Masterson E, Edelhauser HF, Van Horn DL. The role of thyroid hormone in the development of the chick corneal endothelium and epithelium. Invest Ophthalmol Vis Sci 1977; 16:105–15.
393. Matsuda M, Suda T, Manabe R. Quantitative analysis of endothelial mosaic pattern changes in anterior keratoconus. Am J Ophthalmol 1984; 98:43–9.
394. Matsui M, Ito K, Akiya S. Histochemical and electron microscopic examinations and so-called gelatinous drop-like dystrophy of the cornea. Folia Ophthalmol Jap 1973; 23:466–73.
395. Matsuo N, Fujiwara H, Ofuchi Y. Electron and light microscopic observations of a case of Groenouw's nodular corneal dystrophy. Nippon Ganka Kiyo 1967; 18:436–47 [Japanese].
396. Matte U, Leistner S, Lima L, et al. Unique frequency of known mutations in Brazilian MPS I patients. Am J Med Genet 2000; 90:108–9.
397. Mauchart. Staphyloma Vexatum Nomen 1748. Tübingen, Typis Erhardtianis. Ref Type: Thesis/Dissertation.
398. Maumenee IH. The cornea in connective tissue diseases. Ophthalmology 1978; 85:1014–7 [Review].

399. Maurice DM. The location of the fluid pump in the cornea. J Physiol (Lond) 1972; 221:43–54.
400. Maxwell E. Crystalline degeneration of the cornea. Trans Ophthalmol Soc (UK) 1953; 73:697–9.
401. McCarthy M, Innis S, Dubord P, White V. Panstromal Schnyder corneal dystrophy. A clinical pathologic report with quantitative analysis of corneal lipid composition. Ophthalmology 1994; 101:895–901.
402. McCartney AC, Kirkness CM. Comparison between posterior polymorphous dystrophy and congenital hereditary endothelial dystrophy of the cornea. Eye 1988; 2:63–70.
403. McCartney MD, Robertson DP, Wood TO, McLaughlin BJ. ATPase pump site density in human dysfunctional corneal endothelium. Invest Ophthalmol Vis Sci 1987; 28:1955–62.
404. McCartney MD, Wood TO, McLaughlin BJ. Freeze-fracture label of functional and dysfunctional human corneal endothelium. Curr Eye Res 1987; 6:589–97.
405. McCartney MD, Wood TO, McLaughlin BJ. Immunohistochemical localization of ATPase in human dysfunctional corneal endothelium. Curr Eye Res 1987; 6: 1479–86.
406. McCartney MD, Wood TO, McLaughlin BJ. Moderate Fuchs' endothelial dystrophy ATPase pump site density. Invest Ophthalmol Vis Sci 1989; 30:1560–4.
407. McKusick VA. Mendelian Inheritance in Man. In: McKusick VA, ed. Catalogs of Autosomal Dominant, Autosomal Recessive and X-linked Phenotypes. 10th ed. Baltimore: Johns Hopkins University Press, 1992.
408. McPherson SD Jr, Kiffney GT Jr. Some histologic findings in keratoconus. Arch Ophthalmol 1968; 79:669–73.
409. McPherson SD Jr, Kiffney GT Jr, Freed CC. Corneal amyloidosis. (Also in Am J Ophthalmol 1966; 62:1024–33). Trans Am Ophthalmol Soc 1966; 64:148–62.
410. McTigue JW. The human cornea: a light and electron microscopic study of the normal cornea and its alterations in various dystrophies. Trans Am Ophthalmol Soc 1967; 65:591–660.
411. Meek KM, Quantock AJ, Elliott GF, et al. Macular corneal dystrophy: the macromolecular structure of the stroma observed using electron microscopy and synchrotron X-ray diffraction. Exp Eye Res 1989; 49:941–58.
412. Meesmann A. Über eine bisher nicht beschriebene dominant verterbte Dystrophia epithelialis corneae. Ber Dtsch Ophthalmol Ges 1938; 52:154.
413. Meesmann A, Wilke F. Klinische und anatomische Untersuchungen uber eine bisher unbekannte, dominant vererbte Epitheldystrophie der Hornhaut. Klin Monatsbl Augenheilkd 1939; 103:361.
414. Meisler DM, Fine M. Recurrence of the clinical signs of lattice corneal dystrophy (type I) in corneal transplants. Am J Ophthalmol 1984; 97:210–4.
415. Meretoja J. Familial systemic paramyloidosis with lattice dystrophy of the cornea, progressive cranial neuropathy, skin changes and various internal symptoms. A previously unrecognized heritable syndrome. Ann Clin Res 1969; 1:314–24.
416. Meretoja J. Comparative histopathological and clinical findings in eyes with lattice corneal dystrophy of two different types. Ophthalmologica 1972; 165:15–37.
417. Meretoja J. Genetic aspects of familial amyloidosis with corneal lattice dystrophy and cranial neuropathy. Clin Genet 1973; 4:173–85.
418. Meretoja J, Teppo L. Histopathological findings of familial amyloidosis with cranial neuropathy as principal manifestation. Report on three cases. Acta Pathol Microbiol Scand.[A]. 1971; 79:432–40.
419. Midura RJ, Hascall VC, MacCallum DK, et al. Proteoglycan biosynthesis by human corneas from patients with types 1 and 2 macular corneal dystrophy. J Biol Chem 1990; 265:15947–55.
420. Miller KH, Green WR, Stark WJ, et al. Immunoprotein deposition in the cornea. Ophthalmology 1980; 87:944–50.
421. Millin JA, Golub BM, Foster CS. Human basement membrane components of keratoconus and normal corneas. Invest Ophthalmol Vis Sci 1986; 27:604–7.
422. Moestrup B. Tenuity of cornea with Ehlers–Danlos syndrome. Acta Ophthalmol (Copenh) 1969; 47:704–8.
423. Møller HU. Granular corneal dystrophy Groenouw type I (GrI) and Reis–Bücklers' corneal dystrophy (R-B). One entity? Acta Ophthalmol (Copenh) 1989; 67:678–84.
424. Møller HU. Inter-familial variability and intra-familial similarities of granular corneal dystrophy Groenouw type I with respect to biomicroscopical appearance and symptomatology. Acta Ophthalmol (Copenh) 1989; 67:669–77.
425. Møller HU. Granular corneal dystrophy Groenouw type I 115 Danish patients. An epidemiological and genetic population study. Acta Ophthalmol (Copenh) 1990; 68: 297–303.
426. Møller HU. Granular corneal dystrophy Groenouw type I. Clinical aspects and treatment. Acta Ophthalmol (Copenh) 1990; 68:384–9.
427. Møller HU. Granular corneal dystrophy Groenouw type I. Clinical and genetic aspects. Acta Ophthalmol Suppl 1991; 1–40.
428. Møller HU, Ridgway AE. Granular corneal dystrophy Groenouw type I. A report of a probable homozygous patient. Acta Ophthalmol (Copenh) 1990; 68:97–101.
429. Moore TE Jr, Aronson SB. Results of penetrating keratoplasty in keratoconus. Adv Ophthalmol 1978; 37: 106–8.
430. Mortelmans L. Forme familiale de la dystrophie cornéene de Fuchs. Ophthalmologica 1952; 123:88–99.
431. Morton K, Hutchinson C, Jeanny JC, et al. Colocalization of fibroblast growth factor binding sites with extracellular matrix components in normal and keratoconus corneas. Curr Eye Res 1989; 8:975–87.
432. Munier FL, Frueh BE, Othenin-Girard P, et al. BIGH3 mutation spectrum in corneal dystrophies. Invest Ophthalmol Vis Sci 2002; 43:949–54.
433. Munier FL, Korvatska E, Djemai A, et al. Kerato-epithelin mutations in four 5q31-linked corneal dystrophies. Nat Genet 1997; 15:247–51.
434. Nagataki S, Tanishima T, Sakimoto T. A case of primary gelatinous drop-like corneal dystrophy. Jpn J Ophthalmol 1972; 16:107–16.
435. Nakamura T, Nishida K, Dota A, et al. Gelatino-lattice corneal dystrophy: clinical features and mutational analysis. Am J Ophthalmol 2000; 129:665–6.
436. Nakanishi I, Brown SI. Clinicopathologic case report: ultrastructure of the epithelial dystrophy of Meesmann. Arch Ophthalmol 1975; 93:259–63.
437. Nakayasu K, Tanaka M, Konomi H, Hayashi T. Distribution of types I, II, III, IV and V collagen in normal and keratoconus corneas. Ophthal Res 1986; 18:1–10.
438. Nakazawa K, Hassell JR, Hascall VC, et al. Defective processing of keratan sulfate in macular corneal dystrophy. J Biol Chem 1984; 259:13751–7.
439. Nash IS, Greene PR, Foster CS. Comparison of mechanical properties of keratoconus and normal corneas. Exp Eye Res 1982; 35:413–24.
440. Natt E, Kida K, Odievre M, et al. Point mutations in the tyrosine aminotransferase gene in tyrosinemia type-IIi. Proc Natl Acad Sci U.S.A. 1992; 89:9297–301.

441. Negris R. Floppy eyelid syndrome associated with keratoconus. J Am Optom Assoc 1992; 63:316–9.
442. Newsome DA, Foidart JM, Hassell JR, et al. Detection of specific collagen types in normal and keratoconus corneas. Invest Ophthalmol Vis Sci 1981; 20:738–50.
443. Nicholson DH, Green WR, Cross HE, et al. A clinical and histopathological study of Francois-Neetens speckled corneal dystrophy. Am J Ophthalmol 1977; 83:554–60.
444. Niel F, Ellies P, Dighiero P, et al. Truncating mutations in the carbohydrate sulfotransferase 6 gene (CHST6) result in macular corneal dystrophy. Invest Ophthalmol Vis Sci 2003; 44:2949–53.
445. Nirankari VS, Karesh J, Bastion F, et al. Recurrence of keratoconus in donor cornea 22 years after successful keratoplasty. Br J Ophthalmol 1983; 67:23–8.
446. Nishida K, Honma Y, Dota A, et al. Isolation and chromosomal localization of a cornea-specific human keratin 12 gene and detection of four mutations in Meesmann corneal epithelial dystrophy. Am J Hum Genet 1997; 61:1268–75.
447. Norins A, Field L. Atopic dermatitis, atopic cataracts, and keratoconus in one patient. Arch Dermatol 1964; 90:102–3.
448. Nottingham F. In: Nottingham F, ed. Practical Observations on Conical Cornea and on the Short Sight, and Other Defects of Vision Connected with it. London: John Churchill, 1854.
449. Nucci P, Brancato R. Keratoconus and congenital hip dysplasia. Am J Ophthalmol 1991; 111:775–6.
450. Nucci P, Trabucchi G, Brancato R. Keratoconus and Turner's syndrome: a case report. Optomet Vis Sci 1991; 68:407–8.
451. Offret G, Pouliquen Y, Coscas G. A case of familial corneal dystrophy. Clinical, histological and ultrastructural study. Arch Ophtalmol Rev Gen Ophtalmol 1969; 29:537–50.
452. Okada M, Yamamoto S, Tsujikawa M, et al. Two distinct kerato-epithelin mutations in Reis–Bucklers corneal dystrophy. Am J Ophthalmol 1998; 126:535–42.
453. Okada M, Yamamoto S, Watanabe H, et al. Granular corneal dystrophy with homozygous mutations in the kerato-epithelin gene. Am J Ophthalmol 1998; 126:169–76.
454. Orr A, Dubé M-P, Marcadier J, et al. Mutations in the UBIAD1 gene, encoding a potential prenyltransferase, are causal for Schnyder crystalline corneal dystrophy. PLoS ONE 2(8):e685 doi:10.1371/Journal.phone. 0000685.
455. Oxlund H, Simonsen AH. Biochemical studies of normal and keratoconus corneas. Acta Ophthalmol (Copenh) 1985; 63:666–9.
456. Paik KH, Song SM, Ki CS, et al. Identification of mutations in the GNPTA (MGC4170) gene coding for GlcNAc-phosphotransferase alpha/beta subunits in Korean patients with mucolliplidoslis type II or type IIIA. Hum Mutat 2005; 26:308–14.
457. Pameijer JK. Ueber eine fremdartige familiäre oberflächliche Hornhautveränderung. Klin Monatsbl Augenheilkd 1935; 95:516–7.
458. Panjwani N, Drysdale J, Clark B, et al. Protein-related abnormalities in keratoconus. Invest Ophthalmol Vis Sci 1989; 30:2481–7.
459. Parunovic A, Ilic B. Floppy eyelid syndrome associated with keratotorus. Br J Ophthalmol 1988; 72:634–5.
460. Patten JT, Hyndiuk RA, Donaldson DD, et al. Fleck (Mouchetee) dystrophy of the cornea. Ann Ophthalmol 1976; 8:25–32.
461. Pattison S, Pankarican M, Rupar CA, et al. Five novel mutations in the lysosomal sialidase gene (NEU1) in type II sialidosis patients and assessment of their impact on enzyme activity and intracellular targeting using adenovirus-mediated expression. Hum Mutat 2004; 23: 32–9.
462. Paufique L, Etienne R. La cornea farinata.. Bull Soc Ophtalmol 1950; 50:522.
463. Paufique L, Ravault MP, Bonnet M, Laurent C. Dystrophie cristalline de Schnyder. Bull Soc Ophtalmol Fr 1964; 64:104.
464. Paunio T, Kiuru S, Hongell V, et al. Solid-phase minisequencing test reveals Asp_{187}–>Asn (G654→A) mutation of gelsolin in all affected individuals with Finnish type of familial amyloidosis. Genomics 1992; 13: 237–9.
465. Pavlin CJ, Harasiewicz K, Foster FS. Ultrasound biomicroscopic assessment of the cornea following excimer laser photokeratectomy. J Cataract Refract Surg 1994; 20: Suppl:206–11.
466. Peiffer RL Jr, Werblin TP, Patel AS. Keratoconus in a rhesus monkey. J Med Primatol 1987; 16:403–6.
467. Perry HD, Buxton JN, Fine BS. Round and oval cones in keratoconus. Ophthalmology 1980; 87:905–9.
468. Perry HD, Fine BS, Caldwell DR. Reis–Bücklers dystrophy: a study of eight cases. Arch Ophthalmol 1979; 97: 664–70.
469. Pettenati MJ, Sweatt AJ, Lantz P, et al. The human cornea has a high incidence of acquired chromosome abnormalities. Human Genetics 1997; 101:26–9.
470. Philipp W. Altered lectin binding sites in keratoconus corneas. Curr Eye Res 1992; 11:397–409.
471. Pippow G. Zur erbbedingheit der cornea farinata (Mehlstaubartige Hornhautedegeneration). Albrecht von Graefes Arch Klin Exp Ophthalmol 1941; 144: 276–9.
472. Plaas AH, West LA, Thonar EJ, et al. Altered fine structures of corneal and skeletal keratan sulfate and chondroitin/dermatan sulfate in macular corneal dystrophy. J Biol Chem 2001; 276:39788–96.
473. Polack FM. The posterior corneal surface in Fuchs' dystrophy. Scanning electron microscope study. Invest Ophthalmol Vis Sci 1974; 13:913–22.
474. Polack FM. Contributions of electron microscopy to the study of corneal pathology. Surv Ophthalmol 1976; 20: 375–414.
475. Porteous ME, Strain L, Logie LJ, et al. Keratosis follicularis spinulosa decalvans: confirmation of linkage to Xp22.13–p22.2. J Med Genet 1998; 35:336–7.
476. Pouliquen Y, Chauvaud D, Savoldelli M. Kératocône aigu: une étude ultrastructurale. J Fr Ophtalmol 1978; 1:111–8.
477. Pouliquen Y, Graf B, Hamada R, et al. Les fibrocytes dans le kératocône. Aspects morphologiques et modifications de l'espace extracellulaire. Étude en microscopice optique et électronique. Arch Ophtalmol (Paris) 1972; 32:571–86.
478. Pouliquen Y, Graf B, Kozak Yd, et al. Étude morphologique et biochimique du kératocône. I. Étude morphologique du kératocone. Arch Ophtalmol (Paris) 1970; 30: 497–532.
479. Price FW Jr, Whitson WE, Marks RG. Graft survival in four common groups of patients undergoing penetrating keratoplasty. Ophthalmology 1991; 98:322–8.
480. Purcell JJ, Jr., Krachmer JH, Weingeist TA. Fleck corneal dystrophy. Arch Ophthalmol 1977; 95:440–4.
481. Quantock AJ, Meek KM, Ridgway AE, et al. Macular corneal dystrophy: reduction in both corneal thickness and collagen interfibrillar spacing. Curr Eye Res 1990; 9:393–8.

482. Quantock AJ, Meek KM, Thonar EJ. Analysis of high-angle synchrotron x-ray diffraction patterns obtained from macular dystrophy corneas. Cornea 1992; 11: 185–90.
483. Raas-Rothschild A, Cormier-Daire V, Bao M, et al. Molecular basis of variant pseudo-Hurler polydystrophy (mucolipidosis IIIC). J Clin Invest 2000; 105:673–81.
484. Rabb MF, Blodi F, Boniuk M. Unilateral lattice dystrophy of the cornea. Trans Am Acad Ophthalmol Otolaryngol 1974; 78:OP440–4.
485. Rabinowitz YS. Keratoconus. Surv Ophthalmol 1998; 42: 297–319.
486. Rabinowitz YS, Dong LJ, Wistow G. Gene expression profile studies of human keratoconus cornea for NEIBank: a novel cornea-expressed gene and the absence of transcripts for aquaporin 5. Invest Ophthalmol Vis Sci 2005; 46:1239–46.
487. Rabinowitz YS, Maumenee IH, Lundergan MK, et al. Molecular genetic analysis in autosomal dominant keratoconus. Cornea 1992; 11:302–8.
488. Rabinowitz YS, McDonnell PJ. Computer-assisted corneal topography in keratoconus. Refract Corneal Surg 1989; 5:400–8.
489. Radda TM, Menzel EJ, Freyler H, Gnad HD. Collagen types in keratoconus. Graefes Arch Clin Exp Ophthalmol 1982; 218:262–4.
490. Rahi A, Davies P, Ruben M, et al. Keratoconus and coexisting atopic disease. Br J Ophthalmol 1977; 61:761–4.
491. Ramsay RM. Familial corneal dystrophy-lattice type. Trans Am Ophthalmol Soc 1957; 65:701–39.
492. Ramsay RM. Familial corneal dystrophy-lattice type. Trans Can Ophthalmol 1960; 23:222–9.
493. Ramsey MS, Fine BS, Cohen SW. Localized corneal amyloidosis: case report with electron microscopic observations. Am J Ophthalmol 1972; 73:560–5.
494. Rawe IM, Zhan Q, Komai Y, et al. Localization and characterization of a novel extracellular matrix protein Big-h3. Invest Ophthalmol Vis Sci (Suppl) 1995; 36:S27.
495. Reed JW, Cashwell F, Klintworth GK. Corneal manifestations of hereditary benign intraepithelial dyskeratosis. Arch Ophthalmol 1979; 97:297–300.
496. Rehany U, Lahav M, Shoshan S. Collagenolytic activity in keratoconus. Ann Ophthalmol 1982; 14:751–4.
497. Reis W. Fämiliare, fleckige Hornhautetartung. Dtsch Med Wochenschr 1917; 43:575.
498. Remler O. Hereditary Recurrent Erosion of the Cornea. Klin Monatsbl Augenheilkd 1983; 183:59.
499. Ren Z, Lin P-Y, Klintworth GK, et al. Mutations of the M1S1 gene on chromosome 1P in autosomal recessive gelatinous drop-like corneal dystrophy. Proc Internat Soc Eye Res 2000; 71:S108P [abstract].
500. Ren Z, Lin PY, Klintworth GK, et al. Allelic and locus heterogeneity in autosomal recessive gelatinous drop-like corneal dystrophy. Human Genetics 2002; 110:568–77.
501. Ricci V, Filocamo M, Regis S, et al. Expression studies of two novel in CIS-mutations identified in an intermediate case of Hunter syndrome. Am J Med Genet Part A 2003; 120A:84–7.
502. Rice NS, Ashton N, Jay B, Blach RK. Reis–Bucklers' dystrophy. A clinico-pathological study. Br J Ophthalmol 1968; 52:577–603.
503. Ridgway AE, Akhtar S, Munier FL, et al. Ultrastructural and molecular analysis of Bowman's layer corneal dystrophies: an epithelial origin? Invest Ophthalmol Vis Sci 2000; 41:3286–92.
504. Ridley F. Contact lenses in treatment of keratoconus. Br J Ophthalmol 1956; 40:295–304.
505. Ridley F. Eye-rubbing and contact lenses, letter to the editor. Br J Ophthalmol 1961; 45:832.
506. Ridley F. Scleral contact lenses in keratoconus. In: Dabezies OH, ed. Contact Lenses, Symposium in Munich-Feldafing, August 13, 1966. Basel: Krager, 1967:163–73.
507. Risen LA, Binder PS, Nayak SK. Intermediate filaments and their organization in human corneal endothelium. Invest Ophthalmol Vis Sci 1987; 28:1933–8.
508. Robb RM, Kuwabara T. The ocular pathology of type A Niemann–Pick disease. Invest Ophthalmol Vis Sci 1973; 12:366–77.
509. Robert L, Schillinger G, Moczar M, et al. Biochemical study of the keratoconus. Arch Ophtalmol Rev Gen Ophtalmol 1970; 30:590–608 [French].
510. Robertson I. A new aspect of keratoconus. Aust J Ophthalmol 1974; 2/3:144–6.
511. Robertson I. Keratoconus and the Ehlers–Danlos syndrome: a new aspect of keratoconus. Med J Aust 1975; 1:571–3.
512. Robin AL, Green WR, Lapsa TP, et al. Recurrence of macular corneal dystrophy after lamellar keratoplasty. Am J Ophthalmol 1977; 84:457–61.
513. Robin SB, Epstein RJ, Kornmehl EW. Band-shaped, whorled microcystic corneal dystrophy. Am J Ophthalmol 1994; 117: 543–4.
514. Rochels R, Nover A, Schmid F. Ophthalmologic symptoms of Down's syndrome.. Albrecht von Graefes Arch Klin Exp Ophthalmol 1977; 205:9–12 [German].
515. Rodrigues MM, Gaster RN, Pratt MV. Unusual superficial confluent form of granular corneal dystrophy. Ophthalmology 1983; 90:1507–11.
516. Rodrigues MM, Krachmer JH, Hackett J, et al. Fuchs' corneal dystrophy. A clinicopathologic study of the variation in corneal edema. Ophthalmology 1986; 93: 789–96.
517. Rodrigues MM, McGavic JS. Recurrent corneal granular dystrophy: a clinicopathologic study. Trans Am Ophthalmol Soc 1975; 73:306–16.
518. Rodrigues MM, Rajagopalan S, Jones K, et al. Gelsolin immunoreactivity in corneal amyloid, wound healing, and macular and granular dystrophies. Am J Ophthalmol 1993; 115:644–52.
519. Rodrigues MM, Streeten BW, Krachmer JH, et al. Microfibrillar protein and phospholipid in granular corneal dystrophy. Arch Ophthalmol 1983; 101:802–10.
520. Rodrigues MM, Sun T, Krachmer J, Newsome D. Posterior polymorphous corneal dystrophy: recent developments. Birth Defects Org Art Series 1982; 18:479–91.
521. Rodrigues MM, Sun TT, Krachmer J, Newsome D. Epithelialization of the corneal endothelium in posterior polymorphous dystrophy. Invest Ophthalmol Vis Sci 1980; 19:832–5.
522. Rodrigues MM, Waring GO, Laibson PR, Weinreb S. Endothelial alterations in congenital corneal dystrophies. Am J Ophthalmol 1975; 80:678–89.
523. Rosenberg ME, Tervo TM, Gallar J, et al. Corneal morphology and sensitivity in lattice dystrophy type II (familial amyloidosis, Finnish type). Invest Ophthalmol Vis Sci 2001; 42:634–41.
524. Rosenblum P, Stark WJ, Maumenee IH, et al. Hereditary Fuchs' dystrophy. Am J Ophthalmol 1980; 90:455–62.
525. Roth SI, Mittelman D, Stock EL. Posterior amorphous corneal dystrophy. An ultrastructural study of a variant with histopathological features of an endothelial dystrophy. Cornea 1992; 11:165–72.
526. Roth SI, Stock EL, Jutabha R. Endothelial viral inclusions in Fuchs' corneal dystrophy. Hum Pathol 1987; 18:338–41.

527. Rowsey JJ, Reynolds AE, Brown R. Corneal topography. Corneascope. Arch Ophthalmol 1981; 99: 1093–100.
528. Rozzo C, Fossarello M, Galleri G, et al. A common beta ig-h3 gene mutation (delta f540) in a large cohort of Sardinian Reis–Bucklers corneal dystrophy patients. Mutations in brief no 180. Online. Hum Mutat 1998; 12: 215–6.
529. Rubsamen PE, McLeish WM. Keratoconus with acute hydrops and perforation. Brief case report. Cornea 1991; 10:83–4.
530. Ruusuvaara P, Setala K, Liesto K, Tarkkanen A. Acute bilateral corneal hydrops caused by high temperature and high moisture in the Finnish sauna. A clinical and histological case report of a patient with keratoconus. Acta Ophthalmol (Copenh) 1989; 67:310–4.
531. Ruusuvaara P, Setala K, Tarkkanen A. Granular corneal dystrophy with early stromal manifestation. A clinical and electron microscopical study. Acta Ophthalmol (Copenh) 1990; 68:525–31.
532. Santo RM, Yamaguchi T, Kanai A, et al. Clinical and histopathologic features of corneal dystrophies in Japan. Ophthalmology 1995; 102:557–67.
533. Sasaki Y, Tuberville AW, Wood TO, McLaughlin BJ. Freeze fracture study of human corneal endothelial dysfunction. Invest Ophthalmol Vis Sci 1986; 27:480–5.
534. Sawaguchi S, Twining SS, Yue BY, et al. Alpha-1 proteinase inhibitor levels in keratoconus. Exp Eye Res 1990; 50:549–54.
535. Sawaguchi S, Yue BY, Chang I, et al. Proteoglycan molecules in keratoconus corneas. Invest Ophthalmol Vis Sci 1991; 32:1846–53.
536. Sawaguchi S, Yue BY, Sugar J, Gilboy JE. Lysosomal enzyme abnormalities in keratoconus. Arch Ophthalmol 1989; 107:1507–10.
537. Sayegh FN, Ashouri M. Incidence of keratoconus in spring catarrh. Fortschr Ophthalmol 1987; 84:414–7.
538. Schappert-Kimmijser J. Rezidivierende Hornhauterosion und familiäre Hornhautentartung. Klin Monatsbl Augenheilkd 1933; 90:655–61.
539. Scheie HG, Yanoff M, Kellogg WT. Essential iris atrophy. Report of a case. Arch Ophthalmol 1976; 94:1315–20.
540. Schmid E, Lisch W, Philipp W, et al. A new, X-linked endothelial corneal dystrophy. Am J Ophthalmol 2006; 141:478–87.
541. Schmitt-Bernard CF, Guittard C, Arnaud B, et al. BIGH3 exon 14 mutations lead to intermediate type I/IIIA of lattice corneal dystrophies. Invest Ophthalmol Vis Sci 2000; 41:1302–8.
542. Schnyder W. Mitteilung übereinen neuen Typus von familiärer Hornauterkrankung. Schwiez Med Wochenmschr 1929; 59:559.
543. Schnyder WF. Scheibenformige kristalleinlagerungen in der hornhautmitte als erbeiden. Klin Monatsbl Augenheilkd 1939; 103:494.
544. Sédan J, Vallès A. Dégénérescence cornéenne cristalline congénitale de Schnyder. Bull Soc Ophtalmol Fr 1966;436–9.
545. Seitz B, Weidle E, Naumann GO. Einseitige gittrige stromale Hornhautdystrophie Typ III (Hida). Klin Monatsbl Augenheilkd 1993; 203:279–85.
546. Seitz R, Goslar HG. Über das Verhalten von transplantiertem Hornhautgewebe im Empfängerauge: ein klinischer, morphologischer und histochemischer Beitrag. Klin Monatsbl Augenheilkd 1963; 142:943–69.
547. Seitz R, Goslar HG. Beitrag zur Klinik, Hornhautdystrophie. Klin Monatsbl Augenheilkd 1965; 147:673–91.
548. Sekundo W, Lee WR, Kirkness CM, et al. An ultrastructural investigation of an early manifestation of the posterior polymorphous dystrophy of the cornea. Ophthalmology 1994; 101:1422–31.
549. Shapiro MB, France TD. The ocular features of Down's syndrome. Am J Ophthalmol 1985; 99:659–63.
550. Shapiro MB, Rodrigues MM, Mandel MR, Krachmer JH. Anterior clear spaces in keratoconus. Ophthalmology 1986; 93:1316–9.
551. Sharif KW, Casey TA. Penetrating keratoplasty for keratoconus: complications and long- term success [see comments]. Br J Ophthalmol 1991; 75:142–6.
552. Shearman AM, Hudson TJ, Andresen JM, et al. The gene for Schnyder's crystalline corneal dystrophy maps to human chromosome 1p34.1–p36. Hum Mol Genet 1996; 5:1667–72.
553. Sidrys LA. Hereditary Fuchs' dystrophy. Am J Ophthalmol 1981; 91:277–8.
554. Siemens HW. Keratosis follicular spinulosa decalvans. Arch Dermatol Syphilol 1926; 151:384–7.
555. Singh G, Mathur JS. Atopic erythroderma with bilateral cataract, unilateral keratoconus and iridocyclitis, and undescended testes. Br J Ophthalmol 1968; 52:61–3.
556. Skonier J, Bennett K, Rothwell V, et al. beta ig-h3: a transforming growth factor-beta-responsive gene encoding a secreted protein that inhibits cell attachment in vitro and suppresses the growth of CHO cells in nude mice. DNA Cell Biol 1994; 13:571–84.
557. Skonier J, Neubauer M, Madisen L, et al. cDNA cloning and sequence analysis of beta ig-h3, a novel gene induced in a human adenocarcinoma cell line after treatment with transforming growth factor-beta. DNA Cell Biol 1992; 11: 511–22.
558. Slusher MM, Laibson PR, Mulberger RD. Aucte keratoconus in Down's syndrome. Am J Ophthalmol 1968; 66: 1137–43.
559. Small KW, Mullen L, Barletta J, et al. Mapping of Reis–Bucklers' corneal dystrophy to chromosome 5q. Am J Ophthalmol 1996; 121:384–90.
560. Smith RE, McDonald HR, Nesburn AB, Minckler DS. Penetrating keratoplasty: changing indications, 1947 to 1978. Arch Ophthalmol 1980; 98:1226–9.
561. Smith SG, Rabinowitz YS, Sassani JW, Smith RE. Keratoconus and lattice and granular corneal dystrophies in the same eye. Am J Ophthalmol 1989; 108:608–10.
562. Smith VA, Easty DL. Matrix metalloproteinase 2: involvement in keratoconus. European Journal of Ophthalmology 2000; 10:215–26.
563. Smith VA, Hoh HB, Littleton M, Easty DL. Over-expression of a gelatinase A activity in keratoconus. Eye 1995; 9:429–33.
564. Snip RC, Kenyon KR, Green WR. Macular corneal dystrophy: ultrastructural pathology of corneal endothelium and Descemet's membrane. Invest Ophthalmol Vis Sci 1973; 12: 88–97.
565. Snyder M, Bergsmanson J, Doughty M. Keratocytes: no more the quite cells. J Am Optom Assoc 1998; 69:180–7.
566. Sommer A. Keratoconus in contact lens wear. Am J Ophthalmol 1978; 86:442–4 [letter].
567. Spencer WH, Fisher JJ. The association of keratoconus with atopic dermatitis. Am J Ophthalmol 1959; 47:332–4.
568. Stankovic I, Stojanovic D. L'hérédo-dystrophie mouchetée du parenchyme cornéen. Ann Ocul (Paris) 1964; 197: 52–7.
569. Stansbury FC. Lattice type of hereditary corneal degeneration: report of five cases, including one of a child of two years. Arch Ophthalmol 1948; 40:189–217.

570. Starck T, Kenyon KR, Hanninen LA, et al. Clinical and histopathologic studies of two families with lattice corneal dystrophy and familial systemic amyloidosis (Meretoja syndrome). Ophthalmology 1991; 98:1197–206.
571. Steahly LP. Keratoconus following contact lens wear. Ann Ophthalmol 1978; 10:1177–9.
572. Stern GA, Knapp A, Hood CI. Corneal amyloidosis associated with keratoconus. Ophthalmology 1988; 95:52–5.
573. Stewart H, Black GC, Donnai D, et al. A mutation within exon 14 of the TGFBI (BIGH3) gene on chromosome 5q31 causes an asymmetric, late-onset form of lattice corneal dystrophy. Ophthalmology 1999; 106:964–70.
574. Stewart HS, Parveen R, Ridgway AE, et al. Late onset lattice corneal dystrophy with systemic familial amyloidosis, amyloidosis V, in an English family. Br J Ophthalmol 2000; 84:390–4.
575. Stewart HS, Ridgway AE, Dixon MJ, et al. Heterogeneity in granular corneal dystrophy: identification of three causative mutations in the TGFBI (BIGH3) gene-lessons for corneal amyloidogenesis. Hum Mutat 1999; 14:126–32.
576. Stirling R, Pitts J, Galloway NR, et al. Congenital hereditary endothelial dystrophy associated with nail hypoplasia. Br J Ophthalmol 1994; 78:77–8.
577. Stock EL, Feder RS, O'Grady RB, et al. Lattice corneal dystrophy type IIIA. Clinical and histopathologic correlations. Arch Ophthalmol 1991; 109:354–8.
578. Stock EL, Kielar RA. Primary familial amyloidosis of the cornea. Am J Ophthalmol 1976; 82:266–71.
579. Stocker FW. The endothelium of the cornea and its clinical implications. Trans Am Acad Ophthalmol Otolaryngol 1953; 51:669–786.
580. Stocker FW, Holt LB. A rare form of hereditary epithelial dystrophy of the cornea. A genetic, clinical and pathologic study. Trans Am Ophthalmol Soc 1954; 52:133–44.
581. Stocker FW, Holt LB. Rare form of hereditary epithelial dystrophy: genetic, clinical and pathologic study. Arch Ophthalmol 1955; 53:536.
582. Stone DL, Kenyon KR, Stark WJ. Ultrastructure of keratoconus with healed hydrops. Am J Ophthalmol 1976; 82:450–8.
583. Stone EM, Mathers WD, Rosenwasser GO, et al. Three autosomal dominant corneal dystrophies map to chromosome 5q. Nat Genet 1994; 6:47–51.
584. Strachan IM. Cloudy central corneal dystrophy of Francois. Five cases in the same family. Br J Ophthalmol 1969; 53:192–4.
585. Street DA, Vinokur ET, Waring GO III, et al. Lack of association between keratoconus, mitral valve prolapse, and joint hypermobility. Ophthalmology 1991; 98:170–6.
586. Streeten BW, Falls HF. Hereditary fleck dystrophy of the cornea. Am J Ophthalmol 1961; 51:275.
587. Streeten BW, Qi Y, Klintworth GK, et al. Immunolocalization of beta ig-h3 protein in 5q31-linked corneal dystrophies and normal corneas. Arch Ophthalmol 1999; 117:67–75.
588. Streiff EB. Kératocône et rétinite pigmentaire. Bull Soc Fr Ophtalmol 1952; 65:323–6.
589. Stuart JC, Mund ML, Iwamoto T, et al. Recurrent granular corneal dystrophy. Am J Ophthalmol 1975; 79:18–24.
590. Sultana A, Sridhar MS, Jagannathan A, et al. Novel mutations of the carbohydrate sulfotransferase-6 (CHST6) gene causing macular corneal dystrophy in India. Molecular Vision 2003; 9:730–4.
591. Sultana A, Sridhar MS, Klintworth GK, et al. Allelic heterogeneity of the carbohydrate sulfotransferase-6 (CHST6) gene in patients with macular corneal dystrophy. Clin Genet 2005; 68:454–60.
592. Sun M, Goldin E, Stahl S, et al. Mucolipidosis type IV is caused by mutations in a gene encoding a novel transient receptor potential channel. Hum Mol Genet 2000; 9:2471–8.
593. Sunada Y, Nakase H, Shimizu T, et al. Gene analysis of Japanese patients with familial amyloidotic polyneuropathy type IV. Rinsho Shinkeigaku 1992; 32:840–4 [Japanese].
594. Sunada Y, Shimizu T, Nakase H, et al. Inherited amyloid polyneuropathy type IV (Gelsolin Variant) in a Japanese family. Ann Neurol 1993; 33:57–62.
595. Sundin OH, Broman KW, Chang HH, et al. A common locus for late-onset Fuchs corneal dystrophy maps to 18q21.2–q21.32. Invest Ophthalmol Vis Sci 2006; 47: 3919–26.
596. Sundin OH, Jun AS, Broman KW, et al. Linkage of late-onset Fuchs corneal dystrophy to a novel locus at 13pTel–13q12.13. Invest Ophthalmol Vis Sci 2006; 47: 140–5.
597. Swensson O, Swensson B, Nolle B, et al. Mutations in the keratin gene as a cause of Meesman-Wilke corneal dystrophy and autosomal dominant skin cornification disorders. Klin Monatsbl Augenheilkd 2000; 217:43–51.
598. Sysi R. Xanthoma corneae as hereditary dystrophy. Br J Ophthalmol 1950; 34:369–74.
599. Tabbara KF, Butrus SI. Vernal keratoconjunctivitis and keratoconus. Am J Ophthalmol 1983; 95:704–5 [letter].
600. Takacs L, Boross P, Tozser J, et al. Transforming growth factor-beta induced protein, betaIG-H3, is present in degraded form and altered localization in lattice corneal dystrophy type I. Exp Eye Res 1998; 66:739–45.
601. Takagi M, Ishizu M, Suzuki H. An electron microscopic and histochemical study on a corneal granular dystrophy (Groenouw type I). Nippon Ganka Kiyo 1971; 22:479–84 [Japanese].
602. Takahashi A, Nakayasu K, Okisaka S, Kanai A. [Quantitative analysis of collagen fiber in keratoconus]. [Japanese]. Nippon Ganka Gakkai Zasshi 1990; 94: 1068–73.
603. Takahashi K, Murakami A, Okisaka S. Kerato-epithelin mutation (R555Q) in a case of Reis–Bucklers corneal dystrophy (see comments). Nippon Ganka Gakkai Zasshi—Acta Soc Ophthalmol Jpn 1999; 103:761–4 [Japanese].
604. Takeuchi T, Furihata M, Heng HH, et al. Chromosomal mapping and expression of the human B120 gene. Gene 1998; 213:189–93.
605. Takiguchi K, Itoh K, Shimmoto M, et al. Structural and functional study of K453E mutant protective protein/ cathepsin A causing the late infantile form of galactosialidosis. J Hum Genet 2000; 45:200–6.
606. Tang YG, Rabinowitz YS, Taylor KD, et al. Genomewide linkage scan in a multigeneration Caucasian pedigree identifies anovel locus for ketatoconus on chromosome 5q14.3–q21.1. Genet Med 2005; 7:397–405.
607. Tasa G, Kals J, Muru K, et al. A novel mutation in the M1S1 gene responsible for gelatinous droplike corneal dystrophy. Invest Ophthalmol Vis Sci 2001; 42:2762–4.
608. Teng CC. Electron microscope study of the pathology of keratoconus: part 1. Am J Ophthalmol 1963; 55:18–47.
609. Teng CC. Granular dystrophy of the cornea. A histochemical and electron microscopic study. Am J Ophthalmol 1967; 63:772–91.
610. Thalasselis A, Selim AA. Keratoconus-tetany-menopause: the new association. Optomet Vis Sci 1991; 68:357–63.
611. Theodore FH. Congenital type of endothelial dystrophy. Arch Ophthalmol 1939; 21:626–38.

612. Thiel HJ, Behnke H. Ein bisher unbekannte subepitheliale hereditare Hornhautdystrophie. Klin Monatsbl Augenheilkd 1967; 150:862–74.
613. Thomas CI. The Cornea. Springfield, IL: Charles C. Thomas, 1955.
614. Thonar EJ, Lenz ME, Klintworth GK, et al. Quantification of keratan sulfate in blood as a marker of cartilage catabolism. Arthrit Rheum 1985; 28:1367–76.
615. Thonar EJ, Meyer RF, Dennis RF, et al. Absence of normal keratan sulfate in the blood of patients with macular corneal dystrophy. Am J Ophthalmol 1986; 102:561–9.
616. Toma NMG, Ebenezer ND, Inglehearn CF, et al. Linkage of congenital hereditary endothelial dystrophy to chromosome 20. Human Mol Genet 1995; 4:2395–8.
617. Toselli C, Volpi U, Pirodda A. Contributo alla conoscenza della distrofia maculata del parenchima corneale. (Dystrophie mouchetee di Francois e Neetens). Ann Ottalmol Clin Ocul 1966; 92:770–4.
618. Traboulsi EI, Lustbader JM, Lemp MA. Keratoconus in Alagille's syndrome. Am J Ophthalmol 1989; 108:332–3.
619. Traboulsi EI, Weinberg RJ. Familial congenital cornea guttata with anterior polar cataracts. Am J Ophthalmol 1989; 108:123–5.
620. Tremblay M, Dubé I. Macular dystrophy of the cornea; ultrastructure of two cases. Can J Ophthalmol 1973; 8: 47–53.
621. Tripathi RC, Casey TA, Wise G. Hereditary posterior polymorphous dystrophy: an ultrastructural and clinical report. Trans Ophthalmol Soc (UK) 1974; 94:211.
622. Tripathi RC, Garner A. Corneal granular dystrophy. A light and electron microscopical study of its recurrence in a graft. Br J Ophthalmol 1970; 54:361–72.
623. Tsuchiya S, Tanaka M, Konomi H, Hayashi T. Distribution of specific collagen types and fibronectin in normal and keratoconus corneas. Jpn J Ophthalmol 1986; 30:14–31.
624. Tsujikawa M, Kurahashi H, Tanaka T, et al. Identification of the gene responsible for gelatinous drop-like corneal dystrophy. Nat Genet 1999; 21:420–3.
625. Tsujikawa M, Kurahashi H, Tanaka T, et al. Homozygosity mapping of a gene responsible for gelatinous drop-like corneal dystrophy to chromosome 1p. Am J Hum Genet 1998; 63:1073–7.
626. Tsujikawa M, Tsujikawa K, Maeda N, et al. Rapid detection of M1S1 mutations by the protein truncation test. Invest Ophthalmol Vis Sci 2000; 41:2466–8.
627. Twining SS, Everse SJ, Wilson PM, et al. Localization and quantification of alpha-1-proteinase inhibitor in the human cornea. Curr Eye Res 1989; 8:389–95.
628. Tyynismaa H, Sistonen P, Tuupanen S, et al. A locus for autosomal dominant keratoconus: linkage to 16q22.3–q23.1 in Finnish families. Invest Ophthalmol Vis Sci 2002; 43:3160–4.
629. van Osch LD, Oranje AP, Keukens FM, et al. Keratosis follicularis spinulosa decalvans: a family study of seven male cases and six female carriers. J Med Genet 1992; 29: 36–40.
630. van Went M, Wibaut F. Een zeldzame erfelijke hoornvliesaandoening. Ned Tijdschr Geneeskd 1924; 68:2996–3003.
631. Vance JM, Jonasson F, Lennon F, et al. Linkage of a gene for macular corneal dystrophy to chromosome 16. Am J Hum Genet 1996; 58:757–62.
632. Verdi GP, Filippone A. Osservazione di un caso di degenerazione eredofamiliare della cornea, tipo Reis–Bücklers. Boll Oculist 1958; 37:410–30.
633. Verin P, Gendre P, Bertrand B. A propos de deux cas de kératocône familial. Bull Soc Ophtalmol Fr 1984; 84: 951–2.
634. Vithana EN, Morgan P, Sundaresan P, et al. Mutations in sodium-borate cotransporter SLC4A11 cause recessive congenital hereditary endothelial dystrophy (CHED2). Nat Genet 2006; 38:755–7.
635. Vogt A. Keratoconus congenitus in Kombination mit Retinitis pigmentosa bei Blutsverwandtschaft der Eltern. [One page only]. Klin Monatsbl Augenheilkd 1936; 97: 670.
636. Vogt A, Wagner H, Richner H, Meyer G. Das Senium bei eineiigen und zweieiigen Zwillingen. Die Erbenstehung bisher exogen und durch 'Abnützung' erklärter Altersleiden. Arch Klaus-Stift Vererb-Forsch 1939; 14: 475–597.
637. Waardenburg PJ, Jonkers GH. A specific type of dominant progressive dystrophy of the cornea, developing after birth. Acta Ophthalmol (Copenh) 1961; 39:919–23.
638. Waisberg Y. Keratoconus in a patient with somnambulism and eye-pressing. CLAO J 1991; 17:79 [letter].
639. Wales HJ. A family history of corneal erosions. Trans Ophthalmol Soc (NZ) 1955; 8:77–8.
640. Waring GO, Font RL, Rodrigues MM, Mulberger RD. Alterations of Descemet's membrane in interstitial keratitis. Am J Ophthalmol 1976; 81:773–85.
641. Waring GO, Laibson PR, Rodrigues MM. Clinical and pathologic alteration of Descemet's membrane with emphasis on endothelial metaplasia. Surv Ophthalmol 1974; 18:325–68.
642. Waring GO, III, Rodrigues MM, Laibson PR. Corneal dystrophies. II. Endothelial dystrophies. Surv Ophthalmol 1978; 23:147–68.
643. Waring GO, III, Rodrigues MM, Laibson PR. Corneal dystrophies. I. Dystrophies of the epithelium, Bowman's layer and stroma. Surv Ophthalmol 1979; 23:71–122.
644. Waring GO3, Bourne WM, Edelhauser HF, Kenyon KR. The corneal endothelium. Normal and pathologic structure and function. Ophthalmology 1982; 89: 531–90.
645. Warren JF, Aldave AJ, Srinivasan M, et al. Novel mutations in the CHST6 gene associated with macular corneal dystrophy in southern India. Arch Ophthalmol 2003; 121:1608–12.
646. Watanabe H, Hashida Y, Tsujikawa K, et al. Two patterns of opacity in corneal dystrophy caused by the homozygous BIG-H3 R124H mutation. Am J Ophthalmol 2001; 132:211–6.
647. Weber FL, Babel J. Gelatinous drop-like dystrophy. A form of primary corneal amyloidosis. Arch Ophthalmol 1980; 98:144–8.
648. Weidel EG. Granular corneal dystrophy: two variants. In: Ferraz de Oliveira LN, ed. Ophthalmology Today. New York: Elsevier, 1988:617–9.
649. Weidle EG. Differentialdiagnose der Hornhautdystrophien vom Typ Groenouw I, Reis–Bücklers und Thiel–Behnke. Fortschr Ophthalmol 1989; 86:265–71.
650. Weidle EG. Die wabenförmige Hornhautdystrophie (Thiel–Benke). Neubewrtung und Abrenzung gegenuber der Reis–Bücklers'schen Hornhautdystrophie. Klin Monatsbl Augenheilkd 1999; 214:125–35.
651. Weissman BA, Ehrlich M, Levenson JE, Pettit TH. Four cases of keratoconus and posterior polymorphous corneal dystrophy. Optomet Vis Sci 1989; 66:243–6.
652. Welch RB. Bietti's tapetoretinal degeneration with marginal corneal dystrophy: crystalline retinopathy. Trans Am Ophthalmol Soc 1977; 75:176.
653. Wentz-Hunter K, Cheng EL, Ueda J, et al. Keratocan expression is increased in the stroma of keratoconus corneas. Molecular Medicine 2001; 7:470–7.

654. Whitelock RB, Li YH, Zhou LL, et al. Expression of transcription factors in keratoconus, a cornea-thinning disease. Biochemical and Biophysical Research Communications 1997; 235:253–8.
655. Whitley D, Garcia A, Samelson D, et al. Scanning electron microscopy of the corneal endothelium in the avian keratoconus model.? Whitly need to check. Invest Ophthalmol Vis Sci (Suppl) 1989; 30:230.
656. Wilson DJ, Weleber RG, Klein ML, et al. Bietti's crystalline dystrophy. A clinicopathologic correlative study. Arch Ophthalmol 1989; 107:213–21.
657. Wilson SE, Bourne WM. Fuchs' dystrophy. Cornea 1988; 7:2–18.
658. Wilson SE, Bourne WM, Maguire LJ, et al. Aqueous humor composition in Fuchs' dystrophy. Invest Ophthalmol Vis Sci 1989; 30:449–53.
659. Wilson SE, Bourne WM, O'Brien PC, Brubaker RF. Endothelial function and aqueous humor flow rate in patients with Fuchs' dystrophy. Am J Ophthalmol 1988; 106:270–8.
660. Wilson SE, Lin DT, Klyce SD. Corneal topography of keratoconus. Cornea 1991; 10:2–8.
661. Wilson SE, Lin DT, Klyce SD, et al. Topographic changes in contact lens-induced corneal warpage. Ophthalmology 1990; 97:734–44.
662. Witschel H, Fine BS, Grutzner P, McTigue JW. Congenital hereditary stromal dystrophy of the cornea. Arch Ophthalmol 1978; 96:1043–51.
663. Wittebol-Post D, Pels E. The dystrophy described by Reis and Bucklers. Separate entity or variant of the granular dystrophy? Ophthalmologica 1989; 199:1–9.
664. Wittebol-Post D, Van Schooneveld MJ, Pels E. The corneal dystrophy of Waardenburg and Jonkers. Ophthal Paediatr Genet 1989; 10:249–55.
665. Woillez M, Razemon P, Constantinides G. A propos d'un nouveau cas de keratocone chez jumeaux univitellins. Bull Soc Ophtalmol Fr 1976; 76:279–81.
666. Wollensak J. Chemische befunde bei keratokonus. In Symposium on Biochemistry of the Eye, Tutzing Castle, 1966. Basel: Karger; 1968:43–6.
667. Wollensak J, Buddecke E. Biochemical studies on human corneal proteoglycans—a comparison of normal and keratoconic eyes. Graefe's Arch Clin Exp Ophthalmol 1990; 228:517–23.
668. Wolter JR. Secondary cornea guttata. A late change in luetic interstitial keratopathy. Am J Ophthalmol 1960; 50: 17–25.
669. Wolter JR. Secondary cornea guttata in interstitial keratopathy. Ophthalmologica 1964; 148:289–95.
670. Wolter JR. Bilateral keratoconus in Crouzon's syndrome with unilateral acute hydrops. J Pediatr Ophthalmol 1977; 14:141–3.
671. Wolter JR, Henderson JW. Neurohistology of lattice dystrophy of the cornea. Am J Ophthalmol 1963; 55: 475–84.
672. Wolter JR, Larson BF. Pathology of cornea guttata. Am J Ophthalmol 1959; 48:161–9.
673. Woodard G. Keratoconus, dissertation 1980. University of London.
674. Woodward EG. Keratoconus: maternal age and social class. Br J Ophthalmol 1981; 65:104–7.
675. Woodward EG. Keratoconus: epidemiology. J Br Contact Lens Assoc 1984; 7:64–76.
676. Woodward EG, Morris MT. Joint hypermobility in keratoconus. Ophthal Physiol Opt 1990; 10:360–2.
677. Yamada M, Mochizuki H, Kamata Y, et al. Quantitative analysis of lipid deposits from Schnyder's corneal dystrophy. Br J Ophthalmol 1998; 82:444–7.
678. Yamamoto S, Okada M, Tsujikawa M, et al. The spectrum of βig-h3 gene mutations in Japanese patients with corneal dystrophy. Cornea 2000; 19:S21–S23.
679. Yang CJ, SundarRaj N, Thonar EJ, Klintworth GK. Immunohistochemical evidence of heterogeneity in macular corneal dystrophy. Am J Ophthalmol 1988; 106: 65–71.
680. Yanoff M, Fine BS, Colosi NJ, Katowitz JA. Lattice corneal dystrophy. Report of an unusual case. Arch Ophthalmol 1977; 95:651–5.
681. Yassa NH, Font RL, Fine BS, Koffler BH. Corneal immunoglobulin deposition in the posterior stroma. A case report including immunohistochemical and ultrastructural observations. Arch Ophthalmol 1987; 105: 99–103.
682. Yee RW, Sullivan LS, Lai HT, et al. Linkage mapping of Thiel–Behnke corneal dystrophy (CDB2) to chromosome 10q23–q24. Genomics 1997; 46:152–4.
683. Yue BY, Baum JL. The synthesis of glycosaminoglycans by cultures of rabbit corneal endothelial and stromal cells. Biochem J 1976; 158:567–73.
684. Yue BY, Baum JL, Smith BD. Collagen synthesis by cultures of stromal cells from normal human and keratoconus corneas. Biochem Biophys Res Commun 1979; 86:465–72.
685. Yue BY, Sugar J, Benveniste K. Heterogeneity in keratoconus: possible biochemical basis. Proc Soc Exp Biol Med 1984; 175:336–41.
686. Yue BY, Sugar J, Benveniste K. RNA metabolism in cultures of corneal stromal cells from patients with keratoconus. Proc Soc Exp Biol Med 1985; 178:126–32.
687. Yue BY, Sugar J, Schrode K. Histochemical studies of keratoconus. Curr Eye Res 1988; 7:81–6.
688. Zabala M, Archila EA. Corneal sensitivity and topogometry in keratoconus. CLAO J 1988; 14:210–2.
689. Zhou LL, Sawaguchi S, Twining SS, et al. Expression of degradative enzymes and protease inhibitors in corneas with keratoconus. Invest Ophthalmol Vis Sci 1998; 39: 1117–24.
690. Zimmermann DR, Fischer RW, Winterhalter KH, et al. Comparative studies of collagens in normal and keratoconus corneas. Exp Eye Res 1988; 46:431–42.

33

Molecular Genetics of Cataracts

Alan Shiels
Department of Ophthalmology and Visual Sciences, Washington University School of Medicine, St. Louis, Missouri, U.S.A.

INTRODUCTION

Genetic causes of cataracts are well recognized. For example, if the keyword "cataract" is used to search McKusick's Online Mendelian Inheritance in Man over 280 entries are retrieved, many of which include animal, mostly mouse, models of human cataracts (70). Although genetic types of cataracts can present at any age, most are congenital, infantile or childhood, and may be divided into two broad categories based on their association with other phenotypes. Non-syndromic cataracts present as an isolated lens defect in the absence of systemic and/or other ocular phenotypes. In certain cases, however, microcornea may accompany these cataracts in part reflecting the "organizer" role of the lens in anterior eye development (7). In contrast, syndromic cataracts present as a secondary, often inconsistent, feature of over 100 genetically diverse disorders involving systemic and/or other ocular phenotypes.

In terms of genetic diversity, syndromic cataracts are associated with chromosome abnormalities (e.g., Down syndrome), recessive inborn errors of metabolism (e.g., galactosemia) (see Chapter 45), dominant triplet repeat-disorders (e.g., myotonic dystrophy), loss of heterozygosity (e.g., neurofibromatosis type 2), X-linked disorders (e.g., Nance–Horan cataract-dental syndrome), mitochondrial disorders (e.g., myopathy, encephalopathy, lactic acidosis and stroke-like syndrome), and genetically complex disorders (e.g., diabetes mellitus) (see Chapter 31).

Syndromic cataracts can also present with a constellation of systemic abnormalities including mental retardation (25). Severe systemic cataract phenotypes include: galactosemia (*GALT*, 9p), Lowe oculocerebrorenal syndrome (*OCRL*, Xq), branchio-oto-renal syndrome (*EYA1*, 8q), myotonic dystrophy (*DMPK/SIX5*, 19q), and Werner premature aging syndrome (*WRN*, 8p). Less severe systemic cataract phenotypes include: galactokinase-1-deficiency (16), hyperferritinemia cataract syndrome (91), and the adult i blood-group phenotype (122,168), which result from mutations in the genes for a glucose metabolizing enzyme galactokinase-1 (*GALK1*, 17q), an iron-storage molecule ferritin-light chain (*FTL*, 19q), and the glycosylation enzyme glucosaminyl (*N*-acetyl) transferase 2 (*GCNT2*, 6p), respectively.

Other ocular defects associated with syndromic cataracts can also vary widely affecting the retina, optic nerve and anterior segment (e.g., Norrie disease, Marfan syndrome, Weill–Marchesani syndrome, Cockayne syndrome, and Walker–Warburg syndrome). In particular, mutations in several genes for transcription factors including the homeobox genes *PAX6*, *PITX3*, *FOXE3*, *CHX10*, and the bZIP transcription factor *MAF* (Table 1) have been associated with microphthalmia and anterior segment development disorders often associated with glaucoma (58,83). Similarly in the mouse, mutations in *Pax6*, *Pitx3*, *Foxe3*, *Chx10* and *Maf* have been shown to underlie small-eye (*Sey*), aphakia (*ak*), dysgenetic lens (*dyl*), ocular retardation (*or-J*), and opaque flecks in lens (*Ofl*), respectively (58,97). In addition, another homeobox gene, *SIX5*, has been implicated in the characteristic adult-onset cataracts associated with myotonic dystrophy (88,160). A more detailed discussion of syndromic cataracts is beyond the scope of this chapter. Rather, this chapter reviews recent progress made in identifying and characterizing the genetic mutations underlying non-syndromic cataracts in humans and mice, and considers the implications of these findings for the genetic etiology of age-related cataracts.

GENES FOR NON-SYNDROMIC CATARACTS

All three classical types of Mendelian inheritance have been described for non-syndromic cataracts and the possible existence of Y-linked cataracts (40) remains to be confirmed. X-linked isolated cataracts are rare and may represent minimal expression of the Nance–Horan cataract-dental syndrome in man (19,22), which is syntenic with the *Xcat* mutation in mice (79). Autosomal recessive cataracts are more prevalent in consanguineous human populations; however, autosomal dominant cataracts with high penetrance are the most commonly reported form in out-bred populations (67).

The pioneering genetic linkage of autosomal dominant cataracts with the polymorphic Duffy blood group in 1963 (129), and the subsequent assignment of Duffy to chromosome 1 in 1968 (36), represented a landmark in human genetics, as cataracts became the first human disease to be assigned to one of the 22 autosomes (128). During the next ~20 years a few family studies linked Mendelian cataracts with other polymorphic blood groups, including Rh (78) and Ii (99), along with the serum protein haptoglobin (38). With the advent of the human genome project and the development of genome-wide short-tandem-repeat microsatellite markers, genetic linkage studies of over 60 families worldwide (mostly since 1995), have mapped at least 22 independent loci for clinically diverse forms of non-syndromic cataracts on 14 human chromosomes (Table 2). For simplicity, non-syndromic cataracts have been divided into two groups based on their association with crystallin genes or non-crystallin genes (Fig. 1).

Crystallin Genes and Cataracts

According to the National Center for Biotechnology Information, over 14 functional crystallin genes have been located in the human genome and 10 of these are abundantly expressed in the fetal lens (92). Combined, these genes encode >90% of cytoplasmic proteins in the lens, accounting for ~30% of its mass, and establishing its glass-like optical transparency (34) and high refractive index (41). Crystallins are evolutionarily related to stress-response proteins (see Chapter 36) and may be subdivided into two distinct groups; the α-crystallins are members of the small heat-shock protein (sHSP) family that function as molecular chaperones (77), whereas, the β/γ-crystallins

Table 1 A Gene Map of Transcription Factors Associated with Syndromic Cataracts

Chromosome	Gene	Cataract morphology	Other ocular/systemic phenotypes	Mouse (mutant)
1p32	*FOXE3*	Anterior polar?	Anterior segment dysgenesis	4*Foxe3* (*dyl*)
10q25	*PITX3*	Anterior cortical, total posterior polar	Anterior segment dysgenesis	19*Pitx3* (*ak*)
11p13	*PAX6*	Cortical, posterior polar lamellar, anterior capsular, posterior subcapsular	Aniridia, Peters anomaly, foveal hypoplasia, nystagmus	2*Pax6* (*sey*)
14q24.33	*CHX10*	Total?	Microphthalmia, anophthalmia, iris coloboma	12*Chx10* (*or-J*)
16q22–q23	*MAF*	Cortical lamellar, nuclear pulverulent	Microcornea, iris coloboma	8*Maf* (*Ofl*, null)
19q13.32	*SIX5*	"Christmas tree"	Myotonic dystrophy	7*Six5*, (null)

Table 2 A Genetic Map of Non-Syndromic Cataracts in Humans and Mice

Chromosome	Locus/ gene	Mutation	Mode of inheritance	Cataract morphology	Mouse synteny (mutants)
1p36	CCV		AD	Progressive lamellar	
	CTPP1		AD	Posterior polar	
	?		AD	Total	
1q21.1	*GJA8*	p.R23T	AD	Nuclear	3*Gja8* (*No2, Aey5, Lop10,* null)
		p.E48K	AD	Zonular nuclear pulverulent	
		p.V64G	AD	Nuclear	
		p.P88S	AD	Zonular pulverulent	
		p.I247M	AD	Zonular pulverulent	
2p24–pter	?		AD	Coralliform	
2p12	?		AD	Nuclear	
2q33–q35	*CRYGC*	p.T5P		Central zonular pulverulent	1*Crygc* (*Chl13, MNU-8*)
		c.117–118ins5bp		Variable zonular pulverulent	
		p.R168W		Lamellar	
	CRYGD	p.R14/15C	AD	Punctate	1*Crygd* (*ENU4011, Aey4, ENU910, K10, Lop12*)
		p.P23/24T	AD	Lamellar	
		p.P23/24T	AD	Cerulean	
		p.P23/24T	AD	Flaky	
		p.P23/24T	AD	Coral-like	
		p.P23/24T	AD	Fasciculiform	
		p.R36/37S	AD	Crystal-like	
		p.R36/37S	AD	Nuclear golden crystal	
		p.R58/59H	AD	Aculeiform	
		p.W156/157X	AD	Central nuclear	
	CCP		AD	Polymorphic	
3p26.2	?		t(3;4)	Total	
3p21.3–p22.3	?		AR	?	
3q21–q22	*BFSP2*	p.delE233	AD	Nuclear sutural stellate	9*Bfsp2* (null)
		p.delE233	AD	Y-sutural	
		p.R287W	AD	Nuclear sutural lamellar	
3q25–qter	*CRYGS*	p.G18V	AD	Cortical progressive	16*Crygs* (*Opj, rncat*)
9q13–q22	CAAR		AR	Progressive pulverulent	
11q22.1–q23.2	*CRYAB*	p.R120G		"Discrete" (myopathy)	9*Cryab* (null)
		c.450delA		Posterior polar	
12q13–q14	*MIP*	p.E134G	AD	Lamellar sutural	10*Mip* (Cat^{Fr}, Cat^{lop}, Cat^{hfi}, Cat^{Tohm}, null)
		p.T138R	AD	Progressive punctate polymorphic	
13q11–q12	*GJA3*	p.V28M	AD	Variable total	14*Gja3* (null)
		p.F32L	AD	Nuclear pulverulent	
		p.W45S	AD	Nuclear	
		p.P59L	AD	Nuclear punctate	
		p.N63S	AD	Variable pulverulent	
		p.R76H	AD	Nuclear lamellar pulverulent	
		p.R76G	AD	Total	
		p.P187L	AD	Zonular pulverulent	
		p.N188T	AD	Nuclear pulverulent	
		c.1137insC	AD	Punctate	
14q24–qter	CTAA1		t(2;14)	Anterior polar	
15q21–q22	CCSSO		AD	Central saccular sutural	
16q22.1	*HSF4*	p.A20D	AD	?	8*Hsf4* (null)
		p.I87V	AD	Cortical lamellar	

(*Continued*)

Table 2 A Genetic Map of Non-Syndromic Cataracts in Humans and Mice (*Continued*)

Chromosome	Locus/ gene	Mutation	Mode of inheritance	Cataract morphology	Mouse synteny (mutants)
16q22.1	*HSF4*	p.L115P	AD	Lamellar	
		p.R120C	AD	Zonular stellate anterior polar (Marner)	
		g.IVS12+4A>G	AR	Total	
		p.R175P	AR	Nuclear cortical	
		c.595–599del5bp	AR	?	
17p13–p12	CTAA2		AD	Anterior polar	
17q11.2–q12	*CRYBA3/ A1*	g.IVS3+1G>A	AD	Zonular sutural	11*Cryba3/a1* (*Po1*)
		g.IVS3+1G>C	AD	Pulverulent nuclear sutural	
		g.IVS3+1G>A	AD	Sutural nuclear cortical	
		p.G91del	AD	Nuclear	
		p.G91del	AD	Nuclear suture-sparing	
		p.G91del	AD	Lamellar	
17q24	CCA1		AD	Cerulean	
19q13	?		AR	Nuclear	
19q13.4	*LIM2*	p.F105V	AR	Pulverulent cortical sutural	7*Lim2* (*To3*, null)
20p12–q12	CTPP3		AD	Posterior polar	
21q22.3	*CRYAA*	p.W9X	AR	?	17*Cryaa* (*lop18*, *Aey7* null)
		p.R49C	AD	Central nuclear	
		p.R116C	AD	Zonular central nuclear	
22q11.2	*CRYBB1*	p.G220X	AD	Central sutural pulverulent	5*Crybb1*
		p.X253R	AD	Nuclear cortical riders	
	CRYBB2	p.Q155X	AD	Cerulean	5*Crybb2* (*Phil*, *Aey2*)
		p.Q155X	AD	Central zonular pulverulent	
		p.Q155X	AD	Sutural cerulean	
		p.Q155X	AD	Progressive polymorphic	
		p.W151C	AD	Central nuclear	
	CRYBB3	p.G165R	AR	Nuclear cortical riders	*5Crybb3*

Abbreviations: AD, autosomal dominant; AR, autosomal recessive; ?, unknown.

belong to the family of epidermis-specific differentiation proteins, and share a common two-domain β-sheet protein structure composed of four "Greek key" motifs (14). Currently, over 20 mutations in nine crystallin genes, including those for both α-crystallins, four β-crystallins and three γ-crystallins, have been identified (Table 2), making them the most common genes for non-syndromic cataracts.

α-Crystallins

The genes for αA-crystallin (*CRYAA*) and αB-crystallin (*CRYAB*) have a 3-exon structure and encode cytosolic proteins, which share ~55% identity mostly in the phylogenetically conserved "α-crystallin/ sHSP" core domain (exons 2 to 3). In vivo, CRYAA and CRYAB monomers (M_r ~20 kDa) combine in a stoichiometric 3:1 ratio to form a large α-crystallin-complex (M_r ~800 kDa), which accounts for a substantial portion of lens refractive power (77). Three of the five known mutations in *CRYAA* and *CRYAB* are located within the α-crystallin/sHSP core domain (~100 amino acids), and the other two mutations are located outside this domain in exon 1.

CRYAA

CRYAA on human chromosome 21 (21q) encodes a 173-amino-acid protein accounting for ~20% of fetal lens soluble protein (92). Two missense mutations (Arg49Cys, Arg116Cys) and a nonsense mutation (Trp9X) in *CRYAA* (Fig. 2A) have been linked with autosomal dominant (95,101) and recessive cataracts (119), respectively (Table 2). The dominant Arg49Cys and Arg116Cys substitutions are associated with opacities affecting the nucleus, and peri-nuclear cortex of the juvenile lens. Functional expression studies of the Arg49Cys (101) and Arg116Cys (4,30) mutant proteins in bacteria and cultured cells, have shown that both mutants display reduced carboxy-terminal arm of CRYBB1 by 26 amino-acids before terminating at an alternative in-frame stop-codon located downstream in the 3′-untranslated region.

CRYBB2

CRYBB2 lies adjacent to *CRYBB1* on human chromosome 22 (22q) and encodes a 205-amino-acid protein accounting for ~14% of fetal lens soluble protein (92). Two mutations (Gln155X, Trp151Cys) in exon 6 of *CRYBB2* (Fig. 2B) have accompanied autosomal dominant cataracts. A missense substitution (Trp151Cys) has been associated with central nuclear opacities in an Indian family, and modeling of the Trp151Cys mutant protein point to reduced solubility possibly resulting from abnormal intramolecular disulfide-bridge formation (133). Remarkably, a nonsense mutation (Gln155X) has arisen in four geographically distinct regions, associated with cerulean opacities in an American family (94), central and/or zonular pulverulent opacities in a Swiss family (53), sutural cerulean opacities in an Indian family (151) and progressive polymorphic opacities in a Chinese family (164). One plausible explanation for recurrence of the Gln155X mutation is that it represents a gene conversion event between *CRYBB2* and its adjacent pseudogene (*CRYBB2P1*), which also harbors the Gln155X mutation (151). At the translational level, the Gln155X mutation is expected to truncate 51 of the last 55 amino-acids of CRYBB2 encoded by exon 6 including, the carboxy-terminal arm and ~90% of the fourth Greek-key motif. Functional expression studies of recombinant CRYBB2 in bacteria and a mammalian-two-hybrid system indicate that the Gln155X mutant is partially unfolded and exhibits impaired protein-protein interactions (96). It is noteworthy that a member of an American family with cataracts associated with a homozygous Gln155X mutation (94) manifest bilateral microphthalmia, microcornea and a totally opaque dysplastic lens in the absence of systemic abnormalities (15). The increased phenotype severity in the homozygous state suggests that the Gln155X allele does not exert dominant negative effects on the wild-type allele in the lenses of heterozygous individuals, and that other pathologic gain-of-function effects trigger cataracts.

Similarly, in the mouse two mutations in exon 6 of *Crybb2* (Fig. 2B) have been associated with dominant progressive nuclear sutural cataracts. A spontaneous in-frame deletion of 12-bp encoding four amino acids (del185GlnSerValArg188) has been identified in the *Philly* mutant (26) (see Chapter 22), whereas, an N-ethyl–N-nitrosourea (ENU)-induced missense substitution (Val187Glu) has been reported in the *Aey2* mutant (62). The Val187Glu substitution lies within the *Philly* deletion region close to the carboxy-terminus of Crybb2. Both mutations are likely to impair the formation of the fourth Greek-key motif, which may partly explain the loss of heat-stability and abnormal aggregation properties associated with the *Philly* Crybb2 mutant.

CRYBB3

CRYBB3 is clustered with *CRYBB1* and *CRYBB2* on human chromosome 22 (22q) and encodes a 211-amino-acid-protein accounting for up to ~6% of fetal lens soluble protein (92). A single missense mutation (Gly165Arg) in exon 6 has been associated with recessive congenital cataracts in two consanguineous Pakistani families (130). The opacities were described as nuclear with cortical riders, and molecular modeling of CRYBB3 predicts that the Gly165Arg substitution may cause instability of the fourth Greek-key motif, which ultimately, may destabilize the entire protein.

γ-Crystallins

Six functional genes for γ-crystallins (*CRYGA*, *CRYGB*, *CRYGC*, *CRYGD*, *CRYGN*, *CRYGS*) have been identified in the human genome, however, only three (*CRYGC*, *CRYGD*, *CRYGS*) appear to be expressed at significant levels in the human lens, accounting for 15% to 30% of soluble protein (92). Unlike the *CRYB* genes, the *CRYG* genes have a three-exon structure with exons 2 and 3 each encoding a pair of Greek-key domains, and the resulting proteins (M_r ~20 kDa) function as monomers rather than dimers. Currently, nine mutations in *CRYGC*, *CRYGD* and *CRYGS* have been associated with autosomal dominant cataracts in man (Table 2).

At least 20 mutations have been reported in the mouse *Cryg* genes (64); however, the majority of these are linked with *Cryga*, *Crygb*, *Cryge* and *Crygf*. The human counterparts of these genes are either expressed at trace levels in the lens and have not yet been associated with hereditary cataracts (*CRYGA*, *CRYGB*), or have evolved into pseudogenes (*CRYGEP1*, *CRYGFP1*).

CRYGC

CRYGC maps to human chromosome 2 (2q) and encodes a 174-amino-acid-protein accounting for ~14% of lens soluble protein (92). So far, three mutations in *CRYGC* (Thr5Pro, Cys42fs, Arg168Trp) have been associated with autosomal dominant cataracts. A 5-bp duplication in exon 2 has been reported in a large Caucasian pedigree segregating variable zonular pulverulent opacities (127). The insertion mutation is predicted to cause a frame-shift at codon 42 (Cys42fs), which may result in a truncated translation product containing 38 amino-acids of the first Greek-key motif followed by 62 novel amino-acids before an in-frame stop codon is met. A missense substitution (Thr5Pro), also located in exon 2, has been identified in the historically important Coppock-like cataract family segregating central zonular pulverulent opacities (75). Biophysical studies of recombinant CRYGC expressed in bacteria show that the Thr5Pro mutant was mostly insoluble, and when re-natured exhibited thermal instability, consistent with significant conformational changes (48). A second missense substitution (Arg168Trp) located in exon 3 of *CRYGC* has also been shown to co-segregate with lamellar opacities in an Indian pedigree (134).

In the mouse, 2 chemically-induced *Crygc* mutations have been shown to underlie semi-dominant cataracts. A 6-bp deletion in exon 3 has been associated with nuclear radial opacities in the *Chl3* mutant (65). The in-frame deletion is predicted to result in the loss of 2 amino-acids (del141GlyArg142) preventing formation of the fourth Greek-key motif. In the *MNU-8* mutant a nonsense mutation (Trp157X) in *Crygc* has been found to underlie total lens opacities with vacuoles (64). The Trp157X mutation lies in exon 3 and is predicted to truncate the final 15 amino-acids comprising the carboxy-terminal arm but may not prevent formation of the fourth Greek-key motif.

CRYGD

CRYGD lies next to *CRYGC* on human chromosome 2 (2q) and also encodes a 174-amino-acid-protein representing ~2% of lens soluble protein (92). Currently, four missense mutations (Arg14Cys, Pro23Thr, Arg36Ser, Arg58His) in exon 2, and a nonsense mutation (Trp156X) in exon 3 of *CRYGD* (Fig. 2C) have been linked with dominant, mostly nuclear, cataracts. Remarkably, the same Pro23Thr substitution has been independently identified in five families of Indian, Moroccan, European, and Chinese origins, segregating lamellar (134), cerulean (110), flakey silica-like (23), coral-like (102) and fasciculiform (135) opacities. The other mutations are associated with aculeiform (needle-like) opacities (Arg58His) in European (75) and Mexican (169) families, progressive pulverulent opacities (Arg14Cys) in an American family (148), crystal-like opacities (Arg36Ser) in a Czech boy (89) and a Chinese family (66), and central nuclear opacities (Trp156X) in an Indian family (134).

Biophysical studies of recombinant CRYGD harboring each of the four missense substitutions (Arg14Cys, Pro23Thr, Arg36Ser, Arg58His) have detected deleterious gain-of-function effects, which manifest as insolubility and/or crystal-nucleation in the absence of significant protein conformational or thermal stability changes. Thus, the Arg14Cys mutant, associated with progressive punctate opacities, forms disulfide-linked oligomers in vitro culminating in aggregation of this normally monomeric protein (117), whereas, the Arg36Ser and Arg58His mutants, associated with crystal-like and aculeiform cataracts respectively, promote deposition of CRYGD-protein crystals both in vitro (116) and within the lens (89,135). Similarly, the Pro23Thr mutant exhibits dramatically reduced solubility resulting from aberrant clustering of the mutant protein in a condensed phase (39,115).

In the mouse, two missense mutations (Leu45Pro, Val76Asp) in exon 2, along with a missense mutation (Ile90Phe) and two nonsense mutations (Tyr144X, Trp157X) in exon 3 of *Crygd* (Fig. 2C) have been associated with semi-dominant cataracts in the *ENU4011* (Leu45Pro), *Aey4* (Val76Asp), *ENU910* (Ile90Phe), *K10* (Tyr144X), and *Lop12* (Trp157X) mutants (63,64,143). Four of these mutants (*ENU4011*, *Aey4*, *ENU910*, *K10*) were induced with mutagens and descriptions of their cataracts include nuclear and total opacities with increased severity in homozygotes. The *Lop12* mutant likely arose spontaneously and also presents with progressive nuclear cataracts, which have been speculated to resemble the human Coppock cataract first documented in 1910 (143). Coincidentally, the *Lop12* mouse harbors the same missense substitution (Trp156/157X) as that found in *Crygc* in the *MNU-8* mouse and in *CRYGD* in an Indian family with central nuclear cataracts (134).

CRYGS

CRYGS on human chromosome 3 (3q) encodes a 178-amino acid-protein and so far only one dominant missense mutation (Gly18Val) has been linked with progressive cortical cataracts in man (149). Similarly, missense (Phe9Ser) and nonsense (Trp163X) mutations in the mouse *Crygs* gene underlie dominant progressive cataracts in the *Opj* (*opacity due to poor fiber cell junctions*) mutant (141), and recessive nuclear cataracts in the *rncat* mutant (21), respectively. Biophysical studies of recombinant *Crygs* indicate that the Phe9Ser mutant exhibits a marked temperature and concentration dependent decrease in solubility compared with wild-type Crygs (141).

Non-Crystallin Genes and Cataracts

In addition to the six crystallin loci above, at least 16 other loci have been linked with non-syndromic cataracts (Table 2). Currently, no causative genes have been identified at the dominant loci on chromosome 1 (1p) (37,80,106), chromosome 2 (2p) (51,87), chromosome 2 (2q) (132), chromosome 15 meaning (ox eyed) (Fig. 1B). The sclera and cornea of infants and young children are more elastic than those of adults and their eyes enlarge with increased intraocular pressure (IOP) in contrast to adult eyes that typically do not. Enlargement of the cornea produces breaks in Descemet membrane (Haab striae) (Fig. 1C,D). The iris insertion is often very anterior (Fig. 1E) and tissue studies of surgically excised TM specimens from patients with PCG have disclosed thickening of the juxtacanalicular area with layers of spindle cells and surrounding extracellular matrix (ECM) (64) (Fig. 2).

Most cases of PCG are sporadic; in familial cases, autosomal recessive inheritance is most common. Loci have been identified for the infantile form of congenital glaucoma on chromosome 2 (2p21) (50) and chromosome 1 (1p36) (1). The *CYP1B1* gene within the 2p21 locus, which accounts for the majority of familial cases, encodes cytochrome P450B1 (59), a member of a family of mixed-function monooxygenases suspected of being involved in steroid metabolism (51).

Cytochrome P450

CYP1B1 is expressed in the trabecular meshwork, iris, and retina, as well as many non-ocular human tissues. In the mouse eye, expression of this enzyme is limited to the pigmented ciliary epithelium and it is possible that in human it is secreted from the ciliary epithelium to reach the TM (63). Although the ocular substrate for cytochrome P450B1 remains unknown, the enzyme is likely to play an important role in ocular development.

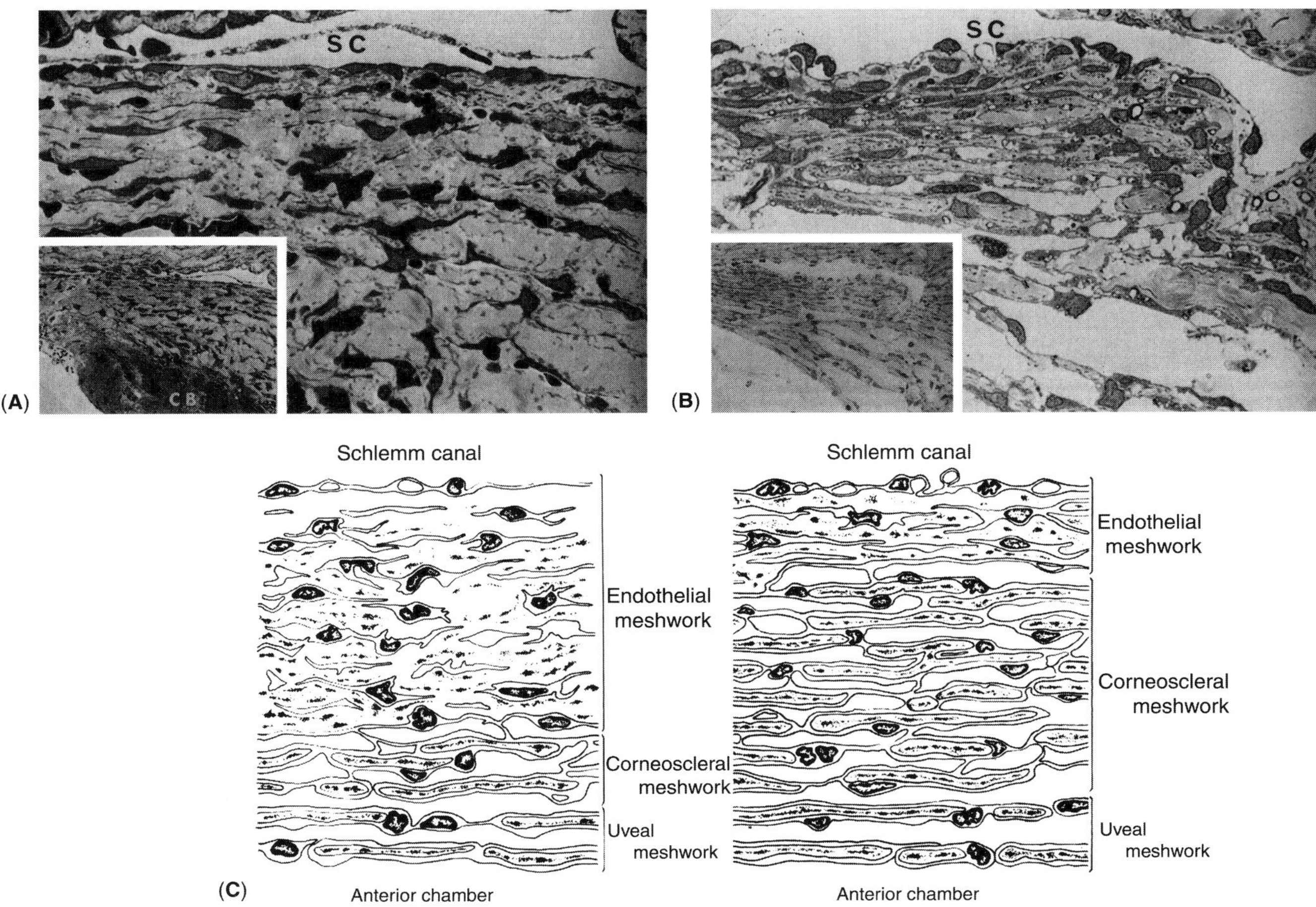

Figure 2 Histopathology of trabecular meshwork in primary congenital glaucoma. (**A**) Trabecular meshwork in a 4-month-old male with early-onset congenital glaucoma in his left eye. Cells in the trabecular area are embedded in extracellular substances. There is no giant vacuole formation at the inner wall of Schlemm canal (SC). CB, ciliary body (toluidine blue, ×1000; inset ×200). (**B**) Tissue of chamber angle in a 4-month-old girl studied as a control. Uveal and corneoscleral meshworks appear to be well differentiated. A thin endothelial meshwork is present beneath the inner wall of SC (toluidine blue, ×1000; inset ×200). (**C**) Schematic drawing of trabecular meshwork. (*Left*) Congenital glaucoma. Endothelial meshwork remains thick because of underdevelopment of trabecular meshwork. (*Right*) Normal trabecular meshwork. The thin meshwork is composed of two to four layers of endothelial cells and surrounding extracellular substances. *Source*: Adapted from Ref. 64.

Table 1 Glaucoma Loci and Genes

Glaucoma type	MIM[a] number	Locus symbol	Locus/loci	Gene
Juvenile OAG	# 137750	GLC1A	1q23–25	*MYOC*
			6p25	*FKHL7*
			10p15–14	*OPTN*
			9q22	
			20p12	
Adult OAG	# 137750	GLC1A	lq23–25	*MYOC*
	# 137760	GLC1B	2cen–q13	
	% 601682	GLC1C	3q21–24	
	% 602429	GLC1D	8q23	
	# 602432	GLC1E	10p15–14	*OPTN*
	% 603383	GLC1G	5q22.1	*WDR36*
		GLC1F	7q35–36	
			3p21–22	

[a]References can be obtained from Online Mendelian Inheritance in Man: http://www.ncbi.nlm.nih.gov/entrez/query.fcgi?db=OMIM

Aside from PCG mutations in *CYP1B1* have also been associated with Peters anomaly and other forms of glaucoma (Table 1).

Libby et al. (34) have shown that mutant *Cyp1b1*$^{-/-}$ mice deficient in cytochrome P450B1 develop focal defects in the anterior chamber angle including an increase in basal lamina of the trabecular meshwork and a small or absent Schlemm canal. Other experiments testing for genes that enhance or suppress angle abnormalities in *Cyp1b1* identified the tyrosinase gene (*Tyr*) as a modifier whose deficiency exacerbates defects in *Cyp1b1* mutant mice (34). Eyes lacking cytochrome P450B1 and tyrosinase demonstrated severe dysgenesis that was alleviated by the administration of L-DOPA, a normal product of tyrosinase. Thus, a pathway involving tyrosinase appears to be important in anterior chamber angle development.

Other

Recently, Kaur et al. (29) implicated the *MYOC* gene in PCG by identifying a patient who was doubly heterozygous for mutations in both the *CYP1B1* and *MYOC* genes, which might be mediated via interaction with *CYP1B1* and/or a yet unidentified locus associated with the disease.

Juvenile Onset Open-Angle Glaucoma

Juvenile open angle glaucoma (JOAG) is an autosomal dominant, early-onset form of POAG, characterized by extremely high IOP with subsequent damage to the optic nerve and visual field. Affected eyes are often myopic. This disease usually begins between the ages of 4 and 35 years and affected individuals often have a strong family history of glaucoma. JOAG generally responds poorly to current therapy.

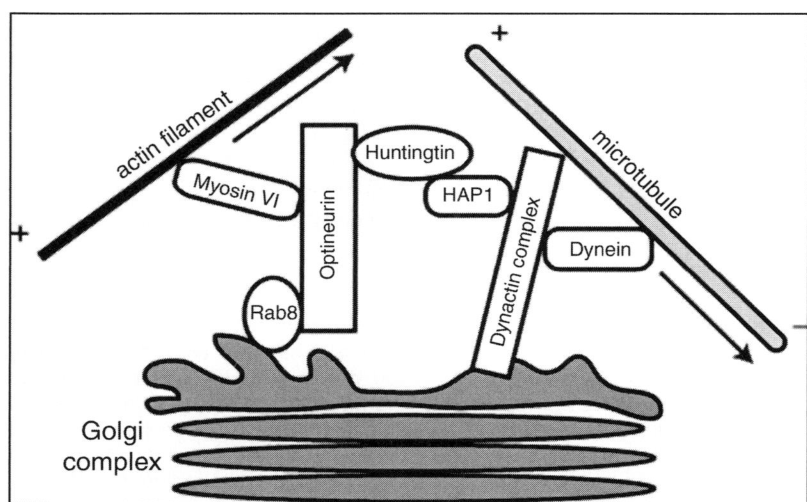

Figure 3 Possible interaction of optineurin with motor protein complexes at the Golgi complex. Optineurin may play a central role in coordinating actin-based and microtubule-based motor function for maintaining the morphology of the Golgi apparatus. *Source*: Adapted from Ref. 49.

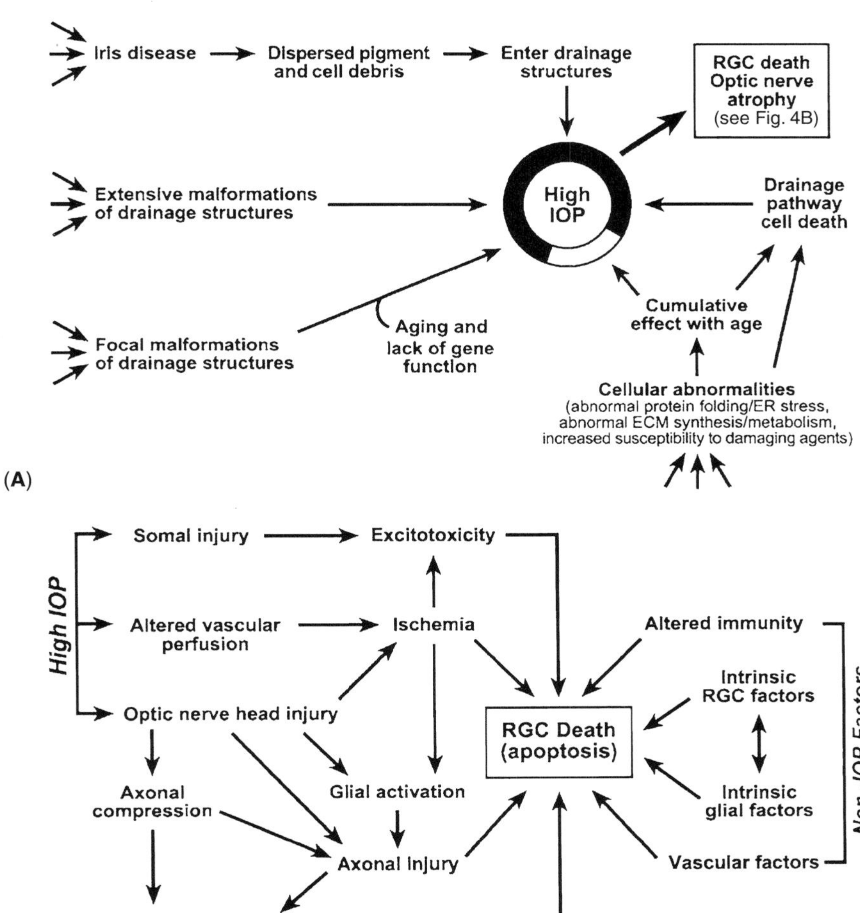

Figure 4 (**A**) Diverse insults can lead to IOP elevation or (**B**) retinal ganglion cell death. Examples of these factors are shown. An array of these factors may conspire additively or synergistically to cause glaucoma in an individual. *Abbreviations*: RGC, retinal ganglion cell; IOP, intraocular pressure; ECM, extracellular matrix. *Source*: Adapted from Ref. 33.

JOAG was first linked to chromosome 1 (1q21–31) by Sheffield et al. in 1993 (56). Four years later, mutations were found in the responsible gene, which was designated the TM glucocorticoid response gene (*TIGR*) (60). The protein product of this gene was later renamed *myocilin*.

Myocilin

Myocilin was first identified in human TM cells that had been exposed to glucocorticoids. The encoding *MYOC* gene has been cloned and isolated from TM, ciliary body, and retina (30,63). Myocilin has a molecular weight of approximately 55 to 57 kDa (80T) and consists of 504 amino acids. The N-terminus contains a motif characteristic of a leucine zipper or coiled-coil domain as well as a myosin-like domain. The C-terminus contains an olfactomedin-like domain. Mutations in *MYOC* that are associated with glaucoma are largely clustered in exon 3 in the olfactomedin domain and are responsible for 2% to 5% of POAG. The onset of glaucoma in persons with these mutations range from young childhood to late adulthood, but occurs most often between 20 and 45 years of age. The Pro370Leu mutation is responsible for very early onset glaucoma, occurring as early as age three to four years (39) while the more common Gly368Stop mutation causes onset of glaucoma in the sixth or seventh decade of life (5).

Myocilin has been found in the sclera, keratocytes and corneal endothelium, TM, ciliary epithelium and in smooth muscle cells of the iris and ciliary body. Considerable amounts of myocilin have also been noted in the aqueous humor (63). In the posterior segment of the eye, myocilin has been localized to the vitreous, the ciliary rootlet and basal body of the connecting cilia of the photoreceptors, optic nerve axons, and astrocytes in the lamina cribrosa.

Myocilin is also found in a variety of non-ocular tissues, including the heart, thymus, prostate, intestine, as well as Schwann cells of peripheral nerves (63), but its physiological function remains poorly understood. It may serve a structural function within the cytoplasm, or may be associated with other molecules within the cell, perhaps as a chaperone protecting vital cellular proteins or enzymes during times of stress (27). Recent evidence indicates that

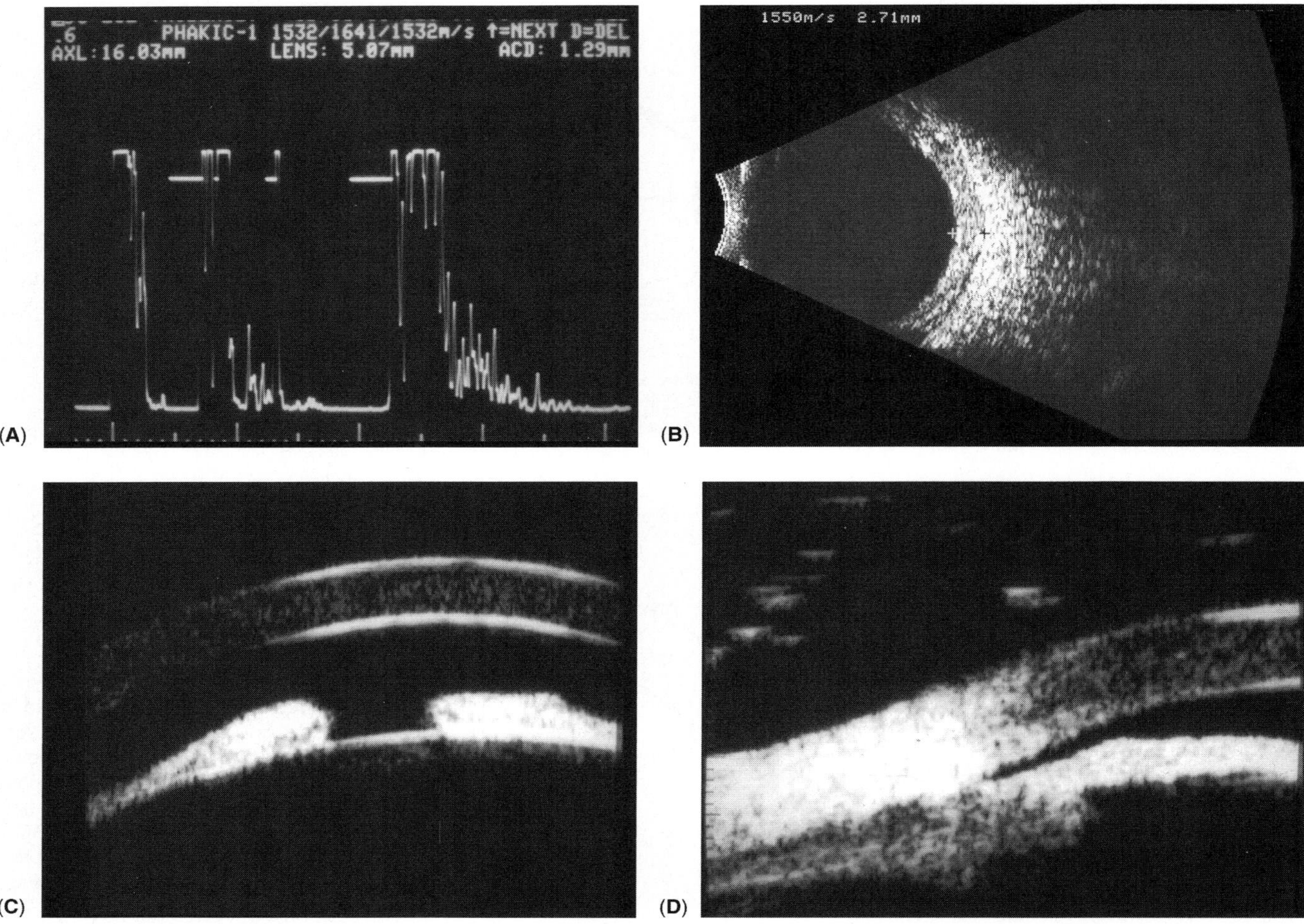

Figure 5 Ultrasound features of an eye with nanophthalmos. Note (**A**) short axial length and (**B**) thick sclera on B scan, as well as (**C**) shallow anterior chamber and (**D**) extremely narrow angle on ultrasound biomicroscopy. *Source*: Courtesy of Ms. Diane Chialant.

myocilin interacts with certain intracellular proteins such as gamma-synuclein, the c-terminal of hevin, and flotillin-1 (25,31,62).

How mutations in *MYOC* cause glaucoma is unknown, but in humans, mutated myocilin appears to cause an elevation in IOP by obstructing conventional outflow passages of the TM (58). It is noteworthy that, haploinsufficiency or loss-of-function appear unlikely to cause glaucoma as mice which are deficient in myocilin do not develop ocular abnormalities or glaucoma (47,63). Furthermore, individuals who are hemizygous or homozygous for glaucoma-associated mutations in myocilin do not appear to develop glaucoma (42,69). Data from Zillig et al. indicate that mutated myocilin is not secreted but retained in the rough endoplasmic reticulum (RER) (72). This may lead to RER dysfunction and cell death, but whether or not this is the mechanism that leads to aqueous humor outflow obstruction remains to be determined.

Studies of transgenic mice examining the effect of mutant myocilin have provided conflicting results. Overexpression of the Tyr437His mutation failed to demonstrate phenotypic changes consistent with glaucoma (74). Interestingly, a more recent study investigating overexpression of the same mutation in the mouse model found significantly elevated IOP and loss of ganglion cells consistent with the glaucoma phenotype (55). Clearly, future studies are needed to sort out the role of this protein in the animal model.

Gradually more is being learned how myocilin causes glaucoma. Myocilin protein is secreted by TM cells in culture. TM cells that are transfected with disease-associated *MYOC* mutations do not secrete this protein. It has been found that myocilin protein with disease-associated mutations misfolds and is prone to aggregation in the RER (35). In cell culture this process is associated with cell death. Similarly, myocilin normally found in the aqueous

Table 2 Glaucoma in Various Disorders of the Eye

Disorder	MIM[a] number	Locus symbol	Locus/loci	Gene
Pseudoexfoliation syndrome	#177650		15q22	*LOXL1*
Pigment dispersion syndrome	%600510	GPDS1	7q35–36	
		GPDS2	18q11–21	
Congenital glaucoma	#231300	GLC3A	2p22–21	*CYP1B1*
	%600975	GLC3B	1p36.2–36.1	
Rieger syndrome	#180500	RIEG1	4q25	*PITX2*
	%601499	RIEG2	13q14	
			11p13	*PAX 6*
Axenfeld–Rieger syndrome	#601631		6p25	*FOXC1 (FKHL7)*
			4q25	*PITX2*
			10q25	*PITX3*
Iridogoniodysgenesis anterior segment mesenchymal dysgenesis	#601631	IRIDI	6p25	*FOXC1 (FKHL7)*
	#107250		10q25	*PITX3*
Autosomal dominant iris hypoplasia	#137600	IRID2	4q25	*PITX2*
Nanophthalmos	%600165	NNO1	11p	*?VMD2*
		NNO2	11q23.3	*MFRP*
Aniridia	#106210	AN2	11p13	*PAX6*
Peters anomaly	*607108		11p13	*PAX6*
	*601542		4q25–q26	*PITX2*
	*601771		2p22–p21	*CYP1B1*
	*601090		6p25	*FOXC1*
Congenital microcoria	%156600		13q31–32	
Microphthalmos (AR)	%251600		14q32	
Ectopia lentis (simple)	#129600		15q21	*FBN1* (*Fibrillin*)
Wagner syndrome	#143200	WGN1	5q13–14	

[a]Reference can be obtained from Online Mendelian Inheritance in Man: http://www.ncbi.nlm.nih.gov/entrez/query.fcgi?db=OMIM. *Abbreviations*: AR, autosomal recessive.

humor is absent in some patients with myocilin-associated glaucoma (24). Recent evidence suggests that myocilin is associated with secretory vesicles. Data derived from cell culture supports the hypothesis that myocilin may function in the secretion of exosomal vesicles (20). Myocilin-associated exosomes, recently identified in human aqueous humor samples, is consistent with this theory. Although much remains to be determined, these data suggest that myocilin may exert its pathological effects through intracellular and extracellular mechanisms (44).

Adult Onset Primary Open-Angle Glaucoma

There is compelling evidence to indicate that the susceptibility to POAG is inherited and that POAG is a highly heterogeneous disorder (57). The prevalence of POAG in first-degree relatives of affected patients is 7 to 10 times higher than the general population and there is also a high concordance rate for POAG between monozygotic twins. Studies have shown that patients with POAG and their family members also have a much higher tendency towards a rise in IOP with use of corticosteroids, indicating a possible hereditary association between steroid response and glaucoma. In addition, the higher prevalence of POAG in African Americans compared to Caucasians may reflect a genetic susceptibility.

The high prevalence of POAG, variability in age of onset, and non-penetrance (lack of phenotypic expression of a disease despite carrying the genetic mutation) in some pedigrees indicate that most cases of POAG are not inherited as a single gene defect but as a "complex" trait that does not demonstrate simple Mendelian inheritance. Interplay between various environmental and genetic factors, or between multiple genes, results in a high degree of variability in phenotypic expression and disease severity that makes linkage analysis extremely challenging. To date, linkage studies on families with POAG provide strong evidence for genetic heterogeneity. At least eight loci and three genes (*MYOC*, *OPTN*, and *WDR36*) (Table 1) have been identified and together these genes are associated with 5% to 10% of all POAG. A recent report also suggests that common polymorphisms in the *NOELIN 2* gene (*OLFM2*) and *OPTN* may interactively contribute to the development of OAG, indicating a polygenic etiology (17).

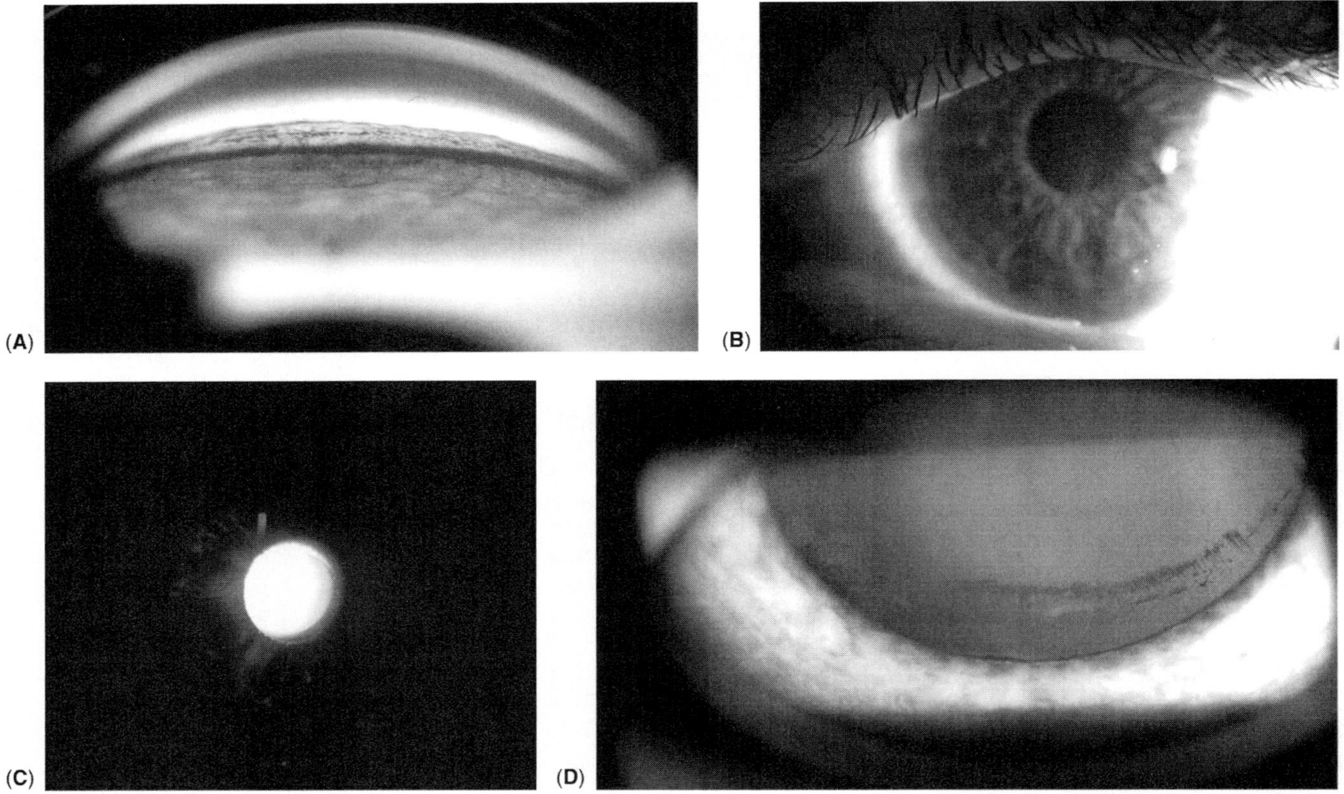

Figure 6 Clinical features of pigment dispersion syndrome: (**A**) Heavy (mascara like) trabecular meshwork pigment; (**B**) Krukenberg spindle—dispersion of pigment granules on the endothelial surface of the cornea; (**C**) peripheral iris transillumination defects; and (**D**) pigment accumulation on the posterior lens surface.

MYOC

Mutations in the *MYOC* gene account for 3% to 5% of adult onset POAG. This gene and its encoded product myocilin is reviewed in the earlier section on JOAG.

OPTN

Optineurin was first discovered as a binding partner of an adenoviral protein (14.7K-interacting protein-2) and was named FIP-2 (32). It was shown to protect infected cells from tumor necrosis factor alpha (TNFα)

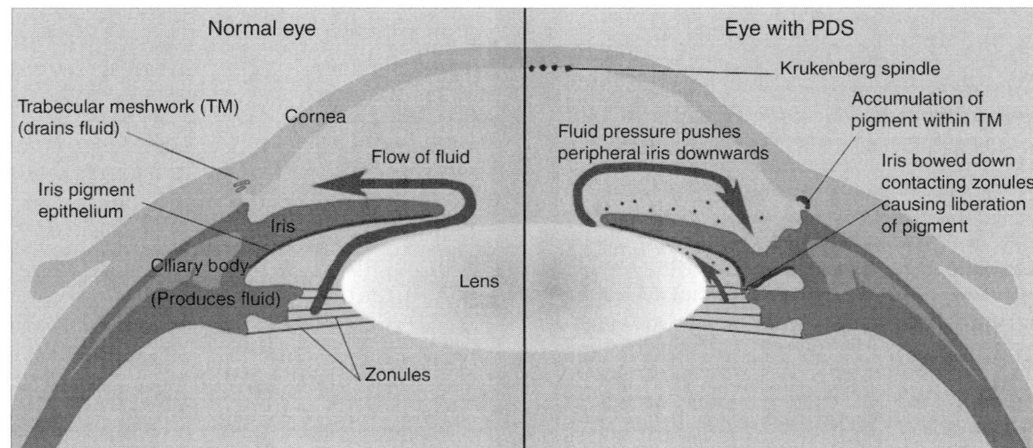

Figure 7 Schematic diagram showing normal eye and eye with pigment dispersion syndrome (PDS). Note the peripheral iris concavity in the eye with PDS. This represents "reverse pupillary block."

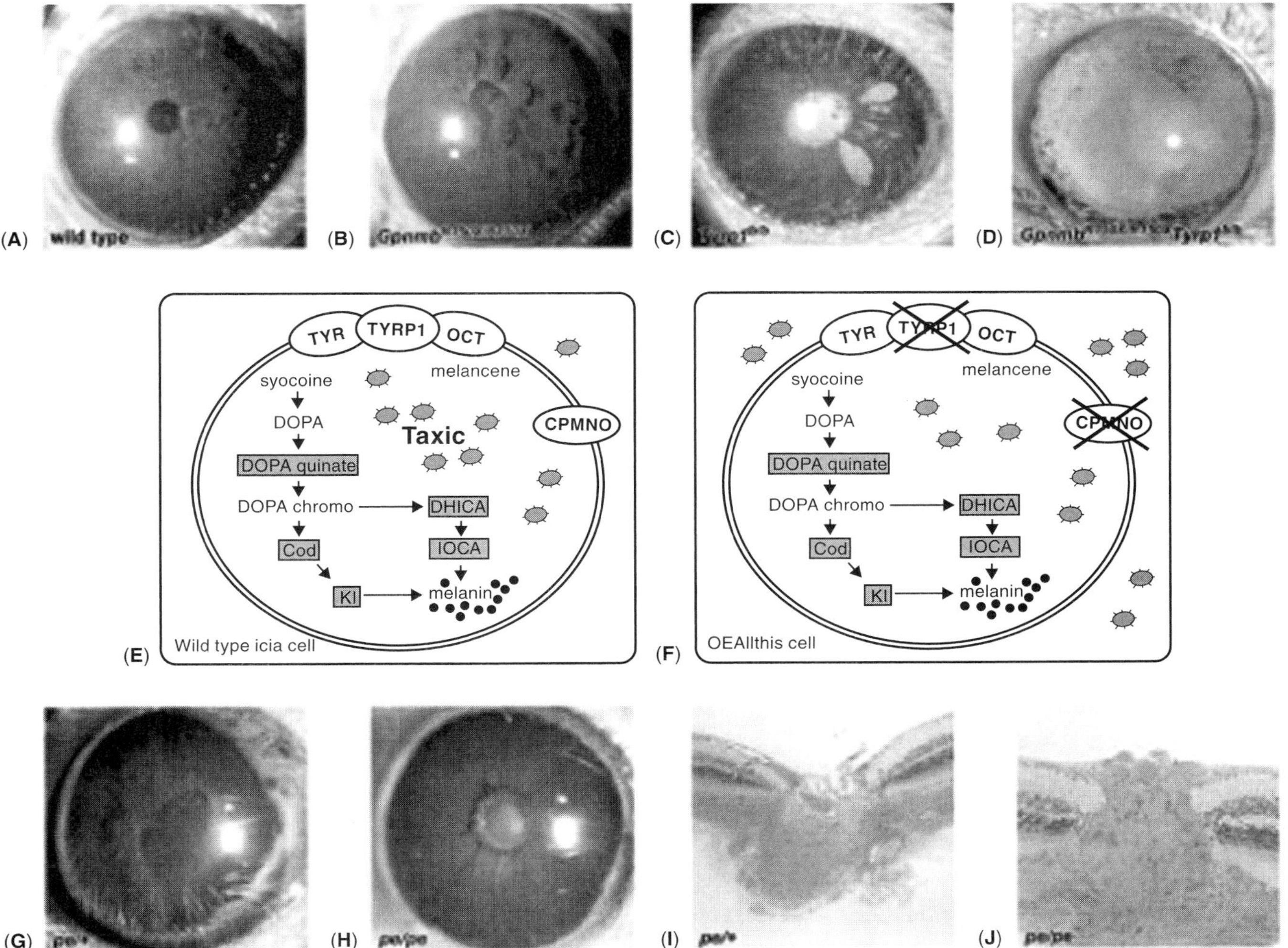

Figure 8 (**A–D**) Melanosomes contribute to pigment dispersion in the DBA/2J mouse. All images are from 24-month-old mice. Mutations in the genes encoding melanosomal proteins *TYRP1* and *GPNMB* cause iris disease. DBA/2J mice are homozygous mutant for both genes and have the most severe disease as shown in (**D**). (**E,F**) Potentially toxic intermediates of melanin production (*shaded*) are largely sequestered inside melanosomes and are converted into pigment (**E**). The Tyrp1 and Gpnmb mutations appear to allow toxic molecules to escape from the melanosomes and damage iris cells (**F**). (**G–J**) Heterozygotes for the *pe* mutation are not hypopigmented and have typical DBA/2J disease (**G,I**). In contrast, homozygosity for this recessive hypopigmentation mutation prevents iris disease (**H**) and glaucomatous nerve excavation (**J**). *Source*: (**A–D**, **G–J**) Adapted from Ref. 8; (**E,F**) adapted from Ref. 26.

induced apoptosis (see Chapter 2). Optineurin has significant homology (53% identity) with NF-B essential modulator and was therefore also called NEMO-related protein (53).

The *OPTN* gene codes for optineurin, which is a conserved 66 kDa protein of unknown function. It has been localized to the Golgi complex (53) where it interacts with a diverse group of proteins that includes Huntingtin and the Ras-associated protein RAB8, which appear to play a role in membrane trafficking pathways. Optineurin also links myosin type VI to the Golgi complex and plays a central role in Golgi ribbon formation and exocytosis (Fig. 3) (49).

Similar to myocilin, optineurin is expressed in a variety of tissues including the TM, non-pigmented ciliary epithelium, retina, brain, placenta, liver, skeletal muscle, and pancreas. Antibodies raised against optineurin can be detected in aqueous humor suggesting that this protein is secreted.

In 2002, sequence alterations in OPTN were found in 16.7% of families with hereditary POAG at the GLC1E locus. The majority of families with OPTN sequence variations have a normal tension glaucoma phenotype (46) and for this reason the encoded protein was named "optic neuropathy inducing" protein or *optineurin*. Recent studies suggest that *OPTN* mutations are a rare cause of POAG and are

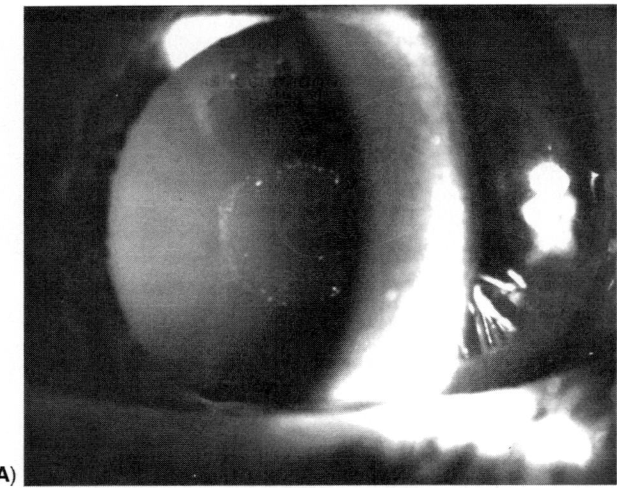

(A)

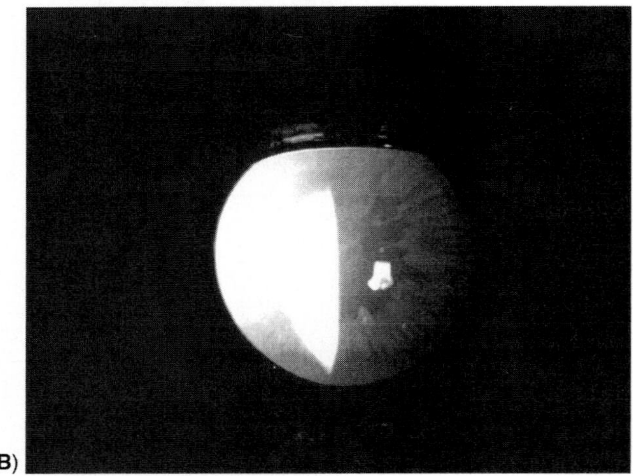

(B)

Figure 9 Clinical appearance of pseudoexfoliation material on the lens capsule. (**A**) White dandruff-like particles visible as a central disc and peripheral band. The material can also be seen well with transillumination following dilation. (**B**) The sawtooth-like peripheral band can easily be seen.

responsible for <1% of normal tension glaucoma, although this frequency may vary according to the population being studied (6).

The pathophysiology of optineurin-associated glaucoma remains largely unknown. TNFα has been shown to facilitate apoptosis of retinal ganglion cells (65). In addition, in glaucomatous optic nerve heads the expression of both TNFα and its receptor, TNFR1 may be upregulated, and appear to parallel the progression of optic nerve degeneration (71). Given that optineurin is induced by TNFα, and the links between TNFα and retinal ganglion cell death, it has been speculated that optineurin may play a neuroprotective role (46,62).

WDR36

WDR36 is a novel gene with 23 exons located on chromosome 5 (5q22.1) (GLC1G locus) that encodes for a 951 amino acid protein with multiple G-beta WD40 repeats (tyrptophan-aspartate repeats). By northern blotting, two distinct mRNA transcripts of 5.9 and 2.5 kb have been observed in human heart, placenta, liver, skeletal muscle, kidney and pancreas and gene expression in lens, iris, sclera, ciliary body, TM, retina and optic nerve has been established by reverse transcription- polymerase chain reaction (RT-PCR) (41). The function of WDR36 remains unknown but it is the third recognized causative gene for adult-onset POAG (41). DNA sequence variants are more common in POAG than in controls but do not segregate within families. It appears that disease-associated sequence variants of WDR36 are not in themselves sufficient to cause disease but may make the disease phenotype more severe (21).

Other

Diverse insults that may lead to IOP elevation and retinal ganglion cell death in glaucoma are summarized in Fig. 4 (33). Apoptosis of TM and retinal ganglion cells may play a role in the pathophysiology of POAG (26) and changes in the ECM of the lamina cribrosa may be important in retinal ganglion cell damage. Although there are many associations between specific TM, retinal ganglion cell and optic nerve genes and POAG, little evidence exists for a pathogenic role for these genes (67). Susceptibility genes may permit other genes and/or environmental factors to lead to glaucoma. For example, the *OPA1* gene and *APOE* gene have been associated with normal tension glaucoma and POAG, respectively (9,15).

Primary Angle Closure Glaucoma

PACG is a leading cause of blindness among certain populations such as the Inuit, and Mongolian populations from East and Southeast Asia. It is far less common in Caucasians, Native Americans, Australian Aborigines, and those of African descent (14). This geographic and racial variation in PACG prevalence most likely reflects structural differences in the eyes in these ethnic groups that manifest in smaller more crowded anterior segments that predispose to pupillary block and subsequent anterior chamber angle closure. These predisposing anatomical differences include shallow anterior chamber depth, thick lens, a more anterior lens position, small corneal diameter, shortened axial length of the globe, and small radius of corneal curvature (36). In addition, the iris insertion into the scleral wall is more anterior in Asians, slightly more posterior in African Americans and most posterior in Caucasians (43).

Very few studies have explored the familial basis of PACG, although Hu found a six fold increased risk

Table 3 Loci and Genes for Systemic Diseases with Associated Glaucoma

Glaucoma type	MIM[a] number	Locus symbol	Locus/loci	Gene
Nail patella syndrome	#161200	NPS	9q34.1	*LMX1B*
Neurofibromatosis type I	+162200	NF1	17q11.2	*NFI*
Charcot–Marie tooth disease type 4	#604563	CMT4B	11p15	*SBF2*
Rubinstein syndrome	#180849	RSTS	16p13.3	*CREBBP* *EP300*
Mucopolysaccharid-osis type VI	+253200	MPS6	5q11–13	*ARSB*
Ehlers–Danlos syndrome type VI	#225400	EDS6	1p36.3–36.2	*PLOD*
Basal cell nevus syndrome	#109400	BCNS	9q22.3	*PCTH1*
Marfan syndrome	#154700	MFS1	15q21.1	*FBN1*
Wiessenbacher–Zweymuller syndrome	#277610	WZS	6p21.3	*COL11A2*
Lowe oculocerebrorenal syndrome	#309000	OCRL1	Xq26.1	*OCRL1*
Marshall syndrome	#154780		1p21	*COL11A1*
Stickler syndrome				
Type I	#108300	STL1	12q13.11–13.2	*COL2A1*
Type II	#184840	STL2	6p21.3	*COL11A2*
Type III	#108300	STL3	1p21	*COL11A1*

[a]References can be obtained from Online Mendelian Inheritance in Man: http://www.ncbi.nlm.nih.gov/entrez/query.fcgi?db=OMIM

for subjects with a family history of PACG in a population-based survey in Shunyi County, Beijing (23). A study of axial anterior chamber depth in twins (without PACG) indicated that about 70% of the variance in dizygotic twins could be attributable to a genetic component (67) and a biometric study showed a relatively shallow anterior chamber depth in siblings, children, nephews, nieces and grandchildren of PACG probands (3). A heritability of 70% was found in this study by Alsbirk indicating that about two thirds of the age and sex independent variation of anterior chamber depth seems to be genetic.

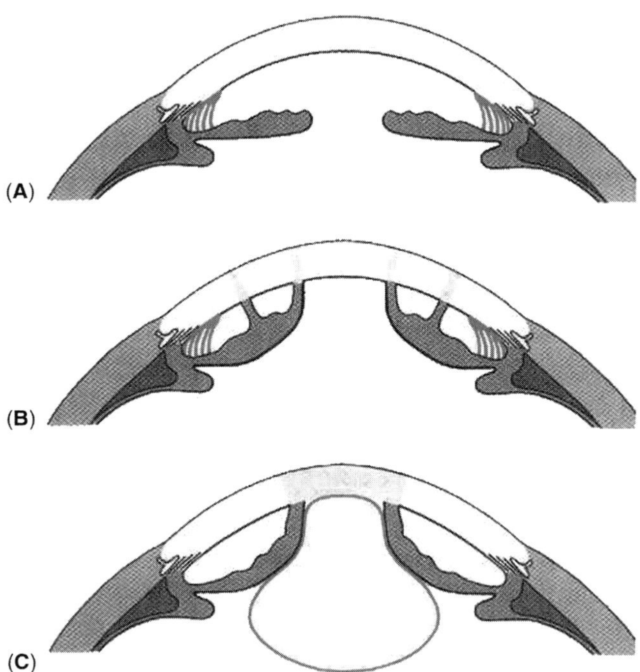

Figure 10 Typical phenotypes seen in the spectrum of anterior segment dysgenesis. (**A**) Axenfeld anomaly—iris strands traverse the chamber angle and insert into a prominent Schwalbe line (posterior emryotoxon). (**B**) Rieger anomaly—midperipheral adhesions from iris to corneal ares seen in addition to Axenfeld anomaly. (**C**) Peters anomaly—central corneal opacification (leukoma) with the local absence of the corneal endothelium. *Source*: Adapted from Ref. 63.

Lowe suggested that the inheritance of a shallow anterior chamber is polygenic with a threshold effect so that the action of numerous grouped or independently inherited genes results in anterior chamber shallowness (36). Environmental factors, such as neural and/or humoral responses to fatigue, mental stress, infection, and trauma, may trigger altered anterior chamber depth and/or degree of pupillary block in PACG. Alsbirk has proposed that in the Inuit population genes for a small, crowded anterior segment are the result of pressure selection to protect the cornea which is vulnerable to freezing in the Arctic climate (4).

Nanophthalmos

Nanophthalmos is a rare disorder of eye development characterized by extreme hyperopia, with a refractive error in the range of +8.00 to +25.00 D (see Chapter 52). Nanophthalmic eyes often have an axial length of <20 mm and a considerably thickened choroidal vascular bed and scleral coat retina (Fig. 5). Sundin et al. (60) have mapped autosomal recessive nanophthalmos to a unique locus on chromosome 11 (11q23.3) and have identified four independent mutations in the *MFRP* gene that is

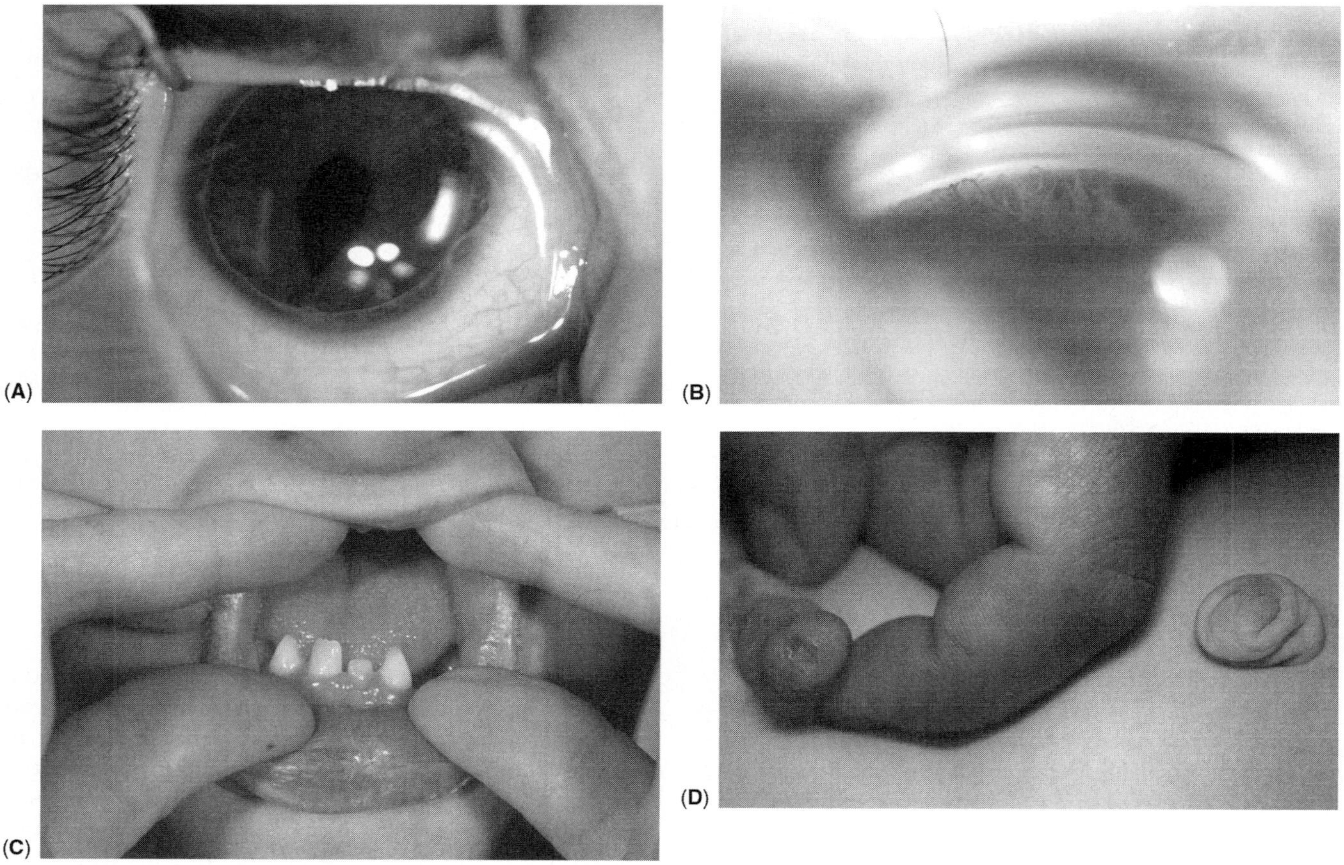

(A) (B) (C) (D)

Figure 11 Slit lamp appearance of patient with Axenfeld–Rieger syndrome. (**A**) Corectopia and prominent Schwalbe line (posterior embryotoxon). (**B**) Iridocorneal adhesions visible to Schwalbe line. (**C**) Hypodontia (fewer teeth) and oligodontia (missing teeth). (**D**) Umbilical anomaly and hypospadia. *Source*: Courtesy of Dr. Wallace L.M. Alward.

selectively expressed in the eye. *MFRP* encodes a protein with homology to the Tolloid metalloproteases and the Wnt-binding domain of the transmembrane receptors that are related to gene product of the *fz* (frizzled) gene of Drosphila. *MFRP* appears primarily devoted to regulating the axial length of the eye.

Another locus has been identified for autosomal dominant nanophthalmos on chromosome 11. Three pathogenic sequence alterations in the gene *VMD2* were identified in five families with nanophthalmos associated with autosomal dominant vitreoretinochoroidopathy (ADVIRC) (see Chapter 29) (70) and some family members developed angle closure glaucoma. *VMD2* encodes bestrophin, a transmembrane protein located at the basolateral membrane of the RPE, that is also mutated in Best macular dystrophy (38) (see Chapter 35). The data show that *VMD2* mutations cause defects of ocular patterning, supporting the hypothesized role for the RPE, and specifically VMD2, in the normal growth and development of the eye.

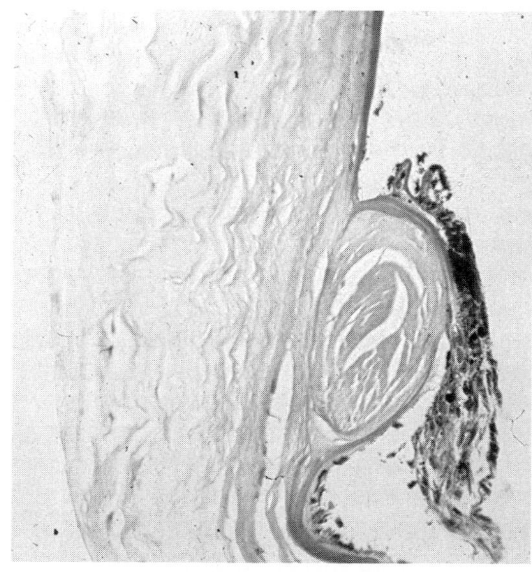

Figure 12 Histopathology of iris adhesion to prominent Schwalbe line (posterior embyotoxon). *Source*: Courtesy of Dr. Wallace L.M. Alward.

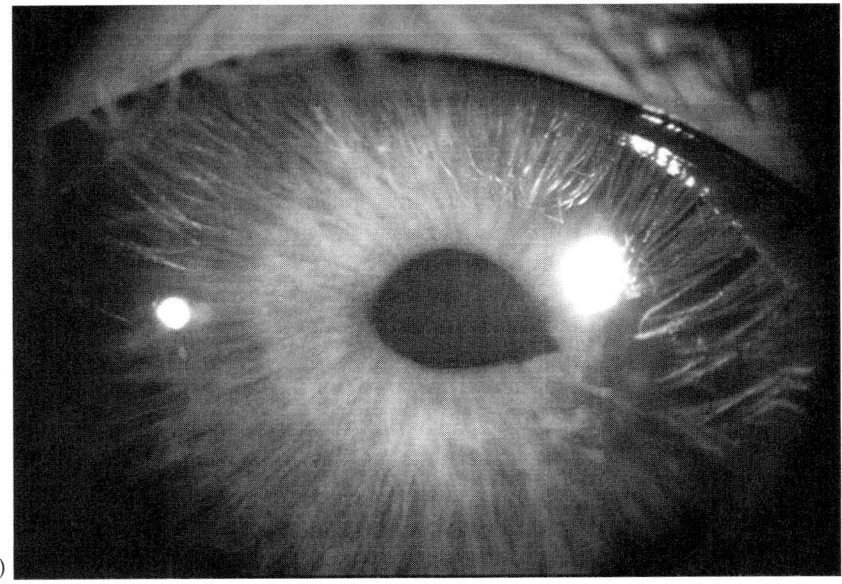
(A)

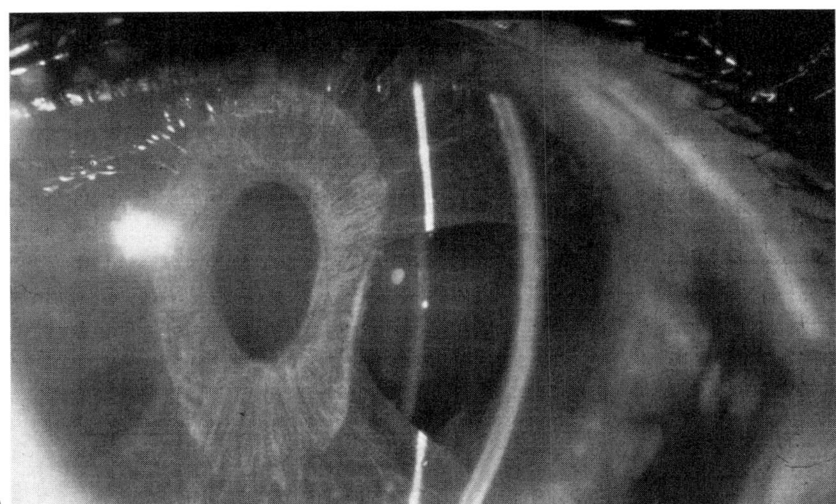
(B)

Figure 13 Variant of anterior segment dysgenesis. Iris hypoplasia with prominent sphincter muscle visible around the pupil. (**A**) Corectopia. (**B**) Polycoria. *Source*: Courtesy of Dr. Wallace L.M. Alward.

SECONDARY GLAUCOMAS

A number of genetically determined ocular disorders are associated with open angle forms of glaucoma as part of their phenotype (Table 2).

Pigmentary Glaucoma

The pigment dispersion syndrome (PDS) is characterized by the dispersion of melanin granules from the iris with deposition in the anterior segment of the eye, including the TM (Fig. 6). It typically affects Caucasian individuals and is more common in young, myopic males. Up to half of the affected individuals with pigmentary glaucoma (PG) develop glaucomatous optic nerve damage over a 10- to 15-year period. Several investigators have demonstrated an autosomal dominant inheritance for PDS (7,10,28,37). In 1997, Andersen et al. mapped a gene for PDS to chromosome 7 (7q35–36), but the disorder is likely to be genetically heterogenous and further studies are underway to determine if additional loci exist.

Although the mechanism of pigment release is unknown, reverse pupillary block has been proposed. In this aqueous humor is "trapped" in the anterior chamber by a lens-induced "flap valve" mechanism. The increased volume of aqueous humor forces the iris to move posteriorly, causing the typical concave iris seen in patients with pigment dispersion syndrome (Fig. 7) (12). In PG, iris cells are damaged resulting in dispersal of iris pigment into the ocular drainage structures, which may in turn elevate IOP in susceptible individuals. A mouse model raises the possibility that mutant melanosomal protein genes contribute to PG. BA/2J mice appear to develop a

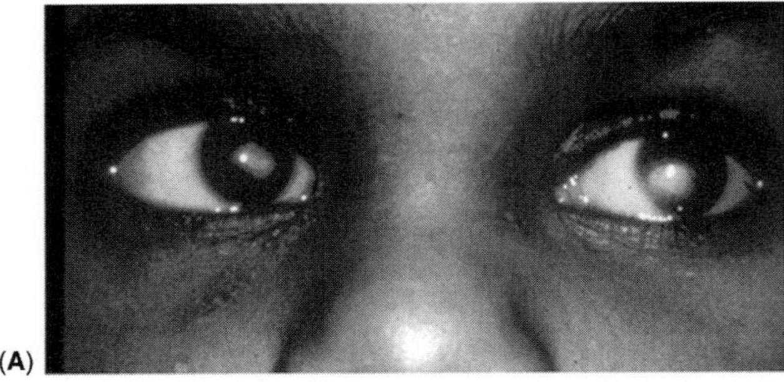
(A)

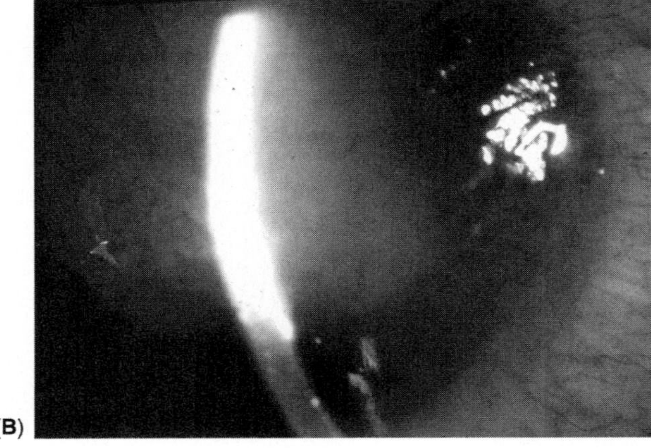
(B)

Figure 14 Peters anomaly showing bilateral white corneas (**A**) and slit lamp view of corneal leukoma (**B**). *Source*: Courtesy of Dr. Wallace L.M. Alward.

form of PG caused by mutations in the glyocoprotein (transmembrane) nmb gene, *Gpnmb*, and the tyrosinase-related protein 1 gene, *Tyrp1* (63). Since both genes encode melanosomal proteins, it has been hypothesized that these mutations permit toxic intermediates of pigment production to leak from melanosomes (Fig. 8). In support of this hypothesis albino and hypopigmentation mutations prevent disease development (8).

Bone marrow-derived cells and inflammatory processes appear to contribute to PG (40). The *Gpnmb* gene is expressed in dendritic cells that control immune responses. Mutated *Gpnmb* appears to disturb ocular immune privilege allowing immune cells to attack the iris and propagate the iris disease that induces glaucoma. Interleukin-18 (IL18) is an important regulator of innate and acquired immune responses and plays an important role in inflammatory and autoimmune diseases. Using the DBA/2J mouse Zhou et al. (73) demonstrated that the expression of both *IL18* and its encoded IL18 in the iris/ciliary body and the level of IL18 in the aqueous humor of DBA/2J mice dramatically increase with age. This increase precedes the onset of clinical evidence of PG, implying a pathogenetic role.

Pseudoexfoliation Syndrome

Patients with pseudoexfoliation syndrome (PEX) have distinct pseudoexfoliated material on their lens capsule (see Chapter 25) (Fig. 9). PEX has been reported to be a stress induced elastic fiber microfibrillopathy (72). In a landmark study, the genetic etiology of PEX and glaucoma in Iceland and Sweden was identified (66). Single nucleotide polymorphisms (SNPs) in the coding region of the lysyl oxidase-like 1 gene (*LOXL1*) are associated with PEX and glaucoma in these populations. *LOXL1*, located on chromosome 15(15q24), encodes for one of many enzymes that are essential for the formation of elastin fibers; they modify tropoelastin, the basic building block of elastin, and catalyze the process for monomers to cross-link and form elastin.

The disease-associated SNPs appear to account for all PEX within the studied populations. Three SNPs in the protein coding portion of *LOXL1* were specifically associated with PEX glaucoma risk. A person homozygous for both of the highest-risk haplotypes was 700 times more likely than those homozygous for the low-risk variants to develop PEX glaucoma. There are likely to be other genes and possible environmental factors that play an important role for the development of PEX and the glaucoma associated with this syndrome. There may also be other important contributing factors in non-Scandinavian populations that remain to be determined. However, this remarkable finding will provide major insights into the pathophysiology of PEX, providing an opportunity for novel treatment approaches to this common and aggressive form of open-angle glaucoma.

Other Developmental Glaucomas

Developmental glaucomas are secondary to morphological malformations of the anterior segment involving the ocular drainage structures and are relatively rare (see Chapter 52). Importantly these developmental abnormalities are not always clinically detectable and may affect the metabolism and function of the drainage structures without disturbing morphology. Glaucomas and known genes associated with ocular developmental disorders are listed in Table 2.

Anterior Segment Dysgenesis

Anterior segment dysgenesis (ASD) is a spectrum of disorders arising from an abnormal migration and differentiation of neural. crest-derived cells (Fig. 10) (63). These include Axenfeld anomaly (anteriorly displaced Schwalbe line with no additional risk of glaucoma), iris hypoplasia and iridogoniodysgenesis (50–75% risk of associated glaucoma), Axenfeld–Rieger anomaly (variable findings ranging from iris adhesions to Schwalbe line to iris hypoplasia with corectopia and polycoria, associated with a 50% risk of glaucoma), and

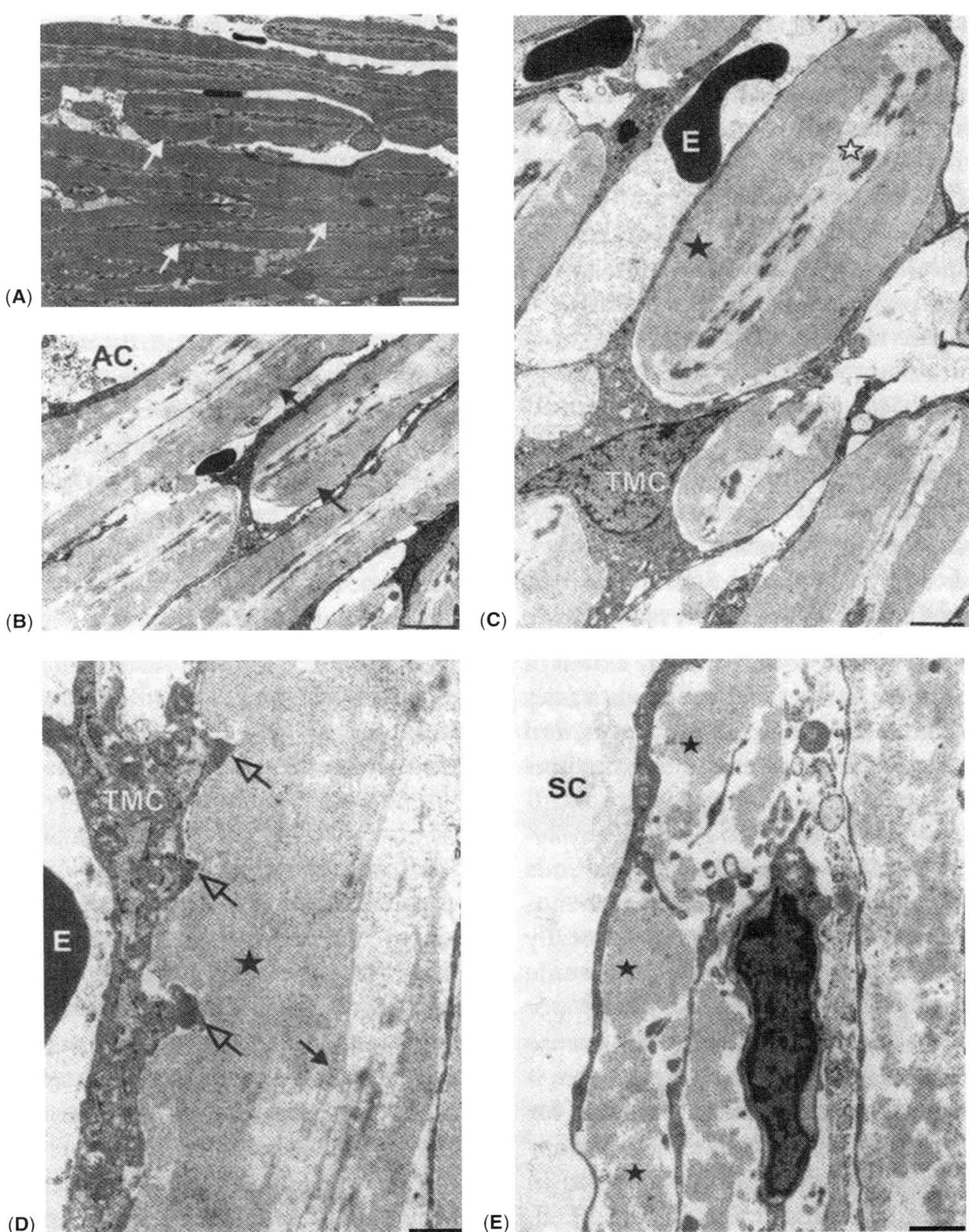

Figure 15 Light (**A**) and electron microscopy (**B**) of the trabecular meshwork (TM) in a 24-year-old patient with Axenfeld syndrome and glaucoma. The intertrabecular spaces are markedly narrow because of an abnormally thickened basement membrane in the TM lamellae (*arrows*). (**C**) The basement membrane (*black star*) surrounds the central core of the TM lamellae (*white star*), which is of normal thickness. (**D**) Processes of TM cells (*open arrows*) protrude into the thickened basement membrane (*star*) which appears granular and contains aggregates of broad-banded material (*solid arrow*). (**E**) The extracellular spaces of the juxtacanalicular meshwork contains numerous aggregates of sheath-derived plaque material (*stars*). *Abbreviations*: AC, anterior chamber; TMC, trabecular meshwork; SC, Schlemm canal; E, erythrocyte. Magnification bars: (**A**) 4 μm; (**B**) 1.7 μm; (**C,E**) 1 μm; (**D**) 0.7 μm.

Peters anomaly (which includes adhesion of the lens to the cornea) (Figs. 11–14). If systemic features such as redundant umbilical skin, dental or skeletal abnormalities are present, then the term Axenfeld–Rieger syndrome (ARS) is used. It is noteworthy that the clinical findings in ASD overlap considerably, even within families, and mutations in the same gene can cause a range of phenotypes. Studies of disease-associated mutant protein products have provided insights into the cause of associated malformations.

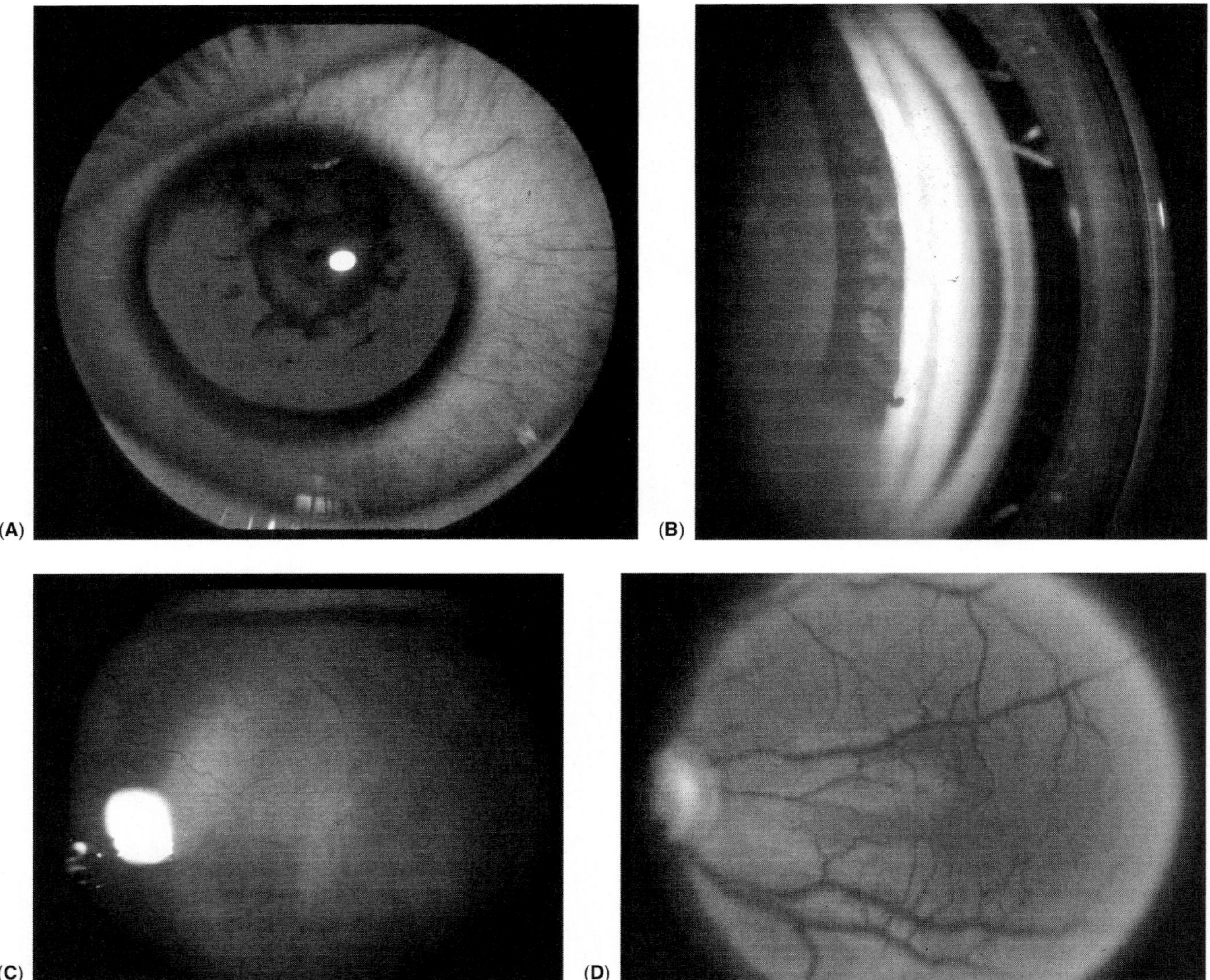

Figure 16 Constellation of ocular findings in aniridia. (**A**) Residual iris stump and cataract visible against red reflex. (**B**) Gonioscopy view demonstrating ease with which ciliary processes can be seen. (**C**) Red reflex view of peripheral cornea demonstrating significant pannus formation. (**D**) Foveal hyoplasia with absence of the foveal avascular zone. *Source*: Courtesy of Dr. Wallace L.M. Alward.

Patients with ASD presumably develop glaucoma because of an impaired drainage of aqueous humor from the anterior chamber angle. However, an ultrastructural analysis of the TM from a 24-year-old patient with ARS and glaucoma disclosed thickening of the basement membrane surrounding the trabecular lamellae of the corneoscleral and uveal TM, as well as large aggregates of plaque material within the extracellular spaces of the juxtacanalicular tissue. Similar findings have been observed in POAG and juvenile-onset forms of OAG (Fig. 15) (18,48).

The primary causative genes that have been identified in varying ASD phenotypes are *PITX2*, *PITX3*, *FOXC1*, and *PAX6*, which encode transcription factors. It is possible that haploinsufficiency of the involved transcription factors may lead to abnormal ECM turnover in the juxtacanalicular meshwork during development, that continues during childhood and adolescence (63).

PITX2

The product of the *PITX2* gene is a paired-like homeodomain transcription factor. The sequences within the homeodomains permit the proteins to regulate the expression of other genes. Both hypomorphic and over-activating alleles of *PITX2* cause human ASD, including ARS, iris hypoplasia, iridogoniodysgenesis, and Peters anomaly (Table 1). PITX2

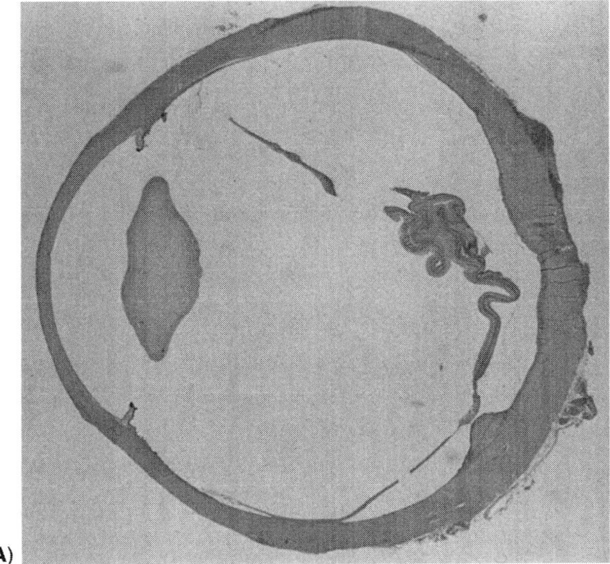

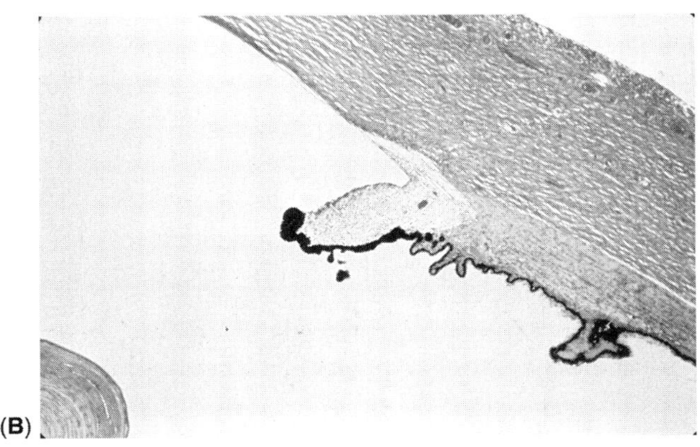

Figure 17 Histopathology of aniridia. (**A**) View of globe demonstrating small iris stump. (**B**) Anomalous iris with ectropion uveae, and abnormal angle structures trabecular meshwork and underdeveloped Schlemm canal. *Source*: From Ref. 63.

therefore appears to play a critical role in development of the anterior segment (see Chapter 51).

PITX3

Like PITX2 PITX3 is paired-like homeodomain transcription factor that causes ASD, including cataracts, corneal opacities and iridocorneal adhesions, when mutated (54).

FOXC1

FOXC1 (forkhead box C1, formerly known as FKHL7) is another transcription factor. It has a DNA binding domain and turns other genes on during development. Mutations in *FOXC1* cause a spectrum of ASD and glaucoma phenotypes (Table 1) (see Chapter 52). Some mutations can lead to dental, jaw, umbilical, and other ocular abnormalities.

Foxc1$^{+/-}$ mice have milder anterior segment defects than *Foxc1*$^{-/-}$ mice (19) Abnormalities in *Foxc1*$^{+/-}$ mice include iris malformations, iridocorneal adhesions and corneal opacification. They also have a variety of anterior chamber angle malformations, including a small or absent Schlemm canal and a hypoplastic, compressed TM. The angle structures have a paucity of ECM, including collagen and elastic tissue, and the cells resemble undifferentiated precursor cells. Not all mice develop clinically detectable abnormalities, although all have histologically detectable malformations of the anterior chamber angle structures.

Proteins interacting with FOXC1, such as the actin-binding protein filamin A (FLNA), have been identified in human nonpigmented ciliary epithelial cells (11). Berry et al. (11) have hypothesized that, given the resemblance of the skeletal phenotypes

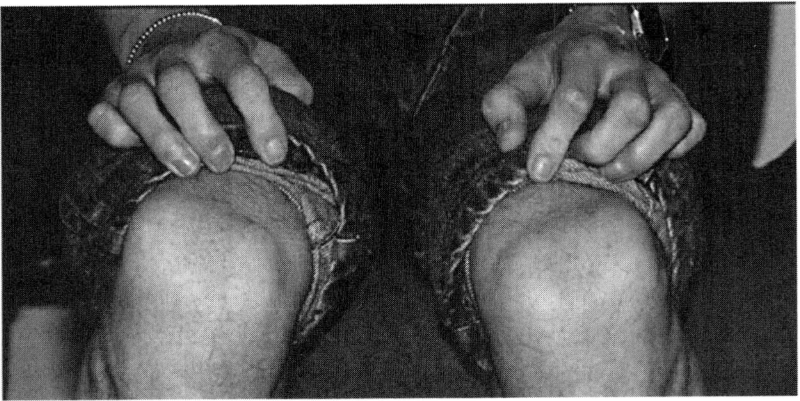

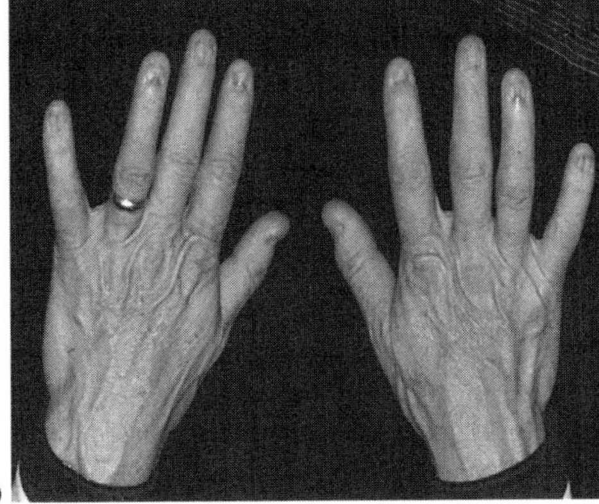

Figure 18 (**A**) Appearance of dysplastic fingernails and (**B**) hypoplastic and frequently subluxed patella in nail patella syndrome. *Source*: Courtesy of Dr. Paul R. Lichter and the University of Michigan W.K. Kellogg Eye Center.

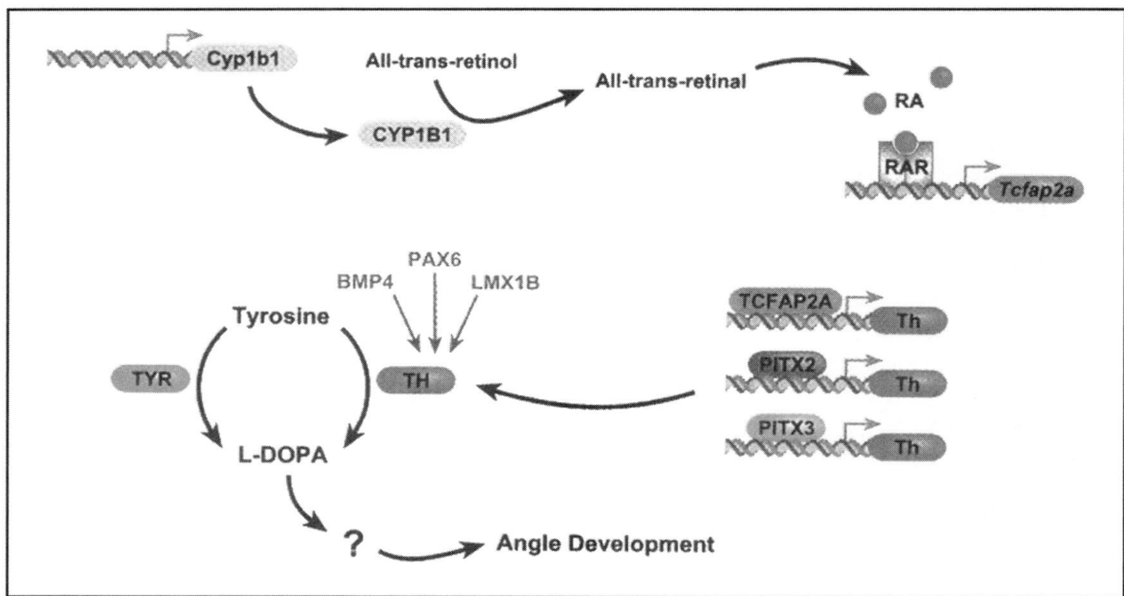

Figure 19 Multiple genes implicated in anterior segment development and glaucoma may modulate L-dopa levels. Many of the genes implicated in anterior segment dysgenesis, elevated IOP, and glaucoma may affect L-dopa levels. Most can be linked to L-dopa through tyrosine hydroxlase (TH). How L-dopa modulates angle development also is not known. It is possible that either L-dopa itself or a catecholamine metabolite(s) of L-dopa mediates an important signaling event(s). *Source*: From Ref. 19.

caused by *FOXC1* loss-of-function mutations and *FLNA* gain-of-function mutations, the effect of *FLNA* on *FOXC1* may contribute to the pathogenesis of skeletal disorders.

PAX6

PAX6 is a key regulator of eye development and it is essential for eye formation in different organisms. It encodes for a transcription factor with homeobox and paired-class DNA binding domains. Mutations in *PAX6* are associated with several phenotypes including aniridia (Figs. 16–18), Peters anomaly and Rieger syndrome. Null mutations or duplications of PAX6 can cause severe anterior segment dysgenesis indicating the importance of PAX6 for normal development (19).

The small eye mutant mouse has a null allele of *Pax6*. Homozygous *Pax6 null* mice have morphological abnormalities of the optic vesicle and failure of lens induction (19). The ocular defects in mice heterozygous for the *Pax6* null allele include microphthalmos, small anterior chambers, corneal haze, iris hypoplasia, iridocorneal adhesions, a hypoplastic and undifferentiated TM and an absence of Schlemm canal (19).

SYSTEMIC DISEASES ASSOCIATED WITH GLAUCOMA

Some inherited systemic disorders are associated with open angle forms of glaucoma and the genes for many of these disorders have been identified and are mapped to specific chromosomal loci. (Table 3) Several of these genetically determined disorders are discussed elsewhere; basal cell nevus syndrome (see Chapter 55), Ehlers-Danlos syndrome type VI (see Chapter 44), Marfan syndrome (see Chapter 36), Lowe oculocerebrorenal syndrome (see Chapter 43), neurofibromatosis type I (see Chapter 55), mucopolysaccharidosis type VI (see Chapter 40), Stickler syndrome (see Chapter 29).

Nail-Patella Syndrome

In addition to dysplastic nails and hyopoplastic patellas, the nail-patella syndrome (NPS) is also associated with nephropathy and primary open angle glaucoma (Fig. 18A,B). Mutations in LMX1B, a LIM homeodomain class transcription factor cause the syndrome (19,63). In Lmx1b$^{-/-}$ mice, there is a lack of expression of keratocan and other ECM molecules. These mice also have loss of two subtypes of collagen type IV, COL4A3 and COL4A4 from the glomerular basement membrane (19).

INSIGHTS INTO MECHANISMS

Although several glaucoma associated genes have been identified, much more research is necessary before the genetic or physiological factors that create a susceptibility to glaucoma are understood. In an initial attempt to link the actions of known genes and pathways in anterior segment formation, Gould et al. (19) have proposed a relationship between TGFβ family signaling and ECM regulation. They have also suggested how various genes involved in anterior segment formation may converge to affect signaling by a common molecule/pathway, e.g., L-dopa (Fig. 19).

Identification of genes, as well as mouse model systems, is helping to elucidate biochemical pathways that ultimately cause glaucoma (26). To reach an in depth understanding of these pathways, however, it will be essential to combine the tools of genomics, molecular biology, developmental biology, bioinformatics and computational biology (19). This should ultimately lead to a better understanding of the normal physiology of the TM, optic nerve, ganglion cells, and other associated tissues. Improved understanding of the state if the eye in disease and health will facilitate the rational development of drugs tailored to specific subtypes of glaucoma (13).

REFERENCES

1. Akarsu AN, Turacli ME, Aktan SG, et al. A second locus (GLC3B) for primary congenital glaucoma (Buphthalmos) maps to the 1p36 region. Hum Mol Genet 1996; 5:1199–203.
2. Allingham RR, Loftsdottir M, Gottfredsdottir MS, et al. Pseudoexfoliation syndrome in Icelandic families. Br J Ophthalmol 2001; 85:702–7.
3. Alsbirk PH. Anterior chamber depth and primary angle-closure glaucoma. II. A genetic study. Acta Ophthalmol (Copenh) 1975; 53:436–49.
4. Alsbirk PH. Primary angle-closure glaucoma: oculometry, epidemiology, and genetics in a high-risk population. Acta Ophthalmol (Suppl) 1976; 127:5–31.
5. Alward WL, Fingert JH, Coote MA, et al. Clinical features associated with mutations in the chromosome 1 open-angle glaucoma gene (GLC1A). N Engl J Med 1998; 338: 1022–7.
6. Alward WL, Kwon YH, Kawase K, et al. Evaluation of optineurin sequence variations in 1,048 patients with open-angle glaucoma. Am J Ophthalmol 2003; 136:904–10.
7. Andersen J, Pralea A, Delbono A, et al. A gene responsible for the pigment dispersion syndrome maps to chromosome 7q35-q36. Arch Ophthalmol 1997; 115:384–8.
8. Anderson MG, Smith RS, Hawes NL, et al. Mutations in genes encoding melanosomal proteins cause pigmentary glaucoma in DBA/2J mice. Nat Genet 2002; 30:81–5.
9. Aung T, Ocaka L, Ebenezer ND, et al. A major marker for normal tension glaucoma: association with polymorphisms in the OPA1 gene. Hum Genet 2002; 110:52–6.
10. Becker B, Podos SM. Krukenberg's spindles and primary open-angle glaucoma. Arch Ophthalmol 1966; 76:635–47.
11. Berry FB, O'Neill MA, Coca-Prados M, Walter MA. FOXC1 transcriptional regulatory activity is impaired by PBX1 in a filamin A-mediated manner. Mol Cell Biol 2005; 25:1415–24.
12. Breingan PJ, Esaki K, Ishikawa H, et al. Iridolenticular contact decreases following laser iridotomy for pigment dispersion syndrome. Arch Ophthalmol 1999; 117:325–8.
13. Challa P. Glaucoma genetics: advancing new understandings of glaucoma pathogenesis. Int Ophthalmol Clin. 2004; 44:167–85.
14. Congdon N, Wang F, Tielsch JM. Issues in the epidemiology and population-based screening of primary angle-closure glaucoma. Surv Ophthalmol 1992; 36:411–23.
15. Copin B, Brezin AP, Valtot F, et al. Apolipoprotein E-promotor single-nucleotide polymorphisms affect the phenotype of primary open-angle glaucoma and demonstrate interaction with the myocilin gene. Am J Hum Genet 2002; 70:1575–81.
16. Damji KF, Stefansson E, Bains HS, et al. Is pseudoexfoliation syndrome inherited? A review of genetic and nongenetic factors and a new observation. Ophthalmic Genetics 1998; 19:175–85.
17. Funayama T, Mashima Y, Ohtake Y, et al. SNPs and interaction analyses of Noelin 2, myocilin, and optineurin genes in Japanese patients with open-angle glaucoma. Invest Ophthalmol Vis Sci 2006; 47:5368–75.
18. Furuyoshi N, Furuyoshi M, Futa R., et al. Ultrastructural changes in the trabecular meshwork of juvenile glaucoma. Ophthalmologica 1997; 211:140–6.
19. Gould DB, Smith RS, John SWM. Anterior segment development relevant to glaucoma. Int J Dev Biol. 2004; 48:1015–29.
20. Hardy KM, Hoffman EA, Gonzalez P. Extracellular trafficking of myocilin in human trabecular meshwork cells. J Biol. Chem 2005; 280:28917–26.
21. Hauser MA, Allingham RR, Linkroum K, et al. Distribution of WDR36 DNA sequence variants in patients with primary open-angle glaucoma. Investigative Ophthalmology & Visual Science. 2006; 47(6):2542–6.
22. Ho CL, Walton DS. Primary congenital glaucoma: 2004 update. J Pediatr Ophthalmol Strabismus 2004; 41:271–88.
23. Hu CN. An epidemiologic study of glaucoma in Shunyi county, Beijing. Chung Hua Yen Ko Tsa Chih 1989; 25:115–9.
24. Jacobson N, Andrews M, Shepard AR, et al. Non-secretion of mutant proteins of the glaucoma gene myocilin in cultured trabecular meshwork cells and in aqueous humor. Hum Mol Genet 2001; 10:117–25.
25. Joe MK, Sohn S, Choi YR, et al. Identification of flotillin-1 as a protein interacting with myocilin: implications for the pathogenesis of primary open-angle glaucoma. Biochem Biophys Res Commun 2005; 336:1201–6.
26. John SW. Mechanistic insights into glaucoma provided by experimental genetics the cogan lecture. Invest Ophthalmol Vis Sci 2005; 6:2649–61.
27. Johnson DH. Myocilin and glaucoma: A TIGR by the tail? Arch Ophthalmol 2000; 118:974–8.
28. Kaiser-Kupfer MI, Kupfer C, McCain L. Asymmetric pigment dispersion syndrome. Trans Am Ophthalmol Soc 1983; 81:310–24.
29. Kaur K, Reddy AB, Mukhopadhyay A, et al. Myocilin gene implicated in primary congenital glaucoma. Clin Genet 2005; 67:335–40.
30. Kubota R, Noda S, Wang Y., et al. A novel myosin-like protein (myocilin) expressed in the connecting cilium of the photoreceptor: molecular cloning, tissue expression, and chromosomal mapping. Genomics 1997; 41:360–9.
31. Li Y, Aroca-Aguilar JD, Ghosh S, et al. Interaction of myocilin with the C-terminal region of hevin. Biochem Biophys Res Commun. 2006; 339:797–804.
32. Li Y, Kang J, Horwitz MS. Interaction of an adenovirus E3 14.7-kilodalton protein with a novel tumor necrosis factor alpha--inducible cellular protein containing leucine zipper domains. Mol Cell Biol 1998; 18:1601–10.
33. Libby RT, Gould DB, Anderson MG, John SW. Complex genetics of glaucoma susceptibility. Annu Rev Genomics Hum Genet 2005; 6:15–44.
34. Libby RT, Smith RS, Savinova OV, et al. Modification of ocular defects in mouse developmental glaucoma models by tyrosinase. Science 2003; 299:1578–81.

35. Liu Y, Vollrath D. Reversal of mutant myocilin non-secretion and cell killing: implications for glaucoma. Hum Mol Genet 2004; 13:1193–204.
36. Lowe RF. Primary angle-closure glaucoma. Inheritance and environment. Br J Ophthalmol 1972; 56:13–9.
37. Mandelkorn R, Hoffman M, Olander K, et al. Inheritance of the pigmentary dispersion syndrome. Ann Ophthalmol 1983; 15:577–82.
38. Manson FD, Black GC. Mutations of VMD2 splicing regulators cause nanophthalmos and autosomal dominant vitreoretinochoroidopathy (ADVIRC). Invest Ophthalmol Vis Sci 2004; 45:3683–9.
39. Michels-Rautenstrauss KG, Mardin CY, Budde WM, et al. Juvenile open angle glaucoma: fine mapping of the TIGR gene to 1q24.3-q25.2 and mutation analysis. Hum Genet 1998; 102:103–6.
40. Mo JS, Anderson MG, Gregory M, et al. By altering ocular immune privilege, bone marrow-derived cells pathogenically contribute to DBA/2J pigmentary glaucoma. J Exp Med 2003; 197:1335–44.
41. Monemi S, Spaeth G, DaSilva A, et al. Identification of a novel adult-onset primary open-angle glaucoma (POAG) gene on 5q22.1. Hum Mol Genet 2005; 14:725–33.
42. Morissette J, Clepet C, Moisan S et al. Homozygotes carrying an autosomal dominant TIGR mutation do not manifest glaucoma. Nature Genetics 1998; 19:319–21.
43. Oh YG, Mineli S, Spaeta G, Steinman WC. The anterior chamber angle is different in different racial groups: a gonioscopic study. Eye 1994; 8:104–8.
44. Perkumas KM, Hoffman EM, McKay BS, et al. Myocilin-associated exosomes in human ocular samples. Exp Eye Res 2007; 84:209–12.
45. Quigley HA, Broman AT. Number of people with glaucoma worldwide in 2010 and 2020. Br J Ophthalmol. 2006; 90:262–7.
46. Rezaie, TA., Child, R. Hitchings, G, et al. Adult-onset primary open-angle glaucoma caused by mutations in optineurin. Science. 2002; 295:1077–9.
47. Ricard CS, Tamm ER. Focus on molecules: Myocilin/TIGR. Exp Eye Res 2005; 81:501–2.
48. Rohen JW, Lutjen-Drecoll E, Flugel C, et al. Ultrastructure of the trabecular meshwork in untreated cases of primary open-angle glaucoma (POAG). Exper Eye Res 1993; 56:683–92.
49. Sahlender DA, Roberts RC, Arden SD, et al. Optineurin links myosin VI to the Golgi complex and is involved in Golgi organization and exocytosis. J Cell Biol 2005; 169:285–95.
50. Sarfarazi M, Akarsu AN, Hossain A, et al. Assignment of a locus (GLC3A) for primary congenital glaucoma (buphthalmos) to 2p21 and evidence for genetic heterogeneity. Genomics 1995; 30:171–7.
51. Sarfarazi M. Recent advances in molecular genetics of glaucomas. Human Mol Genet 1997; 6:1667–77.
52. Schlotzer-Schrehardt U, Lommatzsch J, Kuchle M, et al. Matrix metalloproteinaseses and the inhibitors in aqueous humor of patients with pseudoexfoliation syndrome/glaucoma and primary open-angle glaucoma. Invest Ophthalmol Vis Sci 2003; 44:1117–25.
53. Schwamborn KR, Weil G, Courtois ST, et al. Phorbol esters and cytokines regulate the expression of the NEMO-related protein, a molecule involved in a NF-kappa B-independent pathway. J Biol Chem 2000; 275:22780–9.
54. Semina EV, Ferrell RE, Mintz-Hittner HA, et al. A novel homeobox gene PITX3 is mutated in families with autosomal-dominant cataracts and ASMD. Nature Genet 1998; 19:167–70.
55. Senatorov V, Malyukova I, Fariss R, et al. Expression of mutated mouse myocilin induces open-angle glaucoma in transgenic mice. J Neurosci 2006; 26:11903–14.
56. Sheffield VC, Stone EM, Alward WLM, et al. Genetic linkage of familial open angle glaucoma to chromosome 1q21-1q31. Nature Genet 1993; 4:47–50.
57. Shields MB, Allingham RR, Damji KF, et al. Molecular genetics of the glaucomas. In: Allingham RR, Damji KF, Friedman S, et al, eds. Shields' Textbook of Glaucoma, 5th edition. Philadelphia, PA: Lippincott Williams & Wilkins, 2005:163–9.
58. Stamer WD, Perkumas KM, Hoffman EA, et al. Coiled–coil targeting of myocilin to intracellular membranes. Exp Eye Res, 2006; 83:1386–95.
59. Stoilov I, Akarsu AN, Sarfarazi M. Identification of three different truncating mutations in cytochrome P4501B1 (CYP1B1) as the principal cause of primary congenital glaucoma (Buphthalmos) in families linked to the GLC3A locus on chromosome 2p21. Hum Mol Genet 1997; 6:641–7.
60. Stone EM, Fingert JH, Alward WL, et al. Identification of a gene that causes primary open angle glaucoma. Science 1997; 275:668–70.
61. Sundin OH, Leppert GS, Silva ED, et al. Extreme hyperopia is the result of null mutations in MFRP, which encodes a Frizzled-related protein. Proc Natl Acad Sci U S A. 2005; 102:9553–8.
62. Surgucheva I, Park BC, Yue BY, et al. Interaction of myocilin with gamma-synuclein affects its secretion and aggregation. Cell Mol Neurobiol 2005; 25:1009-33.
63. Tamm ER. Glaucomas in developmental disorders. In: Krieglstein GK, Weinreb RN (series eds.). Essentials in Ophthalmology—Glaucoma volume; Grehn F, Stamper R (chapter eds.) Glaucoma. 1st edition, Springer, Berlin, Heidleberg, New York: Springer, 2004;1–21.
64. Tawara A, Inomata H. Developmental immaturity of the trabecular meshwork in congenital glaucoma. Am J Ophthalmol 1981; 92:508–25.
65. Tezel G, Wax MB. Increased production of tumor necrosis factor-alpha by glial cells exposed to simulated or elevated hydrostatic pressure induces apoptosis in cocultured retinal ganglion cells. J Neurosci 2000; 20:8693–700.
66. Thorleifsson G, Magnusson KP, Sulem P, et al. Common sequence variants in the *LOXL1* gene confer susceptibility to exfoliation glaucoma. Science 2007; 317:1397–400.
67. Tornquist R. Shallow anterior chambers in acute glaucoma. Acta Ophthalmol 1953; 31:1–74.
68. Vittitow J, Borras T. Genes expressed in the human trabecular meshwork during pressure-induced homeostatic response. J Cell Physiol 2004; 201:126–37.
69. Wiggs JL, Vollrath D. Molecular and clinical evaluation of a patient hemizygous for TIGR/MYOC. Arch Ophthalmol. 2001; 119:1674–8.
70. Yardley J, Leroy BP, Hart-Holden N, et al. Mutations of VMD2 splicing regulators cause nanophthalmos and autosomal dominant vitreoretinochoroidopathy (ADVIRC). Invest Ophthalmol Vis Sci 2004; 45:3683–9.
71. Yuan L, Neufeld AH. Tumor necrosis factor-alpha: a potentially neurodestructive cytokine produced by glia in the human glaucomatous optic nerve head. Glia 2000; 32: 42–50.
72. Zenkel M, Poschl E, von der Mark K, et al. Differential gene expression in pseudoexfoliation syndrome. Invest Ophthalmol Vis Sci 2005; 46:3742–52.
73. Zhou X, Li F, Kong L, Tomita H, et al. Involvement of inflammation, degradation, and apoptosis in a mouse model of glaucoma. J Biol Chem 2005; 280:31240–8.
74. Zillig M, Wurm A, Grehn FJ, et al. Overexpression and properties of wild-type and Tyr437His mutated myocilin in the eyes of transgenic mice. Invest Ophthalmol Vis Sci 2005; 46:223–34.

35

Genetic Disorders of the Retina and Optic Nerve

Pelin Atmaca-Sönmez and John R. Heckenlively
Kellogg Eye Institute, University of Michigan, Ann Arbor, Michigan, U.S.A.

INTRODUCTION

The retina is a relatively inaccessible, complex tissue that poses challenges for researchers who attempt to unravel pathogenic events causing diseases. Nevertheless, there has been substantial progress in elucidating the molecular and genetic basis of hereditary retinal diseases during the past 15 years. As of December 19, 2007, 190 genes have been mapped and 138 have been cloned for retinal diseases (http://www.sph.uth.tmc.edu/Retnet/). These advances are exciting since with further research this information holds the promise for treatments. It is now more important than ever to correctly diagnose and genotype patients with hereditary retinal disease.

The inherited optic neuropathies comprise a group of disorders in which cell death is confined to the retinal ganglion cells. It is important to differentiate primary retinal degenerations with accompanying optic atrophy from the primary optic neuropathies since there are overlapping features. For instance, in patients with cone dystrophy, retinal findings may be subtle and optic nerve pallor may be the initial finding. In hereditary retinal degenerations where the bipolar layer of the retina is affected, transsynaptic degeneration may affect the ganglion cells. Nevertheless, optic nerve and retinal disease may also coexist (244). Optic neuropathy can be confirmed clinically by virtue of normal electroretinography (ERG), and abnormal visual evoked potential (VEP) response. The inherited optic neuropathies may be sporadic or familial, in which case the mode of inheritance may be Mendelian (autosomal dominant, autosomal recessive, X-linked recessive) or non-Mendelian (mitochondrial).

PROTEINS INVOLVED IN RETINAL FUNCTION

General Remarks

Retinal degenerations have been found to be due to mutations in the genes that encode proteins involved in functions such as phototransduction, the visual cycle, membrane structure and polarity, intracellular transport, and transcription at the RNA level. Encoded proteins with unknown function have been identified for mutated genes, or in other cases only parts of a gene have been identified and the protein may be unknown. To better understand retinal disease mechanisms, the main systems known to be effected by disease-causing mutations will be mentioned briefly. Among the first identified processes known to be effected by mutations were proteins in the phototransduction cascade and the visual cycle (Fig. 1) (154,224). The chemical reaction that mediates the process by which light is converted into nerve signals (phototransduction) takes place in the outer segments of the photoreceptors. The outer segments are basically flattened sacs made by a lipid membrane whose structure provides extensive surface area for capturing incoming photons. The visual pigments, rhodopsin for rods and red, green or blue opsins for cones, as well as many other functional and structural proteins are located in the outer segments. Rhodopsin consists of an opsin molecule (a seven transmembrane G-protein-coupled receptor) covalently attached to the chromophore 11-*cis* retinal, a vitamin A derivate. Rhodopsin is embedded in high concentrations in the disc membranes and to a lesser extent in the plasma membrane covering the discs. Rhodopsin is predominantly located in the rod outer segment disc membranes and comprises more than 70% of the total rod outer segment protein. It is a major structural protein of the rod outer segments, and is a crucial element of the phototransduction cascade.

Phototransduction Cascade

The activation of rhodopsin by light activates the transducin α-subunit, which in turn activates cyclic guanosine monophosphate (cGMP) phosphodiesterase (PDE), an enzyme that hydrolyses cGMP. When the cGMP levels fall, cGMP-gated cation channels close resulting in hyperpolarization of the photoreceptor cell membrane and a decreased neurotransmitter release at the synaptic region with second order retinal neurons. Cytoplasmic levels of cGMP are restored by retinal-specific guanylate cyclases the

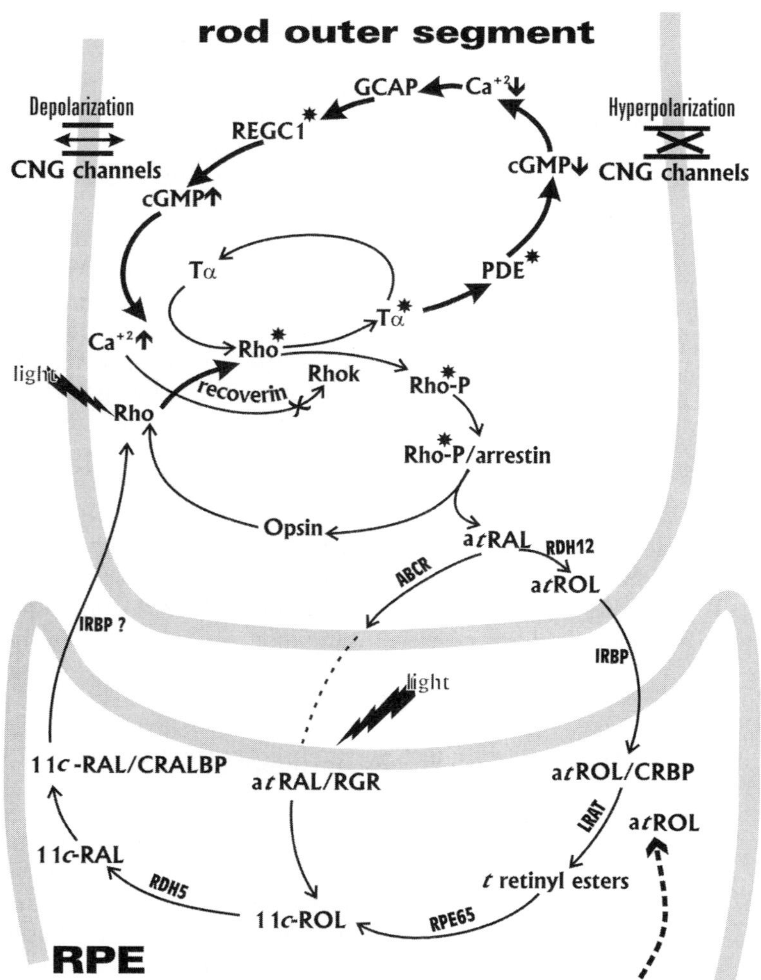

Figure 1 Phototransduction cascade and visual cycle. *Abbreviations*: CNG channels, cyclic nucleotide-gated channels; Rho, rhodopsin; *, activated; T, Transducin; PDE, cGMP-phosphodiesterase; GCAP, guanylate cyclase activation protein; REGC1, retinal-specific guanylate cyclase; Rhok, rhodopsin kinase; Rho-P, phosphorylated rhodopsin; atRAL, all-*trans* retinal; atROL, all-*trans* retinol; 11 c-RAL, 11 *cis*-retinal; 11 c-ROL, 11 *cis*-retinol; ABCR, ATP-binding cassette transporter-retinal; IRBP, interstitial retinol-binding protein; CRALBP, cellular retinaldehyde-binding protein; RDH, retinol dehydrogenase; LRAT, lecithin retinol acyltransferase; RPE65, retinal pigment epithelium-specific 65 kDa protein; RGR, RPE-retinal G protein-coupled receptor; CRBP, cellular retinol-binding protein.

activity of which is modulated by a calcium-sensitive enzyme, guanylate cyclase activation protein (GCAP). As the cGMP concentration increases, the cGMP-gated channels open, and the photoreceptor cell is returned to its depolarized state.

Activation Deactivation of Rhodopsin

The activated form of rhodopsin must be deactivated so that subsequent light can be detected. This deactivation process begins by multiple phosphorylations catalyzed by rhodopsin kinase, followed by the binding of arrestin that terminates the activation properties of rhodopsin, resulting in the splitting of all-*trans* retinal from opsin.

Retinoid Metabolism and the Visual Cycle

The visual cycle, the light-induced movement and transformations of retinoids between the photoreceptors and the retinal pigment epithelium (RPE), is an essential complex process. The all-*trans* retinal that forms as a result of rhodopsin activation by light in the outer segments takes one of two pathways. In the direct pathway, all-*trans* retinal is converted to all-*trans* retinol by retinol dehydrogenase 12 (RDH12), which is then transported to the RPE. Interstitial retinol-binding protein (IRBP) is believed to facilitate this transport (154). In addition to the regeneration of the chromophore, new all-*trans* retinol from the diet is transported to the RPE via the choriocapillaris. Within the RPE, all-*trans* retinol is bound to cellular retinol-binding protein (CRBP), and is converted to all-*trans* retinyl esters by lecithin retinol acyltransferase (LRAT). The conversion of all-*trans* retinyl esters to 11-*cis* retinol requires RPE65. Then, 11-*cis* retinol is converted into 11-*cis* retinal by RDH5 and also possibly by other RDHs. The second scavenger pathway for all-*trans* retinal from the outer segments to the RPE is facilitated by retina-specific ATP-binding cassette transporter (ABCR). In RPE, RPE-retinal G-protein coupled receptor (RGR) appears to play a role in the conversion of all-*trans* retinal to 11-*cis* retinal. Once 11-*cis* retinal is formed, it is bound to cellular retinaldehyde-binding protein (CRALBP) and then IRBP facilitates its transport back to the outer segments where it binds to opsin. The hydrophobic nature and chemical instability of the retinoids necessitate the help of retinoid binding proteins in their transport and also to protect them from oxidation or degradation. CRBP and CRALBP also appear to promote isomerization of all-*trans* retinol in RPE.

Outer Segment Renewal

Outer segments shed their tips which are then phagocytozed by the RPE apical tips to be degraded in the RPE. The RPE ingests approximately one-tenth of each rod outer segment per day (21). New discs are formed at the base of the outer segments. The proteins and other cellular components necessary for outer segment renewal are synthesized in the rod inner segments before being transported to the outer segment through the cilium. This internalization is mediated by the MER tyrosine kinase protooncogene (*MERTK*), and partially by myosin VIIa. At the end of the disc generation, the disc becomes separated from the plasma membrane. This step requires cytoskeletal proteins such as actin and actin-binding proteins.

Hereditary retinal degenerations are both phenotypically and genetically heterogeneous. Different mutations in the same gene may result in clinically different diseases (Table 1), and conversely, mutations in different genes may result in a similar clinical phenotype (Table 2). Secondary expression from other genes may play a role in some varied phenotypes. Histopathologic findings support the idea that in some cases, factors other than the primary gene mutation itself, such as modifier genes, diet, and environment, are responsible for the heterogeneity (228).

INHERITED DISORDERS OF THE RETINA

Retinitis Pigmentosa

General Remarks

Retinitis pigmentosa (RP) is the term used for a group of hereditary disorders associated with diffuse, progressive, primary photoreceptor and in some cases concomitant RPE degeneration, with an estimated prevalence of 1 in 3700 (25). This section delineates the non-syndromic, primary forms of RP and only Usher syndrome (USH) of the syndromic RPs.

Clinical Features

Night blindness and a slowly progressive visual field loss are the major symptoms in RP. Hereditary forms of RP are bilateral and symmetric, and when marked asymmetry is detected old chorioretinitis should be suspected rather than a hereditary condition (Figs. 2–7). The typical fundus features of RP are a pigmentary retinopathy often resembling pigmented "bone-spicules," diffuse mottling of the RPE, thinning and atrophy of the retina and RPE, with relative preservation in the macula, and arteriolar attenuation. Gliotic "waxy-pallor" of the optic nerve head is commonly mentioned in texts, but is typically a feature of a more advanced disease. The central vision is often preserved until later stages of the disease. Cataract, vitreous degeneration, macular changes, and optic nerve head drusen are features commonly associated with RP. The overall incidence of cataract in RP

Table 1 Genes Associated with Phenotypic Heterogeneity in Hereditary Retinal Degenerations

Gene	Protein	Phenotype
RHO	Rhodopsin	adRP; arRP; adCSNB
PDE6B	Rod cGMP phosphodiesterase beta subunit	arRP; adCSNB
ABCA4 (*ABCR*, *RP19*, *STGD1*)	ATP-binding cassette transporter retinal	arStargardt disease; arRP; arCORD
RPE65 (*LCA2*, *RP20*)	Retinal pigment epithelium-specific 65 kDa protein	arLCA; arRP
SEMA4A	Semaphorin 4A	adRP; adCORD
CRB1 (*RP12*)	Crumbs homolog 1	PPRPE; arRP; arLCA; PPCRA
SAG	Arrestin (S-antigen)	arOguchi disease; arRP
LRAT	Lecithin retinol acyltransferase	arRP; arLCA
TULP1 (*RP14*)	Tubby-like protein 1	arRP; arLCA
RDS (*RP7*)	Peripherin 2	adRP; digenic RP with ROM1; dominant adult vitelliform MD
GUCA1A (*COD3*, *GCAP1*)	Guanylate cyclase activator 1A	adCOD; adCORD
GUCA1B (*GCAP2*)	Guanylate cyclase activator 1B	adRP; adMD
RDH5 (*RDH1*)	11-*cis* retinol dehydrogenase 5	ar fundus albipunctatus; arCOD
NR2E3 (*ESCS*, *PNR*)	Nuclear receptor subfamily 2 group E member 3	ESCS; arRP; Goldmann-Favre syndrome
RLBP1 (*CRALBP*)	Cellular retinaldehyde-binding protein	arRP; retinitis punctata albescens; Bothnia dystrophy; recessive Newfoundland rod–cone dystrophy
AIPL1 (*LCA4*)	Arylhydrocarbon-interacting receptor protein-like 1	arLCA; adCORD
GUCY2D (*CORD6*, *LCA1*, *RETGC1*)	Retinal-specific guanylate cyclase	arLCA; adCORD
FSCN2 (*RP30*)	Retinal fascin homolog 2, actin binding protein	adRP; adMD
CRX (*CORD2*)	Cone–rod otx-like photoreceptor homeobox transcription factor	adCORD; ar, ad, de novo LCA; adRP
RPGR (*RP3*)	Retinitis pigmentosa GTPase regulator	X-linked recessive RP; X-linked dominant RP; X-linked CSNB; X-linked cone dystrophy 1; X-linked atrophic MD

Abbreviations: ar, autosomal recessive; ad, autosomal dominant; RP, retinitis pigmentosa; CSNB, congenital stationary night blindness; CORD, cone–rod dystrophy; LCA, Leber congenital amaurosis; PPRPE, recessive RP with para-arteriolar preservation of the RPE; PPCRA, pigmented paravenous chorioretinal atrophy; MD, macular dystrophy; COD, cone dystrophy; ESCS, enhanced S-cone syndrome.
Source: http://www.sph.uth.tmc.edu/Retnet/

patients is approximately 46%; although it increases with age, 43% of RP patients younger than 40 years of age have cataracts (190). The vitreous gel is universally abnormal with several characteristics: tiny, dust-like pigment, posterior vitreous detachment, liquefaction, a posterior matrix of dense white opacities and interconnecting fibers (190). Macular changes are common such as surface wrinkling of the internal limiting membrane (20%), bull eye appearance (36%), and atrophic changes (17%). Cystoid macular edema occurs in approximately 15% of RP patients during the course of their disease (190). There is a very high correlation of circulating anti-retinal antibodies to cystoid edema in RP, and immunosuppression may be appropriate for selected patients with severe cystoid macular edema (89). Carbonic anhydrase inhibitors have also been successful in the management of some patients with cystoid edema and RP (79).

The most relevant ancillary tests in the clinical diagnosis are Goldmann visual field (GVF) test, dark adaptation test and ERG. Standardized full-field ERG is the gold standard for the diagnosis typically showing a loss or marked reduction of amplitudes and eventually the signals become non-detectable for both rod and cone responses. The ERG will vary in detail depending on the stage and severity of the disease, and the pathophysiology of the particular type of RP.

RP can be classified clinically as rod–cone or cone–rod degenerative pattern, according to the ERG responses and visual field patterns (Table 3) (86,127,219). In the rod–cone pattern, rods are affected more severely and earlier than cones and accounts for about 70% of RP. Patients manifest with night blindness and scotomatous or tunnel vision. In contrast, cone–rod pattern patients have better vision at dusk and more complaints of glare, problems in transition from night to day time conditions.

The majority of RP patients present with a rod–cone degeneration pattern, but up to 30% of new cases can present with cone–rod dysfunction and RP visual fields. A point of confusion is that a small number of families have affected individuals who

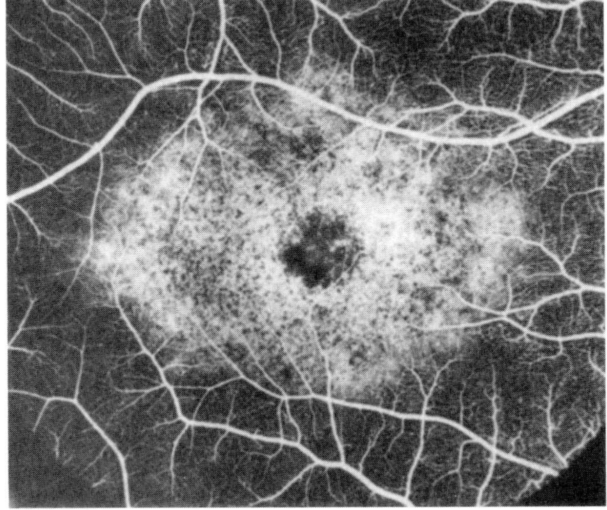

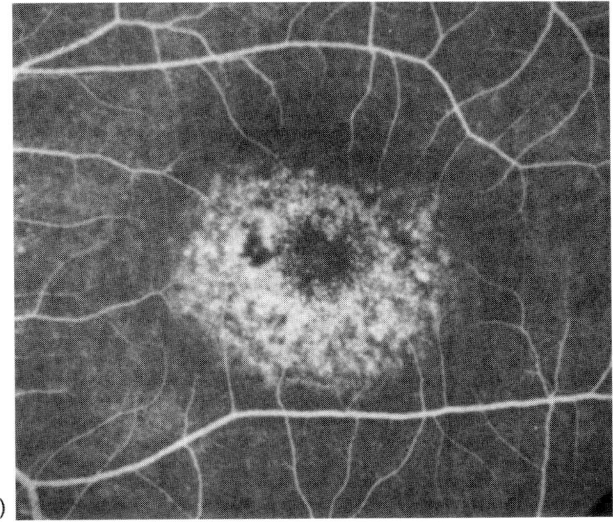

Figure 7 Bull eye dystrophy. Fluorescein angiography in bull eye dystrophy may show retinal dilation and a "dark choroid" (**A**), or the choroid and retinal capillaries may be normal (**B**). *Source*: Courtesy of Professors Alan C. Bird and John Marshall.

confirmed by the study of Chuang et al. (39). Their study shows that Arg135 mutant rhodopsins are hyperphosphorylated and bind with high affinity to arrestin. Mutant rhodopsin recruits the cytosolic arrestin to the plasma membrane, and the rhodopsin–arrestin complex is internalized into the endocytic pathway. The rhodopsin–arrestin complexes alter the morphology of endosomal compartments and severely impair receptor-mediated endocytic functions.

Retinal Degeneration Slow Mutations

Retinal degeneration slow (*RDS*; RP7) encodes peripherin-2, an abundant protein localized to the membrane of the outer segment disc rims in both cones and rods (142). RDS plays an important role in maintaining the rim curvature and possibly in anchoring rod discs to adjacent plasma membrane. In mammalian photoreceptors, peripherin-2 associates with other RDS homodimers and with retinal outer segment membrane protein 1 (ROM1) homodimers, a related tetraspanin protein, to form tetramers (142). Tetramer formation is required for the transport and incorporation of peripherin-2 into nascent discs. The mutant protein is misfolded and defective in its ability to form core tetramers, thus inhibiting its transportation from the translation site in the inner segment to the outer segment. Two mechanisms were suggested for the resulting retinal degeneration: Tetramerization-defective mutants (Cys214Ser, Cys167Tyr, Leu185Pro) cause adRP through a deficiency in wild-type peripherin-2, whereas tetramerization-competent mutant peripherin-2 (Pro216Leu) causes adRP through a dominant negative effect, possibly arising from the introduction of a new oligosaccharide chain that destabilizes discs (142). In homozygous mice with the *rds* mutation, the outer segments fail to develop; whereas in heterozygous mice the outer segments are produced but are shortened and disorganized (42). *RDS* mutations have also been reported in adult vitelliform macular dystrophy (60).

RP1 Mutations

Mutations in the *RP1* gene, along with *RHO* and *RDS*, are among the most common causes of adRP. It is also rarely associated with arRP. The RP1 protein plays a major role in the photoreceptor axoneme in the connecting cilium and a photoreceptor-specific microtubule-associated protein, which participates in controlling the length and stability of the photoreceptor axoneme, and in keeping newly formed outer segment discs in the correct orientation and in the stacking of discs into mature outer segments thus controlling the outer segment disc alignment (138). Disruption of the *Rp1* gene in mice causes disorientation of outer segment discs. Microtubule-associated protein 2, which regulates cytoskeletal dynamics, is phosphorylated by c-Jun N-terminal kinases (JNKs), a subfamily of the mitogen-activated protein kinases. It was shown that JNK signaling cascades are specifically compromised in $Rp1^{-/-}$ mice retinas and that Rp1 and JNK cascades play integral roles in photoreceptor development and maintenance (136). There is also evidence suggesting that Rp1 may also play a role in rhodopsin transport to the outer segments (73). Oxygen levels in the retina are thought to regulate the expression of RP1 (187).

FSCN2 Mutations

A mutation in the *FSCN2* gene is associated with adRP type 30 and autosomal dominant macular dystrophy. The 208delG mutation is the only disease-causing mutation to be identified so far, and it results in a lack of retinal fascin homolog 2 (FSCN2) protein, which is a structural protein that has a pivotal role in assembling actin-based structures in the plasma membrane of the connecting cilium of photoreceptors (254). Haploinsufficiency of *FSCN2* may alter the maintenance and/or elongation of outer segment discs and induce photoreceptor degeneration.

CRX Mutations

The cone–rod homeobox (CRX) gene is expressed in rod and cone photoreceptors, horizontal cells and inner nuclear layer neurons in the retina and cells within the photosensitive pineal gland in mammals. It is a member of the Otx/orthodentical family of transcription factors and functions as a key transcriptional regulator of photoreceptor-specific gene expression such as PDE6A (188), and possibly RP1, GUCY2D, and ABCA4 (192). The expressions of rhodopsin, cone opsins, rod transducin α-subunit, cone arrestin and recoverin are diminished in $Crx^{-/-}$ mice (68). On the other hand, some genes specific to the photoreceptor, such as *Cnga3* and *Neurod*, were upregulated in $Crx^{-/-}$ mice. It should be noted that some mutations such as Arg90Trp reduce but do not abolish the transcriptional regulatory activity of CRX (220). Although neural leucine-zipper (NRL) and CRX are each individually able to induce rhodopsin promoter activity, when expressed together, they exhibit transcriptional synergy in rhodopsin promoter activation (161). However, mutations in *CRX* may alter promoter binding or *NRL* interaction. *Crx* is not essential for photoreceptor cell fate determination, as there are cells that express some photoreceptor-specific genes in $Crx^{-/-}$ animals (68). However, CRX is involved in the terminal differentiation and the functional maintenance of rods and cones. CRX is also required for the elongation of the photoreceptor outer segments (68). There is evidence suggesting that some mutations in *CRX* may interrupt nuclear trafficking of the protein in photoreceptor cells (59).

Mutations in *CRX* have been associated with adRP, dominant and recessive cone–rod dystrophy, and autosomal dominant, autosomal recessive, and de novo Leber congenital amaurosis (LCA) depending on the type of mutation (http://www.sph.uth.tmc.edu/Retnet/).

NRL Mutations

The *NRL* gene which encodes for a retina-specific DNA-binding transcription factor is expressed in rod photoreceptors where it functions synergistically with CRX to regulate the expression of several proteins of the phototransduction cascade such as rhodopsin and rod-specific PDE (175). In addition, NRL is necessary for the expression of an orphan-nuclear receptor, NR2E3, where mutations result in enhanced S-cone syndrome (33). *NRL* is also essential for rod differentiation and normal development of photoreceptor cells. Mutations in NRL have been associated with adRP and arRP. $Nrl^{-/-}$ mice have no rod photoreceptors and an increased number of S-cones (156). Autosomal recessive *NRL* mutations have been associated with a specific type of RP, clumped pigmentary retinal degeneration (175), whose prognosis may be worse than the dominant *NRL* mutations. The different phenotypes produced by dominant versus recessive *NRL* mutations suggest that different mechanisms are responsible.

Mutations in the Precursor mRNA-processing (PRPF) Genes

Three genes that participate in pre-messenger RNA (pre-mRNA) splicing have been associated with different types of adRP. They are *PRPF8* (RP13), *PRFPF31* (RP11) and *PRPF3* (RP18). Pre-mRNA splicing is an essential process in gene expression that removes intron sequences from pre-mRNA between transcription and protein synthesis that would otherwise disrupt the coding potential of intron-containing transcripts. This process takes place in the outer segment nucleus, catalyzed by a large RNA–protein complex called the spliceosome. Expression of the mutant PRPF31 protein was shown to significantly reduce rhodopsin expression in cultured retinal cells and induce apoptosis (255). PRPF8 functions as the catalytic core of the spliceosome, either by facilitating the formation of the core and/or by stabilizing RNA interactions (43). It is noteworthy that these three ubiquitously expressed genes only cause RP and apparently not a more widespread abnormality, and variable expressivity is seen in different families.

IMPDH1 Mutations

IMPDH1 mutations have been linked to one variety of adRP (RP10). *IMPDH1* encodes inosine monophosphate dehydrogenase type 1, a protein that is ubiquitously expressed. It is the rate-limiting enzyme of the de novo pathway of guanine nucleotide biosynthesis. It converts inosine monophosphate into xanthosine monophosphate, which is then converted into guanosine diphosphate and guanosine triphosphate (GTP). Photoreceptors have particularly high requirement for GTP in visual transduction processes. Recent studies show that the majority of the mutations in *IMPDH1* alter the affinity and/or the specificity of single-stranded nucleic acid binding (26).

MERTK Mutations

MERTK mutations have been reported in a few patients with arRP, who had severe retinal degeneration with macular involvement (69). Uniparental disomy, in which a diploid offspring carries a chromosomal pair from a single parent, has been reported in patients with *MERTK* mutations (227). The encoded protein, MERTK, is a member of the receptor tyrosine kinase family of cell-surface receptors that consists of an intracellular kinase-containing domain, a transmembrane region, and a cell-adhesion molecule–related extracellular domain and is expressed in a number of tissues (155). MERTK is involved in the recognition and binding of outer segment debris, possibly due to the appearance of phosphatidylserine in the outer leaflet of the plasma membrane of the shed discs (46,62). In the absence of the functional protein outer segment material accumulates in the subretinal space and this is accompanied by a loss of photoreceptor cells and retinal degeneration as is the case in Royal College of Surgeons rats and c-mer mice that have *Mertk* mutations (229). The disease mechanism for some mutations could be the decreased protein stability which disrupts MERTK signaling (155).

Mutations in Cyclic Nucleotide-Gated Channel Genes

In spite of a similar function, rod and cone cells express different cyclic nucleotide-gated channel (CNGA) genes. Mutations in the *CNGA1* and *CNGB1* genes have been associated with arRP, whereas mutations in the cone channel subunit genes (CNGA3 and CNGB3) have been associated with achromatopsia.

CNGA1 and *CNGB1* encode the rod cGMP-gated (CNG) channel alpha and beta subunits respectively. CNG channels are a group of non-selective ion channels present in different tissues. They are important mediators in the phototransduction cascade and are located in the outer segment plasma membrane. In darkness, CNG channels are opened by cGMP, maintaining an inward current. Light induces a hydrolysis of cGMP, thus resulting in closure of the channels and hyperpolarization of the cell as the response. Native CNG channels are heterotetramers composed of homologous A and B subunits. The product of CNGA1 forms a functional channel by itself and is considered the main functional subunit, whereas the protein encoded by CNGB1 modulates the activity of the channel, but is unable to promote ion transfer by itself (97).

Mutations in PDE Genes

PDE6A mutations have been associated with arRP, whereas *PDE6B* mutations were linked to both arRP and adCSNB. *PDE6A* and *PDE6B* encode α- and β-subunits of cGMP PDE, which participate in the phototransduction cascade by hydrolyzing cGMP. A decrease in intracellular cGMP causes the cGMP-gated cation channels in the outer segment membrane to close. Mutations in *PDE6B* result in abnormally high concentrations of cGMP in the retina presumably due to an absent activity of PDE in the mutant photoreceptor cells in animal studies (5,57). The elevated levels of cGMP are toxic to photoreceptors although as yet the exact mechanism is unknown (52). It is possible that the high cGMP levels result in a higher than normal proportion of open channels which would increase the influx of sodium and calcium ions into the cytoplasm. A genotype and phenotype correlation in a mouse model of *Pde6b* mutation suggests that more severe mutations result in more rapid and severe retinal degeneration (84).

CERKL Mutations

A mutation in *CERKL* (Arg257End) has also been associated with one variety of arRP (RP26). It encodes a ceramide kinase homolog, CERK-like (CERKL) protein. Ceramide kinases convert the sphingolipid metabolite ceramide into ceramide-1-phosphate, both of which are key mediators of cellular apoptosis and survival, playing an essential role in the viability of neuronal cells (230). *CERKL* is predominantly expressed in the retinal ganglion cell layer, although a faint signal is also detected in the inner nuclear and photoreceptor cell layers (230). A cell-culture study suggests that the mutant, truncated CERKL protein accumulates in the nucleus which may yield to retinal degeneration (24).

RLBP1 Mutations

Recessive mutations of *RLBP1* have been associated with several phenotypes: RP, Bothnia dystrophy, retinitis punctata albescens, and Newfoundland rod–cone dystrophy (http://www.sph.uth.tmc.edu/Retnet/). *RLBP1* encodes CRALBP, which is mainly expressed not only in RPE but also in Müller cells, ciliary epithelium, iris, cornea, pineal gland and oligodendrocytes of the optic nerve and brain (204). CRALBP functions in RPE as a major acceptor of 11-*cis*-retinal and 11-*cis*-retinol, and interacts with ezrin, radixin, moesin-binding phosphoprotein 50 suggesting a mechanism for localizing CRALBP to RPE plasma membrane for export of 11-*cis*-retinal to rod outer segments for visual pigment regeneration (173). It also serves as a substrate carrier for 11-*cis*-RDH (also known as RDH5 and formerly as RDH1), facilitating the oxidation of 11-*cis*-retinol to 11-*cis*-retinal (76,205,216). Both rod and cone resensitizations after bleaching are delayed in humans with *RLBP1* mutations and in $Rlbp1^{-/-}$ mice.

RGR Mutations

RGR encodes an integral membrane protein, RGR, that shows considerable overall homology to rhodopsin (106). Different mutations in *RGR* have been reported in patients with adRP, and dominant choroidal sclerosis. RGR is a member of a large family of G protein-coupled receptors and is expressed in the cytoplasm of RPE and Müller cells. RGR binds to all-*trans* retinal in the RPE and photons of light convert all-*trans* retinal within the RGR to 11-*cis* retinal (81); the reverse reaction occurs in rhodopsin by light activation.

Mutations in RP2 and RPGR

Two genes associated with XLRP have been identified to date, RP2 and the retinitis pigmentosa GTPase regulator (*RPGR*) gene. In addition, chromosomal loci have been mapped for three other kinds of XLRP: and Xp21.3-21.2 (RP6), Xp22 (RP23), and Xq26-27 (RP24) (http://www.ncbi.nlm.nih.gov/omim). RP2 mutations account for 10% to 20% of XLRP in the Caucasian population. The RP2 protein is ubiquitously expressed and has functional dual acylation sites at its N-terminus and a region of homology to tubulin-specific cofactor C, a protein involved in the ultimate step of β-tubulin folding, suggesting that it may be involved in the structure or function of the cilium (207). Immunohistochemical analyses of human retina revealed that RP2 is localized to the plasma membranes of all retinal cell types (77). RP2 seems to play a role in arranging the interactions between the plasma membrane and cytoskeleton in photoreceptors as part of the cell signaling or vesicular transport machinery (77).

Mutations in the *RPGR* gene, which encodes several distinct alternatively spliced transcripts of the GTPase regulator causes RP type 3 (RP3). *RPGR* mutations account for 70% to 90% of XLRP and up to 15% to 20% of all RP cases (27). In addition, 29% of single affected males were found to have mutations in either in *RPGR* or the *RPGR-ORF15*, being the most common (27). Mutations in *RPGR* have been linked to various ocular manifestations other than XLRP, such as cone–rod and cone dystrophies, and recessive atrophic macular degeneration. Several non-ocular diseases have been associated inconsistently with *RPGR* mutations such as hearing loss, sinusitis and chronic recurrent respiratory tract and ear infections (99,100). Mutations have been found in all exons and in the alternatively spliced *RPGR-ORF15* isoform. In addition to the axoneme, the RPGR-ORF15 protein is localized to the basal bodies of the photoreceptor connecting cilium (153). Studies suggest that RPGR-ORF15 is involved in microtubule organization and in the regulation of transport in primary cilia (117). The N-terminal half of the protein shows homology to the regulator of chromosome condensation 1 (RCC1), which is a guanine nucleotide exchange factor for the small nuclear GTPase Ran, a GTPase involved in nucleocytoplasmic transport. This enzyme is essential for nucleo-cytoplasmic transport. These findings indicate that RPGR may also be an exchange factor for an unknown GTPase. All affected males have shown evidence of both rod and cone ERG loss consistent with the expression of RPGR in both rods and cones.

The large majority of RP2 and *RPGR* mutations result in truncated encoded proteins and lead to RP with an early age of onset and rapid disease progression. Patients with RP2 and *RPGR* mutations are generally considered to be more severely affected compared to many other types of RP (27,63). One study suggests that patients with RP2 mutations have a significantly lower visual acuity, on average, than do patients with *RPGR* mutations (211). However, the two groups were similar in terms of visual field area and 30-Hz ERG amplitude.

Usher Syndrome

General Remarks

Usher syndrome (USH) is the most frequent cause of combined hereditary deafness and blindness and is also the most common RP syndrome, constituting about 10% of RP patients.

Clinical Features

Based on the clinical features USH is classified into three types, USH1, USH2 and USH3 defined according to the severity and age at onset of the hearing loss, and the presence or absence of vestibular dysfunction (Table 4). These types are divided into further subtypes based on genetic heterogeneity. RP with variable age at onset occurs in all three USH types. USH1 accounts for approximately 30% to 40% of all cases in Caucasians (67), whereas USH2 is the most common form of USH and may account for 40% to 50% of USH2 cases.

USH is recessively inherited and genetically heterogeneous; eight genes and three loci have been identified to date (Table 5). The presence of USH1 proteins at the photoreceptor synaptic active zone strongly suggests that they contribute to the trafficking of synaptic vesicles (55). USH1 proteins are also localized within growing stereocilia and the kinocilium that make up the developing auditory hair bundle, a structure receptive to sound stimulation. Myosin VIIA (USH1B) is an intracellular motor molecule that moves along actin filaments using actin-activated ATPase activity. Cadherin 23 (USH1D) and protocadherin 15 (USH1F) are intracellular adhesion proteins. SANS (USH1G) is a scaffold-protein which controls the hair bundle cohesion and proper development by regulating the traffic of USH1 proteins en route to the stereocilia via its binding to

Table 4 Clinical Characteristics of Usher Syndrome Retinitis Pigmentosa (RP)

Clinical variables	Usher syndrome Type 1	Type 2	Type 3
Retina	RP	RP	RP
Hearing loss			
Onset	Birth	Birth	Late-onset
Severity	Moderate–profound	Mild–moderate	Mild–Moderate
Progressive	No	Rarely; Partial	Yes
Speech abnormality	Moderate–severe	Mild–moderate	Absent
Vestibular dysfunction	Present	Absent/minimal	Variable

myosin VIIa and/or harmonin (3). Harmonin (USH1C) is a scaffold protein that integrates all five USH1 proteins in a protein network via a specific domain (PDZ domain). Harmonin also has an essential central role in the supramolecular network of all known USH1 and USH2 molecules, providing the first molecular link between USH types 1 and 2 (200).

USH2A encodes usherin, a protein that has homology to the thrombospondin family of extracellular matrix proteins, laminin-type epidermal growth factor, and to fibronectin type III (20). These sequence similarities suggest that usherin may function as a cell adhesion molecule or an extracellular matrix protein (208). Usherin is expressed in the cochlea and the outer segments of the retina as well as in the basement membranes of several tissues. *V*ery *L*arge *G*-protein coupled *R*eceptor-*1* (VLGR1, also known as *M*onogenic *A*udiogenic *S*eizure Susceptibility 1 homolog, Mass1) is the largest known cell surface protein localized to the optic nerve and central nervous system. The extracellular portion of the VLGR1 protein contains repeated units resembling calcium-exchanger β motifs, which distinguish it from other G protein-coupled receptors. VLGR1 may also participate in cell adhesion and protein–protein interaction. There seems to be a female predominance with *VLGR1* mutations (246).

Usher type 3 is uncommon. It is the only known type of USH with a slow progressive hearing loss and RP. The causative gene (*USH3A*) encodes Clarin-1 which has been hypothesized to have a role in hair cell and photoreceptor cell synapses (4).

Congenital Stationary Night Blindness

General Remarks

Congenital stationary night blindness (CSNB) is a heterogeneous group of diseases defined by a congenital onset and a stationary course of night blindness. Retinal degeneration does not occur in CSNB. Forms of this condition differ in their inheritance pattern (autosomal dominant, autosomal recessive, or X linked). Most cases of CSNB occur in males, and these X-linked forms have been referred to as complete and incomplete CSNB (162). All cases of CSNB have characteristic findings on ERG with normal visual fields (consistent with myopia) and despite subnormal visual acuity, a relatively good visual prognosis.

CSNB also has been classified by fundus appearance; i.e., those cases with an abnormal and normal fundus, the latter of which can further be classified according to the ERG findings (34).

CSNB with Normal Fundus

CSNB with normal fundus have an absent scotopic ERG. The CSNB phenotype is caused by mutations in the *NYX*, *CACNA1F*, *RHO* (Gly90Asp, Thr94Ile, and Ala292Glu), *GNAT1*, and *PDE6B* genes. The most

Table 5 Genes and Proteins Associated with Usher Syndrome

Usher syndrome: genetic types	Gene	Protein	Chromosomal location
USH1A	Unknown	Unknown	14q32
USH1B	*MYO7A*	Myosin VIIa	11q13
USH1C	*USH1C*	Harmonin	11p15
USH1D	*CDH23*	Cadherin-23	10q22
USH1E	Unknown	Unknown	21q21
USH1F	*PCDH15*	Protocadherin-15	10q21
USH1G	*SANS*	Sans	17q24
USH2A	*USH2A*	Usherin	1q41
USH2B	Unknown	Unknown	3p24
USH2C	*VLGR1*	Very large G-protein coupled receptor 1	5q14
UH3A	*USH3A*	Clarin-1	3q21–25

Source: http://www.sph.uth.tmc.edu/Retnet/

common forms of CSNB by far occur in the X-linked inherited forms in males. Complete CSNB type 1 is characterized by high myopia, mild nystagmus; very poor to flat scotopic ERG; no scotopic threshold response; and recordable oscillatory potentials. The gene for the complete form, *NYX*, encodes a glycosylphosphatidyl-anchored protein called nyctalopin, which is a unique member of the small leucine-rich proteoglycan (SLRP) family (see Chapter 40). The role of other SLRP proteins suggests that mutant nyctalopin disrupts developing retinal interconnections involving the ON-bipolar cells (17).

The X-linked CSNB type 2 is associated with mild myopia. Affected individuals often have a cone–rod dysfunction pattern on ERG. There is a recordable scotopic threshold response and oscillatory potentials are almost nonrecordable. Both forms have negative waveforms in the dark-adapted, bright flash ERG, which consists of a well formed a-wave, and a b-wave that does not return to the isoelectric point. This unique electrophysiologic finding occurs in a limited number of retinal conditions and its presence aids in identification of these disorders (245).

CSNB type 2 is caused by *CACNA1F* mutations. It is thought that aberrations in a voltage-gated calcium channel decreases neurotransmitter release from photoreceptor presynaptic terminals thus presumably affecting both the on pathway and even more the off pathway of the bipolar cells (218).

CSNB with Abnormal Fundus

Oguchi disease is characterized by a mottled gray-white discoloration of the retina with a greenish metallic sheen, abnormally dark macula disappearing after dark adaptation (Mizuo-Nakamura phenomenon), a prolonged dark adaptation (4 hours) also resulting in improvement of rod thresholds to a normal level, normal cone responses, and abnormal rod responses on ERG. Mutations in either the *RHOK* or *SAG*, both of which play a role in deactivating rhodopsin, cause Oguchi disease, a recessive form of CSNB. Unlike the dominant CSNB mutations, these recessive mutations are null alleles leading to no gene products or to mutant proteins that are inactive (116).

Fundus albipunctatus is typified by yellow-white round flecks-dots scattered in a radial pattern from the fovea throughout the retina. Initially there is a poor scotopic ERG response that improves with prolonged dark adaptation. This disorder is caused by a mutation in the *RDH5* gene.

Fleck retina of Kandori has deep gray-yellow irregular subretinal deposits, delayed scotopic ERG responses and b-wave amplitudes that become normal with time.

Nine genes, all of which are cloned, have been linked to CSNB (Table 6). Five of these genes—*RHO*, *GNAT1*, *PDE6B*, *SAG*, and *RHOK*—normally encode proteins in the rod phototransduction cascade.

Similar to the disease mechanism of some of the *RHO* mutations seen in patients with RP, the *RHO* mutations associated with CSNB are thought to result in mutant rhodopsin molecules that can activate the phototransduction cascade even without exposure to light (196).

GNAT1 encodes rod transducin α-subunit that is essential for PDE activation. An in vitro study showed that the mutation alters the interaction of activated transducin with cGMP-PDE (168).

Mutations in the *RDH5* gene, encoding 11-*cis* RDH have been found in patients with a distinct form of CSNB called fundus albipunctatus; 11-*cis* RDH plays a role in the conversion of 11 *cis*-retinol to 11 *cis*-retinal in the RPE. The mutation compromises the 11-*cis* retinal production in the RPE which delays the photoreceptor recovery rate after bleaching. The relatively benign course of the disease may be explained by the fact that a loss of 11-*cis* RDH

Table 6 Genes and Proteins Involved in Congenital Stationary Night Blindness (CSNB)

Inheritance pattern	Chromosomal location	Protein
Autosomal dominant		
RHO (Specific mutations)	3q22.1	Rhodopsin[a]
GNAT1 (Nougaret type)	3p21.31	Rod transducin α subunit
PDE6B (CSNB3)	4p16.3	Rod cGMP phosphodiesterase β subunit
Autosomal recessive		
RHOK, GRK1 (Oguchi type)	13q34	Rhodopsin kinase
SAG (Oguchi type)	2q37.1	Arrestin (s-antigen)
GRM6	5q35.3	Metabotropic glutamate receptor 6
RDH5 (fundus albipunctatus)	12q13.2	11-*cis* retinol dehydrogenase 5
X-linked		
CACNA1F (CSNB2)	Xp11.23	L-type voltage-gated calcium channel α-1 subunit
NYX (CSNB1)	Xp11.4	Nyctalopin
RPGR	Xp11.4	Retinitis pigmentosa GTPase regulator

[a] Most rhodopsin mutations result in retinitis pigmentosa.
Source: http://www.sph.uth.tmc.edu/Retnet/

activity seems to compensated through other dehydrogenases in the RPE (41).

Recently, mutations in *GRM6* (metabotropic glutamate receptor 6) gene have been reported in patients with CSNB. This gene belongs to a G-protein-coupled receptor family (256). Mice lacking *Grm6* show defect in signal transmission from the photoreceptors to ON-bipolar cells with no obvious changes in the retinal organization at the cellular level (151,256). ERGs of patients with *GRMD* mutations show a markedly reduced ON response and a nearly normal OFF response to 6.25-Hz middle-wavelength sawtooth flickering light (51).

Leber Congenital Amaurosis

General Remarks

LCA is characterized by profound visual impairment at birth or within the first year of life.

Clinical Features

Infants present with nystagmus, sluggish pupillary responses to light and on testing extinguished ERGs. A second group reported later by Leber has been termed juvenile LCA, and is characterized by an onset at 2 to 5 years and generally has a severe course (65). Nevertheless, a considerable overlap between juvenile arRP and LCA exists both clinically and genetically (23). This overlap can be explained by different mutations in the same gene, some of which are more severe, leading to an earlier onset and a congenital or very early onset of the retinal degeneration. Less severe mutations result in the same genes in an onset at age 2 to 6 years. Other modifiers such as genetic and environmental factors are also thought to play roles. Most infants show a normal fundus appearance initially, which typically is very blond with diffuse atrophy. Clinical findings include subtle RPE granularity, hypoplastic or slightly swollen optic discs, wrinkling of the inner retinal membrane and a mild vascular attenuation. Pigment deposits usually develop later. So-called macular coloboma (staphylomatous areas of macular atrophy), "salt and pepper" retinopathy, retinitis punctata albescens and nummular pigmentation have been described in cases with LCA.

Eye-rubbing (oculodigital sign), high hyperopia and keratoconus are common associations. LCA can be divided into uncomplicated and complicated types (65). Uncomplicated LCA is described as congenital blindness, nystagmus, high hyperopia and extinguished ERG responses. Complicated LCA is similar to uncomplicated LCA, but an association with other ocular or systemic features such as neurologic abnormalities, mental retardation, deafness, renal anomalies, hepatic dysfunction and skeletal abnormalities exist. Specific syndromes that meet the criteria for complicated LCA include Zellweger syndrome (MIM #214100), Moore-Taylor syndrome, Senior-Loken syndrome (MIM #610189), and Mainzer–Saldino syndrome (MIM 266920). The clinical presentation of infantile neuronal ceroid lipofuscinosis (MIM #256730) is occasionally similar to LCA. Poor visual levels tend to remain stable in most patients, despite progressive retinal pigmentary changes (93).

Histopathology

Tissue studies of eyes obtained from a 16-month-old girl with LCA revealed subretinal deposits corresponding to the white spots and lines in the fundus deposits (163). Light and electron microscopic examination showed distinctive changes in the outer retinal layers and choroid, while the inner retinal layers were nearly normal. The early lesions of LCA are thought to be deposits of loose outer segments and apical processes of the RPE and macrophages.

Differential Diagnosis

The differential diagnosis of LCA includes juvenile RP, cortical blindness, CSNB, infantile phytanic acid storage disease (MIM #266510), early infantile neuronal ceroid lipofuscinosis (Batten diseases) (MIM #256730), and congenital rubella. Patients with juvenile RP often have good central vision sometimes into adulthood, in contrast to the age of onset of severe visual impairment in LCA which ranges from birth to the first year of life.

Genetics

LCA is a genetically heterogenous disease. Mutations in nine genes (*AIPL1, CRB1, CRX, GUCY2D, LRAT, RDH12, RPE65, RPGRIP1, TULP1*) and three loci (LCA3, LCA5, LCA9) have been associated with LCA (Table 7) (http://www.sph.uth.tmc.edu/Retnet/). The inheritance is autosomal recessive in all but *CRX* mutations, which may be inherited in the autosomal recessive or autosomal dominant fashion.

GUCY2D Mutations

The *GUCY2D* gene, expresses the protein retinal-specific guanylate cyclase in the outer segments of cones and to a lesser degree in rods. This enzyme is an essential component of the phototransduction cascade, and is particularly important in maintaining intracellular cGMP levels. Mutations in *GUCY2D* impair the recovery of the dark state after photo-excitation of photoreceptor cells probably by not maintaining sufficient cytosolic cGMP levels. This leads to a reduced opening of the cation channels, impairing the depolarization of the cell and therefore, retinal dysfunction (184). Carriers of *GUCY2D* mutations may have abnormal cone responses and normal rod responses, consistent with the predominant expression of the protein in cones (126). An 11-year-old subject with LCA

Table 7 Associated Gene Mutations with Leber Congenital Amaurosis (LCA)

Gene	Chromosomal location	Protein	Function
GUCY2D (*LCA1*, *CORD6*, *RETGC1*)	17p13.1	Retinal-specific guanylate cyclase (RETGC1)	Phototransduction cascade
RPE65 (*LCA2*, *RP20*)	1p31.2	Retinal pigment epithelium-specific 65 kDa protein	Visual cycle
LCA3	14q24	Unknown	Unknown
AIPL1 (*LCA4*)	17p13.2	Arylhydrocarbon-interacting receptor protein-like 1	Nuclear transport or chaperone activity
LCA5	6q14.1	Unknown	Unknown
RPGRIP1 (*LCA6*)	14q11.2	RPGR-interacting protein 1	Structural component of the ciliary axoneme, anchors RPGR within the cilium
TULP1 (*RP14*)	6p21.31	Tubby-like protein 1	Actin cytoskeletal functions
RDH12	14q24.1	Retinol dehydrogenase	Visual cycle
LCA9	1p36	Unknown	Unknown
LRAT	4q32.1	Lecithin retinol acyltransferase;	Visual cycle
CRB1 (*RP12*)	1q31–q32.1	Crumbs homolog 1	Cell–cell interactions and cell polarity
CRX (*CORD2*)	19q13.3	Cone–rod otx-like photoreceptor homeobox transcription factor	Transcription factor

Abbreviations: PPRPE, para-arteriolar preservation of the RPE; PPCRA, pigmented paravenous chorioretinal atrophy; dCORD, dominant cone–rod dystrophy.
Source: http://www.sph.uth.tmc.edu/Retnet/

caused by mutant *GUCY2D* who had only light perception retained substantial numbers of cones and rods in the macula and far periphery, suggesting the possibility that intervention by gene therapy might be possible in such cases with photoreceptor preservation (159).

RPE65 Mutations

RPE65 encodes a RPE-specific 65 kDa protein which is located in the smooth endoplasmic reticulum (ER) of the RPE and is necessary for the isomerization of all-*trans*-retinylester to 11-*cis*-retinol, and hence the regeneration of the chromatophore 11-*cis*-retinal (198). Mutations in the *RPE65* gene result in decreased visual pigment production. Histological material from a 33-week LCA retina with homozygous mutations in *RPE65* revealed an absence of detectable RPE65 staining and prenatal ocular degeneration. Cell loss and thinning of the outer nuclear photoreceptor layer was evident, the outer segments of the fetal rod photoreceptors were stunted and had decreased immunoreactivity for rhodopsin. Labeling of the cone outer segments with peanut agglutinin was sparse and punctuate (189). *RPE65* mutations have also been found in patients with arRP. Gene therapy has been successfully applied in mice and dogs with mutations in RPE65 (2,251).

AIPL1 Mutations

AIPL1 encodes arylhydrocarbon-interacting protein-like receptor, which is expressed in both developing cone and rod photoreceptors, but it is restricted to rod photoreceptors in the adult human retina. This protein shares sequence similarity with arylhydrocarbon receptor-interacting protein (AIP), a member of a family of peptidylprolyl isomerases that accelerate protein folding by catalyzing the *cis–trans* isomerization of proline imidic peptide bonds in oligopeptides. AIPL1 interacts with and modulates the nuclear translocation of NEDD8 ultimate buster-1, a protein that targets substrates implicated in the regulation of the cell cycle or cell growth for proteasomal degradation (6,233). AIPL1 is also thought to function as a potential chaperone for PDE, as PDE levels were decreased by a post-transcriptional mechanism in mouse models of LCA that both extinguished and reduced AIPL1 levels (139,195). There is a report of an LCA patient heterozygous for a putative *AIPL1* mutation (His82Tyr), who was diagnosed at age 5 months with no light perception and had both eyes enucleated at 22 years of age because of pain (92). In this patient, the retinal photoreceptors were described as being almost totally absent but with remnants of photoreceptor outer segments.

While recessive mutations of *GUCY2D* and *AIPL1* have been associated with LCA, dominant mutations in these genes have been found in patients with cone–rod dystrophy.

RPGRIP1 Mutations

RPGRIP1 encodes *R*etinitis *P*igmentosa *G*TPase *I*nteracting *P*rotein 1 (RPGRIP1), which interacts with the *RPGR* gene for X-linked RP. Both proteins co-localize to the photoreceptor connecting cilium and RPGRIP1 appears to be a structural component of the ciliary axoneme of the connecting cilium of both rods and cones and functions to anchor RPGR within the cilium (125,153). In addition, RPGRIP1 is uniquely expressed in amacrine cells of the inner retina. RPGRIP1 contains a C-terminal RPGR interacting domain and a coiled-coil domain, which is homologous to proteins involved in vesicular trafficking. Knockout mice studies have shown that RPGRIP1 is required for disc morphogenesis of the outer segments in the mouse, perhaps by regulating cytoskeleton dynamics (125).

TULP1 Mutations

TULP1 is a member of the *tubby* gene family, defined by its C-terminal half, which is highly conserved between the mouse *Tub* gene and the human ortholog *TUB*. *TULP1* is found exclusively in photoreceptor cells, localizing primarily in the inner segments and connecting cilium and to a lesser extent in the perinuclear cytoplasm and synaptic termini (250). TULP1 is a cytoplasmic protein that associates with cellular membranes and the cytoskeleton. TULP1 and actin appear to interact and colocalize in photoreceptor cells of the retina, suggesting that TULP1 may be involved in actin cytoskeletal functions such as protein trafficking that takes place at or near the plasma membrane from the inner segment through the connecting cilium into the outer segment of photoreceptor cells (250). *TULP1* mutations have also been associated with arRP.

RDH12 Mutations

RDH12 encodes RDH12 which is involved in the visual cycle and has unusual dual specificity for all-*trans*-retinols and *cis*-retinols. Retinoid dehydrogenases/reductases catalyze key oxidation–reduction reactions in the visual cycle that converts vitamin A to 11-*cis* retinal. RDH12 loss-of-function due to recessive mutations in the gene disrupts the cycle of synthesis of the visual pigment chromophore, 11-*cis* retinal, possibly due to decreased protein stability (225). While mutations in *RDH12* have been associated with LCA, mutations in another retinol dehydrogenase gene, *RDH5*, result in fundus albipunctatus, a much milder dystrophy associated with white dots and delayed dark adaptation.

LRAT Mutations

LRAT encodes LRAT, which is broadly expressed in tissues and at relatively high levels in the intestine, liver, and RPE, where it is involved in the conversion of all-*trans* retinol to all-*trans* retinyl esters. Cell culture studies showed that at least one of the mutations (Ser175Arg) results in lack of acyltransferase activity (226). However, the literature suggests the existence of an additional enzymatic activity within cells and tissues that is able to esterify retinol in an acyl-CoA-dependent manner (177). It was suggested that $[Lrat]^{-/-}$ mice are more susceptible to vitamin A deficiency (137), which may be important in patients with this gene mutation. Mutations of LRAT and RPE65 each block the visual cycle in different ways. With LRAT loss, no vitamin A accumulates in the RPE, obviating retinoid metabolism (15). However, with RPE65 loss, *all-trans*-retinyl ester accumulates to very high levels, but 11-*cis*-retinoids are not formed (199). *LRAT* mutations have also been associated with arRP.

CRB1 Mutations

CRB1 mutations have been found in patients with early onset arRP (RP12) (also known as, Preserved Pararteriolar Retinal Pigment Epithelial RP, or PPRPE RP) (86). Up to 30% of these patients may develop Coats disease in one eye, some of which may become proliferative (49). Coats disease has been noted in 10% to 13% of patients with LCA (http://www.sph.uth.tmc.edu/Retnet/). CRB1 is expressed in the retina and central nervous system and is homologous to *Drosophila* crumbs protein, crumbs homolog 1. CRB1 is involved in cell–cell interactions and cell polarity (49). Most reported *CRB1* mutations truncate the encoded protein; some may result in low levels of protein expression, and a few may disrupt protein folding (49). In contrast to other inherited retinal degenerations, retinas of patients with *CRB1* mutations are remarkably thick in cross-section and lack the distinct layers of normal adult retina, resembling those of immature normal retina (102). It has been suggested that the CRB1 disease pathway disturbs the development of normal human retinal organization by interrupting naturally occurring apoptosis. Animal studies suggest that patients with *CRB1* mutations may benefit from light that is reduced in amount and in intensity (108).

CRX Mutations

CRX is covered in detail above under RP.

Genotype–Phenotype Correlations

A study on genotype–phenotype correlation in LCA patients with mutations in the responsible genes (*AIPL1*, *CRB1*, *CRX*, *GUCY2D*, *RPE65*, and *RPGRIP1*) suggest that patients with *AIPL1* or *RPGRIP1* mutations develop severely decreased vision at a younger age (71). A wide range of visual acuities from 20/40 to no light perception was observed. The widest range of vision was noted for patients with *CRB1* or *RPE65* mutations. Drusen-like deposits were more selectively observed in patients with mutations in the *AIPL1*, *CRB1*, *RPE65*, and *RPGRIP1*, whereas focal regions of peripheral chorioretinal atrophy were observed only in patients with *AIPL1* or *RPE65* mutations.

Table 8 Genes Mutated in Various Inherited Cone Disorders

Disorder	Gene	Chromosomal location	Inheritance
Early onset			
Achromatopsia	*CNGA3*	2q11.2	AR
	CNGB3	8q21–q22	AR
	GNAT2	1p13.3	AR
Blue cone monochromatism	Mutations in red and green opsin genes *OPN1LW, OPN1MW*	Xq28	XR
Late onset			
Cone dystrophy	*GUCA1A* (*COD3*)	6p21.1	AD
	RDH5	12q13–q14	AR
	RPGR (*COD1*)	Xp11.4	XR
	COD2 (not cloned)	Xq27	XR
Cone–rod dystrophy	*AIPL1*	17p13.1	AD
	CRX	19q13.3	AD
	GUCY2D	17p13.1	AD
	RIMS1	6q12–q13	AD
	SEMA4A	1q22	AD
	UNC119	17q11.2	AD
	CORD4 (not cloned)	17q	AD
	ABCA4	1p22.1–p21	AR
	CORD8 (not cloned)	1q12–q24	AR
	CORD9 (not cloned)	8p11	AR
	RPGR (*CORDX*)	Xp11.4	XR
	CORDX2 (not cloned)	Xq27–28	XR
	CORDX3 (not cloned)	Xp11–q13	XR
	COD4 (not cloned)	Xp11–q13.1	XR

Abbreviations: AR, autosomal recessive; XR, X-linked recessive; AD, autosomal dominant.
Source: http://www.sph.uth.tmc.edu/Retnet/

Rod–Cone Interaction

Why and how do cones die in dystrophies where the mutant gene is expressed only in rods such as rhodopsin and PDE6B? Various models have been proposed; one involves a toxin, the other a trophic factor (35). The toxin model suggests that (*i*) the degenerating rods produce a toxin that kills cones, (*ii*) the collapse of the outer nuclear layer leads to physical pressure on the cone outer segments, (*iii*) oxygen levels cannot be reduced enough to keep oxidation products under control, and (*iv*) support cells are affected and make toxins. On the other hand, the trophic factor model suggests that rods and support cells release neurotrophic factors under physiological conditions, which would be impaired under pathological conditions (164).

A rod-derived cone viability factor has been cloned, which may enable cone survival in at least a subset of patients with retinal degeneration (133).

Cone Disorders

The cone dystrophies are diagnosed by standardized ERG testing. Patients typically present with bilateral visual acuity loss, variable color vision abnormalities dependent on the patients' foveal cone function, central scotomata, and variable photosensitivity. Congenital and juvenile onset forms often present with nystagmus. Cone dystrophies can be stationary or progressive. Achromatopsia and cone monochromatism are the major stationary forms, in which abnormalities present at or near birth, and rods remain normal. In contrast, the progressive cone dystrophies are not usually symptomatic until later childhood or early adult life and rods may be affected in the later stages of the disease (158). As in congenital LCA the severity of the mutation in juvenile LCA in a given gene may give variable onset, so congenital and juvenile cone dystrophies may occur in the same genes. Table 8 summarizes the genes involved in hereditary cone disorders.

Congenital Achromatopsia

Patients with congenital achromatopsia also called rod monochromatism, present with poor vision from birth, nystagmus, and variable amounts of color vision loss. Fundus examination initially is normal, but central or mid-peripheral RPE abnormalities such as granularity may be seen. Later, foveal atrophy is detected. Congenital achromatopsia can be classified into *complete* and *incomplete* forms according to cone function. In incomplete achromatopsia (atypical achromatopsia) cone responses can be detected on

ERG to some degree, resulting in mildly better visual acuity (20/80–20/200) and color vision compared to complete achromatopsia, which is characterized by a severe loss of cone function with visual acuity in the 20/200 range and poor color vision. Stable and subnormal rod function is detected on ERG. Care must be taken in using these classifications since some patients' disease will be evolve and photopic function may change over time.

Genetics

The inheritance of congenital achromatopsia is autosomal recessive and mutations in three genes (*CNGA3*, *CNGB3*, and *GNAT2*), all of which are involved in the cone phototransduction cascade, have been associated with congenital achromatopsia: *CNGA3* and *CNGB3* encode the α- and β-subunits of cone cyclic nucleotide-gated (CNG) channels, and *GNAT2* encodes the α-subunit of cone-specific transducin. CNG channels are involved in the entry of calcium into the photoreceptor outer segment. In the dark, cGMP levels are high in cone photoreceptors, therefore enabling cGMP to bind to the α- and β-subunits of CNG channels, resulting in an influx of cations, with consequent cone depolarization (157). However, in light conditions, activated photopigment initiates a cascade culminating in increased cGMP PDE activity, thereby lowering the concentration of cGMP in the photoreceptor which results in closure of CNG cation channels and consequent cone hyperpolarization (157). Mutations in the genes encoding the cone CNG channel subunits are particularly prevalent in achromatopsia; *CNGB3* (40–50%), *CNGA3* (20–30%) and less commonly in *GNAT2*. Both the complete and the incomplete forms of achromatopsia have been associated with *CNGA3* and *GNAT2* mutations, whereas *CNGB3* mutations have been found only in patients with complete achromatopsia.

Most *CNGA3* mutations identified to date are missense mutations (amino acid changing), indicating that there is little tolerance for substitutions with respect to functional and structural integrity of the channel polypeptide (157). *CNGA3* mutations result in loss of channel function, as determined by the failure of cGMP to activate wild-type currents in excised patches (180). Full-length mutant proteins are synthesized but retained in the ER.

In contrast, the majority of *CNGB3* alterations are nonsense (stop codon) mutations. At least some *CNGB3* mutations produce gain-of-function effects on channel gating (29). This may increase the number of open channels, thus increasing the intracellular calcium levels resulting in cone dysfunction or degeneration. A sustained elevation of intracellular calcium is suspected of being a crucial step for apoptosis in general (see Chapter 2) and has been linked specifically to rod photoreceptor degeneration via apoptosis.

GNAT2 mutations result in premature translation termination and truncation of the encoded protein at the carboxy terminus (157). *GNAT2* in cones is the counterpart of *GNAT1* in rods, which causes CSNB when mutated.

Cone Monochromatism

Cone monochromatism is a rare form of congenital color blindness, in which two of the three cone opsins are nearly or completely absent or nonfunctioning.

Blue Cone Monochromatism

Blue cone monochromatism (BCM) presents in a fashion similar to complete achromatopsia, except that there appears to be an intact S (blue) cone function with the absence of both L (red) and M (green) cone functions. The genes coding L and M pigment are located on the long arm of the X- chromosome (Xq28), whereas the S cone (blue) pigment is encoded by a gene located on chromosome 7. Therefore, BCM is X-linked recessive. Some mechanisms responsible for BCM are mutations in L and M pigment genes that result in a lack of functional pigments. The most frequent inactivating mutation disrupts the folding of cone opsin molecules. Another mechanism is a deletion in an upstream region that controls the transcriptional regulation of the L and M visual pigment genes (239). A third molecular genetic mechanism has been described in a single family where exon 4 of an isolated red pigment gene had been deleted (172).

Cone Dystrophy

Patients with cone dystrophy typically present with mild vision loss that progresses over time, which may have an onset in adulthood. An early color vision abnormality may present even before the visual acuity is compromised. This latter may distinguish cone dystrophy from Stargardt disease or other macular dystrophies. The age when visual loss begins and the rate of progression vary widely, but visual acuity usually deteriorates over time to 20/200 or worse. Early in the disease process, the fundus appearance in a cone dystrophy often appears normal; fovea centralis atrophy and a bull eye appearance (Fig. 9) typically develops with time and invariably will be present in later stages. Standardized ERG testing is central to establishing the diagnosis of cone dystrophy.

Cone dystrophy has different modes of inheritance (autosomal dominant, autosomal recessive, and X-linked recessive) and three genes (*GUCA1A*; *RDH5*; *RPGR*); and two more loci (*COD2* and *COD4*) have been identified.

Autosomal Dominant Cone Dystrophy

GUCA1A Mutations

The *GUCA1A* gene, which causes autosomal dominant cone dystrophy, encodes GCAP1, a Ca^{2+}-binding protein involved in the replenishment of cGMP in rods and cones. Activation of the phototransduction cascade leads to a reduction of Ca^{2+} concentration within rod and cone photoreceptors. As Ca^{2+} concentration falls, retinal guanylate cyclase-1 (RetGC1) is activated by the Ca^{2+}-sensitive GCAPs to regenerate cGMP (Fig. 1). Of the three isoforms of GCAP, the function of GCAP1 (GUCA1A) seems to be more important than GCAP2 (GUCA1B) and GCAP3 (GUCA1C). The main functional consequence of three dominant mutations (Tyr99Cys, Glu155Gly, and Ile143NT) has been shown to be a loss of Ca^{2+} sensitivity as a result of cGMP overproduction (176). Therefore, mutant GCAP1 protein activates RetGC1 (also known as GUCY2D) at low Ca^{2+} concentrations but fails to inactivate at high Ca^{2+} concentrations, thereby leading to the constitutive activation of RetGC1 in photoreceptors, even at the high Ca^{2+} concentrations of the dark-adapted state (247). The consequent dysregulation of intracellular Ca^{2+} and cGMP levels is believed to lead to cell death. However, it is currently not known why *GCAP1* mutations result in cone dystrophy, while *RetGC1* mutations result in cone–rod dystrophy, when both of these proteins are expressed in both rods and cones. One possible explanation may be the higher concentrations of RetGC1 and GCAP1 in cone photoreceptors.

Histopathology

A histopathologic examination of eyes from a 75-year-old man with autosomal dominant cone degeneration and a *GCAP1* mutation showed loss of both rods and cones in the fovea and an attenuated RPE (18). Reduced numbers of cones were observed in the parafovea, and only occasional cones were visible in the periphery, whereas rods were preserved in the periphery. Another histopathological study of donor eyes from an 85-year-old affected member of a well-characterized family with an autosomal dominant cone dystrophy, but without a known mutation revealed normal cone pedicles in the macula and peripheral retina (22). An abnormal distribution of cone red and green opsins was observed, and the blue cone opsin displayed restricted distribution to the cone outer segments compared to an age-matched control eye. Rhodopsin staining and the RPE appeared normal.

Autosomal Recessive Cone Dystrophy

Autosomal recessive cone dystrophy is caused by mutations in the *RDH5* gene in which mutations cause fundus albipunctatus in younger individuals which progresses to a cone dystrophy picture in cases older than 40 years of age. Clinically, the patients have stationary night blindness with subretinal spots and delayed dark adaptation. The RDH5 protein is an RPE microsomal enzyme involved in converting 11-*cis* retinol to 11-*cis* retinal; this causes delayed rod and cone resensitization, and is the same pathway involved in RDH12 (170).

X-Linked Recessive Cone Dystrophies

Mutations in the *RPGR* gene causes an X-linked recessive cone dystrophy. Other genes for X-linked recessive cone dystrophy have been mapped to chromosome X (Xq27) (COD2). Yang et al. (252) reported two families with X-linked cone dystrophy who mapped to the COD1 locus in the Xp11.4 region. They identified two distinct mutations in *ORF15* in the *RPGR* gene (ORF15+1343_1344delGG and ORF15+694_708del15). They noted that the phenotype in their patients was distinctly different from RP, the other disease associated with mutations in *ORF15* (252). A second X-linked cone dystrophy has been mapped to Xq27 but the gene has not been identified (19). Finally, there are patients with an adult onset X-linked cone dystrophy with tapetal sheen and the Mizuo-Nakamura effect in which no genetic information has been reported (91).

Cone–Rod Dystrophies

The term "cone–rod" dystrophy refers to inherited conditions that affect both the cones and rods, where the cones are proportionately more affected. Involvement of both types of photoreceptors is based on the ERG amplitudes of the rods and cones. This finding is in distinct contrast to RP patients who typically have rod–cone dysfunction. Numerous retinal diseases manifest cone–rod dysfunction patterns. The four main diagnostic categories which can show cone–rod dysfunction patterns are cone dystrophies (often called cone–rod dystrophy), cone–rod dystrophy (often with bull-eye or full macular lesions and full peripheral visual fields), RP with cone–rod dysfunction who have progressive visual field loss, and some patients with inflammatory diseases of the retina and choroid. Many patients with cone–rod dystrophy are relatively stationary in terms of peripheral visual field loss, although central scotomata may show progression. A review of RP cone–rod degeneration with comparison to cone–rod dystrophy was reported by Heckenlively and colleagues (86,88,127).

Retinitis Pigmentosa with Cone–Rod Dysfunction

Individuals with RP and cone–rod dysfunction patterns typically do not suffer from night blindness until they reach advanced stages of their disease. This category of RP, namely cone–rod RP degeneration has been found in all three Mendelian inheritance patterns. Affected individuals develop a progressive loss of visual field, ring scotomata tighter to fixation than patients with rod–cone RP, and in many cases the different isopters on the GVF are lined up to each other like an onion ring.

The fourth group patients with cone–rod dysfunction changes who need to be considered in the differential diagnosis are those with histories of chorioretinitis or inflammatory insults to their retina. They often have asymmetric findings between eyes, both on the ERG and visual field. Cone–rod ERG dysfunction patterns are common. Most of these patients have a more stable course, but the GVF over time will delineate the progressive cases.

It needs to be emphasized that the GVF will differentiate between RP cone–rod and cone–rod dystrophy. Static perimetry will seldom give the necessary information. The genes involved in cone–rod dystrophies are listed in Table 8.

Autosomal Dominant Cone–Rod Dystrophy

RIMS1 Mutations

A mutation in the *RIMS1* C_2A-domain has been implicated in autosomal dominant cone–rod dystrophy (CORD7). *RIMS1* encodes a rab3A-interacting molecule named synaptic membrane exocytosis protein 1, that is expressed at presynaptic zones in brain and photoreceptors, where neurotransmitters are released (109). The protein localizes to ribbon synapses and interacts with RAB3A, a protein that regulates synaptic vesicle exocytosis. RIM is specifically involved in the regulation of glutamate release at the ribbon synapse of photoreceptors. The location of the mutation site and the pattern of sequence conservation suggest that, in contrast to most C_2-domains, the RIM C_2A-domains may function through Ca^{2+}-independent interactions (47). *RIMS1* is localized in a region where it partially overlaps a locus for one variety of arRP (RP25).

UNC119 Mutations

A heterozygous mutation in another gene, *UNC119*, whose protein is also highly enriched in photoreceptor ribbon synapses and hologous to *Caenorhabditis elegans* neuroprotein, has been associated with late-onset cone–rod dystrophy. This mutation in *UNC119* leads to a premature termination codon associated with late-onset macular atrophy, with bilateral pericentral ring scotomatous visual fields (124). The ERG showed subnormal rod and cone responses with prolonged cone b-wave implicit times to 30.3-Hz flicker and single photopic flash with severe loss of oscillatory potentials. Transgenic mice carrying the identical mutation developed age-dependent fundus lesions accompanied by ERG changes consistent with defects in photoreceptor synaptic transmission such as a depressed b-wave and normal c-wave (124).

SEMA4A Mutations

Different mutations in the *SEMA4A* gene have been associated with adRP as well as cone–rod dystrophy (1). SEMA4A is a member of a large transmembrane protein family known as semaphorins that are involved in angiogenesis, organ development, and immune system functions. *Sema4A* is expressed in ganglion cells, inner retinal neurons, and RPE cells and functions as a transmembrane ligand for a receptor present on photoreceptors (201). Recently, the first human case of adRP and arRP with mutations in *SEM4A* were reported (1,201).

X-Linked Cone–Rod Dystrophy

RPGR-ORF15 Mutations

RPGR-ORF15, which has been associated with XLRP, has also been linked to X-linked cone–rod dystrophy. Cone–rod dystrophy patients with *RPGR-ORF15* mutations tend to have a later onset of visual loss compared to individuals with *CORDX2* and *CORDX3* mutations. In addition, a parafoveal ring of increased fundus autofluorescence was reported to be an early sign of this phenotype (54). As in XLRP, carriers of X-linked cone–rod dystrophy may manifest subtle fundus changes, color vision and ERG abnormalities (19). A histopathologic study of a 69-year-old man with X-linked cone–rod dystrophy caused by a mutation in the *RPGR-ORF15* gene disclosed an atrophic macula with a bull eye appearance, a focal absence of RPE in the macula, and pigmentary changes elsewhere in the retina (48). Cones and rods were absent at the perifovea and were reduced in number with shortened outer segments elsewhere in the macula. The remainder of the retina contained fewer cones than normal and all photoreceptor outer segments were shortened.

X-Linked Retinoschisis

General Remarks

Retinoschisis refers to splitting of the neurosensory retina. Congenital X-linked retinoschisis (XLRS or RS1) is a progressive, bilateral disease that is present at birth. It affects males exclusively and carrier females almost never exhibit fundus changes or visual symptoms.

Clinical Features

Spoke wheel-like linear cystoid structures that extend from the fovea are characteristic, and with rare exception this macular schisis pattern is uniform in XLRS males under the age of thirty. However, with age, macular degeneration occurs, which may obsure this diagnostic feature. Parafoveal cysts may be present and can coalesce and lead to retinal atrophy. Rarely, the schisis spares the macula, but the ERGs of these individuals still have diagnostic waveforms. Peripheral retinoschisis is very common, particularly inferotemporally (11). Other ophthalmoscopic findings include the areas of a golden-yellow sheen and lattice-like regional degeneration. The sheen may disappear when the patient is dark-adapted (Mizuo-Nakamura phenomenon). Other retinal changes include grayish-white dendriform structures, perivascular silver-gray cuffs, vitreous veils with or without retinal blood vessels. The initial discovery of retinoschisis is frequently in young males, who present with vitreous hemorrhage resulting from unsupported retinal vessels bridging a schisis cavity. The vitreous hemorrhage usually clears without intervention. Visual acuity is compromised variably, but the visual acuity loss progresses slowly in most patients. Visual field testing often discloses peripheral and midequatorial scotomas corresponding to areas of schisis and a relative central scotoma. A reduction in the upper nasal quadrant of the peripheral visual field is frequently encountered. Color vision is often impaired and dark adaptation may be mildly affected. Electroculography (EOG) is normal in young affected individuals and in patients with macular-only involvement. However, subnormal EOG responses may be detected in advanced cases. The loss of the ERG dark-adapted, bright flash b-wave amplitude, reflects the middle retinal layer damage, and with the typical macular schisis and X-linked inheritance pattern, confirms the diagnosis of X-linked retinoschisis. The ERG may become extinguished in advanced stages of the disease, and older patients can develop a pigmentary retinopathy similar to RP (86).

Optical coherence tomography (OCT) findings suggest that the primary abnormality of the fovea in juvenile retinoschisis starts in the outer plexiform layer of the retina, unlike the peripheral retina, where the schisis manifests in the nerve fiber layer, though clinical areas of retinoschisis are typically seen in the periphery (72). Studies of the retina by transmission electron microscopy (TEM) in XLRS has revealed numerous extracellular filaments within the retina and vitreous (44). These intraretinal filaments merged with the Müller cell plasma membrane and may represent an extrusion or degeneration of Müller cells which have been suspected of being primarily involved in the pathogenesis of XLRS. However, the identification of the responsible gene and the recognition of the function of its encoded protein as a putative extracellular binding protein have made this concept debatable.

RS1 Mutations

The *XLRS* gene (*RS1*), responsible for congenital X-linked retinoschisis, is located on the short arm of the X-chromosome (Xp22). It is expressed only in the retina and encodes for a retinal specific protein, retinoschisin. All major classes of adult retinal neurons, with the possible exception of horizontal cells, express retinoschisin and its mRNA (222). Retinoschisin is localized within rods and bipolar cell axons that run tightly parallel and immediately adjacent to Müller processes, but to date, have not been found within Müller cells or their processes (222). These findings suggest that Müller cell involvement is secondary.

The discoidin domain in retinoschisin is present in a wide range of membrane and extracellular proteins and it is thought to mediate a variety of cell adhesion and cell signaling processes (249). Retinoschisin is generally believed to function as a retinal cell adhesion protein as mice deficient in retinoschisin have a highly disorganized retina with displacement of bipolar cells into the outer retinal layer, gaps between bipolar cells within the inner retina, disruption of the photoreceptor-bipolar synapses, and progressive degeneration of rod and cone photoreceptors (249). In addition to its discoidin domain, retinoschisin contains a leader or signal sequence, which plays an essential role in the insertion of the nascent retinoschisin polypeptide chain into the membrane of the ER. It is subsequently cleaved in the lumen of the ER by a signal peptidase as a key step in the secretion of retinoschisin from cells. Most disease-linked missense mutations in *RS1* result in severe misfolding of the encoded protein and its retention in the ER (249). Mutations in the leader sequence prevent the insertion of retinoschisin into the ER membrane resulting in mislocalization of these mutant polypeptides in the cytoplasm and their rapid proteolytic degradation. Two disease-linked cysteine mutations (Cys59Ser and Cys223Arg) outside the discoidin domain cause a failure to assemble into a normal multisubunit complex suggesting that oligomerization is crucial for the functioning of retinoschisin as an extracellular adhesion protein (249).

The *Rs1* knock-out mouse mimics structural and electrophysiologic features of human X-linked juvenile retinoschisis. Gene therapy within the adult Rs1h-KO mouse restored a normal ERG configuration (257), which indicates that gene therapy is a viable strategy of therapeutic intervention in XLRS.

Enhanced S-Cone Syndrome

General Remarks

Enhanced S-cone syndrome (ESCS) (MIM #268100) is a rare retinal degenerative disease that was described based on specific ERG findings. The affected retinas have an overabundance of S-cone photoreceptors at birth, a reduced number of L- and M-cones, and few, if any, functional rod photoreceptors (240).

Clinical Features

ESCS manifests as night blindness at an early age, maculopathy that is often cystic, hyperopia, and annular pigmentary retinopathy in the vascular arcade to the midperipheral retina. Unlike typical RP, peripheral retinal vessels are generally not attenuated. Visual acuity ranges from 20/20 to 20/200. Color vision is mostly unaffected. Despite the early onset, the progression is usually slow.

Goldmann–Favre Disease

General Remarks

Goldmann–Favre syndrome is a rare inherited vitreoretinal dystrophy that has similar manifestations to ESCS such as night blindness, hyperopia, macular changes, pigmentary chorioretinal degeneration, and abnormal ERG but differs by having degenerative vitreous with strands, and peripheral and central retinoschisis. In advanced cases, both rod and cone ERGs are markedly diminished and may be non-detectable. When detectable, full-field ERG findings are similar to those in ESCS (104).

Clinical Features

ESCS, Goldmann–Favre disease, and arRP with clumped pigmentation share several phenotypic and genotypic similarities and hence may be different clinical manifestations of the same genetic disorder. All have an autosomal recessive mode of inheritance, and some share mutations in the retinal nuclear receptor subfamily 2 group E3 (*NR2E3*) gene on chromosome 15 (15q24) (210).

NR2E3 Mutations

NR2E3 gene (formerly called photoreceptor-specific nuclear receptor or *PNR*) is a member of the family of ligand-activated nuclear receptor transcription factors. Its encoded protein (NR2E3) is expressed exclusively in rod photoreceptors. Figure 8 depicts NR2E3 function in concert with the neural retina leucine zipper (*NRL*) and cone–rod homeobox containing (*CRX*) genes. NR2E3 activates the expression of rod genes by CRX interaction, in cells that have already been directed toward a rod photoreceptor fate rather than preventing cone generation (33). Several mutations in *NR2E3* have been identified in ESCS.

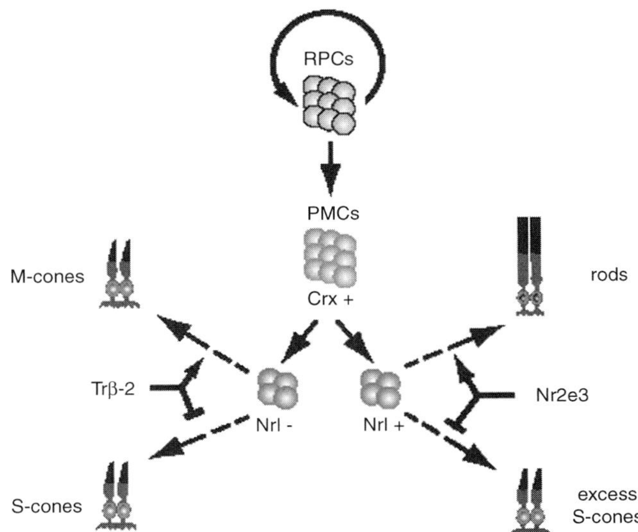

Figure 8 Transcription factors controlling photoreceptor development. At specific times during development, pools of retinal progenitor cells (RPCs) undergo terminal mitosis. The postmitotic cells (PMCs) that express the homeodomain transcription factor Crx are committed to become photoreceptors. PMCs that do not express the basic motif-leucine zipper transcription factor Nrl may produce M-cones if the thyroid hormone receptor-β (Trβ2) is expressed. Crx+, Nrl-, and Trβ2- cells will generate S-cones. The expression of Nrl in Crx+ PMCs induces rod photoreceptor differentiation. Nr2e3, an orphan nuclear receptor that is regulated by Nrl, is needed to produce normal rods. *Source*: Modified from Ref. 156.

Some of them do not normally interact with *CRX* and/or in a transcriptional regulatory function (183). There is a time gap between the birth of rods and rod opsin expression. The nuclear localization of NR2E3 and NRL in rod opsin-negative cells whose nuclei lie in the inner outer nuclear layer at the level of mature rods suggests that these transcription factors are expressed at a time when rods still have some plasticity or competence to acquire a different photoreceptor cell fate (36,134,140). During this period, NR2E3 and NRL guide the postmitotic precursor cells toward a rod fate and away from an S-cone fate.

Full-field ERG is the key test for diagnosis and shows no response to dim light in the dark-adapted state, but a hyperabnormal, slow response to bright light that persists with light adaptation (95). Using high intensity flashes and a cone photoreceptor activation model, it has been shown that the hyperabnormal a-waves are driven almost entirely by S-cones (95). Under standardized ERG conditions the findings in ESCS are: (*i*) a severely reduced or non-detectable rod response to scotopic dim flash, (*ii*) a subnormal slow a-wave and a much reduced slow b-wave for both the scotopic bright-flash response and for the photopic flash cone response, (*iii*) reduced oscillatory potentials, and (*iv*) reduced photopic flicker responses. These ERG findings are not unique to ESCS as they can also be seen in Goldmann–Favre syndrome.

The assumption that there are more S-cones in the retina in ESCS than in normal individuals based on ERG findings was confirmed in a retina from a 77-year-old patient with mutations in *NR2E3*. This eye had no detectable rods and a twofold increase in the number of cones, 92% of which were S-cones (160). The number of long- and medium-wavelength (L/M) cones was reduced as well, and some ESCS cones expressed both S and L/M opsin.

Stargardt Disease and Fundus Flavimaculatus

General Remarks

It is widely accepted that Stargardt disease (STGD) and fundus flavimaculatus (FFM) are different clinical manifestations of the same genetic disease. STGD originally was reported as a juvenile onset macular degeneration in which severe vision loss occurs, whereas FFM was one of the fleck retina disorders with scattered pisciform yellow lesions scattered throughout the posterior pole. In more advanced cases there were more severe deposits in the macula with subsequent atrophy. There is great variability from case to case with both FFM and STGD.

Clinical Features

STGD is a bilateral, progressive maculopathy presenting commonly with decreased central visual acuity. The majority of STGD patients have acuities between 20/40 and 20/200. The condition is characterized by a granularity and atrophy of the outer macula, flattening of the foveal reflex. The RPE changes commonly produce a bull eye maculopathy or a beaten bronze appearance. Adjacent soft yellow-white subretinal flecks, due to focal collections of swollen RPE with intracellular lipofuscin are often seen. The macula progressively atrophies and in some cases may resemble central areolar choroidal atrophy with extensive and well demarcated atrophy. Pigment clumps and local atrophic areas may also be observed in the peripheral retina. Central and paracentral scotomas are common; however, despite the widespread accumulation of lipofuscin in the RPE, peripheral vision is preserved in most patients.

The full-field ERG documents dysfunction of both rods and cones usually with a cone–rod pattern, but can be variable, and are not diagnostic for the disease. Initially doing an ERG and GVF are important to differentiate early cases of RP or cone dystrophy that occasionally resemble STGD clinically. Focal and multifocal ERG is almost always reduced (74,143) and the pattern ERG, a measure of ganglion cell activity, is severely reduced in almost all individuals with STGD regardless of visual acuity (143). Neither test is diagnostic for the condition.

Fluorescein angiography (FA) is extremely valuable in establishing a clinical diagnosis of STGD/FFM. The silent or dark choroids on FA, representing a diffuse blockage of choroidal fluorescence through the pigment epithelium due to accumulated intracellular RPE lipofuscin, is the hallmark of the disease (53). FA is also useful in detecting a subtle maculopathy. Lipofuscin accumulation can also be detected by fundus autofluorescence (40). Ultrahigh-resolution OCT has been used to document the photoreceptors in patients with STGD and central atrophy has been found to be consistent with a complete loss of the central photoreceptor layer (56). The major histopathologic abnormality in STGD is extensive intracellular accumulation of lipofuscin or lipofuscin-like material within the RPE.

STGD can be diagnosed on the clinical findings together with the dark choroid effect on FA, but a precise molecular genetic diagnosis can be obtained by finding a mutation in the *ABCA4* or *ELOVL4* genes.

Genetics

STGD has been mapped to three loci and mutations in two genes have been identified. All autosomal recessive inherited cases have been linked to the *ABCA4* gene (STGD1) on chromosome 1 (1p22). The phenotype due to autosomal dominant inheritance referred to as Stargardt-like macular dystrophy is associated with mutations in the *ELOVL4* gene (STGD3) on chromosome 6 (6q14). In autosomal dominant STGD associated with *ELOVL4* mutations, the ELOVL4 protein is predominantly expressed in ganglion cells of embryonic and postnatal retina (258).

ABCA4 Mutations

ABCA4 is a member of the ATP-binding cassette (ABC) transporter gene superfamily that encodes membrane proteins involved in the translocation of substrates across membranes. It is a complex gene composed of 50 exons spanning an area of approximately 150 kb, which complicates mutational analysis. The protein, ABCR, is also called the rim protein since it is exclusively expressed in the rims of the rod and cone outer segment discs (165). All-*trans* retinal formed as a result of rhodopsin activation by light is released to the intradiscal space, where it reacts with phosphatidylethanolamine to form *N*-retinylidine-phosphatidylethanolamine. ABCR moves this phospholipid complex out of the disc membrane into the cytoplasm. This function of moving a phospholipid from one leaflet of a lipid bilayer to another leaflet is called "flippase" (21). In mutant *Abca4* mice, *N*-retinylidine-phosphatidylethanolamine accumulates in the photoreceptor outer segments. When the shed outer segments are ingested by the RPE, the *N*-retinylidine-phosphatidylethanolamine is converted into a toxic detergent-like molecule, vitamin A-based fluorophore (A2E), within the lysosomes of the RPE. In the presence of oxygen, A2E is oxidized, producing epoxides, which are even more toxic. The accumulation of A2E contributes to lipofuscin formation in the RPE and once formed, A2E cannot be eliminated (152). It is noteworthy that a mutation in a gene that is expressed in photoreceptors yields to apoptosis in the RPE via photooxidative damage (214), leading to subsequent photoreceptor death. The accumulation of the toxic A2E in the RPE ultimately depends on the level of all-*trans* retinal that is formed by the isomerisation of 11-*cis* retinal following light exposure. There is evidence showing that light-deprivation reduces the retinal degeneration in autosomal recessive STGD (152), and, therefore, these patients should avoid excessive light exposure.

Specific *ABCA4* mutations detrimental to protein function, such as deletions, nonsense mutations and insertions, have been found almost exclusively in persons with the severe clinical phenotype of STGD (212). Extreme allelic heterogeneity exists within the *ABCA4* gene when compared to other genetic diseases. Aside from disease producing mutations a large number of non-disease causing single nucleotide polymorphisms (SNPs) have been identified in almost every exon. In addition, many affected individuals with *ABCA4* mutations carry at least two variants of the gene on the same or different alleles (241). It is noteworthy that mutations in *ABCA4* have also been associated not only with STGD, but also with CORD and RP, and that rarely persons within the same family can manifest these different phenotypes (123).

ELOVL4 Mutations

Autosomal dominant STGD has been found to be associated with mutations in *ELOVL4* (elongation of very long chain fatty acids-like 4), a photoreceptor-specific gene, which encodes a protein predominantly localized to the ER, the site of very long chain fatty acid biosynthesis. ELOVL4 is likely to play a central role in the biosynthesis of lipid components within the photoreceptor outer segment membrane, particularly, docosahexaenoic acid from dietary linolenic acid (215). ELOVL4 also seems to contribute to the retention of transmembrane proteins in the ER through its dilysine motif at the C-terminus. Mutations in *ELOVL4* result in premature termination of protein translation and loss of the ER retention signal. When the mutant ELOVL4 protein cannot localize to the ER, it is misrouted into the perinuclear region (9) and alters the trafficking of the wild-type protein by direct physical interactions (234). The mutant ELOVL4 forms higher molecular mass complexes with the wild-type protein that accumulate in aggresomes. It is likely that a residual amount of wild-type ELOVL4 protein escapes the interaction with mutant ELOVL4, which may be sufficient for the normal development and maintenance of retina in early stages of life (234). However, there seems to be a greater demand for ELOVL4 later in life as shown in normal adult mice which may explain the late-onset in some patients. Studies indicate that pathogenic ELOVL4 mutants exert a dominant negative effect on wild type ELOVL4, and this mechanism is responsible for the autosomal dominant inheritance pattern of Stargardt-like macular dystrophy (78). The loss in ELOVL4 may also adversely affect the activity of ABCA4 in disc membranes and thereby leading to the production of A2E-containing lipofuscin deposits in the RPE (78). This may explain the phenotype similarity of patients with mutations in the *ELOVL4* and *ABCA4*.

Best Disease

General Remarks

Best disease (juvenile-onset vitelliform macular dystrophy) (MIM #153700) is an early-onset macular dystrophy characterized by large deposits of lipofuscin-like material in the subretinal space. It is an autosomal dominantly inherited disorder with variable expressivity.

Clinical Features

The maculopathy is usually bilateral and asymmetric and the fundus appearance is variable, depending on the stage of the disorder. The earliest visible lesion, called previtelliform stage, appears to be a yellow subfoveal pigment. The characteristic vitelliform (resembling an egg yolk) lesion is a yellow-orange, round or oval subretinal deposit, which may be single or multiple and 0.5 to 3.0 optic disc diameters in size, frequently in the macular region (Fig. 9). The accumulated material may disintegrate, becoming deeply and irregularly pigmented to give a scrambled-egg appearance. The subretinal material may settle creating a layer, resembling a hypopyon, which is called a pseudohypopyon stage. Subretinal fluid and neurosensory detachment may also be evident. As the disease progresses from the "scrambled egg" stage, the macular RPE shows atrophic changes and clumps of variable size pigment, but surprisingly good vision is maintained unless choroidal neovascularization (CNV) with a disciform scar occurs. The risk of CNV appears to be about 20% for one eye during the course of the disease. The abnormal fundus findings usually first become evident within the first decade, but it can be highly variable. The visual field may show subtle central

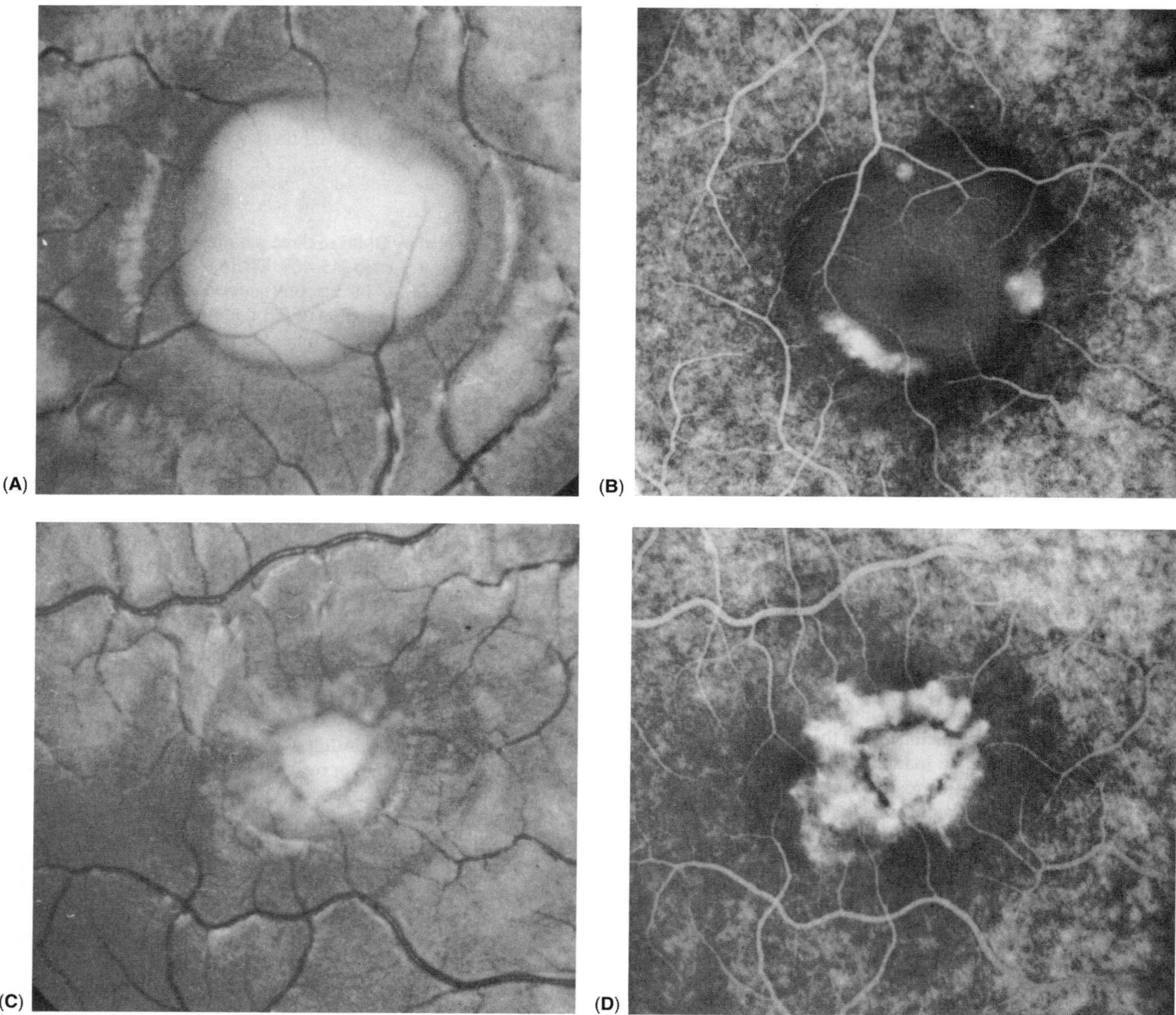

Figure 9 Best disease. A well-defined submacular deposit of yellow material (**A**) with invasion of the material with new blood vessels (**B**). The other eye of the same patient has subretinal fibrosis in which there was vascular tissue (**C, D**) (Courtesy of Professors Alan C. Bird and John Marshall).

sensitivity losses. Pattern, macular and multifocal ERG studies showed that the inner neurosensory retina in the foveal area may be affected in spite of normal visual acuity (105). Color vision can be affected. Aside from Best disease, several other retinal diseases may present clinically with a vitelliform lesion in the fundus, e.g., accumulated subretinal hemorrhage that liquefies, exudates from choroidal vascular lesions, and adult vitelliform dystrophy. However, an abnormal EOG (Arden ratio < 1.3) and a normal to supranormal full-field ERG are characteristics of Best disease and help distinguish it from other vitelliform diseases. Molecular diagnosis for mutations in the *VMD2* gene will help to distinguish Best macular dystrophy cases.

The EOG is abnormal even in the asymptomatic carriers of the disease, which indicates a widespread dysfunction of the photoreceptor–RPE complex. Nevertheless, in some cases of RPE-based diseases such as pattern dystrophies and STGD, a combination of a normal ERG but a mildly abnormal EOG may be seen. A few patients do not develop any macular lesions, but will have an abnormal EOG and the gene mutation.

Histopathology

Histopathologic studies demonstrated severe photoreceptor degeneration at the macula of an 80-year-old patient with Best disease who had bilateral macular scarring (66). In a 28-year-old patient with Best disease who had bilateral scrambled egg lesion with some features of pseudohypopyon in the macula, the ganglion cell layer and inner and outer plexiform layers of the central retina were edematous, and the outer segments showed focal atrophy (242). There was aberrant accumulation of lipofuscin-like material in and under the flattened and enlarged RPE, prominently in the macula (242). Bruch membrane changes such as disruption or thickening were also observed along with CNV. The subretinal and sub-RPE accumulation was also documented on OCT (186). Most best disease patients maintain fairly good central vision if CNV does not occur.

VMD2 Mutations

Best disease has been associated with mutations in the *VMD2* gene localized at 11q13, which encodes the transmembrane protein bestrophin (185). Bestrophin is predominantly localized to the basolateral plasma membrane of RPE (148), and functions as a Ca^{2+}-sensitive Cl^- channel (193). The disease-causing mutations result in loss of Cl^- channel function, with a dominant negative effect. Mutations have also been shown to alter the L-type Ca^+ channel activity in RPE (202). The light peak has been thought to be generated by depolarization of the RPE basolateral plasma membrane due to activation of Cl^- conductance possibly via a Ca^{2+}-sensitive Cl^- channel (70); however, it was recently suggested that either the rate-limiting step for generating light peak amplitude occurs before activation of bestrophin or bestrophin does not directly generate the light peak conductance (148). On the other hand, mistargeting of the mutant bestrophin may also play a role in the pathogenesis (167).

Doyne Honeycomb Retinal Dystrophy

General Remarks

Doyne honeycomb retinal dystrophy (DHRD) (MIM #126600), familial drusen and Malattia levantinese were considered separate entities until 1999 when a single missense mutation in the *EFEMP1* (epidermal growth factor-containing fibrillin-like extracellular matrix protein 1) gene was found in these conditions (217). It is a rare autosomal dominant macular degenerative disease with high penetrance that is asymptomatic in the early stages.

Clinical Features

Onset of DHRD is generally in midlife but it can vary from childhood to old age. Drusen in the macula and the peripapillary area is the hallmark of DHRD, and is usually found in routine ophthalmic examination. Over time, drusen increase in number and size and coalesce to form a plaque at the level of Bruch membrane, along with the atrophic changes at which stage patients complain of symptoms such as decreased visual acuity, metamorphopsia and a scotoma. Pigment clumps, CNV, and subretinal hemorrhage may occur. Occasionally, drusen resolve when the atrophic changes settle. Full-field ERG is usually normal; however, EOG is commonly abnormal. The manifestations are similar to those of drusen seen in age-related macular degeneration (AMD) (see Chapter 18), but the age of onset is much younger.

EFEMP1 Mutations

The *EFEMP1* (fibulin-3) is a member of fibulin gene family and is broadly expressed in extracellular matrix, secreted from RPE. The function of this protein is still unknown. The Arg345Trp mutation has been found in all affected individuals to date, and it causes the protein to be misfolded, inefficiently secreted, and retained within the RPE pattern. Macular and multifocal ERG studies have shown that the inner neurosensory retina in the foveal area may be affected in spite of normal visual acuity (105). This may occur between the RPE and drusen, in addition to being in the nerve fiber layer and interphotoreceptor matrix, but not within drusen (150). An accumulation of misfolded proteins within the ER activates a signaling pathway termed the unfolded protein response. This pathway, which is conserved from yeast to mammals, leads to the activation of stress-responsive gene expression resulting in increased ER protein processing capacity, an increased ability to degrade aggregated proteins, and increased expression of vascular endothelial growth factor (VEGF), an angiogenic chemokine (83). Thus, ER stress may contribute to the retinal dysfunction, and the increased expression of VEGF and subsequent development of CNV (203). The vast majority of the patients with the *EFEMP1* mutation are heterozygous (217). Another suggested mechanism is that the aggregation of the mutated protein from one allele may also cause misfolding of the protein from the unaffected allele, thus causing aberrant extracellular matrix (ECM) deposition (150). Therefore, the mutant protein does not appear to be a major component of drusen but rather seems to contribute to the disease pathogenesis.

Sorsby Fundus Dystrophy

General Remarks

Sorsby fundus dystrophy (SFD) (MIM #136900) is a rare autosomal dominant disorder typically leading to loss of central vision between the third and fifth decades. In the early stages of the disease there is an abnormal accumulation of confluent, widespread, drusen-like material at the level of Bruch membrane along with Bruch membrane thickening, which is believed to impair the metabolic activity of the choriocapillaris and RPE.

Clinical Features

Patients often present with choroidal neovascular membranes that give rise to a hemorrhagic and exudative maculopathy. Atrophy of the RPE/choriocapillaris complex to bare sclera may be the predominant finding in some cases. The disease manifestations show considerable interfamilial, intrafamilial and even variations between individuals. The disease begins in the posterior pole and progresses into the periphery of the retina, leaving the patients with very poor visual acuity. Full-field ERG studies reveal depressed scotopic responses, indicating a defect in the rod photoreceptor system. EOG may also be affected and show decreased EOG light to dark ratios. A TEM study from SFD eyes showed that the elastic layer of Bruch membrane was irregular, thickened, and fragmented in many areas (38).

TIMP3 Mutations

Mutations in the *TIMP3* (tissue inhibitor of metalloproteinases) gene, located on chromosome 22 (22q13), have been associated with SFD (58,240). The encoded protein, TIMP3, localizes to Bruch membrane (236), and was found to be increased in large subretinal deposits in the eye of one patient with SFD (58). TIMPs regulate the ECM composition in equilibrium with matrix metalloproteinases (MMPs), therefore affecting a wide range of physiological processes such as cell growth and migration, angiogenesis, and apoptosis (28). The RPE actively synthesizes and degrades ECM molecules. RPE also synthesizes and secretes MMPs as well as TIMPs at their apical domain. TIMPs have two major domains: N-terminal domain which has been shown to be sufficient for matrix metalloproteinase inhibition and a C-terminal domain responsible for the adhesion of TIMP3 to ECM. TIMP3 is distinguished from other members of the TIMP family by its ability to bind to the ECM. Almost all mutations associated with SFD have been identified in the C-terminus of the protein, leading to the formation of unpaired cysteine residues, which may lead to erroneous disulfide bond formation and abnormal tertiary protein structure (128). A specific mutation of this gene has been investigated in cell culture and showed to retain its function of MMP inhibition. Therefore, the accumulation of the mutant protein and altered cell adhesion is the proposed mechanism in SDF rather than loss of function such as the MMPs inhibition (128,253). The mutant protein forms abnormal complexes (probably dimers), which may not be degraded as rapidly as the normal TIMP3, and may therefore accumulate in Bruch membrane impairing the nutrition and metabolism of the outer retina. This finding was confirmed in a study which showed improvement in visual function tests after high-dose vitamin A in patients with SFD, while reduction in vitamin A dosage reversed the condition (103,104). In addition to its MMP activity, TIMP3 inhibits VEGF-mediated angiogenesis, by blocking the binding of VEGF to vascular endothelial growth factor receptor 2 (VEGFR2) and therefore inhibiting downstream signaling and angiogenesis. This unique function of TIMP3 is independent of its MMP-inhibitory activity (191). Mutant TIMP3 may not exhibit anti-angiogenic properties or the RPE atrophy may lead to a decrease in TIMP3 expression, which would allow VEGF to bind its receptors and therefore, promote CNV (223). The altered structure of Bruch membrane may contribute to this process. It was shown that the overexpression of TIMP3 successfully inhibited the experimental CNV (233). TIMP3 was shown to express apoptotic properties when overexpressed in vitro (14), and an alternative mechanism, particularly in patients with an atrophic maculopathy, could be apoptosis of photoreceptor and RPE induced by an accumulation of dimerized TIMP3. Although no other retinal disease has been found to be associated with heritable mutations in TIMP3 (61), abnormal expression of TIMP3 in Bruch membrane was also observed in eyes with AMD and RP (58,111).

Bietti Crystalline Dystrophy

General Remarks

Bietti crystalline dystrophy (BCD) (MIM #21370) is an autosomal recessive dystrophy characterized by glistening intraretinal dots scattered over the ocular fundus, and corneal crystals. Later RPE atrophy, pigment clumps, and sclerosis of the choroidal blood vessels. In more advanced cases, the crystals often appear at the edges of scalloped retinal lesions. These crystals may also be seen at the corneoscleral limbus about 50% of the time.

Clinical Features

Most patients develop decreased vision, nyctalopia, and central/paracentral scotoma between the second and fourth decades of life. BCD is a progressive disease with patients developing a peripheral visual field loss and marked visual impairment by the fifth or sixth decades of life. It is a rare disease in the West but a relatively common one in Far East (107). ERG findings are markedly variable, even in patients with similar ophthalmoscopic, fluorescein angiographic, and visual field findings. FA discloses a characteristic scalloped loss of RPE in the posterior pole. Unlike RP, retinal vessels appear normal, suggesting that the retinal degeneration occurs secondary to RPE and choricapillaris atrophy.

Histopathology

Histopathologic studies of patients with BCD have disclosed crystals and complex lipid inclusions in fibroblasts of the choroid, cornea, conjunctiva and skin, and in circulating lymphocytes along with advanced panchorioretinal atrophy supporting the biochemical data (113).

CYP4V2 Mutations

The *CYP4V2* gene on chromosome 4q35 has been linked to BCD (107). It is a member of the cytochrome P450 gene and is ubiquitously expressed in the retina, RPE and elsewhere (135). This gene is thought to play a role in fatty acid and corticosteroid metabolism. Biochemical studies show that abnormal lipid metabolism is present in patients with BCD, with a lower than normal conversion of fatty acid precursors into n-3 polyunsaturated fatty acids (131), and two fatty acid-binding proteins are absent or nonfunctional (130). In addition, cells cultured from patients with BCD have abnormally high levels of triglycerides and cholesterol storage.

Choroideremia

General Remarks

Choroideremia (CHM) (MIM #303100) is an X-linked retinal disorder that leads to a diffuse, progressive degeneration of RPE, choriocapillaris and photoreceptors.

Clinical Features

As in RP patients with choroideremia generally present in their first or second decades with night blindness and peripheral vision loss. Equatorial photoreceptors, primarily the rods, are affected earliest and most severely. As the disease progresses, the degeneration involves the anterior retina and posterior pole. The macular area is more resistant to the disease process and central vision is usually preserved until late in the course. Even in the presence of mild ophthalmoscopic changes, there is already a significant visual dysfunction that can be documented with ERG. When recordable, the ERG indicates a rod–cone degeneration. The EOG is abnormal, and the dark adaptation test discloses elevated rod thresholds.

Occasionally female carriers become symptomatic and most have subretinal pigment clumping and a granular appearance of the RPE. With age, many carriers develop focal areas of retinal atrophy. Visual field, ERG and dark adaptation tests are usually normal in choroideremia carriers. The mechanism by which the carriers are affected is explained by the Lyon hypothesis (see Chapter 31) (145). The intracellular distribution of proteins, compartments, substrates and products is an active process called intracellular trafficking. The intracellular trafficking is controlled by GTP-binding proteins, called Rab proteins. Rab proteins need to bind to geranylgerany groups to be activated. However, this activation requires a presenting protein called Rab escort protein (REP-1), which presents Rab to Rab geranylgeranyl transferase (10). The gene responsible for choroideremia (*REP-1*), on Xq21, encodes the widely expressed REP-1 protein. Almost all mutations in the *REP-1* result in a truncation or absence of the protein. Uncommonly some mutations cause a defect in protein folding. Showing the absence of REP-1 protein in leukocytes serves as a practical diagnostic test for choroideremia (146), but mutation analysis gives the definitive diagnosis. Mutations in *REP-1* are not lethal and result in choroideremia because a related gene product, REP-2, serves the needs of all tissues except those of the eye (209). The mutation intervenes with the prenylation of Rab proteins, resulting in unprenylated Rab protein accumulation, particularly Rab27A. Although Rab27A can be prenylated by REP-2, this reaction can be effectively inhibited by other Rab proteins (194). The accumulation of unprenylated Rab27A may contribute to retinal degeneration by impairing photoreceptor opsin transport, RPE phagocytosis, lysosomal degradation or melanin granule transport (8).

Histopathology

A histopathologic examination of the eyes of an 88-year-old symptomatic female carrier of CHM suggests the rod photoreceptors or RPE as the initial sites of pathologic abnormalities (221). The choriocapillaris was normal except where the retina had degenerated severely. REP1 was localized in the cytoplasm of rods but not cones. The CHM carrier retina showed patchy degeneration, but the photoreceptor and RPE loss appeared to be independent (64).

Gyrate Atrophy

General Remarks

Gyrate atrophy (GA) (MIM +258870) is a rare autosomal recessive disease characterized by a scalloped chorioretinal degeneration. The disease is associated with hyperornithinemia due to ornithine-delta-aminotransferase (OAT) deficiency.

Clinical Features

Patients generally present within the first decade of life with night blindness, high myopia and astigmatism. Lesions of the ocular fundus start in the midperiphery as circular, well-circumscribed areas of atrophy while the RPE is generally hyperpigmented. These isolated areas coalesce to form larger areas that are scalloped in appearance, and that spread anteriorly and posteriorly in a gyrate pattern, eventually affecting the macula. Visual loss starts as a progressive constriction of peripheral vision by the second decade followed by central visual acuity loss in the fourth to fifth decades. Photoreceptor dysfunction precedes the ophthalmoscopic evidence of the disease. Visual fields are markedly abnormal and both scotopic and photopic responses are highly impaired even with few areas of choroidal atrophy. The ERG is extinguished as the disease progresses. It was originally thought that the effects of hyperornithinemia were restricted to retinal degeneration, but mild systemic effects such as subclinical skeletal muscle changes, abnormalities on electroencephalography, premature atrophy and white matter lesions of the brain and peripheral nervous system involvement suggest that GA is a systemic disease (182,231,232).

The diagnosis of GA is based on the characteristic fundus findings, supported by plasma amino acid analysis, which shows ornithine levels 10 to 12 times greater than normal and low levels of lysine, glutamate, glutamine, creatine and guanidinoacetate, and an enzyme assay which confirms OAT deficiency.

Genetics

Gyrate atrophy occurs due to mutations in *OAT* gene on chromosome 10 (10q26). The mutation causes deficient OAT, which catalyzes the conversion of ornithine to pyrroline-5 carboxylate, an intermediate in the biosynthesis of glutamate and proline. The mutation results in ornithine accumulation which can be detected in the plasma amino acid analysis.

Histopathology

The ultrastructural analysis of a postmortem eye revealed mitochondrial enlargement with disruption of the cristae in several sites (the corneal endothelium, smooth muscle of the iris and ciliary body, and to a lesser degree in the photoreceptor inner segments) (248). However, mitochondrial abnormalities were not found in the RPE.

Pathogenesis

The pathophysiology of GA is most likely due to high levels of ornithine. Nevertheless, a deficiency of pyrroline-5 carboxylate or other metabolites may also play a role. An animal model of GA (237) and a histopathological analysis of a postmortem eye with choroideremia (248) suggest the RPE as the initial site of insult. The disease mechanism is not clear; ornithine-delta aminotransferase is present in the mitochondrial matrix of most tissues and mitochondrial abnormalities have been found in cells that are clinically not affected in GA.

Reducing plasma ornithine levels by arginine-restricted (precursor of ornithine) diet slows or prevents progression of the disease (112,238). The OAT enzyme is dependent on pyridoxal phosphate and in a subset of patients, a high dose of vitamin B6 (pyridoxine) has also been shown to reduce the plasma ornithine levels which slows retinal degeneration (243). An in vitro study suggests that the L-type amino acid transporters may be involved in the protection against ornithine cytotoxicity in human RPE (170). Thus, amino acid transportation in RPE may be a good target for a new treatment in GA (171).

GENETIC DISORDERS OF THE OPTIC NERVE

Dominant Optic Atrophy

General Remarks

Autosomal dominant optic atrophy (ADOA) is the most frequent form of hereditary optic neuropathy, with an estimated prevalence of approximately 1 in 12,000 (120).

Clinical Features

ADOA has an insidious onset variable visual loss, central, paracentral or cecocentral visual field scotoma, color vision deficits, and symmetric optic atrophy. The optic atrophy may be subtle, being temporal only or involving the entire optic disc. Visual acuity ranges widely from 20/20 to light perception, with the vast majority of the patients having a visual acuity better than 20/200 throughout life. In most patients, visual acuity remains stable (121). Peripapillary atrophy, an absent foveal reflex, mild macular pigmentary changes and nonglaucomatous cupping of the optic nerve head with an absence of a healthy neuroretinal rim can also be seen. Electrophysiologic findings document nonspecific optic nerve dysfunction. Pattern ERG shows preferential N95 waveform reduction early in the disease with P50 reduction as the disease progresses, a feature of typical ganglion cell dysfunction. However, pattern ERG remains detectable even in advanced cases. The VEP responses may be non-detectable in more advanced cases, and when detectable, they are mildly to moderately delayed (13).

Histopathology

Histopathologic studies have shown a primary degeneration of the retinal ganglion cell layer, accompanied by ascending atrophy of the optic nerve (110,122).

Genetics

Mutations in the *OPA1* gene on chromosome 3 (3q29) have been found in 30% to 50% of cases with ADOA. Two more loci for ADOA have been mapped to chromosome 18 (18q12.2–q12.3) (OPA4) and chromosome 5 (22q12.1–q12.3) (OPA5). The *OPA1* gene is widely expressed and abundant in retina. Its encoded protein is a dynamin-related GTPase which localizes to mitochondria. Although *OPA1* is a nuclear gene, the fact that its encoded product localizes in mitochondria suggests that a dysfunction of this cytoplasmic organelle may be the final common pathway for many forms of syndromic and nonsyndromic optic atrophy (181). Defective OPA1 function perturbs mitochondrial inner membrane structure and integrity and leads to cytochrome *c* release and caspase-dependent apoptotic cell death (179). Oxidative phosphorylation is defective in patients with ADOA having *OPA1* mutations shown by the significantly increased time constant of postexercise phosphocreatine resynthesis, indicating a reduced rate of mitochondrial ATP production in the patients (141). These events are also accompanied by profound changes in mitochondrial morphology. Similar findings have also been observed in patients with Leber hereditary optic neuropathy (LHON) (discussed later). Linkage analysis of patients with normal tension glaucoma has shown an association with polymorphisms of the *OPA1* gene, raising the question of whether normal tension glaucoma is a type of hereditary optic neuropathy (12). *OPA1* mutations result in decreased numbers of mitochondrial organelles via apoptosis. Mitochondrial DNA content was found to be lower in the blood of patients with ADOA compared to controls (118). Because mitochondria are a major source of ATP, a reduced cellular mitochondrial content may lead to deficient ATP production and a subsequent degeneration of retinal ganglion cells. However, the pure energy-depletion model does not explain why other energy-dependent cell types such as the RPE and the photoreceptors are not involved in ADOA, since the photoreceptor layer is the richest in enzymes for oxidative metabolism (114). A possible explanation could be that retinal ganglion cells are more vulnerable to free radicals and oxidative stress. It is also possible that mitochondrial network remodeling, especially frequent in retinal ganglion cells, or that reduced expression of OPA1 impairs metabolic pathways that are critical to these cells (114).

Leber Hereditary Optic Neuropathy

Genetics

Leber hereditary optic neuropathy (MIM #535000) is transmitted by non-Mendelian, mitochondrial inheritance and associated with point mutations in mitochondrial DNA, which encode subunits of the respiratory chain (see Chapter 70) (129). Three mutations in mitochondrial DNA, MTND1-3460, MTND4-11778 and MTND6-14484, account for more than 90% of LHON cases. They are most often found in a homoplasmic (100% mutant) state, though heteroplasmy (a mixture of mutant and normal mtDNAs) is not uncommon (30). The remaining LHON mutations are so-called "secondary" mutations, as they generally are not strong risk factors as autonomous entities. Many mutations occur in combination with each other and the primary mutations. LHON shows variable penetrance and a primary mitochondrial DNA mutation is essential but not sufficient to manifest the disease as some individuals harboring homoplasmic LHON mutations remain asymptomatic throughout life (235). An intriguing feature of LHON is that only 50% of men and 10% of women harboring one of the three primary mutations develop optic neuropathy (147). This incomplete penetrance and the preference for male individuals suggest that nuclear or mitochondrial genes, and/or environmental factors, play a role in the pathogenesis of the disease.

All primary LHON mutations alter mtDNA-encoded, inner membrane proteins which contribute to NADH: ubiquinone oxidoreductase or different subunits of complex I, the first site of the respiratory chain. In oxidative phosphorylation, electrons can enter the mitochondrial electron transport chain by oxidation of NADH at the proximal region of complex I (30). Electrons are transferred through complex I-associated electron carriers including a flavoprotein and five to seven iron–sulfur centers, and ultimately reduce ubiquinone to ubiquinol at the distal region of complex I. Electrons are subsequently passed through complex III (ubiquinol:cytochrome *c* oxidoreductase) to complex IV (cytochrome *c* oxidoreductase), and finally to oxygen. Concurrent with electron transfer, protons are translocated from the matrix to the inner membrane space at complexes I, III, and IV, thus generating an electrochemical gradient which is utilized by complex V (ATP synthase) to condense ADP and inorganic phosphate to ATP (30). All mutations show a 15 to 40% reduction in complex I-linked respiration rates; however, metabolic threshold theory suggests that complex I activity must be more than 70% reduced to perturb oxygen consumption or ATP production (132). Therefore, LHON does not appear to be a simple result of decreased complex I activity in mitochondrial electron transfer (31). Although the primary LHON mutations predispose carriers to the disease, it still remains unclear how the amino acid substitutions caused by LHON mutations, which induce only subtle changes in complex I electron-transport function, lead to retinal ganglion cell death.

Impaired complex I-linked respiration alone cannot be the only answer because other mtDNA mutations alter respiration but do not result in LHON. It is possible, however, that LHON mutations may increase mitochondrial reactive oxygen species and this could lead to oxidative stress and apoptosis (16). Experimental studies suggest that an inverse association exists between the activity of complex I and reactive oxygen species, indicating that reactive oxygen species play a pivotal role in the pathogenesis of LHON (45). The apoptotic retinal ganglion cell death in LHON supports these findings (75). In addition, lymphocytes from patients with LHON treated with the oxidizing agent showed a significant increase in the percentage of apoptotic cells with respect to controls (16). These findings are not surprising since mitochondria play a key role in apoptosis. Therefore, a combination of complex I subunit mutations, a partial deficiency of oxidative phosphorylation and an increased production of reactive oxygen species seem to be the mechanisms causing the optic neuropathy (80).

Mitochondria are maternally inherited; therefore, there is no male to male transmission in an LHON pedigree. However, men are more affected with an estimated male to female ratio between 3:1 and 5.6:1, and up to 80% to 90% of patients with LHON are males in some series (174). This may be explained by a modifying factor on the X chromosome (32). Affected women are more likely to have affected children, especially daughters, than unaffected female carriers (82).

Clinical Features

The onset of visual loss typically occurs between the ages of 15 and 35 years but has been observed as early as age 1 to as late as the eighth decade. Vision loss often begins painlessly in one eye, but may also be simultaneous. The second eye is usually affected weeks to months later. The progression of visual loss is acute or subacute, stabilizing after months. Visual acuity ranges between light perception to 20/20. Color vision is affected severely in the early course of the disease. Pupillary light responses may be relatively preserved when compared with the responses in patients' with other forms of optic neuropathies. Visual field defects are typically central or cecocentral. During the acute phase of visual loss, retinal nerve fiber layer swelling, peripapillary telangiectasia, optic disc swelling or hyperemia, retinal vascular tortuosity, retinal and optic disc hemorrhages, macular edema, exudates, and retinal striations can be observed. However, optic atrophy with nerve fiber layer dropout, most pronounced in the papillomacular bundle, eventually develops (96). A triad of signs was suggested to be pathognomonic for LHON: circumpapillary telangiectatic microangiopathy, swelling of the nerve fiber layer around the optic nerve head, and absence of leakage from the optic disc or papillary region on FA (213). In most patients, visual loss remains profound and permanent; however, spontaneous visual recovery can occur depending on which primary mutation is present in the patient. The 11778A mutation is associated with a less than 5% visual recovery frequency, while 40% to 50% of patients harboring the 14484C mutation experience some degree of visual recovery, especially if they had an early age of onset (30).

Histopathology

A histopathologic study of eyes of an 81-year-old woman with LHON from a pedigree characterized by mutations at nucleotide positions 4160 and 14484 revealed marked atrophy of the nerve fiber and retinal ganglion cell layers and optic nerve (115). TEM demonstrated electron-dense, double-membrane-bound inclusions consisting of calcium in retinal ganglion cells suggesting intramitochondrial calcification. The optic nerve was homoplasmic for mutations 4160 and 14484 as was the leukocyte/platelet fraction of whole blood.

LHON may be associated with cardiac abnormalities (such as Wolff-Parkinson-White syndrome, (MIM #194200) Lown-Ganong-Levine syndrome) and neurologic abnormalities such as cerebellar ataxia, tremor, and seizures. The differential diagnosis of LHON includes optic neuritis, ischemic optic neuropathy, compressive optic neuropathy, infiltrative optic neuropathy and optic nerve neoplasm. A definitive diagnosis is established by a genetic analysis of mitochondrial DNA.

ACKNOWLEDGMENTS

The authors thank Foundation Fighting Blindness and the TUBITAK Foundation for their support. RetNet edited by Dr. Stephen Daiger greatly assisted the authors. We would like to thank Debra A. Thompson, PhD, Anand Swaroop, PhD, and Hong Cheng, PhD for useful discussions and assistance in figures.

REFERENCES

1. Abid A, Ismail M, Mehdi SQ, Khaliq S. Identification of novel mutations in SEMA4A gene associated with retinal degenerative diseases. J Med Genet 2006; 43:378–81.
2. Acland GM, Aguirre GD, Ray J, et al. Gene therapy restores vision in a canine model of childhood blindness. Nat Genet 2001; 28:92–5.
3. Adato A, Michel V, Kikkawa Y, et al. Interactions in the network of Usher syndrome type 1 proteins. Hum Mol Genet 2005; 14:347–56.

4. Adato A, Vreugde S, Joensuu T, et al. USH3A transcripts encode clarin-1, a four-transmembrane-domain protein with a possible role in sensory synapses. Eur J Hum Genet 2002; 10:339–50.
5. Aguirre G, Farber D, Lolley R, et al. Retinal degeneration in the dog. III. Abnormal cyclic nucleotide metabolism in rod–cone dysplasia. Exp Eye Res 1982; 35:625–42.
6. Akey DT, Zhu X, Dyer M, Li A, et al. The inherited blindness associated protein AIPL1 interacts with the cell cycle regulator protein NUB1. Hum Mol Genet 2002; 11: 2723–33.
7. Alfinito PD, Townes-Anderson E. Activation of mislocalized opsin kills rod cells: a novel mechanism for rod cell death in retinal disease. Proc Natl Acad Sci U S A 2002; 99:5655–60.
8. Alory C, Balch WE. Organization of the Rab-GDI/CHM superfamily: the functional basis for choroideremia disease. Traffic 2001; 2:532–43.
9. Ambasudhan R, Wang X, Jablonski MM, et al. Atrophic macular degeneration mutations in ELOVL4 result in the intracellular misrouting of the protein. Genomics 2004; 83:615–25.
10. Andres DA, Seabra MC, Brown MS, et al. cDNA cloning of component A of Rab geranylgeranyl transferase and demonstration of its role as a Rab escort protein. Cell 1993; 73:1091–9.
11. Apushkin MA, Fishman GA, Rajagopalan AS. Fundus findings and longitudinal study of visual acuity loss in patients with X-linked retinoschisis. Retina 2005; 25: 612–8.
12. Aung T, Ocaka L, Ebenezer ND, et al. A major marker for normal tension glaucoma: association with polymorphisms in the OPA1 gene. Hum Genet 2002; 110:52–6.
13. Bach M, Hoffmann MB. The origin of the pattern ERG. In: Heckenlively JR, Arden GB, eds. Principles and Practice of Clinical Electrophysiology of Vision. Chapter 13. Cambridge, MA: MIT Press, 2006:185–96.
14. Baker AH, Zaltsman AB, George SJ, Newby AC. Divergent effects of tissue inhibitor of metalloproteinase-1, -2, or -3 overexpression on rat vascular smooth muscle cell invasion, proliferation, and death in vitro. TIMP-3 promotes apoptosis. J Clin Invest 1998; 101:1478–87.
15. Batten ML, Imanishi Y, Maeda T, et al. Lecithin-retinol acyltransferase is essential for accumulation of all-trans-retinyl esters in the eye and in the liver. J Biol Chem 2004; 279:10422–32.
16. Battisti C, Formichi P, Cardaioli E, et al. Cell response to oxidative stress induced apoptosis in patients with Leber's hereditary optic neuropathy. J Neurol Neurosurg Psychiatry 2004; 75:1731–6.
17. Bech-Hansen NT, Naylor MJ, Maybaum TA, et al. Mutations in NYX, encoding the leucine-rich proteoglycan nyctalopin, cause X-linked complete congenital stationary night blindness. Nat Genet 2000; 26:319–23.
18. Ben-Arie-Weintrob Y, Berson EL, Dryja TP. Histopathologic-genotypic correlations in retinitis pigmentosa and allied diseases. Ophthalmic Genet 2005; 26: 91–100.
19. Bergen AA, Pinckers AJ. Localization of a novel X-linked progressive cone dystrophy gene to Xq27: evidence for genetic heterogeneity. Am J Hum Genet 1997; 60:1468–73.
20. Bhattacharya G, Cosgrove D. Evidence for functional importance of usherin/fibronectin interactions in retinal basement membranes. Biochemistry 2005; 44:11518–24.
21. Bok D. Cellular mechanisms of retinal degenerations: RPE65, ABCA4, RDS, and bicarbonate transporter genes as examples. Retina 2005; 25:S18–20.
22. Bonilha VL, Hollyfield JG, Grover S, Fishman GA. Abnormal distribution of red/green cone opsins in a patient with an autosomal dominant cone dystrophy. Ophthalmic Genet 2005; 26:69–76.
23. Booij JC, Florijn RJ, ten Brink JB, et al. Identification of mutations in the AIPL1, CRB1, GUCY2D, RPE65, and RPGRIP1 genes in patients with juvenile retinitis pigmentosa. J Med Genet 2005; 42:e67.
24. Bornancin F, Mechtcheriakova D, Stora S, et al. Characterization of a ceramide kinase-like protein. Biochim Biophys Acta 2005; 1687:31–43.
25. Boughman JA, Conneally PM, Nance WE. Population genetic studies of retinitis pigmentosa. Am J Hum Genet 1980; 32:223–35.
26. Bowne SJ, Sullivan LS, Mortimer SE, et al. Spectrum and frequency of mutations in IMPDH1 associated with autosomal dominant retinitis pigmentosa and leber congenital amaurosis. Invest Ophthalmol Vis Sci 2006; 47:34–42.
27. Breuer DK, Yashar BM, Filippova E, et al. A comprehensive mutation analysis of RP2 and RPGR in a North American cohort of families with X-linked retinitis pigmentosa. Am J Hum Genet 2002; 70:1545–54.
28. Brew K, Dinakarpandian D, Nagase H. Tissue inhibitors of metalloproteinases: evolution, structure and function. Biochim Biophys Acta 2000; 1477:267–83.
29. Bright SR, Brown TE, Varnum MD. Disease-associated mutations in CNGB3 produce gain of function alterations in cone cyclic nucleotide-gated channels. Mol Vis 2005; 11:1141–50.
30. Brown MD. The enigmatic relationship between mitochondrial dysfunction and Leber's hereditary optic neuropathy. J Neurol Sci 1999; 165:1–5.
31. Brown MD, Trounce IA, Jun AS, et al. Functional analysis of lymphoblast and cybrid mitochondria containing the 3460, 11778, or 14484 Leber's hereditary optic neuropathy mitochondrial DNA mutation. J Biol Chem 2000; 275: 39831–6.
32. Bu XD, Rotter JI. X chromosome-linked and mitochondrial gene control of Leber hereditary optic neuropathy: evidence from segregation analysis for dependence on X chromosome inactivation. Proc Natl Acad Sci U S A 1991; 88:8198–202.
33. Bumsted O'Brien KM, Cheng H, Jiang Y, et al. Expression of photoreceptor-specific nuclear receptor NR2E3 in rod photoreceptors of fetal human retina. Invest Ophthalmol Vis Sci 2004; 45:2807–12.
34. Carr RE. Congenital stationary night blindness. In: Heckenlively JR, Arden GB, eds. Principles and Practice of Clinical Electrophysiology of Vision. St. Louis, MO: Mosby, 1991:713–20.
35. Cepko CL. Effect of gene expression on cone survival in retinitis pigmentosa. Retina 2005; 25:S21–4.
36. Cepko CL, Austin CP, Yang X, et al. Cell fate determination in the vertebrate retina. Proc Natl Acad Sci U S A 1996; 93:589–95.
37. Chang GQ, Hao Y, Wong F. Apoptosis: final common pathway of photoreceptor death in rd, rds, and rhodopsin mutant mice. Neuron 1993; 11:595–605.
38. Chong NH, Alexander RA, Gin T, et al. TIMP-3, collagen, and elastin immunohistochemistry and histopathology of Sorsby's fundus dystrophy. Invest Ophthalmol Vis Sci 2000; 41:898–902.

39. Chuang JZ, Vega C, Jun W, Sung CH. Structural and functional impairment of endocytic pathways by retinitis pigmentosa mutant rhodopsin–arrestin complexes. J Clin Invest 2004; 114:131–40.
40. Cideciyan AV, Aleman TS, Swider M, et al. Mutations in ABCA4 result in accumulation of lipofuscin before slowing of the retinoid cycle: a reappraisal of the human disease sequence. Hum Mol Genet 2004; 13:525–34.
41. Cideciyan AV, Haeseleer F, Fariss RN, et al. Rod and cone visual cycle consequences of a null mutation in the 11-cis-retinol dehydrogenase gene in man. Vis Neurosci 2000; 17:667–78.
42. Cohen AI. Some cytological and initial biochemical observations on photoreceptors in retinas of rds mice. Invest Ophthalmol Vis Sci 1983; 24:832–43.
43. Collins CA, Guthrie C. The question remains: is the spliceosome a ribozyme? Nat Struct Biol 2000; 7:850–4.
44. Condon GP, Brownstein S, Wang NS, et al. Congenital hereditary (juvenile X-linked) retinoschisis. Histopathologic and ultrastructural findings in three eyes. Arch Ophthalmol 1986; 104:576–83.
45. Cortopassi G, Wang E. Modelling the effects of age-related mtDNA mutation accumulation; complex I deficiency, superoxide and cell death. Biochim Biophys Acta 1995; 1271:171–6.
46. D'Cruz PM, Yasumura D, Weir J, et al. Mutation of the receptor tyrosine kinase gene Mertk in the retinal dystrophic RCS rat. Hum Mol Genet 2000; 9:645–51.
47. Dai H, Tomchick DR, Garcia J, et al. Crystal structure of the RIM2 C(2)A-domain at 1.4 A resolution. Biochemistry 2005; 44:13533–42.
48. Demirci FY, Gupta N; Radak AL, et al. Histopathologic study of X-linked cone–rod dystrophy (CORDX1) caused by a mutation in the RPGR exon ORF15. Am J Ophthalmol 2005; 139:386–8.
49. den Hollander AI, Davis J, van der Velde-Visser SD, et al. CRB1 mutation spectrum in inherited retinal dystrophies. Hum Mutat 2004; 24:355–69.
50. Dryja TP, Hahn LB, Kajiwara K, Berson EL. Dominant and digenic mutations in the peripherin/RDS and ROM1 genes in retinitis pigmentosa. Invest Ophthalmol Vis Sci 1997; 38:1972–82.
51. Dryja TP, McGee TL, Berson EL, et al. Night blindness and abnormal cone electroretinogram ON responses in patients with mutations in the GRM6 gene encoding mGluR6. Proc Natl Acad Sci U S A 2005; 102:4884–9.
52. Dryja TP, Rucinski DE, Chen SH, Berson EL. Frequency of mutations in the gene encoding the alpha subunit of rod cGMP-phosphodiesterase in autosomal recessive retinitis pigmentosa. Invest Ophthalmol Vis Sci 1999; 40:1859–65.
53. Eagle RC Jr, Lucier AC, Bernardino VB Jr, Yanoff M. Retinal pigment epithelial abnormalities in fundus flavimaculatus: a light and electron microscopic study. Ophthalmology 1980; 87:1189–200.
54. Ebenezer ND, Michaelides M, Jenkins SA, et al. Identification of novel RPGR ORF15 mutations in X-linked progressive cone–rod dystrophy (XLCORD) families. Invest Ophthalmol Vis Sci 2005; 46:1891–8.
55. El-Amraoui A, Petit C. Usher I syndrome: unravelling the mechanisms that underlie the cohesion of the growing hair bundle in inner ear sensory cells. J Cell Sci 2005; 118: 4593–603.
56. Ergun E, Hermann B, Wirtitsch M, et al. Assessment of central visual function in Stargardt's disease/fundus flavimaculatus with ultrahigh-resolution optical coherence tomography. Invest Ophthalmol Vis Sci 2005; 46:310–6.
57. Farber DB, Lolley RN. Cyclic guanosine monophosphate: elevation in degenerating photoreceptor cells of the C3H mouse retina. Science 1974; 186:449–51.
58. Fariss RN, Apte SS, Luthert PJ, et al. Accumulation of tissue inhibitor of metalloproteinases-3 in human eyes with Sorsby's fundus dystrophy or retinitis pigmentosa. Br J Ophthalmol 1998; 82:1329–34.
59. Fei Y, Hughes TE. Nuclear trafficking of photoreceptor protein crx: the targeting sequence and pathologic implications. Invest Ophthalmol Vis Sci 2000; 41: 2849–56.
60. Felbor U, Schilling H, Weber BH. Adult vitelliform macular dystrophy is frequently associated with mutations in the peripherin/RDS gene. Hum Mutat 1997; 10:301–9.
61. Felbor U, Doepner D, Schneider U, et al. Evaluation of the gene encoding the tissue inhibitor of metalloproteinases-3 in various maculopathies. Invest Ophthalmol Vis Sci 1997; 38:1054–9.
62. Feng W, Yasumura D, Matthes MT, et al. Mertk triggers uptake of photoreceptor outer segments during phagocytosis by cultured retinal pigment epithelial cells. J Biol Chem 2002; 277:17016–22.
63. Ferreira PA. Insights into X-linked retinitis pigmentosa type 3, allied diseases and underlying pathomechanisms. Hum Mol Genet 2005; 14(Spec No. 2):R259–67.
64. Flannery JG, Bird AC, Farber DB, et al. A histopathologic study of a choroideremia carrier. Invest Ophthalmol Vis Sci 1990; 31:229–36.
65. Foxman SG, Heckenlively JR, Bateman JB, Wirtschafter JD. Classification of congenital and early onset retinitis pigmentosa. Arch Ophthalmol 1985; 103:1502–6.
66. Frangieh GT, Green WR, Fine SL. A histopathologic study of Best's macular dystrophy. Arch Ophthalmol 1982; 100: 1115–21.
67. Friedman TB, Schultz JM, Ahmed ZM. Usher syndrome type 1: genotype–phenotype relationships. Retina 2005; 25:S40–2.
68. Furukawa T, Morrow EM, Li T, et al. Retinopathy and attenuated circadian entrainment in Crx-deficient mice. Nat Genet 1999; 23:466–70.
69. Gal A, Li Y, Thompson DA, Weir J, et al. Mutations in MERTK, the human orthologue of the RCS rat retinal dystrophy gene, cause retinitis pigmentosa. Nat Genet 2000; 26:270–1.
70. Gallemore RP, Steinberg RH. Light-evoked modulation of basolateral membrane Cl^- conductance in chick retinal pigment epithelium: the light peak and fast oscillation. J Neurophysiol 1993; 70:1669–80.
71. Galvin JA, Fishman GA, Stone EM, Koenekoop RK. Evaluation of genotype–phenotype associations in leber congenital amaurosis. Retina 2005; 25:919–29.
72. Gao H, Kusumi R, Yung CW. Optical coherence tomographic findings in X-linked juvenile retinoschisis. Arch Ophthalmol 2005; 123:1006–8.
73. Gao J, Cheon K, Nusinowitz S, et al. Progressive photoreceptor degeneration, outer segment dysplasia, and rhodopsin mislocalization in mice with targeted disruption of the retinitis pigmentosa-1 (Rp1) gene. Proc Natl Acad Sci U S A 2002; 99:5698–703.
74. Gerth C, Andrassi-Darida M, Bock M, et al. Phenotypes of 16 Stargardt macular dystrophy/fundus flavimaculatus patients with known ABCA4 mutations and evaluation of genotype-phenotype correlation. Graefes Arch Clin Exp Ophthalmol 2002; 240:628–38.

75. Ghelli A, Zanna C, Porcelli AM, et al. Leber's hereditary optic neuropathy (LHON) pathogenic mutations induce mitochondrial-dependent apoptotic death in transmitochondrial cells incubated with galactose medium. J Biol Chem 2003; 278:4145–50.
76. Golovleva I, Bhattacharya S, Wu Z, et al. Disease-causing mutations in the cellular retinaldehyde binding protein tighten and abolish ligand interactions. J Biol Chem 2003; 278:12397–402.
77. Grayson C, Bartolini F, Chapple JP, et al. Localization in the human retina of the X-linked retinitis pigmentosa protein RP2, its homologue cofactor C and the RP2 interacting protein Arl3. Hum Mol Genet 2002; 11:3065–74.
78. Grayson C, Molday RS. Dominant negative mechanism underlies autosomal dominant Stargardt-like macular dystrophy linked to mutations in ELOVL4. J Biol Chem 2005; 280:32521–30.
79. Grover S, Fishman GA, Fiscella RG, Adelman AE. Efficacy of dorzolamide hydrochloride in the management of chronic cystoid macular edema in patients with retinitis pigmentosa. Retina 1997; 17:222–31.
80. Guy J, Qi X, Pallotti F, Schon EA, et al. Rescue of a mitochondrial deficiency causing Leber Hereditary Optic Neuropathy. Ann Neurol 2002; 52:534–42.
81. Hao W, Fong HK. The endogenous chromophore of retinal G protein-coupled receptor opsin from the pigment epithelium. J Biol Chem 1999; 274:6085–90.
82. Harding AE, Sweeney MG, Govan GG, Riordan-Eva P. Pedigree analysis in Leber hereditary optic neuropathy families with a pathogenic mtDNA mutation. Am J Hum Genet 1995; 57:77–86.
83. Harding HP, Calfon M, Urano F, et al. Transcriptional and translational control in the Mammalian unfolded protein response. Annu Rev Cell Dev Biol 2002; 18: 575–99.
84. Hart AW, McKie L, Morgan JE, et al. Genotype-phenotype correlation of mouse pde6b mutations. Invest Ophthalmol Vis Sci 2005; 46:3443–50.
85. Heckenlively JR. Preserved para-arteriole retinal pigment epithelium (PPRPE) in retinitis pigmentosa. Br J Ophthalmol 1982; 66:26–30.
86. Heckenlively JR. RP cone–rod degeneration. Trans Am Ophthalmol Soc 1987; 85:438–70.
87. Heckenlively JR. Hereditary forms of pseudoretinitis pigmentosa. In: Retinitis Pigmentosa. Lippincott, 1987: 194–5.
88. Heckenlively JR, Feldman K, Wheeler NC. Retinitis pigmentosa: cone–rod degenerations. A comparison of clinical findings to electrophysiologic parameters contrasted to the rod–cone degeneration. In: Heckenlively JR, Arden GB, eds. Principles and Practice of Clinical Electrophysiology of Vision. Chicago: Mosby Year Book, 1991:510–27.
89. Heckenlively JR, Jordan BL, Aptsiauri N. Association of antiretinal antibodies and cystoid macular edema in patients with retinitis pigmentosa. Am J Ophthalmol 1999; 127:565–73.
90. Heckenlively JR, Rodriguez JA, Daiger SP. Autosomal dominant sectoral retinitis pigmentosa. Two families with transversion mutation in codon 23 of rhodopsin. Arch Ophthalmol 1991; 109:84–91.
91. Heckenlively JR, Weleber RG. X-linked recessive cone dystrophy with tapetal-like sheen: a newly recognized entity with Mizuo-Nakamura phenomenon. Arch Ophthalmol 1986; 104:1322–28.
92. Heegaard S, Rosenberg T, Preising M, et al. An unusual retinal vascular morphology in connection with a novel AIPL1 mutation in Leber's congenital amaurosis. Br J Ophthalmol 2003; 87:980–3.
93. Heher KL, Traboulsi EI, Maumenee IH. The natural history of Leber's congenital amaurosis. Age-related findings in 35 patients. Ophthalmology 1992; 99:241–5.
94. den Hollander AI, Heckenlively JR, van den Born LI, et al. Leber congenital amaurosis and retinitis pigmentosa with Coats-like exudative vasculopathy are associated with mutations in the crumbs homologue 1 (CRB1) gene. Am J Hum Genet 2001; 69:198–203.
95. Hood DC, Cideciyan AV, Roman AJ, Jacobson SG. Enhanced S cone syndrome: evidence for an abnormally large number of S cones. Vision Res 1995; 35:1473–81.
96. Hung HL, Kao LY, Huang CC. Clinical features of Leber's hereditary optic neuropathy with the 11778 mitochondrial DNA mutation in Taiwanese patients. Chang Gung Med J 2003; 26:41–7.
97. Huttl S, Michalakis S, Seeliger M, et al. Impaired channel targeting and retinal degeneration in mice lacking the cyclic nucleotide-gated channel subunit CNGB1. J Neurosci 2005; 25:130–8.
98. Iakhine R, Chorna-Ornan I, Zars T, et al. Novel dominant rhodopsin mutation triggers two mechanisms of retinal degeneration and photoreceptor desensitization. J Neurosci 2004; 24:2516–26.
99. Iannaccone A, Breuer DK, Wang XF, et al. Clinical and immunohistochemical evidence for an X linked retinitis pigmentosa syndrome with recurrent infections and hearing loss in association with an RPGR mutation. J Med Genet 2003; 40:e118.
100. Iannaccone A, Wang X, Jablonski MM, et al. Increasing evidence for syndromic phenotypes associated with RPGR mutations. Am J Ophthalmol 2004; 137:785–6; author reply 786.
101. Illing ME, Rajan RS, Bence NF, Kopito RR. A rhodopsin mutant linked to autosomal dominant retinitis pigmentosa is prone to aggregate and interacts with the ubiquitin proteasome system. J Biol Chem 2002; 277:34150–60.
102. Jacobson SG, Cideciyan AV, Aleman TS, et al. Crumbs homolog 1 (CRB1) mutations result in a thick human retina with abnormal lamination. Hum Mol Genet 2003; 12:1073–8.
103. Jacobson SG, Cideciyan AV, Regunath G, et al. Night blindness in Sorsby's fundus dystrophy reversed by vitamin A. Nat Genet 1995; 11:27–32.
104. Jacobson SG, Roman AJ, Roman MI, et al. Relatively enhanced S cone function in the Goldmann–Favre syndrome. Am J Ophthalmol 1991; 111:446–53.
105. Jarc-Vidmar M, Popovic P, Hawlina M, Brecelj J. Pattern ERG and psychophysical functions in Best's disease. Doc Ophthalmol 2001; 103:47–61.
106. Jiang M, Pandey S, Fong HK. An opsin homologue in the retina and pigment epithelium. Invest Ophthalmol Vis Sci 1993; 34:3669–78.
107. Jiao X, Munier FL, Iwata F, et al. Genetic linkage of Bietti crystalline corneoretinal dystrophy to chromosome 4q35. Am J Hum Genet 2000; 67:1309–13.
108. Johnson K, Grawe F, Grzeschik N, Knust E. Drosophila crumbs is required to inhibit light-induced photoreceptor degeneration. Curr Biol 2002; 12:1675–80.
109. Johnson S, Halford S, Morris AG, et al. Genomic organisation and alternative splicing of human RIM1, a gene implicated in autosomal dominant cone–rod dystrophy (CORD7). Genomics 2003; 81:304–14.
110. Johnston PB, Gaster RN, Smith VC, Tripathi RC. A clinicopathologic study of autosomal dominant optic atrophy. Am J Ophthalmol 1979; 88:868–75.

111. Jomary C, Neal MJ, Iwata K, Jones SE. Localization of tissue inhibitor of metalloproteinases-3 in neurodegenerative retinal disease. Neuroreport 1997; 8:2169–72.
112. Kaiser-Kupfer MI, Caruso RC, Valle D, Reed GF. Use of an arginine-restricted diet to slow progression of visual loss in patients with gyrate atrophy. Arch Ophthalmol 2004; 122:982–4.
113. Kaiser-Kupfer MI, Chan CC, Markello TC, et al. Clinical biochemical and pathologic correlations in Bietti's crystalline dystrophy. Am J Ophthalmol 1994; 118:569–82.
114. Kamei S, Chen-Kuo-Chang M, Cazevieille C, et al. Expression of the Opa1 mitochondrial protein in retinal ganglion cells: its downregulation causes aggregation of the mitochondrial network. Invest Ophthalmol Vis Sci 2005; 46:4288–94.
115. Kerrison JB, Howell N, Miller NR, et al. Leber hereditary optic neuropathy. Electron microscopy and molecular genetic analysis of a case. Ophthalmology 1995; 102: 1509–16.
116. Khani SC, Nielsen L, Vogt TM. Biochemical evidence for pathogenicity of rhodopsin kinase mutations correlated with the oguchi form of congenital stationary night blindness. Proc Natl Acad Sci U S A 1998; 95:2824–7.
117. Khanna H, Hurd TW, Lillo C, et al. RPGR-ORF15, which is mutated in retinitis pigmentosa, associates with SMC1, SMC3, and microtubule transport proteins. J Biol Chem 2005; 280:33580–7.
118. Kim JY, Hwang JM, Ko HS. Mitochondrial DNA content is decreased in autosomal dominant optic atrophy. Neurology 2005; 64:966–72.
119. Kisselev OG. Focus on molecules: rhodopsin. Exp Eye Res 2005; 81:366–7.
120. Kjer B, Eiberg H, Kjer P, Rosenberg T. Dominant optic atrophy mapped to chromosome 3q region. II. Clinical and epidemiological aspects. Acta Ophthalmol Scand 1996; 74:3–7.
121. Kjer P. Infantile optic atrophy with dominant mode of inheritance: a clinical and genetic study of 19 Danish families. Acta Ophthalmol (Copenh) 1959; 164:1–147.
122. Kjer P, Jensen OA, Klinken L. Histopathology of eye, optic nerve and brain in a case of dominant optic atrophy. Acta Ophthalmol (Copenh) 1983; 61:300–12.
123. Klevering BJ, Maugeri A, Wagner A, et al. Three families displaying the combination of Stargardt's disease with cone–rod dystrophy or retinitis pigmentosa. Ophthalmology 2004; 111:546–53.
124. Kobayashi A, Higashide T, Hamasaki D, et al. HRG4 (UNC119) mutation found in cone–rod dystrophy causes retinal degeneration in a transgenic model. Invest Ophthalmol Vis Sci 2000; 41:3268–77.
125. Koenekoop RK. RPGRIP1 is mutated in Leber congenital amaurosis: a mini-review. Ophthalmic Genet 2005; 26: 175–9.
126. Koenekoop RK, Fishman GA, Iannaccone A, et al. Electroretinographic abnormalities in parents of patients with Leber congenital amaurosis who have heterozygous GUCY2D mutations. Arch Ophthalmol 2002; 120:1325–30.
127. Krauss HR, Heckenlively JR. Visual field changes in cone–rod degenerations. Arch Ophthalmol 1982; 100: 1784–90.
128. Langton KP, McKie N, Curtis A, et al. A novel tissue inhibitor of metalloproteinases-3 mutation reveals a common molecular phenotype in Sorsby's fundus dystrophy. J Biol Chem 2000; 275:27027–31.
129. Larsson NG. Leber hereditary optic neuropathy: a nuclear solution of a mitochondrial problem. Ann Neurol 2002; 52:529–30.
130. Lee J, Jiao X, Hejtmancik JF, et al. Identification, isolation, and characterization of a 32-kDa fatty acid-binding protein missing from lymphocytes in humans with Bietti crystalline dystrophy (BCD). Mol Genet Metab 1998; 65:143–54.
131. Lee J, Jiao X, Hejtmancik JF, et al. The metabolism of fatty acids in human Bietti crystalline dystrophy. Invest Ophthalmol Vis Sci 2001; 42:1707–14.
132. Letellier T, Heinrich R, Malgat M, Mazat JP. The kinetic basis of threshold effects observed in mitochondrial diseases: a systemic approach. Biochem J 1994; 302: 171–4.
133. Leveillard T, Mohand-Said S, Lorentz O, et al. Identification and characterization of rod-derived cone viability factor. Nat Genet 2004; 36:755–9.
134. Levine EM, Fuhrmann S, Reh TA. Soluble factors and the development of rod photoreceptors. Cell Mol Life Sci 2000; 57:224–34.
135. Li A, Jiao X, Munier FL, et al. Bietti crystalline corneoretinal dystrophy is caused by mutations in the novel gene CYP4V2. Am J Hum Genet 2004; 74:817–26.
136. Liu J, Huang Q, Higdon J, et al. Distinct gene expression profiles and reduced JNK signaling in retinitis pigmentosa caused by RP1 mutations. Hum Mol Genet 2005; 14: 2945–58.
137. Liu L, Gudas LJ. Disruption of the lecithin:retinol acyltransferase gene makes mice more susceptible to vitamin A deficiency. J Biol Chem 2005; 280:40226–34.
138. Liu Q, Zuo J, Pierce EA. The retinitis pigmentosa 1 protein is a photoreceptor microtubule-associated protein. J Neurosci 2004; 24:6427–36.
139. Liu X, Bulgakov OV, Wen XH, et al. AIPL1, the protein that is defective in Leber congenital amaurosis, is essential for the biosynthesis of retinal rod cGMP phosphodiesterase. Proc Natl Acad Sci U S A 2004; 101: 13903–8.
140. Livesey FJ, Cepko CL. Vertebrate neural cell-fate determination: lessons from the retina. Nat. Rev. Neurosci. 2: 109–18, 2001.
141. Lodi R, Tonon C, Valentino ML, et al. Deficit of in vivo mitochondrial ATP production in OPA1-related dominant optic atrophy. Ann Neurol 2004; 56:719–23.
142. Loewen CJ, Moritz OL, Tam BM, et al. The role of subunit assembly in peripherin-2 targeting to rod photoreceptor disk membranes and retinitis pigmentosa. Mol Biol Cell 2003; 14:3400–13.
143. Lois N, Holder GE, Bunce C, et al. Phenotypic subtypes of Stargardt macular dystrophy-fundus flavimaculatus. Arch Ophthalmol 2001; 119:359–69.
144. Lolley RN, Rong H, Craft CM. Linkage of photoreceptor degeneration by apoptosis with inherited defect in phototransduction. Invest Ophthalmol Vis Sci 1994; 35: 358–62.
145. Lyon MF. Sex chromatin and gene action in the mammalian X-chromosome. Am J Hum Genet 1962; 14: 135–48.
146. MacDonald IM, Mah DY, Ho YK, et al. A practical diagnostic test for choroideremia. Ophthalmology 105: 1637–40, 1998.
147. Man PY, Turnbull DM, Chinnery PF. Leber hereditary optic neuropathy. J Med Genet 2002; 39:162–9.
148. Marmorstein AD, Marmorstein LY, Rayborn M, et al. Bestrophin, the product of the Best vitelliform macular dystrophy gene (VMD2), localizes to the basolateral plasma membrane of the retinal pigment epithelium. Proc Natl Acad Sci U S A 2000; 97:12758–63.
149. Marmorstein LY, Munier FL, Arsenijevic Y, et al. Aberrant accumulation of EFEMP1 underlies drusen formation in

Malattia Leventinese and age-related macular degeneration. Proc Natl Acad Sci U S A 2002; 99:13067–72.
150. Masu M, Iwakabe H, Tagawa Y, et al. Specific deficit of the ON response in visual transmission by targeted disruption of the mGluR6 gene. Cell 1995; 80:757–65.
151. Mata NL, Weng J, Travis GH. Biosynthesis of a major lipofuscin fluorophore in mice and humans with ABCR-mediated retinal and macular degeneration. Proc Natl Acad Sci U S A 2000; 97:7154–9.
152. Mavlyutov TA, Zhao H, Ferreira PA. Species-specific subcellular localization of RPGR, RPGRIP isoforms: implications for the phenotypic variability of congenital retinopathies among species. Hum Mol Genet 2002; 11: 1899–907.
153. McBee JK, Palczewski K, Baehr W, Pepperberg DR. Confronting complexity: the interlink of phototransduction and retinoid metabolism in the vertebrate retina. Prog Retin Eye Res 2001; 20:469–529.
154. McHenry CL, Liu Y, Feng W, et al. MERTK arginine-844-cysteine in a patient with severe rod–cone dystrophy: loss of mutant protein function in transfected cells. Invest Ophthalmol Vis Sci 2004; 45:1456–63.
155. Mears AJ, Kondo M, Swain PK, et al. Nrl is required for rod photoreceptor development. Nat Genet 2001; 29: 447–52.
156. Michaelides M, Hunt DM, Moore AT. The cone dysfunction syndromes. Br J Ophthalmol 2004; 88:291–7.
157. Michaelides M, Wilkie SE, Jenkins S, et al. Mutation in the gene GUCA1A, encoding guanylate cyclase-activating protein 1, causes cone, cone–rod, and macular dystrophy. Ophthalmology 2005; 112:1442–7.
158. Milam AH, Barakat MR, Gupta N, et al. Clinicopathologic effects of mutant GUCY2D in Leber congenital amaurosis. Ophthalmology 2003; 110:549–58.
159. Milam AH, Rose L, Cideciyan AV, et al. The nuclear receptor NR2E3 plays a role in human retinal photoreceptor differentiation and degeneration. Proc Natl Acad Sci U S A 2002; 99:473–8.
160. Mitton KP, Swain PK, Chen S, et al. The leucine zipper of NRL interacts with the CRX homeodomain. A possible mechanism of transcriptional synergy in rhodopsin regulation. J Biol Chem 2000; 275:29794–9.
161. Miyake Y. Incomplete-type congenital stationary night blindness. In: Heckenlively JR, Arden GB, eds. Principles and Practice of Clinical Electrophysiology of Vision. St. Louis, MO: Mosby, 1991:721–5.
162. Mizuno K, Takei Y, Sears ML, et al. Leber's congenital amaurosis. Am J Ophthalmol 1977; 83:32–42.
163. Mohand-Said S, Deudon-Combe A, Hicks D, et al. Normal retina releases a diffusible factor stimulating cone survival in the retinal degeneration mouse. Proc Natl Acad Sci U S A 1998; 95:8357–62.
164. Molday LL, Rabin AR, Molday RS. ABCR expression in foveal cone photoreceptors and its role in Stargardt macular dystrophy. Nat Genet 2000; 25:257–8.
165. Molthagen M, Schachner M, Bartsch U. Apoptotic cell death of photoreceptor cells in mice deficient for the adhesion molecule on glia (AMOG, the beta 2-subunit of the Na, K-ATPase). J Neurocytol 1996; 25:243–55.
166. Mullins RF, Oh KT, Heffron E, et al. Late development of vitelliform lesions and flecks in a patient with best disease: clinicopathologic correlation. Arch Ophthalmol 2005; 123:1588–94.
167. Muradov KG, Artemyev NO. Loss of the effector function in a transducin-alpha mutant associated with Nougaret night blindness. J Biol Chem 2000; 275:6969–74.
168. Naash ML, Peachey NS, Li ZY, et al. Light-induced acceleration of photoreceptor degeneration in transgenic mice expressing mutant rhodopsin. Invest Ophthalmol Vis Sci 1996; 37:775–82.
169. Nakamura M, Hotta Y, Tanikawa A, et al. A high association with cone dystrophy in fundus albipunctatus caused by mutations of the RDH5 gene. Invest Ophthalmol Vis Sci 2000; 41:3925–32.
170. Nakauchi T, Ando A, Ueda-Yamada M, Yamazaki Y, Uyama M, Matsumura M, Ito S. Prevention of ornithine cytotoxicity by nonpolar side chain amino acids in retinal pigment epithelial cells. Invest Ophthalmol Vis Sci 2003; 44:5023–8.
171. Nathans J, Maumenee IH, Zrenner E, et al. Genetic heterogeneity among blue-cone monochromats. Am J Hum Genet 1993; 53:987–1000.
172. Nawrot M, West K, Huang J, et al. Cellular retinaldehyde-binding protein interacts with ERM-binding phosphoprotein 50 in retinal pigment epithelium. Invest Ophthalmol Vis Sci 2004; 45:393–401.
173. Newman NJ, Lott MT, Wallace DC. The clinical characteristics of pedigrees of Leber's hereditary optic neuropathy with the 11778 mutation. Am J Ophthalmol 1991; 111:750–62.
174. Nishiguchi KM, Friedman JS, Sandberg MA, et al. Recessive NRL mutations in patients with clumped pigmentary retinal degeneration and relative preservation of blue cone function. Proc Natl Acad Sci U S A 2004; 101:17819–24.
175. Nishiguchi KM, Sokal I, Yang L, et al. A novel mutation (I143NT) in guanylate cyclase-activating protein 1 (GCAP1) associated with autosomal dominant cone degeneration. Invest Ophthalmol Vis Sci 2004; 45:3863–70.
176. O'Byrne SM, Wongsiriroj N, Libien J, et al. Retinoid absorption and storage is impaired in mice lacking lecithin:retinol acyltransferase (LRAT). J Biol Chem 2005; 280:35647–57.
177. Oh KT, Longmuir R, Oh DM, et al. Comparison of the clinical expression of retinitis pigmentosa associated with rhodopsin mutations at codon 347 and codon 23. Am J Ophthalmol 2003; 136:306–13.
178. Olichon A, Baricault L, Gas N, et al. Loss of OPA1 perturbates the mitochondrial inner membrane structure and integrity, leading to cytochrome c release and apoptosis. J Biol Chem 2003; 278:7743–6.
179. Patel KA, Bartoli KM, Fandino RA, et al. Transmembrane S1 mutations in CNGA3 from achromatopsia 2 patients cause loss of function and impaired cellular trafficking of the cone CNG channel. Invest Ophthalmol Vis Sci 2005; 46:2282–90.
180. Payne M, Yang Z, Katz BJ, et al. Dominant optic atrophy, sensorineural hearing loss, ptosis, and ophthalmoplegia: a syndrome caused by a missense mutation in OPA1. Am J Ophthalmol 2004; 138:749–55.
181. Peltola KE, Jaaskelainen S, Heinonen OJ, et al. Peripheral nervous system in gyrate atrophy of the choroid and retina with hyperornithinemia. Neurology 2002; 59: 735–40.
182. Peng GH, Ahmad O, Ahmad F, Liu J, Chen S. The photoreceptor-specific nuclear receptor Nr2e3 interacts with Crx and exerts opposing effects on the transcription of rod versus cone genes. Hum Mol Genet 2005; 14: 747–64.
183. Perrault I, Rozet JM, Calvas P, et al. Retinal-specific guanylate cyclase gene mutations in Leber's congenital amaurosis. Nat Genet 1996; 14:461–4.

184. Petrukhin K, Koisti MJ, Bakall B, et al. Identification of the gene responsible for Best macular dystrophy. Nat Genet 1998; 19:241–7.
185. Pianta MJ, Aleman TS, Cideciyan AV, et al. In vivo micropathology of Best macular dystrophy with optical coherence tomography. Exp Eye Res 2003; 76:203–11.
186. Pierce EA, Quinn T, Meehan T, et al. Mutations in a gene encoding a new oxygen-regulated photoreceptor protein cause dominant retinitis pigmentosa. Nat Genet 1999; 22: 248–54.
187. Pittler SJ, Zhang Y, Chen S, et al. Functional analysis of the rod photoreceptor cGMP phosphodiesterase alpha-subunit gene promoter: Nrl and Crx are required for full transcriptional activity. J Biol Chem 2004; 279: 19800–7.
188. Porto FB, Perrault I, Hicks D, et al. Prenatal human ocular degeneration occurs in Leber's congenital amaurosis (LCA2). J Gene Med 2002; 4:390–6.
189. Pruett RC. Retinitis pigmentosa: clinical observations and correlations. Trans Am Ophthalmol Soc 1983; 81:693–735.
190. Qi JH, Ebrahem Q, Moore N, et al. A novel function for tissue inhibitor of metalloproteinases-3 (TIMP3): inhibition of angiogenesis by blockage of VEGF binding to VEGF receptor-2. Nat Med 2003; 9:407–15.
191. Qian J, Esumi N, Chen Y, et al. Identification of regulatory targets of tissue-specific transcription factors: application to retina-specific gene regulation. Nucleic Acids Res 2005; 33:3479–91.
192. Qu Z, Wei RW, Mann W, Hartzell HC. Two bestrophins cloned from Xenopus laevis oocytes express Ca(2+)-activated Cl(–) currents. J Biol Chem 2003; 278:49563–72.
193. Rak A, Pylypenko O, Niculae A, et al. Structure of the Rab7:REP-1 complex: insights into the mechanism of Rab prenylation and choroideremia disease. Cell 2004; 117: 749–60.
194. Ramamurthy V, Niemi GA, Reh TA, Hurley JB. Leber congenital amaurosis linked to AIPL1: a mouse model reveals destabilization of cGMP phosphodiesterase. Proc Natl Acad Sci U S A 2004; 101:13897–902.
195. Rao VR, Cohen GB, Oprian DD. Rhodopsin mutation G90D and a molecular mechanism for congenital night blindness. Nature 1994; 367:639–42.
196. Rao VR, Oprian DD. Activating mutations of rhodopsin and other G protein-coupled receptors. Annu Rev Biophys Biomol Struct 1996; 25:287–314.
197. Redmond TM, Poliakov E, Yu S, et al. Mutation of key residues of RPE65 abolishes its enzymatic role as isomerohydrolase in the visual cycle. Proc Natl Acad Sci U S A 2005; 102:13658–63.
198. Redmond TM, Yu S, Lee E, et al. Rpe65 is necessary for production of 11-cis-vitamin A in the retinal visual cycle. Nat Genet 1998; 20:344–51.
199. Reiners J, van Wijk E, Marker T, et al. Scaffold protein harmonin (USH1C) provides molecular links between Usher syndrome type 1 and type 2. Hum Mol Genet 2005; 14:3933–43.
200. Rice DS, Huang W, Jones HA, et al. Severe retinal degeneration associated with disruption of semaphorin 4A. Invest Ophthalmol Vis Sci 2004; 45:2767–77.
201. Rosenthal R, Bakall B, Kinnick T, et al. Expression of bestrophin-1, the product of the VMD2 gene, modulates voltage-dependent Ca^{2+} channels in retinal pigment epithelial cells. FASEB J 2006; 20:178–80.
202. Roybal CN, Marmorstein LY, Vander Jagt DL, Abcouwer SF. Aberrant accumulation of fibulin-3 in the endoplasmic reticulum leads to activation of the unfolded protein response and VEGF expression. Invest Ophthalmol Vis Sci 2005; 46:3973–9.
203. Saari JC, Crabb JW. Focus on molecules: cellular retinaldehyde-binding protein (CRALBP). Exp Eye Res 2005; 81:245–6.
204. Saari JC, Nawrot M, Kennedy BN, et al. Visual cycle impairment in cellular retinaldehyde binding protein (CRALBP) knockout mice results in delayed dark adaptation. Neuron 2001; 29:739–48.
205. Sandberg MA, Weigel-DiFranco C, Dryja TP, Berson EL. Clinical expression correlates with location of rhodopsin mutation in dominant retinitis pigmentosa. Invest Ophthalmol Vis Sci 1995; 36:1934–42.
206. Schwahn U, Lenzner S, Dong J, et al. Positional cloning of the gene for X-linked retinitis pigmentosa 2. Nat Genet 1998; 19:327–32.
207. Schwartz SB, Aleman TS, Cideciyan AV, et al. Disease expression in Usher syndrome caused by VLGR1 gene mutation (USH2C) and comparison with USH2A phenotype. Invest Ophthalmol Vis Sci 2005; 46:734–43.
208. Seabra MC. New insights into the pathogenesis of choroideremia: a tale of two REPs. Ophthalmic Genet 1996; 17:43–6.
209. Sharon D, Sandberg MA, Caruso RC, et al. Shared mutations in NR2E3 in enhanced S-cone syndrome, Goldmann–Favre syndrome, and many cases of clumped pigmentary retinal degeneration. Arch Ophthalmol 2003; 121:1316–23.
210. Sharon D, Sandberg MA, Rabe VW, et al. RP2 and RPGR mutations and clinical correlations in patients with X-linked retinitis pigmentosa. Am J Hum Genet 2003; 73: 1131–46.
211. Simonelli F, Testa F, Zernant J, et al. Genotype–phenotype correlation in Italian families with Stargardt disease. Ophthalmic Res 2005; 37:159–67.
212. Smith JL, Hoyt WF, Susac JO. Ocular fundus in acute Leber optic neuropathy. Arch Ophthalmol 1973; 90:349–54.
213. Sparrow JR, Nakanishi K, Parish CA. The lipofuscin fluorophore A2E mediates blue light-induced damage to retinal pigmented epithelial cells. Invest Ophthalmol Vis Sci 2000; 41:1981–9.
214. Sprecher H, Luthria DL, Mohammed BS, Baykousheva SP. Reevaluation of the pathways for the biosynthesis of polyunsaturated fatty acids. J Lipid Res 1995; 36: 2471–7.
215. Stecher H, Gelb MH, Saari JC, Palczewski K. Preferential release of 11-cis-retinol from retinal pigment epithelial cells in the presence of cellular retinaldehyde-binding protein. J Biol Chem 1999; 274:8577–85.
216. Stone EM, Lotery AJ, Munier FL, et al. A single EFEMP1 mutation associated with both Malattia Leventinese and Doyne honeycomb retinal dystrophy. Nat Genet 1999; 22: 199–202.
217. Strom TM, Nyakatura G, Apfelstedt-Sylla E, et al. An L-type calcium-channel gene mutated in incomplete X-linked congenital stationary night blindness. Nat Genet 1998; 19:260–3.
218. Sunness JS, Carr RE. Abnormalities of cone and rod function. In: Ryan SJ, ed. Retina. Vol. 1. Philadelphia: Elsevier Mosby, 2006:512–7.
219. Swaroop A, Wang QL, Wu W, et al. Leber congenital amaurosis caused by a homozygous mutation (R90W) in the homeodomain of the retinal transcription factor CRX: direct evidence for the involvement of CRX in the development of photoreceptor function. Hum Mol Genet 1999; 8:299–305.

220. Syed N, Smith JE, John SK, et al. Evaluation of retinal photoreceptors and pigment epithelium in a female carrier of choroideremia. Ophthalmology 2001; 108:711–20.
221. Takada Y, Fariss RN, Tanikawa A, et al. A retinal neuronal developmental wave of retinoschisin expression begins in ganglion cells during layer formation. Invest Ophthalmol Vis Sci 2004; 45:3302–12.
222. Takahashi T, Nakamura T, Hayashi A, et al. Inhibition of experimental choroidal neovascularization by overexpression of tissue inhibitor of metalloproteinases-3 in retinal pigment epithelium cells. Am J Ophthalmol 2000; 130:774–81.
223. Thompson DA, Gal A. Vitamin A metabolism in the retinal pigment epithelium: genes, mutations, and diseases. Prog Retin Eye Res 2003; 22:683–703.
224. Thompson DA, Janecke AR, Lange J, et al. Retinal degeneration associated with RDH12 mutations results from decreased 11-cis retinal synthesis due to disruption of the visual cycle. Hum Mol Genet 2005; 14:3865–75.
225. Thompson DA, Li Y, McHenry CL, et al. Mutations in the gene encoding lecithin retinol acyltransferase are associated with early-onset severe retinal dystrophy. Nat Genet 2001; 28:123–4.
226. Thompson DA, McHenry CL, Li Y, et al. Retinal dystrophy due to paternal isodisomy for chromosome 1 or chromosome 2, with homoallelism for mutations in RPE65 or MERTK, respectively. Am J Hum Genet 2002; 70:224–9.
227. To K, Adamian M, Dryja TP, Berson EL. Histopathologic study of variation in severity of retinitis pigmentosa due to the dominant rhodopsin mutation Pro23His. Am J Ophthalmol 2002; 134:290–3.
228. Tso MO, Zhang C, Abler AS, et al. Apoptosis leads to photoreceptor degeneration in inherited retinal dystrophy of RCS rats. Invest Ophthalmol Vis Sci 1994; 35: 2693–9.
229. Tuson M, Marfany G, Gonzalez-Duarte R. Mutation of CERKL, a novel human ceramide kinase gene, causes autosomal recessive retinitis pigmentosa (RP26). Am J Hum Genet 2004; 74:128–38.
230. Valtonen M, Nanto-Salonen K, Heinanen K, et al. Skeletal muscle of patients with gyrate atrophy of the choroid and retina and hyperornithinaemia in ultralow-field magnetic resonance imaging and computed tomography. J Inherit Metab Dis 1996; 19:729–34.
231. Valtonen M, Nanto-Salonen K, Jaaskelainen S, et al. Central nervous system involvement in gyrate atrophy of the choroid and retina with hyperornithinaemia. J Inherit Metab Dis 1999; 22:855–66.
232. van der Spuy J, Cheetham ME. The Leber congenital amaurosis protein AIPL1 modulates the nuclear translocation of NUB1 and suppresses inclusion formation by NUB1 fragments. J Biol Chem 2004; 279:48038–47.
233. Vasireddy V, Vijayasarathy C, Huang J, et al. Stargardt-like macular dystrophy protein ELOVL4 exerts a dominant negative effect by recruiting wild-type protein into aggresomes. Mol Vis 2005; 11:665–76.
234. Votruba M. Molecular genetic basis of primary inherited optic neuropathies. Eye 2004; 18:1126–32.
235. Vranka JA, Johnson E, Zhu X, et al. Discrete expression and distribution pattern of TIMP-3 in the human retina and choroid. Curr Eye Res 1997; 16:102–10.
236. Wang T, Milam AH, Steel G, Valle D. A mouse model of gyrate atrophy of the choroid and retina. Early retinal pigment epithelium damage and progressive retinal degeneration. J Clin Invest 1996; 97:2753–62.
237. Wang T, Steel G, Milam AH, Valle D. Correction of ornithine accumulation prevents retinal degeneration in a mouse model of gyrate atrophy of the choroid and retina. Proc Natl Acad Sci U S A 2000; 97:1224–9.
238. Wang Y, Macke JP, Merbs SL, et al. A locus control region adjacent to the human red and green visual pigment genes. Neuron 1992; 9:429–40.
239. Weber BH, Vogt G, Pruett RC, et al. Mutations in the tissue inhibitor of metalloproteinases-3 (TIMP3) in patients with Sorsby's fundus dystrophy. Nat Genet 1994; 8:352–6.
240. Webster AR, Heon E, Lotery AJ, et al. An analysis of allelic variation in the ABCA4 gene. Invest Ophthalmol Vis Sci 2001; 42:1179–89.
241. Weingeist TA, Kobrin JL, Watzke RC. Histopathology of Best's macular dystrophy. Arch Ophthalmol 1982; 100: 1108–14.
242. Weleber RG, Kennaway NG. Clinical trial of vitamin B6 for gyrate atrophy of the choroid and retina. Ophthalmology 1981; 88:316–24.
243. Weleber RG, Miyake Y. Familial optic atrophy with negative electroretinograms. Arch Ophthalmol 1992; 110:640–5.
244. Weleber RG, Francis PJ. Differential diagnosis of the electronegative electroretinogram. In: Heckenlively JR, Arden GB, eds. Priniciples and Practice of Clinical Electrophysiology of Vision. Cambridge: MIT Press, 2006:809–22.
245. Weston MD, Luijendijk MW, Humphrey KD, et al. Mutations in the VLGR1 gene implicate G-protein signaling in the pathogenesis of Usher syndrome type II. Am J Hum Genet 2004; 74:357–66.
246. Wilkie SE, Li Y, Deery EC, et al. Identification and functional consequences of a new mutation (E155G) in the gene for GCAP1 that causes autosomal dominant cone dystrophy. Am J Hum Genet 2001; 69:471–80.
247. Wilson DJ, Weleber RG, Green WR. Ocular clinicopathologic study of gyrate atrophy. Am J Ophthalmol 1991; 111: 24–33.
248. Wu WW, Wong JP, Kast J, Molday RS. RS1, a discoidin domain-containing retinal cell adhesion protein associated with X-linked retinoschisis, exists as a novel disulfide-linked octamer. J Biol Chem 2005; 280: 10721–30.
249. Xi Q, Pauer GJ, Marmorstein AD, et al. Tubby-like protein 1 (TULP1) interacts with F-actin in photoreceptor cells. Invest Ophthalmol Vis Sci 2005; 46:4754–61.
250. Yanez-Munoz RJ, Balaggan KS, MacNeil A, et al. Effective gene therapy with nonintegrating lentiviral vectors. Nat Med 2006; 12:348–53.
251. Yang Z, Peachey NS, Moshfeghi DM, et al. Mutations in the RPGR gene cause X-linked cone dystrophy. Hum Mol Genet 2002; 11:605–11.
252. Yeow KM, Kishnani NS, Hutton M, et al. Sorsby's fundus dystrophy tissue inhibitor of metalloproteinases-3 (TIMP-3) mutants have unimpaired matrix metalloproteinase inhibitory activities, but affect cell adhesion to the extracellular matrix. Matrix Biol 2002; 21:75–88.
253. Yokokura S, Wada Y, Nakai S, et al. Targeted disruption of FSCN2 gene induces retinopathy in mice. Invest Ophthalmol Vis Sci 2005; 46:2905–15.
254. Yuan L, Kawada M, Havlioglu N, et al. Mutations in PRPF31 inhibit pre-mRNA splicing of rhodopsin gene and cause apoptosis of retinal cells. J Neurosci 2005; 25: 748–57.
255. Zeitz C, van Genderen M, Neidhardt J, et al. Mutations in GRM6 cause autosomal recessive congenital stationary night blindness with a distinctive scotopic 15-Hz flicker

electroretinogram. Invest Ophthalmol Vis Sci 2005; 46: 4328–35.

256. Zeng Y, Takada Y, Kjellstrom S, et al. RS-1 Gene delivery to an adult Rs1h knockout mouse model restores ERG b-wave with reversal of the electronegative waveform of X-linked retinoschisis. Invest Ophthalmol Vis Sci 2004; 45: 3279–85.

257. Zhang XM, Yang Z, Karan G, et al. Elovl4 mRNA distribution in the developing mouse retina and phylogenetic conservation of Elovl4 genes. Mol Vis 2003; 9:301–7.

Abbreviations

when used as a prefix with a Mendelian Inheritance in Man (MIM number) it indicates a descriptive entry and not a unique locus
+ when used as a prefix with a Mendelian Inheritance in Man (MIM number) it indicates that the entry contains a description of known sequence and a phenotype
% when used as a prefix with a Mendelian Inheritance in Man (MIM number) it indicates that the entry describes a confirmed mendelian phenotype or phenotypic locus for which the underlying molecular basis is not known
***** when used as a prefix with a Mendelian Inheritance in Man (MIM number) it indicates a gene of known sequence
αβ T-cell a subset of T cells with a distinct T cell receptor on their surface with one α cahin and one β
γδ T-cell a subset of T cells with a distinct T cell receptor on their surface with one γ chain and one δ
α-MSH α-melanocyte-stimulating hormone
α-SYN α-synuclein
A adenine and anisotropic
Aβ amyloid beta
A2B5 a type 2 astrocyte precursor marker
A2E a vitamin A-based fluorophore in lipofuscin
A3AR the gene for adenosine receptor A3
AA amyloid protein A, apparent anisotrophy
AANF atrial natriuric factor
AApoAI apolipoprotein AI derived amyloid
AApoAII apolipoprotein AII derived amyloid
AApoAIV apolipoprotein AIV derived amyloid
AASS a gene on chromosome 7 (7q31.3) that codes for α-aminoadipic semialdehyde synthase
AASV ANCA-associated vasculitides
AAV adeno-associated virus
Aβ Aβ protein precursor
Aβ_2M β_2-microglobulin derived protein
ABCA4 the ATP-binding cassette transporter retinal gene on chromosome 1 (1p22.1–p21) (also known as *ABCR*, *RP19*, and *STGD1*)
Abca4 the murine ATP-binding cassette transporter retinal gene
ABCA7 adenosine triphoshate binding cassette protein A7
ABCC6 a gene on chromosome 16 (16p13.1) that causes pseudoxanthoma elasticum when mutated
ABCD1 the gene for ATP-binding cassette subfamily D member 1 on the X chromosome (Xq28)
ABCG5 the ATP-binding cassette subfamily G member 5 gene on chromosome 2 (2p21)
ABCG8 a ATP-binding cassette subfamily G member 8 gene on chromosome 2 (2p21)
ABCR ATP-binding cassette transporter
ABCR the ATP-binding cassette gene on chromosome 1 (1p21–p13) (also known as *ABCA4*, *RP19*, and *STGD1*)
AC anterior chamber
ACA anticentromere antibody
ACAID anterior chamber associated immune deviation
ACal calcitonin derived amyloid
ACE angiotensin-converting enzyme
ACE gene for angiotensin-converting enzyme on chromosome 17 (17q23)
ACL **A**cromegaloid features, **C**utis verticis gyrata and **L**eukoma syndrome
ACR acetylcholine receptor and American College of Rheumatology
ACTA1 the α-actin sketetal muscle gene on chromosome 1 (1q42.1)
ACTA2 the α-2 actin smooth muscle gene on chromosome 10 (10q22–q24)
ACTB the β-actin gene on chromosome 7 (7p22–p12)
ACTC the α-actin cardiac muscle gene on chromosome 15 (15q14) (also known as *ACTC1)*
ACTG1 the γ-1 actin gene on chromosome 17 (17q25.3)
ACTG2 the γ-2 actin gene on chromosome 2 (2p13.1)
ACTH adrenocorticotrophin
ACys cystatin C derived amyloid
AD autosomal dominant, Alzheimer disease
AD1 an autosomal dominant familial type of Alzheimer disease
AD2 a type of Alzheimer disease associated with the APOE*4 allele on chromosome 19
AD3 a type of Alzheimer disease caused by *PSEN1* mutations
AD4 a type of Alzheimer disease caused by *PSEN2* mutations
Ad5E1 early region 1 of human adenovirus type 5
Ad5E1A early region 1A of human adenovirus type 5
ADAID anterior chamber associated immune deviation
ADAMTS10 the gene on chromosome 19 (19p13.3–p13.2) that codes for a disintegrin-like and metalloproteinase with thrombospondin type 1 motif
ADC apparent diffusion coefficient
ADCC antibody-dependent cell mediated cytotoxicity
adCOD autosomal dominant cone dystrophy
adCORD autosomal dominant cone-rod dystrophy
adCSNB autosomal dominant congenital stationary night blindness
ADEN acute disseminated epidermal necrosis
ADH aldehyde dehydrogenase
ADM2 adrenomodulin 2; also known as intermedin
adMD autosomal dominant macular dystrophy
ADOA autosomal dominant optic atrophy
ADP adenosine diphosphate

ADR adverse drug reaction
adRP autosomal dominant retinitis pigmentosa
ADTB3A the gene on chromosome 5 (5q14.1) that causes Hermansky–Pudlak syndrome type 2 when mutated (also known as *HPS1* and *AP3B1)*
ADVIRC **A**utosomal **D**ominant **Vi**treo **R**etino **C**horoidopathy
AEC ankyloblepharon-ectodermal dysplasia-cleft lip/palate
AEF amyloid enhancing factor
AEI/AE3 a pancytokeratin antibody
aFGF acidic fibroblast growth factor
AFib fibrinogen α-chain derived amyloid
AGA the aspartlglycosaminidase gene on chromosome 4 (4q32–q33)
AGC1 the aggregan gene on chromosome 15 (15q26.1)
AGE advanced glycation end-product
AGel gelsolin derived amyloid
AgKS antigenic keratan sulfate
AGL the glycogen debranching enzyme gene on chromosome 1 (1p21)
AGRN the tenascin gene on chromosome 1 (1pter–p32)
AH gamma globulin heavy chain derived amyloid
AHC acute hemorrhagic conjunctivitis
AIAPP islet amyloid polypeptide derived amyloid
AIDS acquired immune deficiency syndrome
AIF apoptosis inducing factor
AIMP2B intergral membrane protein derived amyloid
AIns insulin derived amyloid
AIPL1 the arylhydrocarbon-interacting receptor protein-like 1 gene on chromosome 17 (17p13.1) (also known as *LCA4)*
AKC acute keratoconjunctivitis
AKAP2 the gene for A-kinase anchor protein 2 on chromosome 9 (9q31–q33)
AKAP2 A-kinase anchor protein 2
AKer kerato-epithelin (transforming growth factor beta induced protein) derived amyloid
AKT a protein kinase product of an oncogene
AKT1 an oncogene on chromosome 14 (14q32.3)
AL amyloid protein L (amyloid light chain protein)
Ala alanine
ALac lactoferrin derived amyloid
ALCL anaplastic large cell lymphoma
ALDH aldehyde dehydrogenase
ALDH1A1 aldehyde dehydrogenase family 1 , subfamily A, member 1
ALDH3A1 aldehyde dehydrogenase family 3 , subfamily A, member 1
ALDOA the fructose 1,6-biphosphate aldolase A gene on chromosome 16 (16q22–q24)
ALK anterior lamellar keratectomy
ALL acute lymphoblastic leukemia
ALSG aplasia of the lacrimal and salivary glands
ALV avian leukosis virus
ALys lysozyme derived amyloid
AMD age-related macular degeneration
AMed medin amyloid (lactadherin derived amyloid)
AMP adenosine monophosphate
AMS ablepharon–macrostomia syndrome
An adult nucleus of crystalline lens
ANA antinuclear antibodies
ANCA anti-neutrophil cytoplasmic antibody
ANCL adult neuronal ceroid-lipofuscinosis
ANG1 angiopoetin-1
ANG2 angiopoetin-2
Ank the mouse gene for progressive ankylosis
ANKH a gene on chromosome 5 (5q15.2–p14.1) that is a homolog of the murine *Ank* gene
ANS 8-anilino-l-naphthalenesulfonate
ANT adenine translocator, adenosine nucleotide translocator (also known as ADP/ATP translocator)
Anti-CCP anti-cyclic citrullinated peptide
Anti-La an antibody to SS-B
Anti-Ro an antibody to SS-A
ANVOs abortive neovascular outgrowths
Anx1 annexin 1
AP amyloid p-component
AP sites apurinic/pyrimidinic sites
Apaf-1 apoptotic protease activating factor 1
AP3B1 the gene on chromosome 5 (5q14.1) that causes Hermansky–Pudlak syndrome type 2 when mutated (also known as *HPS2* and *ADTB3A)*
APC antigen presenting cell; adenomatous polyposis coli; and the encoded product of the *APC* gene
APC the gene responsible for adenomatous polyposis coli
APECED **A**utoimmune, **P**oly**E**ndocrinopathy, **C**andidiasis, and **E**ctodermal dystrophy
aPL anti-phospholipid
APO1 cell surface death receptor 2 (also known as CD95)
APO2 death receptor 4 (DR4) (also known as tumor necrosis factor related apoptosis-inducing ligand receptor 1[TRAILR1])
APO2L tumor necrosis factor-related apoptosis inducing ligand (TRAIL)
APO3 death receptor 3 (DR3) (also known as LARD, TRAMP and WSL1)
apoA apolipoprotein A
APOA1 the gene for apolipoprotein AI on chromosome 11 (11q23)
APOA2 the gene for apolipoprotein AII on chromosome 1 (1q21–q23)
APOA4 the gene for apolipoprotein AIV on chromosome 11 (11q23)
apoB apolipoprotein B
APOB the gene for apolipoprotein B on chromosome 2 (2p24–p23)
APOD the gene for apolipoprotein D on chromosome 3 (3q26.2–qter)
apoE apolipoprotein E
APOE the gene for apolipoprotein E on chromosome 19 (19q13.2)
APP a amyloid precursor protein gene on chromosome 21 (21q)
APro prolactin derived amyloid
APrP prion protein derived amyloid
APS antiphospholipid syndrome
APUD cells **A**mine **P**recursor **U**ptake and **D**ecarboxylation cells
AqH aqueous humor
AQP aquaporin
AQP0 aquaporin 0

AR autosomal recessive or aldose reductase
ARA American Rheumatism Association (a former name for the American College of Rheumatology)
ARAT retinal acyltransferase
arCOD autosomal recessive cone dystrophy
arCORD autosomal recessive cone-rod dystrophy
AREDS age-related eye disease study
AREDSII age-related eye disease study II
Arf the murine gene for a protein that stabilizes p53
ARF cyclin-dependent kinase inhibitor 2A (also known as p14)
Arg arginine
ARIX a homolog of the Drosophila aristaless homeobox gene on chromosome 11 (11q13.3–q13.4)
arLCA autosomal recessive Leber congenital amaurosis
ARN acute retinal necrosis
arRP autosomal recessive retinitis pigmentosa
ARS Axenfeld–Rieger syndrome
ARSA the arylsulfatase A gene on chromosome 22 (22q13.31)
ARSB the arylsulfatase B gene on chromosome 5 (5q11–q13)
AS ankylosing spondylitis
ASA the reduced form of ascorbic acid and arylsulfatase A
ASAH the ceramidase gene on chromosome 8 (8p22–p21.3)
ASD anterior segment dysgenesis
Ash a murine gene that is expressed in retinal progenitor cells
ASM acid sphingomyelinase
ASMD anterior segment mesenchymal dysgenesis
Asn asparagine
Asp aspartate
ASPA the aspartocyclase gene on chromosome 17 (17pter–p13)
ASPN the asporin gene on chromosome 9 (9q21.3–q22)
AT ataxia telangiectasia
Ath3 a murine gene that is expressed in retinal progenitor cells
Ath5 a murine gene that is expressed in retinal progenitor cells
ATM the gene on chromosome 11 (11q22.3) that causes ataxia-telangiectasia when mutated
ATP adenosine triphosphate
ATP7A a copper transport P-type adenosine triphosphatase gene on the X chromosome (Xq13)
ATP7B a copper transport P-type adenosine triphosphatase gene on chromosome 13 (13q14.3)
ATPase adenosine triphosphatase
ATTR transthyretin derived amyloid
ATV acute transforming viruses
AUG the codon for methionine
AVM arteriovenous malformation

B2M the β_2-microglobulin gene on chromosome 15 (15q21–q22)
b-HLH-Zip a family of transcription factors that bind to DNA as dimers
β2GP1 β2 glycoprotein 1
βTG β-thromboglobulin
B7 family a group of immunoadjuvant molecules
BAD/Bad BCL2 antagonist of cell death
BAER brainstem evoked response
BALT bronchus associated lymphoid tissue
Bax BCL2-associated X protein
Bak BCL2 antagonist killer 1, also known as BAK1, BCL2L7
BAK benzalkonium chloride
BB an airgun with a smooth bore barrel
BCC basal cell carcinoma
B cell B lymphocyte
BCD Bietti crystalline dystrophy
BCG Bacillus Calmette-Guérin
BCL-1 cyclin D1 (also known as PRAD1)
Bcl-2 an anti-apoptotic factor (also known as B-cell lymphoma 27
Bcl-3 oncogene B-cell lymphoma 3 (formerly Bcl-4)
Bcl-XL a regulator of apoptosis found in mitochondrial membranes
Bcl-w a member of the bcl-2 family
BCL2 the Bcl-2 gene on chromosome 18 (18q21.3)
BCNU bis (chloroethyl) -1-nitrosourea
BCOR the BCL6 corepressor gene on the X chromosome (Xp11.4)
BCR/ABL a fusion gene at the breakpoint cluster region on chromosome 22 (22q11.27)
BCS brittle cornea syndrome
BCSH a gene that codes a component of the mitochondrial respiratory chain complex III
BD Behçet disease
BDNF brain-derived neurotrophic factor
BDUMP bilateral diffuse uveal melanocytic proliferation
BE receptors binding apo-E lipoprotein
BED Bornholm eye disease
bFGF basic fibroblast growth factor (also known as FGF2)
BFP biologic false-positive
BGN the biglycan gene on the X chromosome (Xq28)
BH domains a fragment of the Rho family (RhoGAPS) with guanosine triphoshate hydrolase activity
bHLH basic helix–loop–helix
bHLHZip basic-helix–loop/leucine zipper
Bid/BID BH3-interacting domain death agonist
BIGH3 a former abbreviation for the *TGFBI* gene
BIM/Bim a portion of the Bcl-2 family produced by the *BIM* gene
BIR baculoviral inhibitor of apoptosis (IAP) repeats
BIR2 the second domain of baculoviral inhibitor of apoptosis repeat
BIR3 the third domain of baculoviral inhibitor of apoptosis repeat
BKV a human polyomavirus
BLD basal laminar deposit (basal linear deposit)
BLOC1S3 the gene on chromosome 19 (19q13) that causes Hermansky–Pudlak syndrome type 8 when mutated
bp base pairs
BMI body mass index
BMPR1A the gene for bone morphogenetic protein receptor type IA on chromosome 10 (10q22.3)
BMPR2 the bone morphogenetic protein receptor type II gene on chromosome 2 (2q33)
BMT bone marrow transplantation

Bok a BCL2 related protein involved in apoptosis
BP benzo(a)pyrene, blood pressure
BPAG1 bullous pemphigoid antigen 1
BPES blepharophimosis-ptosis-epicanthus inversus syndrome
BRCA1 breast cancer 1 gene on chromosome 17 (17q21)
BRCA1 the growth inhibitory factor secreted by breast epithelium that is encoded by the *BRCA1* gene
BRCA2 breast cancer 2 gene on chromosome 13 (13q12.3)
Brn3b a murine gene for a transcription factor needed for retinal ganglion cell differentiation
Brn3b a murine transcription factor needed for retinal ganglion cell differentiation
BRUCE baculoviral inhibitor of apoptosis (BIR) repeat containing ubiquitin-conjugating enzyme
BSA bovine serum albumin
BSE bovine spongioform encephalopathy (also known as "mad cow disease")
bZIP basic region leucine zipper

c crystalline lens cortex
C cytosine
C1 first component of complement
C1q q subfraction of first component of complement
C1r r subfraction of first component of complement
C1s s subfraction of first component of complement
C2 second component of complement
C2a a fragment of second component of complement
C2b b fragment of second component of complement
C3 third component of complement
C3a a fragment of third component of complement
C3b b fragment of third component of complement
C3d d fragment of third component of complement
C4 fourth component of complement
C4b b fragment of fourth component of complement
C4S chondroitin-4-sulfate
C5 fifth component of complement
C5a a fragment of fifth component of complement
C5b b fragment of fifth component of complement
C5b67 complex of C5b with C6 and C7
C6 sixth component of complement
C6S chondroitin-6-sulfate
C7 seventh component of complement
C8 eighth component of complement
C9 ninth component of complement
Ca^{2+} calcium ions
Ca^{2+}-stimulated ATPase calcium stimulated adenosine triphosphatase
CA cytosine-adenine dinucleotide
CA15.3 cancer antigen 15.3 (an ocofetal antigen)
CA4 the carbonic anhydrase IV gene on chromosome 17 (17q23.2) (also known as *RP17*)
CACNA1F the calcium channel-voltge dependent alpha-IF subunit on the X chromosome (Xp11.23) (also known as *CSNB2*)
CaGC calgranulin C
CAK chronic actinic keratopathy
CALCA the (pro)calcitonin gene on chromosome 11 (11p15.2–p15)
CALLA common acute lymphoblastic antigen
CALT conjunctiva associated lymphoid tissue
CAM 5.2 an antibody that recognizes low molecular weight cytokeratin
CAMAK Cataract, **M**icrocephaly, **A**rthrogryposis and **K**yphosis
CAMFAK Cataract, **M**icrocephaly, **F**ailure to thrive, **A**rthrogryposis and **K**yphosis
cAMP cyclic adenosine monophosphate
CAM cell adhesion molecule
CAM5.2 a pancytokeratin antibody
cANCA cytoplasmic staining anti-neutrophil cytoplasmic antibody
Cap capsule
CAR cancer-associated retinopathy
CARD caspase recruitment domain
CASR a gene on chromosome 3 (3q13.3–q21) that codes for an extracellular calcium-sensing receptor
CATT cytosine-adenine-thymine-thymine
CBH cutaneous basophil hypersensitivity
CBS the cystathionine beta-synthase gene on chromosome 21 (21q22.3)
CCP cyclic citrullinated peptide
CCR2 the chemokine CC motif receptor 2 gene on chromosome 3 (3p21)
CCR3 the chemokine CC motif receptor 3
CCR4 the chemokine CC motif receptor 4
CCR5 the chemokine CC motif receptor 5 gene on chromosome 3 (3p21)
CCRG cooperative cataract research group
CCS Churg Strauss syndrome
CD cluster of differentiation antigen
CD4 marker for helper T lymphocytes
CD8 marker for suppressor T lymphocytes
CD11b receptor for C3bi (also known as CR3, Mac-1 antigen)
CD11c receptor for C3bi and C3dg (also known as CR4)
CD14 monocyte differentiation antigen (also known as myeloid cell-specific leucine-rich glycoprotein)
CD18 a leucocyte cell adhesion molecule (also known as integrin-beta 2)
CD19 CD19 B lymphocyte antigen
CD19 the gene on chromosome 16(16p11.2) for the CD19 B lymphocyte antigen
Cd21 receptor for C3d (also known as CR2)
CD25 interleukin 2 receptor alpha (also known as TAC antigen)
CD26 a T-cell activation antigen (also known as adenosine deaminase complexing protein 2)
CD31 platelet-endothelial cell adhesion molecule 1; a vascular emdothelial cell marker
CD34 hematopoietic progenitor cell antigen; a vascular emdothelial cell marker
CD35 receptor for C3b (also known as CR1)
CD36 leukocyte differentiation antigen
CD40 an immunoadjuvant molecule
CD46 membrane cofactor protein; the measles virus receptor

CD55 decay-accelerating factor for complement (also known as Cromer blood group)
CD59 protectin (also known as human leukocyte antigen MIC11)
CD62 also known as GMP-140 and granule membrane protein
CD68 a macrophage antigen (also known as macrosialin)
CD80 an immunoadjuvant molecule
CD86 an immunoadjuvant molecule
CD91 low density lipoprotein receptor-related protein 1 (also known as apolipoprotein receptor)
CD95 FAS (also known as aopotosis antigen 1 and FAS antigen)
CD99 surface antigen MIC2
CD117 stem cell factor receptor (also known as c-kit)
CDB corneal dystrophy of Bowman layer and the superficial stroma
CDC Centers for Disease Control and Prevention
Cdc27 cell division cycle 27 homolog
CDH11 the cadherin 11 gene on chromosome on 17 (17q21–q22.1))
CDH23 the cadherin 23 gene on chromosome on 10 (10q22)
Cdk cyclin-dependent kinase
CDK climatic droplet keratopathy
CDK4 cyclin-dependent kinase 4
CDKN2A the cyclin-dependent kinase inhibitor 2A gene on chromosome 9 (9p21)
cDNA complimentary deoxyribonucleic acid
CDP cytidine diphosphate
CEA carcinoembryonic antigen
CERKL the ceramide kinase-like protein gene on chromosome 2 (2q31.3) (also known as *RP26*)
CETP cholesterol ester transfer protein
CEV cell-associated virus
CF complement fixation
CFEOM congenital fibrosis of the extraocular muscles
CFEOM1 congenital fibrosis of the extraocular muscles type 1
CFEOM2 congenital fibrosis of the extraocular muscles type 2
CFH complement factor H
CFH the gene for complement factor H on chromosome 1 (1q32)
CG cytosine-guanine dinucleotide
cGMP cyclic guanosine monophosphate
CGRP calcitonin gene-related peptide
CHARGE association coloboma, heart defects, choanal atresia, mental retardation, genitourinary defects, and ear anomalies
CHED congenital hereditary endothelial dystrophy
CHED1 congenital hereditary endothelial dystrophy type 1
CHED2 congenital hereditary endothelial dystrophy type 2
CHIP 28 aquaporin 1 (also known as aquaporin-CHIP)
CHM choroideremia
CHRNA1 the gene for the α subunit of the acetylcholine receptor on chromosome 2 (2q24–q32)
CHRNB1 the gene for the β subunit of the acetylcholine receptor on chromosome 17 (17p12–p11)
CHRND the gene for the δ subunit of the acetylcholine receptor chromosome 2 (2q33–q34)
CHRND1 the gene for the δ subunit of the acetylcholine receptor on chromosome 2 (2q33–q34)
CHRNE the gene for the ε subunit of the acetylcholine receptor on chromosome 17 (17p13–p12)
CHRNE1 the gene for the ε subunit of the acetylcholine receptor on chromosome 17 (17p13–p12)
CHRPE congenital hypertrophy of the retinal pigment epithelium
CHS1 the gene on chromosome 1 (1q34) that causes Chédiak–Higashi syndrome when mutated
CHST5 the carbohydrate sulfotransferase 5 gene on chromosome 16 (16q22)
CHST6 the carbohydrate sulfotransferase 6 gene on chromosome 16 (16q22)
CHX10 a gene that is abundantly expressed in the retina (also known as the homeobox 10 gene)
C-Fos a proto-oncogene involved in cellular proliferation
c-IAP2 an inhibitor of apoptosis
CIAS1 the gene on chromosome 1 (1q44) that is mutated in familial cold hypersensitivity and the Muckel–Wells syndrome
c-Jun a proto-oncogene
CIN conjunctival intraepithelial neoplasm
CI-MPR cation-independent mannose-phosphate receptor
CJD Creutzfeldt-Jakob disease
Ckd4 cyclin-dependent kinases 4
CLDN19 the claudin 12gene on chromosome 1 (1p34.2)
CLL chronic lymphocytic leukemia
CLN ceroid lipofuscinosis, neuronal
CLN1 ceroid lipofuscinosis, neuronal type 1 (also known as infantile neuronal ceroid lipofuscinosis)
CLN1 the palmitoyl-protein thioesterase-1 gene on chromosome 1 (1p32)
CLN2 ceroid lipofuscinosis, neuronal type 2 (also known as late infantile neuronal ceroid lipofuscinosis)
CLN2 the gene on chromosome 11 (11p15.5) that is responsible for ceroid lipofuscinosis, neuronal type 2
CLN3 ceroid lipofuscinosis, neuronal type 3; also known as juvenile neuronal ceroid lipofuscinosis
CLN3 the gene on chromosome 16 (16p12.1) that is responsible for ceroid lipofuscinosis, neuronal type 3
CLN4 ceroid lipofuscinosis, neuronal type 4 (also known as adult neuronal ceroid lipofuscinosis)
CLN5 ceroid lipofuscinosis, neuronal type 5 (also known as variant late infantile neuronal ceroid lipofuscinosis)
CLN5 the gene on chromosme 13 (13q21.1–q32) that is responsible for ceroid lipofuscinosis, neuronal type 5
CLN6 ceroid lipofuscinosis, neuronal type 6 (also known as variant late infantile neuronal ceroid lipofuscinosis)
CLN6 the gene on chromosome 15 (15q21–q23) that is responsible for ceroid lipofuscinosis, neuronal type 6
CLN7 ceroid lipofuscinosis, neuronal type 7
CLN8 ceroid lipofuscinosis, neuronal type 8 (also known as Turkish variant late infantile neuronal ceroid lipofuscinosis)
CLN8 the gene on chromosome 8 (8pter–p22) that is responsible for ceroid lipofuscinosis, neuronal type 8
CLN9 ceroid lipofuscinosis, neuronal type 9

CLU gene for clusterin on chromosome 8 (8p21–p12)
cm centimeter
cM centimorgan
CME cystoid macular edema
CMV cytomegalovirus
CNBr cyanogen bromide
CNCG the gene on chromosome 4 (4p12) that codes for the alpha subunit of the rod cyclic guanosine monophosphate-gated channel (also known as *CNGA1 and CNCG1*)
CNCG1 the gene on chromosome 4 (4p12) that codes for the alpha subunit of the rod cyclic guanosine monophosphate-gated channel (also known as *CNCG and CNGA1*)
CNGA cyclic nucleotide-gated channel
CNGA1 the gene on chromosome 4 (4p12) that codes for the alpha subunit of the rod cyclic guanosine monophosphate-gated channel (also known as *CNCG and CNCG1*)
CNGA3 the cyclic nucleotide-gated channel alpha-3 gene on chromosome 2 (2q11.2)
CNGB3 the cyclic nucleotide-gated channel beta-3 gene on chromosome 8 (8q21–q22)
CNS central nervous system
CNV choroidal neovascularization
CO2 carbon dioxide
CoA coenzyme A
CO-Ag a cornea associated antigen (also known as corneal calgranulin C)
COI a mitochondrial DNA cytochrome c oxidase subunit I gene of respiratory Complex IV (also known as *MTCO1*)
COII a mitochondrial DNA cytochrome c oxidase subunit II gene of respiratory Complex IV (also known as *MTCO2*)
COIII a mitochondrial DNA cytochrome c oxidase subunit III gene of respiratory Complex IV (also known as *MTCO3*)
COD cone dystrophy
COD1 the gene on the X chromosome (Xp11.4) for retinitis pigmentosa guanosine triphosphate hydrolase regulator (also known as *RP3, CORDX and RPGR*)
COD2 a locus for cone dystrophy on the X chromosome (Xq27)
COD3 the gene for guanylate cyclase activator 1A on chromosome 6 (6p21.1) (also known as *GUCA1A* and *GCAP1*)
COD4 a locus for cone and cone-rod dystrophy on the X chromosome(Xq11–q13.1)
COG Children's Oncology Group
COL1A1 the collagen type 1 alpha-1 gene on chromosome 17 (17q21.31–q22)
COL2A1 the collagen type II alpha-1 polypeptide gene on chromosome 7 (7q22.1)
COL3A1 the collagen type III alpha-1 polypeptide gene on chromosome 2 (2q31)
COL4A1 the collagen type IV alpha-1 polypeptide gene on chromosome 13 (13q34)
COL4A2 the collagen type IV alpha-2 polypeptide gene on chromosome 13 (13q34)
COL4A3 the collagen type IV alpha-3 polypeptide gene on chromosome 2 (2q36–q37)
COL4A4 the collagen type IV alpha-4 polypeptide gene on chromosome 2 (2q36–q37)
COL4A5 the collagen type IV alpha-5 polypeptide gene on the X chromosome(Xp22.3)
COL4A6 the collagen type IV alpha-6 polypeptide gene on the X chromosome(Xp22.3)
Col5a1 the murine collagen type V alpha-1 polypeptide gene
COL5A1 the collagen type V alpha-1 polypeptide gene on chromosome 9 (9q34.2–q34.3)
COL5A2 the collagen type V alpha-2 polypeptide gene on chromosome 2 (2q31)
COL5A3 the collagen type V alpha-3 polypeptide gene on chromosome 19 (19p13.2)
COL6A1 the collagen type VI alpha-1 polypeptide gene on chromosome 21(21q22.3)
COL6A2 the collagen type VI alpha-2 polypeptide gene on chromosome 21(21q22.3)
COL6A3 the collagen type VI alpha-3 polypeptide gene on chromosome 2 (2q37)
COL7A1 the collagen type VII alpha-1 polypeptide gene on chromosome 3 (3p21.3)
COL8A1 the collagen type VIII alpha-1 polypeptide gene on chromosome 3 (3q12–q13)
COL8A2 the collagen type VIII alpha-2 polypeptide gene on chromosome 1 (1p34.3–p32.3)
Col8a1 the murine collagen type 8 alpha-1 polypeptide gene
Col8a2 the murine gene for collagen type 8 alpha-2 polypeptide
COL9A1 the collagen type IX alpha-1 polypeptide gene on chromosome 6 (6q13)
COL9A2 the collagen type IX alpha-2 polypeptide gene on chromosome 1 (1p33–p32.2)
COL10A1 the collagen type X alpha-1 polypeptide gene on chromosome 6 (6q21–q22.3)
COL11A1 a collagen type XI alpha-1 polypeptide gene on chromosome 1 (1p21)
COL11A2 a collagen type XI alpha-2 polypeptide gene on chromosome 6 (6p21.3)
COL12A1 a collagen type XII alpha-1 polypeptide gene on chromosome 6 (6q12–q13)
COL13A1 the collagen type XIII alpha-1 polypeptide human gene on chromosome 10 (10q22)
COL14A1 a collagen type XIV alpha-1 polypeptide gene on chromosome 8 (8q23)
COL15A1 a collagen type XV alpha-1 polypeptide gene on chromosome 9 (9q21–q22)
COL16A1 a collagen type XVI alpha-1 polypeptide gene on chromosome 1 (1p34)
COL17A1 a collagen type XVII alpha-1 polypeptide gene on chromosome 10 (10q24.3)
COL18A1 a collagen type XVIII alpha-1 polypeptide gene on chromosome 21 (21q22.3)
COL19A1 a collagen type XIX alpha-1 polypeptide gene on chromosome 6 (6q12–q14)
COL20A1 a collagen type XX alpha-1 polypeptide gene on chromosome 20 (20q13.33)

COL21A1 a collagen type XXI alpha-1 polypeptide gene on chromosome 6 (6p12.3–11.2)
COL22A1 a collagen type XXII alpha-1 polypeptide gene on chromosome 8 (8q24.3)
COL23A1 a collagen type XXIII alpha-1 polypeptide gene on chromosome 5 (5q35)
COL24A1 the collagen type XXIV alpha-1 polypeptide gene on chromosome 1 (1p22.3)
COL25A1 a collagen type XXV alpha-1 polypeptide gene on chromosome 4 (4q25)
COL26A1 the collagen type XXVI alpha-1 polypeptide gene on chromosome 7 (7q22.1)
COL27A1 the collagen type XXVII alpha-1 polypeptide gene on chromosome 9 (9q32)
COL28A1 the collagen type XXVIII alpha-1 polypeptide gene on chromosome 7 (7p21.3)
COMP cartilage oligomeric matrix protein
COMS Collaborative Ocular Melanoma Study
ConA concanavalin-A
CORD cone-rod dystrophy
CORD2 the gene on chromosome 19 (19q13.3) that codes for cone-rod otx photoreceptor homeobox transcription factor (also known as *CRX*)
CORD4 a locus for cone-rod dystrophy on chromosome 17 (17q)
CORD6 the retinal-specific guanylate cyclase gene on chromosome 17 (17p13.1) (also known as *LCA1, GUCY2D, and RETGC1*)
CORD7 autosomal dominant cone-rod dystrophy
CORD8 a locus for cone-rod dystrophy on chromosome 1 (1q12–q24)
CORD9 a locus for cone-rod dystrophy on chromosome 8 (8p11)
CORDX the retinitis pigmentosa guanosine triphosphate hydrolase regulator gene on the X chromosome (Xp11.4) (also known as *RP3, RPGR and COD1*)
CORDX2 a locus for cone-rod dystrophy on the X chromosome (Xq27–28)
CORDX3 a locus for cone-rod dystrophy on the X chromosome (Xp11–q13)
CoQ Coenzyme Q also known as ubiquinone
COX10 a nuclear gene on chromosome 17 (17p12–p11.2) that codes a component of the mitochondrial respiratory chain complex IV
COX15 a nuclear gene on chromosome 10 (10q24) that codes a component of the mitochondrial respiratory chain complex IV
CP cicatricial pemphigoid
CP49 an early name for phkinin in the lens
CP115 an early name for filensin; also known as cytoskeletal protein 115 kD
CPE ciliary pigmented epithelium; cyopathic effect
CpG cytosine phosphate guanine dinucleotide
C/PL cholesterol phospholipid ratio
CR1 receptor for C3b (also known as CD35)
CR2 receptor for C3d (also known as CD21)
CR3 receptor for C3bi (also known as CD11b)
CR4 receptor for C3bi and C3dg (also known as CD11c)
CRALBP cellular retinaldehyde-binding protein
CRALBP the cellular retinaldehyde-binding protein gene on chromosome 15 (15q26) (also known as *RLBP1*)
CRB1 a gene on chromosome 1 (1q31–q32.1) that codes for a homolog of Drosophila Crumbs 1 (also known as *RP12*)
CRB(II) intestinal intracytoplasmic retinol-binding protein
CRBP cellular retinol-binding protein; also known as retinol-binding protein 1 (RBP1)
CRBP2 cellular retinol-binding protein 2
CREBBP a gene on chromosome 16 (16p13.3) that codes for a transcription factor for a cAMP-response element binding protein
CREST syndrome calcinosis, Raynaud phenomenon, esophageal dysmotility, sclerodactyly, and telangiectasia syndrome
CRP C-reactive protein
CRP the gene for C-reactive protein
Crry complement receptor related protein
CRS congenital rubella syndrome
C-Rel a member of the Rel/NFκB family of transcription factors
CRX the gene on chromosome 19 (19q13.3) that codes for cone-rod otx photoreceptor homeobox transcription factor (also known as *CORD2*)
CRYAA the alpha-A crystallin gene on chromosome 21 (21q22.3)
CRYAB the B-crystallin gene on chromosome 11 (11q22.1–q23.2)
Cryab the murine gene for αB-crystallin
CRYBB1 the beta-B1 crystallin gene on chromosome 22 (22q11.2–q12.1)
CRYBB2 the gene for βB2-crystallin on chromosome 22 (22q11.2)
CRYBB3 the gene for βB3-crystallin on chromosome 22 (22q11.2)
CRYGC the gene for γC-crystallin on chromosome 2 (2q33–q35)
CRYGD the gene for γD-crystallin on chromosome 2 (2q33–q35)
CRYGS the gene for γS-crystallin on chromosome 3 (3q25–qter)
CS chondroitin sulfate
CSF cerebrospinal fluid
CSNB congenital stationary night blindness
CSNB the calcium channel-voltge dependent alpha-IF subunit on the X chromosome (Xp11.23) (also known as *CACNA1F*)
CSNB1 the nyctalopin gene on the X chromosome (Xp11.4) (also known as *NYX*)
CSNB3 the rod cyclic guanosine monophosphate phosphodiesterase beta subunit gene on chromosome 4 (4p16.3) (also known as *PDE6B*)
CSPG2 the versican gene on chromosome 5 (5q13–q14)
CSPG6 the bamacan gene on chromosome 10 (10q25)
CSS Churg–Strauss syndrome
CST3 the cystatin C gene on chromosome 20 (20p11.2)
CT computed tomography
CTG a cytosine-thymine-guanine trinucleotide
CTAP connective tissue activating protein
CTGF connective tissue growth factor
CTH ceramide trihexoside
CTL cytotoxic T lymphocyte
CTLA4 cytotoxic T lymphocyte-associated antigen 4 (also known as CD152)

CTNS a cystine transporter gene on chromosome 17(17p)
CtmPrP a transmembrane form of prion protein
CTRP5 a collagen–like member of the C1q/tumor necrosis factor superfamily gene on chromosome 11 (11q23.3)
CTRP5 a collagen–like member of the C1q/tumor necrosis factor superfamily
CXCL12 chemokine CXC motif ligand 12 (also known as stromal cell-derived factor 1 (SDF-1)
CXCR2 chemokine (C-X-R) receptor 2 (also known as beta interleukin 8 receptor)
CXCR4 chemokine (C-X-R) receptor 4
Cu2+ cupric ions
CU18 an antibody that recognizes breast carcinoma associated antigen 225
CVD cardiovascular disease
CVS chorionic villous sample
cw cataract webbed (a mutant deer mouse)
Cyclin A2 a cyclin encoded by a gene on chromosome 4 (4q27)
Cyclin B1 a cyclin encoded by a gene on chromosome 5 (5q12)
Cyclin C a cyclin encoded by a gene on chromosome 6 (6q21)
Cyclin E2 a cyclin that controls the initiation of DNA synthesis
Cyclin G1 a cyclin encoded by a gene on chromosome 5 (5q32–q34)
Cyclin T2 a cyclin encoded by a gene on chromosome 2 (2p14–q21.3)
CYP1B1 the cytochrome p450 subfamily 1 polypeptide 1 gene on chromosome 2 (2p22–p21)
CYP4V2 the cytochrome p450 family 4 subfamily V polypeptide 2 gene on chromosome 4 (4q35.1)
CYP27A1 the sterol 27-hydroxylase (also known as cytochrome p450 subfamily XXVIIA polypeptide 1 gene on chromosome 2 (2q33–qter)

1D one-dimensional
1D SDS-PAGE one-dimensional sodium dodecyl sulfate-polyacrylamide gel electrophoresis
2D DIGE two-dimensional difference gel electrophoresis
2D PAGE two-dimensional polyacrylamide gel electrophoresis
3D three dimensional
5D4 an anti-keratan sulfate antibody
D diopter
D2-40 a lymphatic-endothelial marker recognizing podoplanin
Da Dalton
DAF decay-accelerating factor
DAG diaminoglycol
DBS dried blood spot
DC dendritic cell
DCC the "delete in colon cancer" gene on chromosome 18 (18q21.3)
DCN the biglycan gene on chromosome 12(12q13.2)
DCR1 decoy receptor 1 (also known as TRAIL3, tumor necrosis factor related apoptosis-inducing ligand receptor 3 [TRAILR3], death receptor 3 [DR3], and TRAIL receptor without an intracellular domain [TRID], and tumor necrosis factor receptor superfamily member 10C [TNFRSF10C])
DcR2 tumor necrosis factor-related apoptosis inducing ligand 4 (TRAIL4)
DcR3 tumor necrosis factor-related apoptosis inducing ligand (TRAIL) (also known as APO2L)
Dct a murine gene involved in melanin production
DED death effector domains
DES the desmin gene on chromosome 2 (2q35)
DESK Descemet stripping endothelial keratoplasty
DG diacylglycerol
DH delayed hypersensitivity
DHA dehydroascorbic acid
DHEAS dehydroepiandrosterone sulfate
DHICA 5,6-dihydroxyindole-2-carboxylic acid
DHRD Doyne honeycomb retinal dystrophy
DHS dehydroascorbic acid
Diablo direct IAP-binding protein with low PI; also known as second mitochodria-derived activator of caspase (SMAC)
DIDMOAD diabetes insipidus, diabetes mellitus, optic atrophy, and deafness
DIF direct immunofluorescence
DLBCL diffuse large B cell lymphoma
DLD a gene that codes for a component of the pyruvate dehydrogenase complex
DLEK deep lamellar endothelial keratoplasty
dLGN dorsal lateral geniculate nucleus
DLN draining lymph node
DM1 myotonic dystrophy type 1 (also known as classic myotonic dystrophy)
DM2 myotonic dystrophy type 2 (also known as proximal myotonic dystrophy)
DMD the dystrophin gene on the X chromosome (Xp21.2) that causes Duchenne muscular dystrophy when mutated
DMN dimethylnitrosamine
DMPK the dystrophia myotonica protein kinase gene on chromosome 19 (19q13.3)
DMS dimethylsulfate
DNA deoxyribonucleic acid
DNMT3B DNA methyltransferase 3B
DR1 death receptor 1 (also known as TNFR1 and CD120a)
DR2 death receptor 2
DR3 death receptor 3 (also known as lymphocyte-associated receptor of death [LARD],TRAMP, WSL1 decoy receptor 1 [DCR1]; TRAIL3, tumor necrosis factor related apoptosis-inducing ligand receptor 3 [TRAILR3], TRAIL receptor without an intracellular domain [TRID], and tumor necrosis factor receptor superfamily member 25 [TNFRSF25])
DR4 death receptor 4 (also known as tumor necrosis factor - related apoptosis-inducing ligand receptor 4 [TRAILR4], DCR2, TRUNDD, and decoy receptor 2)
DR5 death receptor 5 (also known tumor necrosis factor receptor superfamily, member 10B [TNFR10B], tumor necrosis factor-related apoptosis-inducing ligand receptor 2 [TRAIL2], KILLER and TRICK2)

DR6 death receptor 6 (also known as tumor necrosis factor receptor superfamily member 21, osteoprotegenin [OPG], osteoclastogenesis inhibitory factor, and interleukin 1-beta convertase)
DRM desmin-related myofibillar myopathy
DRP-1 dynanim- related protein 1
DS dermatan sulfate
DS PG dermatan sulfate proteoglycan
dsDNA double stranded DNA
DsrNA-RT single standed desoxyribonucleic acid-reverse transcriptase
DSPG3 the epiphycan gene on chromosome 12 (12q21)
dsRNA double stranded RNA
DTI diffusion tensor imaging
DTH delayed type hypersensitivity
DTNBP1 the gene on chromosome 6 (6p22.3) that causes Hermansky–Pudlak syndrome type 7 when mutated
DTT dithiothreitol
dUTP 2′-deoxyuridine 5′-triphosphate

E1A an adenovirus oncoprotein
E1B a gene in adenovirus
E2F a transcription factor that binds to the retinoblastoma gene (*RB1*)
E6 a gene in papillomaviruses
E7 a gene in papillomaviruses
EAF2 a component of the ELL-mediated RNA polymerase II elongation factor
EAU experimental autoimmune uveitis
EB elementary body
EBV Epstein-Barr virus
EC vascular endothelial cell
ECD1 an autoantigen with extracellular domains in Sjögren syndrome
ECF-A eosinophilic chemotactic factor of anaphylaxis
ECG electrocardiograph
ECM extracellular matrix
ECM1 the extracellular matrix protein 1 gene on chromosome 1 (1q21)
ECM2 the extracellular matrix protein 2 gene on chromosome 9 (9q21.3–q22)
ECP eosinophil cationic protein
ECS extracellular space
EDAR ectodysplasin A receptor
EDRF endothelial dependendent relaxation factor
EDS Ehlers–Danlos syndrome
EDS1 Ehlers–Danlos syndrome type 1
EDTA ethylenediaminetetraacetic acid
EDN eosinophil derived neurotoxin
EDN1 gene for endothelin 1 on chromosome 6 (6p24–p23)
EDN1 endothelin 1
EDNRA endothelin receptor type A
EDNRA a gene for endothelin receptor type A on chromosome 4 (4q31.2)
EDNRB a gene for endothelin receptor type B on chromosome 13 (13q22)
EDNRB endothelin receptor type B
EEC syndrome ectodactyly, ectodermal dysplasia, and cleft lip/palate syndrome
EEG electroencephalography; electroencephalograph; electroencephalogram
EEP EDTA-extractable protein
EETs epoxyeicosatrienoic acid
EEV extracellular enveloped virus
EFEMP1 the fibulin 3 gene on chromosome 2 (2p16) (also known as FBLN3)
EFTF eye field transcription factor
e.g. for example
EGF epidermal growth factor
EGFR the gene for epidermal growth factor receptor on chromosome 7 (7p12.3–p12.1)
EIA enzyme-linked immunoassay
EJ-ras an oncogene
EKC epidemic keratoconjunctivitis
EKG electrocardiogram
EKH4 monoclonal antikeratin antibody predominantly expressed in basal epithelial cells
EKH5 monoclonal antikeratin antibody predominantly expressed in eccrine secretory part of structures
EKH6 monoclonal antikeratin antibody predominantly expressed in normal eccrine and ductal structures
ELAM-1 endothelial leukocyte adhesion molecule-1
ELISA enzyme-linked immunosorbent assay
ENA extractable nuclear antigen
ELN the elastin gene on chromosome 7 (7q11.2)
ELOVL4 elongation of very long chain fatty acids-like 4
ELOVL4 the elongation of very long chain fatty acids-like 4 gene on chromosome 6 (6q14)
EM erythema multiforme; electron microscopy
EMA epithelial membrane antigen
EMG electromyograph
EMT epithelial-mesenchymal transition
Endo endothelial cells
ENOS the β-enolase gene on chromosome 17 (17pter–p12)
ENPP2 the ectonucleotide pyrophosphatase/ phosphodiesterase gene on chromosome 8 (8q24.1)
en embryonic nucleus of crystalline lens
env a gene in Rous sarcoma virus
Eo eosinophils
EOG electro-oculography
EOM extraocular muscle
ep epithelium
EP300 a gene on chromosome 22 (22q13) that codes for a histone acetyltransferase (p300) that regulates transcription
Epi epithelial cells
EPMR epilepsy with mental retardation (also known as neuronal ceroid lipofuscinosis type 8)
EPR electron spin resonance
ER endoplasmic reticulum
Erb-B an oncogene
ERCC1 group 1 excision-repair cross-complemeting protein
ERCC6 group 6 excision-repair cross-complemeting protein
ERCC8 group 8 excision-repair cross-complemeting protein
ERG electroretinogram
ERK extracellular signal-regulated kinase (a subgroup of mitogen activated protein kinases, MAPKs)

ERM epiretinal membrane
ERP early receptor potential
ERT enzyme replacement therapy
ESAF endothelial cell angiogenesis factor
ESCB enhanced S-cone syndrome
ESCS a gene on chromosome 15 (15q23) that codes for nuclear receptor subfamily 2, group E, member 3 (also known as *NR2E3* and *PNR*)
ESI electrospray ionization
ESI-LC-MS/MS electrospray ionization liquid chromatography tandem mass spectrometry
ESR erythrocyte sedimentation rate
EST expressed tags
EVR1 exudative vitreoretinopathy type 1
EVR2 exudative vitreoretinopathy type 2
EVR3 exudative vitreoretinopathy type 3
EVR4 exudative vitreoretinopathy type 4

5-Fu 5-fluoruracil
F6H8 perfluorohexyloctane
FA fluorescein angiography
Fab fragment antigen binding
Factor VIII an essential blood clotting factor; a vascular cell marker
FACS fluorescence activated cell sorter
FAD flavin adenine dinucleotide
FADD Fas-assciated death domain
FADH2 reduced flavin adenine dinucleotide
FAH the fumarylacetoacetate hydrolase gene on chromosome 15 (15q23–q25)
FAP familial amyloid polyneuropathy, familial adenomatous polyposis
FAS/Fas apoptosis antigen 1 (APO1) (also known as CD95, cell surface death receptor 2, and FAS antigen)
FASL/Fasl Fas ligand
Fb fibroblasts
FBLN3 the fibulin 3 gene on chromosome 2 (2p16) (also known as *EFEMP1*)
FBLN5 the fibulin 5 gene on chromosome 14 (4q32.1)
FBLN6 the fibulin 6 gene on chromosome 1 (1q24–q25)
FBN1 the fibrillin-1 gene on chromosome 15 (15q21.1)
FBN2 the fibrillin-2 gene on chromosome 5 (5q23–q31)
FBN3 the fibrillin-3 gene on chromosome 19 (19p13.3–p13.2)
Fc constant fragment of immunoglobulin; crystallizable fragment of immunoglobulin
FCD Fuchs corneal dystrophy
fCJD familial Creutzfelt-Jakob disease
FCMD Fukuyama congenital muscular dystrophy
FCMD the fukudin gene on chromosome 9(9q31)
FD fleck corneal dystrophy
Fe^{2+} ferrous ions
Fe^{3+} ferric ions
FEVR familial exudative vitreoretinopathy
FFA fundus fluorescein angiogram
FFI fatal familial insomnia
FMM fundus flavimaculatus
FGA the fibrinogen α-chain gene on chromosome 4 (4q28)
FGF fibroblast growth factor
FGF1 the fibroblast growth factor 1 (acidic fiboblast growth factor) gene on chromosome 5 (5q31)
FGF2 fibroblast growth factor 2 (also known as basic fibroblast growth factor [bFGF])
FGF2 the gene for fibroblast growth factor 2 (basic fibroblast gowth factor) on chromosome 4 (4q25–q27)
Fgf2 the murine gene for fibroblast growth factor 2 (basic fibroblast gowth factor)
FGF8 fibroblast growth factor 8
FGF8 the gene for fibroblast growth factor 8 on chromosome 10 (10q24)
FGF9 fibroblast growth factor 9
FGF9 the gene for fibroblast growth factor 9 on chromosome 13 (13q11–q12)
Fgf10 the murine gene for fibroblast growth factor 10
FGF10 the gene for fibroblast growth factor 10 on chromosome 5 (5p13–p12)
FGFR1 fibroblast growth factor receptor 1
FH familial hypercholesterolemia
FHI Fuchs heterochromic iridocyclitis
FIP-2 an adenoviral protein
FIS1 homolog of *S. cerevisiae*, also known as tetratricipeptide repeat domain 11
FISH fluorescent in situ hybridization
FKH7 the former term for forkhead box C1 transcription factor now known as FOXC1
FKH7 a former term for the gene on chromosome 6 (6p25) that codes for forkhead box C1 transcription factor; now known as *FOXC1*
FKRP4 the fukutin-related protein gene on chromosome 19 (19q13.3)
FLAIR fluid attenuated inversion recovery
FLICE caspase 8 apoptosis-related cysteine protease
FLIP FLICE inhibitory protein
$FLIP_L$ FLICE-like inhibitory protein long-form
$FLIP_S$ FLICE-like inhibitory protein short-form
Flk1 vascular endothelial growth factor receptor 2
Flt-1 fms-like tyrosine kinase-1
FLNA the actin-binding protein filamin A
FMN flavin mononucleotide
FMOD the fibromodulin gene on chromosome 1 (1q32.1)
fn fetal nucleus of the crystalline lens
FN1 the fibronectin gene on chromosome 2 (2q31)
FOXC1 the forkhead box C1 transcription factor gene on chromosome 6 (6p25) (formerly known as *FKHL7)*
Foxc1 the murine forkhead box C1 gene that codes for transcription factor
FOXC1 the forkhead box C1 gene on chromosome 6 (6p25)
Foxc2 the murine forkhead box C2 gene that codes for transcription factor
FOXC2 the forkhead box C2 gene on chromosome 16 (16q24.3)
Foxd1 a transcription factor
FOXE3 the gene for forkhead box E3 on chromosome 1 (1p32)
FOXL2 the forkhead transcription factor
FOXL2 the forkhead transcription factor FOXL2 gene on chromosome 3 (3q23)
FOXP1 the glutamine-rich factor 1 gene on chromosome 3 (3p14.1)

FRAS1 the gene on chromosome 4 (4q) that is responsible for Fraser syndrome
FREM2 the FRAS1-related extracellular matrix protein 2 gene on chromosome 13 (13q13.3)
FSCN2 the retinal fascin homolog 2 actin binding protein gene on chromosome 17 (17q25) (also known as *RP30*)
Fuc fucose
FUCA1 the α-L-fucosidase gene on chromosome 1 (1p34)
FZD4 the gene on chromosome 11 (11q14–q21) that codes a homolog of Drosophila frizzled 4 a member of the"frizzled" gene family
FZD6 the gene coding a homolog of Drosophila frizzled 6 a member of the"frizzled" gene family

g gram
G guanine
G protein a glycoprotein on the surface of rhabdoviruses
G-protein a guanine nucleotide binding protein
G0 the resting phase of the cell cycle
G1 the presynthetic phase of the cell cycle
G2 the phase in the cell cycle between the S and M phases
G3P glyceraldehyde 3-phosphate
G3PD glyceraldehyde 3-phosphate dehydrogenase
G6P glucose-6-phosphate
G6PC the glucose-6-phosphatase gene on chromosome 17 (17q21)
G6PD glucose 6-phosphate dehydrogenase
G6PT1 the glucose 6 phosphate transporter 1 gene on chromosome 11 (11q23)
GA geographic atrophy and gyrate atrophy
GA733-1 a former name for the *TACSTD2* gene on chromosome 1 (1P32)
GAA an acid α-glucosidase gene on chromosome 17 (17q25.2–q25.3)
GABA gamma aminobutyric acid
Gadd45 the gene product of the growth arrest and DNA damage–inducible gene (GADD45A)
GADD153 a DNA repair protein
GADD153 a DNA repair protein gene on chromosome 12 (12q13.1–q13.2)
gag a gene in Rous sarcoma virus
GAG glycosaminglycan; codon for glutamic acid
GAGs glycosaminoglycans
Gal galactose
Gal6ST galactose-6-sulfotransferase
GALC galactosylceramidase
GALC the galactosylceramidase gene on chromosome 14 (14q31)
GalCer galactosylceramide
GalNAc N-acetylgalactosamine
GALNS the galactose 6-sulfatase gene on chromosome 16 (16q24.3)
GALT gut associated lymphoid tissue
GAPO growth retardation, alopecia, pseudoanodontia and optic atrophy syndrome
GAS6 growth arrest-specific 6
GB3 globotriaosylyceramide
GBA the glucocerebrosidase gene on chromosome 1 (1q21)
GBC globotribosyl ceramide
GBE1 the glycogen branching enzyme gene on chromosome 3 (3p12)
GBM glomerular basement membrane
GCA giant cell arteritis and a guanine-cytosine-adenine trinucleotide
GCAP guanylate cyclase activation protein
GCAP1 an isoform of a calcium-binding protein involved in the replenishment of cyclic guanosine monophosphate in rods and cones (also kown as GUCA1A)
GCAP1 the gene for guanylate cyclase activator 1A on chromosome 6 (6p21.1) (also known as *GUCA1A* and *COD3*)
GCAP2 an isoform of a calcium-binding protein involved in the replenishment of cyclic guanosine monophosphate in rods and cones (also known as GUCA1B)
GCAP2 the gene for guanylate cyclase activator 1B on chromosome 6 (6p21.1) (also known as *GUCA1B*)
GCAP3 an isoform of calcium-binding protein involved in the replenishment of cyclic guanosine monophosphate in rods and cones (also known as GUCA1C)
GCD granular corneal dystrophy
GCG a guanine-cytosine-guanine trinucleotide
GCP the gene for green visual pigment on the X chromosome (Xq28)
GD Gaucher disease
GDLD gelatinous drop-like corneal dystrophy
GDP guanosine diphosphate
GFAP glial fibrillary acidic protein
GH growth hormone
GHMP an enzyme superfamily that includes galactokinase, homoserine kinase, mevalonate kinase and phosphomevonate kinase
GIT gastrointestinal tract
GJ gap junction
GJA8 the gap junction protein alpha-8 gene on chromosome 1 (1q21.1)
GJB2 the gap junction protein beta-2 (connexin 26) gene on chromosome 13 (13q11–q12)
GLA the α-galactosidase A gene on the X chromosome (Xq22–24)
Glb1 the murine gene that codes β-galactosidase
GLB1 β-galactosidase
GLB1 the acid β-galactosidase gene on chromosome 3 (3p21.33)
Glc glucose
GLC3A the locus for primary congenital glaucoma type 3 on chromosome 2 (2p21–2p25), where there are homozygous mutations in the cytochrome P4501B1 gene (*CYP1B1*)
GLI glioma associated oncogene
GLRX the glutaredoxin gene on chromosome 5 (5q14)
Glu glutamate
GluCer glucosylceramide
GLUT1 the glucose transporter 1 gene on chromosome 1 (1p35–p31.3)
Gly glycine
GlyNAc6St N-acetylglucosamine 6-O-sulfotransferase
GM2A the GM_2-activator protein gene on chromosome 5 (5q31.3–q33.1)

GM-CSF granulocyte-macrophage colony stimulating factor
GMP-140 granule membrane protein
GNA the *N*-acetylglucosamine 6-sulfatase gene on chromosome 12 (12q14)
GNAS the guanine nucleotide-binding protein, alpha-stimulating activity polypeptide 1 gene on chromosome 20 (20q13.2)
GNAS1 the guanine nucleotide-binding protein, alpha-stimulating activity polypeptide 1 gene on chromosome 20 (20q13.2)
GNAT1 the guanine nucleotide-binding protein alpha-transducing activity polypeptide 1 gene on chromosome 3 (3p21)
GNAT2 the guanine nucleotide-binding protein alpha-transducing activity polypeptide 2 gene on chromosome 1 (1p13.1)
GNPTAB the N-acetylglucosamine-1-phosphotransferase gene on chromosome 12 (12q23.3)
GNPTG the gene on chromosome 16 (16q) for the gamma subunit of N-acetylglucosamine-1-phosphotransferase
gp75 a differentiation antigen of melanocytes
GP100 a melanocyte protein (also known as melanocyte protein 17)
GPC1 the glypican 1 gene on chromosome 2 (2q35–q37)
GPC2 the glypican 2 gene on chromosome 7 (7q22.1)
GPC3 the glypican 3 gene on the X chromosome (Xq26)
GPC4 the glypican 4 gene on the X chromosome (Xq26)
GPC5 the glypican 5 gene on chromosome 13 (13q32)
GPC6 the glypican 6 gene on chromosome 13 (13q32)
GPCR G-protein coupled receptor
Gpr2a a murine gene on chromosome 16
GRIPs glypican-related integral membrane proteoglycans
GRK1 the rhodopsin kinase gene on chromosome 13 (13q34) (also known as *RHOK*)
GRM6 the metabotropic glutamate receptor 6 gene on chromosome 5 (5q35.3)
GRO (MGSA) a cytokine
GRODS granular osmiophilic deposits
GSD glycogen storage diseases
GSH glutathione reduced form
GSL glycosphingolipids
GSN the gelsolin gene on chromosome 9 (9q34)
GSS Gerstmann–Stäussler-Scheinker disease
GSSG oxidized glutathione
GST glutathione S-transferase
GST 5.6 an isoenzyme of glutathione S-transferase
GST 7.4 an isoenzyme of glutathione S-transferase
GSTM1 the glutathione S-transferase mu 1(mGST-1) gene on chromosome 1 (1p13.3)
GSTP1 the gene for glutathione S-transferase pi 1 on chromosome 11 (1q13)
GSTT1 glutathione S-transferase theta 1
GSTT1 the gene for glutathione S-transferase theta 1 (GST-T1) on chromosome 22 (22q11.2)
GTM3 a transformed/immortalized trabecular meshwork cell strain
GTP guanosine triphosphate
GTPase guanosine triphosphate hydrolase
GUCA1A an isoform of a calcium-binding protein involved in the replenishment of cyclic guanosine monophosphate in rods and cones (also kown as GCAP1)
GUCA1A the gene for guanylate cyclase activator 1A on chromosome 6 (6p21.1) (also known as *COD3* and *GCAP1*)
GUCA1B an isoform of a calcium-binding protein involved in the replenishment of cyclic guanosine monophosphate in rods and cones (also known as GCAP2)
GUCA1C an isoform of calcium-binding protein involved in the replenishment of cyclic guanosine monophosphate in rods and cones (also known as GCAP3)
GUG codon for valine
GUSB the β-D-glucuronidase gene on chromosome 7 (7q21.11)
GUCY2D retinal guanylate cyclase-1 (also known as RetGC1)
GUCY2D the retinal-specific guanylate cyclase gene on chromosome 17 (17p13.1) (also known as *CORD6*, *LCA1*, and *RETGC1*)
GVF Goldmann visual field
Gy grey ($1GY=100rad=J/kg=m^2/s^2$)
GYS2 the glycogen synthase gene on chromosome 12 (12p12.3)

5-HT 5-hydroxytryptamine
5-HETE 5-hydroxyeicosatetraenoic acid
12-HETE 12-hydroxyeicosatetraenoic acid
12(R)-HETE 12(R)-hydroxyeicosatetraenoic acid
15-HETE 15-hydroxyeicosatetraenoic acid
H heparin
H_2O_2 hydrogen peroxide
HA hyaluronic acid (also known as hyaluran)
HAMP a gene on chromosome 19 (19q13) that causes hemochromatosis when mutated
HAV hepatitis A virus
HbA adult hemoglobin
HbC hemoglobin C
HB-EGF heparin-binding epidermal growth factor-like growth factor
HbF fetal hemoglobin
HBID hereditary benign intraepithelial dyskeratosis
HBO hyperbaric oxygen
HbS hemoglobin S (sickle cell hemoglobin)
HbSC hemoglobin SC
HBV hepatitis B virus
HBVcAg hepatitis B virus core antigen
HBVsAg hepatitis B virus surface antigen
HCV hepatitis C virus
HD homeodomain
HDL high density lipoprotein
HBV hepatitis B virus
HBVsAg hepatitis B virus surface antigen
HCS hyperferritinemia-cataract syndrome
HDM2 double minute gene (also known as MDM2)
HDM2 the double minute 2 gene, also known as *MDM2*
HDV hepatitis D virus
HEP high-energy phosphates

Hes1 a murine gene that is expressed in retinal progenitor cells

HESX1 a gene on chromosome 3 (3p21.2–p21.1) known as the homeobox gene expressed in ES cells and as the Rathke pouch homeobox gene

HETEs hydroxyeicosatetraenoic acids

HEXA the α-subunit of β-hexosaminidase gene on chromosome 15 (15q23–q24)

HEXA an isoform of β-hexosaminidase consisting of an α- and β-subunit

HEXB the β-subunit of β-hexosaminidase gene on the chromosome 5 (5q13)

HEXB an isoform of β-hexosaminidase consisting of two β-subunits

HFE a gene on chromosome 6 (6p) that causes hemochromatosis when mutated

HFMD hand-foot and mouth disease

Hg mercury

HGF hepatocyte growth factor

HGF the gene for hepatocyte growth factor on chromosome 7 (7q21.1)

HGD the homogentisate 1,2-dioxygenase gene on chromosome 3 (3q21–q23)

HGSNAT the acetyl-CoA-glucosamine *N*-acetyltransferase gene on chromosome 8 (8p11.1)

HHV8 human herpes virus 8

HI hemagglutination inhibition

HIF hypoxia-inducible factor

HIF the hypoxia-inducible transcription factor-1 gene on chromosome 14 (14q21–q24)

HIF_α hypoxia–inducible factor alpha

His histidine

HIV human immunodeficiency virus

HDL high density lipoprotein

HDL-1 high density lipoprotein fraction 1

HDL-2 high density lipoprotein fraction 2

HDL-3 high density lipoprotein fraction 3

HEP high energy phosphates

HGD the homogentisate 1,2 dioxygenase gene on chromosome 3 (3q21–q23)

HHV-6 human herpes virus 6

HHV-8 human herpes virus 8

HK hexokinase

HLA human leukocyte antigen

HLA-A11 haplotype of human leukocyte antigen (HLA)

HLA-B40 haplotype of human leukocyte antigen (HLA)

HLA-B51 haplotype of human leukocyte antigen (HLA)

HLA-B87 haplotype of human leukocyte antigen (HLA)

HLA-DR class II histocompatibility antigen

HLA-DR2 haplotype of class II histocompatibility antigen

HLA-DR4/DRW53 haplotype of class II histocompatibility antigen

HLA-DR15 haplotype of class II histocompatibility antigen

HLA-DR17 haplotype of class II histocompatibility antigen

HLA-DR51 haplotype of class II histocompatibility antigen

HLA-DRB1 haplotype of class II histocompatibility antigen

HLE human lens epithelium

HLOD hierachical level of detail; heterogeneity likelihood of the odds (lod) score

HMB45 antibody that reacts with a neuraminidase sensitive oligosaccharide side chain of a glycoconjungate in immature melanosomes

HMB50 antibody that recognizes a different epitope on the same antigen in melanoctes as HMB45

HMG hydroxymethylglutaryl

HMW kininogen high molecular weight kininogen

HNK-1 human natural killer-1; a marker for the astrocyte type 1 precursor

HPETEs hydroperoxyeicosatetraenoic acids

HPF high power field

HPLC high pressure liquid chromatography

HPS1 the gene on chromosome 10 (10q23.1) that causes Hermansky–Pudlak syndrome type 1 when mutated

HPS2 the gene on chromosome 5 (5q14.1) that causes Hermansky–Pudlak syndrome type 2 when mutated (also known as *ADTB3A* and *AP3B1*)

HPS3 the gene on chromosome 3 (3q24) that causes Hermansky–Pudlak syndrome type 3 when mutated

HPS4 the gene on chromosome 22 (22q11.2–q12.2) that causes Hermansky–Pudlak syndrome type 4 when mutated

HPS5 the gene on chromosome 11 (11p15–p13) that causes Hermansky–Pudlak syndrome type 5 when mutated

HPS6 the gene on chromosome 10 (10q24.32) that causes Hermansky–Pudlak syndrome type 6 when mutated

HPV human papilloma virus

HPV16 human papilloma virus type 16

hr hour

HRP horseradish peroxidase

HRPT2 hyperparathyroidism-2

HRPT2 the gene on chromosome 1 (1q25–q31) responsible for hyperparathyroidism-2

HS heparan sulfate

HSF4 the gene for heat shock transcription factor-4 on chromosome 16 (16q22.12)

HSK herpetic stromal keratitis

HSP heat shock protein

HSP27 heat shock protein 27

HSP40 heat shock protein 40

HSP60 heat shock protein 60

HSPB1 the heat shock protein 27 gene on chromosome 7 (7q11.23)

HSPD1 the heat shock protein 60 gene on chromosome 2 (2q33.1)

HSPF1 the heat shock protein 40 gene on chromosome 19 (19p13.2)

HSPG2 the perlecan gene on chromosome 1 (1p36.1)

HSV herpes simplex virus

HSV-1 herpes simplex virus type 1

HSV-2 herpes simplex virus type 2

HTGL hepatic triglyceride lipase

HTLV-1 human T cell leukemia virus 1

HTLV-2 human T cell leukemia virus 2

HtrA2 HtrA serine peptidase 2 (also known as serine proteinase 25)

HUMARA human androgen-receptor gene on the X chromosome (Xq11.2–q12)

HV-B herpes virus B

HYAL1 the hylauronidase gene on chromosome 3 (3p21.3–p21.2)

I isotropic
IAP inhibitor of apoptosis
IAPP the islet amyloid polypeptide gene on chromosome 12 (12p12.3–p12.1)
IBD identity by descent
ICA internal carotid artery
ICAM intercellular adhesion molecule
ICAM-1 intercellular adhesion molecule-1
ICAM-2 intercellular adhesion molecule-2
ICAM-3 intercellular adhesion molecule-3
ICE syndrome the irido-corneal-endothelial syndrome that includes iris nevus syndrome, Chandler syndrome, and essential iris atrophy
ICZ inner collagenous zone
ID3 A transcription factor inhibitor of DNA binding 3
IDL intermediate density lipoproteins
IDO indoleamine pyrrole 2,3 dioxygenase
IDS the iduronate-2 sulfatase gene on the X chromosome (Xq28)
IDUA the α-L-iduronidase gene on chromosome 4 (4p16.3)
IEF isoelectric focusing
IEV intracelluar enveloped virus
IF immunofluorescence
IFA indirect fluorescent antibody (also immunofluoresecent antibody)
IFκ B nuclear factor of kappa light chain enhancer in B cells inhibitor
IFN interferon
IFNα interferon alpha
IFNβ interferon beta
IFNγ interferon gamma
Ig immunoglobulin
IgA immunoglobulin A
IgD immunoglobulin D
IgE immunoglobulin E
IGF insulin-like growth factor
IGF1 insulin like growth factor 1
IGF2 insulin like growth factor 2
IgG immunoglobulin G
IgG_1 a subgroup of immunoglobulin G
IgG_2 a subgroup of immunoglobulin G
IgG_3 a subgroup of immunoglobulin G
IgG_4 a subgroup of immunoglobulin G
IgGκ immunoglobulin G kappa
IGHD the immunoglobulin delta heavy chain gene on chromosome 14 (14q32.33)
IGHE the immunoglobulin epsilon heavy chain gene on chromosome 14 (14q32.33)
IGHG1 the gamma immunoglobulin heavy chain gene on chromosome 14 (14q32.33)
IGHM the immunoglobulin mu heavy chain gene on chromosome 14(14q32.33)
IGLJ the gene for immunoglobulin κ or λ light chain on chromosome 22 (22q11.2)
IgM immunoglobulin M
IHA indirect hemagglutination
IIH idiopathic intracranial hypertension (also known as pseudotumor cerebri)
IIRC International Intraocular Retinoblastoma Classification
iNOS inducible nitric oxide synthase
IL interleukin
IL1 interleukin 1
IL1α interleukin 1 alpha
IL1β interleukin 1 beta
IL2 interleukin 2
IL2 the interleukin 2 gene on chromosome 4 (4q26–q27)
IL3 interleukin 3
IL4 interleukin 4
IL5 interleukin 5
IL6 interleukin 6
IL7 interleukin 7
IL8 interleukin 8
IL9 interleukin 9
IL10 interleukin 10
IL12 interleukin 12
IL18 interleukin 18
IL1A the interleukin 1 alpha gene on chromosome 2 (2q14)
IL1B the interleukin 1 beta gene on chromosome 2 (2q14)
IL1RN the interleukin 1 receptor antagonist gene on chromosome 2 (2q14.2)
IL2R interleukin 2 receptor
IL18 the interleukin 18 gene on chromosome 11 (11q22.2–q22.3)
IL8RB IL 8 receptor beta gene on chromosome 2 (2q35)
Ile isoleucine
ILGF2 insulin-like growth factor 2
ILL inner limiting lamina of retina
ILM inner limiting membrane of retina
IMPDH1 the inosine monophosphate dehydrogenase 1 gene on chromosome 7 (7q32.1) (also known as *RP10*)
IMV intracellular mature virus
INCL infantile neuronal ceroid-lipofuscinosis
iNOS inducible nitric acid oxide synthase
INS the insulin gene on chromosome 11 (11p15.5)
$InsP_3$ inositol 1,4,5-triphosphate
IOL prosthetic intraocular lens
IOP intraocular pressure
IPCV idiopathic polypoidal choroidal vasculopathy
IP1 inositol phosphate
IP2 inositol biphosphate
IP3 inositol triphosphate
IPE iris pigmented epithelium
IPM interphotoreceptor matrix
IRBP interphotoreceptor cell-binding protein (also known as interstitial retinol-binding protein)
IRE iron-responsive element
IRMA intraretinal microvascular abnormality
IRP iron regulatory protein
ISCOM immunostimulatory complexes
ISSD infantile sialic acid storage disease
ISSVA Internatioanl Society for the Study of Vascular Anomalies
ITM2B the integral membrane protein 2B gene on chromosome 13 (13q14)

JA juvenile rheumatoid arthritis
j-Bid a cleavage product of BH3-interacting domain death agonist (BID)
JCT juxtacanalicular connective tissue

JCV a human polyomavirus
JIA juvenile idiopathic arthritis
JNCL juvenile neuronal ceroid-lipofuscinosis
JOAG juvenile open angle glaucoma
JNK c-Jun N-terminal protein kinase
JNKK1 mitogen-activated protein kinase 4 (also known as MAP2K4)

K^{+} potassium ion
K cell killer T lymphocyte
kb kilobase
KC keratoconus
KCS keratoconjunctivitis sicca
KD Kawasaki disease
kDa kilodalton
Ker keratinocyte
KERA the keratocan gene on chromosome 12 (12q22)
Ki-67 a marker for cell cycle proliferation (also known as Mib-1)
KID **K**eratitis, **I**chthyosis, **D**eafness syndrome
KIF21A the kinesin family member 21A gene on chromosome 12 (12q12)
KGF keratocyte growth factor
Ki-ras a family of retrovirus-associaited DNA sequences (ras) originally isolated from Kirsten murine sarcoma virus
KLHL7 an antigen that elicits autoantibodies in Sjögren syndrome
KLHL12 an antigen that elicits autoantibodies in Sjögren syndrome
KM Michaelis constant
KP keratic precipitate
KRT3 the cytokeratin 3 gene on chromosome 12 (12q13)
KRT12 the cytokeratin 12 gene on chromosome 17 (17q12)
KS keratan sulfate; Kaposi sarcoma
KS-I corneal keratan sulfate
KS-II cartilaginous keratan sulfate
KS-IIA cartilaginous keratan sulfate containing α-(1,3)-fucose and α-(2,6)-linked *N*-acetyl-neuraminic acid residues
KS-IIB cartilaginous keratan sulfate lacking α-(1,3)-fucose and α-(2,6)-linked *N*-acetyl-neuraminic acid residues
KSHV Kaposi sarcoma associated herpesvirus
KSPG keratan sulfate proteoglycan

L lutein
L cone red cone
LADD syndrome lacrimo-auriculo-dento-digital syndrome
LAK lymphokine activated killer cell
LAMP lysosome associated membrane protein
LANA latency-associated nuclear antigen
LAR a transmembrane phosphotyrosine phosphatase
LARD lymphocyte-associated receptor of death (also known as death receptor 3 [DR3])
LASER light amplication by stimulated emission of radiation
LASIK laser assisted *in situ* keratomileusis
LATs latency-associated transcripts
LBL lymphobastic B cell lymphoma
LC liquid chromatography
LCA leukocyte common antigen and Leber congenital amaurosis
LCA1 the retinal-specific guanylate cyclase gene on chromosome 17 (17p13.1) (also known as *CORD6, GUCY2D, and RETGC1*)
LCA2 the retinal pigment epithelium-specific 65 kDa protein gene on chromosome 1 (1p31) (also known as *RPE65* and *RP20*)
LCA3 a locus for Leber congenital amaurosis on chromosome 14 (14q23.3)
LCA4 the arylyhydrocarbon-interacting receptor protein-like 1 gene on chromosome 17 (17p13.1) (also known as *AIPl1*)
LCA5 a locus for Leber congenital amaurosis on chromosome 6 (6q14.1)
LCA6 the RPGR-interating protein 1 gene on chromosome 14 (14q11) (also known as *RPGRIP1*)
LCA9 a locus for Leber congenital amaurosis on chromosome 1 (1p36)
LCAT lecithin-cholesterol-acyltransferase
LCAT the lecithin-cholesterol-acyltransferase gene on chromosome 16 (16q22.1)
LCD lattice corneal dystrophy
LC-MS/MS liquid chromatography–mass spectrometry/mass spectrometry
LD linkage disequilibrium
LD syndrome lymphadema-trichiasis syndrome
LDH lactic dehydrogenase
LDH the lactate dehydrogenase gene on chromosome 11 (11p15.4)
LDL low density lipoprotein
LE lupus erythematosus
LEC CAMs lectin-epithelial growth factor-complement binding adhesion molecules
LECAM-1 lectin-EGF-complement adhesion molecule
LEF lymphoid enhancer-binding factor
LEMNDS a gene on chromosome 12 (12q14) that causes the Buschke–Ollendorff syndrome when mutated
Lens1 a murine gene involved in the induction of the lens placode
LEOPARD multiple lentigines, electrocardiographic conduction abnormalities, ocular hypertelorism, pulmonary stenosis, abnormal genitalia, retardation of growth, sensorineural deafness
Leu leucine
LeY Lewis Y antigen
LFA-1 synonym for CD18
LFB luxol fast blue
LGL large granular lymphocytes
L-GPs lactosaminoglycan-glycoproteins
LGV lymphogranuloma venereum
LHON Leber hereditary optic neuropathy
Lhx2 a murine eye field transcription factor
LI labelling index
LINCL late infantile neuronal ceroid-lipofuscinosis
LIPA an acid lipase gene on chromosome 10 (10q24–q25)
LMW low molecular weight

LMX1B a gene on chromosome 9 (9q34.1) that causes nail patella syndrome when mutated
LMYC an oncogene on chromosome 1 (1p32) with homology to a small region of bothMYC and NMYC (also known as MYCL1)
LN lymph node
LOCS lens opacities case-control classification system
LOCS III lens opacity classification system III
LOD logarithm of the odds
lop a mutant mouse with lens opacities
LORD late-onset retinal degeneration
LOX-1 lectin like oxidized low-density lipoprotein receptor-1
LOXL1 the gene for lysyl oxidase-like 1 on chromosome 15 (15q22)
LPL lipoprotein lipase
LPS lipopolysaccharide
LRAT lecithin retinol acyltransferase
LRAT the lecithin retinol acyltransferase gene on chromosome 4 (4q31.1)
LRN laboratory response network
LRP5 low density lipoprotein receptor-related protein 5
LRP5 the low density lipoprotein receptor-related Protein 5 on chromosome 11 (11q13.4)
LRR leucine-rich repeat
LSC long-space collagen
LSD lysosomal storage disease
LTB_4 leukotriene B_4
LTBP1 the latent TGFβ binding protein 1 gene on chromosome 2 (2p12–q22)
LTBP2 the latent TGFβ binding protein 2 gene on Chromosome 14 (14q24)
LTBP-1 latent TGFβ binding protein 1
LTBP-2 latent TGFβ binding protein 2
LTC_4 leukotriene C_4 (previously known as SRS-A)
LTD_4 leukotriene D_4
LTE_4 leukotriene E_4
LTF the lactoferrin gene on chromosome 3 (3q21–q23)
LTR long terminal repeat, log-transformed refraction
LUM the lumican gene on chromosome 12 (12q21.3–q22)
Lys lysine
LYVE-1 lymphatic vessel endothelial receptor 1
LYZ the gene for lysozyme

4MUGS 4-methylumbelliferyl-*N*-acetylglucosamine-6-sufate
5mc 5-methylcytosine
7MG methylation of guanine on nitrogen in the 7th position
m meter
M molar; also the phase of mitosis in the cell cycle
M1S1 a former name for the *TACSD2* gene on chromosome 1 (1p32)
M-cell a special epithelial cell in the gut
Mab monoclonal antibody
Mab21L1 a murine gene for a homologue of *C. elegans* cell fate-determinng protein mab21 that is expressed in the retina
MAC membrane attack complex
MadCAM1 mucosal addressin cell adhesion molecule
MAF the gene for v-maf avian musculoaponeurotic fibrosarcoma oncogene homolog on chromosome 16 (16q22–q23)
Maf a murine gene that codes for a transcription factor involved in the regulation of crystalline lens induction and development
MAGE melanoma antigen gene
MAGE-3 melanoma-specific antigen 3
MAGP-1 microfibril- associated glycoprotein
MALDI matrix-assisted laser desorption ionization
MALDI-TOF MS matrix-assisted laser desorption ionization-time of flight mass spectrometry
MALT mucosa associated lymphoid tissue
Man mannose
MAN2B1 the α-mannosidase class 2B1-gene on chromosome 19 (19cen–q12)
MANBA the β-mannosidase gene on chromosome 4 (4q22–q25)
Man-6-P mannose 6-phosphate
MAP mitogen-activated protein
MAP2K mitogen-activated protein kinase kinase
MAP3K mitogen-activated protein kinase kinase kinase
MAPK mitogen-activated protein kinase
MAPK14 the gene for mitogen-activated protein kinase p38
MART-1 melanoma antigen recognized by T cells (also known as Melan-A)
MAS McCune–Albright syndrome
Mash1 a murine gene involved in retinal differentiation
Math3 a murine gene involved in retinal development
Math5 a murine gene involved in retinal development
MATP a membrane-associated transporter protein gene on chromosome 5 (5p13.3)
MBP major basic protein (product of eosinophils); myelin basic protein
MBL mannose-binding lectin
MBP myelin basic protein
MC mast cells
MCAF macrophage/monocyte chemotactic and activating factor
MCB membranous cytoplasmic body
MCD macular corneal dystrophy
mcg microgram; same as μg
MCL mantle cell lymphoma
MCL1 a gene on chromosome 1 (1q21) originally isolated from the ML-1 myeloid leukemia cell line
MCOLN1 the mucolipin 1 gene on chromosome 19 (19p13.3–p13.2)
M cone green cone
MCOPS5 microphthlamia syndromic 5
MCP metacarpophalangeal
MCP-1 monocyte chemotactic protein-1
Md myelin-deficient
MD macular dystrophy
MDA malondialdehyde
MDP muramyl dipeptide
MDPF 2-methoxy-2,4-diphenyl-3(2*H*)-furanone
MDM2 double minute 2 gene on chromosome 12 (12q14.3–q15) (also known as *HDM2*)
MEB Muscle-Eye-Brain

MECD Meesmann corneal dystrophy
MEI metastatic efficiency index
MEFV the Mediterranean fever gene on chromosome 16 (16p13)
MEK MARK/ERK kinase
MEL-14 lymphocyte homimg receptor in mice
Melan-A melanoma antigen recognized by T cells (also known as MART-1)
MELAS myoclonic epilepsy, lactic acidosis, and stroke-like episodes
MEN multiple endocrine neoplasia
MEN1 the gene on chromosome 11 (11q13) that is responsible for multiple endocrine neoplasia syndrome type 1A
MEN2A multiple endocrine neoplasia syndrome type 2A
MEN2B multiple endocrine neoplasia syndrome type 2B
MER A novel tyrosine kinase
MERRF myoclonic epilepsy with red ragged fibers
MERTK the MER tyrosine kinase proto-oncogene on chromosome 2 (2q14.1)
MFG–E8 milk-fat-globule-EGF-factor 8
MFGE8 the lactadherin gene on chromosome 15 (15q25)
MFN1 mitofusin 1
MFN2 mitofusin 2
MFRP the membrane-type frizzled-related protein gene on chromosome 11 (11q23.3)
MFRP membrane-type frizzled-related protein
Mg magnesium
Mg^{2+} magnesium ions
MGSA (GRO) a cytokine
mGST-1 glutathione S-transferase mu
MHC major histocompatibility complex
MIA melanoma inhibitory activity
Mib-1 a marker for cell cycle proliferation; also known as Ki-67
MICA the major histocompatibility complex class 1 chain related gene A on chromosome 6 (6p21.3)
MIF macrophage migration inhibitory factor
MIP major intrinsic protein of lens (also known as MP26 and aquaporin-0)
MIP the MIP (aquaporin-0) gene on chromosome 12 (12q13)
MITF microphthalmia transcription factor
Mitf the murine gene that codes for microphthalmia transcription factor
MitfA a major isoform of microphthalmia transcription factor found in the retinal pigment epithelium
MitfD a major isoform of microphthalmia transcription factor found in the retinal pigment epithelium
MitfH a major isoform of microphthalmia transcription factor found in the retinal pigment epithelium
Mkk7 mitogen-activated protein kinase 7 (also known as MAP2K7)
ML-I mucolipidosis I
ML-II mucolipidosis II
ML-III mucolipidosis III
ML-IV mucolipidosis IV
MLB multilamellar body
MLCRD syndrome microcephaly-lymphedema-chorioretinal dysplasia syndrome
MLD metachromatic leukodystrophy
MLGAPC mucin-like glycoprotein associated with photoreceptor cells
MLH1 a DNA repair protein
MLS mucolipidosis
mm millimeter
mM millimolar
MMACHC the gene on chromosome 1 (1p34.1) that causes homocystinemia and methylmalonic aciduria when mutated
MMP matrix metalloproteinase [Zn(2+)-binding endopeptidase] and mitochondrial permeability
MMP-1 matrix metalloproteinase 1 (also known as collagenase)
MMP-2 matrix metalloproteinase 2 (also known as gelatinase, collagenase type IV, collagenase type IV A, and gelatinase A)
MMP-3 matrix metalloproteinase 3 (also known as stromelysin)
MMP-7 matrix metalloproteinase 7
MMP-9 matrix metalloproteinase 9
MMP-14 matrix metalloproteinase 14 (also known as MTI-MMP)
MMP1 the matrix metalloproteinase 1 gene on chromosome 11 (11q22–q23)
MMP2 matrix metalloproteinase 2 gene on chromosome 16 (16q13)
MMP3 matrix metalloproteinase 3 gene on chromosome 11 (11q23)
MMP9 matrix metalloproteinase 9 gene on chromosome 20 (20q11.2–q13.1)
Mn manganese
MNGIE mitochondrial neurogastointestinal encephalopathy syndrome
Mn^{2+} manganese ion
MØ macrophages/monocytes
MOCS1 the molybdenum cofactor synthesis 1 gene on chromosome 6 (6p21.3)
MOCS2 the molybdopterin synthase gene on chromosome 5 (5q11)
MOMP major outer membrane protein
MP macular pigment
MPA microscopic polyangiitis
MP17 a lens membrane protein with calmodulin binding properties
MP20 a lens plasma membrane protein
MP22 a truncated product MP70
MP26 the highly conserved major intrinsic protein of the crystalline lens (also known as aquaporin 0)
MP38 a cleavage product of MP70
MP64 a lens plasma membrane protein
MP70 an outer cortical lens fiber protein now known as connexin 50
MPO myeloperoxidase
MPR a mannose-6-phosphate receptor in the Golgi membranes
MPNST malignant peripheral nerve sheath tumor
MPS mucopolysaccharidosis
MPS I mucopolysaccharidosis type I
MPS IH mucopolysaccharidosis type IH (Hurler syndrome)
MPS IS mucopolysaccharidosis type IS (Scheie syndrome)

MPS IH/S mucopolysaccharidosis type IH/S
MPS II mucopolysaccharidosis type II (Hunter syndrome)
MPS III mucopolysaccharidosis type III (Sanfillipo syndrome)
MPS IIIA mucopolysaccharidosis type IIIA (Sanfillipo syndrome type A)
MPS IIIB mucopolysaccharidosis type IIIB (Sanfillipo syndrome type B)
MPS IIIC mucopolysaccharidosis type IIIC (Sanfillipo syndrome type C)
MPS IIID mucopolysaccharidosis type IIID (Sanfillipo syndrome type D)
MPS IV mucopolysaccharidosis type IV (Morquio syndrome)
MPS IVA mucopolysaccharidosis type IVA (Morquio syndrome type A)
MPS IVB mucopolysaccharidosis type IVB (Morquio syndrome type B)
MPS V mucopolysaccharidosis type V (former term for mucopolysaccharidosis type IS)
MPS VI mucopolysaccharidosis type VI (Maroteaux–Lamy syndrome)
NPS VII mucopolysaccharidosis type VII (Sly syndrome)
MPS VIII mucopolysaccharidosis type VIII (an entity that is no longer recognized)
MPS IX mucopolysaccharidosis type IX (Natowicz disease)
M_r molecular radius/relative molecular mass
MRCS syndrome microcornea, rod-dystrophy, cataract and posterior staphyloma syndrome
MRI magnetic resonance imaging
mRNA messenger ribonucleic acid
MRS magnetic resonance spectroscopy
MS multiple sclerosis
MSA muscle specific actin
MSD multiple sulfatase deficiency
m/sec meters/second
MSH2 aberrant mismatched repair gene
MTCO1 a mitochondrial DNA cytochrome c oxidase subunit I gene of respiratory complex IV (also known as *COI*)
MTCO2 a mitochondrial DNA cytochrome c oxidase subunit II gene of respiratory complex IV (also known as *COII*)
MTCO3 a mitochondrial DNA cytochrome c oxidase subunit III gene of respiratory complex IV (also known as *COIII*)
MTATP6 a gene that codes a component of the mitochondrial respiratory chain complex V
MtDNA mitochondrial DNA
MTHFR 5,10-methlenetetrahydrofolate reductase
MTHFR the gene for 5,10 methylenetetrahydrofolate reductase on chromosome 1 (1p36.3)
MTM1 the myotubularin gene on the X chromosome (Xq28)
MTI-MMP matrix metalloproteinase 14 (also known as MMP14)
MTND1 the subunit 1 of the mitochondrial DNA that codes for nicotinamide adenine dinucleotide dehydrogenase (complex I of the mitochondrial respiratory chain)
MTND2 the subunit 2 of the mitochondrial DNA that codes for nicotinamide adenine dinucleotide dehydrogenase (complex I of the mitochondrial respiratory chain)
MTND3 the subunit 3 of the mitochondrial DNA that codes for nicotinamide adenine dinucleotide dehydrogenase (complex I of the mitochondrial respiratory chain)
MTND4 the subunit 4 of the mitochondrial DNA that codes for nicotinamide adenine dinucleotide dehydrogenase (complex I of the mitochondrial respiratory chain)
MTND5 the subunit 5 of the mitochondrial DNA that codes for nicotinamide adenine dinucleotide dehydrogenase (complex I of the mitochondrial respiratory chain)
MTND6 the subunit 6 of the mitochondrial DNA that codes for nicotinamide adenine dinucleotide dehydrogenase (complex I of the mitochondrial respiratory chain)
MTND7 the subunit 7 of the mitochondrial DNA that codes for nicotinamide adenine dinucleotide dehydrogenase (complex I of the mitochondrial respiratory chain)
MTTK the gene that codes mitochondrial tRNA lysine from mitochondrial nucleotides 8295–8364
MTTL1 the gene that codes mitochondrial tRNA leucine from mitochondrial nucleotides 3230–3304
MTTV the gene that codes mitochondrial tRNA valine from mitochondrial nucleotides 1602–1670
MTTW the gene that codes mitochondrial tRNA tryptophan from mitochondrial nucleotides 5512–5576
mTOR mammalian target of rapamycin. It is a serine/threonine protein kinase
MudPIT multidimensional protein identification technology
MuSK muscle specific kinase
MVD microvascular density
MW molecular weight
MYC an oncogene on chromosome 8 (8q24.12–q24.13)
MYOC the myocilin gene on chromosome 1 (1q21-31)
MYO7A the myosin VIIa gene on chromosome 11 (11q13)
MYP a locus for myopia
MYP1 a locus for myopia on the X chromosome (Xq28)
MYP2 a locus for myopia on chromosome 18 (18p11.31)
MYP3 a locus for myopia on chromosome 12 (12q21–23)
MYP4 a locus for myopia on chromosome 7 (7q36)
MYP5 a locus for a myopia on chromosome 17 (17q21–23)
m/z mass-to-charge ratio where m is the mass and z is the charge)
MZL marginal zone lymphoma

Na^+ sodium ion
NA nucleic acid
NAA N-acetyl aspartic acid
NAAT nucleic acid amplification test
Na^+, K^+-ATPase sodium-potassium adenosine triphosphatase

NaCl sodium chloride
NAD^+ nicotinamide adenine dinucleotide (oxidized form)
NADH nicotinamide adenine dinucleotide (reduced form)
$NADP^+$ nicotinamide adenine dinucleotide phosphate (oxidized form)
NADPH nicotinamide adenine dinucleotide phosphate (reduced form)
NAGA the α-*N*-acetylgalactosaminidase gene on chromosome 22 (22q11)
NAGLU the α-N-acetylglucosaminidase gene on chromosome 17 (17q21)
NAION non-arteritic anterior ischemic optic neuropathy
NAIP neuronal apoptosis inhibiting protein
NARP neurogenic muscle weakness, ataxia and retinitis pigmentosa
NB84 a marker of neuroblastoma
NBCCS nevoid basal cell carcinoma syndrome
NB-DGJ N-butyldeoxygalactonojirimycin
NC nucleocapsid
N-CAM neural cell adhesion molecule
NCL neuronal ceroid-lipofuscinosis
ND Norrie disease
nDNA nuclear DNA
NDP the norrin gene on the X-chromosome (Xp11.4)
NDUFS1 a nuclear gene on chromosome 2 (2q33–q34) that codes a component of the mitochondrial respiratory chain complex I
NDUFS3 a nuclear gene on chromosome 11 (11p11.11) that codes a component of the mitochondrial respiratory chain complex I
NDUFS4 a nuclear gene on chromosome 5 (5q11.1) that codes a component of the mitochondrial respiratory chain complex I
NDUFS7 a nuclear gene on chromosome 19 (19p13) that codes a component of the mitochondrial respiratory chain complex
NDUFS8 a nuclear gene on chromosome 11 (11q13) that codes a component of the mitochondrial respiratory chain complex I
NDUFV1 a nuclear gene on chromosome 11 (11q13) that codes a component of the mitochondrial respiratory chain complex I
NDV Newcastle disease virus
Nd:YAG neodymium-doped yttrium aluminum garnett laser
NEDD8
NEU1 the neuraminidase 1 gene on chromosome 6 (6p21.3)
NeuroD a murine gene that is expressed in retinal progenitor cells
NF neurofilaments
NF1 neurofibromatosis type 1
NF1 the gene responsible for neurofibromatosis type 1
NF2 neurofibromatosis type 2
NF2 the gene for neurofibromatosis type 2 on chromosome 22 (22q12.2)
NFκB nuclear factor of kappa light chain gene enhancer in B cells
NFκB1 nuclear factor kappa-B subunit 1
NFκB2 nuclear factor kappa-B subunit 2
N-FKyn 3-hydroxykynurenine
NGF nerve growth factor
NGFR nerve growth factor receptor
Ngn2 a murine gene that is expressed in retinal progenitor cells
NH_4OH ammonia hydroxide
NHL non-Hodgkin lymphoma
NHS the gene on the X-chromosome (Xp22.13) that is responsible for Nance–Horan syndrome
NICH non-involuting cogenital hemangioma
NIH National Institutes of Health
NK cell natural killer cell
nm nanometer
NMYC an oncogene on chromosome 2 (2p24.1) that homologous with the *MYC* oncogene that was amplified in neuroblastoma cell line (also known as *MYCN*)
NMDA N-methyl-D-aspartate
NMR nuclear magnetic resonance
NO nitric oxide
NOEV N-acyl beta-valienamine
nop nuclear opacification (a mutant mouse)
NOS1 the gene for nitric oxide synthase on chromosome 12 (12q24.2–q24.31)
NPC1 a lipid trafficking protein gene on chromosome 18 (18q11–q12)
NPC2 the gene on chromosome 14 (14q24.3) that is responsible for Niemann-Pick disease type C2
NPCE nonpigmented ciliary epithelium
NPD Niemann-Pick disease
NP-A Niemann-Pick disease type A
NP-B Niemann-Pick disease type B
NP-C1 Niemann-Pick disease type C1; formerly designated Niemann-Pick disease type D
NP-C2 Niemann-Pick disease type C2
NP-D Niemann-Pick disease type D
NPL non-parametric linkage
NPPA the atrial natriuretic factor gene on chromosome 1 (1p36.2)
NPS nail patella syndrome
NR2E3 the nuclear receptor subfamily 2, group E, member 3 gene on chromosome 15 (15q23) (also known as *ESCS* and *PNR*)
NRAMP1 the natural resistance-associated macrophage protein 1 gene on chromosome 2 (2q35)
NRAMP2 the natural resistance-associated macrophage protein 2 gene on chromosome 12 (12q13)
NRL the neural retina leucine zipper gene on chromosome 14 (14q11.2) (also known as *RP27*)
NSAIDs non-steroidal anti-inflammatory drugs
NSC nuclear sclerotic cataract
NSE neuron specific enolase
NTF3 neurotrophin 3
NTF4 neurotrophin 4
NTF5 neurotrophin 5
NYX the nyctalopin gene on the X chromosome (Xp11.4) (also known as *CSNB1*)

3-OH Kyn N-formylkynurenine
O_2 oxygen radical also known as superoxide anion
O^4MT methylation of thymine on oxygen in 4th position
O^6MG methylation of guanine on oxygen in 6th position

OA ocular albinism
OAT L-ornithine:2-oxoacid aminotranferase
OCA oculocutaneous albinism
OCA1 oculocutaneous albinism type 1
OCA1A oculocutaneous albinism type 1A
OCA1B oculocutaneous albinism type IB
OCA2 oculocutaneous albinism type 2
OCA2 the gene on chromosome 15 (15q11.2–q12) that causes oculocutaneous albinism type 2 when mutated
OCA3 oculocutaneous albinism type 3
OCA4 oculocutaneous albinism type 4
Ocl-2 protoncogene which inhibits apoptosis
OCP ocular cicatricial pemphigoid
OCRL1 a gene on the X chromosome (Xq26.1) that codes for phosphatidylinositol 4,5-bisphosphate 5-phosphatase in the trans Golgi network
OCSS oculocraniosomatic syndromes
OCT optical coherent tomography
OCZ outer collagenous zone
ODFR oxygen-derived free radicals
OGN the osteoglycin gene on chromosome 9 (9q21.3–q22)
OH• hydroxyl radical
OI osteogenesis imperfecta
OLM outer limiting membrane of retina; also ocular larva migrans
OMD the osteomodulin gene on chromosome 9 (9q22)
Omi HTRA serine peptidase 2; also known as HTRA2 and serine protease 25
OMIM Online Mendelian Inheritance in Man
OMNTI oral melanotic neuroectodermal tumor of infancy
OMP1 the gene for MOMP
Omp1 a single copy gene on the *C. trachamatis* chromosome
OPA1 optic atrophy 1
OPA4 optic atrophy 4
OPA5 optic atrophy 5
OPG osteoprotegerin (also known as death receptor 6 (DR6), tumor necrosis factor receptor superfamily member 21, osteoclastogenesis inhibitory factor, and interleukin 1-beta convertase)
OPMD oculopharyngeal muscular dystrophy
OPN1LW an opsin 1 red cone pigment gene on the X chromosome (Xq28)
OPN1MW an opsin 1 green cone pigment gene on the X chromosome (Xq27)
OPTC the opticin gene on chromosome 1 (1q32.1)
OPTN the optoneurin gene on chromosome 10 (10p15–p14)
ORF open reading frame
ORF15 open eading frame 15
ORF73 protein encoded by Kaposi sarcoma associated herpes virus (KSHV)
Otx the family of murine genes that code for orthodenticle-related transcription factors
OTX2 the gene on chromosome 14 (14q21–q22) that is the homolog of the Drosophila orthodentide gene
Otx2 a murine eye field transcription factor that is the homolog of the *Drosophila* orthodentide gene
OVA ovalbumin
OXYS oxidation sensitive
6PGD 6-phosphogluconate dehydrogenase
P platelets, probability, short arm of a chromosome
P16 cyclin-dependent kinase inhibitor 2A (also known as CDKN2A and INK4)
p21 cyclin-dependent kinase inhibitor 1A (also known as CDKN1A)
p27 cyclin-dependent kinase inhibitor 1B (also known as CDKN1B)
P30/32$^{\mathrm{MIC2}}$ a cell surface antigen that reacts with antibodies against CD99 (surface antigen MIC2)
p50 nuclear factor kappa-B subunit 1 (also known as transcription factor NFKB1)
p52 repressor of the inhibitor of protein kinase 52-KDa
P53 the protein product of the *TP53* gene on chromosome 17 (17p13.1)
P63 the protein product of the *TP73L* gene on chromosome 3 (3q27)
P65 Golgi peripheral membrane protein P65 (also known as Golgi reassembly stacking protein 1)
PA polyarteritis nodosa
PABN1 polyadenylate-binding nuclear protein 1
PABN1 polyadenylate-binding nuclear protein 1 gene
PACAP pituitary adenylate cyclase-activating protein
PACG primary angle closure glaucoma
PAF platelet activating factor
PADGEM platelet activation-dependent granule external membrane protein
PAGE polyacrylamide gel electrophoresis
PAM primary acquired melanosis
PAMP pathogen–associated molecular pattern
pANCA perinuclear staining anti-neutrophil cytoplasmic antibody
PAP1 the PIM1-kinase associated protein 1 gene on chromosome 7 (7p14.3) (also known as *PIM1* and *RP9*)
PARK1 the α-SYN gene on chromosome 4 (4q21)
PARK2 the ubiquitin E3 ligase gene on chromosome 6 (6q25.2–q27)
PARK3 the ubiquitin C-terminal hydrolase L1 gene on chromosome 2 (2p13)
PARP poly (ADP-ribose) polymerase
PAS periodic acid Schiff
PAX2 the paired box gene 2 on chromosome 10 (10q24)
Pax2 the murine gene for paired box-2
PAX6 the gene for paired box-6 on chromosome 11 (11p13)
Pax6 the murine gene for paired box-6
PC phosphatidylcholine
PCDH15 the protocadherin-15 gene on chromosome 10 (10q21)
PCF pharyngeal conjunctival fever
PCG primary congenital glaucoma
PCR polymerase chain reaction
PCTH1 a gene on chromosome 9 (9q22.3)that codes for a transmembrane protein that suppresses TGFβ and Wnt families of signally proteins
PD polyol dehydrogenase, pseudoefficiency and Parkinson disease
PDCD1 the programmed cell death 1 gene on chromosome 2 (2q37.3)
PDE phosphodiesterase

PDE6A the rod cyclic guanosine monophosphate phosphodiesterase alpha subunit gene on chromosome 5 (5q33.1)
PDE6B the rod cyclic guanosine monophosphate phosphodiesterase beta subunit gene on chromosome 4 (4p16.3) (also known as *CSNB3*)
PDGF platelet derived growth factor
PDHA1 a gene on the X chromosome (Xp22.2–p22.1) that codes for a component of the pyruvate dehydrogenase complex
PDR proliferative diabetic retinopathy
PDS pigment dispersion syndrome
PDZ domain a structural domain of 80-90 amino acids that is found in certain signaling proteins
PE phosphatidylethanolamine
PEDF pigment epithelium-derived growth factor
PET positron emission tomography
PEX pseudoexfoliation syndrome
PEX1 the peroxisome biogenesis factor 1 (peroxin-1) gene on chromosome 7 (7q21–q22)
PEX10 the peroxisome biogenesis factor 10 (peroxin-10) gene on chromosome 1 (1p36.32)
PEX13 the peroxisome biogenesis factor 13 (peroxin-13) gene on chromosome 2 (2p15)
PEX26 the peroxisome biogenesis factor 26 (peroxin-26) gene on chromosome 22 (22q11.21)
PF-4 platelet factor 4
PFKM the muscle phosphofructokinase gene on chromosome 12(12q13.3)
PFV persistent fetal vasculature
PG proteoglycan; prostaglandin, pigmentary glaucoma
PGAM2 the muscle phosphoglycerate mutase gene on chromosome 7 (7p13–p12.3)
PGD_2 prostaglandin D2
PGE_2 prostaglandin E2
PGF placenta growth factor
PGF_2 prostaglandin F2
PGG_2 prostaglandin G2
PGH_2 prostaglandin H2
PGI_2 prostacyclin
PGP 9.5 ubiquitin carboxyl-terminal esterase L1
pH a measure of the of the acidity of a solution in terms of the hydrogen ions
PHA phytohemaglutinin
Phako phacoemulsification
PHKA1 the muscle isoform of the α-subunit of phosphorylase kinase gene on the X chromosome (Xq13)
PHKA2 the α-subunit of phosphorylase kinase gene on the X chromosome (Xp22.2–p22.1)
PHKB the β-subunit of liver and muscle phosphorylase kinase gene on chromosome 16 (16q12–q13)
PHKG2 the gene on the chromosome 16 (16q11–p12) that codes for the testis/liver isoform of the γ-subunit of phosphorylase kinase
PHLDA1 the gene on chromosome 12 (12q15) for pleckstrin homology-like domain Family A member 1 (also known as T cell death–associated gene 51)
PHPV persistent hyperplastic primary vitreous
Pi inorganic phosphate
PI phosphatidylinositol
pI isoelectric point
PI3K phosphoinositide-3 kinase
PIK3R3 phosphatidylinositol 3 kinase
PIM1 the PIM1-kinase associated protein 1 gene on chromosome 7 (7p14.3) (also known as *PAP1 and RP9*)
PIP proximal interphalangeal
PIP_2 phosphatidylinositol 4, 5-bisphosphate
PIP5K3 the phosphatiditylinositol-3-phosphate 5 kinase type III gene on chromosome 2 (2q35)
PITC phenylisothiocyanate
PITX2 the paired-like homeodomain transcription factor 2
PITX2 the paired-like homeodomain transcription factor 2 gene on chromosome 4 (4q25–q26)
Pitx2 the murine paired-like homeodomain transcription factor 2 gene
PITX3 the paired-like homeodomain transcription factor 3
PITX3 the paired-like homeodomain transcription factor 3 gene on chromosome 10 (10q25)
PLOD the lysyl hydroxylase gene on chromosome 1 (1p36.3–36.2)
PLP1 the main integral protein of myelin (proteolipid protein 1) gene on the X chromosome (Xq22)
PLXND1 the plexin D1 gene on chromosome 3 (3q21.3)
PM plasma membrane
PMMA polymethylmethacrylate
PML progressive multifocal leukoencephalopathy
PMN polymorphonuclear leukocyte/polymorphonuclear neutrophils
PMR polymyalgia rheumatica
PN polyarteritis nodosa
PNET primitive neuroectodermal tumor
PNR photoreceptor cell-specific nuclear receptor
PNR a gene on chromosome 15 (15q23) that codes for nuclear receptor subfamily 2, group E, member 3 (also known as *NR2E3* and *ESCS*)
PNS peripheral nervous system
POAG primary open angle glaucoma
Pol a gene of Rous sarcoma virus
POLA Pathologies Ocularies Liees a l'Age
POMGnT1 protein O-linked mannose beta 1,2-N-acetylglucosaminyltransferase 1
POMT1 the protein O-mannosyltransferase gene on chromosome 9 (9q34.1)
PORN progressive outer retinal necrosis
POU the gene for POU proteins (a family of proteins that are transcription factors with a bipartite DNA binding domain (POU domain); named after three mammalian transripton factors (Pit-1, Oct-1/Oct-2, and Unc-86)
PPAR peroxisome proliferator-activated receptor
PPCD posterior polymorphous corneal dystrophy
PPCRA pigmented paravenous chorioretinal atrophy
PPD purified protein derivative of tuberculin
PPGB the cathepsin protective protein gene on chromosome 20 (20q13.1)
PPP pentose phosphate pathway
PPP2CA the protein phosphatase 2A gene on chromosome 5 (5q23–q31)
PPRPE recessive retinitis pigmentosa with para-arteriolar preservation of the retinal pigment epithelium
PPT1 palmitoyl-protein thioesterase 1

PRAD1 parathyroid adenomatosis 1 (also known as cyclin D1 and BCL-1)
pRb retinoblastoma gene product
PRELP a small interstitial proteoglycan with proline arginine-rich end leucine rich repeats
PRELP the gene on chromosome 1 (1q32) that codes for the proteoglycans known as PRELP
pre-mRNA precursor messenger mRNA
PRG1 the serglycin gene on chromosome 10 (10q22.1)
PRKAR1A the protein kinase cAMP-dependent regulatory type 1 alpha gene on chromosome 17 (17q23–q24)
PRL the prolactin gene on chromosome 6 (6p22.2–p21.3)
PRNP the gene for prions on chromosome 20 (20pter–p12)
PROMM proximal myotonic myopathy
ProMMP-2 promatrix metalloproteinase-2
Prox1 the prospero-related homeobox 1 murine gene that codes for a transcription factor that is involved in the regulation of crystalline lens induction and development
PrP the normal cellular isoform of prion protein
PrP^c wildtype prion protein
PRPF3 a gene for human homolog of yeast pre-mRNA splicing factor 3 on chromosome 1 (1q21.2) (also known as *RP18*)
PRPF8 a gene for the human homolog of yeast pre-mRNA splicing factor C8 on chromosome 17 (17p13.3) (also known as *RP13*)
PRPF31 a gene for human homolog of yeast pre-mRNA splicing factor 31 on chromosome 19 (19q13.42) (also known as *RP11*)
PRPH2 the peripherin 2 gene on chromosome 6 (6p21.1–cen) (also known as *RDS* and *RP7*)
PrP^{sc} mutated prion protein (also known as PrPSC)
PrPSC mutated prion protein (also known as PrP^{SC})
PrPSc the abnormal disease-causing isoform of prion protein
PRR pattern recognition receptor
PSAP the saposin sulfatide activator gene on chromosome 10 (10q22.1)
PSC posterior subcapsular cataract
PSEN1 the presenilin-1 gene on chromosome 14 (14q)
PSEN2 the presenilin-2 gene on chromosome 1 (1q31–q42)
PSH proteinthiol
pSS primary Sjögren syndrome
PSH protein thiol
PTC phenylthiocarbamoyl
PTCH the human homolog of the *Drosophila* patch gene on chromosome 22 (23–q31)
PtdSer phosphatidylserine
PTEN a phosphatase and tensin homolog gene on chromosome 10 (10q23.31) that is mutated in Cowden syndrome
PTH phenylthiohydantoin; parathyroid hormone
PTLD post-transplant lymphoproliferative disease
PTMs post-translational modifications
PTP permeability transition pore
PTPN22 protein tyrosine phosphatase non-receptor 22
PTPRC protein kinase phosphatase receptor type C gene on chromosome 1(1q31–q32)
PU phacoantigenic uveitis
PUFA polyunsaturated fatty acid
PUK peripheral ulcerative keratitits
PVD posterior vitreous detachment
pVHLD the von Hippel-Lindau disease protein
PVR proliferative vitreoretinopathy
PYGL the liver phosphorylase gene on chromosome 14 (14q21–q22)
PYGM the muscle phosphorylase gene on chromosome 11 (11q13)
^{31}P-NMR phosphorous 31-nuclear magnetic resonance

q long arm of a chromosome
QTL quantitative trait locus

R rad
RA rheumatoid arthritis
Rab a family of small guanosine triphosphate (GTP)-binding proteins within the Ras superfamily that regulates vescicular trafficking pathways
RAB3A a protein that regulates synaptic vesicle exocytosis
RAB8A a Ras-associated protein
RAD51 a gene on chromosome 15 (15q15.1) that codes a homolog of *S. cerevisiae* RAD51
RAG1 recombination activating gene 1 on chromosome 11 (11p13)
RAG2 recombination activating gene 2 on chromosome 11 (11p13)
RANTES a cytokine (**R**egulated on **A**ctivation, **N**ormal **T** **E**xpressed and **S**ecreted)
RAR retinoic acid receptor
RARE retinoic acid-response element
Ras retrovirus-associated DNA sequences originally isolated from murine sarcoma virus; the Ras superfamily of small guanosine triphosphate (GTP)-binding proteins regulates vescicular trafficking pathways and includes the Rab family
^{86}Rb rubidium 86
Rb retinoblastoma
RB reticulate body
RB1 the retinoblastoma gene on chromosome 13 (13q14)
RBC red blood cell
RBP retinol binding protein
RBP1 retinol-binding protein 1 (also known as cellular retinol-binding protein [CRBP])
RCP the gene for red visual pigment on the X chromosome (Xq28)
RCS Royal College of Surgeons
RD retinal detachment
RDH1 the 11-*cis* retinol dehydrogenase 5 gene on chromosome 12 (12q13–q14) (also known as *RDH5*)
RDH5 retinol dehydrogenase 5
RDH5 the 11-*cis* retinol dehydrogenase 5 gene on chromosome 12 (12q13–q14) (also known as *RDH1*)
RDH12 retinol dehydrogenase 12
RDH12 the retinol dehydrogenase 12 gene on chromosome 14 (14q24.1)
rDNA ribosomal deoxyribonucleic acid
RDS the peripherin 2 gene on chromosome 6 (6p21.1–cen) (also known as *PRPH2* and *RP7*)

RDH5 the 11-*cis* retinol dehydrogenase 5 gene on chromosome 12 (12q13–q14) (also known as *RDH1)*

REAL classification Revised European American Lymphoma Classification

RECQL2 the recq protein-like 2 gene on chromosome 8 (8p12–p11.2)

RELA the A homolog of V-REL avian reticuloendotheliosis viral oncogene on chromosome 11 (11q12–q13)

RELB the B homolog of V-REL avian reticuloendotheliosis viral oncogene on chromosome 19 (19q13.32)

REP-1 Rab excort protein 1

REP-2 Rab excort protein 2

RER rough endoplasmic reticulum

RET the rearranged during transfection proto-oncogene on chromosome 10 (10q11.2)

RetGC1 retinal guanylate cyclase-1 (also known as GUCY2D)

RETGC1 the retinal-specific guanylate cyclase gene on chromosome 17 (17p13.1) (also known as *CORD6, GUCY2D*, and *LCA1*)

RF rheumatoid factor

RGC reinal ganglion cell

RGD an integrin-binding motif (ArgGlyAsp)

RGR retinal pigment epithelium-retinal G-protein coupled receptor

RGR the retinal pigment epithelium-retinal G-protein Coupled receptor gene on chromosome 10 (10q23.1)

Rho a family of small guanosine triphosphate (GTP) binding proteins

RHO the rhodopsin gene on chromosome 3 (3q21–q24) (also known as *RP4*)

RHOK the rhodopsin kinase gene on chromosome 13 (13q34) (also known as *GRK1*)

RICH rapidly involuting congenital hemangioma

RIM a protein involved in the regulation of glutamate release at the ribbon synapse of photoreceptors

RIMS1 protein regulating synaptic membrane exocytosis 1 gene on chromosome 6 (6q12–q13)

RK radial keratotomy

RLBP1 the cellular retinaldehyde-binding protein gene on chromosome 15 (15q26) (also known as *CRALBP*)

RNFLI retinal nerve fiber layer infarct (also known as "cotton wool" spot)

Ro Sjögren syndrome related antigen

ROBO3 a gene on chromosome 11 (11q23–q25) that codes a homolog of *Drosophila* roundabout 3

ROI reactive oxygen intermediates

ROM1 the rod outer segment protein 1 gene on chromosome 11 (11q13)

ROP retinopathy of prematurity

ROS reactive oxygen species

RP retinitis pigmentosa, refractive power, and relapsing polychondritis

RP1 the oxygen-regulated photoceptor protein 1 gene on chromosome 8(8q12.1)

RP3 the gene on the X chromosome (Xp11.4) for retinitis pigmentosa guanosine triphosphate hydrolase regulator (also known as *RPGR, CORDX* and *COD1*)

RP4 the rhodopsin gene on chromosome 3 (3q21–q24) (also known as *RHO*)

RP7 the peripherin 2 gene on chromosome 6 (6p21.1–cen) (also known as *RDS* and *PRPH2)*

RP9 the PIM1-kinase associated protein 1 gene on chromosome 7 (7p14.3) (also known as *PAP1 and PIM1*)

RP10 the inosine monophosphate dehydrogenase 1 gene on chromosome 7 (7q32.1) (also known as *IMPDH1*)

RP11 a gene on chromosome 19 (19q13.42) that codes for human homolog of yeast pre-mRNA splicing factor 31 (also known as *PRPF31*)

RP12 a gene on chromosome 1 (1q31–q32.1) that codes for a homolog of *Drosophila* Crumbs 1 (also known as *CRB1*)

RP13 a gene on chromosome 17 (17p13.3) that codes for human homolog of yeast pre-mRNA splicing factor C8 (also known as *PRPF8*)

RP14 the tubby–like protein 1 gene on chromosome 6 (6p21.3) (also known as *TULP1*)

RP17 the gene for carbonic anhydrase IV on chromosome 17 (17q23.2) (also known as *CA4*)

RP18 a gene on chromosome 1 (1q21.2) that codes for human homolog of yeast pre-mRNA splicing factor 3 (also known as *PRPF3*)

RP19 the ATP-binding cassette transporter retinal gene on chromosome 1 (1p21–p13) (also known as *ABCA4, ABCR*, and *STGD1*)

RP20 a gene on chromosome 1 (1p31) that codes for retinal pigment epithelium-specific 65 kDa protein (also known as *RPE65* and *LCA2*)

RP22 a locus for retinitis pigmentosa on chromosome 16 (16p12.3–p12.1)

RP25 a locus for retinitis pigmentosa on chromosome 6 (6cen–q15)

RP26 the gene for ceramide kinase-like protein on chromosome 2 (2q31.3) (also known as *CERKL*)

RP27 a gene on chromosome 14 (14q11.2) that codes for neural retina leucine zipper (also known as *NRL*)

RP28 a locus for retinitis pigmentosa on chromosome 2 (2p16–p11)

RP29 a locus for retinitis pigmentosa on chromosome 4 (4q32–q34)

RP30 the gene on chromosome 17 (17q25) that codes for retinal fascin homolog 2 actin bindig protein (also known as *FSCN2*)

RP31 a locus for retinitis pigmentosa on chromosome 9 (9p22–p13)

RP32 a locus for retinitis pigmentosa on chromosome 1 (1p34.3–p13.3)

RPE retinal pigment epithelium

RPE65 retinal pigment epithelium-specific 65 kDa protein

RPE65 a gene on chromosome 1 (1p31) that codes for retinal pigment epithelium-specific 65 kDa protein (also known as *LCA2* and *RP20*)

RPED retinal pigment epithelium detachment

RPGR the gene on the X chromosome (Xp11.4) for retinitis pigmentosa guanosine triphosphate hydrolase regulator (also known as *RP3, CORDX* and *COD1*)

RPGR-ORF15 a highly repetitive purine-region in the open reading frame 15 of the *RRGR* gene

RPGRIP1 the RPGR-interating protein 1 gene on chromosome 14 (14q11.2) (also known as *LCA6*)

RRD rhegmatogenous retinal detachment
RS Reiter syndrome
RS1 the retinoschism gene on the X chromosome (Xp22.2–p22.1)
RSV Rous sarcoma virus
RT-PCR reverse transcription-polymerase chain reaction
RVFV rift valley fever virus
RX the retina and anterior neural fold homeobox gene on chromosome 18 (18q21.3) (also known as *RAX*)
Rx1 a murine eye field transcription factor
RYR1 the ryanodine receptor 1 gene on chromosome 19 (19q13.1)

^{35}S sulfur isotope 35
S sulfur and the phase of synthesis in the cell cycle
S-antigen arrestin
S100 a calcium binding protein
SAA serum amyloid protein A
SAA1 the serum amyloid A1 gene on chromosome 11 (11p15.1)
SAA1 serum amyloid A1
SAA2 the serum amyloid A2 gene on chromosome 11 (11p15.1)
SAA2 serum amyloid A2
SAA3 the serum amyloid A3 gene on chromosome 11 (11p15.1–p14))
SAA3 serum amyloid A3
SAA4 the serum amyloid A4 gene on chromosome 11 (11p15.1)
SAA4 serum amyloid A4
SAAL an acute phase reactant protein; a precursor of SAA
SAC seasonal allergic conjunctivitis
SAG the arrestin gene on chromosome 2 (2q37.1)
SAGE serial analysis of gene expression
SALT skin associated lymphoid tissue
SAM senescence accelerated mouse; also sterile alpha motif
SANS the sans gene on chromosome 17 (17q24)
SAP serum amyloid protein
SAP-A saposin A
SAP-B saposin B
SAP-C saposin C
SAP-D saposin D
SAPK stress-activated protein kinase
SARA2 a gene on chromosome 5 (5q31.10 that causes chylomicron retention disease when mutated
SAT1 the spermidine/spermine N(1)-acetyltransferase-1 gene on the X chromosome (Xp22.1)
SBF2 a gene on chromosome 17 (17q11.2) that causes Charcot-Marie Tooth disease type 4 when mutated
SCC squamous cell carcinoma
S cone blue cone
SCD Schnyder corneal dystrophy
SCID severe combined immune deficiency
sCJD sporadic Creutzfelt-Jakob disease
SC02 a nuclear gene on chromosome 22 (22q13) that codes for a component of the mitochondrial respiratory chain complex IV
SDC1 the syndecan 1 gene on chromosome 2 (2p24.1)
SDC2 the syndecan 2 gene on chromosome 8 (8q22–q24)
SDC3 the syndecan 3 gene on chromosome 1 (1p32)
SDC4 the syndecan 4 gene on chromosome 20 (20q12–q13)
SDF-1 stromal cell-derived factor 1 (also known as chemokine CXC motif ligand 12)
SDHA a gene on chromosome 5 (5p15) that codes a component of the mitochondrial respiratory chain complex II
SDS sodium dodecyl sulfate
SDS-PAGE sodium dodecyl sulfate-polyacrylamide gel electrophoresis
Se selenium
sec second
SED spondyloepiphyseal dysplasia with dwarfism
SEER **S**urveillance, **E**pidemiology, and **E**nd **R**esults
SEGA subependymal giant cell astrocytoma
SELDI-TOF surface-enhanced laser desorption ionization time-of flight
SEM scanning electron microscopy and standard error of the mean
SEMA4A semaphorin 4A (also known as SEMAB)
SEMA4A the semaphorin 4A gene on chromosome 1 (1q22) (also known as *SEMAB*)
SEMAB the semaphorin 4A gene on chromosome 1 (1q22) (also known as *SEMA4A*)
SEN subependymal nodules
SEPN1 the selenoprotein N gene on chromosome 1 (1p36–p35)
Ser serine
SFAs semifluorinated alkanes
SFD Sorsby fundus dystrophy
SGSH the heparan *N*-sulfatase gene on chromosome 17 (17q25.3)
SH sulfhydryl group
SH3BP2 SH3 domain-binding protein 2
SHH the sonic hedgehog gene on chromosome 7 (7q36)
Shh the murine sonic hedgehog gene
sHSPs small heat shock proteins
SIAT9 the sialyltransferase-9 gene on chromosome 2 (2p11.2)
sICAM-1 soluble form of ICAM-1
SIgA sectory component of immunoglobulin A
sIL-2r soluble interleukin 2 receptor
SILAC stable isotope labelling with amino acids in cell culture
Sip1 a murine gene that codes a transcription factor that is involved in crystalline lens induction and develpment
Six3 a murine eye field transcription factor that is the homolog of the Drosophila sine oculis homeobox 3 gene
SIX5 the gene for sine oculis-5 on chromosome 19 (19q13.3)
SIX6 a gene on chromosome 14 (14q23) that is the homolog of the Drosophila sine oculis homeobox 6 gene
Six6 a murine eye field transcription factor that is the homolog of the Drosophila sine oculis homeobox 6 gene
SJS Stevens Johnson syndrome
Ski a murine proto-oncogene
SLC4A11 the sodium borate cotransporter gene on chromosome 20 (20p13–p12)

SLC39A4 a gene on chromosome 8 (8q24.3) that controls zinc absorption from the intestine
SLC40A1 a gene on chromosome 2 (2q32) that causes hemochromatosis when mutated
SLC1745 a gene on chromosome 6 (6q14–q15)that codes for a transporter of sialic acid into the lysosome
SLE systemic lupus erythematosus
SLEB2 a locus for systemic lupus erythematosus susceptibility on chromosome 2 (2q37)
SLIPS syndecan-like integral membrane proteoglycans
SLL small lymphocytic lymphoma
SLRR a superfamily of small proteoglycans containing tandem arrays of leucine-rich repeats
SLS segment long spacing
Smac/SMAC second mitochondria-derived activator of caspases
SMADs a group of related intracellular proteins critical for transmitting to the nucleus signals from TGFβ
SMPD1 a sphingomyelinase gene on chromosome 11 (11p15.4–p15.1)
SNAILs a family of zinc finger transcription factors first identified in *Drosophila*
SNAP-25 a protein involved in the regulation of acetylcholine release
SNP single nucleotide polymorphism
SO sympathetic ophthalmia
SOC53 suppressor of cytokine signaling
SOD superoxide dismutase
SOD2 the manganese superoxide dismutase gene on chromosome 6 (6q25.3)
SOX1 the Sry-box 1 gene on chromosome 13 (13q34)
Sox1 the murine Sry-box 1 gene
SOX2 the Sry-box 2 gene on chromosome 3 (3q26.3–q27)
Sox2 the murine Sry-box 2 gene
SOX3 the Sry-box 3 gene on the X chromosome 3 (Xq26.3)
Sox3 the murine Sry-box 3 gene
SOX9 SRY-Box 9 the product of the SRY-related HMG-box gene 9
sp. species
SPARC secreted protein, acidic, cysteine-rich (also known as osteonectin)
SPK superficial punctate keratitis
SRBC sheep red blood cell
Src a gene in Rous sarcoma virus
SRP signal recognition particle
SRS-A slow reacting substance of anaphylaxis (currently known as leukotreine C_4)
SRT substrate reduction therapy
SS Sjögren syndrome
SS-A an antigen to Sjögren syndrome
SS-B an antigen to Sjögren syndrome
SSc systemic sclerosis
SSCP single-stranded conformational polymorphism
ssDNA single standed deoxyribonucleic acid
SSH suppression subtraction hybridization
SSPE subacute sclerosing panencephalitis
ssRNA-RT single standed ribonucleic acid-reverse transcriptase
sSS secondary Sjögren syndrome
ST sulfotransferase
STGD Stargardt disease
STGD1 Stargardt disease type 1
STGD1 the ATP-binding cassette transporter retinal gene on chromosome 1 (1p21–p13) (also known as RP19, *ABCA4*, and *ABCR*)
STGD2 Stargardt disease type 3
STGD3 Stargardt disease type 3
STS serologic test for syphilis
STS a gene for steroid sulfatase on the X chromosome (Xp22.32)
SUMF1 the gene on the chromosome 3 (3p26) that codes for a sulfatase that acts on all substates
SUOX the sulfite oxidase gene on chromosome 12
SubRPE subretinal pigment epithelium
SURF1 a nuclear gene on chromosome 9 (9q34) that codes a component of the mitochondrial respiratory chain complex IV
SV systemic vasculidides
SV40 simian virus 40
SWS Sturge–Weber syndrome
SYPRO™ a registered tradename of Molecular Probes

T thymine
T1-weighted image a magnetic resonance image using short TE and TR times; it has greater signal intensity from fat containing tissues
T2-weighted image a magnetic resonance image made with a sequence with long TR and TE to show contrast in tissues with varying T2 relaxation times; water gives a strong signal
T3 triiodothyronine
T4 thyroxine
TA Takayasu arteritis
TACSTD2 the current name for the gene on chromosome 1 (1p32) that was formerly called *M1S1, TROP2*, and *GA733-1*
TALL1 tumor necrosis factor and Apo1-related leukocyte-expressed ligand 1 (also known as tumor necrosis factor ligand, member 13B [TNFSF13B] and B cell activating factor, and zTNF4)
TAP transporter associated with antigen processing
TAT the tyrosine aminotransferase gene on chromosome 16 (16q22.1–q22.3)
TATA thymine-adenine-thymine-adenine
TBA thiobarbituric acid
TBD Thiel-Behnke corneal dystrophy
tBid truncated Bid
Tc phase separation temperature
Tc cytotoxic T-cell
TCA tricarboxylic acid cycle (also known as Krebs cycle and citric acid cycle)
T cell T lymphocyte
TCF8 a transcription factor 8 gene on chromosome 10 (10p11.2)
TCR T-cell receptor
TCR Vβ variable region of the T-cell receptor β chain
TdT terminal deoxynucleotidyl transferase
TDT transmission disequilibrium test
TEK gene encoding endothelial cell-specific tyrosine kinase receptor
TEM transmission electron microscopy

TEN toxic epidermal necrolysis
TEWL transepithelial water loss
TFR2 a gene on chromosome 7 (7q22) that causes hemochromatosis when mutated
TG thymine-guanine dinucleotide
TGase transglutaminase
TG2 tissue transglutaminase
TG3 epidermal transglutaminase
TGF transforming growth factor
TGFα transforming growth factor α
TGFβ transforming growth factor β
TGFB the transforming growth factor β1 gene on chromosome 19 (19q13.1), also known as *TGFB1*
TGFβ1 transforming growth factor β1
TGFB1 the transforming growth factor β1 gene on chromosome 19 (19q13.1)
TGFβ2 transforming growth factor β2
TGFBI the transforming growth factor beta induced gene on chromosome 5 (5q31)
TGFBIp transforming growth factor beta induced protein
TGFBR2 the TGFβ receptor 2 gene on chromosome 3 (3p22)
TGIF the transforming growth factor beta-induced factor gene on chromosome 18 (18p11.3)
TGM2 the transglutaminase-2 gene on chromosome 20 (20q11.2–q12)
Th helper T cell
Th0 precursors of other helper T cells
Th1 helper T cell type 1 that is involved in cell-mediated immunity (also known as Th1-cell)
Th2 helper T cell type 2 that stimulates antibody production by B-cells (also known as Th2-cell)
Thr threonine
Thy-1 a major cell surface protein of T lymphocytes
TIGR an former term for the *MYOC* gene on chromosome 1 (1q21–31) that codes for myocilin
TIL tumor infiltrating lymphocytes
TIMP tissue inhibitor of metalloproteinase
TIMP1 the tissue inhibitor of metalloproteinase 1 gene on the X chromosome (Xp11.3–p11.23)
TIMP2 the tissue inhibitor of metalloproteinase 2 gene on chromosome 17 (17q25)
TIMP3 the tissue inhibitor of metalloproteinase 3 gene on chromosome 22 (22q12.1–q13.2)
TIMP1 tissue inhibitor of metalloproteinase 1
TIMP2 tissue inhibitor of metalloproteinase 2
TIMP3 tissue inhibitor of metalloproteinase 3
tk thymine kinase
TKT transketolase
Tll the murine paired box-6 gene
TLR Toll-like receptor
TM trabecular meshwork
TMS triple-membrane structure
TNC the tenascin C gene on chromosome 9 (9q33)
TNF tumor necrosis factor
TNF the tumor necrosis factor gene on chromosome 6 (6p21.3)
TNFα tumor necrosis factor α
TNFβ tumor necrosis factor β
TNR the tenascin R gene on chromosome 1 (1q24)
TNFR tumor necrosis factor receptor
TNFR1 tumor necrosis factor receptor 1 (also known as tumor necrosis factor receptor superfamily member 1A, death receptor 1 and CD120a)
TNFR2 tumor necrosis factor receptor 2 (also known as CD120b)
TNFRSF1A tumor necrosis factor receptor superfamily, member 1A
TNFRSF1B tumor necross factor receptor superfamily, member 1B
TNFRSF12 tumor necrosis factor receptor superfamily member 12 (also known as death receptor 3 [DR3], lymphocyte-associated receptor of death [LARD], TRAMP, and WSL1)
TNFR25 tumor necrosis factor receptor 1
TNFSF13B tumor necrosis factor ligand, member 13B (also known as B cell activating factor, TALL1 and zTNF4)
TNM tumor-nodes-metastases
TP53 the tumor protein p53 gene on chromosome 17 (17p13.1)
TP73L the gene on chromosome 3 (3q27) that codes for tumor protein p73-like (also known as tumor protein p63)
TPA 12-O-tetradecanoylphobol-13-acetate
TPO thyroid peroxidase
TRADD tumor necrosis factor receptor associated death domain
TRAF1 tumor necrosis factor receptor associated factor 1
TRAR2 tumor necrosis factor receptor associated factor 2
TRAIL tumor necrosis factor-related apoptosis inducing ligand (also known as APO2L)
TRAIL3 tumor necrosis factor-related apoptosis inducing ligand 3 (also known as DCR1)
TRAIL4 tumor necrosis factor-related apoptosis inducing ligand 4 (also known as DCR2)
TRAILR1 Tumor necrosis factor (TNF)-related apoptosis-inducing ligand receptor 1 (also known as death receptor 4 [DR4] and APO2)
TRAILR2 Tumor necrosis factor (TNF)-related apoptosis-inducing ligand receptor 2 (also known as death receptor 5 [DR5], KILLER and TRICK2)
TRAILR3 Tumor necrosis factor (TNF)-related apoptosis-inducing ligand receptor 3 (also known as death receptor 3 [DR3], tumor nerosis factor receptor superfamily member 10C [TNFRSF10C], decoy receptor 1 [DCR1] and TRAIL receptor without an intracellular domain [TRID])
TRAILR4 Tumor necrosis factor (TNF)-related apoptosis-inducing ligand receptor 4
TRAP150 the thyroid hormone receptor associated protein 3 gene on chromosome 1 (1p34.3)
TRB trilateral retinobastoma
Treg regulatory T-cells
TRH thyrotropin releasing hormone
TRIC trachoma and inclusion conjunctivitis
TRICK 2 death receptor 5 (DR5) also known as tumor necrosis factor-related apoptosis-inducing ligand receptor 2 [TRAIL2] and KILLER)
TRKA tyrosine kinase receptor A
TRKB tyrosine kinase receptor B
TRKC tyrosine kinase receptor C

TROP2 a former name for the *TACSTD2* gene on chromosome 1 (1p32–p31)
TRP1 a tyrosinase-related protein enzyme that catalyzes DHICA polymerization
TRP1 the tyrosinase-related protein 1 gene on chromosome 9 (9q23)
TRYP-1 enzyme that catalyzes the polymerization of 5,6-dihydroxyindole-2-carboxylic acid
tRNA transfer RNA
Ts suppressor T-cell
TSC tuberous sclerosis complex
TSC1 a gene for tuberous sclerosis complex on chromosome 9 (9q34)
TSC2 a gene for tuberous sclerosis complex on chromosome 16 (16p13.3)
TSD Tay-Sachs disease
TSH thyroid stimulating hormone
TSTA tumor-specific transplantation antigens
TTF-1 thyroid transcription factor 1
TTP1 tripeptidyl peptidase 1
TTP1 the tripeptidyl peptidase 1 gene on chromosome 8 (8q13.1–q13.3)
TTR the transthyretin gene on chromosome 18 (18q11.2–q12.1)
TTT transpupillary thermotherapy
Try a murine gene involved in melanin production
TUCAN tumor-up-regulated caspase recruitment domain (CARD)-containing antagonist
TULP1 Tubby–like protein 1
TULP1 the tubby–like protein 1 gene on chromosome 6 (6p21.3) (also known as *RP14*)
TUNEL terminal deoxynucleotidyl transferase (TdT) mediated 2′-deoxyuridine 5′-triphosphate (dUTP) nick-end labelling
Tyr tyrosine
TYR the tyrosinase gene on chromosome 11 (11q14-21)
Tyrp1 a murine gene involved in melanin production
TWIST a transcription factor
TXA_2 thromboxane A_2

U uracil
UBE2A the ubiquitin conjugating enzyme E2A gene on the X chromosome (Xq24–q25)
UBE2B the ubiquitin conjugating enzyme E2B gene on chromosome 5 (5q23–q31)
UBIAD1 a gene on chromosome 1 (1p34–1p36) that encodes a potential prenyltransferase
UDP uridine diphosphate
UGH uveitis-glaucoma-hyphema
U.K. United Kingdom
UNC119 the retinal gene 4 on chromosome 17 (17q11.2)
UNICEF Unted Nations International Children's Emergency Fund
UP ubiquinated proteins
UPS ubiquitin-proteasome system
US$ US dollars
U.S. United States
USH syndrome Usher syndrome
USH1 a type of Usher syndrome that has been mapped to chromosome 14 (14q32)
USH1B a type of Usher syndrome due to a mutation in the *MYO7A* gene
USH1C a type of Usher syndrome due to a mutation in the *USH1C* gene
USH1C the harmonin gene on chromosome 11 (11p15)
USH1D a type of Usher syndrome due to a mutation in the *CDH23* gene
USH1E a type of Usher syndrome that has been mapped to chromosome 21 (21q21)
USH1F a type of Usher syndrome due to a mutation in the *PCDH15* gene
USH1G a type of Usher syndrome due to a mutation in the *SANS* gene
USH2 a type of Usher syndrome
USH2A a type of Usher syndrome due to a mutation in the *USH2A* gene
USH2A the usherin gene on chromosome 1 (1q41)
USH2B a type of Usher syndrome that has been mapped to chromosome 3 (3p24)
USH2C a type of Usher syndrome due to a mutation in the *VLGR1* gene
USH3 a type of Usher syndrome
USH3A a type of Usher syndrome due to a mutation in the *USH3A* gene
USH3A a clarin-1 gene on chromosome 3 (3q21–25)
USP6 ubiquitin-specific protease 6
USP6 the ubiquitin-specific protease 6 gene on chromosome 17 (17p13)
UV ultraviolet
UVA ultraviolet A (100–290 nm)
UVA1 ultraviolet A1 (340–400 nm)
UVA2 ultraviolet A2 (320–340 nm)
UVB ultraviolet B (290–320 nm)

−ve negative
+ve positive
VDAC voltage-dependent anion channel
Val valine
Vax1 a murine ventral anterior homeobox gene
Vax2 a murine ventral anterior homeobox gene
VCAM-1 vascular cell adhesion molecule-1
vCJD variant Creutzfeldt-Jakob disease
VDAC voltage dependent anion channel (also known as porin)
VDR the vitamin D receptor gene on chromosome 12 (12q–q14)
VEGF vascular endothelial growth factor
$VEGF_{120}$ an isoform of vascular endothelial growth factor with 120 amino acids
$VEGF_{145}$ a human isoform of vascular endothelial growth factor with 145 amino acids
$VEGF_{165}$ a human isoform of vascular endothelial growth factor with 165 amino acids
$VEGF_{164}$ a murine isoform of vascular endothelial growth factor with 165 amino acids

$VEGF_{188}$ a murine isoform of vascular endothelial growth factor with 189 amino acids
$VEGF_{189}$ a human isoform of vascular endothelial growth factor with 189 amino acids
$VEGF_{206}$ a human isoform of vascular endothelial growth factor with 206 amino acids
VEGF-A vascular endothelial growth factor A
VEGF-B vascular endothelial growth factor B
VEGF-C vascular endothelial growth factor C
VEGF-D vascular endothelial growth factor D
VEGF-E vascular endothelial growth factor E
VEGFR1 vascular endothelial growth factor receptor 1
VEGFR2 vascular endothelial growth factor receptor 2
VEGFR3 vascular endothelial growth factor receptor 3
VEP visual evoked potential
VER visual evoked response
VHL von Hippel-Lindau protein
VHL the gene on chromosome 3 (3p25–26) that causes von Hippel-Lindau disease when mutated
VHLD von Hippel-Lindau disease
VIP vasoactive intestinal peptide
VIPR vasoactive intestinal peptide receptor
vJNCL variant juvenile neuronal ceroid lipofuscinosis
VKC vernal keratoconjunctivitis
VKH Vogt–Koyanagi–Hirada syndrome or disease
VLCFA very long chain fatty acid
VLDL very low density lipoproteins
VLGR1 the very large G-protein coupled receptor 1 gene on chromosome 5 (5q14)
vLINCL variant late infantile onset neuronal ceroid lipofuscinosis
VLM visceral larva migrans
VMD2 the bestrophin gene on chromosome 11 (11q13)
VSX1 the visual system homeobox gene 1 on chromosome 20 (20p11.2)
VSV vesicular stomatitis virus
VTNS the gene on chromosome 17 (17p13) that codes for a transporter of cystine
VWF von Willebrand factor
VZV varicella zoster virus

WAGR syndrome Wilms tumor-aniridia-genitourinary anomalies-mental retardation syndrome
WD repeat-containing protein 36
WDR36 a gene on chromosome 5 (5q22.1) that causes primary open glaucoma when mutated
WEE1 the Wee1 tyrosine kinase gene on chromosome 11 (11p15.3–p15.1)
WG Wegener granulomatosis
WHO World Health Organization
WNTs a family of highly conserved developmental control genes involved in signaling pathways that were first identified in *Drosophila*
Wnt4 a murine developmental control gene involved in signaling pathways that were first identified in *Drosophila*
WRD-36 an unusual extracellular matrix protein
WT1 a gene on chromosome 11 (11p13) for a zinc finger DNA–binding protein
WTV weak transforming viruses

XIAP X-linked inhibitor of apoptosis protein
XLRP X linked recessive retinitis pigmentosa
XLRS X-linked retinoschisis
XP xeroderma pigmentosum
XR x-linked recessive
xRP X-linked recessive retinitis pigmentosa

Z zeaxanthin and Zwischenscheibe
Z band a perpendicularly arranged band in striated muscle
ZIP a family of metal ion transporters
Zip4 the protein product of the *SLC39A4* gene
zTNF4 tumor necrosis factor ligand, member 13B (also known as B cell activating factor [TNFSF13B])
ZNF9 the zinc finger protein 9 gene on chromosome 3 (3q21.3)

Index

Note: Page numbers followed by F indicate figures; page numbers followed by T indicate tables.